MEDICAL MICROBIOLOGY

113915

KT-231-963

Commissioning Editor: Timothy Horne
Project Development Manager: Siân Jarman
Project Manager: Nancy Arnott
Designer: Erik Bigland
New illustrations by: MTG

MEDICAL MICROBIOLOGY

A GUIDE TO MICROBIAL INFECTIONS:
PATHOGENESIS, IMMUNITY, LABORATORY DIAGNOSIS AND CONTROL

EDITED BY

David Greenwood BSc PhD DSc FRCPath
Emeritus Professor of Antimicrobial Science, University of Nottingham Medical School, Nottingham, UK

Richard C. B. Slack MA MB BChir FFPHM MRCPath DRCOG
Senior Lecturer, Division of Microbiology, University of Nottingham Medical School, Nottingham, UK; Consultant in Communicable Disease Control, Nottingham Health Authority; Honorary Consultant, Public Health Laboratory Service

John F. Peutherer BSc MB ChB MD FRCPath FRCPE
Formerly Senior Lecturer, Department of Medical Microbiology, University of Edinburgh Medical School; Honorary Consultant, The Royal Infirmary of Edinburgh NHS Trust, Edinburgh, UK

SIXTEENTH EDITION

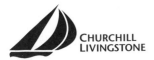
CHURCHILL LIVINGSTONE

EDINBURGH LONDON NEW YORK OXFORD PHILADELPHIA ST LOUIS SYDNEY TORONTO 2002

CHURCHILL LIVINGSTONE
An imprint of Elsevier Science Limited

© E & S Livingstone 1960, 1965
© Longman Group Limited 1973, 1975, 1978
© Longman Group UK Limited 1992,
   assigned to Pearson Professional Limited 1995
© Pearson Professional Limited 1997
© 2002, Elsevier Science Limited. All rights reserved.

No part of this publication may be reproduced, stored in a retrieval
system, or transmitted in any form or by any means, electronic,
mechanical, photocopying, recording or otherwise, without either
the prior permission of the publishers or a licence permitting
restricted copying in the United Kingdom issued by the Copyright
Licensing Agency, 90 Tottenham Court Road, London W1T 4LP.
Permissions may be sought directly from Elsevier's Health Sciences
Rights Department in Philadelphia, USA: phone: (+1) 215 238 7869,
fax: (+1) 215 238 2239, e-mail: healthpermissions@elsevier.com.
You may also complete your request on-line via the Elsevier Science
homepage (http://www.elsevier.com), by selecting 'Customer
Support' and then 'Obtaining Permissions'.

First edition 1925
Second edition 1928
Third edition 1931
Fourth edition 1934
Fifth edition 1938
Sixth edition 1942
Seventh edition 1945
Eighth edition 1948
Ninth edition 1953
Tenth edition 1960

Eleventh edition 1965
Twelfth edition (Vol. 1) 1973
Twelfth edition (Vol. 2) 1975
Thirteenth edition (Vol. 1) 1978
Thirteenth edition (Vol. 2) 1980
Fourteenth edition 1992
Fifteenth edition 1997
Sixteenth edition 2002
Reprinted 2003 (twice)

ISBN 0-443-07077-6

International Student Edition ISBN 0-443-07078-4
Reprinted 2003 (twice)

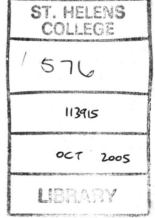

ST. HELENS
COLLEGE

576

113915

OCT 2005

LIBRARY

British Library Cataloguing in Publication Data
A catalogue record for this book is available from the British
Library

Library of Congress Cataloging in Publication Data
A catalog record for this book is available from the Library of
Congress

Note
Medical knowledge is constantly changing. As new information
becomes available, changes in treatment, procedures, equipment
and the use of drugs become necessary. The editors and the
publishers have taken care to ensure that the information given in
this text is accurate and up to date. However, readers are strongly
advised to confirm that the information, especially with regard to
drug usage, complies with the latest legislation and standards of
practice.

 ELSEVIER SCIENCE your source for books,
journals and multimedia
in the health sciences
www.elsevierhealth.com

The
publisher's
policy is to use
paper manufactured
from sustainable forests

Printed in China
P/03

PREFACE

In the course of the preparation of this new edition the book reached the notable landmark of 75 years of uninterrupted publication: the original version, T. E. Mackie and J E. McCartney's *An Introduction to Practical Bacteriology as Applied to Medicine and Public Health*, first appeared in 1925. It would be a fascinating exercise to chart the history of medical microbiology through the successive editions. When the book first appeared the ground-breaking work of the microbiological pioneers had matured into an established science and practitioners were confident that their knowledge of the relationship of microbes to disease was secure, if incomplete. It was also a time when the curricula of Medical Schools included many hours of practical microbiology, and young doctors were expected to be familiar with the techniques involved in the laboratory diagnosis of microbial disease.

Since that time, microbiological knowledge has expanded beyond all recognition. Virology, immunology, antimicrobial chemotherapy and the epidemiology of infectious disease — even infectious diseases as a medical specialty — have blossomed into fields of study in their own right, each with its own specialized language and literature. Mycology and parasitology, which have always maintained a sturdy independence, have similarly continued to flourish; molecular biology, unknown when Mackie and McCartney first wrote, has established a dominant presence. It is no longer possible for any one textbook to cover all aspects of medical microbiology in depth, nor for medical students and laboratory scientists to become fully conversant during their training with each topic and the laboratory skills that accompany them. Details of laboratory procedures are now the subject of an excellent sister volume (*Mackie and McCartney: Practical Medical Microbiology*; 14th edition, edited by J. G. Collee, A. G. Fraser, B. P. Marmion and A. Simmons, 1996) and for this edition we have continued to dispense with technical details that are of minor relevance to student doctors, leaving only sufficient information to allow an intelligent use of laboratory services.

As always, the text has been thoroughly updated to include the latest developments, which proceed unabated. We continue to be concerned that the needs of medical students and other health care workers in all geographical areas are fully catered for. A new chapter on medical entomology is included in recognition of the importance of arthropods in their own right and in the transmission of infectious disease. The authorship of the book — originally written by Edinburgh teachers primarily for the use of their students — has once more been expanded and now includes international experts from around the world. The contributions have been carefully edited to ensure consistency of style and coverage. For the first time authors have been encouraged to recommend relevant electronic information sources. This decision was not taken without some trepidation, since accurate citation is problematic given the internet's state of flux and some sites are poorly maintained. Moreover, we recognize that today's students are often more adept at exploiting electronic information than are their mentors and there are those who believe that the electronic revolution has rendered textbooks redundant. However, the world of electronic information is so vast, so unregulated and so variable in quality, that we believe that students will continue to welcome a compact authoritative digest of essential information and explanation that can be accessed at will — portable, easy to annotate, independent of electricity, not subject to sudden inexplicable failure and with viruses confined to their proper medical context!

That infection continues to have a major impact on human well-being and medical practice throughout the world scarcely needs emphasizing: hardly a day goes by without a microbiological story being given high prominence in the world press. The need for young health care professionals throughout the world to be offered a synoptic view of the broad discipline of microbiology during their formative years and beyond is greater than ever. The continuing aim of this book is to provide such an overview.

Once again our sincere thanks go to our contributors who have given unstintingly of their time and expertise to provide an authoritative text, and to the editorial staff of Elsevier Science in Edinburgh, for their unfailing courtesy and efficiency in seeing the book through to publication.

Nottingham and Edinburgh
May 2002

D.G.
R.C.B.S.
J.F.P.

SOURCES OF ELECTRONIC INFORMATION

In addition to the specific suggestions provided at the end of individual chapters, the following internet sites, most of which offer diverse links to sources of further information, are recommended as the starting point for searches of information on microbial topics.

American Society for Microbiology:
www.asmusa.org

Centers for Disease Control and Prevention:
www.cdc.gov

CDC National Center for Infectious Diseases:
www.cdc.gov/ncidod/index.htm

Medscape: www.medscape.com/Home/Topics/ID/
InfectiousDiseases.html

Oregon Health Sciences University:
www.ohsu.edu/clinweb

Public Health Laboratory Service:
www.phls.co.uk

PubMed (National Library of Medicine):
www.ncbi.nlm.nih.gov/PubMed/

Society for General Microbiology:
www.socgenmicrobiol.org.uk

University of Leicester:
www.micro.msb.le.ac.uk/

World Health Organization:
www.who.int/home-page/

The Wellcome Trust Tropical Medical Resource produces excellent CD-ROMs under the general title *Topics in International Health*. They are marketed by CABI Publishing (www.cabi.org) with special reduced rates for students and developing countries. Presently available titles include:

Acute Respiratory Infection
Diarrhoeal Diseases
HIV/AIDS
Leishmaniasis
Leprosy
Malaria (2nd edn)
Schistosomiasis
STDs
Trachoma
Tuberculosis

CONTRIBUTORS

D. Ala'Aldeen
Division of Microbiology and Infectious Diseases
University Hospital
Queen's Medical Centre
Nottingham
NG7 2UH

R. P. Allaker
Department of Clinical and Diagnostic Oral Sciences
Barts and the London Queen Mary's School of
Medicine and Dentistry
Turner Street
London
E1 2AD

M. R. Barer
Department of Microbiology and Immunology
University of Leicester
University Road
Leicester
LE1 9HN

A. D. T. Barrett
Department of Pathology
University of Texas Medical Branch at Galveston
Galveston TX 77555-0609
USA

S. M. Burns
Royal Infirmary of Edinburgh
Little France
51 Little France Crescent
Edinburgh
EH16 4SA

E. O. Caul
Public Health Laboratory
Myrtle Road
Kingsdown
Bristol
BS2 8EL

H. Chart
Laboratory of Enteric Pathogens
Central Public Health Laboratory
61 Colindale Avenue
London
NW9 5HT

A. Cockayne
Institute of Infections and Immunity
Queen's Medical Centre
Nottingham
NG7 2UH

T. J. Coleman
PHLS Leptospira Reference Unit
Public Health Laboratory
County Hospital
Hereford
HR1 2ER

M. J. Corbel
National Institute for Biological Standards and Control
Blanche Lane
South Mimms
Potters Bar
Herts
EN6 3QG

H. A. Cubie
Royal Infirmary of Edinburgh
Little France
51 Little France Crescent
Edinburgh
EH16 4SA

D. Cubitt
Department of Microbiology
Great Ormond Street Hospital
London
WC1N 3JH

J. M. Darville
Department of Medical Microbiology
Southmead Hospital
Westbury-on-Trym
Bristol
BS10 5NB

U. Desselberger
Public Health Laboratory
Level 6
Addenbrooke's Hospital
Hills Road
Cambridge
CB2 2QW

G. F. S. Edwards
Scottish Legionella Reference Unit
Stobhill NHS Trust
133 Balornorck Road
Glasgow
G21 3UW

E. G. V. Evans
Welsh Mycology Reference Unit
Department of Medical Microbiology and PHL
University of Wales College of Medicine
Heath Park
Cardiff
CF14 4XN

J. R. W. Govan
Medical Microbiology
University of Edinburgh Medical School
Teviot Place
Edinburgh
EH8 9AG

J. M. Grange
Centre for Infectious Disease and International Health
Windmeyer Institute for Medical Science
46 Cleveland Street
London
W1P 6DB

D. Greenwood
11 Perry Road
Sherwood
Nottingham
NG5 3AD

J. M. Hardie
Department of Clinical and Diagnostic Oral Sciences
Barts and the London Queen Mary's School of
Medicine and Dentistry
Turner Street
London
E1 2AD

C. A. Hart
Department of Medical Microbiology
University of Liverpool
Duncan Building
Daulby Street
Liverpool
L69 3GA

J. Hood
Department of Bacteriology
Glasgow Royal Infirmary
Glasgow
G4 0SF

H. Humphreys
Royal College of Surgeons in Ireland
Education and Research Centre
Smurfit Building
Beaumont Hospital
Dublin 9
Ireland

J. W. Ironside
National Creutzfeld–Jakob
Disease Surveillance Unit
Western General Hospital
Crewe Road
Edinburgh
EH4 2XU

M. Kilian
Department of Medical Microbiology and Immunology
University of Aarhus
The Bartholin Building
DK-800 Aarhus C
Denmark

J. McLauchlin
Food Safety Laboratory
Central Public Health Laboratory
61 Colindale Avenue
London
NW9 5HT

C. R. Madeley
Burnfoot
Stocksfield
Northumberland
NE43 7TN

R. C. Matthews
Department of Medical Microbiology
Clinical Sciences Building
Manchester Royal Infirmary
Manchester
M13 9WL

P. Morgan-Capner
Royal Preston Hospital
Sharoe Green Lane
Fulwood
Preston
PR2 9HT

M. Norval
Medical Microbiology
University of Edinburgh Medical School
Teviot Place
Edinburgh
EH8 9AG

M. M. Ogilvie
Medical Microbiology
University of Edinburgh Medical School
Teviot Place
Edinburgh
EH8 9AG

J. S. M. Peiris
Department of Microbiology
Pathology Building
Queen Mary
Hospital Compound
University of Hong Kong
Hong Kong

T. H. Pennington
Department of Bacteriology
Medical School
Foresterhill
Aberdeen
AB25 2ZD

J. F. Peutherer
44 Bridge Road
Colinton
Edinburgh
EH13 OLQ

T. L. Pitt
Laboratory of Hospital Infection
Central Public Health Laboratory
61 Colindale Road
London
NW9 5HT

N. W. Preston
36 Queen's Drive
Stockport
SK4 3JW

D. Reid
29 Arkleston Road
Paisley
PA1 3TE

P. Riegel
Institut de Bacteriologie
3 Rue Koeberle
6700 Strasbourg
France

T.V. Riley
Department of Microbiology
Queen Elizabeth II Medical Centre
Nedlands
W. Australia 6009
Australia

P. Simmonds
Laboratory for Molecular and Clinical Virology
University of Edinburgh
Summerhall
Edinburgh
EH9 1QH

R. A. Simpson
Health Care Science Ltd
Unit 5
North End Industrial Estate
Burymead Road
Hitchin
Herts
SG5 1RT

M. B. Skirrow
Western Lodge
Hanley Swan
Worcester
WR8 0DL

M. P. E. Slack
Department of Microbiology
John Radcliffe Hospital
Headington
Oxford
OX3 9DU

R. C. B. Slack
Division of Microbiology and Infectious Diseases
University of Nottingham Medical School
Queen's Medical Centre
Nottingham
NG7 2UH

J. Stewart
Medical Microbiology
University of Edinburgh Medical School
Teviot Place
Edinburgh
EH8 9AG

S. Sutherland
Medical Microbiology
University of Edinburgh Medical School
Teviot Place
Edinburgh
EH8 9AG

D. Taylor-Robinson
6 Vache Mews
Vache Lane
Chalfont St Giles
Buckinghamshire
HP8 4UT

K. J. Towner
Public Health Laboratory
University Hospital
Queen's Medical Centre
Nottingham
NG7 2UH

D. H. Walker
Department of Pathology
University of Texas Medical Branch at Galveston
Galveston, TX 77555-0609
USA

M. E. Ward
Molecular Microbiology
Mailpoint 814
Southampton General Hospital
Southampton
SO16 6YD

S. C. Weaver
Department of Pathology
University of Texas Medical Branch at Galveston
Galveston TX 77555-0609
USA

Xue-Jie Yu
Department of Pathology
University of Texas Medical Branch at Galveston
Galveston, TX 77555-0609
USA

CONTENTS

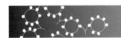

PART 1
MICROBIAL BIOLOGY

1   Microbiology and medicine   2
    D. Greenwood

2   Morphology and nature of micro-
    organisms   9
    M. R. Barer

3   Classification and identification of
    micro-organisms   25
    T. L. Pitt

4   Bacterial growth and physiology   37
    M. R. Barer

5   Antimicrobial agents   46
    D. Greenwood and M. M. Ogilvie

6   Bacterial genetics   61
    K. J. Towner

7   Sterilization and disinfection   73
    R. A. Simpson and R.C.B. Slack

8   Bacterial pathogenicity   83
    D. Ala'Aldeen

9   Virus–cell interactions   93
    M. Norval

PART 2
INFECTION AND IMMUNITY

10 Immunological principles: antigens and
    antigen recognition   110
    J. Stewart

11 Innate and acquired immunity   121
    J. Stewart

12 Immunity in viral infections   146
    J. Stewart

13 Parasitic infections: pathogenesis and
    immunity   154
    J. Stewart

14 Immunity in bacterial infections   161
    J. Stewart

PART 3
BACTERIAL PATHOGENS AND ASSOCIATED DISEASES

15 Staphylococcus   168
    Skin infections; osteomyelitis; food
    poisoning; foreign body infections
    H. Humphreys

16 Streptococcus and enterococcus   174
    Pharyngitis; scarlet fever; skin and
    soft tissue infections; streptococcal
    toxic shock syndrome; pneumonia;
    meningitis; urinary tract infections;
    rheumatic fever; post-streptococcal
    glomerulonephritis
    M. Kilian

17 Coryneform bacteria, listeria and
    erysipelothrix   189
    Diphtheria; listeriosis; erysipeloid
    J. McLauchlin and P. Riegel

18 Mycobacterium   200
    Tuberculosis; leprosy
    J. M. Grange

19 Environmental mycobacteria   215
    Opportunist disease
    J. M. Grange

20 Actinomyces, nocardia and
    tropheryma   221
    Actinomycosis; nocardiasis;
    Whipple's disease
    J. M. Grange

21 Bacillus   225
    Anthrax; food poisoning
    R. C. B. Slack

22 Clostridium   231
    Gas gangrene; tetanus; food poisoning;
    pseudomembranous colitis
    T. V. Riley

23 Neisseria and moraxella 242
Meningitis; gonorrhoea; respiratory
infections
R. C. B. Slack

24 Salmonella 250
Food poisoning; enteric fever
H. Chart

25 Shigella 260
Bacillary dysentery
H. Chart

26 Escherichia 265
Urinary tract infection; travellers' diarrhoea;
haemorrhagic colitis; haemolytic uraemic
syndrome
H. Chart

27 Klebsiella, enterobacter, proteus and other
enterobacteria 275
Pneumonia; urinary tract infection;
opportunist infection
H. Chart

28 Pseudomonads and non-fermenters 282
Opportunist infection; cystic fibrosis;
melioidosis
J. R. W. Govan

29 Campylobacter and helicobacter 288
Enteritis; gastritis; peptic ulcer
M. B. Skirrow

30 Vibrio, mobiluncus, gardnerella and
spirillum 296
Cholera; vaginosis; rat bite fever
H. Chart

31 Haemophilus 304
Respiratory infections; meningitis;
chancroid
M. P. E. Slack

32 Bordetella 311
Whooping cough
N. W. Preston and R. C. Matthews

33 Legionella 318
Legionnaires' disease; Pontiac fever
J. Hood and G. F. S. Edwards

34 Brucella, bartonella and streptobacillus 322
Brucellosis; Oroya fever; trench fever; cat
scratch disease; bacillary angiomatosis;
rat-bite fever
M. J. Corbel

35 Yersinia, pasteurella and francisella 329
Plague; pseudotuberculosis; mesenteric
adenitis; pasteurellosis; tularaemia
M. J. Corbel

36 Non-sporing anaerobes 337
Wound infection; periodontal disease;
abscess; normal flora
R. P. Allaker and J. M. Hardie

37 Treponema and borrelia 343
Syphilis; yaws; relapsing fever; Lyme disease
A. Cockayne

38 Leptospira 352
Leptospirosis; Weil's disease
T. J. Coleman

39 Chlamydia 358
Genital and ocular infections; infertility;
atypical pneumonia
M. E. Ward

40 Rickettsia, orientia, ehrlichia and
coxiella 369
Typhus; spotted fevers; scrub typhus;
ehrlichioses; Q fever
D. H. Walker and Xue-Jie Yu

41 Mycoplasmas 379
Atypical pneumonia; genital tract infection
D. Taylor-Robinson

PART 4
VIRAL PATHOGENS AND ASSOCIATED
DISEASES

42 Adenoviruses 392
Respiratory disease; conjunctivitis; gut
infections
J. S. M. Peiris and C. R. Madeley

43 Herpesviruses 399
Herpes simplex; varicella and zoster;
infectious mononucleosis; B cell
lymphomas; cytomegalovirus disease;
roseola infantum; Kaposi's sarcoma;
herpes B
M. M. Ogilvie

44 Poxviruses 421
Smallpox; molluscum contagiosum;
parapoxvirus infections
T. H. Pennington

45 Papovaviruses 429
Warts: warts and cancers; progressive
multifocal leuco-encephalopathy
H. Cubie

46 Hepadnaviruses 438
Hepatitis B infection; deltavirus infection
P. Simmonds and J. F. Peutherer

47 Parvoviruses 448
B19 infection; erythema infectiosum
H. A. Cubie

48 Picornaviruses 455
Meningitis; paralysis; rashes; intercostal
myositis; myocarditis; infectious hepatitis;
common cold
S. M. Burns

49 Orthomyxoviruses 468
Influenza
S. Sutherland

50 Paramyxoviruses 475
Respiratory infections; mumps; measles
J. S. M. Peiris and C. R. Madeley

**51 Arboviruses: alphaviruses, flaviviruses and
bunyaviruses** 484
Encephalitis; yellow fever; dengue;
haemorrhagic fever; miscellaneous tropical
fevers; undifferentiated fever;
A. D. T. Barrett and S. C. Weaver

52 Togavirus and hepacivirus 501
Rubella and hepatitis C viruses
P. Morgan-Capner and P. N. Simmonds

53 Arenaviruses and filoviruses 513
Lassa, Junin, Machupo, Sabia and Flexal
virus haemorrhagic fevers;
Marburg and Ebola Fevers
C. A. Hart

54 Reoviruses 521
Gastroenteritis
U. Desselberger

55 Retroviruses 527
Acquired immune deficiency syndrome;
lymphoma
P. Simmonds and J. F. Peutherer

56 Caliciviruses and astroviruses 539
Diarrhoeal disease
D. Cubitt

57 Coronaviruses 546
Upper respiratory tract disease
J. M. Darville and E. O. Caul

58 Rhabdoviruses 551
Rabies
S. Sutherland

**59 Transmissible spongiform
encephalopathies (prion diseases)** 558
Scrapie; BSE; Creutzfeldt–Jakob disease;
variant Creutzfeldt-Jakob disease
J. W. Ironside

**PART 5
FUNGAL PATHOGENS, PARASITIC INFECTIONS
AND MEDICAL ENTOMOLOGY**

60 Fungi 568
Thrush; ringworm; subcutaneous and
systemic mycoses
E. G. V. Evans

61 Protozoa 589
Malaria; toxoplasmosis; cryptosporidiosis;
amoebic dysentery; sleeping sickness;
Chagas' disease; leishmaniasis; giardiasis;
trichomoniasis
D. Greenwood

62 Helminths 601
    Intestinal worm infections; filariasis;
    schistosomiasis; hydatid disease
    D. Greenwood

63 Arthropods 615
    Arthropod-borne diseases; ectoparasitic
    infections; allergy
    D. Greenwood

PART 6
**DIAGNOSIS, TREATMENT AND CONTROL OF
INFECTION**

64 Infective syndromes 624
    R. C. B. Slack

65 Diagnostic procedures 635
    R. C. B. Slack

66 Strategy of antimicrobial
    chemotherapy 642
    R. C. B. Slack

67 Epidemiology and control of community
    infections 653
    D. Reid

68 Hospital infection 662
    R. C. B. Slack

69 Immunization 670
    R. C. B. Slack

INDEX 680

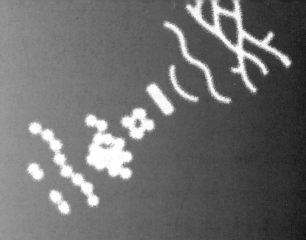

PART 1
MICROBIAL BIOLOGY

1

Microbiology and medicine

D. Greenwood

Applications of microbiology have transformed the diagnosis, prevention and cure of disease. Along with improved nutrition and living conditions, they have – at least in developed communities – revolutionized human health, doubled the average length of life and ensured the safe upbringing of most children born, where before only a minority survived. The conquest of epidemic and fatal infections has sometimes seemed so conclusive that the main challenges in medicine are often seen to lie in other fields, such as those of the mental illnesses and degenerative diseases.

However, infection is far from defeated. For example, in the poorer countries of the world, an estimated 10 million young children die each year from the effects of infectious diarrhoeas, measles, malaria, tetanus, diphtheria and whooping cough alone. The tragedy is that we have the means to hand to prevent nearly all these deaths. Many other infections continue to take their toll: tuberculosis still claims about 3 million victims each year; classic diseases such as cholera, typhoid and leprosy are far from being under control.

Even in the developed world, infection is still extremely common: at least a quarter of all illnesses for which patients consult their doctors are infective; a substantial proportion of patients acquire infection while in hospital, sometimes with multiresistant organisms. Intensive farming methods and a shift in eating habits to pre-prepared 'fast foods' have led to a sharp increase in food-related infection. In hospitals, new approaches to therapy that deplete the competence of the patient's immune system to cope with infection, as well as the increasing use of shunts, intravenous cannulae and prosthetic devices, all provide the ever-resourceful microbes with new opportunities to invade the host. Previously unsuspected links between microbes and diseases such as cancer, peptic ulcer, inflammatory bowel disease and rheumatoid arthritis have been uncovered. Surprisingly, 'new' agents of infectious disease continue to be recognized (Table 1.1). The rise and spread of the human immunodeficiency virus (HIV), the causative agent of acquired immune deficiency syndrome (AIDS), provides

a sobering reminder of the potential impact of microbial disease.

The relative freedom of society from fatal infections depends on the continued, informed deployment of complex countermeasures, including:

- alert epidemiological surveillance;
- rigorous environmental sanitation and infection control;
- full implementation of immunization programmes;
- correct diagnosis and treatment of infections.

It is as essential now as it ever was that adequate resources are provided for these purposes, and that

Table 1.1 Some newly recognized infectious agents, 1980–2000

Agent	Disease
Balamuthia mandrillaris	Granulomatous amoebic encephalitis
Bartonella henselae	Cat scratch disease
Borrelia burgdorferi	Lyme disease
Chlamydophila pneumoniae	Pneumonia
Cyclospora cayetanensis	Diarrhoea
Ehrlichia chafeensis	Human ehrlichiosis
Escherichia coli O157	Haemolytic uraemic syndrome
Helicobacter pylori	Gastritis
Hepatitis C virus	Hepatitis
Hepatitis E virus	Hepatitis
Hepatitis G virus	Hepatitis
Human herpesvirus 6	Exanthem subitum
Human herpesvirus 8	Kaposi's sarcoma
Human immunodeficiency virus	Acquired immune deficiency syndrome (AIDS)
Human T cell lymphotropic virus	Adult T cell leukaemia; tropical spastic paraparesis
Microspora (various genera)	Diarrhoea
Mobiluncus spp.	Bacterial vaginosis
New variant CJD agent	Spongiform encephalopathy
Nipah virus	Encephalitis
Tropheryma whippelii	Whipple's disease

CJD, Creutzfeldt–Jakob disease.

health care personnel should be well trained in matters relating to infection.

DEVELOPMENT OF MICROBIOLOGY

Microbiology is the study of living organisms of microscopic size. The term was introduced by the French chemist Louis Pasteur, whose demonstration that fermentation was caused by the growth of bacteria and yeasts (1857–60) provided a main impetus for the development of the science.

Micro-organisms were first seen about 1675 by the Dutchman Antony van Leeuwenhoek. His microscopes consisted of a single biconvex lens that magnified about ×200 and resolved bodies with diameters down to about 1 μm. He found many micro-organisms in materials such as water, mud, saliva and the intestinal contents of healthy subjects, and he recognized them as living creatures ('animalcules') because they swam about actively. That he saw bacteria as well as the larger microbes is known from his measurements of their size ('one-sixth the diameter of a red blood corpuscle') and his drawings of the forms we now recognize as cocci (spheres), bacilli (rods) and spirochaetes (spiral filaments).

Leeuwenhoek observed that very large numbers of bacteria appeared in watery infusions of animal or vegetable matter that were left to stand for a week or two at room temperature. He believed that these huge populations were the progeny of a few parental organisms, or seeds, that were originally present in the materials of the infusion or had entered it from the air. Other scientists suggested that the organisms arose by spontaneous generation from dead organic matter, and this began a controversy that lasted for 200 years.

The French microscopist Louis Joblot first described the prototype of the experiment that was ultimately to settle the matter (1718). He boiled a flask of an infusion of hay for 15 min to kill any microbes originally present, covered it with a parchment cap to prevent the later entry of other microbes from the air and showed that, on subsequent standing, it remained free from microbial growth. Similar experiments, notably those of John Needham (1749), showed, by contrast, that heated, covered infusions allowed the growth of organisms and so appeared to demonstrate the occurrence of spontaneous generation. It was not at first realized how exacting were the conditions needed to kill all micro-organisms, and maintain sterility. The necessary techniques were perfected by Lazzaro Spallanzani (1765 and 1776) and Louis Pasteur (1860–64). Pasteur's flasks of infusions, sterilized by autoclaving at 115–120°C, always remained sterile despite the entry of unheated air through a dust-stopping 'swan neck' or cotton wool stopper, and so finally proved the absence of spontaneous generation.

The controversy over spontaneous generation had the valuable outcome of establishing many of the basic techniques of bacteriology. Convenient nutrient media for preparing cultures of bacteria in the laboratory were derived from meat and vegetable infusions, and reliable methods were developed for the sterilization and maintenance of sterility of culture media and equipment. The need for high temperatures for sterilization was explained by Ferdinand Cohn's (1876) discovery that certain bacteria form heat-resistant spores. Other techniques essential for the rapid progress of bacteriology were developed by the German bacteriologist Robert Koch, who in 1877 described methods for the easy microscopic examination of bacteria in dried, fixed films stained with aniline dyes. Koch also devised a simple method for isolating pure cultures of bacteria by plating out mixed material on a solid culture medium – originally nutrient gelatine, later agar – on which the progeny of single bacteria grow in separate colonies.

MICRO-ORGANISMS AND DISEASE

Few of the micro-organisms that abound in nature are disease-producing, or *pathogenic*, for man. Most are free-living in soil, water and similar habitats, and are unable to invade the living body. Some free-living micro-organisms obtain their energy from daylight or by the oxidation of inorganic matter, but the majority feed on dead organic matter, and are termed *saprophytes*. In contrast, a parasite lives in or on, and obtains its nourishment from, a living host. In medical usage, the term *parasite* is nowadays usually reserved for parasitic protozoa, helminths and arthropods. The last usually affect the outside of the body, and are termed *ectoparasites*. *Commensal* micro-organisms constitute the normal flora of the healthy body. They live on the skin and on the mucous membranes of the upper respiratory tract, intestines and vagina, and obtain nourishment from the secretions and food residues. They are generally harmless, but under certain circumstances – such as when the body's defences are impaired – they may invade the tissues and cause disease, thus acting as *opportunist* pathogens. True pathogens are the micro-organisms that are adapted to overcoming the normal defences of the body and invading the tissues; their growth in the tissues, or their production of poisonous substances (*toxins*), damages the tissues and causes the manifestations of disease. The process of microbial invasion of the body is called *infection*. Those infective diseases that are readily communicable from person to person are called *infectious* or *contagious*.

The germ theory of disease was slow in gaining acceptance, though it was early recognized that epidemic diseases such as smallpox, measles, typhus and syphilis were probably spread from person to person. The Italian scholar Girolamo Fracastoro, in his book *De Contagione* (1546), distinguished three modes of transmission:

- by direct contact, i.e. touching a patient's body;
- by contact with clothing and household goods contaminated by a patient;
- at a distance through the air.

He explained contagion as being caused by the transmission of invisible seeds, or germs, different kinds of which were the specific causes of the different diseases. It is unclear whether he regarded the germs as living, but their ability to multiply in successive hosts would certainly be necessary for their continued spread.

Fracastoro's views were largely forgotten by the time Leeuwenhoek discovered micro-organisms, but speculation then began that these organisms might be the cause of certain diseases.

Bacteria

In 1876, Robert Koch, a country doctor in East Prussia, reported his observations on anthrax. Ten years earlier, C. J. Davaine had shown that the blood of sheep dying from anthrax contained numerous non-motile filaments and that its inoculation into healthy sheep caused them to develop anthrax. These findings, however, did not exclude the possibility that the filaments were inanimate products of the disease rather than its cause. Koch began his work by transmitting anthrax from infected sheep and cattle to the mouse, an unnatural but convenient laboratory host. He observed filaments in the blood and tissues of the infected mouse, and proved that they were living bacteria by watching them grow and form spores in drops of sterile ox serum or aqueous humour seeded with fragments of infected tissue. He showed that the bacteria alone were the cause of the disease by growing them in a series of eight pure cultures in aqueous humour, each seeded with a small proportion of the preceding one, and then reproducing the disease by inoculation of the final culture into a mouse. He thus provided the evidence, now described as *Koch's postulates*, which Jacob Henle had earlier stated would be needed to prove that a particular micro-organism was the cause of a particular disease, namely:

- that the microbe be found in the body in all cases of the disease;
- that it be isolated from a case and grown in a series of pure cultures in vitro;
- that it reproduce the disease on the inoculation of a late pure culture into a susceptible animal.

Koch obtained a research appointment in Berlin and there built up a successful school of bacteriology. He demonstrated the pathogenic roles of the tubercle bacillus (1882) and cholera vibrio (1883), and established the general principle that specific micro-organisms cause different kinds of disease. This principle is not absolute, as demonstrated in 1883 by the Scottish surgeon Alexander Ogston, who showed that *Staphylococcus aureus* and *Streptococcus pyogenes* could each cause various suppurative infections, such as abscesses and wound sepsis.

Fungi

Alongside the discovery of the pathogenic role of bacteria, the involvement of fungi was soon established. The first clear demonstration of a pathogenic role was made by the Italian civil servant Agostino Bassi (1835), who showed that the muscardine disease of silkworms was invariably associated with an invasion of their tissues by a fungus, and that the disease could be transmitted by the inoculation of material from the tissues of an infected worm into those of a healthy one. The discovery set in train a search for fungal agents of human disease. Meticulous microscopical studies enabled David Gruby, an eccentric Hungarian who eventually settled in Paris, to recognize and differentiate the yeasts of thrush and the fungi responsible for the various forms of ringworm (1841–1845). However, characterization of the fungi responsible for systemic mycoses such as histoplasmosis and coccidioidomycosis had to await investigations in central and South America in the early years of the 20th century. Techniques necessary for the systematic study of fungi in pure culture were refined by Raymond Sabouraud in the 1890s.

Protozoa and helminths

Worms visible to the naked eye had been recognized in antiquity and Leeuwenhoek observed protozoa likely to have been *Giardia lamblia* in his own faeces in 1676. Great strides were made in the 19th century, during the course of which most of the protozoal and helminthic parasites that infect man were described. Among many notable events were:

- the discovery by James Paget (while a first-year medical student at St Bartholomew's Hospital, London) of the larvae of *Trichinella spiralis* in muscle during an autopsy (1835);
- the observation by Alfred Donné of *Trichomonas vaginalis* in vaginal secretions (1836);

- the discovery of adult worms of *Schistosoma haematobium* by Theodor Bilharz in Cairo (1851);
- the recognition of the parasites of malaria in human blood by the French Army surgeon Alphonse Laveran (1880).

Painstaking studies by numerous workers, of whom Patrick Manson, Ronald Ross and David Bruce are among the most celebrated, later elucidated the complex life cycles of many parasitic worms and protozoa.

Viruses

The viruses were more difficult to demonstrate, for most were too small to be seen with the light microscope and none could be grown on an inanimate culture medium. At first they could be demonstrated only by observation of the disease they produced when infected tissue was inoculated into a susceptible animal. Thus, in 1881, Pasteur and his colleagues failed to isolate any micro-organism capable of causing rabies, but they were able to reproduce the disease in dogs and rabbits by the intracerebral injection of brain tissue or saliva from a fatal case. They suggested that the causal agent was an organism too small to be seen, although the agent might be a bacterium, or a larger microbe that was present, but undetected. The means of excluding such a possibility was devised by Ivanowski (1892) in experiments with the viral mosaic disease of tobacco; he transmitted the disease to healthy plants by the inoculation of juice from a diseased plant after it had been filtered through a porcelain filter fine enough to prevent the passage of bacteria. Filter-passing viruses were soon demonstrated in foot-and-mouth disease of cattle by Loeffler and Frosch (1898), in yellow fever by Reed, Carroll, Agramonte and Lazear (1900) – who had to test their inoculations in human volunteers – and in other diseases. Virology did not progress rapidly, however, until after the Second World War, when the availability of the electron microscope enabled viruses to be visualized and the use of living human and animal tissue cells for the in-vitro culture of viruses was developed by John Enders (1949) and others from the earlier work of pioneers such as Alexis Carrel.

IMMUNITY AND IMMUNIZATION

It was known from ancient times that persons who had suffered from a distinctive disease, such as smallpox or measles, resisted it on subsequent exposures and rarely contracted it a second time. Such an acquired immunity is generally effective only against the same type of infection as that previously suffered.

Artificial immunization against smallpox was practised in various communities by the unsafe method of inoculating smallpox exudate through the skin (*variolation*). The practice was popularized in England by Lady Mary Wortley Montagu, who had herself suffered from smallpox as a young woman. She observed variolation in Turkey while accompanying her husband as Ambassador in Constantinople, and was sufficiently impressed to submit her own son to the procedure in 1718. In 1796, the safer method of inoculating cowpox exudate (*vaccination*) was discovered by the Gloucestershire doctor Edward Jenner. Present-day vaccinia virus is different from cowpox virus, and its origin is obscure. The introduction of both variolation and vaccination was vigorously opposed in certain quarters, but vaccination has been instrumental in eradicating natural smallpox, the last case of which occurred in Somalia in 1977.

The natural existence of a safe immunizing agent such as vaccinia virus is exceptional, and we owe to Pasteur the development of immunizing strains of pathogenic microbes which are artificially *attenuated* (reduced in virulence) by prolonged or repeated culture under laboratory conditions. Pasteur derived such attenuated live *vaccines* for fowl cholera, anthrax, swine erysipelas and rabies, and called them *vaccines* in honour of Jenner's work with cowpox (Latin *vacca* = cow). In 1881 he made a convincing controlled trial of his anthrax vaccine, in which a vaccinated group of cows and sheep survived a later challenge by the inoculation of virulent anthrax bacilli, while a control group of unvaccinated animals perished from the same challenge. Today, attenuated live vaccines are used with outstanding success against such diseases as tuberculosis, poliomyelitis, measles and yellow fever.

The efficacy of vaccines consisting of killed bacteria was discovered by Salmon and Smith in 1886 in experiments on salmonellosis in pigeons. Today, killed vaccines are used against, for example, typhoid fever, whooping cough and influenza. In about 1900, Loewenstein in Vienna and Glenny in London discovered that toxins responsible for diphtheria and tetanus were effective in immunizing against the diseases after treatment with formaldehyde. The *toxoids* are now used routinely for immunization.

The first step in elucidating the mechanisms of acquired immunity was the discovery of *antibodies* by Behring and Kitasato in 1890. They found that the injection of sublethal doses of diphtheria or tetanus toxin into guinea-pigs rendered the animals immune to the later injection of large doses of the same toxin. The immunity was associated with the appearance in the animals' blood of a substance, *antitoxin*, which specifically neutralized the toxin. Protective antibodies that reacted directly with bacteria and viruses were soon demonstrated by other workers .

Antibodies have a highly specific affinity for the microbial substances, or *antigens*, that have induced their formation, and this property is exploited in the common use of blood serum containing antibodies (*antiserum*) in laboratory tests for the precise identification of micro-organisms. Discovery of the means of perpetuating the growth of single antibody-producing cells has enabled these techniques to be further refined by the use of *monoclonal antibodies* that exhibit absolute specificity for the target antigens.

SEROTHERAPY AND CHEMOTHERAPY

The work of Behring and Kitasato led to the successful use of antisera raised in animals for the treatment of patients with diphtheria, tetanus, pneumonia and other diseases. Because, however, the antisera contained animal proteins foreign to the human body, and were given by injection, serotherapy often caused unpleasant allergic responses, called *serum sickness*. For this reason, and also because serotherapy was unsuccessful against many kinds of infection, further progress depended on the development of drugs that exhibited *selective toxicity* – the ability to inhibit or kill microbes without harming the patient.

Although agents active against bacteria now form the most abundant group of antimicrobial drugs, the earliest therapeutic successes were achieved with antiprotozoal and anthelminthic compounds. Indeed, effective treatments for malaria (cinchona bark), amoebic dysentery (ipecacuanha root), tapeworm (male fern) and roundworm (wormseed) have been known for centuries. In contrast, effective therapy for systemic bacterial disease was unknown before the use of hexamine (methenamine) at the turn of the 20th century and Paul Ehrlich's development of the arsenical Salvarsan (arsphenamine) for spirochaetal disease in 1909. Even these discoveries were of limited value. The true beginning of the therapeutic revolution in infection dates from Gerhard Domagk's description of Prontosil (the forerunner of sulphonamides) in 1935, the development of Alexander Fleming's penicillin by Howard Florey and his colleagues in 1940, and Selman Waksman's exploitation of the potential for antibiotic production among soil micro-organisms in the 1940s. Within 25 years of these discoveries, most of the major groups of antimicrobial agents had been recognized, and more recent developments have chiefly involved chemical alteration of existing molecules.

Progress in the development of antiviral, antifungal and antiparasitic compounds has been much slower. Therapeutic choice in non-bacterial infection consequently remains severely limited, though the HIV pandemic has stimulated much work in the antiviral field that has been rewarded with some success. Meanwhile, the explosion of knowledge in immunology has renewed hopes that it may be possible to manipulate immunological processes triggered by infection to the benefit of the host.

SOURCES AND SPREAD OF INFECTION

The sources of infection from which pathogenic microbes are disseminated to susceptible hosts are listed in Table 1.2. Inanimate objects (*fomites*) may act as passive vehicles of infection, or infection can be passed directly from person to person, sometimes from healthy *carriers* in whom infection is unsuspected. Often pathogens are acquired from food, water or soil. Some infections, such as rabies, bubonic plague, brucellosis and leptospirosis, have their sources in animals, which are the natural hosts of the pathogen, and are called

Table 1.2 Sources of infection			
Environmental sources	Person-to-person[a]	Medical or surgical procedures	Self-infection
Inanimate objects Water, food, soil, etc. Animals (bites and scratches; zoonoses) Arthropod vectors	Airborne infection Direct contact (touching, kissing, etc.) Maternal transmission (intrauterine, transplacental) Sexual transmission	Instrumentation, operations Transfusion (blood and blood products) Transplants (tissues, organs)	Endogenous sources (normal flora) Shared needles Needlestick injuries
[a]Infected persons or healthy carriers.			

zoonoses. They are transmissible from animals to man, but not ordinarily from person to person, so that prevention depends on the control of human contact with the infected animals.

In the late 19th century it was discovered that blood-sucking arthropods spread certain diseases. In 1893, Theobald Smith and F. L. Kilborne showed that ticks that bite an infected cow and transmit its blood to another animal spread Texas fever of cattle. Subsequently, it was shown that malaria was transmitted by *Anopheles* mosquitoes (Ronald Ross, 1898), yellow fever by *Aedes* mosquitoes (Walter Reed and co-workers, 1900), bubonic plague by the rat flea (W. G. Liston and co-workers, 1905) and typhus fever by lice (Charles Nicolle, 1909). Campaigns of vector control by the use of insecticides and other means have since been conducted for the prevention of these diseases.

It is not only arthropods that can transmit micro-organisms by injection. The introduction of syringe needles for medical procedures (and drug abuse) and the development of blood transfusion vastly increased the potential for the spread of blood-borne infections such as hepatitis B and AIDS. This has necessitated the rigorous screening of blood products and the design of policies aimed at preventing the inadvertent transmission of such infections.

Epidemiological observations may suggest the mechanism by which an infection is transmitted and so lead to the formulation of preventive measures even when the causal micro-organism is still unknown. In 1846, for instance, in a maternity clinic in Vienna, Ignaz Semmelweis deduced that puerperal fever was caused by a putrefactive agent that doctors picked up on their hands when attending patients or performing necropsies, and which they then transferred into the birth canal when assisting women at childbirth. He reduced the number of maternal deaths from nearly 10% to about 3.5% by requiring staff to wash their hands in chloride of lime before attending the birth.

In a comparable study in London, John Snow (1849 and 1854) showed that the geographical distribution of cholera was related to the sources of the supplies of drinking water, and concluded that the 'peculiar poison of the disease' was spread in patients' faeces, which contaminated water later drunk by other persons (*faecal-oral transmission*). He personally removed the pump-handle of the supply in Broad Street, Soho – an example of practical infection control which has inspired many students of epidemiology although the evidence that it had any effect on the outcome of the outbreak is sparse. Measures subsequently taken to ensure the purity of drinking water by protection, filtration and chlorination have led to the decline of cholera, typhoid fever and other water-borne infections.

The development of the techniques of antiseptic and aseptic surgery for the prevention of wound sepsis had its origin in the conception by Joseph Lister (1867) that if, as shown by Pasteur, bacteria were the cause of the fermentation and putrefaction of dead organic matter, they might well also be the cause of suppuration in living tissues. By covering operation wounds with dressings soaked in carbolic acid to kill any bacteria present in them and to exclude others from entry, and by disinfecting his hands and instruments, he greatly reduced the incidence of sepsis in his patients.

A major group of infections that have proved largely insusceptible to control by environmental sanitation is those of the respiratory tract, e.g. common colds, sore throats, influenza, whooping cough, pneumonia, tuberculosis, measles and chickenpox. Organisms that enter and leave the body via the respiratory tract may be transmitted by a variety of means, including contact and air-borne secretion droplets. The ease of transmission, as well as the frequency with which urban dwellers share and breathe air polluted by others, explains the continuing high prevalence of respiratory infections. Similar considerations attend the spread of sexually transmitted diseases. Changes in social behaviour have facilitated the ease with which these diseases are maintained in the community despite the availability of effective treatments.

As well as these kinds of *exogenous* infections from external sources, there are also many infections, termed *endogenous*, which are caused by the invasion of tissues by a commensal organism that hitherto grew harmlessly elsewhere in the body, e.g. infections of the lung with pneumococci previously resident in the throat. The prevention of endogenous infections depends on the avoidance of predisposing conditions that impair the tissue defences.

Although infective illness remains common, there has been a phenomenal decrease in the death rate from the classic infections, especially in industrialized countries. Since the steep decline began before preventive and curative medicine became significantly effective, the earlier reduction in deaths must have been due to improvements in nutrition and living conditions that increased the resistance of individuals to infection. The subsequent introduction of immunization programmes and antimicrobial therapy has made a further substantial contribution to the saving of life, but let no-one imagine that microbial disease has been conquered!

RECOMMENDED READING

Brock T D (ed.) 1999 *Milestones in Microbiology*. American Society for Microbiology, Washington, DC

Bulloch W 1938 *The History of Bacteriology*. Oxford University Press, Oxford

Collard P 1976 *The Development of Microbiology*. Cambridge University Press, Cambridge

Cox F E G (ed.) 1996 *Illustrated History of Tropical Diseases*. Wellcome Trust, London

Foster W D 1970 *A History of Medical Bacteriology and Immunology*. Cox and Wyman, London

Grove D I 1990 *A History of Human Helminthology*. CAB International, Wallingford, Oxford

Mann J 1999 *The Elusive Magic Bullet: the Search for the Perfect Drug*. Oxford University Press, Oxford

Waterson A P, Wilkinson L 1978 *An Introduction to the History of Virology*. Cambridge University Press, Cambridge

Zinsser H 1935 *Rats, Lice and History*. Routledge, London

Internet site

United Nations Children's Fund. *The State of the World's Children 2002*: www.unicef.org/sowc02

2

Morphology and nature of micro-organisms

M. R. Barer

Micro-organisms are beyond doubt the most successful forms of life; they have been here longest, they are the most numerous and their distribution defines the limits of the biosphere, encompassing environments previously thought incapable of sustaining life. Here, we are concerned with the tiny fraction of micro-organisms that form associations with humans and these encompass the cellular entities, *bacteria, archaea, fungi*, and *protozoa* and the subcellular entities, viruses, viroids and prions. Whether the last three can be considered organisms or even living entities is a matter for debate. None the less, their transmissible nature, the immune responses they provoke and our inability to detect them with the naked eye place them firmly within the province of microbiology. The first two of these criteria also require us to consider some multicellular macroscopically visible organisms, (members of the *helminths*) as agents of infection (see Chapter 62). Most of this chapter is concerned with bacteria. The subcellular entities are briefly introduced and the remaining medically significant groups are considered in more specialized chapters.

Medical microbiology has been founded on recognizing micro-organisms that are associated with human disease. This recognition has relied predominantly on two techniques:

- microscopy
- propagation in laboratory cultures.

Over the past 30 years, it has become possible to detect, describe and differentiate micro-organisms by biochemical and genetic methods and this has had two profound effects on microbiology. First, largely due to the work of Carl Woese, it is now possible to make a reasonable assessment of the evolutionary relationships between micro-organisms, a task that previously could only be achieved for macro-organisms by examining fossil records (micro-organisms have not left interpretable fossils). Woese's approach led to the recognition of a whole 'new' *domain* (a group ranking above kingdom level) of cellular organisms, the

Archaea, and a fundamental review of microbial classification (Fig. 2.1). Second, the accumulation of molecular data describing microbes (including many complete genome nucleotide sequences) is underpinning the development of molecular detection methods. Thus morphology and cultural characteristics are regarded by many as secondary characteristics in the context of classification and identification, while molecular detection methods are steadily encroaching on microscopy and culture in clinical laboratories.

We are currently in a transitional, information-gathering phase. It seems likely that molecular descriptions and detection methods will come to dominate our view of the microbial world. However, at present it must be emphasized that the morphological classification provides a basic structure that is understood by clinicians and will remain as a basis for communication, at least in the medium term. Moreover, light and fluorescence microscopy remain competitively cheap and rapid compared to molecular methods as means of providing information relevant to the clinical management

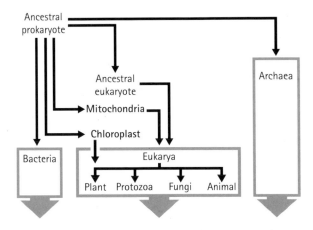

Fig. 2.1 Diagram illustrating proposed evolutionary pathways from a putative common ancestral prokaryote to the present. *The *Archaea* were not recognized as a separate lineage until Woese's work.

of infection. Finally, the discipline of medical microbiology requires the understanding of the basic structural properties and physiology of micro-organisms to underpin our approach to infections.

PROKARYOTIC AND EUKARYOTIC CELLS

Micro-organisms are microscopic in size and are usually unicellular. The diameter of the smallest body that can be resolved and seen clearly with the naked eye is about 100 μm. All medically relevant bacteria are smaller than this and a microscope is therefore necessary to see individual cells. When propagated on solid media, bacteria (and fungi) form macroscopically visible structures comprising at least 10^8 cells, which are known as *colonies*.

Woese's insights provided for the first time a coherent view of the evolutionary pathways behind the diversity of all living organisms. In particular, a satisfactory explanation is offered for the existence and diversity of *prokaryotic* and *eukaryotic* cells and all living forms are seen to fall within three *domains* of life, the *Bacteria*, the *Archaea* or the *Eukarya*. Although the first two of these are both prokaryotes (organisms without a membrane bound nucleus), the *Archaea* share many characteristics with the *Eukarya*. This division is of practical significance since the earlier the point of divergence, the greater the difference in metabolic properties between the present day representatives of the two lineages. These differences can be exploited by directing treatments at processes unique to the target organism. Some key differences between the three domains of life are summarized in Table 2.1.

ANATOMY OF THE BACTERIAL CELL

The principal structures of a typical bacterial cell are shown in Fig. 2.2. The *protoplast*, i.e. the whole body of living material (*protoplasm*), is bounded peripherally by a very thin, elastic and semi-permeable cytoplasmic (or plasma) membrane (a conventional phospholipid bilayer). Outside, and closely covering this, lies the rigid, supporting *cell wall*, which is porous and relatively permeable. Cell division occurs by the development, from the periphery inwards, of a transverse cytoplasmic membrane and a transverse cell wall known as a *septum* or *cross-wall*.

The pattern of cell division and the structures associated with the cell wall and the cytoplasmic membrane (collectively the cell envelope) combine to produce the cell morphology and characteristic patterns of cell arrangement. The recognition of these features by oil-immersion light microscopy remains of great practical value in making presumptive identifications of bacteria associated with human infections. Bacterial cells may have two basic shapes, spherical (*coccus*) or rod-shaped (*bacillus*); the rod-shaped bacteria show variants that are comma-shaped (*vibrio*), spiral (*spirillum* and *spirochaete*) or filamentous (Fig. 2.3).

The *cytoplasm*, or main part of the protoplasm, is a predominantly aqueous environment packed with ribosomes and numerous other protein and nucleotide–protein complexes. The cytoplasmic contents are not normally visible by light microscopy, which can only resolve objects <0.2 μm in diameter. Some larger structures such as spores (see below) or *inclusion granules* of storage products such as volutin (polyphosphate), lipid (poly-β-hydroxybutyrate), glycogen or starch occur in

Table 2.1   General characteristics of cellular micro-organisms in the three domains of life.

	PROKARYOTES		EUKARYOTES
Domains	*Bacteria*	*Archaea*	*Eukarya*
Major groups (examples only)	Gram positives, Proteobacteria	Methanococcus, Thermococcus	Fungi, Entamoebae, Cilliates, Flagellates
Cell diameter	~1 μm	~1 μm	~10 μm
Membrane-bound organelles	–	–	+ (e.g. mitochondria, nucleus, golgi, etc.)
Chromosomes	Single, closed circular	Single, closed circular	Multiple, linear
Introns	Rare	Rare	Common
Transcription/translation	Coupled	Coupled	Compartmentalized
mRNA	Very labile	Very labile	Stable and labile
Ribosomes	70S	70S	80S
Protein synthesis inhibited by:			
chloramphenicol	+	–	–
diphtheria toxin	–	+	+
Peptidoglycan cell wall	+	–	–

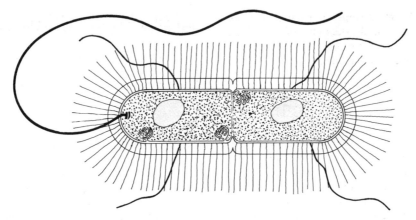

Fig. 2.2 A diagram of a dividing bacterial cell with a single flagellum, four sex pili, numerous common fimbriae, a cell wall, a cytoplasmic membrane, two nuclear bodies, three mesosomes and numerous ribosomes.

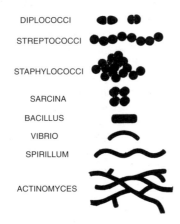

DIPLOCOCCI

STREPTOCOCCI

STAPHYLOCOCCI

SARCINA

BACILLUS

VIBRIO

SPIRILLUM

ACTINOMYCES

Fig. 2.3 The shapes and characteristic groupings of various bacterial cells.

some species under specific growth conditions. Specialized labelling techniques (generally requiring fluorescence imaging) enable visualization of the nuclear material or *nucleoid* and other structures (e.g. the forming cell division annulus). Figure 2.4 is an electron micrograph of a thin section of a dividing bacterial cell. Outside the cell wall there may be a protective gelatinous covering layer called a *capsule* or, when it is too thin to be resolved with the light microscope, a *microcapsule*. Soluble large-molecular material may be dispersed by the bacterium into the environment as *loose slime*. Some bacteria bear, protruding outwards from the cell wall, one or more kinds of filamentous appendages: *flagella*, which are organs of locomotion; *fimbriae*, which appear to be organs of adhesion; and *pili*, which are involved in the transfer of genetic material. Because they are exposed to contact and interaction with the cells and humoral substances of the body of the host, the surface structures of bacteria are the structures most likely to have special roles in the processes of infection.

Bacterial nucleoid

The genetic information of a bacterial cell is mostly contained in a single, long molecule of double-stranded deoxyribonucleic acid (DNA) which can be extracted in the form of a closed circular thread about 1 mm long. The cell solves the problem of packaging this enormous macromolecule by condensing and looping it into a *supercoiled* state. As well as the chromosome, the bacterium may contain one or more additional fragments of *episomal* (extrachromosomal) DNA, known as *plasmids*. Bacteria are essentially haploid organisms with only one allele of each gene per cell, although there may be multiple copies of chromosomes and plasmids. Unlike the mitotic or meiotic divisions of eukaryotic cells, chromosomal segregation in bacteria at the time of cell division (or fission) does not involve structures that can be resolved by light microscopy. None the less, the speed at which replication can occur (cell divisions more frequently than one every 15 min in some cases) and the simultaneous requirement for multiple rounds of chromosome replication in one cell provide a mind-boggling challenge for the segregation machinery. (Imagine unravelling two 1-mm double-stranded threads inside a sphere 1 μm across – scale it up to metre threads and millimetre spheres if you wish).

The bacterial nucleoid lies within the cytoplasm. This means that as DNA-dependent RNA polymerase makes RNA, ribosomes may attach and initiate protein synthesis on the still attached (nascent) messenger RNA. Synthesis of mRNA and protein (transcription and translation) are therefore seen to be directly coupled in bacteria. In contrast, complete transcripts in eukaryotic cells

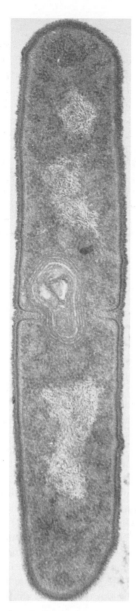

Fig. 2.4 A thin section of a dividing bacillus showing cell wall, cytoplasmic membrane, ribosomes, a developing cross-wall, and a mesosome. (By courtesy of Dr P. J. Highton and the editors of *Journal of Ultrastructure Research.*) ×50 000.

have to be spliced (to remove the non-coding introns) and capped with polyadenine (this rarely occurs with bacterial mRNA) before the post-transcriptionally modified message is translocated to the cytoplasm.

Ribosomes

Bacterial ribosomes are slightly smaller (10–20 nm) than those of eukaryotic cells and they have a sedimen-

tation coefficient of 70S, being composed of a 30S and a 50S subunit (cf. 40S and 60S in the 80S eukaryotic counterparts). They may be seen with the electron microscope, and number tens of thousands in growing cells. Multiple ribosomes attach to single mRNA molecules to form *polysomes*. It was the nucleotide sequencing of DNA encoding small subunit ribosomal RNA (rDNA) that led Woese to postulate the evolutionary pathways shown in Fig 2.1. Essentially all cellular organisms can now be classified at least down to genus level by their small subunit rRNA (SSrRNA) nucleotide sequences. Subsequently it was recognized that, since growing cells contain so many ribosomes, it should be possible to detect unique identifying (or determinative) SSrRNA sequences by complementary in-situ hybridization with fluorescently labelled oligonucleotide probes. Indeed, it is now possible to apply this approach to natural samples and this has enabled us to recognize cells of bacteria that have never been grown in laboratory culture.

Cytoplasmic membrane

The bacterial protoplast is limited externally by a thin, elastic cytoplasmic membrane which is 5–10 nm thick and consists mainly of phospholipids and proteins. Its structure can be resolved in some ultrathin sections examined by electron microscopy. *Membranes* generally appear in suitably stained electron microscope preparations as two dark lines about 2.5 nm wide separated by a lighter area of similar width. The basic structure and composition of the bacterial cytoplasmic membrane shown diagrammatically in Fig. 2.5 is similar to that of all cells (presumably this had already evolved in the 'ancestral prokaryote'). Integral, transmembrane and peripheral or anchored proteins occur in abundance and perform similar functions to those described in eukaryotes (e.g. transport and signal transduction). A key feature differentiating prokaryotic cytoplasmic membranes from those of eukaryotes is their multifunctional

Fig. 2.5 A diagram of a unit membrane. A lipid bilayer with polar (hydrophilic) regions externally orientated towards a layer of protein at each surface has a characteristic appearance when stained and seen in cross-section in the electron microscope.

Cell wall

The cell wall (Fig. 2.6) encases the protoplast and lies immediately external to the cytoplasmic membrane. It is 10–25 nm thick, strong and relatively rigid, though with some elasticity, and openly porous, being freely permeable to solute molecules smaller than 10 kDa in mass and 1 nm in diameter. It supports the weak cytoplasmic membrane against the high internal osmotic pressure of the protoplasm (usually between 5 and 25 atm.) and maintains the characteristic shape of the bacterium in its coccal, bacillary, filamentous or spiral form.

Except under defined osmotic conditions, protoplast survival is dependent on the integrity of the cell wall. If the wall is weakened or ruptured, the protoplasm may swell from osmotic inflow of water and burst the weak

nature. Thus, while in eukaryotic cells the endoplasmic reticulum and Golgi apparatus are involved in protein secretion, packaging and processing, and the mitochondrial inner membrane is the site of electron transport and oxidative phosphorylation, all of these functions must be performed by one membrane in prokaryotes. It is hardly surprising that prokaryotic cell membranes are relatively protein-rich, allowing relatively little space for phospholipids. It should be noted that the proposed endosymbiotic origin of two key organelles in eukaryotes, mitochondria and chloroplasts, has been confirmed by SSrRNA sequencing (Fig. 2.1). Both these organelles are almost certainly derived from free-living bacteria (they contain and encode bacterial 70S ribosomes).

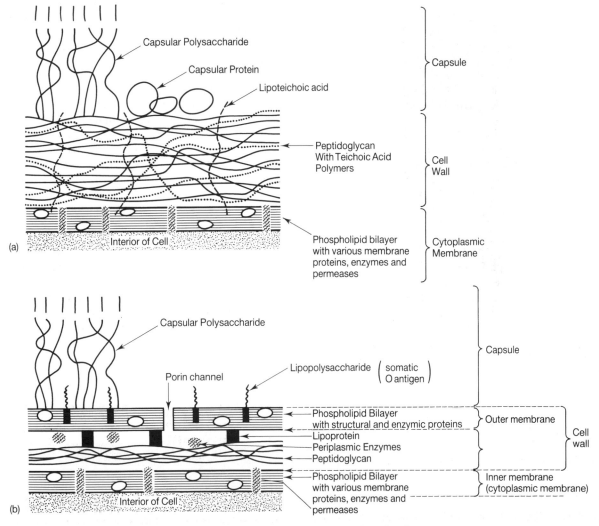

Fig. 2.6 **a** The envelope of the Gram-positive cell wall. **b** The envelope of the Gram-negative cell wall.

cytoplasmic membrane. This process of lethal disintegration and dissolution is termed *lysis*.

The cell wall plays an important part in *cell division*. A transverse partition of cell wall material grows inwards, like a closing iris diaphragm, from the lateral wall at the equator of the cell and forms a complete *septum* (or cross-wall) separating two daughter cells. The cell wall can be demonstrated by electron microscopy; it is seen both in ultrathin sections and, as an empty fold surrounding the shrunken protoplast, in whole cell preparations shadow-cast with heavy metal.

The chemical composition of the cell wall differs considerably between different bacterial species, but in all species the main strengthening component is *peptidoglycan* (syn. *mucopeptide* or *murein*). Peptidoglycan is composed of *N*-acetylglucosamine and *N*-acetylmuramic acid molecules linked alternately in a chain (Fig. 2.7). This heteropolymer forms a single molecular continuous sack around the protoplast (described as the murein sacculus). The thickness of the peptidoglycan layer turns out to be of great practical significance in differentiating medically significant bacteria. In the late 19th century a Danish physician, Christian Gram, immortalized himself by devising a staining procedure that we now know distinguishes bacteria with a thick (Gram-positive) and a thin (Gram-negative) murein sacculus. The traditional classification of bacteria is fundamentally rooted in this dichotomy, which has, fortunately, largely been supported by rRNA-based classification.

The rapid (<5 min) Gram stain procedure remains a cornerstone of day-to-day practice in detecting and identifying bacteria in clinical laboratories (see pp. 21–22).

The *N*-acetylmuramic acid units of peptidoglycan each carry a short peptide, usually consisting of L-alanine, D-glutamic acid, either *meso*-diaminopimelic acid (in Gram-negative bacteria) or L-lysine (in Gram-positive bacteria) and D-alanyl-D-alanine. The wall is given its strength by cross-links that form between adjacent strands. These may be formed directly between the *meso*-diaminopimelic acid or L-lysine of one strand and the penultimate D-alanine of the next, or (the usual form in Gram-positive organisms) through an interpeptide bridge composed of up to five amino acids; in either case, the terminal D-alanine is lost in the cross-linking reaction (Fig. 2.8). Several antibiotics interfere with the construction of the cell wall peptidoglycan (see Chapter 5).

The bacterial cell wall also contains other components whose nature and amount vary with the species. Many Gram-positive bacteria contain relatively large amounts of *teichoic acid* (a polymer of ribitol or glycerol phosphate complexed with sugar residues) interspersed with the peptidoglycan; some of this material (*lipoteichoic acid*) is linked to lipids buried in the cell membrane.

Electron microscopy reveals that Gram-negative bacteria possess a second *outer membrane* external to the peptidoglycan layer. This is essentially another unit membrane in which the outer leaflet is composed of a molecule referred to as lipopolysaccharide (LPS). Like the cytoplasmic membrane, this membrane contains many associated proteins whose functions include select-

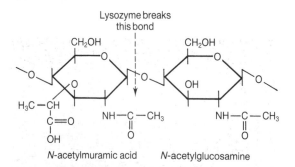

Fig. 2.7 The basic building block of bacterial cell wall peptidoglycan. *N*-Acetylmuramic acid is derived from *N*-acetylglucosamine by the addition of a lactic acid unit. Each *N*-acetylmuramic acid molecule is substituted with a pentapeptide; an *N*-acetylglucosamine molecule is joined to the muramylpentapeptide within the cell membrane and the unit is transferred to growth points in the existing peptidoglycan, where adjacent strands are cross-linked. (See also Fig. 2.8.)

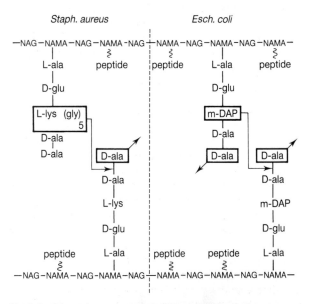

Fig. 2.8 Schematic representation of the peptidoglycan of a representative Gram-positive organism (*Staphylococcus aureus*) and a representative Gram-negative organism (*Escherichia coli*). Note that in the Gram-positive organism cross-linking occurs through a peptide bridge (pentaglycine in *Staph. aureus*), whereas direct cross-linking occurs in *Esch. coli*. In both cases the terminal D-alanine is lost. Not all peptides are engaged in cross-linking in *Esch. coli*, and carboxypeptidases remove redundant D-alanine residues.

ive permeability (porins) and attachment (adhesins). The outer membrane confers several important properties on Gram-negative bacteria:

- it protects the peptidoglycan from the effects of lysozyme (a natural body defence substance which cleaves the link between *N*-acetylglucosamine and *N*-acetylmuramic acid (see Fig. 2.7);
- it impedes the ingress of many antibiotics.

Components of the lipopolysaccharide, in particular the core structure, lipid A, form *endotoxin*, which, when released into the bloodstream, may give rise to *endotoxic shock*.

In addition to the basic Gram-related properties outlined above, a third type of cell envelope is characteristic of mycobacteria, a group that includes the causal agents of tuberculosis and leprosy. Mycobacteria are taxonomically Gram-positive bacteria, though they can rarely be demonstrated as such. The peptidoglycan layer is covalently linked on its outer aspect to arabinogalactan, which is itself substituted with unique lipids known as *mycolic acids*. These β-hydroxy fatty acids range from 60 to 90 carbon residues and, together with non-covalently linked free lipids, form an extremely hydrophobic external layer. This layer has some properties in common with the Gram-negative outer membrane (indeed, porins have recently been detected therein). The whole envelope structure confers the property of *acid-fast staining* by methods such as the Ziehl–Neelsen (ZN), or phenol-auramine procedures (see p. 22). These methods are of great practical significance in the diagnosis of mycobacterial diseases (see Chapters 18 and 19).

The cell envelope is a highly dynamic structure in growing bacterial cultures. Its components are subject to rapid turnover (synthesis, assembly, disassembly and degradation) and there is busy molecular traffic in and out of the cytoplasm. Although the diagrammatic and photographic representations here give it a somewhat monolithic and immutable character, the envelope and other surface structures can change very rapidly (within minutes) in response to environmental signals. The cell surface receives and transmits many signals from the surrounding environment, including those involving other bacteria, particularly those belonging to the same strain. This latter phenomenon is known as *quorum sensing* and appears to be important in regulating gene expression in groups of bacteria.

The structures involved in the molecular traffic through the cell envelope are the subject of intense investigation. In particular, the outward secretion of proteins attracts much current interest. At least four distinct processes have been identified and all involve impressive macromolecular complexes anchored in the cytoplasmic membrane. Of particular interest here are the

Type III secretion systems in Gram-negative bacteria. The fully assembled multiprotein complex spans the cytoplasmic membrane, the periplasmic space, the murein sacculus and the outer membrane and, in some cases, projects from the cell surface into an adjacent host (human) cell. These impressive delivery systems are capable of injecting *effector molecules* into the host cell and thereby subvert the latter's function to the advantage of the microbe.

Extracellular polysaccharides: capsules, microcapsules and loose slime

Many bacteria have been demonstrated to possess a more or less continuous but relatively amorphous layer external to the Gram-negative and Gram-positive envelopes described above. Although these are quite readily detected in some bacteria grown under laboratory conditions, they are somewhat ephemeral in others. These structures appear to be important in mediating contact with potentially hostile environments and may be subject to strict environmental control.

When this layer is fully hydrated and resolvable by light microscopy, it is called a *capsule* (Fig. 2.9). When it is narrower, and detectable only by indirect, serological means, or by electron microscopy, it may be termed a *microcapsule*. The capsular gel consists largely of water and has only a small content (e.g. 2%) of solids. In most species, the solid material is a complex polysaccharide, though in some species its main constituent is polypeptide.

Loose slime, or *free slime*, is an amorphous, viscid colloidal material that is secreted extracellularly by some bacteria. In bacteria that also possess a demonstrable capsule the slime is generally similar in chemical composition and antigenic character to the capsular substance. When slime-forming bacteria are grown on a solid culture medium, the slime remains around the bacteria as a matrix in which

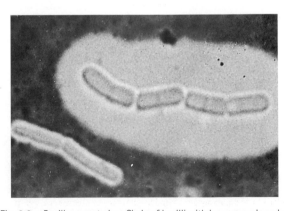

Fig. 2.9 *Bacillus megaterium.* Chain of bacilli with large capsule and pair with very small capsule. Wet film with India ink, ×3500.

they are embedded and its presence confers on the growths a watery and sticky 'mucoid' character. The slime is freely soluble in water and, when the bacteria are grown or suspended in a liquid medium, it passes away from them and disperses through the medium.

All of these features appear to have some role in interactions with the external environment. In some cases capsules have been shown to protect against phagocytosis, the lytic action of complement and bacteriophage invasion. In at least three instances antibodies directed against capsular antigens have been shown to protect against infection and, indeed, capsular preparations are used in several vaccines. Capsules also appear to have a role in protecting cells against desiccation. The production of extracellular polysaccharides in general provides a matrix within which *biofilm* formation can take place.

S-layers

A rather more structured (paracrystalline) protein layer has been demonstrated in some bacteria. This S-layer can be shown by electron microscopy and appears to share at least some functional properties in common with capsules.

Flagella and motility

Motile bacteria possess filamentous appendages known as *flagella*, which act as organs of locomotion. The flagellum is a long, thin filament, twisted spirally in an open, regular wave form. It is about 0.02 μm thick and is usually several times the length of the bacterial cell. It originates in the bacterial protoplasm and the structure projects through the cell envelope. According to the species, there may be one, or up to 20, flagella per cell. In elongated bacteria the arrangement of the flagella may

be *peritrichous*, or *lateral*, when they originate from the sides of the cell, or *polar*, when they originate from one or both ends. Where several occur on a cell, they may function coiled together as a single 'tail'. The external portion of a flagellum is essentially a polymer of a single protein, *flagellin*, while the basal region inserted into the cytoplasmic membrane comprises multiple subunits, which anchor and power the organ. In a remarkably elegant manner, the flagellar motor is powered directly (as opposed to indirectly via ATP) by the proton gradient created across the cytoplasmic membrane by electron transport. In *Escherichia coli,* alternation between the anticlockwise and clockwise motion of the flagella effects, respectively, linear or tumbling motility. The intervals between these two patterns are modulated by chemical signals in the environment and the end result is that the bacterium shows *chemotactic behaviour* (movement towards or away from certain stimuli).

Flagella are invisible in ordinary light microscope preparations, but may be shown by the use of special staining methods, and in special circumstances by darkground illumination. Because of the difficulties of these methods, the presence of flagella is commonly inferred from the observation of motility. They can be demonstrated easily and clearly with the electron microscope, usually appearing as simple fibrils without internal differentiation (Fig. 2.10). In some preparations the flagellum appears as a hollow tube formed of helically twisted fibrils, and the flagella of some bacteria, e.g. vibrios, have an outer sheath. In the spirochaetes the flagellum is located in the periplasm and hence is referred to as an endoflagellum and this presumably underpins their characteristic spiral motion.

Motility is clearly important to many bacteria and probably serves mainly to place the cell in environments favourable to growth and free from noxious influences.

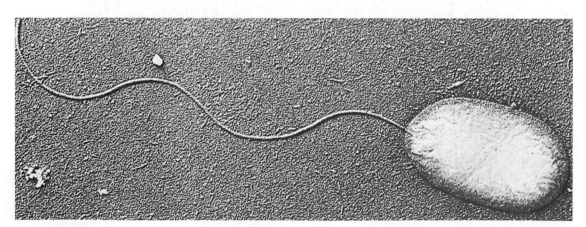

Fig. 2.10 *Pseudomonas aeruginosa.* Bacillus with a single polar flagellum, dried and shadow-cast. Electron micrograph, ×38 000. (From Wilkinson J F, Duguid J P 1960 The influence of cultural conditions on bacterial cytology. *International Review of Cytology* 9: 1–76.)

In some cases possession of flagella is thought to contribute to the pathogenesis of disease.

Fimbriae and pili

Many bacteria possess filamentous appendages termed *fimbriae* or *pili*. These terms are often used interchangeably, although the latter was originally reserved for structures involved in genetic exchange between bacteria (sex pili – see below). Fimbriae are far more numerous than flagella (e.g. 100–500, being borne peritrichously by each cell) and are much shorter and only about half as thick (e.g. varying from 0.1 to 1.5 μm in length and having a uniform width between 4 and 8 nm). They do not have the smoothly curved spiral form of flagella and are mostly more or less straight. They cannot be seen with the light microscope but are clearly seen with the electron microscope in preparations that have been metal-shadowed or negatively stained with phosphotungstic acid (Fig. 2.11).

Multiple types (e.g. types 1 and 2, P type etc.) of fimbriae have been recognized according to their dimensions, antigenic and phenotypic properties. They have been most extensively studied in *Esch. coli*. In the medical and veterinary contexts, fimbriae are recognized to be important in mediating adhesion between the bacterium and host cells (classically this was recognized in the phenomenon of haemagglutination, a property of type 1, mannose-sensitive pili). In contrast, *sex pili* are structurally similar to other fimbriae but are longer and confer the ability to attach specifically to other bacteria that lack these appendages. Sex pili initiate the process of conjugation (see Chapter 6); they also act as receptor sites for certain bacteriophages described as being

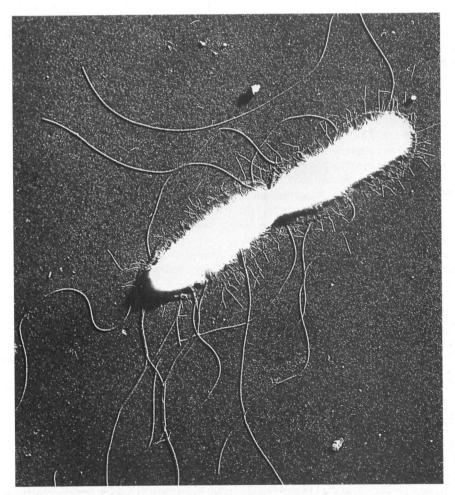

Fig. 2.11 *Salmonella enterica* serotype Typhi. Dividing bacillus from log-phase culture bears about 15 long wavy flagella and over 100 short fimbriae. Note dense (white) shrunken protoplast surrounded by an empty fold of cell wall. Whole bacillus dried and shadow-cast. Electron micrograph, ×16 000. (From Duguid J P, Wilkinson J F 1961 Environmentally induced changes in bacterial morphology. *Symposia of the Society for General Microbiology* 11: 69–99.)

'donor-specific'. In general it appears that the tip of the structure is responsible for a receptor-specific interaction with the cell to which the fimbriate cell is attaching.

It should be noted that fimbriae are not the only means by which bacteria can be involved in specific adhesion events. *Non-fimbrial adhesins* (generally proteins or glycoproteins) are also important in this regard. Receptor-specific interactions are very important in infective disease as they are thought to determine much of the tissue tropism of the pathological process.

THE BACTERIAL 'LIFE CYCLE'

Multicellular organisms have been recognized for many years to pass through many different stages. These may include many immature forms (cf. the larval stages of helminth parasitic worms) or dormant forms (e.g. plant seeds). Even protozoa and fungi may show multiple developmental stages. In contrast, bacteria have been viewed as growing (*vegetative*), stationary or dead. With the exception of spore-forming genera (see below), because they do not undergo morphological differentiation, bacterial cells have been considered essentially uniform in their properties. As indicated above, it is now recognized that all bacteria adapt extensively and rapidly to their environment. This adaptation takes place at both the phenotypic (gene expression) and genotypic (genetic complement and arrangement) levels. It seems clear that there are many more physiological states in which bacteria can exist than previously acknowledged and that these states may influence the capacity of the immune system and antimicrobial agents to eliminate them. In particular, the possibility that non-sporulating bacteria are capable of dormancy, a reversible state of metabolic shutdown, has attracted much interest. Spore formation, however, is the key paradigm of differentiation and dormancy in bacteria.

The different forms taken on by organisms at different stages in the life cycle are of course important in their recognition. The range of basic cellular forms of bacteria was mentioned above. It is difficult to generalize but important to mention that bacterial cell morphology does alter with the physiological state. Characteristically, the cells of bacteria that are growing rapidly are larger than their non- or slowly-growing counterparts. Although this does not alter basic coccal morphology, it may make bacilli appear more intermediate (cocco-bacillary) or spherical (coccoid) in shape. Bacilli exposed to certain noxious influences (notably some antibiotics) may produce extended forms that are sometimes described as filamentous. Bacteria that are characterized as essentially filamentous produce a mat of intertwining filaments known as a mycelium (one

characteristic form of fungal growth). This form of growth is also associated with fragmentation in which coccal forms may be released and this results in highly *pleomorphic* cultures. All of these alternate growth forms are undoubtedly under the influence of environmental signals although their identities have yet to be determined in most cases.

Bacterial spores

Some bacteria, notably those of the genera *Bacillus* and *Clostridium*, develop a highly resistant resting phase or *endospore*, whereby the organism can survive in a dormant state through a long period of starvation or other adverse environmental conditions (resuscitation of spores several thousand years old has been claimed). The process does not involve multiplication: in *sporulation*, each vegetative cell forms only one spore, and in subsequent *germination* each spore gives rise to a single vegetative cell. Geneticists have viewed sporulation as a paradigm of a simple differentiation process and the key molecular processes required in *Bacillus subtilis* are now understood in great detail. In the face of sporulation stimuli, classically starvation or transition from growth to stationary phase, a programme of sequential expression of specific genes is triggered. The end result is a morphologically distinct structure, the endospore, within the *mother cell*.

In unstained preparations the spore is recognized within the parent cell by its greater refractility. It is larger than lipid inclusion granules and is often ovoid, in contrast to the spherical shape of the lipid granules. Mature ungerminated spores are 'phase-bright' when viewed by phase-contrast microscopy; immature or germinated spores are 'phase-dark'. When mature, the spore resists coloration by simple stains, appearing as a clear space within the stained cell protoplasm. Spores are slightly acid-fast and may be stained differentially by a modification of the ZN method. The appearance of the mature spores varies according to the species, being spherical, ovoid or elongated, occupying a terminal, subterminal or central position, and being narrower than the cell, or broader and bulging it (Fig. 2.12). Spores of some species have an additional, apparently loose, covering known as the *exosporium* (Fig. 2.13).

Spores are much more resistant than the vegetative forms to exposure to disinfectants, drying and heating (see Chapter 7). Thus, application of moist heat at 100–120°C or greater for a period of 10–20 min may be needed to kill spores, whereas heating at 60°C suffices to kill vegetative cells. In the dry state, or in moist conditions unfavourable to growth, spores may remain viable for many years. The marked resistance of spores has been attributed to several factors in which they

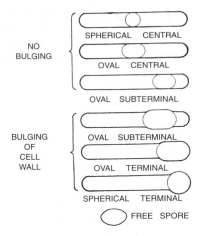

Fig. 2.12 The shape and situation of the spore in the bacterial cell.

NO BULGING
- SPHERICAL CENTRAL
- OVAL CENTRAL
- OVAL SUBTERMINAL

BULGING OF CELL WALL
- OVAL SUBTERMINAL
- OVAL TERMINAL
- SPHERICAL TERMINAL

FREE SPORE

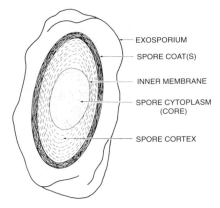

EXOSPORIUM
SPORE COAT(S)
INNER MEMBRANE
SPORE CYTOPLASM (CORE)
SPORE CORTEX

Fig. 2.13 Cross-section of a bacterial spore. The core is surrounded by the inner spore membrane. The cortex, a laminated structure, is protected by a more resistant layer or multiple layers forming the spore coat. In some cases, a loose outer covering (exosporium) can be defined.

differ from vegetative cells: the impermeability of their cortex and outer coat, their high content of calcium and dipicolinic acid, their low content of water, and their very low metabolic and enzymic activity.

Reactivation of the spore is termed *germination* and it should be noted that this is not just a reversal of the process by which the spore was formed. Germination of the spore occurs in response to specific stimuli that are generally related to external conditions favourable to growth. It is irreversible and involves rapid degradative changes. The spore successively loses its heat resistance and its dipicolinic acid; it loses calcium, it becomes permeable to dyes and its refractivity changes. Spores that have survived exposure to severe adverse influences such as heat are much more exacting than normal spores in their requirements for germination. For this reason, specially enriched culture media are used when testing the sterility of materials, such as surgical catgut, that have been exposed to disinfecting procedures. In the process of germination, the spore swells, its cortex disintegrates, its coat is broken open and a single vegetative cell emerges.

The initiation of germination (*activation*) is incompletely understood. It is clear that the state of dormancy of spores may be altered by various treatments, e.g. transient exposure to heat at 80°C, so that germination can then proceed more rapidly in the individual cells or more completely in a spore population. Activation is distinct from germination and is reversible if germination does not proceed.

Following germination, cell growth leading up to the formation of the first vegetative cell and prior to the first cell division is referred to as *outgrowth*. The conditions required for successful outgrowth may differ markedly from those that allow germination.

Conidia (exospores)

Some of the mycelial bacteria (*Actinomycetales*) and many filamentous fungi form *conidia*, resting spores of a kind different from endospores. The conidia are borne *externally* by abstriction from the ends of the parent cells (conidiophores), and are disseminated by the air or other means to fresh habitats. They are not especially resistant to heat and disinfectants.

Pleomorphism and involution

During growth, bacteria of a single strain may show considerable variation in size and shape, or form a proportion of cells that are swollen, spherical, elongated or pear-shaped. This pleomorphism occurs most readily in certain species (e.g. *Streptobacillus moniliformis* and *Yersinia pestis*) in ageing cultures on artificial medium and especially in the presence of antagonistic substances such as penicillin, glycine, lithium chloride, sodium chloride in high concentrations, and organic acids at low pH. The abnormal cells are generally regarded as degenerate or *involution* forms; some are non-viable, whilst others may grow and revert to the normal form when transferred to a suitable environment. In many cases the abnormal shape seems to be the result of defective cell wall synthesis; the growing protoplasm expands the weakened wall to produce a grotesquely swollen cell comparable to a spheroplast (see below) that later usually bursts and lyses.

Spheroplasts and free protoplasts

If bacteria have their cell walls removed or weakened while they are held in a sufficiently concentrated solution such as 0.2–1.0 M sucrose, with 0.01 M Mg^{2+} to prevent them imbibing water by osmosis, they may escape being lysed and, instead, may become converted into viable spherical bodies. If all the cell wall material has been removed from them, the spheres are *free protoplasts*. If they remain enclosed by an intact, but weakened residual cell wall, they are called *spheroplasts*. Protoplasts, for example, are readily liberated from the Gram-positive *Bacillus megaterium* by dissolution of the cell walls with egg-white lysozyme. Spheroplasts are readily produced from Gram-negative bacilli such as *Esch. coli* by growing the organism in the presence of penicillins or other β-lactam antibiotics that specifically inhibit synthesis of the peptidoglycan component of the cell wall. A similar result may be obtained by culturing certain bacteria on media lacking a nutrient, e.g. diaminopimelic acid, lysine or a hexosamine derivative, that they require specifically for cell wall synthesis.

Protoplasts and spheroplasts are osmotically sensitive; they vary in size with the osmotic pressure of the suspending medium and, if the medium is much diluted, they swell up, burst and perish by lysis. If maintained in an osmotically protective nutrient medium, they remain viable and continue to metabolize, synthesize and grow. Protoplasts do not multiply (but see L-forms below). Spheroplasts, when kept in suitable conditions, may multiply by fission or budding and reproduce through many serial subcultures. Protoplasts cannot revert to normal bacterial morphology by re-forming their cell walls, but spheroplasts commonly revert en masse when transferred to a culture medium lacking the cell wall inhibitor.

L-forms of bacteria

These are abnormal growth forms that may arise spontaneously (e.g. in *Streptobacillus moniliformis* and *Bacteroides* spp.) or by the inhibition of cell wall synthesis in bacteria of normal morphology. They are stable in the sense that special conditions of culture, such as the presence of penicillin, are not required to prevent their reversion to the parental bacterial forms. They continue to reproduce as L-forms through repeated subcultures in the absence of cell wall inhibitor, and give rise to revertants of normal bacterial morphology only occasionally. They differ from the parent bacteria in lacking a rigid cell wall and, in consequence, regular size and shape, but unlike protoplasts they are capable of growing and multiplying on a suitable nutrient medium. They range in size from minute bodies about 0.1 μm in diameter to large forms of 10–20 μm. The smallest viable forms are about 0.3 μm in diameter and may pass through bacteria-stopping filters.

Colonies of L-phase organisms on agar media are small and have a characteristic 'fried egg' appearance, rather

like mycoplasmas, which naturally lack peptidoglycan. Because of their fragility, microscopic examination of L-forms is best done in situ on the agar medium, a cover slip being applied to a block of agar bearing the growth. If desired, the organisms can be stained after fixation by a fixative that is allowed to diffuse through the agar.

L-forms should probably be regarded as laboratory artifacts that do not occur or survive to any important extent in natural habitats, although it is possible that they could account for bacterial persistence during therapy with certain antibiotics. L-forms are non-pathogenic to laboratory animals.

MORPHOLOGICAL STUDY OF MICRO-ORGANISMS

Microscopic examination provided our first insights into the microbial world and the practical classification of bacteria is still rooted in observations made on fixed and stained preparations. The information obtained this way has stood the test of time and routine bacteriological analysis is still highly dependent on light microscopy, as are mycological and parasitological analyses. However, in the context of diagnostic work, it must be recognized that these are essentially subjective methods requiring both skill and expertise. In the future, it seems likely that, as soon as they become reliable and economically competitive, molecular methods will come to replace the recognition of morphology in the routine practice of microbiology. In contrast, the role of microscopy in determining the nature, morphology and natural history of micro-organisms has undergone a renaissance in the final two decades of the twentieth century. The range of relevant microscopic techniques and their applications will be briefly surveyed below.

Light microscopy of unstained preparations

The formation of a recognizable image by any form of transmission microscopy depends on differences in light absorption, refractive index and refractility of the preparation studied. Staining can artificially create these differences but in unstained preparations some form of *contrast enhancement* technique is required. The crudest means of enhancing contrast can be achieved by altering the illumination by lowering the condenser so that illumination of the specimen is diffuse or by using a *dark-ground* condenser so that only refracted light is transmitted to the observer. Both these methods are good at detecting refractile boundaries (e.g. membranes) and, particularly in the case of dark-ground illumination, objects below the resolution of conventional light microscopy, notably the slim spiral agent of syphilis (*Treponema pallidum*), can be detected this way. Both these methods achieve contrast at the expense of detail.

Much more detail can be preserved with the more sophisticated methods of illumination used in *phase-contrast* and *Nomarski* (or *differential*) *interference contrast* microscopy. Phase-contrast, developed in the middle of the 20th century, has been the mainstay technique used in the microscopy of bacteria, fungi and protozoa. Phase-contrast is widely used in the preliminary examination of urine specimens. Nomarski microscopy became established in the 1970s and is used extensively in eukaryotic cell biology. Both methods use sophisticated illumination methods to produce interference patterns which result in light and dark zones in the image corresponding to zones with different refractile properties. Nomarski microscopy is slightly more difficult to set up than phase-contrast. However, the latter produces a light halo around objects that makes it very difficult to discern detail. Nomarski is therefore the method of choice for studying detail within eukaryotic cells. Neither method is capable of resolving detail within bacterial cells.

Staining or labelling of micro-organisms

Staining gained the reputation of a quasi-science in the latter half of the 20th century. The established methods reflected the empirical efforts of microbiologists and pathologists working up to a century before to render microbes visible by any means whatsoever. Two basic methods provide foundations for differential staining and detection of bacteria: the Gram stain and the acid-fast stains referred to above. Current understanding of staining processes allows a reasoned explanation for the basis of the labelling reaction in both cases on the basis of staining theory. Moreover, it must be appreciated that many of the difficulties associated with staining methods in the past relate to difficulties in obtaining reliable and chemically defined reagents. In addition to substantial improvements in these areas, the development of immunological reagents and other forms of specific ligands have heralded an era in which we can view modern staining procedures more as specific labelling procedures that locate particular molecules or processes.

Bacteria and blood protozoa like malaria parasites are generally studied when fixed and stained. Smears or films of bacterial cultures and clinical specimens are usually fixed by heat, the slide being first thoroughly dried in air and then heated gently in a flame. Vegetative bacteria are thereby killed, attached to the surface of the slide and preserved from undergoing autolytic changes. Blood films are fixed in methanol. Chemical fixatives such as formalin, mercuric chloride and osmic acid are used for sections of infected tissue.

During staining, the coloured, positively charged cation of basic dyes such as methylene blue combines with negatively charged groups in the cell protoplasm, especially with the phosphate groups in the abundant nucleic acids. Acidic dyes, having coloured anions, do not stain bacteria strongly except at very acid pH values, and thus can be used for 'negative staining' (see below). Cells or structures that stain with basic dyes at normal pH values are described as *basophilic*, and those that stain with acidic dyes as *acidophilic*. It should be noted that the bacterial cell wall is not stained by ordinary methods, and the coloured body seen corresponds to the cell protoplasm only. This is usually much shrunken as a result of drying. Chains of stained bacteria thus show the coloured bodies separated by gaps that are the sites of unstained, connecting cell walls. Certain bacteria do not colour evenly with simple stains, perhaps because of the manner in which the protoplasm shrinks when the cell is dried and fixed. Thus, the diphtheria bacillus shows a 'beaded' appearance, with alternating dark and light bars. The plague bacillus shows 'bipolar staining', the ends being more deeply coloured than the centre.

Negative or *background staining* is of value as a rapid method for the simple morphological study of bacteria and yeasts. The organisms are mixed with a substance such as India ink, or nigrosin, which, after spreading as a film, yields a dark background in which the organisms stand out as bright, unstained objects. Eosin-saline can similarly be used for the negative staining of intestinal protozoa. *Silver impregnation* methods are used to stain spirochaetes, especially in tissues. The slender cells are thickened by a dark deposit of silver on their surface.

Differential staining reactions. For blood protozoa, polychrome dyes such as Giemsa, Leishman or other *Romanowsky stains* are used for differential staining of the characteristic morphological features of the parasites (see Chapter 61). Various stains may be helpful in the diagnosis of fungal disease, depending on the species and its location in the body (see Chapter 60).

In the case of bacteria, *Gram's stain* has the widest application, distinguishing them as 'Gram-positive' or 'Gram-negative', according to whether or not they resist decoloration with acetone, alcohol or aniline oil after staining with a triphenyl methane dye, such as methyl violet, and subsequent treatment with iodine. The Gram-positive bacteria resist decoloration and remain stained a dark purple colour. The Gram-negative bacteria are decolorized, and are then counterstained light pink by the subsequent application of safranin, neutral red or dilute carbol fuchsin. In routine diagnostic work a Gram-stained smear is often the only preparation examined microscopically, since it shows clearly the general morphology of the bacteria as well as revealing their Gram reaction. It should be noted that characteristically Gram-positive species may sometimes appear Gram-negative under certain conditions of growth, especially in ageing cultures on nutrient agar. Gram reactivity appears to reflect a fundamental aspect of cell structure and is correlated with many other biological properties. Thus, the different species of a single genus generally show the same reaction. Gram-positive bacteria are more susceptible than Gram-negative bacteria to the antibacterial actions of penicillin, acids, iodine, basic dyes, detergents and lysozyme, and less susceptible to alkalis, azide, tellurite, proteolytic enzymes, lysis by antibody and complement, and plasmolysis in solutes of high osmotic pressure.

The probable mechanism of the Gram stain is attributed to differences in the permeability of the two essential cell wall types. After staining with methyl violet and treatment with iodine, a dye–iodine complex is formed within the cell; this is insoluble in water but moderately soluble and dissociable in the acetone or alcohol used as the decolorizer. Under the action of the decolorizer, the dye and iodine diffuse freely out of the Gram-negative cell, but not from the Gram-positive cell, presumably because the cell wall of the latter is less permeable. Gram-positive bacteria become Gram-negative when their cell wall is ruptured or removed.

The *acid-fast staining reaction*, as revealed by the ZN method, is of value in the detection of the tubercle bacillus and some other mycobacteria. These 'acid-fast' bacteria have cell walls containing unique lipids (mycolic acids) with chain lengths of up to 90 carbon atoms. They are relatively impermeable to simple aqueous stains, but when permeability is altered by heating or phenol (or both), concentrated solutions of basic fuchsin, and the fluorescent dyes auramine and rhodamine can produce well stained cells that subsequently resist decolorization by 20% sulphuric acid. Any decoloured non-acid-fast organisms are counterstained in a contrasting colour with methylene blue or malachite green. Modifications of the ZN method are useful for the demonstration of organisms such as *Nocardia* spp. and some protozoa, notably *Cryptosporidium parvum*.

THE NATURE AND COMPOSITION OF VIRUSES

Structure

The basic infectious particle of a virus is known as the *virion*. In the simplest viruses this consists of nucleic acid and a surrounding coat of protein called the *capsid*. Some viruses are enclosed within an *envelope*, usually derived from host cell membranes but modified by the inclusion of viral glycoproteins. The capsid is composed

of distinct morphological units or *capsomeres* which are assembled from viral proteins. Depending on the arrangement of these proteins, the capsomeres may be spherical, cylindrical or ring-like in appearance. The *nucleocapsid* is the combination of nucleic acid and capsid. The arrangement of the capsomeres around the nucleic acid determines the *symmetry* of the virion. When the capsomeres are applied directly to the helical nucleic acid this forms a coil-like structure with the appearance of a hollow tube. Viruses with this arrangement are said to have *helical symmetry*. Most helical viruses enclose the nucleocapsid within an envelope and thus do not have a rigid appearance. The other major type is shown by the viruses with *icosahedral symmetry* (Fig. 2.14), in which the capsomeres are arranged as if they lay on the faces of an icosahedron which has 20 equilateral triangular faces and 12 corners or apices (Fig. 2.15). Capsomeres on the faces and edges of this

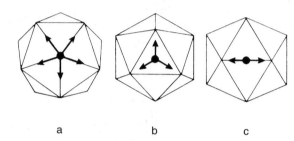

Fig. 2.14 An icosahedron viewed along its **a** five-fold, **b** three-fold and **c** two-fold axes of symmetry.

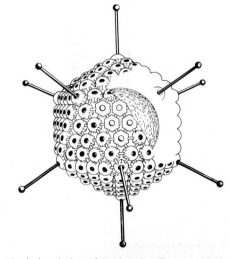

Fig. 2.15 An icosahedron of an adenovirus. The core of DNA is represented by a circular mass. Some of the pentamers at the 12 vertices have been indicated with protruding fibres and terminal knobs. The remaining 240 hexamer capsids are, for the most part, shown as compressed into hollow spheres linked to each other by divalent bonds. The hexagonal shape of a few of the capsomeres is seen in the centre of the diagram.

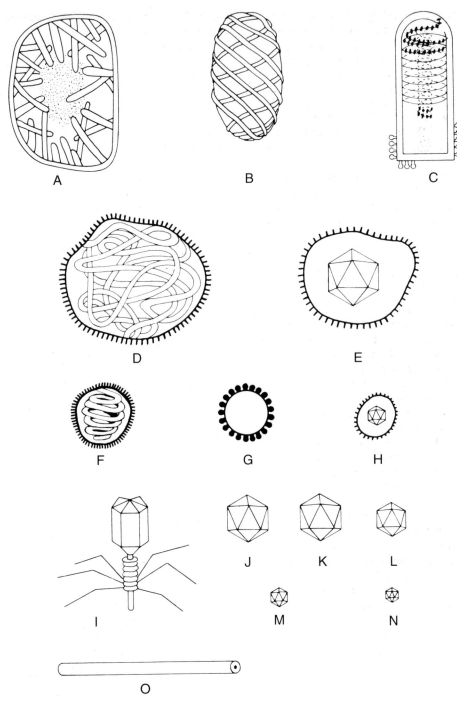

Fig. 2.16 Morphology of viruses.

A Orthopoxvirus
B Parapoxvirus
C Rhabdovirus
D Paramyxovirus

E Herpesvirus
F Orthomyxovirus
G Coronavirus
H Togavirus

I T-even coliphage
J Adenovirus
K Reovirus
L Papovavirus

M Picornavirus
N Parvovirus
O Tobacco mosaic virus

figure are called hexons as they always link with six adjacent capsomeres; those positioned at the apices are the pentons as they always join to five capsomeres. Viruses with icosahedral symmetry have a rigid structure and, under the electron microscope, have a characteristic hexagonal outline with triangular faces. However, if the diameter of the virion is less than about 50 nm the particle will appear spherical. Many viruses with icosahedral symmetry are enclosed by an outer envelope. The poxviruses are large and complex and do not show either type of symmetry; they are referred to as complex. The size of virions varies considerably, from 25 to 300 nm, in different families (Fig. 2.16).

Viral nucleic acid

The commonest types of nucleic acid in viruses of humans are single-stranded RNA and double-stranded DNA. However, both double-stranded RNA and single-stranded DNA occur in the reoviruses and parvoviruses, respectively. The genomes of RNA viruses may be present as a single strand as in paramyxoviruses, or as two copies as in the retroviruses, or exist as a specific number of fragments as in the orthomyxoviruses and reoviruses. Circular molecules of DNA are present in the virions of papovaviruses and hepadnaviruses. The amount of nucleic acid in virions is constant for a particular virus but shows considerable variation; thus the molecular weight can vary from about 1.5 million in the parvoviruses and hepadnaviruses to between 80 million and 240 million for the poxviruses.

Virion enzymes

Several viruses carry essential enzymes in the virion. As discussed in Chapter 9, an RNA-dependent RNA polymerase or transcriptase is an essential component of the virion in several virus families, including the negative-strand RNA viruses. Among DNA viruses only the poxviruses carry a DNA-dependent RNA polymerase. The hepadnaviruses have a virion polymerase complex that has some similarity to the reverse transcriptase complex found in the retroviruses.

Viral proteins

Analysis of the proteins produced in a cell during viral infection shows that some are essential components of the virion; these are the structural proteins and include capsid proteins and enzymes as well as basic core proteins which may be necessary to package the nucleic acid within the capsid. Other proteins such as enzymes are needed for the production of viral components but are not part of the virion; these are the non-structural proteins. The essential steps of virus attachment and penetration of the host cell are known to depend on regions of the outer capsid such as the apical fibres and knobs of adenoviruses or on parts of the envelope glycoproteins of viruses such as influenza A and B and the human immunodeficiency virus.

Viroids, defective viruses and prions

Our concept of the organismal nature of infectious agents is stretched to the limit by these infective entities. Viroids are essentially circular RNA molecules that have been associated with several plant diseases; they do not encode proteins or possess a capsid. The hepatitis delta agent has some features in common with viroids and with defective viruses (viruses that need the help of another virus for the formation of infectious particles). In the case of the delta agent these features result in an infective agent that can be transmitted in parallel with hepatitis B.

Prions are proteinaceous infective agents that are responsible for the transmissible spongiform encephalopathies (see Chapter 59). An increase in the number of prion proteins in a new host seems to result from the capacity of the introduced protein to induce abnormal conformational changes in a closely related host protein rather than by replication. Accumulation of the protein in the induced conformation produces the characteristic pathology of the disease.

RECOMMENDED READING

Armitage J P 1999 Bacterial tactic responses. *Advances in Microbial Physiology* 41: 231–291

Blair D F 1995 How bacteria sense and swim. *Annual Review of Microbiology* 49: 489–522

Frey D, Oldfield R J, Bridger R C 1979 *A Colour Atlas of Pathogenic Fungi.* Wolfe Medical, London

Madeley C R, Field A M 1988 *Virus Morphology,* 2nd edn. Churchill Livingstone, Edinburgh

Moat A G, Foster J W 1995 *Microbial Physiology,* 3rd edn. Wiley-Liss, New York

Neidhardt F C, Ingraham J L, Schaechter M 1990 *Physiology of the Bacterial Cell: A Molecular Approach.* Sinauer, Sunderland, MA

Nikaido H, Vaara M 1985 Molecular basis of bacterial outer membrane permeability. *Microbiological Reviews* 49: 1–32

Olds R J 1975 *A Colour Atlas of Microbiology.* Wolfe Medical, London

Internet sites

www.cellsalive.com/
www.ucmp.berkeley.edu/bacteria/bacteriamm.html

Classification and identification of micro-organisms

T. L. Pitt

Micro-organisms may be classified in the following large biological groups:

1. Algae
2. Protozoa
3. Slime moulds
4. Fungi
5. Bacteria
6. Archaebacteria
7. Viruses.

The algae (excluding the blue-green algae), the protozoa, slime moulds and fungi include the larger and more highly developed micro-organisms; their cells have the same general type of structure and organization, described as *eukaryotic*, as that found in higher plants and animals. The bacteria, including organisms of the mycoplasma, rickettsia and chlamydia groups, together with the related blue-green algae, comprise the smaller micro-organisms, with a simpler form of cellular organization described as *prokaryotic*. The archaebacteria are a distinct phylogenetic group of prokaryotes, which bear only a remote ancestral relationship to other organisms (see Chapter 2). Since the algae, slime moulds and archaebacteria are not thought to contain species of medical or veterinary importance they will not be considered further. Blue-green algae do not cause infection, but certain species produce potent peptide toxins that may affect persons or animals ingesting polluted water.

The viruses are the smallest of the infective agents; they have a relatively simple structure that is not comparable with that of a cell, and their mode of reproduction is fundamentally different from cellular organisms. Even simpler are *viroids*, protein-free fragments of single-stranded circular RNA that cause disease in plants. Another class of infectious particles are *prions*, which are the causative agents of fatal neurodegenerative disorders in animals and humans. These are postulated to be naturally occurring host cell membrane glycoproteins that undergo conformative changes to an infectious isoform (see Chapter 59).

TAXONOMY

Taxonomy consists of three components: *classification, nomenclature* and *identification*. Classification allows the orderly grouping of micro-organisms while nomenclature concerns the naming of these organisms and requires agreement so that the same name is used unambiguously by everyone. Changes in nomenclature may give rise to confusion and are subject to internationally agreed rules. In clinical practice, microbiologists are generally concerned with identification – the correct naming of isolates according to agreed systems of classification. These components, together with taxonomy, make up the overarching discipline of *systematics* which is concerned with evolution, genetics and speciation of organisms, and is commonly referred to as *phylogenetics*.

Protozoa, fungi and helminths are classified and named according to the standard rules of classification and nomenclature that have been developed following the pioneering work of the 18th century Swedish botanist Linnaeus (Carl von Linné). Large subdivisions (class, order, family, etc.) are finally classified into individual *species* designated by a Latin binomial, the first term of which is the *genus*, e.g. *Plasmodium* (genus) *falciparum* (species). Occasionally it is useful to recognize a biological variant with particular properties: thus, *Trypanosoma* (genus) *brucei* (species) *gambiense* (variant) differs from the variant *T. brucei brucei* in being pathogenic for humans.

Bacteria are similarly classified, but the infinite variety of microbial life and the natural capacity of bacteria for variation and adaptation make rigid classification difficult. Identification is performed by the use of keys that allow the organization of bacterial traits based on growth or activity in a biochemical test system. Some tests are definitive of a genus or species, e.g. the universal production of catalase enzyme and cytochrome C, respectively, by *Staphylococcus* spp. and *Pseudomonas aeruginosa*. Other characters may be unique to individual species and serve to differentiate them from organisms with closely similar biochemical activity profiles. The genes for some test characters (e.g. lactose utilization, antibiotic resistance) may be carried on self-replicating extrachromosomal DNA elements, *plasmids*, which may be transferred among unrelated bacteria or be lost from the host strain. Some bacteria do not grow in the laboratory (leprosy bacillus, treponemes), and identification by genetic methods may be necessary. The taxonomic ranks used in the classification of bacteria are (example in parentheses):

- Kingdom (Prokaryotae)
- Division (Gracilicutes)
- Class (Betaproteobacteria)
- Order (Burkholderiales)
- Family (Burkholderiaceae)
- Genus (*Burkholderia*)
- Species (*Burkholderia cepacia*).

Some genera, such as *Acinetobacter*, have been subdivided into a number of genomic species by DNA homology analysis. Some are named and others are referred to only by a number. Many of the genomic species cannot be differentiated with accuracy by phenotypic tests. Another subgenus grouping in current usage is species complexes, which are differentiated into genomovars by polyphasic taxonomic methods. A good example of this is the *Burkholderia cepacia* complex of organisms which includes a very diverse group of organisms ranging from strict plant to human pathogens.

At present no standard classification of bacteria is universally accepted and applied, although *Bergey's Manual of Determinative Bacteriology* is widely used as an authoritative source. Bacterial nomenclature is governed by an international code prepared by the *International Committee on Systematic Bacteriology* and published as *Approved Lists of Bacterial Names* in the *International Journal of Systematic and Evolutionary Microbiology*; most new species are also first described in this journal, and a species is only considered to be validly published if it appears on a validation list in this journal.

The *International Committee on Taxonomy of Viruses* (ICTV) classifies viruses, and publishes its reports in the journal *Archives of Virology*. Latin names are used wherever possible for the ranks family, subfamily and genus, but at present there are no formal categories higher than family, and binomial nomenclature is not used for species. Viruses do not lend themselves easily to classification according to Linnaean principles, and vernacular names still have wide usage among medical virologists. Readers are referred to the standard work on virus taxonomy *Classification and Nomenclature of Viruses* and the ICTV database website.

METHODS OF CLASSIFICATION

Adansonian or numerical classification

In most systems of bacterial classification, the major groups are distinguished by fundamental characters, such as cell shape, Gram-stain reaction and spore formation; genera and species are usually distinguished by properties such as fermentation reactions, nutritional requirements and pathogenicity. The relative 'importance' of different characters in defining major and minor groupings is often purely arbitrary. The uncertainties of arbitrary choices are avoided in the Adansonian system of taxonomy. This system determines the degrees of relationship between strains by a statistical coefficient that takes account of the widest range of characters, all of which are considered of equal weight. It is clear, of course, that some characters, e.g. cell shape or Gram reaction, represent a much wider and permanent genetic commitment than other characters which, being dependent on only one or a few genes, may be unstable. For this reason, the Adansonian method is most useful for the classification of strains within a larger grouping that shares major characters.

By scoring a large number of phenotypic characters it is possible to estimate a *similarity coefficient* when shared positive characters are considered, or a *matching coefficient* when both negative and positive shared characters (matches) are taken into account. This numerical taxonomy is best performed on a computer which calculates degrees of similarity for a group of different organisms and these data are displayed as a *similarity matrix*, or a dendrogram tree (Fig. 3.1).

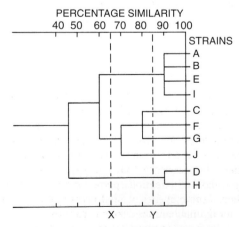

Fig. 3.1 A hierarchic taxonomic tree (*dendrogram*) prepared from similarity matrix data. The broken lines X and Y indicate levels of similarity at which separation into genera and species might be possible.

DNA composition

The hydrogen bonding between guanine and cytosine (G–C) base pairs in DNA is stronger than that between adenine and thymine (A–T). Thus, the melting or denaturation temperature of DNA (at which the two strands separate) is primarily determined by the G + C content. At the melting temperature, the separation of the strands brings about a marked change in the light absorption characteristics at a wavelength of 260 nm, and this is readily detected by spectrophotometry. There is a very wide range in the G + C component of DNA of bacteria, varying from about 25 to 80 mol% in different genera. However, for any one species, the G + C content is relatively fixed, or falls within a very narrow range, and this provides a basis for classification.

DNA homology

Another approach to classification is to arrange individual organisms into groups on the basis of the *homology* of their DNA base sequences. This exploits the fact that double strands re-form (anneal) from separated strands during controlled cooling of a heated preparation of DNA. This process can be readily demonstrated with suitably heated homologous DNA extracted from a single species, but it can also occur with DNA from two related species, so that hybrid pairs of DNA strands are produced. These hybrid pairings occur with high frequency between complementary regions of DNA, and the degree of hybridization can be assessed if labelled DNA preparations are used. Binding studies with messenger RNA (mRNA) can also give information to complement these observations, which provide genetic evidence of relatedness among bacteria. Organisms with different G + C ratios are very unlikely to show significant DNA homology. However, organisms with the same, or close, G + C ratios do not necessarily show homology.

Ribosomal RNA sequencing

The structure of ribosomal RNA (rRNA) appears to have been highly conserved during the course of evolution, and close similarities in nucleotide sequences reflect phylogenetic relationships. Advances in technology have made nucleotide sequencing relatively simple and the rRNA sequences (and other genes) of most medically important bacterial species are available from a number of internet sites, so that investigation of similarities in oligonucleotides derived from rRNA is increasingly used in taxonomic studies. Far fewer full-length gene sequences are known for 23S rRNA than for 16S rRNA. A rapid and universal bacterial identification scheme is possible based on the amplification of the variable length 16S–23S rDNA spacer regions. Nucleotide sequence variation in ribosomal genes is sometimes insufficient to discriminate between closely related species. Other candidate genes have been explored but the *recA* gene, which encodes a protein essential for repair and recombination of DNA, appears to be one of the best suited for phylogenetic analysis in that it defines evolutionary trees consistent with those observed for rRNA genes. Knowledge of the sequence diversity allows the design of species-specific oligonucleotide primers to give specific sized amplicons in single or multiplex polymerase chain reaction (PCR) assays (see p. 71 for description of PCR).

CLASSIFICATION IN CLINICAL PRACTICE

The identification of micro-organisms in routine practice requires a pragmatic approach to taxonomy. Table 3.1 outlines a simple, but practical, classification scheme in which organisms are grouped according to a few shared characteristics. Within these groups, organisms may be further identified, sometimes to species level, by a few supplementary tests. Protozoa, helminths and fungi can often be definitively identified on morphological criteria alone (see appropriate chapters).

Protozoa

These are non-photosynthetic unicellular organisms with protoplasm clearly differentiated into nucleus and cytoplasm. They are relatively large, with transverse diameters mainly in the range 2–100 μm. Their surface membranes vary in complexity and rigidity from a thin, flexible membrane in amoebae, which allows major changes in cell shape and the protrusion of pseudopodia for the purposes of locomotion and ingestion, to a relatively stiff pellicle in ciliate protozoa, which preserves a characteristic cell shape. Most free-living and some parasitic species capture, ingest and digest internally solid particles of food material; many protozoa, for instance, feed on bacteria. Protozoa, therefore, are generally regarded as the lowest forms of animal life, though certain flagellate protozoa are closely related in their morphology and mode of development to photosynthetic flagellate algae in the plant kingdom. Protozoa reproduce asexually by binary fission or by multiple fission (*schizogony*), and some also by a sexual mechanism (*sporogony*). The most important groups of medical protozoa are the *sporozoa* (malaria parasites, etc.), amoebae and flagellates (see Chapter 61).

Table 3.1 A simple classification of some micro-organisms of medical importance

EUKARYOTIC GENERA

Protozoa
Sporozoa: *Plasmodium, Isospora, Toxoplasma, Cryptosporidium*
Flagellates: *Giardia, Trichomonas, Trypanosoma, Leishmania*
Amoebae: *Entamoeba, Naegleria, Acanthamoeba*
Others: *Babesia, Balantidium*

Fungi
Mould-like: *Epidermophyton, Trichophyton, Microsporum, Aspergillus*
Yeast-like: *Candida*
Dimorphic: *Histoplasma, Blastomyces, Coccidioides*
True yeast: *Cryptococcus*

PROKARYOTIC GENERA

Filamentous bacteria
Actinomyces, Nocardia, Streptomyces, Mycobacterium

'True bacteria'
Gram-positive bacilli: Aerobes – *Corynebacterium, Listeria, Bacillus*
   Anaerobes – *Clostridium, Lactobacillus, Eubacterium*
Gram-positive cocci: *Staphylococcus, Streptococcus, Enterococcus*
Gram-negative cocci: Aerobes – *Neisseria*
   Anaerobes – *Veillonella*
Gram-negative bacilli: Aerobes –
   Enterobacteria – *Escherichia, Klebsiella, Proteus, Salmonella, Shigella, Yersinia*
   Pseudomonads – *Pseudomonas, Burkholderia, Stenotrophomonas*
   Parvobacteria – *Haemophilus, Bordetella, Brucella, Pasteurella*
   Anaerobes – *Bacteroides, Fusobacterium*
Gram-negative vibrios: *Vibrio, Spirillum, Campylobacter, Helicobacter*

Spirochaetes
Borrelia, Treponema, Brachyspira, Leptospira

Mycoplasmas
Mycoplasma, Ureaplasma

Rickettsiae and chlamydiae
Rickettsia, Coxiella, Chlamydia

Fungi

These are non-photosynthetic organisms possessing relatively rigid cell walls. They may be saprophytic or parasitic, and take in soluble nutrients by diffusion through their cell surfaces.

Moulds grow as branching filaments (*hyphae*), usually between 2 and 10 μm in width, which interlace to form a meshwork (*mycelium*). The hyphae are coenocytic (i.e. have a continuous multinucleate protoplasm), being either non-septate or else septate with a central pore in each cross-wall. Moulds reproduce by the formation of various kinds of sexual and asexual spores that develop from the vegetative (feeding) mycelium, or from an aerial mycelium that effects their air-borne dissemination (see Chapter 60).

Yeasts are ovoid or spherical cells that reproduce asexually by budding and also, in many cases, sexually, with the formation of sexual spores. They do not form a mycelium, although the intermediate *yeast-like fungi* form a pseudomycelium consisting of chains of elongated cells. The *dimorphic fungi* produce a vegetative mycelium in artificial culture, but are yeast-like in infected lesions. The higher fungi of the class *Basidiomycetes* (mushrooms), which produce large fruiting structures for aerial dissemination of spores, are not infectious for humans or animals, although some species are poisonous.

Bacteria

The main groups of bacteria are distinguished by the microscopic observation of their morphology and staining reactions. The Gram-staining procedure, which reflects fundamental differences in cell wall structure, separates most bacteria into two great divisions: *Gram-positive bacteria* and *Gram-negative bacteria* (see Chapter 2).

Details of structure provide a basis for a separate division into:

1. *Filamentous bacteria (Actinomycetes)*, most of which are capable of true branching and which may produce a type of mycelium.
2. *'True' bacteria*, which multiply by simple binary fission.
3. *Spirochaetes*, which divide by transverse binary fission.
4. *Mycoplasmas*, which lack a rigid cell wall.
5. *Rickettsiae* and *chlamydiae*, which are strict intracellular parasites.

Filamentous bacteria

These are sometimes referred to as 'higher bacteria'. A few are of medical interest as pathogens, and some produce antibiotics.

1. *Actinomyces*. Gram-positive, non-acid-fast, tend to fragment into short coccal and bacillary forms and not to form conidia; anaerobic (e.g. *Actinomyces israelii*).

2. *Nocardia*. Similar to *Actinomyces*, but aerobic and mostly acid-fast (e.g. *Nocardia asteroides*).

3. *Streptomyces*. Vegetative mycelium does not fragment into short forms; conidia form in chains from aerial hyphae (e.g. *Streptomyces griseus*).

4. *Mycobacterium*. Acid-fast; Gram-positive, but does not readily stain by the Gram method; usually bacillary, rarely branching; aerobic (e.g. *Mycobacterium tuberculosis*).

True bacteria

Most medically important bacteria fall into this group. They are classified on the basis of their shape.

1. *Cocci* – spherical, or nearly spherical, cells
2. *Bacilli* – relatively straight, rod-shaped (cylindrical) cells
3. *Vibrios and spirilla* – curved or twisted rod-shaped cells.

Cocci. The main groups of cocci are distinguished by their predominant mode of cell grouping and their reaction to the Gram stain. The different cocci are relatively uniform in size (usually about 1 μm in diameter). Some species are capsulate and a very few are motile.

1. *Streptococcus*. Gram-positive; cells mainly adherent in chains due to successive cell divisions occurring in the same axis (e.g. *Streptococcus pyogenes*); sometimes predominantly diplococcal (e.g. *Streptococcus pneumoniae*).

2. *Staphylococcus* and *Micrococcus*. Gram-positive; cells mainly adherent in irregular clusters due to successive divisions occurring irregularly in different planes (e.g. *Staphylococcus aureus*).

3. *Sarcina*. Gram-positive cells mainly adherent in cubical arrays of eight, or multiples thereof, due to division occurring successively in three planes at right angles (e.g. *Sarcina lutea*).

4. *Neisseria*. Gram-negative; cells mainly adherent in pairs and slightly elongated at right angles to axis of pairs (e.g. *Neisseria meningitidis*).

5. *Veillonella*. Gram-negative; generally very small cocci arranged mainly in clusters and pairs; anaerobic (e.g. *Veillonella parvula*).

Bacilli. The primary subdivision of the rod-shaped bacteria is made according to their staining reaction by the Gram method and the presence or absence of endospores.

1. *Gram-positive spore-forming bacilli*. Apart from some rare saprophytic varieties, the only bacteria to form endospores are those of the genera *Bacillus, Paenibacillus* (aerobic) and *Clostridium* (anaerobic). They are Gram-positive, but liable to become Gram-negative in ageing cultures. The size, shape and position of the spore may assist recognition of the species, e.g. the bulging, spherical, terminal spore ('drumstick' form) of *Clostridium tetani*.

2. *Gram-positive non-sporing bacilli*. These include several genera. *Corynebacterium* is distinguished by a tendency to slight curving, a club-shaped or ovoid swelling of the bacilli, and their arrangement in parallel or angular clusters caused by the snapping mode of cell division. *Erysipelothrix* and *Lactobacillus* are distin-

guished by a tendency to grow in chains and filaments, and *Listeria* by flagella that confer motility.

3. *Gram-negative bacilli*. This large grouping includes numerous genera such as the pseudomonads and the family Enterobacteriaceae ('coliform bacilli') as well as small, often pleomorphic, bacilli represented by *Haemophilus, Brucella*, etc. ('parvobacteria'), and anaerobes such as *Bacteroides* and *Prevotella*.

4. *Vibrios and spirilla*. Vibrios and the related campylobacters are recognized as short, non-flexuous, comma-shaped bacilli (e.g. *Vibrio cholerae*) and spirilla as non-flexuous spiral filaments (e.g. *Anaerobiospirillum*, '*Spirillum minus*'). They are Gram-negative and mostly motile, having polar flagella and showing very active 'darting' motility.

Spirochaetes

These organisms differ from the 'true' bacteria in being slender flexuous spiral filaments which, unlike the spirilla, are motile without possession of flagella. The staining reaction, when demonstrable, is Gram-negative. The different varieties are recognized by their size, shape, wave form and refractility, observed in the natural state in unstained wet films by dark-ground microscopy (Fig. 3.2).

Borrelia. Larger and more refractile than the other pathogenic spirochaetes and more readily stained by ordinary methods; coils large and open, with a wavelength of 2–3 μm; by electron microscopy a leash of between eight and twelve fibrils, each about 0.02 μm thick, is seen twisted round the whole length of the protoplast (e.g. *Borrelia recurrentis*).

Treponema. Thinner filaments in coils of shorter wavelength (e.g. 1.0–1.5 μm), typically presenting a regular 'corkscrew' form; feebly refractile and difficult to stain except by silver impregnation methods; by electron microscopy, a leash of four fibrils is seen wound round the protoplast within the cell wall (e.g. *Treponema pallidum*).

Leptospira. The coils are so fine and close (wavelength about 0.5 μm) that they are barely discernible by dark-ground microscopy, though can clearly be seen winding

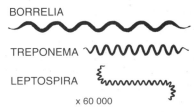

BORRELIA

TREPONEMA

LEPTOSPIRA

x 60 000

Fig. 3.2 Morphology of spirochaetes.

round two axial filaments by electron microscopy. One or both extremities of the organism are hooked, or recurved, so that it may take the shape of a walking-stick, an 'S' or a 'C' (e.g. *Leptospira interrogans*).

Mycoplasmas

These are prokaryotes that differ from 'true' bacteria in their smaller size and their lack of a rigid cell wall, which leads to extreme pleomorphism and sensitivity to external osmotic pressure. The viable elements range from 0.15 to over 1 μm in diameter, the smallest being capable of passing through filters that retain conventional bacteria. Mycoplasmas can be cultivated on cell-free nutrient media, and are the smallest and simplest organisms capable of autonomous growth.

Rickettsiae and chlamydiae

The rickettsiae are rod-shaped, spherical or pleomorphic Gram-negative organisms. They are generally smaller than 'true' bacteria, but are still resolvable in the light microscope. Most are strict parasites that can grow only in the living tissues of a suitable animal host, usually intracellularly (e.g. *Rickettsia prowazekii*). Chlamydiae are similar to rickettsiae, but have a more complex intracellular cycle (e.g. *Chlamydia trachomatis*).

Viruses

Viruses usually consist of little more than a strand of DNA or RNA enclosed in a simple protein shell known as a *capsid*. Sometimes the complete nucleocapsid may be enclosed in a lipoprotein envelope largely derived from the host cell. Viruses are capable of growing only within the living cells of an appropriate animal, plant or bacterial host; none can grow in an inanimate nutrient medium. The viruses that infect and parasitize bacteria are named *bacteriophages* or *phages*. A simple classification of the viruses that are involved in human disease is shown in Table 3.2.

IDENTIFICATION OF MICRO-ORGANISMS

Precise identification of bacteria is time-consuming and contentious, and is best carried out in specialized reference centres. For most clinical purposes, clear, rapid guidance on the likely cause of an infection is required and, consequently, microbiologists usually rely on a few simple procedures, notably microscopy and culture, backed up, when necessary, by a few supplementary tests. Microscopy is the most rapid test of all, but culture

Table 3.2 Principal types of virus causing human disease

Types of virus	Examples
RNA viruses	
Orthomyxoviruses	Influenza A, B, C viruses
Paramyxoviruses	Parainfluenza viruses
	Mumps virus
	Measles virus
	Respiratory syncytial virus
	Hendra virus
Rhabdoviruses	Rabies virus
Arenaviruses	Lassa virus
Filoviruses	Marburg and Ebola viruses
Togaviruses	Many arboviruses
	Rubella virus
Flaviviruses	Yellow fever virus
	Dengue virus
	Japanese encephalitis virus
	West Nile virus
	Hepatitis C virus
Bunyaviruses	Hantaan virus
Coronaviruses	Human coronavirus
Caliciviruses	Norwalk-like viruses
	Hepatitis E
Picornaviruses	Enteroviruses
	Poliovirus (3 types)
	Echovirus (31 types)
	Coxsackie A virus (24 types)
	Coxsackie B virus (6 types)
	Enterovirus types 68–71
	Hepatitis A virus (type 72)
	Rhinovirus, many serotypes
Retroviruses	Human immunodeficiency viruses types 1 and 2
	Human T-lymphotropic virus types I and II
Reoviruses	Rotaviruses
DNA viruses	
Poxviruses	Variola, vaccinia
	Molluscum contagiosum virus
	Orf
Herpesviruses	Herpes simplex virus types 1 and 2
	Varicella zoster virus
	Cytomegalovirus
	Epstein–Barr virus
	Human herpesvirus type 6
Adenoviruses	Many serotypes
Papovaviruses	JC virus
	Human papillomavirus
Hepadnaviruses	Hepatitis B virus
Parvoviruses	B19 virus

inevitably takes at least 24 h, and sometimes longer. More rapid tests are constantly being sought, and some progress has been achieved with antigen detection methods and specific *gene probes* (see below).

Most specimens for bacteriological examination, whether from humans, animals or the environment, contain mixtures of bacteria, and it is essential to obtain *pure cultures* of individual isolates before embarking on identification. Non-cultural methods, such as antigen detection or gene probes, do not have this disadvantage; however, they do have the potential limitation of being highly specific so that the investigator must know beforehand what it is necessary to look for.

Microscopy

Morphology and staining reactions of individual organisms generally serve as preliminary criteria to place an unknown species in its appropriate biological group. A Gram stain smear suffices to show the Gram reaction, size, shape and grouping of the bacteria, and the arrangement of any endospores. An unstained wet film may be examined with dark-ground illumination in the microscope to observe the morphology of delicate spirochaetes; an unstained wet film, or 'hanging-drop', preparation is examined with ordinary bright-field illumination for observation of motility. To identify mycobacteria, or other acid-fast organisms, a preparation is stained by the Ziehl-Neelsen method or one of its modifications (see p. 22). The microscopic characters of certain organisms in pathological specimens may be sufficient for presumptive identification, e.g. tubercle bacilli in sputum, or *T. pallidum* in exudate from a chancre. However, many bacteria share similar morphological features, and further tests must be applied to differentiate them.

Cultural characteristics

The appearance of colonial growth on the surface of a solid medium, such as nutrient agar, is often very characteristic. Attention is paid to the diameter of the colonies, their outline, their elevation, their translucency (clear, translucent or opaque) and colour. Changes brought about in the medium (e.g. haemolysis in a blood agar medium) may also be significant. The range of conditions that support growth is characteristic of particular organisms. The ability or inability of the organism to grow in the presence (aerobe) or absence (anaerobe) of oxygen, in a reduced oxygen atmosphere (microaerophile) or in the presence of CO_2, or on media containing selective inhibitory factors (e.g. bile salt, specific antimicrobial agents, or low or high pH) may also be of diagnostic significance.

Biochemical reactions

Species that cannot be distinguished by morphology and cultural characters may exhibit metabolic differences that can be exploited. It is usual to test the ability of the organism to produce acidic and gaseous end-products when presented with individual carbohydrates (glucose, lactose, sucrose, mannitol, etc.) as the sole carbon source. Other tests determine whether the bacterium produces particular end-products (e.g. indole or hydrogen sulphide) when grown in suitable culture media, and whether it possesses certain enzyme activities, such as oxidase, catalase, urease, gelatinase or lecithinase. Traditionally, such tests have been performed selectively and individually according to the recommendations of standard guides, such as the invaluable *Cowan and Steel's Manual for the Identification of Medical Bacteria*. However, today most diagnostic laboratories use commercially prepared microgalleries of identification tests which, though expensive, combine simplicity and accuracy. Test kits are now available for a number of different groups of organisms, including enterobacteria, staphylococci, streptococci and anaerobes. Other kits facilitate the testing of carbon source utilization, the assimilation of specific substrates and the enzymes produced by an organism.

On occasion, more elaborate procedures may be used for the analysis of metabolic products or whole cell fatty acids. Indeed, a fully automated fatty acid-based identification system, which combines high resolution gas chromatography and pattern recognition software, is increasingly used to identify a wide variety of aerobic and anaerobic bacterial species. New profiles are added to a computerized database, thus increasing the sensitivity of the system.

INDIRECT IDENTIFICATION METHODS

Gene probes

These are cloned fragments of DNA that recognize complementary sequences within micro-organisms (see p. 71). Binding is detected by tagging the DNA with a radioactive label, or with a reagent that can be developed to give a colour reaction, such as biotin. By selecting DNA fragments specific for features characteristic of individual organisms, gene probes can be tailored to the rapid identification of individual species in clinical material. The disadvantages of this approach are that the organism itself may be dead and a viable isolate is not made available for subsequent tests of susceptibility to antimicrobial agents, toxin production or epidemiological investigation.

Culture and preliminary identification of bacteria in the laboratory is time-consuming and relatively labour-intensive. Bacteria may also be uncultivable, slow growing, or fastidious in nutrient requirements. Nucleic acid techniques for the detection and identification of bacteria have evolved against this background and today numerous commercially available systems have been developed and many are in use in diagnostic laboratories. The technologies fall into three basic groups:

- target amplification by PCR, transcription-mediated amplification, nucleic acid sequence-based amplification, etc.
- probe amplification using ligase chain reaction or Q-beta replicase
- signal amplification as in branched DNA assay.

It is possible to detect the presence of an increasing number of species either by PCR of universal or specific gene targets or by hybridization with specific probes. As with conventional methods, nucleic acid technology has its limitations, the most frequent being contamination of a sample by post-amplification products. Other factors include operator skill, primer design, stringency of assay, presence of inhibitory compounds in the specimen and the ubiquity of the organism sought. The latter is fundamental to the interpretation of results as many bacterial pathogens occur naturally as commensals in certain body sites. The new technologies do, however, offer a considerable advantage over phenotypic methods in terms of sensitivity, and many optimized PCR systems claim to be able to detect as few as two to ten bacteria per millilitre of specimen, which is far below the threshold of conventional culture.

Nucleic acid assays for antimicrobial resistance genes are also in use and development. A recently described innovation may have the potential to detect, identify the species, subtype the organism and identify resistance genes on microscope slide smears. The technique uses peptide nucleic acid (PNA, pseudopeptides) with DNA binding capacity. The PNA molecules have a polyamide backbone instead of the sugar phosphate of DNA and RNA, and nucleotide bases attached to this backbone are able to hybridize by specific base pairing with complementary DNA or RNA sequences. PCR amplification of target genes on conventionally stained microscope smears is also possible and this accelerates the prospect of very rapid and sensitive test methods limited only by the specificity of the primer for the target.

In the past 5 years, many prokaryotic genomic sequences have been completed. This has been paralleled by the development of high-density oligonucleotide arrays which consist of many thousands (current limit 500 000) of different probes. These arrays are constructed by in-situ oligonucleotide synthesis on a glass support by photolithography or other methods. Hybridization of the prelabelled target nucleic acids to the bound probe is detected directly with fluorescein or radioactive ligands, or indirectly using enzyme conjugates. Areas of application for high-density arrays include DNA sequencing, strain genotyping, identifying gene functions, location of resistance genes, changes in mRNA expression and phylogenetic related-

ness. A recent and increasingly used development is that of real time PCR which combines sample amplification with a means for detection of the specific product by fluorescence so that both steps take place conveniently in a single reaction tube. The system has significant advantages over conventional PCR in terms of rapidity, simplicity and number of manual procedures, and that contamination is effectively eliminated by the tube being closed after amplification. Quantification of the target DNA is also possible with this system, allowing estimation of viral or bacterial numbers in a specimen.

Antibody reactions

Species and types of micro-organism can often be identified by specific serological reactions. These depend on the fact that the serum of an animal immunized against a micro-organism contains specific antibodies for the homologous species or type that reacts in a characteristic manner (e.g. agglutination or precipitation) with the particular micro-organism. Such simple in-vitro tests have been used for many years in microbiology, notably in the formal identification of presumptive isolates of pathogens (e.g. salmonellae) from clinical material. The specificity and range of antibody tests have been greatly improved by the availability of highly specific *monoclonal antibodies*. These are produced by the *hybridoma* technique in which individual antibody-producing spleen cells are fused with 'immortal' tumour cells in vitro. The progeny of these hybrid cells produce only the type of antibody appropriate to the spleen cell precursor .

Latex agglutination

By adsorbing specific antibody to inert latex particles, a visible agglutination reaction can be induced in the presence of homologous antigen. This principle can be applied in reverse to detect serum antibodies. Latex-based kits are widely used for serological grouping of organisms and detection of toxins produced by bacteria during growth.

Enzyme–linked immunosorbent assay

In enzyme-linked immunosorbent assay (ELISA), a specific antibody is attached to the surface of a plastic well and material containing the test antigen is added. After washing, the presence of the antigen is detected by addition of more of the specific antibody, this time labelled with an enzyme which can initiate a colour reaction when provided with the appropriate substrate. The intensity of the colour change is related to the amount of antigen bound. The ELISA method may also be used in the reverse manner for the quantitative detection of antibodies, by adsorbing purified antigen to the well before adding test serum; in this case the enzyme-linked system used to detect the antigen–antibody reaction is a labelled anti-human globulin. In immunoglobulin (Ig) M antibody capture ELISA (MAC-ELISA), widely used in virological diagnosis for the detection of IgM, anti-human μ chain antibody (usually raised in goats) is bound to the well. The test serum is added, and any IgM binds to the capture reagent; after washing, purified antigen (e.g. rubella antigen) is added, and this can be detected with an appropriate labelled antibody.

Haemagglutination and haemadsorption

Certain viruses, notably the influenza viruses, have the property of attaching to specific receptors on the surface of appropriate red blood cells. In this manner the virus particles act as bridges linking the red cells in visible clumps. In tissue culture, such haemagglutinins may appear on the surface of cells infected with a virus. If red cells are added to the tissue culture, they adhere to the surface of infected cells, a phenomenon known as *haemadsorption*. Red blood cells can also be coated with specific antibody so that they agglutinate in the presence of the homologous virus particle in a manner similar to that described for latex agglutination above.

Fluorescence microscopy and immunofluorescence

When certain dyes are exposed to ultraviolet light, they absorb energy and emit visible light (i.e. they fluoresce). Tissues or organisms stained with such a dye and examined with ultraviolet light in a specially adapted microscope are seen as fluorescent objects; for example, auramine can be used in this way to stain *Mycobacterium tuberculosis*. Antibody molecules can be labelled by conjugation with a fluorochrome dye such as fluorescein isothiocyanate (which fluoresces green) or rhodamine (orange–red). When fluorescent antibody is allowed to react with homologous antigen exposed at a cell surface, this *direct immunofluorescence* procedure affords a highly sensitive method for the identification of the particular antigen. For this procedure it is necessary to have a specific antibody conjugate for each antigen; however, unconjugated antibody can be used and the reaction then detected by addition of an antiglobulin conjugate which will react with any antibody from the species in which the antibody was raised.

Immuno–polymerase chain reaction

This technique arose out of the fusion of antibody technology with PCR methods with the aim of enhancing the capability of antigen detection systems. In immuno-PCR, a linker molecule with bispecific binding affinity for DNA and antibodies is used to attach a DNA molecule (marker) to an antigen–antibody complex. This produces a specific antigen–antibody–DNA conjugate. The attached DNA marker can be amplified by PCR with appropriate primers and the presence of amplification products shows that the marker DNA is attached to antigen–antibody complexes which indicates the presence of antigen. The enhanced sensitivity of immuno-PCR achieved over ELISA is reported to be in excess of 10^5, theoretically allowing as few as 580 antigen molecules (9.6×10^{-22} moles) to be detected.

TYPING OF BACTERIA

A population of bacteria presumed to descend from a single bacterium as found in a natural habitat, in primary cultures from the habitat, and in subcultures from the primary cultures, is called a *strain*. Each primary culture from a natural source is called an *isolate*. The distinction between strains and isolates may be important; for example, cultures of typhoid bacilli isolated from 10 different patients should be regarded simply as 10 different *isolates* unless epidemiological or other evidence indicates that the patients have been infected from a common source with the same *strain*. Strains with demonstrable ancestral lineage have been termed *clones*, but this term should be used with caution as it does not imply that they are identical, as is the case with a cloned cell.

The ability to discriminate between similar strains may be of great epidemiological value in tracing sources or modes of spread of infection in a community or hospital ward, and various typing methods have been devised. Strains may be distinguishable only in minor characters and it is usually simpler to establish differences between isolates from a common source than unequivocally to prove their identity. Demonstration of an identical response by a single reproducible typing method is not proof that two strains are the same. However, the confidence with which similarity can be inferred is greatly increased if more than one typing method is used.

Biotyping

Biochemical test reactions which are not universally positive or negative within a species may define *biotypes* of the species and these may be efficient strain markers. However, in practice biotyping is often less discriminatory than other strain typing methods and may be unstable because of loss of the property. Differences among strains may also be detected by variations in sensitivity to fixed concentrations of chemicals such as heavy metals, a process known as *resistotyping*. The nutritional requirements of the isolate (amino acids) for growth may also be used to define the *auxotype* of an isolate.

Serotyping

Many surface structures of bacteria (lipopolysaccharide and outer membrane, flagella, capsule etc.) are antigenic, and antibodies raised against them can be used to group isolates into defined *serotypes*. Some species are characterized by numerous antigenic types and serotyping for these species is highly discriminatory, while for others conservation of antigen epitopes renders serotyping of little value for epidemiological purposes. Members of the species *Salmonella enterica* are defined by their somatic and flagellar serotypes (see Chapter 24). Capsular antigens may be associated with pathogenicity of the organism and many vaccines protect the individual against infection by stimulating antibodies to capsular antigen epitopes.

Phage typing

Bacteria often show differential susceptibility to lysis by certain bacteriophages. The phage adsorbs to a specific receptor on the bacterial surface and injects its DNA into the host. Phage DNA may become stably integrated into the bacterial chromosome and this state is referred to as *lysogeny*; phages capable of this are called *temperate phages*. In lysogeny, a small proportion of host cells express the phage genes and some cell lysis and liberation of phage progeny occur. Alternatively, the phage DNA may enter a replicative cycle, leading to the death of the host and the production of new phage particles. These *lytic* or *virulent* wild phages lyse the bacterium at the end of the replicative cycle and release a large number of daughter phage particles that infect neighbouring cells. This process leads to visible inhibition of the growth of the host cells. The *phage type* of the culture is identified according to the pattern of susceptibility to a set of lytic and/or temperate phages. Lytic phages may be readily recovered from sewage, waste and river water, and temperate phages may be released from a lysogenic strain by induction with ultraviolet radiation or chemical mutagens. Phage typing is widely used to discriminate among strains of salmonellae and staphylococci. Phages are also useful tools for genetic studies and for the manipulation and transfer of genes between strains.

Bacteriocin typing

Bacteriocins are naturally occurring antibacterial substances, elaborated by most bacterial species, that are active mainly against strains of the same genus as the producer strain. Bacteriocin typing may define the spectrum of bacteriocins produced by field strains, or the sensitivity of these strains to bacteriocins of a standard panel of strains. Patterns of production or susceptibility to bacteriocins allow the division of species into *bacteriocin types*.

Protein typing

Bacteria manufacture thousands of proteins that can be visualized by electrophoresis in acrylamide gels in the presence of a strong detergent. The proteins separate according to molecular size and, after staining with a dye, the pattern of bands from each isolate can be compared. This system has been successfully used for typing many bacterial and fungal species. Investigation of microbial populations by gel electrophoresis of metabolic enzymes, which can then be detected by specific substrates, is also widely applied for clonal analysis within species.

Restriction endonuclease typing

Restriction endonucleases are a family of enzymes that each cut DNA at a specific sequence recognition site, which may be rare or frequent in the DNA of the species being examined. Both plasmid and chromosomal DNA can be analysed by this means. Frequent-cutting endonucleases generate numerous small fragments that can be resolved by conventional electrophoresis in agarose gel and detected by staining with a dye. Rare cutters produce large DNA fragments that need to be separated in special electrical fields with a pulsed current (*pulsed-field gel electrophoresis*). This technique is widely used to size genomes of species and to detect variations in the DNA of individual strains (Fig.3.3).

Gene probe typing

DNA probes (see earlier) for strain typing consist of cloned specific, random or universal sequences that can detect restriction site heterogeneity in the target DNA. The detection of variation in rDNA gene loci is the basis of *ribotyping*, and this method has been universally applied to the typing of various species. Some genera, such as *Mycoplasma*, cannot be ribotyped as they have only a single copy of the rRNA operon. Other commonly used probes are *insertion sequences* (lengths of DNA involved in transposition; see Chapter 6) that may define clonal structures of populations.

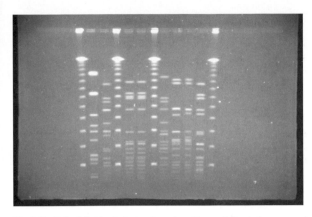

Fig. 3.3 Pulsed-field gel electrophoresis patterns of *Staphylococcus aureus* isolates.

Polymerase chain reaction typing

PCR is a technique that allows specific sequences of DNA to be amplified. Multiple copies of regions of the genome defined by specific oligonucleotide primers are made by repeated cycles of amplification under controlled conditions. Such methods can be used to study DNA from any source. Several variations on the PCR theme have been described, and use of these techniques continues to expand and develop. PCR-mediated DNA fingerprinting makes use of the variable regions in DNA molecules. These may be variable numbers of tandem repeat regions or areas with restriction endonuclease recognition sequences. To perform *PCR typing*, it is necessary to know the sequences of the bordering regions so that specific oligonucleotide primers can be synthesized. Primers may be specific for a known sequence or be random. Random primers are extensively used in the techniques *random applied polymorphic DNA typing* (RAPD) and *arbitrarily primed PCR* (AP-PCR). Amplified fragment length polymorphism is a DNA sequence-based technique which combines restriction endonuclease digestion with PCR. Incorporation of a fluorescent label and the use of a capillary DNA sequencer allows optimal standardization of repro-

ducibility and resolution of single base pair differences between genomes.

Multilocus sequence typing

This technique indexes allelic variation in several housekeeping genes by nucleotide sequencing rather than indirectly from the electrophoretic mobilities of their gene products, as was the case with its parent technique, multilocus enzyme electrophoresis. Housekeeping genes are not subject to selective forces as variable genes and they diversify slowly. Multiple genes (usually seven) are employed to overcome the effects of recombination in a single locus, which might distort the interpretation of the relationship of the strains being compared. Multilocus sequence typing (MLST) can rightly be referred to as definitive genotyping as sequence data are unambiguous and databases of allelic profiles of isolates of individual species are accessible via the internet. The level of discrimination of MLST depends on the degree of diversity within the population to generate alleles at each locus, but some highly uniform species such as *M. tuberculosis* are not amenable to analysis by the technique.

Miscellaneous methods

Bacterial chemotyping or whole cell analysis was formerly performed by pyrolysis mass spectrometry, in which the sample is bombarded with electrons and the resulting charged fragments are recorded according to their mass:charge ratio. In new machines, such as the matrix-assisted laser desorption/ionization time of flight spectrometers (Maldi-ToF-MS), the sample is not destroyed but instead molecular ions from the surface components of intact cells are recorded. The technique is rapid (1–2 min) and said to be able to discriminate between closely related species, and serotypes and phage types of a species. Other methods, such as fatty acid profiles and lipopolysaccharide electrophoretic profiles for Gram-negative species, have also been applied for strain fingerprinting.

RECOMMENDED READING

Barrow GI, Feltham RKA (eds) 1993 *Cowan and Steel's Manual for the Identification of Medical Bacteria*, 3rd edn. Cambridge University Press, Cambridge

Holt JG (editor-in-chief) 1994 *Bergey's Manual of Determinative Bacteriology*, 9th edn. Williams and Wilkins, Baltimore

Murray PR, Baron EJ, Pfaller MA, Tenover FC, Yolken RH (eds) 1995 *Manual of Clinical Microbiology*, 6th edn. ASM Press, Washington DC

Sano T, Smith CL, Cantor CR 1992 Immuno-PCR: very sensitive antigen detection by means of specific antibody–DNA conjugates. *Science* **258**: 120–122

Van Regenmortel MHV, Fauquet CM, Bishop DHL (eds) 2000 *Virus taxonomy. Classification and Nomenclature of Viruses*. Academic Press, San Diego

Woese CR 2000 Interpreting the universal phylogenetic tree. *Proceedings of the National Academy of Sciences USA* **97**: 8392–8396

Internet sites

Genotyping database at Oxford University:
www.mlst.zoo.ac.uk

International Committee on Taxonomy of Viruses:
www.ncbi.ntm.nih.gov/ICTVdB

Sequence Retrieval System: www.embl-heidelberg.de/srs5

Woese's work at National Academy of Sciences: www.pnas.org

4

Bacterial growth and physiology

M. R. Barer

Most of what we know about bacteria derives from their growth. Their ability to propagate may be seen as a supreme achievement which enables them to attain enormous populations at rates which are breathtaking from a human perspective. These properties underpin their capacity for change by mutation and the rapidity with which some infections develop.

Bacterial growth involves both an increase in the size of organisms and an increase in their number. Whatever the balance between these two processes, the net effect is an increase in the total mass (*biomass*) of the culture. Medical microbiologists have traditionally concentrated on the number of individuals in growth studies. Whether this emphasis on cell number is appropriate remains uncertain; none the less, it will be adopted here, since the number of individual bacteria involved is important in the course and outcome of infections and in the measurement of the effects of antibiotics.

Students of medicine may be surprised and even dismayed to hear that organisms as small as bacteria have a physiology. However, the complement of enzymes and the biochemical and biophysical processes occurring in a prokaryotic cell at any one time represent the product of genetic and biochemical control mechanisms which are every bit as sophisticated and tightly regulated as those in eukaryotic cells. Moreover, the recognition and definition of the mechanisms by which bacteria sense and adapt to nutritional and noxious stimuli in their environments have provided insights that are likely to translate into medically significant advances in the foreseeable future.

Although this chapter only discusses bacterial growth and physiology, many of the principles are also applicable to fungi. The central difference between their growth is that cell division is generally achieved in bacteria by *binary fission* to produce identical offspring which cannot be distinguished as parents and progeny, while fungi divide by budding in the case of yeast growth and hyphal septation in the mould form.

BACTERIAL GROWTH

When placed in a suitable nutritious environment and maintained under appropriate physical and chemical conditions, a bacterial cell begins to grow and, when it has manufactured approximately twice the amount of component materials that it started with, divides. The range of specific components which define 'suitable' and 'appropriate' for all known bacteria (and *Archaea*) is so broad that it actually defines the global biosphere (those environments which can sustain life), and includes temperatures and pressures present at the opening of hydrothermal vents on the ocean floor to the outer reaches of the atmosphere. Although these conditions do not regularly occur in humans, they serve to illustrate that no part of the body or medical device with which it may come in contact is too difficult for bacteria to colonize and that bacteria may lurk in surprising environmental niches. Conversely, the conditions required for some organisms to grow are so precise that so far we have not been able to reproduce them in artificial laboratory media. This applies to some well known organisms such as the agents of leprosy and syphilis, but it also applies to many other potential pathogens about which we are beginning to learn through molecular methods which do not depend on growth. In fact, it is estimated that we have not yet isolated more than 1% of all the bacterial species that exist, and it is almost certain that there are many medically important organisms among the 'as yet uncultivated' micro-organisms.

As the central technique in bacteriology, growth in the laboratory has been used to serve many different purposes. From the clinical perspective, growth is used for detection and identification, and for the assessment of antibiotic effects, while scientific and industrial objectives are often served by growth in bulk to obtain sufficient biomass for detailed biochemical analysis and to produce the desirable products of the brewing and biotechnology industries.

Types of growth

In the laboratory bacterial growth can be seen in three main forms:

1. By the development of *colonies*, the macroscopic product of 20–30 cell divisions of a single cell.
2. By the transformation of a clear broth medium to a turbid suspension of 10^7–10^9 cells per millilitre.
3. In *biofilm* formation, in which growth is spread thinly (300–400 μm thick) over an inert surface and nutrition obtained from a bathing fluid.

In natural systems only biofilms, such as those that develop on the surfaces of intravascular cannulae, appear to have the same appearance and properties as growth produced in the laboratory, while colonies, the other form of *sessile* growth, rarely reach macroscopic dimensions. Turbid liquid systems caused by *planktonic* growth of a single organism are also a rarity in nature. However, in spite of these unrepresentative features, growth in macroscopic colonies and growth to high cell densities in broth offer great practical advantages and remain central techniques.

Growth phases in broth culture

Bacterial growth in broth has been studied in great detail and has provided a framework within which the growth state or growth phase of any given pure culture of a single organism can be placed; these phases are summarized in the idealized *growth curve* shown in Fig. 4.1. When growth is initiated by inoculation into appropriate broth conditions, the number of cells present appears to remain constant for the *lag phase*, during which cells are thought to be preparing for growth. Increase in cell number then becomes detectable, and its rate accelerates rapidly until it is established at the maximum achievable rate for the available conditions. This is known as the

exponential phase because the number of cells is increasing exponentially with time. To accommodate the astronomic changes in number, the growth curve is normally displayed on a logarithmic scale which shows a linear increase in log cell number with time (hence the older term *log-phase*). This log-linear relationship is sufficiently constant for a given bacterial strain under one set of conditions that it can be mathematically defined and is often quoted as the *doubling time* for that organism. Doubling times have been measured at anything between 13 min for *Vibrio cholerae* and 24 h for *Mycobacterium tuberculosis*. On this basis it is not surprising that cholera is a disease that can kill within 12 h, while tuberculosis takes months to develop. A further consequence is that, when specimens are submitted to diagnostic laboratories for the detection of these organisms by culture, a result is usually available for *V. cholerae* the next day while several weeks are required for conventional culture of *M. tuberculosis*.

It is often difficult to grasp fully the scale of exponential microbial growth; the message may be strengthened by considering that the progeny of a lecture theatre containing 150 students would exceed the global population of humanity (6×10^9) within $8^1/_2$ h if they were able to breed like *Escherichia coli*!

Exponential growth cannot be sustained indefinitely in a closed (*batch*) system with limited available nutrients. Eventually growth slows down, and the total bacterial cell number reaches a maximum and stabilizes. This is known as the *stationary* or *post-exponential phase*. At this stage it becomes important to know what method has been used to determine the growth curve. If a direct method which assesses the total number of cells present is used then the count remains constant. Such methods include counting cells in a volumetric chamber observed by microscopy, electronic particle counters and measurement of turbidity. If, however, the growth potential of the individual cells present in the culture is assessed by taking regular samples, making 10-fold dilutions of these and inoculating them onto agar, then the number of *colony-forming units* (cfu) per unit volume can be determined at each sample time. Although such cfu counts closely parallel the results obtained by direct counting methods in the exponential and early stationary phases, a divergence begins to emerge towards the end of the latter; the total cell number remains constant while the colony count declines. This marks the beginning of the final, *decline phase*, in the sequence of growth states which can be observed in broth. The discrepancy between the total and cfu counts is conventionally held to represent the death of cells because of nutrient exhaustion and accumulation of detrimental metabolic end-products. However, there is some doubt concerning this interpretation (see below).

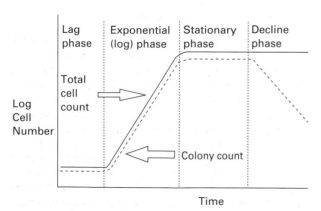

Fig. 4.1 Phases of growth in a broth culture.

The study of bacterial growth in broth provides a valuable point of reference to which practical, experimental and routine diagnostic procedures are often related. For example, the length of the lag phase and rates of exponential growth in different circumstances are used to make predictions and contribute to safety standards for storage in the food industry. An important feature that emerges is that cultures inoculated with cells prepared at different stages in the growth curve yield different results. The exponential phase is the most reproducible and readily identified, and is therefore used most frequently. It can be extended in an open system known as *continuous culture* using a *chemostat* in which cells of a growing culture are continuously harvested and nutrients continuously replenished. Chemostat studies have provided very detailed information on the chemistry of microbial growth and the way in which different organisms convert specific substrates into biomass. The extraordinary efficiency of this process has made natural and genetically manipulated microbes a powerful resource for the biotechnology industry.

In contrast to growth in broth, far less is known about the state of the bacteria in a mature macroscopic colony on an agar plate. Such a colony presents a wide range of environments, from an abundance of oxygen and nutrients at the edge to almost no oxygen or nutrients available to those cells in the centre. It is likely that all phases of growth are represented in colonies, depending on the location of a particular cell and the age of the culture. Although in practice colonies can be used reliably to inoculate routine tests of antimicrobial susceptibility in clinical laboratories, they cannot be considered a defined starting point for experimental work because they comprise such a heterogeneous population of cells. In fact, colonies are complex and dynamic communities in which cells at different locations can show startlingly different phenotypes. In spite of its complexity, the capacity for and quality of colonial growth of specific organisms on specialized media is central to the laboratory description of medically important bacteria.

MEDIA FOR BACTERIAL GROWTH

The media used in a medical diagnostic bacteriology laboratory have their origins, for the most part, back in the 'golden age of bacteriology' in the late 19th and early 20th centuries. A vast amount of experience and knowledge has accrued from their use and, apart from better standardization and quality control in their production, little has changed in their basic design. The objectives of early medium design were to grow pathogenic bacteria, separate them from the other organisms present in samples and, ultimately, differentiate

their phenotypic properties so that they could be identified. A critical development was the introduction of solidifying agents, most particularly the largely indigestible polysaccharide extract of seaweed known as agar. Alternative solidifying agents include gelatine and egg albumen. Before the development of solid media, pure cultures could be achieved only by dilution of inocula so that only one growing cell or clump of cells was present at the initiation of growth, a very laborious and unreliable procedure. In contrast, solid media in Petri dishes provided a growth substrate onto which mixed cultures could be inoculated and, providing the population density could be made low enough to allow development of well separated colonies, the different organisms present could be differentiated and subsequently separated into pure cultures.

Media used for isolation and identification of pathogens

The central features of media in medical bacteriology are:

1. A source of protein or protein hydrolysate, often derived from casein or an infusion of brain, heart or liver obtained from the nearest butcher.
2. Control of pH in the final product (after sterilization).
3. A defined salt content.

Early media often included blood or serum in an attempt to reproduce nutritional features present in the human body. Growth of some pathogens was found to be dependent on such supplements, and it was recognized that these relatively *fastidious* or *nutritionally exacting* organisms were dependent on *growth factors*. The identity of many of the growth factors is now known (e.g. haemin and several coenzymes) but blood often remains their most convenient source.

Selective and indicator media

Tremendous ingenuity has gone into designing growth media that provide information relevant to patient management as early as possible. There are two main approaches, both of which depend on adding supplements to the basal medium. *Selective media* contain substances such as bile salts or antibiotics that inhibit the growth of some organisms but have little or no effect on the organisms for whose isolation they were designed. They are essential for samples containing a normal microbial flora such as faeces. The inclusion of components or specific reagents that show whether the bacteria possess a particular biochemical property characterizes an *indicator medium*. Such media are critical to the rapid presumptive identification of isolates. Combinations of selective and indicator supplements in agar media have led to formulations with some remarkably elegant differential properties which effectively colour-code the colonies according to their biochemical properties, and restrict growth to a desired range of organisms. Broth indicator media tend to be much simpler, since they generally require a pure inoculum of a single organism and reveal only one property per formulation. Broth media with selective properties are usually referred to as *enrichment media* as they change the balance of organisms inoculated in favour of the desired range of organisms, thereby enriching them.

Media for laboratory studies

Most of the objectives of a clinical diagnostic laboratory can be fulfilled with the range of media outlined above. However, the composition of these media is not defined, and this poses problems for some investigations, including the detailed analysis of antibiotic action. Wherever possible, such investigations are based on a *defined* or *synthetic medium* where every chemical component is carefully regulated. In genetic experiments use is often made of a *minimal medium* in which every component is required for the growth of the organism under investigation, so that if one component is removed, growth cannot occur. Minimal media also prevent the growth of mutants that have additional nutritional requirements to those of the parent strain. For some organisms, particularly those which can grow outside the human body, minimal media may comprise as little as an ammonium salt to provide nitrogen, a carbon source, which in some cases can be as simple as carbon monoxide, trace amounts of iron and other essential elements, and pH adjustment to within an appropriate range. Defined and minimal media generally have to be developed for small groups of closely related organisms and should not be used for other organisms.

Relatively well defined media are preferred, even for routine antibiotic tests, because quantitative aspects of bacterial biochemistry, growth and susceptibility to noxious stimuli can be substantially influenced by minor changes in medium composition. The use of fully defined media has underpinned almost all of what we know about bacterial physiology. Rather curiously, however, it is well recognized that defined media are often suboptimal for the recovery of bacteria from environments in which they have been stressed. This may reflect the support provided to injured bacteria by complex media. Defined media can really only be optimized for bacteria in a single physiological state while complex media have greater potential to cope with the diversity of states present in natural samples.

BACTERIAL PHYSIOLOGY

The complement of processes that enables an organism to occupy and thrive in a particular environment places certain requirements on its physiology. Traditional descriptions of bacterial groups emphasize features which place a microbe in particular ecological niches. Thus we have *acidophiles* for organisms such as *Lactobacillus* spp. which grow at lower pH levels than most other organisms, and *halophiles* for organisms which grow at high salt concentrations. The environments which can be colonized by a pathogen are, of course, critical in determining its reservoirs and potential modes of transmission. More recently it has been recognized that individual bacteria are not restricted to a single physiological state. Rather, they respond to environmental stimuli and undergo *adaptive responses* which confer improved capacity for survival in adverse conditions. All these properties sustain the *viability* of the organism. However, it has become apparent that our ability to measure viability by conventional means may be inadequate.

The specific means by which a particular organism obtains energy and raw materials to sustain its growth (its nutritional type) and the physical conditions it requires reflect its fundamental physiological characteristics. Placing an organism into the groups defined by these characteristics is an important step in its conventional classification.

Nutritional types

Traditionally, all living organisms have been divided into two nutritional groups: *heterotrophs* and *autotrophs*. The former depend on the latter to produce organic molecules by fixing carbon dioxide, predominantly by photosynthesis. Bacterial metabolism is now recognized to be so diverse that it cannot be encompassed by these two terms. Three basic features are used in the present terminology: the *energy source*, the *hydrogen donors* and the *carbon source*.

Energy for adenosine triphosphate (ATP) synthesis may be obtained from light in a *phototrophic* organism and from chemical oxidations in the case of a *chemotrophic* organism. The hydrogen donor type characterizes an organism as an *organotroph* if it requires organic sources of hydrogen and as a *lithotroph* if it can use inorganic sources (e.g. ammonia or hydrogen sulphide). Finally, the terms autotroph and heterotroph are reserved for the carbon source; the former can fix carbon dioxide directly while the latter require an organic source. In general, only the energy and hydrogen donor designations are referred to routinely by combining the two terms. Hence we refer to *chemo-organotrophs* (the vast majority of currently recognized medically important organisms) and *chemolithotrophs* (e.g. some *Pseudomonas* spp.). Surprisingly, there are even some *photolithotrophs* with medical significance; the cyanobacteria are now known to produce many toxins that can affect humans.

Physical conditions required for growth

All living organisms use oxidation to transfer energy to compounds which participate in their internal biochemical and biophysical processes. Oxidation of a molecule is equivalent to the removal of hydrogen, and requires another molecule to receive electrons in the process. In *aerobic* respiration the final electron recipient in the oxidation process is molecular oxygen (i.e. O_2) whilst under *anaerobic* conditions (in the absence of oxygen) most medically important organisms use an organic molecule as the final electron recipient, and the oxidative process is referred to as *fermentation*. There are also some forms of anaerobic respiration which use inorganic electron acceptors such as nitrates. Respiration in this context is generally used to denote involvement of a membrane-associated electron transport chain in the oxidation. In the early period of development of life on the earth there was no oxygen in the atmosphere; thus, at this time, all bacteria were *anaerobes*. Subsequently, following the development of photo-autotrophic organisms, atmospheric oxygen became abundant, and organisms capable of using oxygen evolved.

Although aerobic metabolism is a more efficient means of obtaining energy than anaerobiosis, it is not without its cost. Some oxidation–reduction (redox) reactions occurring in the presence of oxygen commonly result in the formation of the reactive superoxide (O_2^-) and hydroxyl (OH^-) radicals as well as hydrogen peroxide (H_2O_2), all of which are highly toxic. To cope with this, aerobic organisms or *aerobes* have developed two enzymes which detoxify these molecules. *Superoxide dismutase* converts superoxide radicals to hydrogen peroxide ($2O_2^- + 2H^+ \rightarrow H_2O_2 + O_2$), while *catalase* converts hydrogen peroxide to water and oxygen in the reaction $2H_2O_2 \rightarrow 2H_2O + O_2$. Possession or lack of these enzymes has the important consequence of defining the atmosphere necessary for growth and survival of different organisms. Moreover, when produced in large amounts, the enzymes also provide protection for pathogenic organisms against the reactive oxygen intermediates deliberately produced as a defence mechanism by phagocytic cells.

Growth atmosphere

These oxygen-related features underpin the major practical grouping of bacteria according to their atmospheric requirements (Table 4.1). Thus, *strict* or *obligate aerobes* require oxygen, usually at ambient levels (~20%) and *strict* or *obligate anaerobes* require the complete absence of oxygen. Many organisms exhibit intermediate properties: *facultative anaerobes* generally grow better in oxygen but are still able to grow well in its absence; *micro-aerophilic* organisms require a reduced oxygen level (~5%); *aerotolerant anaerobes* have a fermentative pattern of metabolism but can tolerate the presence of oxygen because they possess superoxide dismutase. Many medically important organisms are facultative anaerobes. There is a mixture of aerobic and anaerobic micro-environments in the human body and the capacity to replicate in both is clearly advantageous. For obvious reasons, strict anaerobes are particularly associated with infection of tissues where the blood supply has been interrupted.

Among the various physical requirements for the growth of different bacterial groups, atmosphere assumes particular importance because in practice agar cultures from most clinical specimens are set up aerobically and anaerobically. Thus, when growth is first inspected after overnight incubation the isolates can readily be differentiated into strict aerobes, anaerobes and facultative anaerobes according to the conditions under which they have grown. Various atmospheric conditions can also be obtained in broth media. If the medium is unstirred, strict aerobes tend to grow on the surface, micro-aerophiles just under the surface and anaerobes in the body of the medium away from the surface. Growth of anaerobes is often improved by addition of a reducing agent such as cysteine or thioglycollate to mop up any free oxygen.

Growth temperature

The other significant physical condition for bacterial growth from the medical perspective is temperature (see Table 4.1). Pathogens which actually replicate on or in the human body must be able to grow within the temperature range 20–40°C, and are generally referred to as *mesophiles*. Organisms which can grow outside this range are either *psychrophiles* (cold-loving) or *thermophiles* (heat-loving). The former may be capable of growth in food or pharmaceuticals stored at normal refrigeration temperatures (0–8°C), while the latter can be a source of proteins with remarkable thermotolerant properties, e.g. taq polymerase, the key enzyme used in the polymerase chain reaction. Organisms such as the leprosy bacillus that prefer lower growth temperatures are often associated with skin and superficial infections, while organisms which grow in the colon (often a few degrees warmer than normal body temperature) can grow well up to 44°C.

Table 4.1 Key descriptive terms used to categorize bacteria according to their growth requirements

Descriptive term	Property	Example
Growth atmosphere		
Strict (obligate) aerobe	Requires atmospheric oxygen for growth	*Pseudomonas aeruginosa*
Strict (obligate) anaerobe	Will not tolerate oxygen	*Bacteroides fragilis*
Facultative anaerobe	Grows best aerobically, but can grow anaerobically	*Staphylococcus* spp., *Esch. coli*, etc.
Aerotolerant anaerobe	Anaerobic, but tolerates exposure to oxygen	*Clostridium perfringens*
Micro-aerophilic organism	Requires or prefers reduced oxygen levels	*Campylobacter* spp., *Helicobacter* spp.
Capnophilic organism	Requires or prefers increased carbon dioxide levels	*Neisseria* spp.
Growth temperature		
Psychrophile	Grows best at low temperature (e.g. <10°C)	*Flavobacterium* spp.
Thermophile	Grows best at high temperature (e.g. >60°C)	*Bacillus stearothermophilus*[a]
Mesophile	Grows best between 20 and 40°C	Most bacterial pathogens

[a] Not a pathogen; its spores are very heat-resistant and are used for testing the efficiency of heat sterilization.

Extremophiles

Some bacteria require ostensibly bizarre physical conditions for growth. For example, barophiles isolated from the ocean floor may require enormous pressures before they can replicate. Such organisms are often referred to as *extremophiles*. The properties of these organisms serve to remind us that microbes have the potential to occupy any environmental niche where energy and nutrition are available. It should be noted that most extremophiles actually turn out to belong to the *Archaea* (see Chapter 2).

Bacterial metabolism

Although some bacteria are able to obtain their resources for growth in ways that seem alien to us, the core of their metabolism is essentially very similar to that of mammalian cells. The basic details of glycolysis, the tricarboxylic acid cycle, oxidative phosphorylation, ATP biosynthesis and amino acid metabolism are constant. Variations in the pathways that feed into and flow from these core processes are readily detected by what are loosely termed *biochemical tests* in medical laboratories. These detect traits such as the ability to use individual carbohydrate sources to produce acid and the possession of specific enzymes.

The common nature of central catabolic and anabolic pathways in bacteria and higher organisms reflects the economy of biology and evolution. Processes that work well cannot be outcompeted and tend to be preserved in the genetic stock. Thus, many of the specific enzymes involved in bacterial metabolism show remarkable levels of conservation in their amino acid sequences across very substantial distances in evolutionary terms. DNA sequencing has enabled identification of *molecular families* of proteins that have a common evolutionary origin.

In addition to the metabolic enzymes, it has been recognized that many transport proteins responsible for importing and exporting specific substrates into and out of the bacterial cytoplasm are closely related in their structure and mode of function to those present in mammalian cells. Of course, because bacteria generally have only one cell compartment in which to operate, the location of these proteins is often different; for example, since they have no mitochondria, the cytoplasmic membrane contains the components of the electron transport chain, and the proton gradient across the inner mitochondrial membrane is generated across the cytoplasmic membrane instead. This feature actually means that bacteria can perform some energy-requiring processes at the cell surface, notably flagellar rotation (motility), by directly exploiting the proton gradient rather than consuming ATP.

Aside from its role in identification and intrinsic biological interest, bacterial metabolism has real consequences for man. In direct terms, the resident microflora have consequences in human health and disease. For example, the bacteria in dental plaque produce acid when presented with certain carbohydrate sources, and this acid is responsible for tooth decay; on the positive side, bacteria in the intestines deconjugate bile salts and thereby contribute to the enterohepatic circulation. It seems likely that the importance of such bioconversions will be increasingly recognized in the future. In particular, the role of bacteria in recovering nitrogen excreted into the colon in marginal human nutritional states and metabolic activity leading to the formation of carcinogens or other biologically active molecules are both areas where there is much room for further work.

Humans are also indirectly affected by microbial metabolism. At one level, the chemistry of our environment has been extensively shaped by microbes; the original development of oxygen in our atmosphere, the availability of elemental sulphur and the flow of nitrogen are all critically dependent on microbial metabolism. Exploitation of microbial metabolism in industry has, of course, given us ethanol, and many of the other alcohols and acids that result from fermentation have commercial value. Finally, bacteria have been used to combat the deleterious effects of environmental pollution in the process referred to as *bioremediation*.

Adaptive responses in bacteria

The extent to which bacteria respond to environmental stimuli was originally recognized by monitoring gross phenotypic, biochemical and behavioural changes. Much of the genetic basis for how bacteria change their phenotypes was established in the 1960s and 1970s following on from the paradigm established for β-galactosidase regulation in *Esch. coli* by Jacob and Monod. The scale and rapidity (major changes can be seen in seconds) of bacterial responses became apparent through the 1980s and 1990s as the use of global analytical approaches that attempt to characterize the instantaneous expression of every gene the organism carries became established. At the translational level, the use of two-dimensional gel electrophoresis has underpinned the so-called *proteomic* approach. This technique reveals and separates most of the several hundred proteins which are being synthesized by a pure culture at a particular time. The catalogue of different proteins detected represents those proteins that the organism requires to function in the circumstances from which the sample was drawn. Assays of this type have shown that different sets of proteins are made in the exponential and stationary phases of the growth cycle and, indeed, in response to almost any environmental change. This finding underpins the recognition of just how different the phenotype of a single organism can be in different physiological states and reinforces the need to define the inoculum used in laboratory experiments. More recently the development of DNA arrays has enabled global analysis of responses at the transcriptional level by detecting mRNA molecules relating to every gene in the organism in a single analysis. The complement of RNA species present in an organism at a given time is referred to as the *transcriptome*. The basic features of the comparative protein and mRNA analyses are outlined in Fig. 4.2.

The effects of specific sublethal but noxious stimuli on gene expression are the subject of intense current study. Each different stimulus leads to an adaptive *stress response*, which is to some extent specific to the stimulus applied. Heat shock (the effects of raising temperature to 45°C and above for a few minutes) has been studied most extensively. The newly synthesized proteins elicited in this response are referred to as *heat*

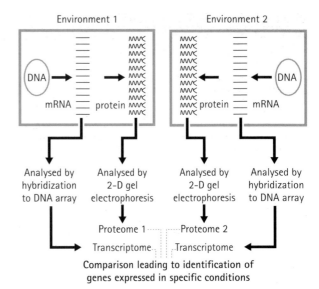

Fig. 4.2 Global strategies for identifying differentially expressed genes. Proteomics leads to the identification of protein spots that are particularly associated with specific environmental conditions. N-terminal amino acid sequencing of material extracted from a spot then allows the responsible gene to be identified and ultimately sequenced. Transcriptome analysis requires a representation of all the genes concerned in a DNA array and therefore needs prior knowledge (ideally a complete sequence) of the genome of the organism to be tested. These two global approaches provide a very comprehensive picture of the physiology of the organism under study.

shock proteins (HSPs). When the amino acid sequences of the principal HSPs were determined they were found to belong to a molecular family now recognized in all prokaryotic and eukaryotic cells. Apart from their role in improving the ability of bacteria to survive heat shock, HSPs, by virtue of their similarity to host cell HSP antigens, seem to be involved in initiating autoimmune damage and immune dysfunction. A very important feature of the stress response in bacteria is that many of the stimuli used are prominent aspects of the stresses applied by the human immune system to an invading pathogen. Thus, acid stress is provided by the stomach and the hostile environment of phagolysosomes includes both oxidative and pH stress.

The information built up from studying stress responses has made it possible to identify sets of proteins which are made in response to several different stresses and those which appear exclusive to one stress. Together with other approaches, this has allowed recognition of *global regulatory systems* or *networks* within bacteria which are responsible for differential gene expression under different circumstances. The hierarchy of specific control mechanisms involved has spawned two important new terms, *stimulon* and *regulon*. A stimulon denotes all those genes whose expression is increased or decreased by a specific external stimulus, while a regulon refers to all those genes under the influence of a specific regulatory protein. A regulon may affect several operons (see Chapter 6), and there may be many regulons in one stimulon.

Regulatory networks have been identified in almost every area of bacterial physiology. Thus, in addition to the stimuli cited above, osmotic stress, cold shock, nutrient limitation (separate responses for carbon, nitrogen and phosphate), anaerobic and many other stimulons are recognized. These control systems are responsible for making sure the organism only synthesizes proteins appropriate to its current circumstances. A particularly important medical example of this is the regulation of proteins concerned with an organism's progress in an infection (virulence factors). Equally important from the scientific perspective is the recognition that chemicals secreted by an organism can themselves act as regulatory stimuli to individuals of the same species in a way analogous to the pheromones released by insects.

Although it is still important to recognize that different organisms are particularly adapted to special environmental niches with descriptive terms such as mesophile, acidophile and halophile, the discovery of adaptive responses in bacteria has pushed us into an uncertain period where much of what has been established about the tolerance of micro-organisms to noxious stresses will have to be re-examined. Furthermore, since the extent to which bacteria modulate their phenotype according to their circumstances is now clear, the need for caution in concluding that any property detected in the laboratory is significant in a natural infection is unavoidably obvious.

Bacterial viability

A central feature of the general and adaptive physiology of bacteria is its capacity to preserve the viability of a particular organism. There is, however, a persistent problem – how do we define viability in practical terms? Traditionally, the operational definition of the capacity of a cell to form a colony on an appropriate agar medium (the colony or cfu count) has been almost universally accepted. It is also often expressed as the proportion of cells within a population which are capable of forming colonies. However, it must be emphasized that viability is not a clearly measurable property. At the individual level, it expresses the expectation that, in a suitable environment, a particular cell has the capacity to grow and undergo binary fission and that its progeny will have the same potential. The key assumption is that colony counts provide an accurate measure of viability.

The central problem can be stated as follows: it is self-evident that if a bacterial cell produces a colony it must have been viable, but to what extent is it true that a cell which fails to do this is non-viable or dead? Immediately contradictions to this proposal can be identified. The bacterial pathogens, such as *Mycobacterium leprae* and *Treponema pallidum*, which cannot be induced to form colonies on available agar media are clearly viable. Similarly, all the 'as yet uncultivated organisms' (possibly as many as 99% of all bacterial species) are clearly able to propagate themselves. They simply have not been sporting enough to do it on our laboratory media. A further exception is the phenomenon of bacterial recovery from injury (e.g. cold or osmotic shock) in which colony counts can be shown to rise in the absence of cell division.

It is possible that some organisms which are readily cultivable may be able to switch to a physiological state in which they cannot be induced to form colonies. The current popular terminology for cells in this putative state is *viable but non-culturable* (VNC).

Epidemiological and laboratory evidence provide some support for the existence of a VNC state. In particular, the occurrence of several infectious diseases acquired from environmental sources, notably cholera, is at variance with our ability to recover the causal organisms from the implicated source. Environmental studies have demonstrated cells with immunological properties compatible with those of the cholera vibrio but failed to recover the organism in culture, and laboratory studies have indicated that the organism can persist in a non-culturable form. There is also evidence that non-culturable forms may revert to their 'normal' culturable state.

A major attraction of the VNC hypothesis is that it may resolve a number of important mysteries in medical microbiology. In general, these are situations in which we know the organism must be present but are unable to culture it. This is particularly so with diseases such as tuberculosis that have latent phases.

The most significant problem for the VNC hypothesis is that it has not been defined in physiological, biochemical or genetic terms. On the face of it, one might expect transition to the VNC state to result from an adaptive response such as those described in the previous section. Alternatively, transition might be the result of a programme of gene expression such as that observed in spore formation or starvation. From this standpoint the stationary and decline phases in the growth cycle outlined above (when spore formation is induced in sporulating bacteria) may represent the initiation of and transition to a non-culturable phase rather than loss of viability (the traditional view). In spite of their popularity, these ideas must presently be viewed as interesting speculations for which there is circumstantial but no conclusive evidence.

Measurement of viability has been of great practical value in medical microbiology. Colony counts performed to investigate the action of antibiotics and other disruptive influences such as heat, and those performed at different stages during experimental infections in animal models of human infections, have provided a wealth of valuable information. Moreover, there is no reason to doubt that this approach will continue to be extremely useful.

None the less, it is necessary to maintain a clear view of the limitations of bacterial culture as a measure of the organisms present in a sample and of their viability. Studies often use the term 'viability' when in fact growth on agar or in broth was measured, and confusion would be prevented if the terms 'culturability' and 'colony counts' were used instead.

We are now entering an era in which many diagnostic and investigational techniques may be replaced by molecular detection procedures. The fact that signals based on such techniques may come from culturable, dead and potentially VNC cells should be recognized. Unravelling these three possibilities presents ample challenge for medical and non-medical microbiologists alike.

RECOMMENDED READING

Barer M R, Harwood C R 1999 Bacterial viability and culturability. *Advances in Microbial Physiology* 41: 94–138

Moat A G, Foster J W 1995 *Microbial Physiology*, 3rd edn. Wiley-Liss, New York

Neidhardt F C, Ingraham J L, Schaechter M 1990 *Physiology of the Bacterial Cell: A Molecular Approach*. Sinauer, Sunderland, MA

Roszaak D B, Colwell R R 1987 Survival strategies of bacteria in the natural environment. *Microbiological Reviews* 51: 365–379

Internet site

www.micro.msb.le.ac.uk/LabWork/bact/bact1.htm

5

Antimicrobial agents

D. Greenwood and M. M. Ogilvie

The study of antimicrobial agents embraces not only antibacterial compounds, but also antiviral, antifungal, antiprotozoal and even anthelminthic agents. The treatment of individual infections is dealt with in the appropriate chapters and the general strategy of antimicrobial chemotherapy, which is crucial to the control of antimicrobial drug resistance, is covered in Chapter 66.

Antibiotics are naturally occurring microbial products; synthetic compounds such as sulphonamides, quinolones, nitrofurans and imidazoles should strictly be referred to as *chemotherapeutic agents*. However, since some antibiotics can be manufactured synthetically while others are the products of chemical manipulation of naturally occurring compounds (*semi-synthetic antibiotics*) the distinction is now ill-defined. Nowadays the term *antibiotic* is used loosely to describe agents (mainly, but not exclusively, antibacterial agents) used to treat systemic infection. Antimicrobial substances that are too toxic to be used other than in topical therapy or for environmental decontamination are referred to as *antiseptics* or *disinfectants* (see Chapter 7).

ANTIBACTERIAL AGENTS

The principal types of antibacterial agent are listed in Table 5.1. Because there are so many of them it is convenient to group them according to their site of action.

Table 5.1 Principal types of antibacterial agent (other than agents used exclusively in mycobacterial infection)

Agent	Site of action	Usual activity[a] against					
		Staphylococci	Streptococci	Enterobacteria	Pseudomonas aeruginosa	Mycobacterium tuberculosis	Anaerobes
Penicillins	Cell wall	(+)	+	v	v	−	+[b]
Cephalosporins	Cell wall	+	+	+	v	−	+[b]
Other β–lactam agents	Cell wall	v	v	+	v	−	v
Glycopeptides	Cell wall	+	+	−	−	−	+[c]
Tetracyclines	Ribosome	(+)	(+)	(+)	−	−	(+)
Chloramphenicol	Ribosome	+	+	+	−	−	+
Aminoglycosides	Ribosome	+	−	+	v	v	−
Macrolides	Ribosome	+	+	−	−	−	+
Lincosamides	Ribosome	+	+	−	−	−	+
Fusidic acid	Ribosome	+	+	−	−	+	+
Oxazolidinones	Ribosome	+	+	−	−	−	+
Streptogramins	Ribosome	+	+[d]	−	−	−	−
Rifamycins	RNA synthesis	+	+	+	−	+	+
Sulphonamides	Folate metabolism	(+)	(+)	(+)	−	−	−
Diaminopyrimidines	Folate metabolism	+	+	(+)	−	−	−
Quinolones	DNA synthesis	v	v	+	v	v	−
Nitrofurans	DNA synthesis	−	−	+	−	−	+
Nitroimidazoles	DNA synthesis	−	−	−	−	−	+

v, variable activity among different agents of the group.
[a] Usual spectrum of intrinsic activity; parentheses indicate that resistance is common.
[b] Poor activity against anaerobes of the *Bacteroides fragilis* group.
[c] Poor activity against most Gram-negative anaerobes.
[d] Poor activity against *Enterococcus faecalis*.

Inhibitors of bacterial cell wall synthesis

Since most bacteria possess a rigid cell wall that is lacking in mammalian cells, this structure is a prime target for agents that exhibit *selective toxicity*, the ability to inhibit or destroy the microbe without harming the host. However, the bacterial cell wall can also prevent access of agents that would otherwise be effective. Thus, the complex outer envelope of Gram-negative bacteria is impermeable to large hydrophilic molecules, which may be prevented from reaching an otherwise susceptible target.

Inhibitors of bacterial cell wall synthesis act on the formation of the peptidoglycan layer (Fig. 5.1). Bacteria that lack peptidoglycan, such as mycoplasmas, are resistant to these agents.

β-Lactam agents

Penicillins, cephalosporins and other compounds that feature a β-lactam ring in their structure fall into this group (Fig. 5.2). All these compounds bind to proteins situated at the cell wall–cell membrane interface. These *penicillin-binding proteins* are involved in cell wall construction, including the cross-linking of the peptidoglycan strands that gives the wall its strength. Opening of the β-lactam ring by hydrolytic enzymes, collectively called *β-lactamases*, abolishes antibacterial activity. Many such enzymes are found in bacteria. Those elaborated by Gram-negative enteric bacilli are particularly diverse in their activity and properties. Most prevalent are the so-called *TEM β-lactamases* (TEM-1, TEM-2, etc.), numerous forms of which have evolved under selective pressure of β-lactam antibiotic use.

Penicillins. Benzylpenicillin (penicillin G) exhibits unrivalled activity against staphylococci, streptococci, neisseriae, spirochaetes and certain other organisms. However, resistance, normally due to the production of β-lactamase, has undermined its activity against staphylococci and, to a lesser extent, gonococci. Bacteria that exhibit reduced susceptibility to penicillin by a non-enzymic mechanism are also encountered. Benzylpenicillin revolutionized the treatment of infection caused by some of the most virulent bacterial pathogens, but it also suffers from several shortcomings:

- breakdown by gastric acidity when given orally
- very rapid excretion by the kidney
- susceptibility to penicillinase (β-lactamase)
- a restricted spectrum of activity.

Further development of the penicillin family has been directed towards improving these properties. Crucial to this was the discovery that removal of the phenylacetic acid side-chain left intact the core structure, 6-aminopenicillanic acid, the starting point for the numerous semi-synthetic penicillins that have been produced (Fig. 5.3). Among the most important penicillins are:

- phenoxymethyl penicillin (penicillin V), which can be given orally
- procaine penicillin, a long-acting salt of benzylpenicillin
- flucloxacillin, an antistaphylococcal compound
- ampicillin and amoxicillin, which are active against some enterobacteria
- ticarcillin, azlocillin and piperacillin, which are active against *Pseudomonas aeruginosa*.

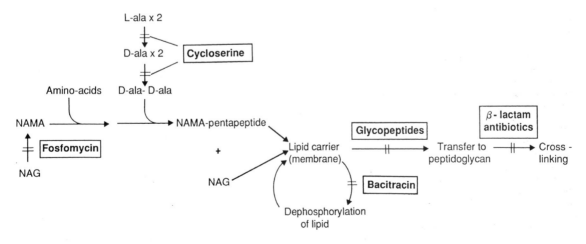

NAG = *N*-acetylglucosamine

NAMA = *N*-acetylmuramic acid

Fig. 5.1 Sites of action of inhibitors of bacterial cell wall synthesis.

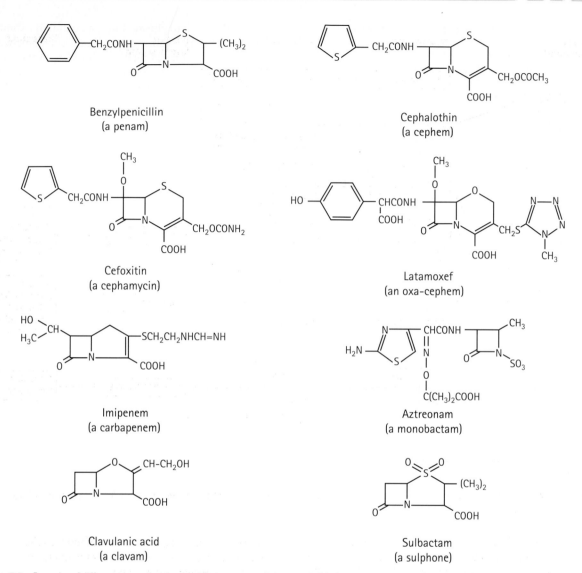

Fig. 5.2   Examples of different types of molecular structure among β-lactam antibiotics.

None of these compounds, with the exception of flucloxacillin (and related antistaphylococcal penicillins), exhibits stability to staphylococcal β-lactamase. *Methicillin-resistant Staphylococcus aureus* (MRSA; a term that has persisted although methicillin is now virtually obsolete) and other staphylococci that owe their resistance to alterations in the target penicillin-binding proteins are resistant to all penicillins and to all other β-lactam antibiotics.

Cephalosporins. Cephalosporins are close cousins of the penicillins, but the β-lactam ring is fused to a six-membered dihydrothiazine ring rather than the five-membered thiazolidine ring of penicillins. The additional carbon carries substitutions that may alter the pharmacological behaviour of the molecule, and sometimes its antibacterial activity. Some cephalosporins (e.g. cephalothin and cefotaxime) carry an acetoxymethyl group on the extra carbon. This can be removed by hepatic enzymes to yield a less active derivative, but it is doubtful whether this has any therapeutic significance. Other cephalosporins (e.g. cefamandole, cefoperazone, and the oxa-cephem, latamoxef) possess a methyltetrazole substituent. Use of compounds with this feature has been associated with hypoprothrombinaemia and bleeding in some patients.

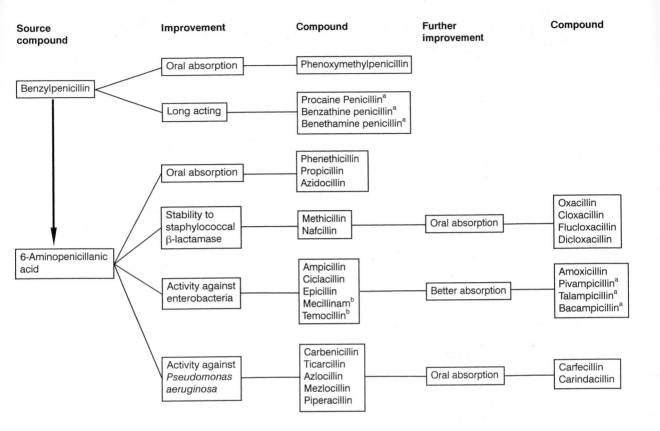

Fig. 5.3 Development of penicillins. 'Improvement' means a qualitative improvement, and is not intended to indicate that compounds listed together are necessarily equivalent.

[a] Pro-drugs that release active penicillins
[b] Inactive against Gram-positive bacteria

Cephalosporins are generally stable to staphylococcal penicillinase (though they are differentially susceptible to hydrolysis by the various types of enterobacterial β-lactamase), but they lack activity against enterococci. They exhibit a broader spectrum than most penicillins and are less prone to cause hypersensitivity reactions. The range of available derivatives is shown in Fig. 5.4. Among the most important are:

- cefalexin and cefaclor, which can be given orally
- cefuroxime and cefoxitin, which are stable to many β-lactamases
- cefotaxime and ceftriaxone, which combine β-lactamase stability with high intrinsic activity
- ceftazidime and cefpirome, which additionally exhibit good activity against *Ps. aeruginosa*.

Other β-lactam agents. Various agents with diverse properties share the structural feature of a β-lactam ring with penicillins and cephalosporins (Fig. 5.2):

- *Monobactams* (e.g. aztreonam) are monocyclic compounds with a spectrum that is restricted to aerobic Gram-negative bacteria.
- *Carbapenems* (e.g. imipenem and meropenem) have an unusually broad spectrum of activity, embracing most Gram-positive and Gram-negative aerobic and anaerobic bacteria. Imipenem is inactivated by a dehydropeptidase in the human kidney, and is co-administered with a dehydropeptidase inhibitor, cilastatin.
- *Oxa-cephems* (e.g. latamoxef) are broad-spectrum β-lactamase-stable compounds.
- The *clavam*, clavulanic acid, exhibits poor antibacterial activity, but has proved useful as a β-lactamase inhibitor when used in combination with β-lactamase-susceptible compounds (e.g. co-amoxiclav, the combination of amoxicillin and clavulanic acid).

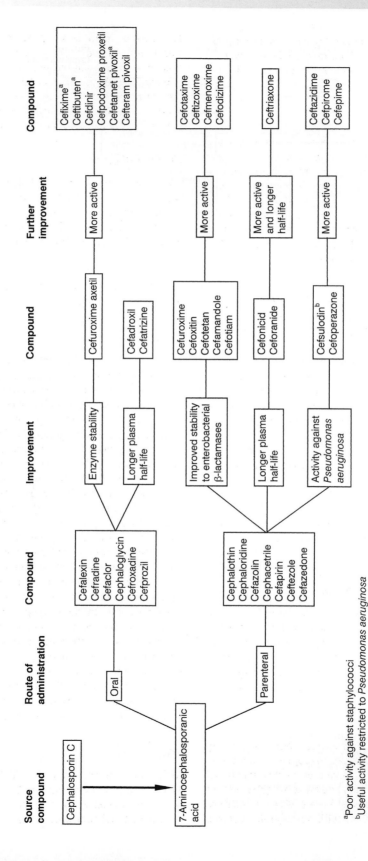

Fig. 5.4 Development of cephalosporins. 'Improvement' means a qualitative improvement, and is not intended to indicate that compounds listed together are necessarily equivalent.

[a]Poor activity against staphylococci
[b]Useful activity restricted to *Pseudomonas aeruginosa*

- The *sulphones*, sulbactam and tazobactam, also act as β-lactamase inhibitors and are marketed combined with ampicillin (or cefoperazone) and piperacillin, respectively.

Glycopeptides

Vancomycin and teicoplanin are large molecules that are unable to penetrate the outer membrane of Gram-negative bacteria, and the spectrum is consequently restricted to Gram-positive organisms. Their chief importance resides in their action against Gram-positive cocci with multiple resistance to other drugs. However, enterococci and staphylococci, including MRSA, that exhibit resistance or reduced sensitivity to glycopeptides are being reported more frequently.

Other inhibitors of bacterial cell wall synthesis

- Fosfomycin is a naturally occurring antibiotic with a simple phosphonic acid structure. It exhibits a fairly broad spectrum, notably against Gram-negative bacilli, and is mainly used for the treatment of urinary tract infection. Resistance arises readily in vitro.
- Bacitracin is active against Gram-positive bacteria, but is too toxic for systemic use. It is found in many topical preparations, and is also used in the laboratory in the presumptive identification of haemolytic streptococci of Lancefield group A (see p. 185).
- Cycloserine is an analogue of D-alanine used only as a second-line agent in infections with multiresistant strains of *Mycobacterium tuberculosis*.
- Isoniazid and some other compounds used in tuberculosis probably act by interfering with formation of the mycolic acids of the mycobacterial cell wall.

Inhibitors of bacterial protein synthesis

Bacterial ribosomes are sufficiently different from those of mammalian cells to allow selective inhibition of protein synthesis. Some of the agents that act at this level do, however, have an effect in eukaryotic cells. Most are true antibiotics (or derivatives thereof) produced by *Streptomyces* species or other soil organisms.

Tetracyclines

These are broad-spectrum agents with important activity against chlamydiae, rickettsiae, mycoplasmas and, surprisingly, malaria parasites, as well as most conventional Gram-positive and Gram-negative bacteria. They prevent binding of amino-acyl transfer RNA (tRNA) to the ribosome and inhibit, but do not kill, susceptible bacteria.

The various members of the tetracycline group are closely related and differ more in their pharmacological behaviour than in antibacterial activity. Doxycycline and minocycline are in most common use. Resistance has limited the value of tetracyclines against many Gram-positive and Gram-negative bacteria, but not against rickettsiae, chlamydiae and mycoplasmas to date.

Chloramphenicol

This compound, and the related thiamphenicol, also possess a very broad antibacterial spectrum. They act by blocking the growth of the peptide chain. Use of chloramphenicol has been limited to typhoid fever, meningitis and a few other clinical indications because of the occurrence of a rare but fatal side-effect, aplastic anaemia. Thiamphenicol is said to lack this disadvantage, but is more likely to cause a reversible type of bone marrow toxicity.

Aminoglycosides

Streptomycin, the first antibiotic to be discovered by random screening of soil organisms, is predominantly active against enterobacteria and *M. tuberculosis*. Like other members of the aminoglycoside family it has no useful activity against streptococci, anaerobes or intracellular bacteria. The group also has in common a tendency to damage the eighth cranial nerve (ototoxicity) and the kidney (nephrotoxicity). The chief properties of aminoglycosides are shown in Table 5.2. They inhibit formation of the ribosomal initiation complex and also cause misreading of messenger RNA (mRNA). They are bactericidal compounds, and some, notably gentamicin and tobramycin, exhibit good activity against *Ps. aeruginosa*. Such compounds have been widely used, often in combination with β-lactam antibiotics, with which they interact synergically, in the 'blind' treatment of sepsis in immunocompromised patients. Resistance may arise from ribosomal changes (streptomycin), or alterations in drug uptake. However, it is more often caused by bacterial enzymes that phosphorylate, acetylate or adenylate exposed amino or hydroxyl groups. Enzymic resistance consequently affects the various aminoglycosides differentially, depending on the possession of exposed groups that can be attacked by the enzyme involved. Amikacin is resistant to most of the common enzymes.

Macrolides

Macrolides are antibiotics in which a large macrocyclic lactone ring is substituted with some unusual sugars. They act by interfering with the translocation of mRNA on the bacterial ribosome. They are mainly used as anti-

Table 5.2 Summary of the important differential properties of aminoglycoside antibiotics

Aminoglycoside	Activity against		Relative susceptibility to inactivation by bacterial enzymes	Relative degrees of	
	Pseudomonas aeruginosa	Mycobacterium tuberculosis		Ototoxicity	Nephrotoxicity
Amikacin	+	+	±	++	+
Gentamicin	+	–	++	++	++
Kanamycin	–	+	++	++	++
Neomycin	–	±	++	+++	++
Netilmicin	+	–	+	+	+
Sissomicin	+	–	++	++	++
Streptomycin	–	+	++	+++	±
Tobramycin	+	–	++	++	++

staphylococcal and antistreptococcal agents, though some have wider applications. They have no useful activity against enteric Gram-negative bacilli. The original macrolide, erythromycin, is unstable in gastric acid and is usually administered orally as the stearate salt or as an esterified *pro-drug* (pharmacological preparations that improve absorption and deliver the active drug into the circulation). Salts suitable for intravenous administration are also available. Certain later macrolides, including clarithromycin, dirithromycin and roxithromycin, offer improved pharmacological properties.

The macrolactone ring of these compounds is composed of 14 atoms, but other macrolides have additional carbons conferring a 16-membered structure. These include oleandomycin, josamycin, midecamycin (the properties of which are similar to those of erythromycin), and spiramycin, which has some useful activity against the protozoan parasite, *Toxoplasma gondii*.

Some newer macrolides feature structural changes in the macrocyclic ring: in azithromycin, a compound distinguished by good tissue penetration and a long terminal half-life, the ring has been expanded by inclusion of a nitrogen atom to form an *azalide*; in telithromycin, a compound that retains activity against macrolide-resistant Gram-positive cocci, a keto function has been introduced to produce a *ketolide*.

Lincosamides

The original lincosamide antibiotic, lincomycin, has been superseded by the 7-deoxy-7-chloro derivative, clindamycin, which is better absorbed after oral administration and is more active against the organisms within its spectrum. These include staphylococci, streptococci and most anaerobic bacteria, against which clindamycin exhibits outstanding activity. Enthusiasm for the use of clindamycin has been tempered by an association with the occasional development of severe diarrhoea, which sometimes pro-

gresses to a life-threatening pseudomembranous colitis (see *Clostridium difficile*, Chapter 22).

Lincosamides bind to the 50S ribosomal subunit at a site closely related to that at which macrolides act. Inducible resistance to macrolides caused by enzymic modification of the ribosomal binding site also renders the cells resistant to lincosamides (and streptogramins; see below), but only in the presence of macrolides, which alone are able to act as inducers.

Fusidic acid

The structure of fusidic acid is related to that of steroids, but the antibiotic is devoid of steroid-like activity. It blocks factor G, which is involved in peptide elongation. Fusidic acid has an unusual spectrum of activity that includes corynebacteria, nocardia and *M. tuberculosis*, but the antibiotic is usually regarded simply as an antistaphylococcal agent. It penetrates well into bone and has been widely used (generally in combination with a β-lactam antibiotic to prevent the selection of resistant variants) in the treatment of staphylococcal osteomyelitis.

Oxazolidinones

Concerns about the spread of resistance in staphylococci, enterococci and pneumococci have revived interest in antibacterial compounds formerly rejected. The oxazolidinones, of which linezolid is the only one in clinical use, is an example of such a renaissance. These compounds prevent the formation of the ribosomal initiation complex and are narrow-spectrum anti-Gram-positive agents.

Streptogramins

This is the collective name for a family of antibiotics that occur naturally as two synergic components. They were formerly used mainly in animal husbandry, though one member of the group, pristinamycin, is available in some countries as an antistaphylococcal agent. Wider use was limited by poor solubility, but derivatives suitable for parenteral administration, quinupristin and dalfopristin, have been developed as a combination product. The combination exhibits bactericidal activity against most Gram-positive cocci, but has poor activity against *Enterococcus faecalis*.

Mupirocin

This is an antibiotic, produced by *Pseudomonas fluorescens*, which blocks incorporation of isoleucine into proteins. Its useful activity is restricted to staphylococci and streptococci, and, since it is inactivated when given systemically, it is used only in topical preparations.

Inhibitors of nucleic acid synthesis

A number of important antibacterial agents act directly or indirectly on DNA or RNA synthesis.

Sulphonamides and diaminopyrimidines

These agents affect DNA synthesis because of their role in folic acid metabolism. Folic acid is used in many one-carbon transfers in living cells, including the conversion of deoxyuridine to thymidine. During this process the active form of the vitamin, tetrahydrofolate, is oxidized to dihydrofolate, and this must be reduced before it can function in further reactions. Sulphonamides are analogues of *para*-aminobenzoic acid, and prevent the condensation of this compound with dihydropteridine during the formation of folic acid. Diaminopyrimidines, which include the broad-spectrum antibacterial agent trimethoprim and the antimalarial compounds pyrimethamine and cycloguanil (the metabolic product of proguanil), prevent the reduction of dihydrofolate to tetrahydrofolate. Sulphonamides and diaminopyrimidines thus act at sequential stages of the same metabolic pathway and interact synergically, but in bacterial infections trimethoprim is generally sufficiently effective, and less toxic, when used alone.

Sulphonamides are broad-spectrum antibacterial agents, but resistance is common and the group also suffers from problems of toxicity. The numerous sulphonamides exhibit similar antibacterial activity, but differ widely in their pharmacokinetic behaviour. They have largely been replaced by safer and more active agents, although the combination of sulphamethoxazole with trimethoprim (co-trimoxazole) is still used. Sulfadoxine or sulphadiazine combined with pyrimethamine are used in malaria and toxoplasmosis, respectively.

Quinolones

These drugs act on the α subunit of DNA gyrase. Their properties allow them to be roughly categorized into three groups (Table 5.3). Nalidixic acid and its early congeners are narrow-spectrum agents active only against Gram-negative bacteria. Their use is virtually restricted to urinary tract infection, although they have also been used in enteric infections and, in the case of acrosoxacin, in gonorrhoea. Later quinolones, such as ciprofloxacin and ofloxacin, which are 6-fluoro derivatives, display much enhanced activity and a broader spectrum, although activity against some Gram-positive cocci, notably *Streptococcus pneumoniae*, is unreliable. Continued development has produced compounds that lack the latter defect and, in some cases, exhibit further broadening of the spectrum and improved pharmacokinetic properties.

Quinolones are quite well absorbed when given orally and are widely distributed throughout the body. Extensive metabolization may occur, particularly with nalidixic acid and the older derivatives. Ciprofloxacin and other fluoroquinolones are widely used despite certain problems of toxicity, and resistance is becoming more prevalent.

Nitroimidazoles

Azole derivatives feature prominently among antifungal, antiprotozoal and anthelminthic agents. Those that exhibit antibacterial activity are 5-nitroimidazoles. At low redox (E_h) values they are reduced to a short-lived intermediate that causes strand breakage in DNA. Because of the requirement for low E_h values, 5-nitroimidazoles are active only against anaerobic (and certain micro-aerophilic) bacteria and anaerobic protozoa. The

Table 5.3 Types of quinolone antibacterial agent

Narrow-spectrum compounds[a]	Broad-spectrum compounds[b]	Compounds with further enhanced spectrum[c]
Acrosoxacin	Ciprofloxacin	Clinafloxacin
Cinoxacin	Enoxacin	Gatifloxacin
Flumequine	Levofloxacin	Gemifloxacin
Nalidixic acid	Lomefloxacin	Moxifloxacin
Oxolinic acid	Norfloxacin	Sparfloxacin
Pipemidic acid	Ofloxacin	Tosufloxacin
Piromidic acid	Pefloxacin	Trovafloxacin
	Rufloxacin	

[a] Spectrum restricted to enteric Gram-negative bacilli.
[b] Improved activity against *Pseudomonas aeruginosa* and Gram-positive cocci.
[c] Further improved activity against Gram-positive cocci and some anaerobes.

representative of the group most commonly used clinically is metronidazole, but similar derivatives include tinidazole, ornidazole and nimorazole.

Nitrofurans

The most familiar nitrofuran derivative is nitrofurantoin, an agent used exclusively in urinary tract infection. Other nitrofurans, including furazolidone, which is used in enteric infections, are marketed for a variety of purposes in some parts of the world. The mode of action of nitrofurans has not been elucidated, but it is probable that a reduced metabolite acts on DNA in a manner analogous to that of the nitroimidazoles.

Novobiocin

This compound acts on the β subunit of DNA gyrase (cf. quinolones). It was once widely used as a reserve antistaphylococcal agent, but is no longer favoured because of problems of resistance and toxicity.

Rifamycins

This group of antibiotics is characterized by excellent activity against mycobacteria, although other bacteria are also susceptible; staphylococci in particular are exquisitely sensitive. These compounds act by inhibiting transcription of RNA from DNA. Rifampicin, the best known member of the group, is used in tuberculosis and leprosy. Wider use has been discouraged on the grounds that it might inadvertently foster the emergence of resistance in mycobacteria. Rifapentine has similar properties, but exhibits a longer plasma half-life. Rifabutin (ansamycin) is used in infections caused by atypical mycobacteria of the avium-intracellulare group (see Chapter 19).

Miscellaneous antibacterial agents

Polymyxins

Polymyxin B and colistin (polymyxin E) act like cationic detergents to disrupt cell membranes. They exhibit potent antipseudomonal activity, but toxicity has limited their usefulness, except in topical preparations and bowel decontamination regimens. If systemic use is contemplated, a sulphomethylated derivative, colistin sulphomethate, is preferred.

Antimycobacterial agents

As well as streptomycin and rifampicin (see above), various agents are used exclusively for the treatment of mycobacterial infection. These include isoniazid, ethambutol and pyrazinamide, which are commonly found in antituberculosis regimens, and diaminodiphenylsulphone (dapsone) and clofazimine, which are used in leprosy. Cycloserine and p-aminosalicylic acid (PAS), which were formerly used in tuberculosis, have now been largely abandoned except for drug-resistant tuberculosis. Some fluoroquinolones and macrolides exhibit activity against certain mycobacteria, and may have a role in treatment.

ANTIFUNGAL AGENTS

Although fungi cause a wide variety of infections (see Chapter 60), relatively few agents are available for treatment, especially for the systemic therapy of serious mycoses. Superficial fungal infections of the skin and mucous membranes can often be treated with topical agents, including *polyenes*, such as nystatin, or *azole* derivatives, of which many (clotrimazole, miconazole, econazole, etc.) are marketed as vaginal pessaries and creams. For dermatophyte infections of the nails, oral therapy with griseofulvin or the allylamine derivative terbinafine is peculiarly suitable, since these agents are deposited in newly formed keratin. Serious systemic disease caused by yeasts and other fungi is often treated with the polyene, amphotericin B, which is extremely toxic. Newer formulations of the drug, in which it is complexed with liposomes or lipids, are better tolerated. The pyrimidine analogue 5-fluorocytosine is active against many types of yeast, and is used in combination with amphotericin B in severe systemic yeast infections. A new agent, caspofungin, is a member of the echinocandin class of agents that interfere with β-glucan synthesis in the fungal cell wall. It is active against various fungi, including *Candida*, *Aspergillus* and *Histoplasma* species (but not *Cryptococcus neoformans*) and is administered by intravenous infusion.

Azole derivatives exhibit the broadest spectrum of activity, embracing yeasts, filamentous fungi and dimorphic fungi, but few are suitable for systemic use. Those that are include the 2-nitroimidazole ketoconazole, and the triazoles itraconazole and fluconazole. Itraconazole is unique in exhibiting useful activity against *Aspergillus fumigatus*; fluconazole is particularly well distributed after oral administration, and has been used successfully in systemic yeast infections, including cryptococcal meningitis.

The fungus, *Pneumocystis carinii*, long thought to be a protozoon, is not susceptible to conventional antifungal agents (see p. 588).

The spectrum of activity of the common antifungal compounds is shown in Table 5.4. Most act by interfering with the integrity of the fungal cell membrane,

Table 5.4 Summary of the spectrum of activity of antifungal agents

Agent	*Candida albicans*	*Cryptococcus neoformans*	Dermatophytes	*Aspergillus fumigatus*	Dimorphic fungi
Amphotericin B	+	+	–	+	+
Flucytosine	+	+	–	–	–
Griseofulvin	–	–	+	–	–
Imidazoles	+	+	+	–	+
Nystatin[a]	+	–	+	–	–
Terbinafine	–	–	+	+[b]	+[b]
Triazoles	+	+	+	(+)[c]	+

[a] For topical use only.
[b] Clinical efficacy not yet established.
[c] Itraconazole is active against *A. fumigatus*, but fluconazole is not.

either by binding to membrane sterols (polyenes), or by preventing the synthesis of ergosterol (azoles and allylamines). Their use in individual fungal diseases is considered in Chapter 60.

ANTIVIRAL AGENTS

Compared with the number of agents available for the treatment of bacterial infection, there are relatively few antiviral agents. However, an increasing number are effective in the treatment and prophylaxis of a range of viral diseases. Those antiviral agents in clinical use are presented in Table 5.5 for agents used for diseases other than human immunodeficiency virus (HIV) infection, and Table 5.6 for the equally long list of antiretroviral agents.

About half of all the antiviral agents presently available are nucleoside (or nucleotide) analogues, which are phosphorylated within cells to an active triphosphate and inhibit viral DNA synthesis. Some important antiviral compounds, representing a range of molecular structures, are illustrated in Fig. 5.5.

Nucleoside analogues

Inhibitors of herpesvirus DNA polymerase

The most widely used antiviral agent, aciclovir (and the related penciclovir), is first phosphorylated to the monophosphate by a virus-encoded thymidine kinase produced in cells infected by the herpes simplex virus (HSV) or by varicella-zoster virus (VZV). Subsequent

Table 5.5 Antiviral agents in clinical use for infections other than HIV

Compound	Mode of action	Indication
Aciclovir[a]	Nucleoside analogue	Herpes simplex; varicella-zoster
Amantadine (and rimantadine)	Viral uncoating	Influenza A
Cidofovir	Nucleotide analogue	Cytomegalovirus retinitis
Famciclovir	Pro-drug of penciclovir	Herpes simplex; zoster
Fomivirsen	Antisense oligonucleotide	Cytomegalovirus retinitis
Foscarnet	Inhibition of DNA polymerase	Cytomegalovirus; aciclovir-resistant herpes simplex or varicella-zoster
Ganciclovir	Nucleoside analogue	Cytomegalovirus
Interferon-α	Immunomodulator	Chronic hepatitis B and C
Lamivudine	Nucleoside analogue	Chronic hepatitis B
Oseltamivir	Neuraminidase inhibitor	Influenza A and B
Penciclovir[a]	Nucleoside analogue	Herpes simplex; zoster
Ribavirin[b]	Nucleoside analogue	Respiratory syncytial virus; hepatitis C
Valaciclovir	Pro-drug of aciclovir	Herpes simplex; zoster
Zanamivir	Neuraminidase inhibitor	Influenza A and B

HIV, human immunodeficiency virus.

[a] Available in pro-drug formulations.
[b] Also known as tribavirin.

Table 5.6 Antiretroviral agents in clinical use
Nucleoside analogue reverse transcriptase inhibitors
Abacavir
Didanosine
Lamivudine
Stavudine
Zalcitabine
Zidovudine
Non-nucleoside reverse transcriptase inhibitors[a]
Delavirdine
Efavirenz
Nevirapine
Protease inhibitors
Amprenavir
Indinavir
Nelfinavir
Ritonavir
Saquinavir
[a] Active against HIV-1 only.

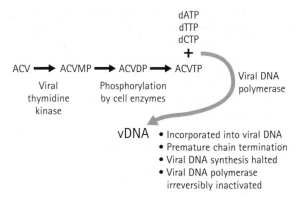

Fig. 5.6 The mode of activation and action of aciclovir (ACV).

growing herpesvirus DNA chain, which is prematurely terminated. The lack of cellular toxicity of aciclovir is caused by two selective features:

- initial phosphorylation takes place only in virus-infected cells
- aciclovir triphosphate inhibits viral (not cellular) DNA polymerase.

Aciclovir has an established record in treatment of HSV and VZV disease, as prophylaxis against HSV reactivation after transplantation, and in the long-term suppression of recurrent genital herpes. Valaciclovir and famciclovir are oral pro-drug formulations of aciclovir and penciclovir, respectively. They provide improved systemic drug levels and require less frequent administration.

phosphorylation steps are completed by cellular kinases to form aciclovir triphosphate. This competes with the natural substrate for the viral DNA polymerase, becomes incorporated into the viral DNA chain and inhibits further DNA polymerase activity (Fig. 5.6). Aciclovir lacks a 3′-hydroxyl group on its acyclic side-chain, and therefore it cannot form a phosphodiester bond with the next nucleotide due to be added to the

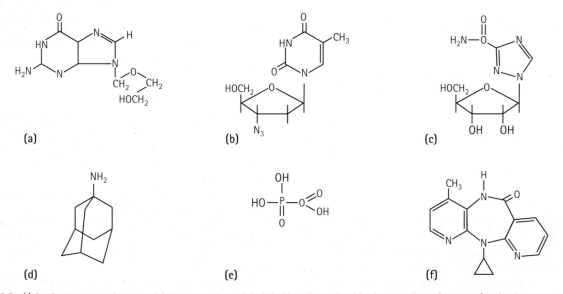

Fig. 5.5 Molecular structures of some antiviral compounds. a aciclovir, b zidovudine, c ribavirin, d amantadine, e foscarnet, f nevirapine.

Ganciclovir, which exhibits preferential activity against another herpesvirus, cytomegalovirus (CMV), is activated by a CMV protein kinase in CMV infected cells, but there is also considerable phosphorylation in uninfected cells, and ganciclovir is much more toxic than aciclovir. Ganciclovir also exhibits antiviral effects against human herpesviruses HHV-6 and HHV-7, which do not respond to aciclovir.

Cidofovir is a nucleoside monophosphate and therefore does not require activation. It is converted in cells into the diphosphate, which inhibits CMV DNA polymerase. It shows activity against a range of DNA viruses, but its main clinical use is for CMV retinitis.

These antiviral agents inhibit only replicating herpesvirus and do not eliminate the latent virus. Reduced susceptibility is occasionally found in isolates of HSV, VZV or CMV from severely immunocompromised hosts.

Other inhibitors of viral RNA or DNA synthesis

Ribavirin (British Approved Name: tribavirin) is a nucleoside analogue that has no useful antiherpes activity, but is used in a nebulized form in the treatment of respiratory syncytial virus infection and intravenously for Lassa fever. It is also used orally in combination with interferon for the treatment of chronic hepatitis C.

Lamivudine, one of the nucleoside analogues active against HIV reverse transcriptase (see below), also inhibits reverse transcriptase activity of hepatitis B virus (HBV), and reduces virus replication. Adefovir, a nucleoside phosphonate presently in development for use in HIV therapy, also exhibits activity against HBV.

Non-nucleoside anti-herpes agents

Foscarnet, a pyrophosphate analogue, inhibits nucleic acid synthesis without requiring any activation, and is an important agent for treatment of those herpesvirus infections that have become resistant to aciclovir or ganciclovir through mutations in the viral thymidine kinase (or protein kinase) gene. Fomivirsen is an antisense oligonucleotide that inhibits translation of messenger RNA into proteins. It has limited use as a local treatment for CMV retinitis.

Agents that block viral uncoating

Amantadine, a symmetrical amine compound, has long been known to inhibit influenza A virus replication, but its mode of action was only discovered much later when resistant mutants could be examined at the molecular level. Amantadine (and rimantadine, a similar drug) blocks an ion channel formed by the integral membrane protein (M2) of influenza A (but not influenza B) virus, preventing uncoating of the virus within cells.

Pleconaril, a capsid-binding agent that inhibits the uncoating of enteroviruses, is under investigation for the treatment of enterovirus meningitis.

Neuraminidase inhibitors

Zanamivir and oseltamivir are agents specifically designed to block the action of the influenza virus enzyme neuraminidase by occupying the catalytic site. They act on influenza A and B viruses. Neuraminidase is found on the surface of influenza virus and these compounds act extracellularly, reducing the spread of influenza viruses locally. Zanamivir is taken by inhalation into the oropharynx; oseltamivir is the oral pro-drug form of a similar agent.

Interferons

Interferons, naturally occurring antiviral compounds produced by mammalian cells in response to viral infection, are now manufactured by genetic recombination. Interferon-α is used to reduce persistent carriage of hepatitis B and C viruses. The mode of action of interferon-α is complex, producing an antiviral state in cells to which it binds, and interfering with the production of virus in those cells. However interferons also act through immune modulation, up-regulating the expression of major histocompatibility complex (MHC) molecules on cell surfaces. This is a significant part of the action in clearing chronic hepatitis B.

Modification by addition of polyethylene glycol to give a compound called *peginterferon* results in sustained effects after just one dose per week. This agent appears to offer an effective treatment for chronic hepatitis C, a common form of chronic hepatitis. New developments in antiviral therapy are expected in this field.

Antiretroviral agents

The human immunodeficiency virus (HIV) pandemic has generated an enormous interest in potential antiviral agents. Three classes of drugs are now generally available (Table 5.6). All inhibit only replicating HIV and do not eliminate the integrated proviral DNA.

When used in the recommended combination regimens (highly active antiretroviral therapy; see Chapter 55), these compounds reduce HIV replication to levels undetectable in the circulation and postpone the appearance of acquired immune deficiency syndrome (AIDS) in infected patients.

Emergence of resistant mutants has been a problem with all classes of anti-HIV agents, and has stimulated developments in the field of antiviral susceptibility testing.

Nucleoside reverse transcriptase inhibitors

The earliest anti-HIV agent, zidovudine (azidothymidine), and several other compounds, including didanosine (dideoxyinosine), zalcitabine (dideoxycytidine), lamivudine and stavudine are nucleoside analogues. They are activated (phosphorylated) by cellular enzymes and inhibit the reverse transcriptase function of the viral polymerase of HIV-1 or HIV-2 by becoming incorporated into the proviral DNA. Phosphorylation rates vary in different cell types, and between resting and replicating cells.

Unlike aciclovir, these nucleoside analogues are associated with some toxicity as there is less selectivity in their activation and action:

- Initial phosphorylation is by cellular kinases.
- Some inhibition of cellular (mitochondrial) DNA polymerase occurs.

Non-nucleoside reverse transcriptase inhibitors

These compounds, which include nevirapine, delavirdine and efavirenz, inhibit HIV-1 only. They bind directly, without activation, away from the catalytic site of reverse transcriptase, but exert a structural change that inhibits its action. They are not incorporated into the DNA chain.

HIV protease inhibitors

Compounds that act at a late stage in the viral cycle by interfering with the cleavage of essential polyprotein precursors have fulfilled their initial promise. Indinavir, saquinavir, ritonavir, nelfinavir and amprenavir are examples of such compounds.

ANTIPARASITIC AGENTS

The choice of agents for the treatment of protozoal and helminthic infections remains extremely limited. Part of the problem is that protozoa and helminths are very varied, reflecting diverse solutions to the problems of their specialized parasitic existence. Consequently, there are few 'broad-spectrum' antiprotozoal or anthelminthic agents, although some compounds exhibit a surprising range of activity. Thus the antiprotozoal nitroimidazoles, such as metronidazole, are active against *Entamoeba histolytica*, *Trichomonas vaginalis* and *Giardia lamblia* (see Chapter 61); benzimidazoles, like mebendazole and albendazole, act against most intestinal nematodes;

Table 5.7 Principal agents used against the major protozoan parasites of man

Species	Agent
Cryptosporidium parvum	(Azithromycin ± paromomycin)
Entamoeba histolytica	Metronidazole Diloxanide furoate (Emetine)
Giardia lamblia	Metronidazole (Mepacrine)
Leishmania spp.	Sodium stibogluconate Amphotericin B
Plasmodium spp.	Chloroquine Quinine Pyrimethamine Proguanil Mefloquine Halofantrine Artemisinin (and derivatives)
Toxoplasma gondii *Trichomonas vaginalis* *Trypanosoma brucei* ssp. *rhodesiense* and *gambiense*	Pyrimethamine + sulphadiazine Metronidazole Melarsoprol (Suramin) (Pentamidine) Eflornithine[a]
Trypanosoma cruzi	(Nifurtimox)

Compounds in brackets are of limited value.
[a] Not active against *T. brucei rhodesiense*.

praziquantel not only exhibits good activity against all human schistosomes but also includes other trematodes and tapeworms in its spectrum (see Chapter 62). Most remarkably of all, ivermectin is active not only against many filarial worms and some intestinal roundworms but also against ectoparasites such as the scabies mite.

Antimicrobial agents commonly used against pathogenic protozoa and helminths are shown in Tables 5.7 and 5.8, respectively.

ANTIMICROBIAL SENSITIVITY TESTS

To establish the activity of an antimicrobial agent, micro-organisms are tested for their ability to grow in the presence of suitable concentrations of the drug. Bacteria are the simplest to test and, in practice, routine sensitivity testing is usually reserved for the common, easily grown bacterial pathogens. Tests of mycobacteria, fungi, viruses and some other organisms are available in certain laboratories and reference centres.

Table 5.8 Spectrum of activity of the principal anthelminthic agents

Agent	Active against
Benzimidazoles[a]	Intestinal nematodes
Diethylcarbamazine	Filariae
Ivermectin	*Onchocerca volvulus*; other filariae
Levamisole	Hookworms; *Ascaris lumbricoides*
Niclosamide	Tapeworms
Metriphonate	*Schistosoma haematobium*
Oxamniquine	*Schistosoma mansoni*
Piperazine	*A. lumbricoides*
	Enterobius vermicularis
Praziquantel	*Schistosoma* spp.; other trematodes; tapeworms
Pyrantel pamoate	*A. lumbricoides*; *E. vermicularis*; hookworms
Trivalent antimonials	*Schistosoma* spp.

[a] Includes mebendazole, thiabendazole and albendazole.

Antibacterial agents

Potency of antibacterial agents is often expressed as the *minimum inhibitory concentration* (MIC): the lowest concentration of the agent that prevents the development of visible growth of the test organism during overnight incubation. Serial dilutions of the agent are prepared in a suitable broth or agar medium and a standard inoculum of the test organism is added. If agar is used, many different isolates can be tested at the same time by spot inoculation of the plate. Broth dilution MIC titrations have the advantage that the *minimum bactericidal concentration* (MBC) can additionally be estimated by subculture of dilutions of the antibiotic above that in which inhibition has occurred overnight. The MBC is usually taken as the lowest concentration able to reduce the original inoculum by a factor of a thousand; e.g. from 10^5 colony-forming units (cfu)/ml to 10^2 cfu/ml or below. To establish the rate of killing, the number of viable organisms in broth cultures is measured at timed intervals after addition of appropriate concentrations of the antibiotic.

Antibiotic titrations are too laborious for the routine assessment of antibiotic activity in clinical practice, although a truncated form of the method, in which isolates are tested at agreed *break points* of sensitivity or resistance, is sometimes used. A common alternative method is the *disc diffusion test*. The culture to be examined is seeded confluently, or semiconfluently, over the surface of an agar plate, and paper discs individually impregnated with different antibiotics are spaced evenly over the inoculated plate. Antibiotic diffuses outwards from each disc into the surrounding agar and produces a diminishing gradient of concentration. On incubation, the bacteria grow on areas of the plate except those around the drugs to which they are sensitive. The width of the *zone of inhibition* is a rough measure of the degree of sensitivity to the drug. A highly standardized version of the disc-diffusion method, the *Bauer–Kirby test*, is favoured in the USA and some other countries.

Characteristics of the growth medium (such as pH or the presence of antagonizing substances), the size of the bacterial inoculum and the conditions of the test may influence the results of sensitivity tests. In disc methods, the size of the inhibition zone is additionally affected by the diffusion characteristics of the antibiotic. It is therefore important that suitable control organisms are tested in parallel in all tests of antibiotic susceptibility. In *Stokes' method*, control is achieved by placing antibiotic discs at the interface between inocula of the test and control bacteria on the same plate. In this way the zone of inhibition obtained with the test organism can be directly compared with that of a known control, and variations in the cultural conditions or in disc content can be avoided.

Antiviral agents

Tests for antiviral susceptibility are still far from routine, being readily available only through reference or specialist laboratories. Experience with these assays is steadily increasing, but the clinical benefits of measuring antiviral susceptibility have still to be established. The detection of resistance may usefully guide therapeutic decisions in the management of HIV infection.

Phenotypic assays

Phenotypic assays measure the inhibitory effect of the antiviral agent on the clinical virus isolate. The plaque reduction assay for inhibition of HSV by aciclovir is one example. An effect is usually considered to be significant when virus replication or product formation is reduced by 50% compared to that found with no drug (50% inhibitory concentration: IC_{50}).

For HIV assays, inhibition of replication in cultures of peripheral blood mononuclear cells is preferred. There are also recombinant virus assays in which HIV genes of interest from the test isolate are put into a laboratory strain to provide a cheaper, faster assay.

Genotypic assays

These tests detect the presence of known resistance-associated mutations in viral genes (e.g. HIV reverse transcriptase or protease), from which reduced susceptibility is predicted. Some of these assays are available in commercial kit format, e.g. a line probe assay using reverse hybridization of amplified viral fragments with a panel of oligonucleotides.

ASSAY OF ANTIMICROBIAL DRUGS

In most clinical circumstances in which antimicrobial agents are used it is not usually necessary to measure the concentrations achieved in blood or other body fluids (see Chapter 65). Such measurements are needed, however, during the development of a new agent to establish the pharmacokinetic behaviour of the drug.

Various techniques are available, including microbiological methods in which the antibiotic-containing material and known dilutions of the drug are titrated in parallel against a susceptible indicator organism. Analytical techniques such as high-pressure liquid chromatography may also be used.

In the few cases in which assays are needed in clinical practice, notably during treatment with aminoglycosides, immunochemical methods are often used with commercially available instrumentation.

RECOMMENDED READING

Finch R G, Greenwood D, Norrby S R, Whitley R J 2002 *Antibiotic and Chemotherapy: Anti-infective Agents and their Use in Therapy*, 8th edn. Churchill Livingstone, Edinburgh

Franklin T J, Snow G A 1998 *Biochemistry and Molecular Biology of Antimicrobial Drug Action*, 5th edn. Kluwer Academic Publishers, Dordrecht

Greenwood D (ed.) 2000 *Antimicrobial Chemotherapy*, 4th edn. Oxford University Press, Oxford

Kucers A, Crowe S M, Grayson M L, Hoy J F 1997 *The Use of Antibiotics: a Clinical Review of Antibacterial, Antifungal and Antiviral Drugs*, 4th edn. Heinemann, London

Lorian V (ed.) 1996 *Antibiotics in Laboratory Medicine*, 4th edn. Lippincott, Williams & Wilkins, Baltimore

Russell A D, Chopra I 1996 *Understanding Antibacterial Action and Resistance*, 2nd edn. Ellis Horwood, Chichester

Internet sites

Encarta: encarta.msn.com (contains a useful entry on antibiotics)

Thomas Jefferson University, Philadelphia, Pennsylvania: jeffline.tju.edu/CWIS/OAC/antibiotics-guide/intro.html

World Health Organization. Essential Drugs and Medicines Policy: www.who.int/medicines/adm-1.htm/

6

Bacterial genetics

K. J. Towner

GENETIC ORGANIZATION AND REGULATION OF THE BACTERIAL CELL

All properties of a bacterial cell, including those of medical importance such as virulence, pathogenicity and antibiotic resistance, are determined ultimately by the genetic information contained within the cell *genome*. This information is normally encoded by the specific sequence of nucleotide bases comprising the deoxyribonucleic acid (DNA) of the cell. There are four common nucleotide bases in DNA: adenine, guanine, cytosine and thymine; it is the linear order in which these bases are arranged that determines the properties of the cell. With only a few exceptions, most of the genetic information required by the bacterial cell is arranged in the form of a single circular double-stranded chromosome. In *Escherichia coli* the chromosome is about 1300 μm long and occurs in an irregular coiled bundle lying free in the cytoplasm. The DNA is not associated with protein or histone molecules as it is in eukaryotic cell chromosomes.

In addition to the single main chromosome, bacterial cells may also carry one or more small circular extra-chromosomal elements. These were originally called episomes, but are now termed *plasmids*. Plasmids replicate independently of the main chromosome in the cell. Although dispensable, they often carry supplementary genetic information coding for beneficial properties (e.g. resistance to antibiotics) that enable the host cell to survive under a particular set of environmental conditions.

A third source of genetic information in a bacterial cell can be provided by the presence of certain types of bacterial viruses, *bacteriophages*. Bacteriophages consist essentially of just a protein coat enclosing the virus genome and, since they are unable to multiply in the absence of their bacterial host, generally they are lethal to their host cell. In some instances, they can enter a potentially long-term state of controlled replication, *lysogeny*, within the bacterial cell without causing lysis. In such a state the bacteriophage genome effectively becomes a temporary part of the total genetic information available to the cell and may consequently bestow additional properties on the cell.

Not all genetic material consists of double-stranded DNA. Some bacteriophages contain single-stranded molecules of either DNA or RNA which can be either circular or linear in configuration. Within the prokaryotic kingdom, and including bacteriophages, genome size varies over more than three orders of magnitude, from about 3 to 5000 kilobases (kb) (Table 6.1).

Processes leading to protein synthesis

The character of a bacterial cell is determined essentially by the specific polypeptides that comprise its enzymes and other proteins. The DNA acts as a template for the *transcription* of RNA by RNA polymerase for subsequent protein production within the cell. In the transcription process the specific sequence of nucleotides in the DNA determines the corresponding sequence of nucleotides in the messenger RNA (mRNA). This, in turn, is then *translated* into the appropriate sequence of amino acids by ribosomes.

Table 6.1 Examples of prokaryotic genetic elements			
Genetic element	Type	Configuration	Size (kb)
Bacterial chromosome			
Escherichia coli	DNA	ds circular	3.8×10^3
Bacillus subtilis	DNA	ds circular	2.0×10^3
Plasmids			
R300B	DNA	ds circular	9.0
RK2	DNA	ds circular	60.0
Bacteriophages			
MS2	RNA	ss linear	3.6
Φ174	DNA	ss circular	5.4
T7	DNA	ds linear	40.4
Abbreviations: ss, single-stranded; ds, double-stranded.			

Finally, the sequence of amino acids in the resulting polypeptide chain determines the configuration into which the polypeptide chain folds itself, which in many cases determines the enzymic properties of the completed protein. A segment of DNA that specifies the production of a particular polypeptide chain is called a *gene*, while the processes of transcription and translation leading to protein synthesis are collectively termed the *central dogma* of molecular biology. These processes are illustrated schematically in Fig. 6.1.

Gene regulation

Most bacteria contain enough DNA to code for the production of between 1000 and 3000 different polypeptide chains, i.e. 1000–3000 different genes. However, during normal bacterial life, some polypeptides will be required only at particular stages, while others will be needed only when the cell is provided with a new or unusual growth substrate, or is confronted with a new challenge

(e.g. an antibiotic). Thus, many antibiotic resistance mechanisms found in bacteria are *inducible* (see below). Protein production is an energy-intensive process, and therefore the expression of many genes is controlled actively within the cell to prevent wasteful energy consumption.

In prokaryotic bacteria the process of gene expression is regulated mainly at the transcriptional level, thereby conserving the energy supply and the transcription–translation apparatus. This is achieved by means of regulatory elements that either inhibit or enhance the rate of RNA chain initiation and termination for a particular gene. Numerous complex regulatory chain mechanisms are involved in co-ordinating the many biochemical reactions that proceed inside a cell, but related genes involved in a common regulatory system are often clustered on the bacterial chromosome. Such functional clusters are known as *operons*, of which the most well known example is the lactose operon of *Esch. coli* (Fig. 6.2).

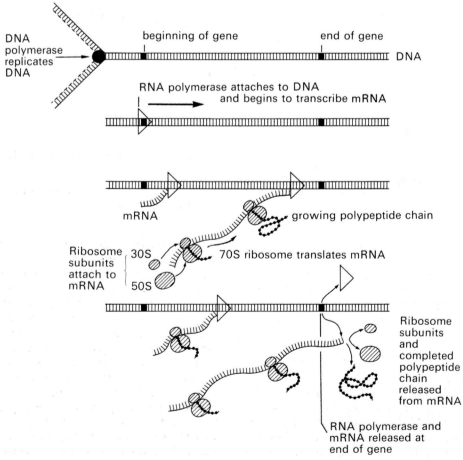

Fig. 6.1 The central dogma of molecular biology.

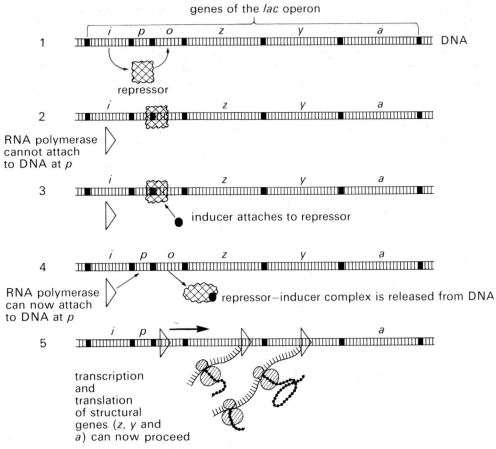

Fig. 6.2 The *lac* operon of *Escherichia coli*.
1 The *lac* repressor is produced from the *i* gene
2 Binding of the repressor to the operator site (*o*) prevents transcription of the genes *z* (β-galactosidase), *y* (galactoside permease) and *a* (transacetylase)
3 The inducer (lactose, or a closely related derivative) can bind specifically to the repressor
4 The repressor molecule is thereby altered at its operator-binding site and the repressor–inducer complex is released from the DNA
5 RNA polymerase can now attach to the promoter site (*p*) and transcribe the structural genes of the *lac* operon.

For transcription to occur as the first stage in protein synthesis, RNA polymerase has to attach to DNA at a specific *promoter* region and transcribe the DNA in a fixed direction. This process can be switched off by the attachment of a *repressor* molecule to a specific region of the DNA, known as the *operator*. This lies between the promoter and the structural gene(s) being transcribed; the repressor then blocks the movement of the RNA polymerase molecule so that the following genes are not transcribed.

The repressor is often an allosteric molecule with two active sites. One recognizes the operator region so that the repressor can bind to it to prevent transcription. The other recognizes an *inducer* molecule. When the inducer is present it binds to the repressor and alters simultaneously the binding specificity at the other site,

so that the repressor no longer binds to the operator and transcription can resume.

There are many different variations on this basic regulatory system. For example, a repressor may be normally inactive, but activated by the end-product of a biosynthetic pathway; thus only when the end-product is present in adequate concentration will the repressor combine with the operator and switch off transcription of the operon. Alternatively, regulation of certain operons involves proteins that bind to the DNA and assist RNA polymerase to initiate transcription. These are just a few examples, and other regulatory systems display both minor and major differences. Finally, it should be stressed that prokaryotic gene regulation frequently involves interwoven regulatory circuits that respond to a variety of different stimuli.

MUTATION

As bacteria reproduce by asexual binary fission, the genome is normally identical in all the progeny. The DNA replication process is therefore very accurate, but occasional rare inaccuracies produce a slightly altered nucleotide sequence in one of the progeny cells. Such a mutation is heritable and will be passed on stably to subsequent generations. One of the fundamental requirements for evolution is that, although gene replication must normally be completely accurate to ensure stability, there must also be occasional variation to produce new or altered characters that could prove to be of selective value to the organism. Mutations may not produce any observable effect on the structure or function of the corresponding protein, but in a small proportion of cases an enzyme with altered specificity for substrates, inhibitors or regulatory molecules may be produced. This is the kind of mutation that is most likely to be of evolutionary value to an organism; indeed, many examples of acquired antibiotic resistance have been shown to be of this type (see Chapter 5). Other mutations may alter a gene so that a non-functional protein is formed; if this protein is essential to the cell then the mutation will be lethal.

Since mutation may occur in any of the several thousand genes of the cell, and different mutations in the same gene may produce different effects in the cell, the number of possible mutations is very large. Particular mutations occur at fairly constant rates, normally between once per 10^4 and once per 10^{10} cell divisions. As a large bacterial colony contains at least 10^9 cells, even a 'pure' bacterial culture will contain many thousands of different mutations affecting many of the genes in the cell. Some of these mutations will be viable and could be selected by particular environmental conditions during subculture. For the same reason, in an infected patient, a variety of mutants will appear spontaneously in the population that grows from the few bacteria originally entering the body. Such mutations may enhance the ability of an organism to grow in the body, e.g. by conferring antibiotic resistance, enhanced virulence, or altered surface antigens. In such a situation, cells with the mutation will rapidly outgrow cells without the mutation, so that selection of the mutant cells occurs and they soon become the predominant type.

Phenotypic variation

The properties of a bacterial cell at a particular time are referred to as the *phenotype* of the cell. These properties are determined not only by its genome (*genotype*), but also by its environment. *Phenotypic variation* occurs when the *expression* of genes is changed in response to the environment, e.g. by the induction or repression of synthesis of particular enzymes. The distinction is important: genotypic mutation is heritable and maintained through changes in environmental conditions, whereas phenotypic variation is reversible, being dependent on environmental conditions and altering when these change. Phenotypic variation is therefore not a form of mutation.

Types of mutation

Mutations can be divided conveniently into *multisite mutations*, involving extensive chromosomal rearrangements such as inversions, duplications and deletions, and *point mutations*, which are defined as only affecting one, or very few, nucleotides. The structure of DNA is such that point mutations can be divided into one of three basic types (Fig. 6.3):

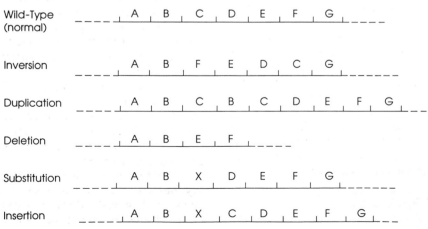

Fig. 6.3 Examples of types of mutations. The top sequence represents a portion of the wild-type chromosome from which the different mutational rearrangements shown below are derived.

- the substitution of one nucleotide for another
- the deletion of one or more nucleotides
- the insertion of one or more nucleotides.

Mutations occur spontaneously during replication of DNA, but most are corrected immediately by the editing apparatus of the cell. Occasional mutations, particularly those conferring a selective advantage to the cell, will be inherited stably by the progeny, but secondary mutations can occasionally restore the original nucleotide sequence. It is important to distinguish this relatively rare event of *back-mutation* from the separate process of *phase variation*, which is readily reversible and occurs with relatively high frequency in either direction, e.g. once per 10^3 cell divisions. The variation of certain Gram-negative bacteria between a fimbriate and a non-fimbriate phase, and the variation of flagellar antigens in *Salmonella enterica* serotypes are examples of phase variation. These seem to involve special genetic regions that are specifically inverted to yield alternative gene products and different phenotypes. In some cases it is known that promoters initiate RNA transcription in different directions to give a flip–flop type of action. The number of such switching systems is probably quite limited, but they have value to the organism in providing a mechanism to switch to a reversible alternative, as opposed to an irreversible change.

Until the invention of the polymerase chain reaction (see below and Chapter 3), the study of bacterial genetics was dependent largely upon the isolation and characterization of mutants in particular genes. Mutations may occur in any gene, but many individual mutations are lethal. Other mutations affect gene products that are essential only under particular cultural conditions. The detailed function and regulation of processes in the bacterial cell can often be analysed only by searching systematically for mutations that affect each separate step in a process. Thus, mutations can be found that produce increased resistance to almost any antimicrobial agent, and the study of such mutants is an essential step in understanding the modes of action of antibiotic agents and mechanisms of resistance to them. Other mutations affect different enzymes in a biosynthetic pathway or enzymes involved in the breakdown of a variety of substances in the bacterial environment, and study of such mutations is vital for the elucidation of these pathways. Similarly, many different types of regulation occur in the co-ordination of all the biochemical reactions that proceed inside a cell, and the isolation of specific mutants is fundamental to their understanding.

GENE TRANSFER

A change in the genome of a bacterial cell may be caused either by a mutation in the DNA of the cell or result from the acquisition of additional DNA from an external source. DNA may be transferred between bacteria by three mechanisms:

- transformation
- conjugation
- transduction.

Each of these mechanisms probably occurs at a low frequency in nature and may therefore have been of value in bacterial evolution. It should, however, be noted that the acquisition by bacteria of new properties following gene transfer is significant, as with mutation, only if the new genetic end-product is subject to favourable selection by the conditions under which the bacteria are growing.

Transformation

Most species of bacteria are unable to take up exogenous DNA from the environment; indeed, most bacteria produce nucleases that recognize and break down foreign DNA. However, bacteria in some genera, notably pneumococci, *Haemophilus influenzae* and certain *Bacillus* species, have been shown to be capable of taking up DNA either extracted artificially or released by lysis from cells of another strain. Cells are *competent* for transformation only under certain conditions of growth, usually in late log phase or, in *Bacillus* species, during sporulation. However, bacterial geneticists have also developed treatments by means of which organisms can be made artificially competent. In the case of *Esch. coli* the treatment involves incubation at a low temperature (4°C) in the presence of calcium ions, followed by a short exposure to a temperature of 42°C. Several other factors, including other metal ions, also stimulate the process. The absolute requirement for calcium ions in producing competent cells of *Esch. coli* indicates that structural alterations in the cell wall, sufficient to allow the passage of DNA molecules, are probably taking place.

Once a piece of DNA has entered the cell by transformation, it has to become incorporated into the existing chromosome of the cell by a process of *recombination* in order to survive. This is a complex molecular process for which the transformed DNA must have been derived from a closely related strain, since pieces of DNA can normally recombine with the chromosome only when there is a high degree of nucleic acid similarity (*homology*).

Any gene may be transferred by transformation, as any fragment of a donor chromosome may be taken up by the recipient cells. However, a piece of DNA introduced into a cell by transformation will normally be relatively short, and will only contain a very small number of genes. For this reason, transformation is of limited use for studying the organization of genes in relation to one another (*genetic mapping*; see later).

Conjugation

Conjugation is a process in which one cell, the *donor* or male cell, makes contact with another, the *recipient* or female cell, and DNA is transferred directly from the donor into the recipient. Certain types of plasmids carry the genetic information necessary for conjugation to occur. Only cells that contain such a plasmid can act as donors; those lacking a corresponding plasmid act as recipients.

Transfer of DNA between cells by conjugation requires direct contact between the donor and recipient cells. Plasmids capable of mediating conjugation carry genes coding for the production of a 1–2 μm-long protein appendage, termed a *pilus*, on the surface of the donor cell. The tip of the pilus attaches to the surface of a recipient cell and holds the two cells together so that DNA can then pass into the recipient cell. It is probable, but not absolutely certain, that transfer actually occurs through the pilus; alternatively, the pilus could act simply as a mechanism by which the donor and female cells are drawn together. Different types of pilus are specified by different types of plasmid and can therefore be used as an aid to plasmid classification.

In the vast majority of cases, the only DNA transferred during the conjugation process is the plasmid that mediates the process. It is thought that one strand of the circular DNA of the plasmid is nicked open at a specific site and the free end is passed into the recipient cell. The DNA is replicated during transfer so that each cell receives a copy. As donor ability is dependent upon having a copy of the plasmid, the recipient strain becomes converted into a donor, able to conjugate with further recipients and convert them in turn. In this way a plasmid may spread rapidly through a whole population of recipient cells; this process is sometimes described as infectious spread of a plasmid.

Mobilization of chromosomal genes by conjugation

Many different types of plasmids have the ability to transfer themselves. Some (but not all) plasmids also have the ability to mobilize the chromosomal genes of bacteria. The prototype plasmid of this type is the 'F factor' (fertility factor) of *Esch. coli*. The F factor is a plasmid that contains the basic genetic information for extrachromosomal existence and for self-transfer. Cells that contain the F plasmid free in the cytoplasm (*F+ cells*) have no unusual characteristics apart from the ability to produce F pili and to transfer the F plasmid to *F− cells* by conjugation. In a very small proportion of F+ cells, the F plasmid becomes inserted into the bacterial chromosome. Once inserted, the entire chromosome behaves like an enormous F plasmid, and hence chromosomal genes can be transferred in the normal manner to a recipient cell at a relatively high frequency. Cultures of cells in which the F plasmid has inserted into the chromosome are consequently termed *high-frequency recombination* (Hfr) strains. One important difference is that the chromosome tends to break randomly during the longer time period required for complete transfer. Only the very rare recipient cell that receives the whole chromosome, complete with the entire integrated F plasmid, will also become F+.

There is an additional mechanism by which chromosomal genes may be mobilized by conjugation to a recipient cell. In any culture of Hfr cells there are a few in which the F plasmid has excised itself from the chromosome and reverted to the free state. The F plasmid is not always excised accurately, and occasionally an F plasmid is excised together with some of the neighbouring chromosomal genes. An F plasmid that has picked up a small portion of the chromosome in this way is known as an *F-prime* (F′). A well known example is the F-*lac* plasmid, which is an F′ carrying the genes of the *Esch. coli* lactose operon. When an F′ transfers itself into a recipient cell, its associated genes function normally on the plasmid in the new host. Thus non-lactose-fermenting organisms become lactose fermenters when they receive F-*lac*. When F-*lac* is transferred into *Esch. coli*, the cells become diploid for the *lac* genes. The particular value of this partial diploidy is that it allows the study of interactions between different *lac* operon mutations within the same cell.

It is important to emphasize that the F plasmid system is confined to *Esch. coli* and other closely related enteric bacteria. Many other plasmids are capable of mediating conjugation, and sometimes chromosome mobilization, not only in *Esch. coli* but also in other bacteria. For example, plasmid RP4 and its relatives have been used to mediate conjugation in a wide range of Gram-negative bacteria, and there have been reports of conjugation systems in Gram-positive bacteria, such as *Enterococcus faecalis*, and several *Streptomyces* species.

Transduction

The third known mechanism of gene transfer in bacteria involves the transfer of DNA between cells by bacteriophages. Most bacteriophages carry their genetic information (the phage genome) as a length of double-stranded DNA coiled up inside a protein coat. Other phages are known in which the phage genome consists of single-stranded DNA or RNA but, as far as is known, transducing phages all contain double-stranded DNA. Two major types of transduction are known to occur in bacteria: *generalized* transduction and *specialized* transduction.

Generalized transduction

When bacteriophages multiply inside an infected bacterial cell, each phage head is normally filled with a copy of the replicated phage genome. However, with certain types of phage a new phage particle is formed, at a frequency of about 1 in 10^6, which accidentally contains a length of bacterial chromosome DNA instead of phage DNA. When such a phage particle subsequently infects a second bacterial cell, the DNA that enters the cell is a short segment of chromosome from the original host. Bacterial genes have been *transduced* by the phage into the second cell. Since phages of this type pick up any portion of the bacterial chromosome at random, they can transduce any chromosomal gene at approximately the same frequency, and are termed *generalized transducing phages*. Genes can be transduced only between fairly closely related strains as particular phages usually attack only a limited range of bacteria. As well as chromosomal genes, generalized transducing bacteriophages may also pick up and transfer plasmid DNA. As an example, the penicillinase gene in staphylococci is usually located on a plasmid, and it may be transferred into other staphylococcal strains by transduction.

Specialized transduction

Bacteriophages that lyse the host cell are known as *virulent* phages, and are said to produce a lytic cycle of infection. In contrast, *temperate* phages are able to infect a cell without necessarily causing immediate cell lysis and death. The surviving bacterial cell (carrying a copy of the bacteriophage genome) is termed a *lysogen*. The cells are said to be *lysogenic*, and the latent phage is called a *prophage*. In such cases the phage DNA is often inserted into the host cell DNA and is replicated stably as part of the host cell chromosome. This is a symbiotic relationship in which the integrated phage DNA imparts *immunity* to the lysogenized cell against superinfection by genetically related phages, as well as certain unrelated phages.

The lysogenic state is stable but not permanent. The prophage may become excised from the chromosome, followed by the replication of phage DNA and lysis of the cell in the normal way. This process of phage induction occurs spontaneously at low frequency (10^{-2}–10^{-5} per cell per generation), but the frequency can be increased artificially, e.g. with ultraviolet light.

Following induction, excision of prophage is usually exact. However, occasionally the prophage picks up DNA adjacent to the phage integration site. Since the phage protein coat can contain only a fixed amount of DNA, a transducing phage that contains a few bacterial genes at one end of its DNA often lacks a few phage genes at the other end. When the defective phage genome is transduced into a second cell, the phage can still integrate into its normal site on the chromosome, but is unable to replicate normally and lyse the cell. The result is that the added piece of bacterial DNA is transduced to the chromosome of the new host cell by the defective phage DNA. Since a temperate phage normally has a specific insertion site on the chromosome, it can pick up and transduce only a short length of DNA containing a few genes on either side of this site. The process is therefore termed *specialized* or *restricted transduction*.

Lysogenic conversion

The presence of prophage DNA constitutes a genetic alteration to the host cell. Usually only the phage repressor gene is expressed, but in certain cases it can be demonstrated that other genes are also expressed by the host cell. For example, *Corynebacterium diphtheriae* only produces diphtheria toxin when it is lysogenized by β phage; the toxin is specified by one of the phage genes. This process is termed *lysogenic conversion*. It is probable that the production of many toxins by staphylococci, streptococci and clostridia is also dependent upon lysogenic conversion by specific bacteriophages. In such cases, lysogenic conversion not only gives the cell superinfection immunity, but also actively influences the virulence of the bacterium for humans.

PLASMIDS

Properties encoded by plasmids

As described earlier, plasmids are circular extrachromosomal genetic elements that may encode a variety of supplementary genetic information, including the information for self-transfer to other cells by conjugation. Not all plasmids can transfer themselves: the *non-conjugative* class of plasmids encodes neither donor pili nor transfer. They can, however, be *mobilized* by other conjugative plasmids present in the same donor cell. Apart from this optional transfer ability, all bacterial plasmids contain the basic genetic information necessary for self-replication and segregation into daughter cells at cell division. Plasmids seem to be ubiquitous in bacteria; many encode genetic information for such properties as resistance to antibiotics, bacteriocin production, resistance to toxic metal ions, enterotoxin production, enhanced pathogenicity, reduced sensitivity to mutagens, or the ability to degrade complex organic molecules.

Plasmid classification

Because of the vast range of plasmids, it is necessary to have a means of classification so that their distribution and epidemiology can be studied.

Plasmids can be grouped initially according to the properties which they encode, but other methods are needed to study their spread and distribution. These methods can be subdivided conveniently into physical and genetic methods.

Physical methods

Since all plasmids are relatively small structures that are normally separate from the bacterial cell chromosome, it is possible to isolate them from the chromosome by physical techniques. Centrifugation and electrophoresis techniques allow the sizes of different plasmids to be compared directly. Plasmids of similar size that confer identical phenotypes on the host cells may, however, be totally unrelated from a molecular viewpoint. Such relationships can be examined by generating *restriction endonuclease fingerprints* from purified plasmid DNA. A restriction endonuclease is an enzyme that cuts the DNA molecule at, or near to, a specific nucleotide sequence to produce discrete DNA fragments which can be separated by gel electrophoresis. The pattern ('fingerprint') of fragments produced is dependent on the distribution of the specific DNA sequences recognized by the enzyme. Closely related plasmids will produce the same, or very similar, fingerprints, while unrelated plasmids will produce different fingerprints (Fig. 6.4). Restriction endonucleases of different specificities may be needed to generate distinctive fingerprints.

Genetic methods

An initial genetic test will distinguish groups of plasmids which are self-transmissible from those that are not. Linked with the question of transferability is the question of host range: for example, some groups can be transferred only between members of the enterobacteria, others can be transferred from the enteric bacteria to the *Pseudomonas* family, while others can be transferred between almost any Gram-negative bacteria. Similar host range relationships exist amongst plasmids of Gram-positive bacteria.

Once the host range of a plasmid has been determined, plasmids may be classified by *incompatibility testing*. This method relies on the fact that closely

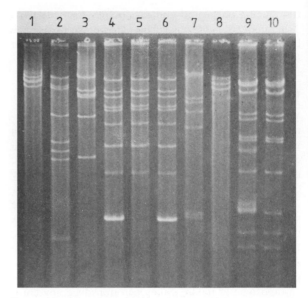

Fig. 6.4 Examples of plasmid fingerprints. Plasmids in tracks 4, 5 and 6 are closely related to each other. Similarly, plasmids in tracks 9 and 10 are closely related. Plasmids in the other tracks appear to be unrelated.

related plasmids are unable to coexist stably in the same bacterial cell. Plasmids which are sufficiently closely related to interfere with each other's replication in this manner are said to be *incompatible* and to belong to the same *incompatibility group*. In contrast, unrelated plasmids can coexist stably and are therefore said to belong to different incompatibility groups.

If the introduction of an unknown plasmid into a host that contains a plasmid of known incompatibility group results in the elimination of the resident plasmid, this is evidence that they are incompatible; the unknown plasmid belongs to the same group as the known plasmid. However, for reproducible results, plasmids must be classified by incompatibility in one chosen host since incompatibility relationships may differ in different hosts.

A final method for plasmid classification involves the use of specific virulent bacteriophages. All members of the same plasmid incompatibility group produce the same type of pilus for conjugation. For some incompatibility groups, specific virulent bacteriophages have been isolated that will adhere only to the type of pilus produced by that particular group of plasmids. Lysis by such a phage shows that a particular type of pilus is being produced, which in turn allows the identification of the group to which the plasmid contained in the cell belongs.

Plasmid epidemiology and distribution

Some plasmid groups have been identified in many different countries of the world, while others have so far been found only in a single bacterial species isolated from a solitary ecological niche. There seem to be two major ways in which plasmids spread:

- by direct transfer from one bacterium to another in a particular micro-environment
- by being carried in a particular host from one environment, e.g. a hospital, to another.

The epidemiological tracing of these pathways requires identification not just of the plasmids involved but also of their host bacterial strains.

GENETIC MAPPING

The location of genes with reference to each other and to their respective control regions by mapping techniques is an essential part of genetic analysis. Historically, this required the transfer of genetic material between different mutants, initially by conjugation to locate the approximate position of an unknown gene on the chromosome or a plasmid, followed by fine structure mapping with generalized transduction. By far the most extensive genetic map available is that of the *Esch. coli* strain K12 chromosome. It is now a relatively simple matter to map an 'unknown' gene on the chromosome of *Esch. coli* K12, but is much more difficult for less intensively studied genera.

A more modern approach that can be used for all bacterial genera makes use of molecular techniques allowing the isolation, cloning and nucleotide sequencing of individual genes (see Chapter 3). Once a particular gene or sequence of DNA has been selected and analysed, it is then possible to label it and use the gene as a *probe* in hybridization experiments. Alternatively, it is possible to synthesize a small stretch of nucleotides, termed an *oligonucleotide*, from within the overall gene sequence for use as a probe. *Hybridization* is a process in which two single strands of nucleic acid come together to form a stable double-stranded molecule. As long as the sequence of bases is complementary on each strand, the two strands will bind together by the formation of hydrogen bonds. Oligonucleotide probes are normally only 10–40 bases in length, and can be synthesized and chemically labelled by automated instruments designed specifically for this purpose. The labelled probe can then be used in hybridization experiments with relatively large fragments ('fingerprints') generated from the entire bacterial chromosome with rare-cutting restriction endonucleases. The probe will hybridize only to the chromosomal DNA fragment containing the original gene from which the probe was derived, and will therefore indicate the precise physical location of the original gene in relation to other known genes and control regions. It is therefore now possible to elucidate the relationship between gene structure and function in the cell at the most fundamental molecular level.

THE GENETIC BASIS OF ANTIBIOTIC RESISTANCE

All of the properties of a micro-organism are determined ultimately by genes located either on the chromosome or on plasmids or on lysogenic bacteriophages. With regard to antibiotic resistance it is important to distinguish between *intrinsic* and *acquired* resistance. Intrinsic resistance is dependent upon the natural insusceptibility of an organism. In contrast, acquired resistance involves changes in the DNA content of a cell, such that the cell acquires a phenotype (i.e. antibiotic resistance) which is not inherent in that particular species.

Intrinsic resistance

Organisms that are naturally insensitive to a particular drug will always exist. The most obvious determinant of bacterial response to an antibiotic is the presence or absence of the target for the action of the drug. Thus, polyene antibiotics such as amphotericin B kill fungi by binding tightly to the sterols in the fungal cell membrane and altering the permeability of the fungal cell. Since bacterial membranes do not contain sterols they are intrinsically resistant to this class of antibiotics. Similarly, the presence of a permeability barrier provided by the cell envelopes of Gram-negative bacteria is important in determining sensitivity patterns to many antibiotics. Intrinsic resistance is usually predictable in a clinical situation and should not pose problems provided that an informed and judicious choice is made of appropriate antimicrobial therapy.

Acquired resistance

A problem of chemotherapy has been the appearance of resistance to particular drugs in a normally sensitive microbial population. An organism may lose its sensitivity to an antibiotic during a course of treatment. In some cases the loss of sensitivity may be slight, but often organisms become resistant to clinically achievable concentrations of a drug. Once resistance has appeared, the continuing presence of an antibiotic exerts a *selective pressure* in favour of the resistant organisms. Three main factors affect the frequency of acquired resistance:

- the amount of antibiotic which is being used
- the frequency with which bacteria can undergo spontaneous mutations to resistance
- the prevalence of plasmids able to transfer resistance from one bacterium to another.

Chromosomal mutations

Random spontaneous mutations occur continuously at a low frequency in all bacterial populations, and some mutations may confer resistance to a particular antibiotic. The rate at which these mutations occur is not influenced by the antibiotic, but in the presence of the drug the resistant mutant can survive, grow and eventually become the predominant, or only, member of the population. The degree of resistance conferred by chromosomal mutation depends upon the biological consequences of the mutation. With *single large-step mutations* the drug target is altered by mutation so that it is totally unable to bind a drug, although it can still carry out its normal biological functions sufficiently well to permit the continued survival of the cell. This type of mutation occurs with streptomycin, but is otherwise not very common clinically. More commonly, the target is altered so that it can no longer bind a drug as efficiently, although it still has some residual affinity. In such a case a higher concentration of antibiotic would be required to produce the same antimicrobial effect: the *minimum inhibitory concentration* (MIC) of the antibiotic for the organism would be increased. Once a slightly resistant organism has been produced, additional mutational events – each conferring an additional small degree of resistance – can eventually lead to the production of organisms that are highly resistant. This is called the *multistep pattern of resistance*. Spontaneous chromosomal mutation is of clinical importance in tuberculosis in which mutants resistant to any single drug, e.g. streptomycin, rifampicin or isoniazid, are likely to be present in the patient before the start of treatment. If only one drug is given to the patient, the few resistant mutant bacteria will multiply and eventually cause a relapse of the disease. Combined therapy with several drugs to which the organism is sensitive is used in the treatment of tuberculosis, so that each drug kills the few mutants that are resistant to the other. The frequency with which double or triple mutations occur spontaneously in the same cell is so low as to be clinically insignificant.

There are many other examples of chromosomal mutations to antibiotic resistance which have assumed clinical importance. Bacterial enzymes called β-lactamases are commonly responsible for resistance to penicillins, cephalosporins and related antibiotics that contain a β-lactam ring (see Chapter 5). Mutations in the genes controlling the production of chromosomally encoded β-lactamases in Gram-negative bacteria can result in overproduction of these enzymes and consequent resistance to the cephalosporin antibiotics normally regarded as stable to β-lactamase.

Chromosomal mutations leading to antibiotic resistance are in many cases just as important clinically as the types of transferable resistance described in the next section.

Transferable antibiotic resistance

Of the three modes of gene transfer in bacteria, it is plasmid-mediated conjugation that is of greatest significance in terms of drug resistance. Plasmids conferring resistance to one or more unrelated groups of antibiotics (*R plasmids*) can be transferred rapidly by conjugation throughout the population.

R plasmids were first demonstrated in Japan in 1959, when it was shown that resistance to several antibiotics could be transferred by conjugation between strains of *Shigella* and *Esch. coli*. Many surveys since then in all parts of the world have shown that R plasmids are common and widespread.

The way in which R plasmids are built up in vivo probably varies from case to case, but it is clear that simple transfer factors can pick up resistance genes and combine them with non-transmissible resistance plasmids to produce complex transmissible R plasmids that encode resistance to as many as eight or more different antimicrobial drugs. This process of plasmid evolution is accelerated considerably by genetic elements termed *transposons*. These are linear pieces of DNA, often including genes for antibiotic resistance, that can migrate between unrelated plasmids and/or the bacterial chromosome independently of the normal bacterial recombination processes. R plasmids can transfer themselves into a wide range of commensal and pathogenic bacteria. Once resistance to an antibiotic appears in any one of these species, the process of *transposition* assists the dissemination of the responsible gene between different R plasmids and subsequent distribution to other bacterial species.

A crucial question remains regarding the mechanism by which transposons acquire the resistance genes in the first place. The answer lies in the existence of a further class of genetic element, termed an *integron*. These elements form an essential 'building block' of many transposons and allow the rapid formation and expression of new combinations of antibiotic resistance genes in response to selection pressures. A detailed description of the properties of integrons lies outside the scope of this text (see Recommended Reading), but suffice it to say that these elements seem to provide the primary mechanism for initial antibiotic resistance gene capture and dissemination, certainly amongst Gram-negative bacteria.

As the prevalence of multiple-resistance R plasmids carrying transposons and integrons continues to increase, infections caused by a wide range of pathogens become more difficult to treat. In addition, R plasmids can also carry genes, e.g. for toxin production, that confer increased virulence on a bacterial cell. Thus, use of antibiotics may select for bacteria carrying plasmids that confer not only multiple drug resistance but also increased pathogenicity.

Control of antibiotic resistance

The major cause of the spread of genes conferring antibiotic resistance is the selection pressure brought about by the increased, and often indiscriminate, use of antibiotics in humans and animals. Plasmid-encoded drug resistance is increased by the widespread use of antibiotics in animal husbandry, where antibiotics are used as animal feed supplements and whole animal populations may be treated, rather than an individual patient as occurs in medical practice. When R plasmids are present, the mass use of antibiotics fails to prevent the spread of resistance and selects R plasmids in the gut flora of the whole population of animals. Such R plasmids, evolved in farm animals, can spread to human commensal *Esch. coli*, followed by transfer to more important human pathogens.

It is important to minimize the use of antibiotics as much as possible and to reduce the chance of cross-infection. Rational use of antibiotics and sensible restriction of their availability in humans and animals could prevent further spread of R plasmids and perhaps reduce their incidence. Some R plasmids are unstable and tend to lose resistance genes when the selection pressure is removed. R plasmids are also lost spontaneously from a small proportion of cells in a culture since plasmid replication and segregation are not always precisely synchronous with chromosome replication and segregation. Cells that lose an R plasmid may have a slight metabolic advantage and may slowly outgrow drug-resistant organisms. Moreover, R plasmids that evolve in one species may be unstable in another or may transfer themselves to other organisms much less efficiently. Similarly, organisms that are adapted to the gut of a calf, pig or chicken may not establish readily in humans. Such factors may help to contain the spread of R plasmids.

APPLICATIONS OF MOLECULAR GENETICS

Specific gene probes

Every properly classified species must, by definition, have somewhere on its chromosome a unique DNA sequence that distinguishes it from every other species. If this sequence can be identified, a specific labelled DNA probe (see earlier) can be used in a hybridization reaction to recognize pathogen-specific DNA released from clinical samples. Initial isolation of the infecting pathogen is not necessary and, consequently, DNA probes can be used to detect pathogens that cannot be cultured easily in vitro.

DNA probes have already been used successfully to identify a wide variety of pathogens, from simple viruses to pathogenic bacteria and parasites. Probes have also been developed which can recognize specific antibiotic resistance genes, so that antimicrobial susceptibility of an infecting organism can be determined directly without primary isolation and growth. Commercial kits incorporating DNA probes are now available to detect a range of bacteria and viruses.

Nucleic acid amplification technology

In the *polymerase chain reaction* (PCR) a thermostable DNA polymerase and two specific oligonucleotide primers are used to produce multiple copies of specific nucleic acid regions quickly and exponentially (Fig. 6.5). The specificity of the reaction is controlled by the oligonucleotide primers that direct replication of the intervening 'target' region. In an exponential reaction, the target sequence is amplified a million-fold or more within a few hours. Although PCR is the most widely used method, other amplification techniques for DNA and RNA molecules are available. Once an amplification reaction has occurred, a variety of methods are available to detect the amplified product, of which the simplest is to identify the product by size after electrophoresis and migration on an agarose gel. For many diagnostic applications, the simple visualization of an amplification product of characteristic size is a significant result since it indicates the presence of the target DNA sequence in the original sample, but confirmation of sequence identity by specific hybridization tests is often required.

Amplification offers an exquisitely sensitive approach to the detection and identification of specific microorganisms in a variety of sample types. Potentially, a characteristic DNA or RNA sequence from a single virus

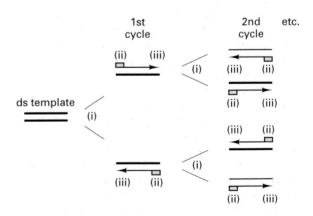

Fig. 6.5 Schematic outline of PCR. Each cycle in the exponential reaction consists of three steps: (i) heat denaturation, typically at 94°C, to dissociate double-stranded (ds) DNA; (ii) annealing of primers (▭) at a temperature determined empirically for each individual PCR; (iii) elongation at an optimal temperature for thermostable polymerase activity, typically 72°C for *Taq* polymerase.

particle or bacterial cell can be amplified to detectable levels within a very short period of time. The method has received particular attention for detecting the presence of low numbers of bacteria or virus particles in clinical and environmental specimens. For example, while a diagnostic antibody response may take up to 8 weeks to develop in an individual infected with human immunodeficiency virus (HIV), specific HIV sequences can be detected in a few hours by PCR, even if present at only 1 part per 100 000 human genome equivalents.

Molecular typing of micro-organisms

Typing of micro-organisms is increasingly important for studying cross-infection and epidemiological relationships, particularly during outbreaks of nosocomial infection (see Chapter 68). Molecular fingerprinting methods are now the most commonly used techniques for assessing the relatedness of individual bacterial isolates in epidemiological studies. These techniques can be used to study any organism from which DNA can be prepared and offer the possibility of a unified approach to microbial typing that can be applied immediately to a new epidemiological problem with no prior knowledge of the organisms being investigated.

DNA sequencing

A complete DNA sequence forms the ultimate reference standard for identifying micro-organisms and their subtypes. Increasing numbers of micro-organisms are now being sequenced and the knowledge gained is of immense value for research purposes. However, even with rapid automated sequencing techniques, it is highly unlikely that routine diagnostic laboratories will ever have the facilities or resources to sequence all their isolates of clinical or epidemiological interest routinely. One possibility might involve the sequencing of small relatively conserved regions of the genome that can provide diagnostic information, and such techniques for sequencing genes encoding 16S ribosomal RNA are sometimes used presumptively to identify 'unknown' or unculturable isolates derived from clinical specimens.

An alternative approach that may become available in the near future involves the use of *DNA microarrays* (sometimes called '*DNA chips*'). These consist of a very large number of evenly spaced spots of DNA fixed to a microscope slide. Each spot is a unique DNA fragment transferred by a gridding robot from 96-well plates on to the slide. Such DNA chips may become commercially available and could then be hybridized in diagnostic laboratories with DNA extracts from 'unknown' isolates to yield distinctive patterns of hybridization on the slide. Such patterns would be readily amenable to computerized analysis and comparison with electronic databases. At the time of writing, this technology remains in the future, but may ultimately revolutionize diagnostic microbiology in the 21st century.

RECOMMENDED READING

Bryan L E (ed.) 1984 *Antimicrobial Drug Resistance*. Academic Press, New York

Erlich H A 1989 *PCR Technology – Principles and Applications of DNA Amplification*. Stockton Press, New York

Goering RV 2000 The molecular epidemiology of nosocomial infection: past, present and future. *Reviews in Medical Microbiology* 11: 145–152

Hall RM, Collis CM 1998 Antibiotic resistance in Gram-negative bacteria: the role of gene cassettes and integrons. *Drug Resistance Updates* 1: 109–119

Innis MA, Gelfand DH, Sninsky JJ, White T 1990 *PCR Protocols – A Guide to Methods and Applications*. Academic Press, San Diego

Mazel D, Davies J 1999 Antibiotic resistance in microbes. *Cellular and Molecular Life Sciences* 56: 742–754

Rowe-Magnus DA, Mazel D 1999 Resistance gene capture. *Current Opinion in Microbiology* 2: 483–488

Schleif R 1986 *Genetics and Molecular Biology*. Addison Wesley, Reading, MA

Tenover F C 1988 Diagnostic deoxyribonucleic acid probes for infectious diseases. *Clinical Microbiology Reviews* 1: 82–101

Towner K J, Cockayne A 1993 *Molecular Methods for Microbial Identification and Typing*. Chapman and Hall, London

7

Sterilization and disinfection

R. A. Simpson and R. C. B. Slack

Procedures that kill micro-organisms have important applications in practical microbiology and in the practice of medicine and surgery. Laboratory work with pure cultures requires the use of apparatus and culture media that have been rendered sterile, while the need to avoid infecting the patient requires the use of equipment, instruments, dressings and parenteral drugs that are free from all living micro-organisms, or at least from those which may give rise to infection.

General definitions

Several terms are used to describe processes for the killing or removal of micro-organisms, and it is important to recognize the difference in meaning.

Sterilization is a process used to achieve sterility, an absolute term meaning the absence of all viable micro-organisms.

Disinfection is a process which reduces the number of contaminating micro-organisms, particularly those liable to cause infection, to a level which is deemed no longer harmful to health. The term *sanitization* is also used, particularly in the USA, to describe disinfection, generally in conjunction with catering and food equipment.

Antisepsis is used to describe disinfection applied to living tissue such as a wound.

Cleaning is a soil-removing process which removes many micro-organisms. The reduction in contamination by cleaning processes is difficult to quantify other than visually. However, it has wide application in the hospital environment and is the necessary prerequisite to sterilization and disinfection.

Decontamination is a general term for the treatment used to make equipment safe to handle, and includes microbiological, chemical, radioactive and other contamination.

STERILIZATION

Sterilization means the freeing of an article from all living organisms, including viruses, bacteria and their spores, and fungi and their spores. In practice, all processes of sterilization have a finite probability of failure. An article may be regarded as sterile if it can be demonstrated that there is a probability of less than 1 in a million of there being viable micro-organisms on it.

Uses

Sterilization is required for instruments and materials used in procedures that involve penetration into normally sterile parts of the body, e.g. in surgical operations, intravenous infusions, hypodermic injections and diagnostic aspirations. It is also required for media, reagents and equipment used in laboratory practice.

Methods

Five main methods are used for sterilization.

Heat. The only method of sterilization that is both reliable and widely applicable is by heating under carefully controlled conditions at temperatures above 100°C to ensure that bacterial spores are killed. There is some concern that even this temperature is insufficient to destroy prions.

Ionizing irradiation. Both β (electrons) irradiation and γ (photons) irradiation are employed industrially for the sterilization of single-use disposable items such as needles and syringes, latex catheters and surgical gloves, and in the food industry to reduce spoilage and remove pathogens.

Filtration. Filters are used to remove bacteria and all larger micro-organisms from liquids that are liable to be spoiled by heating, e.g. blood serum and antibiotic solutions in which contamination with filter-passing viruses is improbable or unimportant. Industrial scale filtration is widely used to reduce bacterial load and remove cysts of protozoa which are not killed by chlorination in the production of drinking water.

Sterilant gases. Ethylene oxide is used mainly by industry for the sterilization of plastics and other thermolabile materials that cannot withstand heating. Formaldehyde in combination with subatmospheric steam is more commonly used in hospitals for reprocessing thermolabile equipment. Both processes carry toxic and other hazards for the user and the patient.

Sterilant liquids. Use of liquids such as glutaraldehyde is generally the least effective and the most unreliable method. Such methods should be regarded as 'high-grade disinfection' only, to be applied when no other sterilization method is available, e.g. for heat-labile fibreoptic instruments such as flexible endoscopes.

DISINFECTION

Disinfection, the freeing of an article from some or all of its burden of contaminating micro-organisms, is a relative term embracing a wide range of efficacy against particular viruses, vegetative bacteria and fungi, but not usually including bacterial spores.

Uses

Disinfection is applied in circumstances in which sterility is unnecessary or sterilizing procedures are impracticable. Thus, in the absence of demonstrable clinical need, it is uneconomic to sterilize bed-pans, eating utensils, bed linen and other items of everyday living which may spread infection within hospitals. Moreover, the pathogens likely to be present on these articles rarely include those that form spores.

Similarly, it is a valuable precaution to treat the skin around the site of an invasive procedure, such as an injection or surgical operation, with an antiseptic that will kill many of the vegetative micro-organisms and reduce the chance of some of them being carried into the wound.

Methods

Disinfection is achieved by means of processes similar to, although less severe than, those used for sterilization.

Heat. Various methods are available using steam or water; some incorporate a cleaning stage within an automatic controlled process.

Ultraviolet radiation. This has limited application for the disinfection of surfaces and some piped-water supplies, but lacks penetrative power for more widespread application.

Gases. Formaldehyde is used as a fumigant in laboratory environments, e.g. before changing a filter in a safety cabinet or in the event of a gross spillage.

Filtration. Air supplied to operating theatres and other critical environments is filtered to remove potentially hazardous micro-organisms.

Chemical. Various chemicals with antimicrobial properties are used as disinfectants. They are all liable to be inactivated by excessive dilution and contact with organic materials such as dirt or blood, or a variety of other materials. Nevertheless, they may provide a convenient method for environmental disinfection and other specific applications.

CHOICE OF METHOD

The choice of method of sterilization or disinfection depends on:

- the nature of the item to be treated
- the likely microbial contamination
- the risk of transmitting infection to patients or staff in contact with the item.

Choice is based on an assessment of risk according to different categories of patient (e.g. immunocompromised), the equipment involved and its application (Table 7.1). The selection of sterilization, disinfection or simple cleaning processes for individual items of equipment and the environment should be agreed as part of the infection control policy of a hospital (see Chapter 68). The preferred option wherever possible, for both sterilization and disinfection, is heat rather than chemicals. This relates not only to the antimicrobial efficacy but to safety considerations, which are more difficult to control in some chemical processes. Wherever chemicals are to be used for disinfection and sterilization, the safety of persons involved directly or indirectly in the procedure must be considered. It should be remembered that all sterilizing and disinfecting agents have some action on human cells. No method should be assumed to be safe unless appropriate precautions are taken.

MEASUREMENT OF MICROBIAL DEATH

Every method used must be validated to demonstrate the required degree of microbial kill. With heat sterilization and irradiation, a biological test may not be required if the physical conditions are sufficiently well defined and controlled. For practical purposes a micro-organism may be regarded as 'dead' when it has lost the ability to reproduce.

Table 7.1 Risks to patients from equipment and the environment

Risk group	Examples	Choice of process
1. High risk (critical) Direct contact with a break in skin or mucous membrane or entering a sterile body area	Surgical instruments; needles, syringes; parenteral fluids; arthroscopes	Must be sterile: heat sterilization, irradiation
2. Intermediate risk (semi–critical) Direct contact with mucous membrane but tissue is intact	Endotracheal tubes; aspirators; gastroscopes	Need not be sterile: disinfection acceptable; thorough cleaning with liquid chemicals
3. Low risk (non–critical) No direct contact with the patient other than via unbroken skin	Bed-pans; urinals; furniture; sinks, drains; walls, floors	Thorough cleaning (with disinfection as necessary) by washer or disinfector with detergents

When micro-organisms are subjected to a lethal process, the number of viable cells decreases exponentially in relationship to the extent of exposure. If the logarithm of the number of survivors is plotted against the lethal dose received (e.g. time of heating at a particular temperature) the resulting curve is described as the *survivor curve*. This is independent of the size of the original population and is approximately linear. The linear survivor curve is an idealized concept and, in practice, minor variations, such as an initial shoulder or final tail, occur (Fig. 7.1).

D value. The *D value* or *decimal reduction value* is the dose required to inactivate 90% of the initial population. From Figure 7.1, it can be seen that the time (dose) required to reduce the population from 10^6 to 10^5 is the same as the time (dose) required to reduce the population from 10^5 to 10^4, i.e. the D value remains constant over the full range of the survivor curve. Extending the treatment beyond the point at which there is one surviving cell does not give rise to fractions of a surviving cell but rather to a statement of the probability of finding one survivor. Thus by extrapolation from the experimental data it is possible to determine the lethal dose required to give a probability of less than 10^{-6} which is required to meet the pharmacopoeial definition of 'sterile'.

FACTORS INFLUENCING RESISTANCE

Many common factors affect the ability of micro-organisms to withstand the lethal effects of sterilization or disinfection processes. Factors specific to individual processes are considered in the description of those processes.

Species or strain of micro-organism

In general, vegetative bacteria and viruses are more susceptible, and bacterial spores the most resistant, to sterilizing and disinfecting agents. However, within different species and strains of species there may be wide variation in intrinsic resistance. For example, within the Enterobacteriaceae, D values at 60°C range from a few minutes (*Escherichia coli*) to 1 h (*Salmonella enterica* serotype Senftenberg). The typical D value for *Staphylococcus aureus* at 70°C is less than 1 min compared with 3 min for *Staph. epidermidis*. However, an unusual strain of *Staph. aureus* has been isolated with a D value of 14 min at 70°C. Such variations may be attributed to morphological or physiological changes such as alterations in cell proteins or specific targets in the cell envelope affecting permeability.

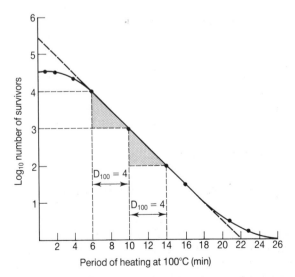

Fig. 7.1 The rate of inactivation of an inoculum of bacterial spores showing the decimal reduction time (*D* value) at 100°C and the non-linear 'shoulder and tail' effects.

Inactivation data obtained for one micro-organism should not be extrapolated to another; thus it should not be assumed that bactericidal disinfectants are also potent against viruses. The inactivation data for scrapie, bovine spongiform encephalopathy and Creutzfeldt–Jakob disease (CJD) suggest that prions are highly resistant agents, requiring six times the normal heat sterilization cycle (134°C for 18 min). This has led to requirements for the mandatory use of disposable instruments which are in direct contact with brain or other nervous tissue (including the retina) or tonsils where the risk of exposure to the prion causing CJD is high.

Physiological state

The conditions under which the micro-organisms were grown before exposure to the lethal process have a marked effect on their resistance. Organisms grown under nutrient-limiting conditions are typically more resistant than those grown under nutrient-rich conditions. Resistance usually increases through the late logarithmic phase of growth of vegetative cells and declines erratically during the stationary phase.

Ability to form spores

Bacterial endospores, formed principally by *Bacillus* and *Clostridium* species, are relatively resistant to most processes. Similarly, fungal spores are more resistant than the vegetative mycelium, although they are not usually as resistant as bacterial spores. Bacterial spores were used to define the sterilization processes in current use, and preparations of bacterial spores (biological indicators) are used to monitor the efficacy of ethylene oxide sterilization, in which physical monitoring is inadequate (see p. 230). In general, disinfection processes have little or no activity against bacterial spores.

Suspending menstruum

The micro-environment of the organism during exposure to the lethal process has a profound effect on its resistance. Thus, micro-organisms occluded in salt have greatly enhanced resistance to ethylene oxide; the presence of blood or other organic material will reduce the effectiveness of hypochlorite solution.

Number of micro-organisms

The higher the initial 'bioburden', the more extensive must be the process to achieve the same assurance of sterility. Stringent washing and cleaning before the process is an essential part of the success of decontamination of instruments.

STERILIZATION BY HEAT

Moist heat is much more effective than dry heat because it kills micro-organisms by coagulating and denaturing their enzymes and structural proteins, a process in which water participates. It is therefore necessary for all parts of the load to be sterilized to be in direct contact with water molecules or steam. Sterilization requires exposure to moist heat at 121°C for 15 min.

Dry heat is believed to kill micro-organisms by causing a destructive oxidation of essential cell constituents. Killing of the most resistant spores by dry heat requires a temperature of 160°C for 2 h. This high temperature causes slight charring of paper, cotton and other organic materials.

Factors influencing sterilization by heat

The factors to be considered include:

1. The temperature
2. The time of exposure
3. The number of vegetative micro-organisms and spores present
4. The species
5. The strain and spore-forming ability of the micro-organisms
6. The nature of the contaminated material.

Temperature and time. These are inversely related, with shorter times sufficing at higher temperatures. The recommended combinations of temperature and holding time are listed in Table 7.2. These do not include time for heating up or cooling the load for safe handling. Thus the total cycle time for processing a sterilized article will be much longer.

Microbial load. The number of micro-organisms and spores affects the rapidity of sterilization. The number of survivors falls exponentially with the duration of heating (see Fig. 7.1) and the time of complete

Table 7.2 Minimum recommended hold times for heat sterilization

Process	Temperature (°C)	Hold time (min)
Dry heat	160	120
	170	60
	180	30
Moist heat	121	15
	126	10
	134	3

sterilization increases in relation to the numbers initially present. In practice it is usual to minimize the number of contaminating bacteria by prior cleaning. If this is not possible, e.g. contaminated laboratory cultures, an extended period of heating to achieve the required temperature will be needed.

Sterilization by moist heat

Moist heat sterilization requires temperatures above that of boiling water. Such conditions are attained under controlled conditions by raising the pressure of steam in a pressure vessel (*autoclave*). At sea level, boiling water at atmospheric pressure (1 bar) will produce steam at 98–100°C, whereas raising the pressure to 2.4 bar increases the temperature to 125°C, and at 3.0 bar to 134°C. Conversely, at subatmospheric pressures, including those at higher altitude, water will boil at lower temperatures.

The quality of steam for sterilization

Steam is non-toxic and non-corrosive, but for effective sterilization it must be *saturated*, which means that it holds all the water it can in the form of a transparent vapour. It must also be *dry*, which means that it does not contain water droplets.

Saturated steam is more efficient than dry heat, partly because of the greater lethal action of moist heat but also because it is quicker in heating up the article to be sterilized. When dry saturated steam meets a cooler surface it condenses into a small volume of water and liberates the latent heat of vaporization. The energy available from this latent heat is considerable, e.g. 6 litres of steam at a temperature of 134°C (and a corresponding pressure of 3 bar absolute) will condense into 10 ml of water and liberate 2162 J of heat energy. By comparison, less than 100 J of heat energy is released to an article by the sensible heat from air at 134°C.

Steam at a higher temperature than the corresponding pressure would allow is referred to as *super-heated steam*, and behaves in a similar manner to hot air. Conversely, steam which contains suspended droplets of water at the same temperature is referred to as *wet steam* and is less efficient. The presence of air in steam affects the sterilizing efficiency by changing the pressure–temperature relationship.

Types of steam sterilizer

Sterilizers for porous loads. These are intended to deal with dressings, textiles, wrapped instruments and wrapped utensils. Such loads are liable to trap air within the fabric, packaging or within narrow lumen instruments. This type of sterilizer must have a vacuum-assisted air removal stage to ensure that adequate air is removed from the load before admission of steam. The vacuum pulsing of air also ensures that the load is dry on completion of the cycle.

Sterilizers for fluids in sealed containers. Sterilizers for pharmaceutical fluids and laboratory media in sealed containers and ampoules must have a safety feature to ensure that the door cannot be opened until the contents of the glass containers have fallen below 80°C. This is because the thermal stress of cold air on opening the door may cause the bottles to explode under pressure, causing serious injury.

Sterilizers for unwrapped instruments and utensils. These simple machines should not be used for wrapped articles. They are recommended for use in dental clinics and in general practice.

Laboratory sterilizers. These are needed for several different types of load, such as culture media in containers, laboratory glassware and equipment.

Monitoring of steam sterilizers

Physical measurements of temperature, pressure and time with thermometers and pressure gauges are recorded for every load, and periodic detailed tests are undertaken with temperature-sensitive probes (thermocouples) inserted into standard test packs. Biological indicators comprising dried spore suspensions of a reference heat-resistant bacterium, *Bacillus stearothermophilus*, are no longer considered appropriate for routine testing, although spore indicators are essential for low-temperature gaseous processes in which the physical measurements are not reliable.

Sterilizers incorporating a vacuum-assisted air removal cycle are fitted with an air detector. In addition, the *Bowie–Dick test* monitors penetration of steam into a wrapped pack and will detect uneven steam penetration by a 'bubble' of residual air in the pack. In the original test, an adhesive indicator tape, in the shape of a cross, was stuck onto a sheet of paper which was placed at the centre of a stack of towels (the test pack). The indicator shows a colour change from colourless to black, which should be even along the entire cross of the tape.

Sterilization by dry heat

Incineration

This is an efficient method for the sterilization and disposal of contaminated materials at a high temperature. It has a particular application for pathological waste materials, surgical dressings, sharp needles and other clinical waste.

Red heat

Inoculating wires, loops and points of forceps are sterilized by holding them in the flame of a Bunsen burner until they are red hot. Disposable loops are sometimes used when highly pathogenic organisms may be encountered because 'splattering' of unburnt material may occur from the burner.

Flaming

Exposure of scalpels and the necks of flasks to a flame for a few seconds is of uncertain efficacy. Inoculating loops and needles are sometimes treated by immersing them in methylated spirit and burning off the alcohol, but this does not produce a sufficiently high temperature for sterilization, and care must be taken to avoid the flammable risk of alcohol.

Hot air sterilizer

Hot air sterilizers are used to process materials which can withstand high temperatures for the length of time needed for sterilization by dry heat (see Table 7.2), but which are likely to be affected by contact with steam. Examples include oils, powders, carbon steel microsurgical instruments and empty laboratory glassware. The overall cycle of heating up and cooling may take several hours.

Microwave ovens

The heating effect in microwave ovens is not uniform and no reliable sterilization process using microwaves is presently available.

STERILIZATION BY IRRADIATION

Ionizing radiations, including γ rays, X-rays and accelerated electrons, are lethal to all cells. Bacterial species differ in their sensitivity to ionizing radiations, although the degree of resistance varies during the growth cycle and bacterial spores are generally more resistant than vegetative cells. Sterilization is achieved by the use of high-speed electrons from a machine such as a linear accelerator or by an isotope source such as cobalt-60; a dose of 255 kGy is generally adequate, which makes this a large-scale industrial process. It is used to sterilize large amounts of prepacked single-use items such as plastic syringes and catheters.

STERILIZATION BY GASEOUS PROCESSES

Ethylene oxide

This is a highly penetrative, non-corrosive and microbicidal gas which is used in industry for the sterilization of single-use, heat-sensitive medical devices such as prosthetic heart valves and plastic catheters. Ethylene oxide sterilization is usually carried out at temperatures below 60°C in conditions of high relative humidity. To ensure sterility, material should be exposed to a gas concentration of 700–1000 mg/l at 45–60°C and a relative humidity above 70% for about 2 h. Care must be taken because of toxicity to personnel, flammability and explosion risk. The sterilized product must be aerated to remove residual ethylene oxide before it can be safely used on the patient, and the turn-round time is consequently slow.

Low-temperature steam and formaldehyde

This combines the thermal effects of steam generated at subatmospheric pressure (73–80°C) and a gaseous agent, formaldehyde, to give an effective sporicidal process. This method is appropriate for the reprocessing of heat-sensitive instruments and items of hospital equipment which can withstand temperatures up to 80°C only. Again, safety requirements make the process inappropriate for routine hospital use.

STERILIZATION BY FILTRATION

Fluids, including bacterial cultures, can be rendered free of bacteria by passage through filters with a pore size of less than 0.45 μm. The method is used in the separation of toxins and other soluble products of bacterial growth, and in the preparation of thermolabile parenteral fluids such as antibiotic solutions, radiopharmaceuticals and blood products which would not withstand the preferred option of sterilization by heat. The efficiency of microbial retention is dependent on many factors, including the initial number of micro-organisms, their type and the composition and pore size of the filter. Most viruses, and certain bacteria such as mycoplasmas, can pass through filters with a pore size as low as 0.22 μm.

Early filter types, including unglazed ceramic *Chamberland* filters, asbestos *Seitz* filters and *sintered glass* filters, have been largely superseded by *membrane* filters made of cellulose esters or other polymers.

DISINFECTION

The efficacy of disinfection depends on the severity of the treatment (temperature and/or chemical concentration) and the process time. There are no methods that are instantaneously effective or that will 'kill all known (household) germs'.

Cleaning

Thorough cleaning is a prerequisite for successful disinfection, and it is also a valuable method for disinfection in its own right. Any process used to kill micro-organisms has a limited capacity and, for both disinfection and sterilization, it is essential that the lowest possible number of organisms are present at the start of the process. Removal of debris dried on instruments or other items that are difficult to clean may be enhanced by the use of *ultrasonic baths*. The detergents used in cleaning have some disinfection properties, and the dilution effect of thorough rinsing further reduces the microbial load.

Disinfection by moist heat

This is the method of first choice. It can be precisely controlled, leaves no toxic residues and does not promote the development of resistant strains. Washing or rinsing laundry or eating utensils in water at 70–80°C for a few minutes will kill most non-sporing micro-organisms present. Similarly, steam maintained at sub-atmospheric pressure at 73°C is used in *low-temperature steam* disinfectors in hospitals to disinfect thermolabile reusable equipment.

Exposure to boiling water for 20 min achieves highly effective disinfection; although this is not a sterilization process it can be useful in emergencies if no sterilizer is available.

Disinfection by ultraviolet radiation

Ultraviolet radiation is a low-energy, non-ionizing radiation with poor penetrating power that is lethal to micro-organisms under optimum conditions. The shortest ultraviolet rays that reach the earth's surface in quantity have a wavelength of about 290 nm, but even more effective radiation of 240–280 nm is produced by mercury lamps. It is used in the treatment of air, water, thin films and surfaces such as laboratory safety cabinets.

Disinfection by gases

Traditionally, formaldehyde gas was used to disinfect rooms previously occupied by patients with contagious diseases such as smallpox. It is still used for disinfection of complex heat-sensitive equipment, including anaesthetic machines and baby incubators, and for periodic decontamination of laboratory safety cabinets.

Disinfection by filtration

This method is used to remove micro-organisms from air supplied to critical sites such as operating theatres, pharmaceutical clean rooms, ultraclean laminar airflow ventilation systems and for the treatment of extracted air from laboratories handling dangerous pathogens. A properly installed *high-efficiency particulate air* (HEPA) filter achieves 99.997% or better arrestance to particles of 0.5 μm, and can produce sterile air at the filter face.

Disinfection by chemicals

Chemicals used in the environment or on the skin (*disinfectants* or *antiseptics*) cannot be relied on to kill or inhibit all pathogenic micro-organisms. The distinction between disinfectants and antiseptics is not clear-cut: an antiseptic can be regarded as a special kind of disinfectant which is sufficiently free from injurious effects to be applied to the surface of the body, though not suitable for systemic administration. Some would restrict the term *antiseptic* to preparations applied to open wounds or abraded tissue and would prefer the term *skin disinfection* for the removal of organisms from the hands and intact skin surfaces.

Factors influencing the performance of chemical disinfectants

These include:

- The concentration and stability of the agent.
- The number, type and accessibility of micro-organisms.
- The temperature and pH.
- The presence of organic (especially protein) or other interfering substances.

In general, the rate of inactivation of a susceptible microbial population in the presence of an antimicrobial chemical is dependent on the relative concentration of the two reactants, the micro-organism and the chemical. The optimum concentration required to produce a standardized microbial effect in practice is described as the *in-use* concentration. Care must always be taken in preparing an accurate in-use dilution of concentrated product. Accidental or arbitrary overdilution may result in failure of disinfection.

The velocity of the reaction depends upon the number and type of organisms present. In general, Gram-positive bacteria are more sensitive to disinfectants than Gram-negative bacteria; mycobacteria and fungal spores are relatively resistant, and bacterial spores are highly resistant. Enveloped or lipophilic viruses are relatively sensitive, whereas hydrophilic viruses such as poliovirus and other enteroviruses are less susceptible. Although difficult to test in vitro, there is evidence that the hepatitis B virus is more resistant than other viruses (including the human immunodeficiency virus) and most vegetative bacteria to the action of chemical disinfectants and heat.

Glutaraldehyde is highly active against bacteria, viruses and spores. Other disinfectants, such as hexachlorophane, have a relatively narrow range of activity, predominantly against Gram-positive cocci. Some disinfectants are more active or stable at a particular pH value; although glutaraldehyde is more stable under acidic conditions, use at a higher pH value (8.0) improves the antimicrobial effect.

Disinfectants may be inactivated by hard tap water, cork, plastics, blood, urine, soaps and detergents, or another disinfectant. Information should be sought from the manufacturer or from reference authorities to confirm that the disinfectant will remain active in the circumstances of use.

Alcohols

Isopropanol, ethanol and industrial methylated spirits have optimal bactericidal activity in aqueous solution at a concentration of 70–90% and have little bactericidal effect outside this range. They have limited activity against mycobacteria and are not sporicidal. Action against viruses is generally good. Because they are volatile, alcohols have been widely recommended as rapidly drying disinfectants for skin and surfaces. However, they may not achieve adequate penetration and kill, particularly if organic matter such as blood or other protein-based contamination is present. Alcohols are suitable for physically clean surfaces such as washed thermometers or trolley tops but not for dirty surfaces. Care must be taken when used on the skin in conjunction with diathermy and other instances of flammable risk. Alcohols or alcohol-based formulations with chlorhexidine or povidone iodine are good choices for hand disinfection; they are applied to dry skin, often with added emollient to counteract the drying effect.

Aldehydes

Most aldehyde disinfectants are based on glutaraldehyde or formaldehyde formulations, alone or in combination. *Glutaraldehyde* has a broad-spectrum action against vegetative bacteria, fungi and viruses, but acts more slowly against spores. It is often used for equipment such as endoscopes that cannot be sterilized or disinfected by heat. It is an irritant to the eyes, skin and respiratory mucosa, and must be used with adequate protection of staff and ventilation of the working environment. This is achieved by wearing protective clothing, working in safety hoods or using air scavenging equipment. In many countries these agents are strictly controlled by Health and Safety officials. It must be thoroughly rinsed from treated equipment with sterile water to avoid carry-over of toxic residues and recontamination. The alkaline buffered solution is claimed to remain active for several days, but this will vary depending on the 'in-use' situation, including the amount of organic material. Special closed washer–disinfector systems are available for decontaminating flexible endoscopes. Alternatives to glutaraldehyde used in these systems include the oxidizing agents peracetic acid, chlorine dioxide and super-oxidized water (see below).

Biguanides

Chlorhexidine. This is commonly used for disinfection of the skin and mucous membranes. It is less active against Gram-negative bacteria such as *Pseudomonas* and *Proteus* species, and in aqueous solution has limited virucidal, tuberculocidal and negligible sporicidal activity. It is often combined with a compatible detergent for handwashing or with alcohol as a hand-rub. Chlorhexidine has low irritancy and toxicity, and is effective even on exposed healing surfaces. It is inactivated by organic matter, soap, anionic detergents, hard water and some natural materials such as the cork liners of bottle closures.

Halogens

Hypochlorites. These broad-spectrum, inexpensive chlorine-releasing disinfectants are the disinfectants of choice against viruses, including hepatitis B virus. For circumstances of heavy soilage such as blood spillage, a concentration of 10 000 ppm of available chlorine is recommended.

They are inactivated by organic matter and corrode metals, so that contact with metallic instruments and equipment should be avoided. The bleaching action of hypochlorites may have a detrimental effect on fabrics, e.g. in treating a spillage on a carpet.

Chlorine-releasing disinfectants are relatively stable in concentrated form as liquid bleach or as tablets (sodium dichloroisocyanurates) but should be stored in well-sealed containers in a cool, dark place. On dilution to the required concentration for use, activity is rapidly lost.

Hypochlorites have widespread application as laboratory disinfectants on bench surfaces and in discard pots. Care should be taken to remove all chlorine-releasing agents from laboratory areas before the use of formaldehyde fumigation to avoid the production of carcinogenic reaction products.

Iodine. Like chlorine, iodine is inactivated by organic matter and has the additional disadvantages of staining and hypersensitivity. The *iodophors*, which contain iodine complexed with an anionic detergent, or *povidone iodine*, a water-soluble complex of iodine and polyvinyl pyrrolidone, are less irritant and cause less staining. Aqueous and alcohol-based povidone iodine preparations are widely used in skin disinfection, including preoperative preparation of the skin.

Phenolics

These have been widely used as general-purpose environmental disinfectants in hospital and laboratory practice. They exhibit broad-spectrum activity and are relatively cheap. Clear soluble phenolics have been used to disinfect environmental surfaces and spillages if organic soil and transmissible pathogens may have been present. As hospital disinfection policies are rationalized, phenolics are being replaced by detergents for cleaning, and by hypochlorites for disinfection of contaminated sources. Most phenolics are stable and not readily inactivated by organic matter, with the exception of the chloroxylenols ('Dettol'), which are also inactivated by hard water and are not recommended for hospital use. Phenolics are incompatible with cationic detergents. Contact should be avoided with rubber and plastics, such as mattress covers, since they are absorbed and may increase the permeability of the material to body fluids. The slow release of phenol fumes in closed environments and the need to avoid skin contact are other reasons for care in use of phenolics.

The bis-phenol *hexachlorophane* has particular activity against Gram-positive cocci, and has been used in powder or emulsion formulations as a skin disinfectant, notably for prophylaxis against staphylococcal infection in nurseries. There has been some concern about the possible toxic effect of absorption across the neonatal skin barrier on repeated exposure. An alternative, which has been used in the control of methicillin-resistant *Staph. aureus* (MRSA) outbreaks is *triclosan.*

Oxidizing agents and hydrogen peroxide

Various agents, including chlorine dioxide, peracetic acid and hydrogen peroxide, have good antimicrobial properties but are corrosive to skin and metals. Hydrogen peroxide is highly reactive and has limited application for the treatment of wounds.

Surface-active agents

Anionic, cationic, non-ionic and amphoteric *detergents* are generally used as cleaning agents. The cationic (*quaternary ammonium compounds*) and amphoteric agents have limited antimicrobial activity against vegetative bacteria and some viruses but not mycobacteria or bacterial spores. Quaternary ammonium compounds disrupt the membrane of the micro-organisms, leading to cell lysis. Care must be taken to avoid overgrowth by Gram-negative contaminants and inactivation by mixing cationic and anionic agents. Disinfection may be enhanced by the appropriate combination of a surface-active agent with disinfectant to improve contact spread and cleansing properties.

Disinfectant testing

A wide range of testing methods has been developed for different products and different applications in the medical, food and veterinary areas. Standardization of test methods within Europe is currently in progress, and will include:

1. Simple screening tests of the rate of kill.
2. Laboratory tests simulating in-use conditions (skin disinfection tests and inanimate surface tests).
3. In-use tests on equipment and solutions.

The purpose of the 'in-use' test is to monitor not only the performance of a particular disinfectant but also how it is being used. Samples of the disinfectant dilutions in use around the hospital are taken to determine the survival and multiplication of contaminating pathogens in a stale or over-diluted formulation.

STERILIZATION AND DISINFECTION POLICY

Each hospital, through the infection control team, should agree a policy to ensure that staff responsible for sterilization and disinfection are familiar with the agents to be used and the procedures involved. The policy should consider the following.

1. The sources (equipment, skin and environment) for which a choice of process is required.
2. The processes and products available for sterilization and disinfection. An effective policy may include a limited number of process options; restrictions on the range of chemical disinfectants will eliminate unnecessary costs, confusion and chemical hazards.
3. The category of process required for each item: sterilization for surgical instruments and needles; heat disinfection for laundry, crockery, bed-pans; cleaning for floors, walls and furniture.
4. The specific products and method to be used for each item of equipment, the site of use and the staff responsible for the procedure.

Effective implementation of the policy requires liaison and training of staff and updating the policy. Safety considerations for staff and patients require a careful assessment of specific procedures to minimize risks, e.g. to avoid skin contact and fumes from disinfectants by the use of protective clothing and local ventilation which must conform to local health and safety regulations. This includes the use of fume cabinets, air scavenging equipment and sealed washer–disinfectors. These requirements take decontamination of medical instruments away from small clinics into specialized sterile supply departments.

RECOMMENDED READING

Ayliffe G A J, Coates D, Hoffman P N 1993 *Chemical Disinfection in Hospitals*, 2nd edn. Public Health Laboratory Service, London

Block S S (ed) 1991 *Disinfection, Sterilization and Preservation*, 4th edn. Lea and Febiger, Philadelphia

Gardner J F, Peel M M 1991 *Introduction to Sterilization and Disinfection*, 2nd edn. Churchill Livingstone, Edinburgh

Medical Devices Agency 1996 *Sterilization, Disinfection and Cleaning of Medical Equipment. Guidance on Decontamination from the Microbiology Advisory Committee to the Department of Health.* Medical Devices Agency, London

Russell A D, Hugo W B, Ayliffe G A J (eds) 1998 *Principles and Practice of Disinfection, Preservation and Sterilisation*, 3rd edn, Blackwell Scientific, Oxford

8

Bacterial pathogenicity

D. Ala'Aldeen

Pathogenicity, or the capacity to initiate disease, is a relatively rare quality among microbes. It requires the attributes of *transmissibility* or communicability from one host or reservoir to a fresh host, *survival* in the new host, *infectivity* or the ability to breach the new host's defences, and *virulence*, a variable that is multifactorial and denotes the capacity of a pathogen to harm the host. Virulence in the clinical sense is a manifestation of a complex parasite–host relationship in which the capacity of the organism to cause disease is considered in relation to the resistance of the host.

TYPES OF BACTERIAL PATHOGEN

Bacterial pathogens can be classified into two broad groups, *opportunists* and *primary pathogens*.

Opportunistic pathogens

These rarely cause disease in individuals with intact immunological and anatomical defences. Only when such defences are impaired or compromised, as a result of congenital or acquired disease or by the use of immunosuppressive therapy or surgical techniques, are these bacteria able to cause disease. Many opportunistic pathogens, e.g. coagulase-negative staphylococci and *Escherichia coli*, are part of the normal human flora and are carried on the skin or mucosal surfaces where they cause no harm and may actually have a beneficial effect by preventing colonization by other potential pathogens. However, introduction of these organisms into anatomical sites in which they are not normally found, or removal of competing bacteria by the use of broad-spectrum antibiotics, may allow their localized multiplication and subsequent development of disease.

Primary pathogens

These are capable of establishing infection and causing disease in previously healthy individuals with intact immunological defences. However, these bacteria may more readily cause disease in individuals with impaired defences.

The above classification is applicable to the vast majority of pathogens. However, there are exceptions and variations within both categories of bacterial pathogens. Different strains of any bacterial species can vary in their genetic make up and virulence. For example, the majority of *Neisseria meningitidis* strains are harmless commensals and are considered to be opportunistic bacteria; however, some hypervirulent clones of the organism can cause disease in the previously healthy individual. Conversely, people vary in their genetic make up and susceptibility to invading bacteria, including meningococci.

VIRULENCE DETERMINANTS

Both opportunistic and primary pathogens possess *virulence determinants* or *aggressins* that facilitate pathogenesis. Possession of a single virulence determinant is rarely sufficient to allow the initiation of infection and production of pathology. Many bacteria possess several virulence determinants, all of which play some part at various stages of the disease process. In addition, not all strains of a particular bacterial species are equally pathogenic. For example, although six separate serotypes of encapsulated *Haemophilus influenzae* are recognized, serious infection is almost exclusively associated with isolates of serotype b. Moreover, even within serotype b isolates, 80% of serious infections are caused by six out of over 100 clonal types.

Different strains of a pathogenic species may cause distinct types of infection, each associated with possession of a particular complement of virulence determinants. Different strains of *Esch. coli*, for example, cause several distinct gastro-intestinal diseases, urinary tract infections, septicaemia, meningitis and a range of other minor infections (see Chapter 26).

Expression and analysis of virulence determinants

Many pathogens produce an impressive armoury of virulence determinants in vitro. However, relatively early in the study of pathogenesis, it was appreciated that a knowledge of the behaviour of the pathogen in vivo is crucial to an understanding of virulence.

Animal models have been used to compare the virulence of naturally occurring variants differing in the expression of a particular determinant, and have provided much useful information, but the possibility that observed differences in virulence may be due to additional cryptic phenotypic or genotypic variations cannot always be excluded. More recently, molecular techniques have been used to construct *isogenic* mutants of bacteria that differ only in the particular determinant of interest, and these constructs have allowed more detailed analysis of the role of such components in pathogenesis.

Most studies of bacterial virulence determinants are by necessity performed in model systems in vitro. However, growth conditions in vitro differ significantly from those found in tissues, and since the expression of many virulence determinants is influenced by environmental factors, it is essential that such studies use cultural conditions that mimic as closely as possible those found in the host.

Genetic studies have shown that expression of several different virulence determinants in a single bacterium is sometimes regulated in a co-ordinated fashion. Iron limitation, the situation encountered in host tissues, is one environmental stimulus which co-ordinately increases production of many bacterial proteins, including virulence determinants such as haemolysin of *Esch. coli* and diphtheria toxin from *Corynebacterium diphtheriae*. In other bacteria, e.g. *Staphylococcus aureus* and *Pseudomonas aeruginosa*, some virulence determinants are expressed exclusively or maximally during the stationary phase of growth. Expression of these factors is associated with production of inducer molecules or pheromones in the bacterial culture which accumulate as the bacteria grow until a threshold level is reached and gene expression is triggered – a process known as *quorum sensing*. The ability to regulate production of virulence determinants may save energy in situations in which expression is not required, e.g. in the environment, and quorum sensing may be important in establishing a sufficiently large population of bacteria in tissue to guarantee survival of the infecting organism. It is also clear that most organisms express some proteins only when in direct contact with host cells.

Molecular studies have also allowed mechanisms of transmission of virulence determinants to be investigated. Virulence determinants encoded by genomic DNA sequences, plasmids, bacteriophages and transposons have been reported. It is interesting that, in nature, these genetic elements can move between related organisms and horizontally transfer virulence factors (e.g. toxins) and transform the recipient bacteria to more adapted or more virulent pathogens. Apart from these genetic elements, there are other mechanisms by which some bacteria can exchange virulence genes. For example, neisseriae recognize and take up DNA fragments that contain specific sequences (uptake sequences) and incorporate them in their own genomes. This way they can either vary the structure of an existing gene or, in the process, acquire a new set of genes. The genome of several bacterial pathogens has recently been fully sequenced. The data reveal that several bacteria have acquired very large stretches of foreign DNA (often called pathogenicity isles) which contain virulence-related genes. This further demonstrates that the microbial population consists of a vibrant, kinetic and highly interactive community. In this community, bacteria will evolve continuously and new pathogens, or old pathogens with newly acquired capabilities, could emerge as a result.

Establishment of infection

Potential pathogens may enter the body by various routes, including the respiratory, gastro-intestinal, urinary or genital tracts. Alternatively, they may directly enter tissues through insect bites, or by accidental or surgical trauma to the skin. Many opportunistic pathogens are carried as part of the normal human flora, and this acts as a ready source of infection in the compromised host. For many primary pathogens, however, transmission to a new host and establishment of infection are more complex processes. Transmission of respiratory pathogens, such as *Bordetella pertussis*, may require direct contact with infectious material since the organism cannot survive for any length of time in the environment. Sexually transmitted pathogens such as *Neisseria gonorrhoeae* and *Treponema pallidum* have evolved further along this route, and require direct person-to-person mucosal contact for transmission. Man is the only natural host for these pathogens, which die rapidly in the environment. The source of infection may be individuals with clinical disease or subclinically infected *carriers*, in whom symptoms may be absent or relatively mild either because the disease process is at an early stage or because of partial immunity to the pathogen.

In contrast, for many gastro-intestinal pathogens such as *Salmonella, Shigella* and *Campylobacter* species the primary source is environmental, and infection follows ingestion of contaminated food or water. Many of these organisms also infect other animals, often without harmful effect, and these act as a *reservoir of infection* and source of environmental contamination.

Colonization

For many pathogenic bacteria, the initial interaction with host tissues occurs at a mucosal surface and colonization – the establishment of a stable population of bacteria in the host – normally requires *adhesion* to the mucosal cell surface. This allows the establishment of a focus of infection that may remain localized or may subsequently spread to other tissues. Adhesion is necessary to avoid innate host defence mechanisms such as peristalsis in the gut and the flushing action of mucus, saliva and urine which remove non-adherent bacteria. For invasive bacteria, adhesion is an essential preliminary to penetration through tissues. Successful colonization also requires that bacteria are able to acquire essential nutrients – in particular iron – for growth.

Adhesion

Adhesion involves surface interactions between specific *receptors* on the mammalian cell membrane (usually carbohydrates) and *ligands* (usually proteins) on the bacterial surface. The presence or absence of specific receptors on mammalian cells contributes significantly to tissue specificity of infection. Non-specific surface properties of the bacterium, including surface charge and hydrophobicity, also contribute to the initial stages of the adhesion process. Several different mechanisms of bacterial adherence have evolved, all utilizing specialized cell surface organelles or macromolecules, that help to overcome the natural forces of repulsion that exist between the pathogen and its target cell.

Fimbrial adhesins

Electron microscopy of the surface of many Gram-negative and some Gram-positive bacteria reveals the presence of numerous thin, rigid rod-like structures called *fimbriae*, or *pili,* that are easily distinguishable from the much thicker bacterial flagella (see p. 17). Fimbriae are involved in mediating attachment of some bacteria to mammalian cell surfaces. Different strains or species of bacteria may produce different types of fimbriae which can be identified on the basis of antigenic composition, morphology and receptor specificity (Table 8.1). A broad division can be made between those fimbriae in which adherence in vitro is inhibited by D-mannose (*mannose-sensitive fimbriae*) and those unaffected by this treatment (*mannose-resistant fimbriae*).

The antigenic composition of fimbriae can be complex. For instance, two fimbrial antigens called col-

Table 8.1 Examples of fimbriae produced by Gram-negative pathogens

Designation	Bacterium
Common (type 1)[a]	Enterobacteriaceae Uropathogenic *Escherichia coli*
CFA I, CFA II (CS1, CS2, CS3) E8775 (CS4, CS5, CS6)	Enterotoxigenic *Esch. coli* from humans
K88 K99 F41	Enterotoxigenic *Esch. coli* from animals
Pap-G, Prs-G	Uropathogenic *Esch. coli*
P fimbriae X-adhesins (S, M)	Pyelonephritogenic *Esch. coli*
N-Methylphenylalanine fimbriae	*Pseudomonas, Neisseria, Moraxella, Bacteroides, Vibrio* species

See text for abbreviations and explanation.
[a] Mannose-sensitive fimbriae.

onization factor antigens (CFA) I and II have been detected in enteropathogenic *Esch. coli* strains. CFA II consists of three distinct fimbrial antigens designated as coli surface (CS) antigens 1, 2 and 3. Another *Esch. coli* strain, E8775, has been found to produce three other CS antigens, CS4, CS5 and CS6. Pyelonephritogenic *Esch. coli* isolates produce a group of adhesins called X-adhesins; two fimbrial types designated S and M on the basis of receptor specificity have been identified in this group.

The evolutionary significance of such heterogeneity may be that the ability of an individual bacterium to express several different types of fimbriae allows different target receptors to be used at different anatomical sites of the infected host. In vitro, production of fimbriae is influenced by cultural conditions such as incubation temperature and medium composition, which may switch off production of fimbriae or induce a phase change from one fimbrial type to another.

For some fimbriae the association with infection is clear. Thus the K88 fimbrial antigen is clearly associated with the ability of *Esch. coli* K88 to cause diarrhoea in pigs; pigs lacking the appropriate intestinal receptors are spared the enterotoxigenic effects of *Esch. coli* strains of this type. In many other instances the association between production of fimbriae and infection remains putative at present. Production of fimbriae is controlled by either chromosomal or plasmid genes.

The structure of one of these fimbrial types – *type 1* or *common fimbriae* – has been studied in detail. These consist of aggregates of a structural protein subunit called *fimbrillin* (or pilin) arranged in a regular helical array to produce a rigid rod-like structure of 7 nm diameter, with a central hole running along its length.

A highly conserved minor protein, located at both the tip and at intervals along the length of the fimbriae, mediates specific adhesion. Type 1 fimbriae bind specifically to D-mannose residues. Their role in vivo remains controversial; however, they may be involved in the pathogenesis of urinary tract infections.

Other Gram-negative bacteria, including those of the genera *Pseudomonas, Neisseria, Bacteroides* and *Vibrio*, produce fimbriae that share some homology, especially in the amino-terminal region of the fimbrillin subunits (the so-called *N-methylphenylalanine fimbriae*). These fimbriae have been shown to act as virulence determinants for *Ps. aeruginosa* and *N. gonorrhoeae*.

Non-fimbrial adhesins

Non-fimbrial adhesins include the filamentous haemagglutinin of *Bord. pertussis*, a mannose-resistant haemagglutinin from *Salmonella* serotype Typhimurium and a fibrillar haemagglutinin from *Helicobacter pylori*. Outer membrane proteins are involved in the adherence of *N. gonorrhoeae* and enteropathogenic *Esch. coli* to cell surfaces.

Exopolysaccharides present on the surface of some Gram-positive bacteria are also involved in adhesion. For example, *Streptococcus mutans*, which is involved in the pathogenesis of dental caries, synthesizes a homopolymer of glucose which anchors the bacterium to the tooth surface and contributes to the matrix of dental plaque. Actinomyces may adhere to other oral bacteria – a process called *co-aggregation*. Teichoic acid and surface proteins of coagulase-negative staphylococci mediate adherence of the bacterium to prosthetic devices and catheters, contributing to increasing numbers of hospital-acquired infections. Continued growth following attachment to these biomaterials may result in formation of a *biofilm* which may hinder successful antibiotic treatment by restricting access of drugs to the bacterium.

Flagella act as adhesins in *Vibrio cholerae* and *Campylobacter jejuni*. Bacterial motility is also thought to be important in chemotaxis of these organisms and *H. pylori* towards intestinal cells and in penetration of these bacteria through the mucous layer during colonization.

Binding to fibronectin

Fibronectin is a complex multifunctional glycoprotein found in plasma and associated with mucosal cell surfaces, where it promotes numerous adhesion functions. Many pathogenic bacteria bind fibronectin at the bacterial surface, and for some organisms fibronectin has been shown to act as the cell surface receptor for bacterial adhesion. In *Streptococcus pyogenes*, lipoteichoic acid mediates attachment of the bacterium to the amino terminus of the fibronectin molecule. Attachment of *Staph. aureus* to cell surfaces also involves the amino terminus of fibronectin, but the bacterial ligand appears to be protein in this instance. *T. pallidum* also binds fibronectin. The significance of the interaction with fibronectin in the pathogenesis of syphilis and many other bacterial diseases needs further clarification. Binding of bacterial pathogens to a number of other connective tissue proteins including collagen, laminin and vitronectin has also been described.

Consequences of adhesion

In addition to preventing loss of the pathogen from the host, adhesion induces structural and functional changes in mucosal cells, and these may contribute to disease. For example, adherence of enteropathogenic *Esch. coli* (EPEC) to epithelial cells induces rearrangements of the cell cytoskeleton causing loss of microvilli and localized accumulation of actin, without subsequent invasion of the host cell. In contrast, adherence of *H. pylori* to gastric epithelial cells causes enhanced production of the pro-inflammatory chemokine interleukin-8 (IL-8), which contributes to gastric pathology. In both cases, these changes involve induction of intracellular signalling pathways triggered following binding of the bacteria to specific receptors on the epithelial cell surface. Adhesion of bacteria to mammalian cells may also induce changes in bacterial protein synthesis.

Invasion

Once attached to a mucosal surface, some bacteria exert their pathogenic effects without penetrating the tissues of the host: toxins, other aggressins and induction of intracellular signalling pathways mediate tissue damage at local or distant sites. For a number of pathogenic bacteria, however, adherence to the mucosal surface represents but the first stage of the invasion of tissues. Examples of organisms that are able to invade and survive within host cells include mycobacteria and those of the genera *Salmonella, Shigella, Escherichia, Yersinia, Legionella, Listeria, Campylobacter* and *Neisseria*. Cell invasion confers the ability to avoid humoral host defence mechanisms and potentially provides a niche rich in nutrients and devoid of competition from other bacteria. However, survival of bacteria in professional phagocytes, such as macrophages or polymorphonuclear leucocytes, depends on subverting intracellular killing mechanisms that would normally result in microbial destruction (see below). For some bacteria, e.g. *Neisseria menin-*

gitidis, penetration through or between epithelial cells allows dissemination from the initial site of entry to other body sites.

Uptake into host cells

The initial phase of cellular invasion involves penetration of the mammalian cell membrane and many intracellular pathogens use normal phagocytic entry mechanisms to gain access.

Shigellae invade colonic mucosal cells but rarely penetrate deeper into the host tissues. Inside the cell, they are surrounded by a membrane-bound vesicle derived from the host cell. Soon after entry, this vesicle is lysed by the action of the plasmid-encoded haemolysin, and the bacteria are released into the cell cytoplasm. *Listeria monocytogenes* produces a heat shock protein with a similar function, termed *listeriolysin*. Once free in the cell cytoplasm, shigellae multiply rapidly with subsequent inhibition of host cell protein synthesis. Several hours later the host cell dies, and bacteria spread to adjacent cells where the process of invasion is repeated.

In contrast to shigellae, most salmonellae proceed through the superficial layers of the gut and invade deeper tissues, in particular cells of the reticuloendothelial system such as macrophages. Salmonellae also occupy a host-derived vesicle, but this does not lyse. Instead, several vesicles coalesce to form large intracellular vacuoles. These vacuoles traverse the cytoplasm to reach the opposite side of the cell and initiate spread to adjacent cells and deeper tissues. For both *Salmonella* and *Shigella* species, bacterial protein and RNA synthesis are required for invasion.

Role of cell receptors

The availability of specific receptors defines the type of host cells that are involved. As a result some pathogens can invade a wide range of cell types whilst others have a much more restricted invasive potential. The receptors for some of the invasive pathogens have been identified. For example, *Legionella pneumophila* and *Mycobacterium tuberculosis* adhere to complement receptors on the surface of phagocytic cells. The receptor for *Yersinia pseudotuberculosis* belongs to a family of proteins termed *integrins* that form a network on the surface of host cells to which host proteins such as fibronectin can bind. Mimicry of the amino acid sequence (Arg-Gly-Asp) of fibronectin that mediates attachment to the integrins may represent a common mechanism of effecting intracellular entry.

The ability to utilize integrins may not be restricted to intracellular bacteria. The filamentous haemagglutinin of *Bord. pertussis* may use the fibronectin integrin to mediate attachment in the respiratory tract.

Avoidance of host defence mechanisms

Colonization by bacterial pathogens results in the induction of specific and non-specific humoral and cell-mediated immune responses designed to eradicate the organism from the site of infection. Products of the organism may be chemotactic for phagocytic cells which are attracted to the site. Moreover, complement components may directly damage the bacterium and release peptides chemotactic for phagocytic cells. Other humoral antibacterial factors include lysozyme and the iron chelators transferrin and lactoferrin. Lysozyme is active primarily against Gram-positive bacteria but potentiates the activity of complement against Gram-negative organisms. Transferrin and lactoferrin chelate iron in body fluids, and reduce the amount of free iron to levels below that necessary for bacterial growth.

Pathogenic bacteria have evolved ways of avoiding or neutralizing these highly efficient clearance systems. Since most of the interactions between the bacterium and the immune effectors involve the bacterial surface, resistance to these effects is related to the molecular architecture of the bacterial surface layers.

Capsules

Many bacterial pathogens need to avoid phagocytosis, and production of an extracellular capsule is the most common mechanism by which this is achieved. Virtually all the pathogens associated with meningitis and pneumonia, including *H. influenzae, N. meningitidis, Esch. coli* and *Str. pneumoniae*, have capsules, and non-capsulate variants usually exhibit much reduced virulence. Most capsules are polysaccharides composed of sugar monomers that vary among different bacteria. Polysaccharide capsules reduce the efficiency of phagocytosis in a number of ways:

1. In the absence of specific antibody to the bacterium, the hydrophilic nature of the capsule may hinder uptake by phagocytes, a process which occurs more readily at hydrophobic surfaces. This may be overcome if the phagocyte is able to trap the bacterium against a surface – a process referred to as *surface phagocytosis*.

2. Capsules prevent efficient opsonization of the bacterium by complement or specific antibody, events that promote interaction with phagocytic cells. Capsules may either prevent complement deposition completely or cause complement to be deposited at a distance from the bacterial membrane where it is unable to damage the organism.

3. Capsules tend to be weakly immunogenic and may mask more immunogenic surface components and reduce interactions with both complement and antibody. In some cases, e.g. serogroup B *N. meningitidis* and serotype K1 *Esch. coli*, the capsular polysaccharide may mimic host polysaccharides moieties (e.g. brain sialic acid) and be seen as self-antigen.

Streptococcal M protein

The M protein present on the surface of *Str. pyogenes* is not a capsule but functions in a similar manner to prevent complement deposition at the bacterial surface. The M protein binds both fibrinogen and fibrin, and deposition of this material on the streptococcal surface hinders the access of complement activated by the alternative pathway.

Resistance to killing by phagocytic cells

Some pathogens not only survive within macrophages and other phagocytes, but may actually multiply intracellularly. The normal sequence of events following phagocytosis involves fusion of the *phagosome* in which the bacterium is contained with *lysosomal granules* present in the cell cytoplasm. These granules contain enzymes and cationic peptides involved in oxygen-dependent and oxygen-independent bacterial killing mechanisms (see p. 128).

Different organisms use different strategies for survival (Table 8.2). *M. tuberculosis* is thought to resist intracellular killing by preventing phagosome–lysosome fusion; other bacteria are able to resist the action of such lysosomal components following fusion. Some organisms stimulate a normal respiratory burst but are intrinsically resistant to the effects of the potentially toxic oxygen radicals produced. Production of catalase by *Staph. aureus* and *N. gonorrhoeae* is thought to protect these organisms from such toxic products. The smooth lipopolysaccharide of many bacterial pathogens is also thought to contribute to their resistance to the effects of bactericidal cationic peptides present in the phagolysosome.

Table 8.2 Some strategies adopted by bacteria to avoid intracellular killing

Species	Method
Mycobacterium tuberculosis	Prevents phago–lysosome fusion
Salmonella serotype Typhi	Fails to stimulate O_2-dependent killing
Staphylococcus aureus	Produces catalase to negate effect of toxic O_2 radicals
Neisseria gonorrhoeae	
Legionella pneumophila	Inhibits phago–lysosome acidification

Antigenic variation

Variation in surface antigen composition during the course of infection provides a mechanism of avoidance of specific immune responses directed at those antigens. This strategy is most highly developed in blood-borne parasitic protozoa, such as trypanosomes, but is also exhibited by bacteria. Pathogenic *Neisseria*, for example, are capable of changing surface antigens using three highly efficient mechanisms. These are mutation of individual amino acids, phase variation (switching genes on and off) and horizontal exchange of DNA material. *N. meningitidis* can avoid the killing effect of antibodies against its major porin (PorA) by mutating amino acids and/or acquiring parts or all of its *porA* gene from another meningococcal strain. The organism can switch off the expression of its capsule or its immunogenic proteins by shifts in the nucleotide sequence encoding them. The latter varies as a result of recombination or mutation during DNA replication.

Another interesting mechanism of antigen variation in *Neisseria* is the genetic rearrangements demonstrated in the fimbriae. Usually only one complete fimbrillin gene is expressed, although there may be several incomplete 'silent' gene sequences present on the chromosome. Movement of the incomplete gene sequences to an expression locus results in synthesis of a protein that may differ antigenically from the original. Alternatively, variant fimbrillin gene DNA may be acquired from other strains of the same species by transformation to allow new genes to be constructed by recombination at the expression site.

The borreliae that cause relapsing fever use a similar strategy to generate antigenic variation in their outer surface proteins. Other bacteria show strain-specific antigenic variability, for example group A streptococci produce up to 75 antigenically distinct serotypes of M protein.

The capacity for variation in surface antigens allows for longer survival of an individual organism in a host and means that antibody produced in response to infection by one strain of a pathogen may not protect against subsequent challenge with a different strain of that bacterium. This makes the variable antigens elusive targets for protective antibodies and development of vaccines based on inhibition of attachment or generation of opsonic or bactericidal antibodies particularly difficult for these organisms.

Immunoglobulin A proteases

Several species of pathogenic bacteria that cause disease on mucosal surfaces produce a protease that specifically cleaves immunoglobulin A (IgA), the principal antibody type produced at these sites. These proteases are specific for human IgA isotype I. Nearly all the pathogens causing meningitis possess an IgA protease and a polysaccharide capsule enabling them to persist on the mucosal surface and resist phagocytosis during the invasive phase of the disease.

Serum resistance

To survive in the bloodstream, bacteria must be able to resist lysis as a result of deposition of complement on the bacterial surface. In the Enterobacteriaceae, resistance is primarily due to the composition of the lipopolysaccharide (LPS) present in the bacterial outer membrane. *Smooth* colonial variants which possess polysaccharide 'O' side-chains in their LPS are more resistant than *rough* colonial variants that lack such side-chains (see below). The side-chains sterically hinder deposition of complement components on the bacterial surface. Conversely, however, some O chain polysaccharides activate complement by an alternate pathway leading to lysis of the bacterial cell. In *N. meningitidis* group B and *Esch. coli* K1, sialic acid capsules prevent efficient complement activation and, in *N. gonorrhoeae*, complement binds but forms an aberrant configuration in the bacterial outer membrane so that it is unable to effect lysis.

Iron acquisition

The concentration of free iron in bodily secretions is below that required for bacterial growth because it is chelated by high-affinity mammalian iron-binding proteins such as transferrin and lactoferrin. To multiply in body fluids or on mucous membranes, bacteria must therefore obtain iron, and many bacterial pathogens have evolved very efficient mechanisms for scavenging iron from mammalian iron-binding proteins. Bacteria such as *Esch. coli, Klebsiella pneumoniae* and some staphylococci produce extracellular iron chelators called *siderophores* for this purpose. Others including *N. meningitidis, Haemophilus parainfluenzae, H. influenzae* type b, *Staphylococcus epidermidis* and *Staph. aureus* have specific receptors for transferrin or lactoferrin, or both, on their surfaces, and are able to bind these proteins and their chelated iron directly from body fluids. Production of siderophores, their cell surface receptors and receptors for transferrin, lactoferrin and other mammalian iron-binding proteins is iron-regulated and mainly occurs under conditions of iron restriction.

Two other mechanisms of iron acquisition from mammalian iron chelators have been described. Some *Bacteroides* species remove iron by proteolytic cleavage of the chelator. In *Listeria monocytogenes*, reduction of

the Fe^{3+} ion to Fe^{2+} reduces the affinity for the chelator sufficiently for it to be removed by the bacterium.

Many bacteria express receptors for binding and/or internalizing other mammalian iron-containing molecules, such as haem, haemoglobin and haemoglobin–haemopexin complexes. These mammalian molecules are located intracellularly and can be released by bacterial haemolysins that lyse the red cells or are directly utilized by intracellular organisms.

Toxins

In many bacterial infections the characteristic pathology of the disease is caused by *toxins*. Toxins may exert their pathogenic effects directly on a target cell or may interact with cells of the immune system resulting in the release of immunological mediators (cytokines) that cause pathophysiological effects. Such effects may not always lead to the death of the target cell but may selectively impair specific functions. Substances that have toxic physiological effects on target cells in vitro do not necessarily exert the same effects in vivo, but a number of toxins have been shown to be responsible for the typical clinical features of bacterial disease.

Two major types of toxin have been described: *endotoxin*, which is a component of the outer membrane of Gram-negative bacteria, and *exotoxins*, which are produced extracellularly by both Gram-negative and Gram-positive bacteria.

Endotoxin

Endotoxin, also called LPS (lipopolysaccharide) or LOS (lipo-oligosaccharide), is a component of the outer membrane of Gram-negative bacteria, and is released from the bacterial surface via outer membrane vesicles (blebs), following natural lysis of the bacterium or by disintegration of the organism in vitro. LPS is anchored into the bacterial outer membrane through a unique molecule termed *lipid A* (Fig. 8.1). Covalently linked to lipid A is an eight-carbon sugar, ketodeoxyoctonate (KDO), in turn linked to the chain of sugar molecules (saccharides) which form the highly variable O antigen structures of Gram-negative bacteria. On bacteriological media, bacteria carrying LPS containing O antigen form *smooth* colonies with hydrophilic surfaces, in contrast to those carrying LOS which lack the O antigen and form *rough* colonies with hydrophobic surfaces.

The term *endotoxin* was originally introduced to describe the component of Gram-negative bacteria responsible for the pathophysiology of *endotoxic shock*, a syndrome with high mortality, particularly in immunocompromised or otherwise debilitated individuals. Endotoxin activates complement via the alternative

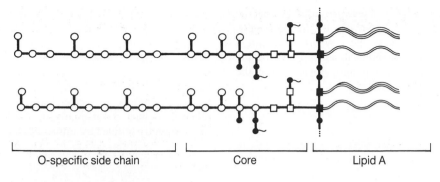

O-specific side chain   Core   Lipid A

O = various sugar residues

□ = ketodeoxyoctonate (KDO)

■ = glucosamine

•⌒ = phosphoethanolamine

⌒⌒ = fatty acid residues

Fig. 8.1 Diagrammatic representation of the structure of bacterial lipopolysaccharide. (After Reitschel E T, Galanos C, Lüderlitz O 1975 Structure, endotoxicity and immunogenicity of the lipid A component of bacterial lipopolysaccharide. In: Schlessinger D (ed.) *Microbiology – 1975*. American Society for Microbiology, Washington DC, pp 307–314.)

pathway, but most of the biological activity of the molecule is attributable to lipid A. Both endotoxin and lipid A are potent activators of macrophages, resulting in the induction of a range of cytokines which are involved in the regulation of immune and inflammatory responses (see Chapter 11).

Exotoxins

Exotoxins, in contrast to endotoxin, are diffusible proteins secreted into the external medium by the pathogen. Most pathogens secrete various protein molecules that facilitate adhesion to, or invasion of, the host. Many others cause damage to host cells. The damage could be physiological, e.g. cholera toxin promotes electrolyte (and fluid) excretion from enterocytes without killing the cells. Or, the damage is pathological where the toxin, e.g. diphtheria toxin, inhibits protein synthesis and induces cell death. Exotoxins vary in their molecular structure, biological function, mechanism of secretion and immunological properties. The list of bacterial exotoxins is now endless and increasing; however, they are often classified by their mode of action on animal cells:

• type I toxins bind surface receptors and stimulate transmembrane signals
• type II toxins act directly on membranes, forming pores or disrupting lipid bilayers
• type III toxins translocate an active enzymatic component into the cell which modifies an intracellular target molecule.

Examples of exotoxins and their effects on target cells are shown in Table 8.3. Bacteria secrete proteins using various mechanisms (again named types I–V), some of which are not clearly understood. Figure 8.2 shows types I and V; these are relatively well characterized. In type I, at least three proteins get together to form a channel through which large molecules (such as haemolysin of *Esch. coli*) are exported. In type V, however, a single precursor protein that consists of three domains will find its way across the inner and outer membranes and cleave itself off the cell. These latter proteins are called *autotransporters*. A typical example is the IgA1 protease of *Neisseria* spp.

Enterotoxins cause symptoms of gastro-intestinal disease, including diarrhoea, dysentery or vomiting. In some cases the disease is caused by ingestion of pre-formed toxin in food, but in most cases colonization of the intestine is required before toxin is made.

Cholera toxin and heat-labile toxins of enterotoxigenic *Esch. coli* (ETEC) do not induce inflammatory changes in the intestinal mucosa, but perturb the processes that regulate ion and water exchange across the intestinal epithelium (see Chapters 26 and 30). In contrast, the enterotoxins of *Clostridium difficile, C. perfringens* type A and *Bacillus cereus* cause structural damage to epithelial cells, resulting in inflammation. Other gastro-intestinal pathogens such as enteropathogenic *Esch. coli* (EPEC) mediate damage by ill-defined mechanisms following close contact between the bacterium and the cell surface.

Table 8.3 Some effects of bacterial exotoxins

Toxic effect	Examples
Lethal action	
Effect on neuromuscular junction	*Clostridium botulinum* toxin A
Effect on voluntary muscle	Tetanus toxin
Damage to heart, lungs, kidneys, etc.	Diphtheria toxin
Pyrogenic effect	
Increase in body temperature	Exotoxins of *Staphylococcus aureus* and *Streptococcus pyogenes*
	Staphylococcal toxic shock syndrome toxin 1
Action on gastro-intestinal tract	
Secretion of water and electrolytes	Cholera and *Escherichia coli* enterotoxins
Pseudomembranous colitis	*Clostridium difficile* toxins A and B
Bacillary dysentery	Shigella toxin
Vomiting	*Staph. aureus* enterotoxins A–E
Action on skin	
Necrosis	Clostridial toxins; staphylococcal α-toxin
Erythema	Diphtheria toxin; streptococcal erythrogenic toxin
Permeability of skin capillaries	Cholera enterotoxin; *Esch. coli* heat-labile toxin
Nikolsky sign[a]	*Staph. aureus* epidermolytic toxin
Cytolytic effects	
Lysis of blood cells	*Staph. aureus* α-, β- and δ-lysins, leucocidin
	Streptolysin O and S
	Clostridium perfringens α and θ toxins
Inhibition of metabolic activity	
Protein synthesis	Diphtheria toxin; shiga toxin

[a] Separation of epidermis from dermis.

Toxins in respiratory infections

The involvement of exotoxins in the pathogenesis of most bacterial respiratory infections is unclear, except for *Bord. pertussis*, the causative agent of whooping cough. This organism produces various extracellular products:

- A tracheal cytotoxin which inhibits the beating of cilia on tracheal epithelial cells;
- Pertussis toxin, which exhibits several systemic effects;
- An adenylate cyclase that interferes with phagocyte function.

Toxins acting on subepithelial tissues

Another group of toxins causes damage to subepithelial tissues following penetration and multiplication of the pathogen at the site of infection. Many of these toxins also inhibit or interfere with components of the host immune system. Membrane-damaging toxins such as staphylococcal α and β toxins, streptolysin O and streptolysin S and *C. perfringens* α and θ toxins inhibit leucocyte chemotaxis at subcytolytic concentrations, but cause necrosis and tissue damage at higher concentrations.

Systemic effects of toxins

Some toxins cause damage to internal organs following absorption from the focus of infection. Included in this category are the toxins causing diphtheria, tetanus and botulism, and those associated with streptococcal scarlet fever and staphylococcal toxic shock syndrome. The diphtheria toxin, the gene for which is bacteriophage-encoded, inhibits protein synthesis in mammalian cells. Tetanus toxin, in contrast, exerts its effect by preventing the release of inhibitory neurotransmitters whose function is to prevent overstimulation of motor neurones in the central nervous system, resulting in the convulsive muscle spasm characteristic of tetanus. Diphtheria and tetanus toxins represent the sole determinant of disease and are neutralized by specific antitoxin antibody. As a result, vaccination with diphtheria and tetanus toxoids (formalin-inactivated toxins) is highly effective (see Chapter 69).

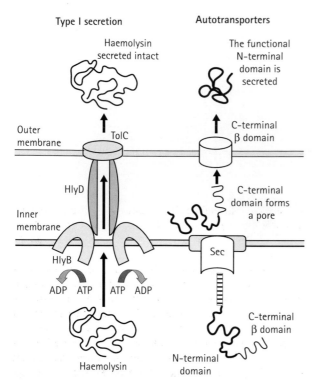

Fig. 8.2 Diagrammatic representation of Type I and Type V (autotransporter) secretion of exotoxins across the bacterial cell membrane. Hly, haemolysin; Tol, special receptor.

toxic shock syndrome caused by certain strains of *Staph. aureus* that produce a toxin designated *toxic shock syndrome toxin 1* (TSST-1). This toxin belongs to a group of functionally related proteins collectively referred to as *superantigens*, which includes the staphylococcal enterotoxins, staphylococcal exfoliative toxin and streptococcal pyrogenic exotoxin A. These molecules are potent T cell mitogens whose reactivity with lymphocytes induces cytokine release, and may initiate tissue damage by mechanisms similar to those postulated to account for Gram-negative endotoxic shock (see p. 164).

Other extracellular aggressins

Many bacteria secrete a range of enzymes that may be involved in the pathogenic processes.

Proteus spp. and some other bacteria that cause urinary tract infections produce *ureases* that break down urea in the urine, and the release of ammonia may contribute to the pathology. The urease produced by the gastric and duodenal pathogen *H. pylori* is similarly implicated in the virulence of the organism. *L. pneumophila* produces a metalloprotease thought to contribute to the characteristic pathology seen in legionella pneumonia.

Many other degradative enzymes, including *mucinases*, *phospholipases*, *collagenases* and *hyaluronidases*, are produced by pathogenic bacteria. Many non-pathogenic bacteria also produce such enzymes, and their role in pathogenesis requires further clarification.

Understanding of the basic mechanisms of pathogenesis is important for the design of new or improved vaccines and appropriate therapies. Such knowledge is also invaluable in the analysis of 'new' bacterial pathogens that are recognized from time to time. However, for some bacterial diseases, e.g. syphilis, such approaches have still not defined the mechanisms of pathogenesis or the virulence determinants involved, and new strategies employed by such successful pathogens may yet be discovered.

Botulism results from the ingestion of preformed toxin produced by *Clostridium botulinum* in food contaminated with this bacterium, and is not a true infectious disease. The toxic activity is due to a family of serologically distinct polypeptide neurotoxins that prevent release of acetylcholine at neuromuscular junctions, resulting in the symptoms of flaccid paralysis. These toxins have been used clinically in treating squints and muscle spasm.

Other toxins cause disseminated multisystem organ damage. Such pathology is seen in staphylococcal

RECOMMENDED READING

Alouf J E, Freer J H 1999 *Bacterial protein toxins*. 2nd edn. Academic Press, London
Mims C, Nash A, Stephen J 2000 *Mims' Pathogenesis of Infectious Disease* 5th edn. Academic Press, London.
Ofek I, Doyle R J 1994 *Bacterial Adhesion to Cells and Tissues*. Chapman and Hall, London

Patrick S, Larkin M J 1995 *Immunological and Molecular Aspects of Bacterial Virulence*. Wiley, Chichester
Salyers A A, Whitt D D 2002 *Bacterial Pathogenesis: a Molecular Approach*. 2nd edn. ASM Press, Washington
Williams P, Ketley J, Salmond G 1998 *Bacterial Pathogenesis* Vol. 28 Academic Press, London

9

Virus–cell interactions

M. Norval

Viruses are totally dependent on the cells they infect to provide the energy, metabolic intermediates and most, in some cases all, of the enzymes required for their replication. With advances in the techniques of molecular virology and modelling, together with the classical methods of electron microscopy, titration and biochemical assay, it has become possible to study virus–cell interactions to a sophisticated level. The picture that has emerged, and is still emerging, is a fascinating one, as viruses are found to associate with, and affect, cells in a wide variety of ways. The range of possible interactions is indicated in Table 9.1. It is possible to divide these into three broad categories that show considerable overlap:

1. Viruses that infect and replicate within cells causing the cells to lyse when the progeny virions are released. This is called a *cytolytic cycle*, the infection is *productive* and the cell culture demonstrates *cytopathic effects*, which are often characteristic of the infecting virus. The host cells are termed *permissive*. In some instances viruses are produced from the infected cells but the cells are not killed by the process, i.e. the infection is *productive* but *non-cytolytic*, and may become *persistent*.

2. Viruses that infect cells but which do not complete the replication cycle. Thus the infection is called *abortive* or *non-productive*. Abortive infections can be due to a mutation in the virus so that some essential function is lost, or to the production of defective interfering particles, or to the action of interferons. It may be

possible to manipulate the conditions in vitro to obtain a *steady state* or *persistent infection* in which infected and uninfected cells coexist and there is some, generally limited, virus production.

3. Viruses that enter cells but are not produced by the infected cell. The virus is maintained within the cell in the form of DNA, which replicates in association with the host cell DNA. The host cell is termed *non-permissive* and the infection is *non-productive*. Occasionally this type of interaction induces cell *transformation*. In other cases a *latent infection* may result in which very little or no viral gene expression occurs and the cell retains its normal properties.

THE LYTIC OR CYTOCIDAL GROWTH CYCLE

While there are large differences in the details of the lytic growth cycle depending on the virus studied and to some extent on the host cell, certain features are common, and a simplified description will be given first. The quantitative aspects of virion production were determined initially using bacteriophages but have now been ascertained for many animal viruses growing in vitro in cell culture. A one-step growth curve is obtained when samples are removed from an infected cell culture at intervals and assayed for the total content of infectious virus after artificial lysis of the cells (Fig. 9.1).

In the early part of the cycle, virus particles come into contact with the cells, and may then *attach* or *adsorb* to them. This marks the start of the *eclipse phase*. The virion then *penetrates* into the host cell and is partially *uncoated* to reveal the viral genome. *Macromolecular synthesis* of viral components follows. Often this can be divided into *early* and *late phases* separated by the replication of the viral nucleic acid. Early messenger RNA (mRNA) is first transcribed and translated into proteins. These are frequently non-structural proteins and enzymes required to undertake nucleic acid synthesis and the later stages of replication. Viral nucleic acid is

Table 9.1 The range of virus–cell interactions	
Type of infection/effect on cells	Comment
Cytolytic	Virus produced
Non-cytolytic (persistent)	Virus produced
Abortive	Virus not produced
Abortive (persistent)	Virus produced
Latency (persistent)	Viral nucleic acid present
Transformation (persistent)	Viral nucleic acid present

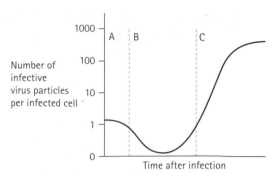

Fig. 9.1 Lytic growth cycle of a virus. Samples are removed from the infected culture at intervals and assayed for the total content of virus. Phase A, adsorption; phase B, eclipse; phase C, assembly and release.

then produced, followed by late mRNA transcription and translation. Most proteins made at this stage are structural ones, and will make up part of the final virion. The eclipse phase ends with the *assembly* and *release* of newly formed virus particles. The cycle is shown in diagrammatic form in Fig. 9.2, and can vary from as little as 8 h for some picornaviruses to more than 40 h for cytomegalovirus, a human herpesvirus.

Attachment (adsorption)

The initial interaction is by random collision, and depends on the relative concentrations of virus particles and cells. The ionic composition of the culture medium is an important factor as both viruses and cells are negatively charged at neutral pH and would tend to repel each other. The presence of cations, such as Mg^{2+}, there-fore helps to promote close contact. Adsorption then takes place through a *specific binding site* on the virus and a *receptor* on the plasma membrane of the cell. It is largely temperature- and energy-independent.

Viruses vary widely in the range of cells to which they can adsorb, depending on the nature of the site to which they attach and how widespread it is amongst cells of different types, tissues and species. Some examples are shown in Table 9.2. Most cellular receptors are glycoproteins, and the number expressed in different cell types and tissues may be a factor in determining susceptibility, i.e. the capacity of a cell or animal to become infected with a particular virus, and symptoms. The number of receptors per cell is generally several thousand. The expression of the receptors may change if the cells are cultured in vitro. Thus, monkey kidney cells are commonly used for the growth of poliovirus in vitro although this virus does not affect the kidney in vivo in infected monkeys. With some viruses, the requirement for specific receptors can be bypassed, experimentally at least, by infection with extracted viral nucleic acid. Cells that are normally resistant can therefore become infected.

Rabies virus binds to the acetylcholine receptor found on neurones. Orthomyxoviruses and paramyxoviruses have envelope glycoproteins protruding from the surface of the virion which have specific binding sites for the oligosaccharide side-chains of glycoproteins or glycolipids terminating in *N*-acetylneuraminic acid (sialic acid). These are found on the membranes of most cells. The haemagglutinin consists of trimers of two polypeptides, HA_1 and HA_2, and the binding site for sialic acid is located on the globular part of HA_1, which is furthest from the envelope of the virus. Poliovirus, a picornavirus, infects only primate cells, and only those of the

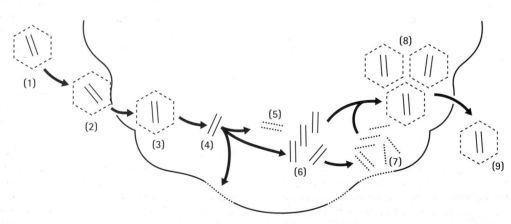

Fig. 9.2 A simplified viral replication cycle showing a hypothetical virus particle (1) attaching to the surface of a susceptible cell (2), penetrating into the cell (3), being uncoated (4), undergoing early transcription and translation (5), then replication of the viral nucleic acid (6), late transcription and translation (7), and, finally, assembly of new virus particles (8) and release from the cell (9).

Table 9.2 Examples of known viral receptors

Virus	Receptor	Distribution
Epstein–Barr virus	CD21 (complement receptor)	B cells, epithelial cells
Human herpesvirus 6	CD46 (regulator of complement activation)	Widely distributed
HIV	CD4 with chemokine receptor	T cells, monocytes, dendritic cells
Measles virus		
Wild	CDw150 (lymphocyte activation)	Some T and B cells
Vaccine	CD46	Widely distributed
Parvovirus B19	P antigen (globoside)	Red blood cells
Poliovirus	Immunoglobulin-like receptor	Widely distributed
Rhinoviruses	Major: intercellular adhesion molecules	Endothelial cells, activated cells
	Minor: low density lipoprotein	Widely distributed

central nervous system or the intestine. The receptor in this case is a member of the immunoglobulin gene superfamily coded by a gene on the human chromosome 19. It has been estimated that there are up to 3×10^3 such receptor sites per cell. The attachment is through an arrangement of the structural proteins VP1, VP2 and VP3 of the virus. Many members of the rhinovirus group also use one of the immunoglobulin gene superfamily proteins as a receptor; in this case intercellular adhesion molecule-1 (ICAM-1), a ligand important in the adhesion of leucocytes. Epstein–Barr virus infects human B lymphocytes and epithelial cells, and is largely selective for them due to the expression in mature B cells of a receptor for one of the complement cleavage fragments to which the virus binds. The attachment of human immunodeficiency virus (HIV) to cells is mediated by the interaction between a glycoprotein, gp120, in the viral envelope and CD4 antigen expressed on T helper cells, monocytes and some dendritic cells. Several co-receptors for HIV have been identified which are members of the chemokine receptor family.

Recent knowledge regarding the details of HIV entry in particular has led to the concept that some cell surface molecules, in addition to the receptor, may be required by many viruses to complete the entry stage of the replication cycle. Indeed, it is likely that there is a complex interaction between different functional domains of the virus and several receptor arrays. First there is the attachment step whereby the virus binds to the receptor, and then entry itself may involve a different set of receptors. For example, cell-bound heparan sulphate acts as an attachment receptor for HIV and the entry receptor, as noted above, is CD4, together with the chemokine receptor acting as co-receptor. This more complicated view of the initial contact between the virus and the cell suggests that the attachment receptor may not be the only determinant of tissue tropism. An illustration is provided by the distribution of ICAM-1 which is broader than the tropism of the rhinoviruses using this molecule as a receptor.

Penetration (uptake)

Penetration occurs immediately after adsorption and, unlike adsorption, requires energy and does not proceed at 0°C. Despite much study, it is still not clear how many viruses enter cells, particularly in vivo, and, furthermore, which route of entry leads to a successful infection. There are probably two main mechanisms.

1. Receptor-mediated endocytosis

This method is used by both enveloped and non-enveloped viruses, and is essentially the same as the normal uptake of macromolecules bound to cell surface receptors. Receptors with adsorbed virus particles move together (patch) to pits coated with clathrin, before moving into the cytosol to form small uncoated vesicles which then fuse together as endosomes. A proton pump in the endosome lowers the pH to about 5. For enveloped viruses, this change causes a rearrangement of the hydrophobic components of selected viral polypeptides leading to their fusion with the endosome membrane. Thus the viral nucleocapsid is released into the cytosol. The endosomes combine with lysosomes, which eventually cause degradation of any viral components contained within. This process is outlined in Fig. 9.3. In the case of influenza virus, a part of the haemagglutinin (the hydrophobic amino (N)-terminal of HA_2) is responsible for the fusion, the fusion sequence being activated by the low pH of the endosome. There is also a contribution from M_2, another membrane glycoprotein of the virus, which forms an ion channel at low pH and allows the liberation of the ribonucleoproteins from the virions into the cytoplasm. Non-enveloped viruses also enter by receptor-mediated endocytosis, but the end-point is not fusion and is ill-defined, as yet. In adenoviruses, a viral protein may be activated at low pH, capable of lysing the endosomal membrane. In other viruses, proteolytic cleavage of the capsid may occur, thus activating a viral

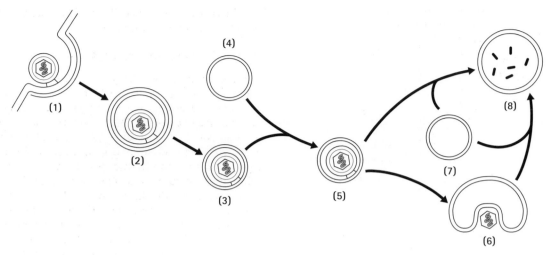

Fig. 9.3 Receptor-mediated endocytosis of an enveloped virus. The virus attaches to specific receptors on the cell membrane (1), which patch at coated pits before being pinched off to form vesicles (2). These lose their coat (3) and fuse with other vesicles (4) to form endosomes (5). At the acid pH of endosomes, fusion of the viral envelope and the endosome membrane occurs, releasing the virus into the cytosol (6). (7) Fusion of the endosome with lysosomes leads to the final degradation of viral components and their return to the surface (8).

component, which may then lyse or permeabilize the endosomal membrane.

2. Fusion with the plasma membrane

This mechanism is used only by certain enveloped viruses, including some paramyxoviruses, retroviruses and herpesviruses. It requires the presence of a specific viral protein in the envelope that facilitates the fusion between the envelope and the plasma membrane at physiological pH. Subsequently there is release of the nucleocapsid into the cytosol. One example of such a protein is the F (fusion) protein of measles virus, which is activated following attachment of the virus to the cell membrane via the haemagglutinin glycoprotein. The cellular receptor may be internalized following fusion.

Uncoating

Uncoating can take place at several stages and sites in the cell. Some viruses, such as the rhinoviruses, undergo conformational changes on attachment which result in the opening of the capsid and release of selected viral proteins and the viral nucleic acid into the cell. Those enveloped viruses entering by receptor-mediated endocytosis may be affected by the low pH and the action of lysosomal enzymes. Uncoating can also be found in the cytosol and, in the case of some DNA viruses such as herpes simplex virus, this stage occurs at the nuclear pore, allowing the viral DNA to enter the nucleus thereafter. Reoviruses never fully uncoat, the viral genome remaining within a recognizable capsid structure.

Poxviruses become uncoated in two stages. In the first, the outer layers and lateral bodies are removed within endosomal vesicles using host enzymes, and the core lies in the cytosol. Poxviruses carry their own DNA-dependent RNA polymerase, and this enzyme is used in the second stage to transcribe mRNA, which is translated into a special uncoating protein; this enables the final release of viral DNA from the core.

Following uncoating, it is necessary for the viral nucleic acid with, in some instances, viral enzymes or proteins from the capsid to proceed to the correct site in the cell to commence synthesis of the macromolecules which will comprise the new virions. In some cases this happens entirely in the cytosol, e.g. poliovirus; others replicate in the nucleus, e.g. herpesviruses, while a third category has nuclear and cytoplasmic stages, e.g. influenza viruses. In most instances it is not known how the transport is controlled although an important role for the cytoskeleton has been proposed.

Synthesis of viral components

The nucleic acid in viruses is either single- or double-stranded, circular or linear, in one piece or segmented. In addition, viruses vary enormously in their complexity, ranging from those with nucleic acid sufficient to code for only a few proteins, such as the papovaviruses, up to those coding for several hundred proteins, such as the poxviruses. Although every virus has a unique method of replicating and has a strict temporal control on the synthesis of components, each must present functional mRNA to the cell, so that new virally encoded polypep-

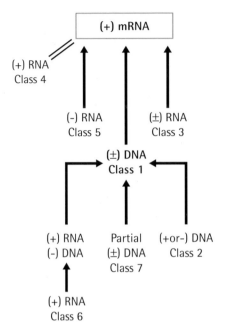

Fig. 9.4 Division of animal viruses into seven classes, based on mechanisms of transcription.

tides and nucleic acid can be synthesized using the normal cellular processes. Thus, only viruses that contain DNA and replicate in the nucleus can use solely cellular enzymes for transcription and translation. All other viruses must synthesize their mRNA by processes other than those found in uninfected cells. Seven different classes, six of which were first described by Baltimore in 1970, can be distinguished (Fig. 9.4). Conventionally in the scheme, nucleic acid of the same polarity or sense as mRNA is called 'positive' (+), while that of the opposite polarity or anti-sense is called 'negative' (−). Rather than

be exhaustive, one or two illustrative examples from each class will now be described.

Class 1. Double-stranded DNA viruses

This comprises a very large group of viruses which contain double-stranded DNA in a linear, e.g. herpesviruses, adenoviruses and poxviruses, or a circular form, e.g. papovaviruses. The poxviruses can be divided from the others as their replication takes place entirely in the cytoplasm, and they can code for all the factors required for their own transcription and genomic replication. In the remaining double-stranded DNA viruses, replication occurs in the nucleus and is dependent to some extent on host cell factors. Herpes simplex virus is used as an example (Fig. 9.5). After uncoating at the nuclear pore, the viral nucleic acid enters the nucleus and, using the normal host cell mechanisms of transcription and translation, three groups of viral polypeptides are synthesized in a strict temporal fashion. They are called immediate early (α), early (β) and late (γ). A component in the virus particle (α-TIF, a γ protein), acting as a transactivator, induces the transcription of the first set of mRNAs. A second component of the viral tegument called VHS inhibits host cell macromolecular synthesis, and all the metabolic energy of the cell is turned towards the production of new virus particles. The genes coding for the α, β and γ proteins have been mapped on the genome, and, while the β and γ genes tend to be scattered, the α genes are located together. Amongst the early gene products are thymidine kinase and a virus-specific DNA polymerase. Most of the late proteins are structural proteins, and they inhibit the synthesis of the α and β proteins. Between β and γ protein synthesis, new viral DNA begins to be made, probably by circularization using a rolling circle model.

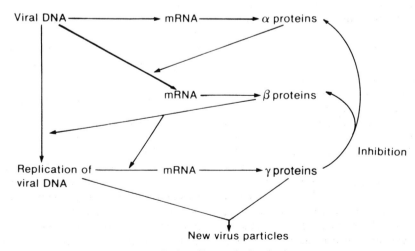

Fig. 9.5 Diagram of macromolecular synthesis during the replication of herpes simplex virus.

Class 2. Single-stranded DNA viruses

Parvoviruses comprise the sole family in this group. They are small, with DNA of molecular weight about 2×10^6. Some parvoviruses contain DNA of '–' polarity, and grow only in rapidly dividing cells; others contain either '+' or '–' DNA, and depend on co-infection with a helper virus for their replication. Parvoviruses use the cellular DNA polymerases to make the viral genome double-stranded, called the replicative form. Priming is by the viral nucleic acid itself forming a loop at the 3′ terminus. This is followed by displacement of the parental DNA strand and synthesis of more DNA complementary to the template strand. Messenger RNAs are made using the appropriate DNA strand as the template, and are translated into viral proteins (Fig. 9.6).

Class 3. Double-stranded RNA viruses

In this group are found the reoviruses and rotaviruses. All members have segmented genomes, and each RNA segment codes for a single polypeptide. Replication of viral nucleic acid, transcription and translation occur solely in the cytoplasm without nuclear involvement at any stage. The virus carries its own RNA-dependent RNA polymerase, an enzyme unique to some RNA viruses and not found in uninfected cells. It enables the transcription of one strand (–) into mRNAs, subsequently translated into viral proteins. The transcription is thus asymmetric and conservative, i.e. only mRNAs are formed, and the parental duplex is not broken apart. Each mRNA is later encapsidated and copied once to form double-stranded molecules (Fig. 9.7). Several hours pass between the '+' and '–' strands of the new virus particles being synthesized. Thus the replication of the double-stranded DNA and RNA viruses is very different.

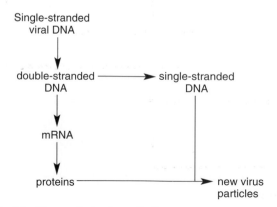

Fig. 9.6 Diagram of parvovirus replication.

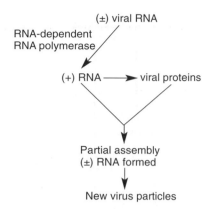

Fig. 9.7 Diagram of double-stranded RNA virus replication.

Class 4. '+' single-stranded RNA viruses

This class comprises a large group of viruses containing RNA of the same polarity as mRNA. Because they code for all the proteins they require during replication, the viral RNA extracted from the virions is infectious by itself. Poliovirus falls into this category, and is used as an example (Fig. 9.8). Macromolecular synthesis of viral components occurs entirely in the cytoplasm. Following entry of poliovirus into the cell, the viral RNA binds to ribosomes, acts as mRNA and is translated in its entirety into one large polypeptide. This is then proteolytically cleaved to give as products RNA polymerase and protease enzymes and new capsid proteins. Using the polymerase enzyme, '–'-strand RNA is synthesized with the genomic RNA as the template, and a temporary double-stranded RNA is formed, called the replicative intermediate. The replicative intermediate consists of complete '+' RNA and numerous partially completed '–' strands. When the '–' strands are ready, they can be used as templates to make more '+'-strand RNA. This is required as genomic RNA for assembly into new virus particles and for transcription into more viral proteins. At the same time as viral replication, host cell protein synthesis and RNA synthesis are inhibited. Initiation of translation of cellular mRNA requires the participation of a cap-binding protein at the 5′ end. Poliovirus induces the cleavage of this protein, and thus halts the synthesis of cellular proteins. The RNA genome of poliovirus does not have such a cap although it has a small protein, called VPg, at the 5′ end. A special region near the 5′ end of the genome directs cap-independent initiation of protein synthesis. Complex interactions between viral and cellular proteins are thought to determine how much viral RNA is used for new virus particles or is translated into protein. The capsid of poliovirus consists of 60 copies of each of four proteins, VP1, VP2, VP3 and VP4, forming the

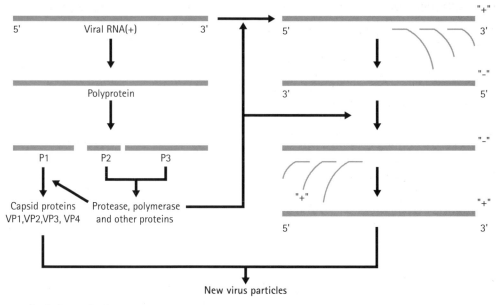

Fig. 9.8   Diagram of poliovirus replication.

icosahedron. One of the first cleavages of the polyprotein produces VP1, which is then broken into VP0, VP3 and VP1. Finally, on assembly, VP0 is cleaved into VP4 and VP2, a process catalysed by VP0 itself.

Class 5. '–' single-stranded RNA viruses

Viruses of this group have single-stranded RNA of '–' polarity, and all must carry their own RNA transcriptase complex to be infectious, as the normal cellular

enzymes are unable to replicate RNA. Influenza virus is an example (Fig. 9.9). It contains eight segments of '–'-strand RNA, plus the RNA transcriptase complex within each virus particle. After entry into the cell by receptor-mediated endocytosis, transcription to viral mRNA occurs in the nucleus. Influenza virus is the only '–'-strand RNA virus to replicate in the nucleus. To initiate transcription, a nucleotide sequence of about 10–13 bases, found at the 5′ end of the cellular mRNAs and already capped, is used. This is cleaved from cellular

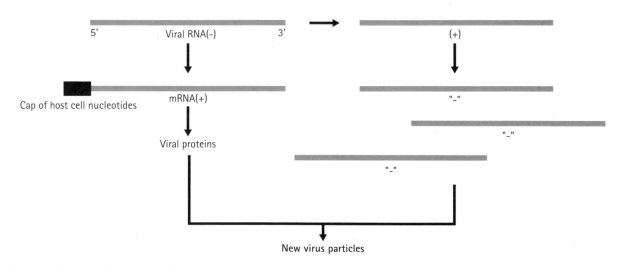

Fig. 9.9   Diagram of influenza virus replication.

mRNAs by an endonuclease activity of the viral RNA transcriptase complex. Thus all the viral mRNAs have a 5′-terminal segment of the host cell mRNA. Once the mRNAs have been generated, they are translated into polypeptides. Each genomic segment produces one mRNA, translated into one polypeptide except in two instances where, by RNA splicing of the original transcript, more than one mRNA is produced and therefore more than one protein. Unlike the transcription of mRNAs, the production of '+'-strand RNAs, required as intermediates to make the progeny '−'-strand RNAs, proceeds without the need for primers. There is much trafficking of viral polypeptides in the cell; the haemagglutinin, neuraminidase and M_2 protein are inserted in the plasma membrane, and the M_1 protein below this point on the membrane, while the nucleocapsid assembles around the viral RNAs in the nucleus.

Class 6. Retroviruses

Viruses of this group are unique as they contain single-stranded RNA (in the form of two identical subunits), yet they replicate via an integrated double-stranded DNA stage. Retroviruses are the only such family and the virus particles contain a reverse transcriptase complex, with RNA-dependent DNA polymerase activity, from which the name 'retrovirus' is derived. This enzyme is not found in normal cells. Following entry, synthesis of DNA complementary to the viral RNA occurs using the reverse transcriptase, originating at a primer binding site near the 5′ end of the viral genome. The primer is a specific transfer RNA (tRNA); for example tRNA^{lys} in human immunodeficiency virus. Transcription proceeds towards the 5′ end, and is probably continued by a jump across to the 3′ end of the same molecule. In addition to RNA-dependent DNA polymerase activity, the reverse transcriptase complex has ribonuclease (RNAase) H activity, i.e. it is able to digest RNA from a DNA–RNA hybrid (Fig. 9.10). The resulting single-stranded DNA is then made double stranded, using the reverse transcriptase as enzyme and starting from a purine-rich sequence. Thus, a linear double-stranded DNA form is produced, first found in the cytoplasm. The viral RNA has a short sequence of about 12–235 bases repeated at each end. During replication there is generation of a longer repeat sequence, from 250 to 1000 nucleotides, at both ends of the DNA molecule. This is called the *long terminal repeat*; it contains the enhancer and promoter sequences controlling the expression of the viral genome as well as the sequence for the initiation of transcription. The linear double-stranded DNA is able to circularize, and is found in this form in the nucleus. The next step is integration of the circular DNA into the host cell DNA. This is catalysed by an integrase carried by the virion. It is thought that the circular viral DNA is cleaved leaving staggered ends, and the cellular DNA similarly, to allow insertion of the viral DNA into the cellular DNA; the viral DNA is now called a *provirus*. The site of insertion is not thought to be specific. The provirus is colinear

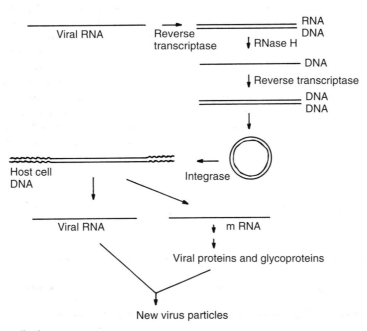

Fig. 9.10 Diagram of retrovirus replication.

with the original viral genome, and is always flanked by a 4–6-base pair direct repeat of the host DNA: this repeat is also found flanking transposons. The integrated state is a stable one and, as the DNA of the cell is replicated during cell growth, so the viral DNA is also replicated. Integration can result, on occasion, in cell transformation (see below). The replication cycle is completed using the normal cellular RNA polymerase II to synthesize viral RNA and viral mRNAs, which are translated into polyproteins and processed into the final proteins found in the virus particle. A viral protease is responsible for many of these cleavages. The control of this stage is complex.

Class 7. Partial double-stranded DNA viruses

Hepadnaviruses are unique amongst the animal viruses in containing partial double-stranded DNA and in replicating via an RNA intermediate, as shown in Fig 9.11. One example of this group is hepatitis B virus. The first stage in the replication cycle is the production of fully double-stranded DNA, which occurs in the nucleus, followed by the synthesis of single-stranded positive-sense RNA using the cellular DNA-dependent RNA polymerase. The RNA is transported into the cytoplasm and is translated into the core protein which encapsidates the RNA, together with newly synthesized viral RNA-dependent DNA polymerase (reverse transcriptase). Then, using this enzyme, a complementary negative strand of DNA is made, while the RNA is degraded. The DNA is next transcribed into positive-sense DNA, and is found as partial double-stranded DNA in the new virus particles.

Assembly and release

Following synthesis of viral proteins and viral nucleic acid, there is a stage of assembly called *morphogenesis*, followed by *release* of virus particles, the productive phase of the infection. The release is either through *cell lysis*, or through *budding* without cell death in many instances. The former method is used by non-enveloped icosahedral viruses, and the latter by enveloped viruses. There is also some evidence for active release without cell lysis for some non-enveloped viruses. Generally the components which will constitute the new virions are produced in high quantities, and the assembly process is probably rather inefficient.

Viruses that are released by killing the cell depend on the cell disintegrating to let them out. For this type of virus, morphogenesis may occur spontaneously once the capsid proteins have been made, the specificity depending on the amino acid sequence of the proteins. Thus the structural proteins of the viruses can form capsomeres by themselves, which then aggregate to form the procapsid, a structure without nucleic acid. Often there is proteolytic cleavage of a capsid protein to form the final virus particle, as has been described for poliovirus. The precise nature of the interaction between the nucleic acid and the structural proteins that make up the capsid is not known, despite extensive study. It is possible that the viral nucleic acid is inserted into the procapsid through a pore, or it might cause a structural reorientation of the procapsid, thereby becoming internalized. Alternatively, the capsomeres may accumulate around a condensed core of nucleic acid as the nucleic acid is being synthesized.

The second method of assembly and release is by budding. This can take place through the plasma membrane, thus releasing the virions from the cell e.g. orthomyxoviruses and retroviruses (Fig. 9.12), or through internal membranes, such as the inner nuclear membrane in the case of the herpesviruses (Fig. 9.13b), followed by fusion of the vesicles containing the viruses with the plasma membrane. Envelope glycoproteins specified by the virus are synthesized by essentially the same mechanism as cellular membrane glycoproteins. The viral proteins destined to become envelope proteins contain a sequence of 15–30 hydrophobic amino acids known as the signal sequence. This sequence binds the growing polypeptide chain to a receptor on the cytoplasmic side of the rough endoplasmic reticulum and

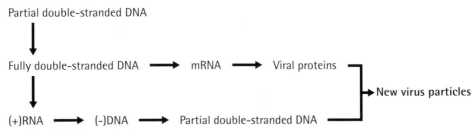

Fig. 9.11 Diagram of hepatitis B virus replication.

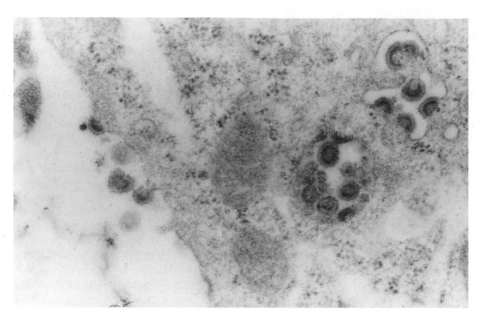

Fig. 9.12 Budding of retroviruses. ×70 000.

enables its passage through the membrane. Glycosylation occurs in the lumen of the rough endoplasmic reticulum, and the proteins are transported to the Golgi apparatus. There they are further glycosylated and acylated before transport to the plasma membrane, the direction probably determined by a sorting signal in the polypeptide sequence. In some cases, the signal directs the viral glycoprotein to one surface of the cell only, e.g. orthomyxoviruses bud only from the outer (apical) surface of epithelial cells, while rhabdoviruses bud only from the inner (basal) surface. The viral glycoproteins are very important in terms of antigenicity as the hydrophilic domains protrude from the surface of the cell, with the N terminus being furthest away, and change its surface structure significantly. They remain anchored in the membrane via a hydrophobic domain near the carboxyl (C) terminus. After insertion into the membrane, the viral glycoproteins accumulate together to form oligomers; at the same time the host cell glycoproteins move away. At the C terminus there is frequently a short hydrophilic sequence which remains inside the cell and is assumed to interact with the internal components of the virus during assembly. The nucleocapsid becomes engulfed by the membrane, forming a bud that matures and eventually pinches off. In some cases, a final cleavage of the glycoprotein is required to make the virus infectious. For example, the haemagglutinin H_0 of influenza virus is cleaved into two peptides, HA_1 and HA_2, linked by disulphide bridges.

Several thousand virus particles can be produced per infected cell, although this number varies considerably with virus type and host cell type. The budding viruses tend to be released slowly over several hours, while the lytic ones are released together. Only a few of the newly formed virus particles are infectious, as indicated by a high ratio of particles to infectious virions. Presumably most do not have the correct complement of proteins, enzymes or viral nucleic acid, or have been assembled incorrectly.

Evidence has accumulated in recent years to indicate that, for some viruses at least, perturbation of the normal cell metabolism during replication can stimulate cell death by *apoptosis*. Several virus-specific factors have been identified as inducers of apoptosis, such as by causing DNA strand breaks in the case of a parvovirus, by stabilization of the tumour suppressor gene product p53 in the case of Epstein–Barr virus, or by receptor signalling in the case of HIV. The advantage to the virus could be that the spread of the infection is enhanced as the entire cellular contents, including the progeny viruses, are packaged into membrane-bound apoptotic bodies that are then taken up by adjacent cells. In contrast, other viral proteins have been revealed which block or delay apoptosis, presumably until sufficient progeny viruses have been produced within the cells. In this case, the factors target specific stages of the apoptotic pathway. For example, caspases are inhibited during poxvirus infections, the action of interferon is downregulated during influenza virus infections and p53 is destroyed during some human papillomavirus infections. Therefore the susceptibility of the host cell to apoptosis depends on the acute-death pathways in the cell itself and the range of apoptotic modulators induced by the infecting viruses.

Microscopy of infected cells

It is possible to observe effects on the host cell microscopically. In the first place there may be morphological changes called *inclusion bodies* in the infected cell, seen by altered staining behaviour. The inclusion bodies are nuclear or cytoplasmic and vary in their composition. They can consist of viral factories where morphogenesis occurs, crystalline arrays of virus particles ready for release, over-production of a particular viral protein or proteins, or some aberrant cellular structure, such as clumped chromatin. Some inclusion bodies are shown in Fig. 9.13. Secondly, the cells may be killed by the viral infection. There are several possible reasons for this, including factors produced by the virus which induce apoptosis (see section above). It is likely

that the accumulation of viral structural proteins is toxic for the cells in some cases. In addition, some viruses, such as herpes simplex virus and the poxviruses, inhibit host cell macromolecular synthesis from an early stage in the replication cycle which leads to structural and functional damage. Plasma membrane function and permeability change, and lysosomal membranes begin to break down, allowing leakage of the contents with degradative activity into the cytoplasm. There may also be marked effects on the cyto-skeleton. These changes lead to a *cytopathic effect*, clearly seen in cell culture. It can take several forms, one of the commonest being *cell rounding* and subsequent detachment from the solid surface (Fig. 9.14b). Another is the formation of a *syncytium*, where the membranes of adjacent infected cells fuse and a giant cell is formed containing many nuclei (Fig. 9.14c). In some cases, the nuclei fuse to make hybrid cells, a property that used to be exploited in monoclonal antibody production.

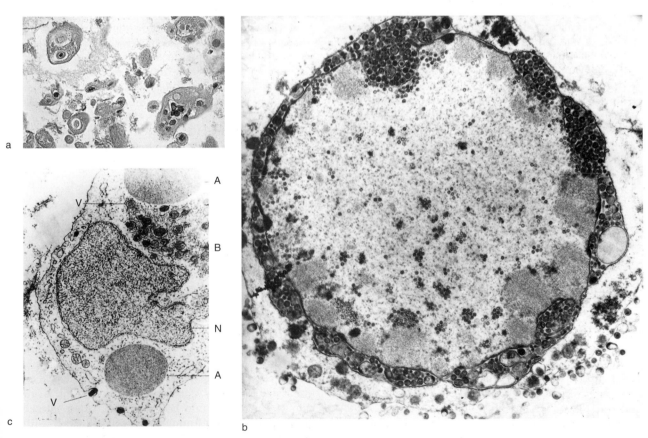

Fig. 9.13 Effects of viruses on cells. **a** Light microscopy of a skin lesion due to herpesvirus to show cell fusion and intranuclear inclusions (Cowdry type A). ×60. **b** Electron micrograph of a cell infected with herpes simplex virus. Assembly of capsids within nucleus – enveloped virus between layers of nuclear membrane. ×9000. **c** Type A (accumulation of viral protein) and type B (virus factory) inclusions (identified as A and B, respectively) in the cytoplasm of a poxvirus-infected cell. V, virus; N, the cell nucleus. ×700.

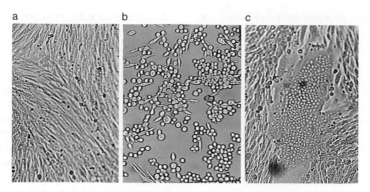

Fig. 9.14 Cytopathic effects: **a** uninfected fibroblast cells; **b** cell rounding due to herpes simplex virus; **c** syncytium formation or cell fusion due to respiratory syncytial virus. All unstained. ×65.

NON-CYTOCIDAL PRODUCTIVE INFECTIONS

Some viruses are able to infect cells productively but the cells are not killed by the replication process. Viruses that are released by budding frequently come into this category. The cell type used for the infection is critical, and, presumably, any inhibitory effect of the virus on the cellular metabolism does not take place. This type of interaction may lead to a *persistent infection* in which infected cells and viruses coexist over a long period of time. There will, however, be antigenic changes in the infected cells, often the insertion of viral glycoproteins in the plasma membrane. This can be exploited for the detection of a virus; e.g. if influenza virus is cultured in monkey kidney cells, virus is produced from the cells but there is no immediate cytopathic effect. However, there is insertion of viral haemagglutinin into the plasma membrane during replication. Thus, when red blood cells of certain species are added to the infected cells, they adhere to the haemagglutinin and can be seen microscopically. This phenomenon is called *haemadsorption*.

ABORTIVE (NON-PRODUCTIVE) INFECTIONS

Some viruses are unable to infect cells because they cannot adsorb to them; the cells are therefore called *resistant*. In other cases viruses are able to infect cells but are not produced from them; the infection is therefore called *non-productive* or *abortive*, and the cells are *non-permissive*. Often there is a block on one stage of the replication cycle due to the absence of a cellular function essential for viral replication. The same interaction can also occur in a permissive cell if the viral genome itself is *defective* in some way, so that the replication cannot be completed. This can happen in two ways.

- First the virus is too small to code for all the proteins required in replication. An example is provided by the adeno-associated viruses belonging to the Parvoviridae family. They are unable to replicate on their own but depend on a second 'helper' virus infecting the same cell and providing the essential function that they lack. Adenoviruses act as the helper viruses and are thought to activate transcription of the parvovirus genome in the infected cell.
- Secondly, abortive infections can arise due to viral mutation. In fact, only a few amino acid substitutions in selected proteins of the virus can change the nature of a lytic infection. In some cases the non-productive infection can be converted into a persistent one where new virus particles are synthesized: three examples follow.

Temperature-sensitive mutants

Here the wild-type virus has mutated to produce a variant – a temperature-sensitive (ts) mutant – lacking an essential gene function at the *non-permissive temperature*, normally above 38°C. This is thought to be due to the thermal instability of the secondary or tertiary structure of a particular protein. The temperature can be lowered, generally to below 35°C, to a level called *permissive* where the defect is no longer functional and the infection becomes productive. However, ts mutants tend to be less cytopathic than the wild type, even at permissive temperatures, probably because they synthesize less mRNA and protein. Thus, within a cell culture, a persistent infection can result with a balance between infected and uninfected cells together with virus production. Ts mutants have been used to identify the gene responsible for a particular replication step and to map where functions lie on the viral genome. It is possible to place ts mutants into complementation groups where, at the non-permissive temperature, the defect in one ts mutant is compensated for by a second ts mutant with a defect in a different gene.

Defective interfering particles

It has been known for many years that, if cells are infected at high multiplicity, then, amongst the progeny, there will be a number of virus particles with genomes shorter than normal, containing at least one deletion – so-called defective interfering particles (DIPs). Thus these particles are not able to replicate themselves although they are able to infect new cells. However, they can replicate in the presence of helper virus, often the parental virus, which compensates for the lack of a particular gene or gene cluster in the DIPs. The DIPs retain an origin of replication and the ability to form capsids. One of their important properties is that they *interfere* with the replication of normal parental viruses because, firstly, it requires less time and energy to replicate the defective genome compared with the full-length genome and, secondly, the transcriptase complex has a greater affinity for the defective genome than the full-length one. Hence DIPs, as their numbers increase, have a greater and greater effect on the replication of parental virus. It is possible to obtain an in-vitro cell culture in which infected and uninfected cells together with infectious virus and DIPs are in balance over a prolonged period of time. Thus a steady state exists and the infection is persistent.

Abortive infections maintained by interferons

The final example of abortive infections arises due to the action of *interferons* in infected cell cultures. Interferons are produced from virally infected cells and can protect other cells from attack by viruses. These molecules, of α or β types, inhibit various stages of the viral replication cycle, especially polypeptide synthesis (see Chapter 12 for details). In cell culture, persistent infections can be obtained where the antiviral effects of interferons protect sufficient cells from the cytolytic effects of viral replication to allow cells and viruses to coexist.

LATENCY

Latency represents a type of persistence where the virus is present in the form of its genome only and there is limited expression of viral genes, occasionally as mRNA only and not at the level of protein. The genome is found either integrated into the host cell chromosome or as a circular non-integrated episome. It is maintained throughout cell division when the host cell replicates. Latent infections are more common with DNA viruses than RNA viruses, perhaps because no mechanisms exist to maintain RNA for long periods of time intracellularly. One example of latency is provided by Epstein–Barr virus, which persists in B lymphocytes as episomal viral DNA with limited transcription of viral genes, probably around 11 protein products being expressed. For herpes simplex virus during latency in neuronal cells, no viral proteins are detected and only a few RNA transcripts from one part of the viral genome, called latency-associated transcripts. In some cases, specific stimuli trigger the *reactivation* of the virus from the latent state, and the infection becomes productive.

TRANSFORMATION

In this type of virus–cell interaction, the virus infects the cell non-productively, and is found in the form of viral DNA, either integrated in the host cell DNA, or non-integrated, or in both states. The properties of the cells are changed dramatically, a process called *transformation*. Transformed cells have similar properties to tumour cells, and a detailed study of the mechanism of viral transformation has led to increased understanding of the molecular basis of cancer. Only members of some virus families are able to transform cells. These include herpesviruses, adenoviruses, hepadnaviruses, papovaviruses and poxviruses of the DNA viruses, and, of the RNA viruses, only retroviruses. The type of cell infected and the species are also important. It should be noted that transformation is a rare event: at most only 1 in 10^5 cells infected by a particular virus will become transformed.

Some of the main properties of transformed cells that distinguish them from normal cells are listed below:

- loss of contact inhibition of growth
- can grow to high saturation density
- less requirement for serum factors
- indefinite number of cell divisions
- viral antigens expressed
- fibronectin absent
- fetal antigens often found
- changes in agglutinability by plant lectins
- induction of tumours in experimental animals.

One of the most striking changes is the loss of contact inhibition of growth, so that cells which normally grow in an ordered fashion beside their neighbours and stop dividing when they touch each other, now grow on top of each other and lose their orientation with respect to each other (Fig. 9.15). As a result they reach much higher densities. They have less requirement for serum factors in

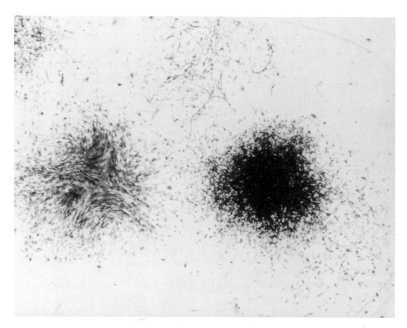

Fig. 9.15 Colonies of human embryo fibroblasts growing normally (left) and following viral transformation (right).

the medium and can be cultured in suspension without being attached to a solid surface (anchorage-independent). Normal cells have a limited number of cell divisions, called the Hayflick limit, which they can undergo in vitro before apoptosis, e.g. for cells taken from a human fetus it is around 60. Transformed cells no longer have this limit and thus can grow and divide indefinitely. There are many changes in the surface properties of transformed cells. Often viral-specific antigens are found, particularly ones synthesized early in the replication cycle. Fibronectin, a surface glycoprotein thought to be important in keeping cells together in a tissue or organ, is no longer found. Commonly fetal antigens are expressed and the agglutinability of cells by plant lectins changes, demonstrating alterations in the distribution of membrane glycoproteins. Finally, some transformed cells form tumours when injected into susceptible animals. Often these animals have to be immunocompromised in some way before tumours are produced, or the cells inserted into an immunologically protected site, such as the cheek pouch of the hamster. In addition, it is important to appreciate that by no means all transformed cells will form tumours. It is thought that there are degrees of transformation and that several stages have to be completed before the cells are fully transformed and equivalent to malignant tumour cells. Viral transformation may represent only the first step or a single step in such a pathway. There are no in-vitro markers that determine the degree of transformation; thus the potential

ability of the transformed cell to produce tumours in experimental animals cannot be predicted, as yet.

All the viruses that cause transformation in vitro have a similar interaction with the host cell (Fig. 9.16). The initial stages are exactly as for the productive infections described earlier in this chapter. There is adsorption, penetration, uncoating and, in most but not all cases, selected viral genes are expressed as proteins, giving the cell new antigenic properties. At this stage the viral nucleic acid becomes integrated in the host cell DNA, probably not at a specific site, or it circularizes and is maintained in a non-integrated episomal form in the nucleus. The association is a stable one, so that when the host cell DNA is replicated, the viral nucleic acid is also replicated and the number of viral genome copies per cell remains constant over many cell generations. Thus, transformation is a heritable alteration. With some viruses, such as Epstein–Barr virus and the papovaviruses, the whole viral genome is normally integrated, while with others, such as herpes simplex virus and adenoviruses, only part of the viral genome is integrated, and the remainder is lost.

Recent work in this area has concentrated on the molecular events surrounding transformation and in analysing the functions of the viral proteins found in transformed cells. Two examples of transforming viruses, one RNA and the other DNA, are briefly described now to illustrate the approaches taken. Both are associated with human tumours.

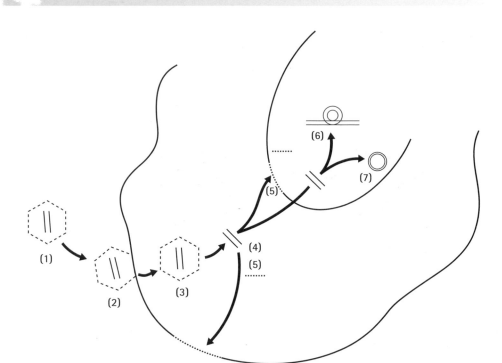

Fig. 9.16 A simplified diagram showing the events of viral transformation. The hypothetical virus (1) adsorbs (2), penetrates (3), is uncoated (4), and usually some early viral proteins are synthesized (5) followed by integration of the viral genome in the host cell DNA (6) or formation of a circular non-integrated genomic DNA (7).

The first is human T lymphotropic or T cell leukaemia virus type I (HTLV-I), a retrovirus, which is found in CD4+ T cells of patients with adult T cell leukaemia. It is able to transform CD4+ lymphocytes in vitro with integration of the DNA provirus. Genetic analysis has revealed that the viral genome can code for several non-structural proteins including one of special interest called Tax, of molecular weight 40 kDa. This protein, which has no cellular homologue, is able to activate transcription in the long terminal repeat of the integrated virus. It may also activate transcription of several cellular genes at more distant sites, which are involved in proliferation, including the genes for interleukin-2 and the interleukin-2 receptor. Interleukin-2 is an important cytokine, and increasing its expression, plus that of its receptor, may have profound implications for the control of T cell activation.

The second example is human papillomavirus type 16 (HPV-16), found as integrated DNA in many cases of carcinoma of the cervix. In vitro this virus is able to transform most types of human epithelial cells including keratinocytes. The viral proteins responsible for transformation are the products of two genes, E6 and E7: E6 protein interacts with p53, and E7 with retinoblastoma protein, thereby inactivating them. As both p53 and retinoblastoma protein act as cellular growth-suppressing proteins, loss of their functions is likely to lead to transformation. In addition, integration of the viral genome normally involves the disruption of the E2 gene, the product of which is required to stop transcription of the E6 and E7 promoter.

RECOMMENDED READING

Ansardi D, Porter D C, Anderson M J, Morrow C D 1996 Poliovirus assembly and encapsidation of genomic RNA. *Advances in Virus Research* 46: 1–68

Bangham C R, Kirkwood T B 1993 Defective interfering particles and virus evolution. *Trends in Microbiology* 1: 260–264

Dalgleish A G 1991 Viruses and cancer. *British Medical Bulletin* 47: 21–46

de la Torre J C, Oldstone M B A 1996 Anatomy of viral persistence: mechanisms of persistence and associated diseases. *Advances in Virus Research* 46: 311–343

Evans D J, Almond J W 1998 Cell receptors for picornaviruses as determinants of cell tropism and pathogenesis. *Trends in Microbiology* 6: 198–202

Fields D N, Knipe D M, Howley P M (eds) 1996 *Virology*, 3rd edn. Lippincott-Raven, Philadelphia

Gaudin Y, Ringrok R W H, Brunner J 1995 Low-pH induced conformational changes in viral fusion proteins: implications for the fusion mechanism. *Journal of General Virology* 76: 1541–1556

Greber U F, Singh I, Helenius A 1994 Mechanism of virus uncoating. *Trends in Microbiology* 2: 52–56

Harper D R 1994 *Molecular Virology*. BIOS Scientific, Oxford

Hay J, Ruyechan W T 1992 Regulation of herpes simplex virus type 1 gene expression. *Current Topics in Microbiology and Immunology* 179: 1–14

Haywood A M 1994 Virus receptors: binding, adhesion strengthening, and changes in viral structure. *Journal of Virology* 68: 1–5

Hobman T C 1993 Targeting of viral glycoproteins to the Golgi complex. *Trends in Microbiology* 1: 124–130

Nomoto A, Kioke S, Aoki J 1994 Tissue tropism and species specificity of poliovirus infection. *Trends in Microbiology* 2: 47–51

Phillips A C, Vousden K H 1998 Human papillomaviruses and cancer. In *Viruses and Human Cancer*, eds J R Arrand and D R Harper, BIOS Scientific, Oxford, pp 39–84

Roulston A, Marcellus R C, Branton P E 1999 Viruses and apoptosis. *Annual Review of Microbiology* 53: 577–628

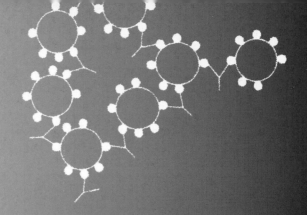

PART 2
INFECTION AND IMMUNITY

10

Immunological principles: antigens and antigen recognition

J. Stewart

An antigen is any substance capable of provoking the lymphoid tissues of an animal to respond by generating an immune reaction specifically directed at the inducing substance and not at other unrelated substances. The response is not to the entire molecule but to individual chemical groups that will have a specific three-dimensional shape. The specificity of the response to these *antigenic determinants* or *epitopes* is an important characteristic of immune responses. The reaction of an animal to contact with antigen, called the *acquired immune response*, takes two forms; first, the *humoral* or *circulating antibody response* and, second, the *cell-mediated response*, and their characteristics are described in Chapter 11. Most of the information available on the specificity of the immune response comes from studies of the interaction of circulating antibody with antigen. An antibody directed against an epitope of a particular molecule will react only with this determinant or other very similar structures. Even minor chemical changes in the conformation of the epitope will markedly reduce the ability of the original antibody to react with the altered material.

The term 'antigen', referring to substances either acting as stimulants of the immune response or reacting with antibody, is used rather loosely by immunologists. Use is made of the functional classification of antigens into:

- substances that are able to generate an immune response by themselves, which are termed immunogens
- molecules that are able to react with antibodies but are unable to stimulate their production directly.

The latter substances are often low molecular weight chemicals, termed *haptens*, that will react with preformed antibodies but only become immunogenic when attached to large molecules, called *carriers*. The hapten forms an epitope on the carrier molecule that is recognized by the immune system and stimulates the production of antibody. In other words, the ability of a chemical grouping to interact with an antibody is not enough to stimulate an immune response. As we will see later, when discussing the sites on molecules recognized by cells of the immune system, all antigens can be considered to be composed of haptens on larger carrier structures.

GENERAL PROPERTIES OF ANTIGENS

A substance that acts as an antigen in one species of animal may not do so in another if it is represented in the tissues or fluids of the second species. This underlines the requirement that an antigen must be a foreign substance to elicit an immune response. For example, egg albumen, whilst an excellent antigen in rabbits, fails to induce an antibody response in fowl. The more foreign and evolutionarily distant a substance is to a particular species, the more likely it is to be a powerful antigen.

A widely recognized requirement for a substance to be antigenic in its own right, without having to be attached to a carrier molecule, is that it should have a molecular weight in excess of 5000. It is, however, possible to induce an immune response to substances of lower molecular weight. For example, glucagon (molecular weight of 3800) can stimulate antibody production but only if special measures are taken such as the use of an *adjuvant* which gives an additional stimulus to the immune system. Very large proteins, such as the crustacean respiratory pigment haemocyanin, are very powerful antigens and are widely used in experimental immunology. Polysaccharides vary in antigenicity, e.g. dextran with a molecular weight of 600 000 is a good antigen, whereas dextran with a molecular weight of 100 000 is not.

Some low molecular weight chemical substances appear to contradict the requirement that an antigen be large. Among these are picryl chloride, formaldehyde and drugs such as aspirin, penicillin and sulphonamides. These substances are highly antigenic, particularly if applied to the skin. The reason for this appears to be that such materials form complexes by means of covalent bonds with tissue proteins. The complex of such a substance, acting as a hapten, with a tissue protein acting as a carrier, forms a complete antigen. This phenomenon has important implications in the development of certain types of hypersensitivity (see Chapter 11).

ANTIGENIC DETERMINANTS

The immune system does not recognize an infectious agent or foreign molecule as a whole but reacts to structurally distinct areas – antigenic determinants or epitopes. Thus, exposure to a micro-organism will generate an immune response to many different epitopes. The antiserum produced will contain different antibodies reactive with each determinant. This will ensure that an individual will be protected from the micro-organism by producing a response to at least a few of the possible determinants. If the host only reacted to the organism as a whole then failure to react to this one site would have dire consequences, i.e. it would not be able to eliminate the pathogen. Certain antibodies may react with an epitope composed of residues that can also be part of two other epitopes recognized by different antibodies (Fig. 10.1).

A response to antigen involves the specific interaction of components of the immune system, antibodies and lymphocytes, with epitopes on the antigen. The lymphocytes have receptors on their surface that function as the recognition units – on B lymphocytes surface-bound immunoglobulin is the receptor and on T lymphocytes the recognition unit is known as the T cell receptor. The interaction between an antibody (or cell-bound receptor) and antigen is governed by the complementarity of the electron cloud surrounding the determinants. The overall configuration of the outer electrons, not the chemical nature of the constituent residues, determines the shape of the epitope and its complementary *paratope* (the part of the antibody or T cell receptor that interacts with the epitope). The better the fit between the epitope and the paratope the stronger the non-covalent bonds formed and consequently the higher the affinity of the interaction.

Antigenic determinants have to be topographical, i.e. composed of structures on the surface of molecules, and can be constructed in two ways. They may be contained within a single segment of primary sequence or assembled from residues far apart in the primary sequence but brought together on the surface by the folding of the molecule into its native conformation. The former are known as *sequential* epitopes, and those formed from distant residues are *conformational* epitopes. The majority of antigenic structures recognized by antibodies depend on the tertiary configuration of the immunogen (conformational), while T cell epitopes are defined by the primary structure (sequential).

ANTIGENIC SPECIFICITY

Foreignness of a substance to an animal can depend on the presence of chemical groupings that are not normally found in the animal's body. Arsenic acid, for example, can be chemically introduced into a protein molecule and, as a hapten, acts as a determinant of antigenic specificity of the molecule. There are many other examples where antibodies are able to distinguish subtle chemical differences between molecules. Thus, antisera can distinguish between glucose and galactose, which differ only by the interchange of a hydrogen atom and a hydroxyl group on one carbon atom.

The ability of antibody (or T cell receptors) to form a high-affinity interaction with an antigen depends on intermolecular forces, which act strongly only when the two molecules come together in a very precise manner. The better the fit, the stronger the bond. An antibody molecule directed against a particularly shaped antigenic determinant might be able to react with another similar but not quite identical determinant, as shown in Fig. 10.2. This type of cross-reaction does occur but the strength of the bond between the two molecules will be diminished in the case of the less well-fitting determinant.

A common source of confusion concerning the specificity of antibodies arises when an antibody to a particular antigen is found to be capable of combining with an apparently unrelated antigen. For example, glucose residues are present in many different types of molecule, and an antibody that binds to a glucose determinant in antigen X-glucose would be likely to react with the glucose group in antigen Y-glucose provided

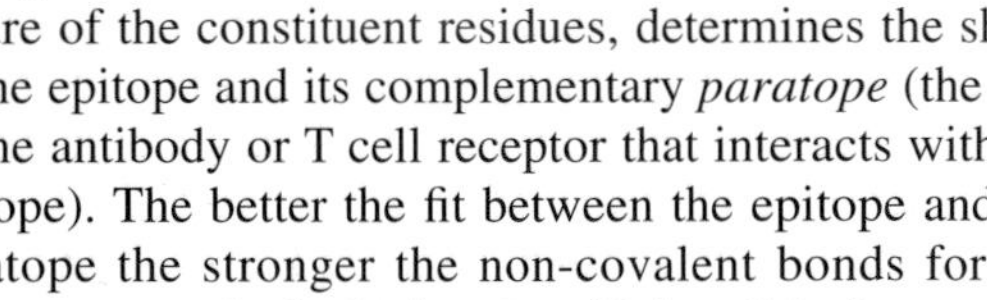

Fig. 10.1 Overlapping epitopes. Two epitopes (1 and 2) on an antigen induce the formation of three antibodies (A, B and C).

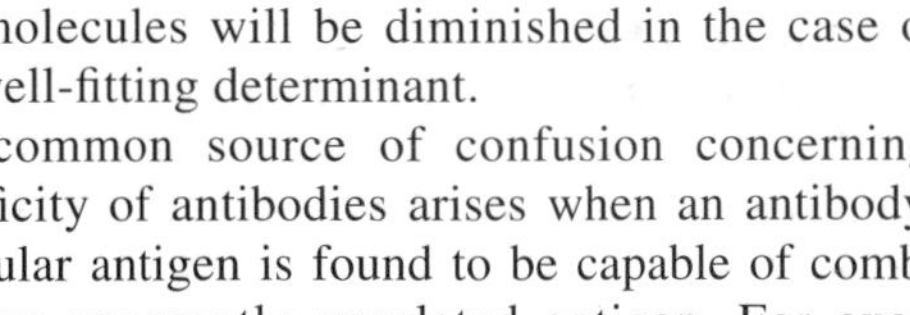

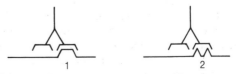

Fig. 10.2 Specificity and cross-reactions. Antibody produced in response to an antigen that contains epitope 1 will also combine with epitope 2.

the two determinants are equally accessible. The antibody directed against the glucose determinant is not a non-specific type of antibody but is simply reacting with an identical chemical determinant in another antigen molecule.

In laboratory practice, cross-reactivity is often found between antisera to certain bacterial antigens and antigens present on cells such as erythrocytes. Antigens shared in this way are known as *heterophile antigens*. The best known of the heterophile antigens is the Forssman antigen, which is present on the red cells of many species as well as in bacteria such as pneumococci and salmonellae. Another heterophile antigen is found in *Escherichia coli* and human red cells of blood group B individuals. These cross-reactivities are probably responsible for the generation of antibodies found in individuals of a certain blood group that bind to the red blood cells of individuals of a different blood group. These antibodies are known as *isohaemagglutinins* because they are able to bind the red blood cells and clump them together, i.e. cause agglutination.

IMMUNOGLOBULINS

Towards the end of the 19th century, von Behring and Kitasato in Berlin found that the serum of an appropriately immunized animal contained specific neutralizing substances or antitoxins. This was the first demonstration of the activity of what are now known as *antibodies* or *immunoglobulins*. Antibodies are:

- Glycoproteins.
- Present in the serum and body fluids.
- Induced when immunogenic molecules are introduced into the host's lymphoid system.
- Reactive with, and bind specifically to, the antigen that induced their formation.

The liquid collected from blood that has been allowed to clot is known as *serum*. It contains a number of molecules but no cells or clotting factors. If serum is prepared from an animal that has been exposed to an antigen then it is known as an *antiserum* since it will contain antibodies reactive to the inducing antigen. When the components of serum are separated electrophoretically then the heterogeneity of immunoglobulins can be seen, i.e. they appear as broad bands (Fig. 10.3). This technique separates serum components into various fractions, labelled α, β and γ. Most of the antibody molecules are present within the γ fraction, and they are sometimes referred to as γ-globulins.

There are five distinct *classes* or *isotypes* of immunoglobulins, namely IgG, IgA, IgM, IgD and IgE. They differ from each other in size, charge, carbohydrate

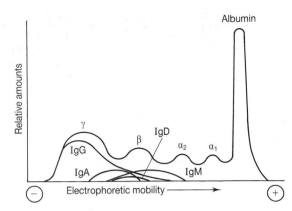

Fig. 10.3 Separation of serum proteins by electrophoresis.

content and, of course, amino acid composition (Table 10.1). Within certain classes there are subclasses that vary slightly in structure and function. These classes and subclasses can be separated from each other serologically, i.e. using antibody. If injected into the correct species they will induce the formation of antibodies that can be used to differentiate between the different isotypes.

Antibody structure

All antibody molecules have the same basic four chain structure composed of two light chains and two heavy chains (Fig. 10.4). The light chains (molecular weight of 25 000) are one of two types designated κ and λ and only one type is found in one antibody. The heavy chains vary in molecular weight from 50 000 to 70 000, and it is these chains that determine the isotype. They are designated α, δ, ε, γ and μ for the respective classes of immunoglobulin (Table 10.1). The individual chains are held together by disulphide bridges and non-covalent interactions.

When individual light chains are studied it is found that they are composed of two distinct areas or *domains* of approximately 110 amino acids. One end of the chain is identical in all members of the same isotype, and is termed the constant region of the light chain, C_L. The other end shows considerable sequence variation, and is known as the variable region, V_L. The heavy chains are also split into domains of approximately the same size, the number varying between the five types of heavy chain. One of these domains will show considerable sequence variation (V_H) while the others (C_H) are similar for the same isotype. The tertiary structure generated by the combination of the V_L and V_H regions determines the shape of the antigen-combining site or paratope. Since the two light and two heavy chains are identical, each antibody unit will have two identical paratopes situated at the amino (*N*)-terminal end of the

Table 10.1 Physicochemical properties of human immunoglobulins. The immunoglobulin serotype is determined by the type of heavy chain present. The different characteristics observed are also controlled by the heavy chain. Variation within a class gives rise to subclasses

Characteristic	Immunoglobulin isotype				
	IgA[a]	IgD	IgE	IgG	IgM[b]
Mean serum concentration (mg/dl)	300	5	0.005	1400	150
Mass (kDa)	160	184	188	160	970
Carbohydrate (%)	7–11	9–14	12	2–3	12
Half-life (days)	6	3	2	21	5
Heavy chain	α	δ	ε	γ	μ

[a] IgA is also found as a dimer, and in secretions IgA is present in dimeric form associated with a protein known as secretory component.
[b] Data for IgM as a pentamer.

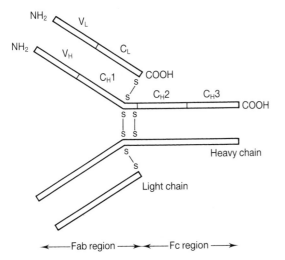

Fig. 10.4 Basic structure of an immunoglobulin molecule. See text for details.

molecule that recognizes the antigen. The carboxyl (C)-terminal end of the antibody will be the same for all members of the same class or subclass, and is involved in the biological activities of the molecule. The area of the heavy chains between the C_H1 and C_H2 domains contains a varying number of interchain disulphide bonds and is known as the *hinge region*. A number of enzymes cleave immunoglobulins at distinct points to generate different peptide fragments. Using these enzymes, antibodies can be divided into a Fab region ('fragment antigen binding') containing the paratope and an Fc region ('fragment crystallizable') that is similar for all antibodies of the same isotype.

Despite the differences between the various isotypes, as shown in Table 10.1, all antibody molecules are composed of the same basic unit structure, with the Fab portion containing the antigen-recognizing paratope and the Fc region carrying out the activities that protect the host, i.e. effector functions. The differences seen in the Fc region between

the various heavy chains are responsible for the different biological activities of the antibody isotypes.

IgG

This is the major immunoglobulin of serum, making up 75% of the total and having a molecular weight of 150 000 in humans. Four subclasses are found in humans – IgG1, IgG2, IgG3 and IgG4 – that differ in their relative concentrations, amino acid composition, number and position of interchain disulphide bonds and biological function. IgG is the major antibody of the secondary response (see Chapter 11) and is found in both the serum and tissue fluids.

IgA

In man, most of the serum IgA occurs as a monomer, but in many other mammals it is mostly found as a dimer. The dimer is held together by a J chain, which is produced by the antibody-producing plasma cells. IgA is the predominant antibody class in seromucous secretions such as saliva, tears, colostrum and respiratory, gastrointestinal and genitourinary secretions. This secretory IgA (sIgA) is always in the dimeric form and is composed of two basic four-chain units (two light chains and two heavy chains), a J chain and the secretory component. The secretory component is part of the molecule that transports the dimer produced by a submucosal plasma cell to the mucosal surface (Fig. 10.5). It facilitates passage through the epithelial cells and protects the secreted molecule from proteolytic digestion. There are two subclasses of IgA – IgA1 and IgA2.

IgM

IgM is a pentamer of the basic unit with μ heavy chains and a single J chain. Because of its large size this isotype is mainly confined to the intravascular pool, and

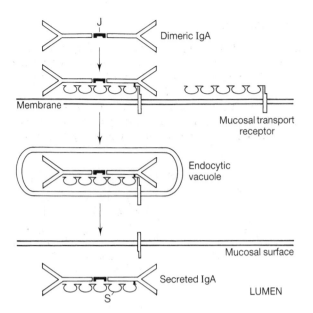

Fig. 10.5 Transport of secretory IgA. J, J chain; S, secretory component.

is the first antibody type to be produced during an immune response.

IgD

Many circulating B cells have IgD present on their surface, but it accounts for less than 1% of the circulating antibody. It is composed of the basic unit with δ heavy chains. The protein is very susceptible to proteolytic attack and therefore has a very short half-life in serum.

IgE

The IgE is present in extremely low levels in the serum. However, it is found on the surface of mast cells and basophils, which possess a receptor specific for the Fc part of this molecule.

Antigen binding

The variability in amino acid sequence in the variable domains of light and heavy chains is not found over their entire length but is restricted to short segments. These segments show considerable variation, and are termed *hypervariable regions*. Hypervariable regions are now known to contain the residues that make direct contact with the antigen, and are referred to as *complementarity determining regions* (CDRs). Although the remaining *framework* residues do not come into direct contact with the antigen, they are essential for the formation of the correct tertiary structure of the variable domain and maintenance of the integrity of the binding site. In both

light and heavy chains there are three CDRs that, in combination, form the paratope.

The antigen and antibody are held together by various individually weak non-covalent interactions. However, the formation of a large number of hydrogen bonds and electrostatic, van der Waals and hydrophobic interactions leads to a considerable binding energy. These attractive forces are only active over extremely short distances and therefore the epitope and paratope must have complementary structures to enable them to combine. If the electron clouds overlap or residues of similar charge are brought together then repulsive forces will come into play. The balance of attraction against repulsion will dictate the strength of the interaction between an antibody and a particular antigen, i.e. the affinity of the antibody for the antigen.

Antibody diversity

It is now known that an antigen selects from the available antibodies those that can combine with its epitopes. It therefore follows that an individual must have an extremely large number of different antibodies to cope with the vast array of different antigens present in the environment.

Immunoglobulin variability

The paratope is produced by the CDRs of the light and heavy chains generating a specific three-dimensional shape. Any light chain can join with any heavy chain to produce a different paratope. Thus, theoretically, with 10^4 different light chains and 10^4 different heavy chains, 10^8 different specificities could be generated.

The germ-line DNA is the structure of the gene as it is inherited. All cells in the body contain all the inherited genes but different genes become active in different cells at different times. Within B lymphocytes, the cells that differentiate to antibody-producing plasma cells, the functional immunoglobulin genes are formed by gene rearrangements and recombinations. These events give rise to the production of different variable domains in each B lymphocyte. Once a functional gene has been constructed no other rearrangements are allowed to take place within this cell. This dictates that one particular cell will produce antibodies with an identical antigen-combining site and is known as *allelic exclusion*. There is evidence that the gene segments for the variable region of immunoglobulins are particularly susceptible to mutations. This can lead to subtle changes in specificity and/or affinity that are important as an immune response develops (see Chapter 11).

When a B lymphocyte is first stimulated by antigen it will produce IgM. As the immune response develops, the class of antibody changes. However, the immunoglobulin produced will have the same variable domain and therefore bind to the same antigen. All that is altered, or *switched*, is the heavy chain constant region. Thus the progeny of a single B cell will produce different immunoglobulin isotypes as the response to a particular antigen develops, but each will have the same paratope.

Secreted and membrane immunoglobulins

At different stages in its development a B cell will produce immunoglobulins that have to be inserted into the membrane or secreted. The membrane-bound immunoglobulin will be used as the antigen receptor of the B cell and a cell that binds antigen through this molecule will then secrete immunoglobulin of the same specificity. The only difference between the two types of antibody is to be found at the C terminus, where the membrane form has an additional part, the transmembrane portion.

Antibody function

Knowledge gained from the structural studies discussed above has gone some way towards an understanding of the biological activities of the immunoglobulin molecule.

The primary function of an antibody is to bind the antigen that induced its formation. Apart from cases where this results in direct neutralization (e.g. inhibition of toxin activity or of microbial attachment) other effector functions must be generated. The binding of antigen is mediated by the Fab portion, and the Fc region controls the biological defence mechanisms. For every antibody the paratope will be different, and it will therefore recognize different epitopes. However, for every antibody of the same isotype the heavy chain constant domains will be the same, and they will therefore all perform the same functions (Table 10.2).

Neutralization

Because antibodies are at least divalent they can form a complex with multivalent antigens. Depending on the physical nature of the antigen these *immune complexes* exist in various forms (Fig. 10.6). If the antibody is directed against surface antigens of particulate material such as micro-organisms or erythrocytes then *agglutination* will occur. This results in a clump or aggregate that

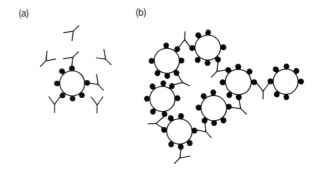

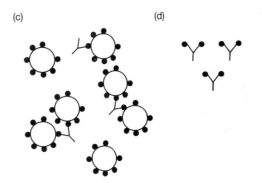

Fig. 10.6 Immune complex formation: **a** antibody excess; **b** equivalence; **c** antigen excess; **d** monovalent antigen.

Table 10.2 Biological properties of human immunoglobulins. These activities are determined by the Fc portion of the molecules

Function	Immunoglobulin isotype							
	IgA	IgD	IgE	IgG1	IgG2	IgG3	IgG4	IgM
Neutralize	++	–	–	+	+	+	+	+++
Complement fixation	±[a]	–	–	++	+	+++	–	+++
Binding to phagocytes	±[b]	–	–	+++	±	+++	+	–
Binding to mast cells	–	–	+++	–	–	–	+	–
Enter tissues	–	–	–	+	+	+	+	–
Placental transfer	–	–	–	+	±	+	+	–
Protects mucosal surfaces	+	–	–	–	–	–	–	–

[a] IgA will activate the alternative pathway.
[b] Receptors for the Fc portion of IgA have been found on neutrophils and alveolar macrophages.

will isolate the potential pathogen, stop its dissemination and stimulate its removal by other mechanisms. If the antigen is soluble then the size of the complex will determine its physical state. Small complexes will remain soluble while large complexes will form *precipitates*.

As might be expected from knowledge of the structure of IgM, its 10 combining sites make it a very efficient agglutinating antibody molecule. Rabbit IgM has been shown to be more than 20 times as active as IgG in bringing about bacterial agglutination. Because of its size, IgM is largely confined to the bloodstream and probably plays an important role in protecting against blood invasion by micro-organisms. Certain sites on micro-organisms are critical to the establishment of an infection. Antibody bound to these sites will interfere with attachment processes and could, therefore, stop infection by the microbe. The binding of an antibody to functionally important residues in toxins will neutralize their harmful effects.

Complement activation

The activation of the complement system is one of the most important antibody effector mechanisms. The complement cascade is a complex group of serum proteins that mediate inflammatory reactions and cell lysis. It is discussed more fully in Chapter 11. The Fc portion of certain isotypes (Table 10.2), once antigen has been bound, will activate complement; this requires that C1q, a subunit of the first complement component, cross-links two antibody Fc portions. For this to happen the two regions must be in close proximity. It has been calculated that a single IgM molecule is 1000 times more efficient than IgG. This is because two IgG molecules must be close together for complement activation. A large number of IgG molecules would be required for this to occur if the epitopes are spread. Not all isotypes activate complement, presumably because they do not have the required amino acid sequence, and therefore tertiary structure, in the Fc portion. C1q binds to residues in the C_H3 domain of IgM and the C_H2 domain of IgG. Some isotypes, when interacting with antigen, can activate the alternative pathway of complement that does not use C1 but gives rise to the same biological activities.

Cell binding and opsonization

The Fc portion of certain immunoglobulin isotypes is able to interact with various cell types (Table 10.2). Antibodies specific for particular antigens, such as bacteria, play a valuable role by binding to the surface and making the antigen more susceptible to phagocyto-sis and subsequent elimination. This process is known as *opsonization*, and is again mediated by the Fc portion of the antibody. A specific conformation on the Fc region of certain isotypes is recognized by *Fc receptors* on the surface of the phagocyte. The important residues are in the C_H2 domain near the hinge region. Individually, the interactions are not strong enough to signal the uptake of the antibody molecule; therefore, free immunoglobulin is not internalized. However, when an antigen is coated by many antibody molecules then summation of all the interactions stimulates phagocytosis or other effector mechanisms.

Certain phagocytic cells have receptors for activated complement components, *complement receptors*. If the binding of antibody to the antigen can activate the complement cascade then various complement components will be deposited on the antigen–antibody complex. Phagocytic cells that have receptors for these complement components will then ingest the complexes.

The above-mentioned processes require that the antibody is first complexed with antigen. However, certain cell types will bind free antibody. Mast cells and basophils have Fc receptors that are specific for IgE. These cells perform a protective function but are also involved in hypersensitivity reactions described in Chapter 11. In humans, IgG has the ability to cross the placenta and reach the fetal circulation. This is a passive process involving specific Fc receptors. This route is limited to primates whereas, in ruminants, immunoglobulin from colostrum is absorbed through the intestinal epithelium. Another Fc-mediated mechanism, already described, is the selective transport of IgA into mucosal secretions.

ANTIGEN RECOGNITION

The immune system has evolved to protect us from potentially harmful material but it must not respond to self molecules. Two separate recognition systems are present:

• humoral immunity
• cell-mediated immunity.

Antibody is the recognition molecule of humoral immunity. This glycoprotein is produced by plasma cells and circulates in the blood and other body fluids. Antibody is also present on the surface of B lymphocytes. The interaction of this surface immunoglobulin with its specific antigen is responsible for the differentiation of these cells into plasma cells. Antibody molecules, whether free or on the surface of a B cell, will recognize free native antigen.

This contrasts dramatically with the situation in cell-mediated immunity; the T lymphocyte antigen receptor will only bind to fragments of antigen that are associated with products of the *major histocompatibility complex* (MHC). T cell recognition of antigen is said to be *MHC-restricted*. These MHC products are present on the surface of cells, therefore T cells only recognize cell-associated antigens. This MHC-restricted recognition mechanism has evolved because of the functions carried out by T lymphocytes. Some T cells produce immuno-regulatory molecules, *lymphokines*, some of which influence the activities of host cells and others that directly kill infected or foreign cells. Therefore, it would be inefficient or dangerous to produce these effects in response to either free antigen or antigen sitting idly on some cell membrane. The joint recognition of MHC molecules and antigen ensures that the T cell makes contact with antigen on the surface of the appropriate target cell.

B cell receptor

Antibody is found free in body fluids and as a trans-membrane protein on the surface of B lymphocytes, i.e. surface immunoglobulin, where it acts as the B cell antigen receptor. The antibody present on the surface of the B cell is exactly the same molecule as will be secreted when the cell develops into a plasma cell except for the extreme C-terminal end as described above. It should be noted that the molecules present on the cell surface are present as monomers even though they are secreted in a polymeric form.

T cell receptor

The complex on T lymphocytes that is involved in antigen recognition is composed of a number of glyco-protein structures. Some of these molecules have been systematically named by CD (cluster of differentiation) nomenclature using antibodies. These generic names will be used in preference to other symbols sometimes found in the literature.

The T cell antigen receptor is a heterodimer composed of an α and a β or a γ and a δ chain. Each chain contains a variable and constant domain, transmembrane portion and cytoplasmic tail. The variable domain folds to form a paratope that will interact with antigenic peptides that are associated with MHC molecules on a cell surface. The majority of T cells use the α/β heterodimer in antigen recognition. The role of cells that possess the γ/δ molecules is unknown but they may be involved in the immune response to particular types of antigens at specific anatomical sites. The T cell receptor is the molecule that is responsible for the recognition of specific MHC–antigen complexes and will be different for every T cell. Genetic rearrangements of germ-line genes, similar to those seen in B cells, produce functional T cell receptors.

CD3 is present on all T cells and is non-covalently linked to the T cell receptor. The CD3 complex is thought to be involved in signal transduction, leading to cell activation, when a ligand binds to the T cell receptor.

CD4 and CD8 are mutually exclusive molecules. They are present on T cells that are restricted in their recognition of antigen by MHC class II and class I molecules, respectively. Due to their almost exclusive correlation with a specific MHC class it is thought that these molecules bind to non-polymorphic determinants on the MHC molecules. This interaction could stabilize the binding of the T cell receptor to the MHC–antigen complex or it may in fact have a co-receptor function. In the former case the CD4 or CD8 molecule could interact with the same MHC molecule as the T cell receptor or with a different one and this interaction does not generate a stimulatory signal, i.e. it solely stabilizes the specific interaction (T cell receptor with antigen–MHC). In the latter case the T cell receptor and CD4 or CD8 bind to the same MHC molecule but at different sites, and the joint signal that is generated leads to the stimulation of the T cell.

MAJOR HISTOCOMPATIBILITY COMPLEX

The MHC is part of the genome that codes for molecules that are important in immune recognition – including interactions between lymphoid cells and other cell types. It is also involved in the rejection of allografts. The MHCs of a number of species have been studied but most is known about those of the mouse and humans.

The gene complex contains a large number of individual genes that can be grouped into three classes on the basis of structure and function of their products. The molecules coded for by the genes are sometimes referred to as *MHC antigens* because they were first defined by serological analysis, i.e. using antibodies.

The MHC of humans is known as *human leucocyte group A* (HLA), and in mice it is referred to as *histocompatibility 2* (H2).

Gene organization

The genes that code for the HLA molecules are found on the short arm of chromosome 6. They are arranged over a region of between 2000 and 4000 kilobases in size containing enough DNA for over 200 genes. The MHC genes are contained within regions known as A, B, C and D (Fig. 10.7).

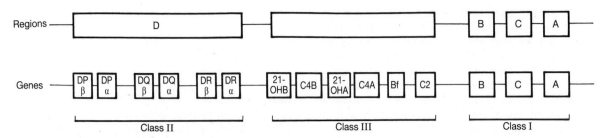

Fig. 10.7 MHC gene map of humans.

MHC class I molecules consist of two non-covalently associated polypeptide chains. A single gene that codes for the larger chain is present in the A, B and C regions while the smaller chain, known as β_2-microglobulin, is coded for elsewhere in the genome.

MHC class II molecules are composed of two chains, both of which are coded for within the D region. There are three class II molecules, DP, DQ and DR. The class III genes are grouped together in a region between D and B. These genes code for a number of complement components but most have nothing to do with the immune system.

MHC antigen structure and distribution

The MHC class I molecule is a dimer composed of a glycosylated transmembrane protein, of molecular weight 45 000, coded for within the MHC, linked to a smaller protein, β_2-microglobulin (Fig. 10.8a). The globular protein formed by these two peptides is present on the surface of all nucleated cells in humans, except neurones. β_2-microglobulin is required for the processing and expression of MHC-encoded molecules on the cell membrane. The MHC-encoded class I glycoprotein folds into three globular domains (α_1, α_2 and α_3) held in place by disulphide bonds and non-covalent interactions. These globular domains are found on the outer surface of the cell. There is a short cytoplasmic tail and a transmembrane portion. β_2-microglobulin is non-covalently associated with the α_3 domain.

The MHC class II molecules consist of two polypeptide chains (α and β) held together by non-covalent interactions (Fig. 10.8b). They have a much more limited cellular distribution, being limited to the surface of certain cells of the immune system. In humans, they are normally found on dendritic cells, B lymphocytes, macrophages, monocytes and activated T lymphocytes. The MHC class II molecule consists of two non-covalently associated peptides, α and β. Each chain is composed of two extracellular domains, a transmembrane portion and a cytoplasmic tail.

These two types of molecule are folded into domains of a similar overall structure to immunoglobulin and, along with other molecules of the immune system involved in recognition processes, are thought to have evolved from a common ancestral molecule. A number of members of this *immunoglobulin supergene family* are depicted in Fig. 10.9. MHC class II molecules, some interleukin receptors and Fc receptors are also included in the family.

The MHC antigens of each class have a similar basic structure. However, fine structural differences can be detected in the α_1 and α_2 domains of class I molecules and in α_1 and β_1 domains of class II molecules. These domains form a cleft on the outermost part of the molecules in which antigen fragments are found. The variations found are due to differences in the amino acid sequence and can be detected serologically. The variable residues will give rise to different three-dimensional shapes on the MHC molecules. This will in turn influence the selection of which antigen fragments can bind to a particular MHC molecule.

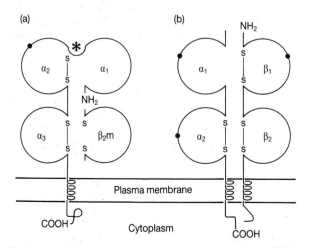

Fig. 10.8 Structure of MHC class I and class II molecules. Schematic representation of **a** class I and **b** class II molecules as found in the plasma membrane. β_2m, β_2-microglobulin ●, carbohydrate moieties; *, antigen-binding cleft.

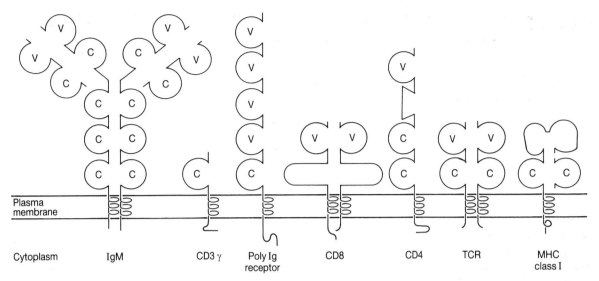

Fig. 10.9 The immunoglobulin supergene family. A number of molecules involved in the immune system display striking similarities in overall structure. Regions similar to immunoglobulin domains are shown as circles; those related to variable and constant domains are designated V and C, respectively.

There are, therefore, many different forms of these molecules that can be identified in a population – they are highly *polymorphic*. Thus, it is highly unlikely that two individuals will have exactly the same MHC antigens. The MHC molecules of a particular individual can be given a designation using tissue-typing reagents. So, on each chromosome of an individual will be the genes that code for an A, B, C, DP, DQ and DR molecule. As the MHC genes are co-dominant, the products of both alleles are expressed on the cell surface. All the nucleated cells in the body will therefore express multiple copies of two HLA-A, two HLA-B and two HLA-C molecules. On certain cell types there will also be HLA-DP, -DQ and -DR molecules that were inherited from both parents.

Function

The MHC class I and class II molecules are essential for immune recognition by T lymphocytes. They can only bind to antigens when they are associated with these molecules. The different classes of molecule are involved in antigen recognition by different T cell types or subsets.

- T lymphocytes that have CD4 molecules on their surface recognize antigen in association with MHC class II molecules.
- T lymphocytes that have CD8 molecules are restricted by MHC class I molecules.

The T lymphocyte subsets perform different functions, but the division is not absolute. The one thing that

they have in common is that they recognize, through their T cell receptor complex (CD3, CD4 or CD8, TCR), antigen fragments in association with MHC molecules (Fig. 10.10). In general terms:

- CD4-positive (CD4$^+$) cells produce molecules, lymphokines, that stimulate and support the production of immune system cells.
- CD8$^+$ positive cells are involved in the destruction of virally infected cells (see Ch.11) and the destruction of tissue grafts from MHC-incompatible donors.

The CD4$^+$ cells produce molecules that stimulate growth and differentiation of cells. These molecules are most effective over short distances since they will be more

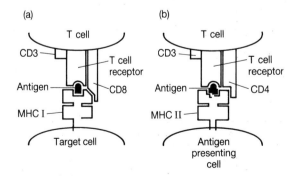

Fig. 10.10 Molecules involved in T cell recognition. **a** Antigen fragments that associate with class I molecules are recognized by T cells that have the CD8 molecule. **b** Antigen fragments that associate with MHC class II are recognized by T cells that have the CD4 molecule on their surface.

concentrated. This will happen when the two cells involved are actually joined together or in close proximity. The stimulation of CD4$^+$ T cells by antigen fragments on the surface of a responsive cell, or on a cell in the vicinity of a responsive cell, will greatly increase the effectiveness of the messenger molecules produced by the T cell.

RECOMMENDED READING

Abbas A K, Lichtman A H, Pober J S 2000 *Cellular and Molecular Immunology*, 4th edn. Saunders, Philadelphia

Weir D M, Stewart J 1997 *Immunology*, 8th edn. Churchill Livingstone, Edinburgh

Janeway C A 1993 How the immune system recognizes invaders. *Scientific American* Sept: 41–47

Internet site

ntri.tamuk.edu/immunology/abproduction.html

11

Innate and acquired immunity

J. Stewart

The environment contains a vast number of potentially infectious organisms – viruses, bacteria, fungi, protozoa and worms. Any of these can cause damage if they multiply unchecked, and many could kill the host. However, the majority of infections in the normal individual are of limited duration and leave very little permanent damage. This fortunate outcome is due largely to the *immune system*.

The immune system is split into two functional divisions. *Innate immunity* is the first line of defence against infectious agents, and most potential pathogens are checked before they establish an overt infection. If these defences are breached, the acquired immune system is called into play. *Acquired immunity* produces a specific response to each infectious agent, and the effector mechanisms generated normally eradicate the offending material. Furthermore, the adaptive immune system remembers the particular infectious agent and can prevent it causing disease later.

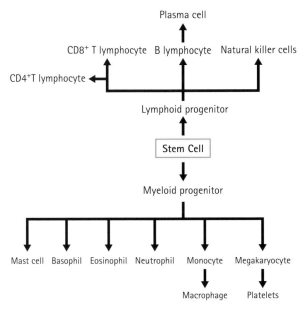

Fig. 11.1   Cells of the immune system.

THE IMMUNE SYSTEM

The immune system consists of a number of organs and several different cell types. All the cells of the immune system, tissue cells and white blood cells or *leucocytes*, develop from pluripotent stem cells in the bone marrow. These haemopoietic stem cells also give rise to the red blood cells or *erythrocytes*. The production of leucocytes is through two main pathways of differentiation (Fig. 11.1). The *lymphoid* lineage produces T lymphocytes and B lymphocytes. Natural killer (NK) cells, also known as large granular lymphocytes, probably also develop from lymphoid progenitors. The *myeloid* pathway gives rise to mononuclear phagocytes, monocytes and macrophages, and granulocytes, basophils, eosinophils and neutrophils, as well as platelets and mast cells. Platelets are involved in blood clotting and inflammation while mast cells are similar to basophils but are found in tissues.

Lymphoid cells

Lymphocytes make up about 20% of the white blood cells present in the adult circulation. Mature lymphoid cells are long-lived and may survive for many years as memory cells. These mononuclear cells are heterogeneous in size and morphology. The typical small lymphocytes are agranular and comprise the T and B cell populations. The larger cells are referred to as large granular lymphocytes because they contain cytoplasmic granules. Cells within this population are able to kill certain tumour and virally infected cells (natural killing) and destroy cells coated with immunoglobulin (antibody-dependent cell-mediated cytotoxicity).

Morphologically it is quite difficult to distinguish between the different lymphoid cells and impossible to differentiate the subclasses of T cell. Since these cells

121

carry out different processes they possess molecules on their surface unique to that functional requirement. These molecules, referred to as cell markers, can be used to distinguish between different cell types and also identify cells at different stages of differentiation. The different cell surface molecules have been systematically named by the CD (cluster of differentiation) system, and some of those expressed by different T cell populations are shown in Table 11.1. These CD markers are identified using specific monoclonal antibodies (see p. 136). The presence of these specific antibodies on the cell surface is then visualized using labelled antibodies that recognize the first antibody.

Myeloid cells

The second pathway of development gives rise to a variety of cell types of different morphology and function.

Mononuclear phagocytes

The common myeloid progenitor in the bone marrow gives rise to *monocytes* that circulate in the blood and migrate into organs and tissues to become *macrophages*. The human blood monocyte is larger than a lymphocyte and usually has a kidney-shaped nucleus. This actively phagocytic cell has a ruffled membrane and many cytoplasmic granules. These *lysosomes* contain enzymes and molecules that are involved in the killing of microorganisms. Mononuclear phagocytes adhere strongly to surfaces and have various cell membrane receptors to aid the binding and ingestion of foreign material. Their activities can be enhanced by molecules produced by T lymphocytes, called *lymphokines*. Macrophages and monocytes are capable of producing various complement components, prostaglandins, interferons and *monokines* such as interleukin (IL)-1 and tumour necrosis factor. Lymphokines and monokines are collectively known as *cytokines*.

Polymorphonuclear leucocytes

These cells are sometimes referred to as *granulocytes* and are short-lived cells (2–3 days) compared to macrophages, which may survive for months or years. They are classified as *neutrophils*, *eosinophils* and *basophils* on the basis of their histochemical staining. The mature forms have a multilobed nucleus and many granules. Neutrophils constitute 60–70% of the leucocytes, but also migrate into tissues in response to injury or infection.

Neutrophils. These are the most abundant circulating granulocyte. Their granules contain numerous microbicidal molecules and the cells enter the tissues when a chemotactic factor is produced, as the result of infection or injury.

Eosinophils. Eosinophils are also phagocytic cells, although they appear to be less efficient than neutrophils. They are present in low numbers in a healthy, normal individual (1–2% of leucocytes), but their numbers rise in certain allergic conditions. The granule contents can be released by the appropriate signal, and the cytotoxic molecules can then kill parasites that are too large to be phagocytosed.

Basophils. These cells are found in extremely small numbers in the circulation (<0.2%) and have certain characteristics in common with tissue *mast cells*. Both cell types have receptors on their surface for the Fc portion of IgE, and cross-linking of this immunoglobulin by antigen leads to the release of various pharmacological mediators. These molecules stimulate an inflammatory response. There are two types of mast cell: one is found in connective tissue and the other is mucosa associated. Mast cells and basophils are both bone marrow derived, but their developmental relationship is not clear.

Platelets

Platelets are also derived from myeloid progenitors. In addition to their role in clotting they are involved in inflammation.

INNATE IMMUNITY

The healthy individual is protected from potentially harmful micro-organisms in the environment by a number of very effective mechanisms, present from birth, that do not depend upon prior exposure to any particular micro-organism. The innate defence mechanisms are non-specific in the sense that they are effective against a wide range of potentially infectious agents. The characteristics and constituents of innate and acquired immunity are shown in Table 11.2.

Table 11.1 Major T lymphocyte markers

Marker	Distribution	Proposed function
CD2	All T cells	Adherence to target cell
CD3	All T cells	Part of T cell antigen–receptor complex
CD4	Helper subset (T_H)	MHC class II-restricted recognition
CD7	All T cells	Unknown
CD8	Cytotoxic subset (T_C)	MHC class I-restricted recognition

MHC, major histocompatibility complex.

Table 11.2 Characteristics and determinants of innate and acquired immunity

Innate immunity	Acquired immunity
Non-specific	Specific
No change with repeat exposure	Memory
Mechanical barriers	
Bactericidal substances	
Natural flora	
Humoral	
Acute phase proteins	Antibody
Interferons	
Lysozyme	
Complement	
Cell-mediated	
Natural killer cells	T lymphocytes
Phagocytes	

Determinants of innate immunity

Species and strains

Marked differences exist in the susceptibility of different species to infective agents. The rat is strikingly resistant to diphtheria whilst the guinea-pig and humans are highly susceptible. The rabbit is particularly susceptible to myxomatosis, and humans to syphilis, leprosy and meningococcal meningitis. Susceptibility to an infection does not always imply a lack of resistance to disease caused by the micro-organism. For example, although humans are highly susceptible to the common cold, the infection is overcome within a few days. In some diseases, it may be difficult to initiate the infection, but once established the disease can progress rapidly – inferring a lack of resistance. For example, rabies occurs in both humans and dogs but is not readily established as the virus does not ordinarily penetrate healthy skin. Once infected, however, both species are unable to overcome the disease. Marked variations in resistance to infection have been noted between different strains of mice, and it is possible to breed, by selection, rabbits of low, intermediate and high resistance to experimental tuberculosis.

Individual differences and influence of age

The role of heredity in determining resistance to infection is well illustrated by studies on tuberculosis in twins. If one homozygous twin develops tuberculosis, the other twin has a 3 to 1 chance of developing the disease compared with a 1 in 3 chance if the twins are heterozygous. Sometimes genetically controlled abnormalities are an advantage to the individual in resisting infection as, for example, in a hereditary abnormality of the red blood cells (sickling). These red blood cells cannot be parasitized by *Plasmodium falciparum*, thus conferring a degree of resistance to malaria in the affected individuals.

Infectious diseases are often more severe in early childhood and in young animals; this higher susceptibility of the young appears to be associated with immaturity of the immunological mechanisms affecting the ability of the lymphoid system to deal with and react to foreign antigens. This is also the time when infectious agents are encountered for the first time (primary exposure), and a memory-acquired immune response cannot be called upon to aid elimination. In certain viral infections, e.g. polio and chickenpox, the clinical illness is more severe in adults than in children. This may be due to a more active immune response producing greater tissue damage. In the elderly, besides a general waning of the activities of the immune system, physical abnormalities (e.g. prostatic enlargement leading to stasis of urine) or long-term exposure to environmental factors (e.g. smoking) are common causes of increased susceptibility to infection.

Hormonal influences and sex

There is decreased resistance to infection in diseases such as diabetes mellitus, hypothyroidism and adrenal dysfunction. The reasons for this decrease have not yet been clarified but may be related to enzyme or hormone activities. It is known that glucocorticoids are anti-inflammatory agents, decreasing the ability of phagocytes to ingest material. They also have beneficial effects by interfering in some way with the toxic effects of bacterial products such as endotoxins.

There are no marked differences in susceptibility to infections between the sexes. Although the overall incidence and death rate from infectious disease are greater in the male than in the female, both infectious hepatitis and whooping cough have a higher morbidity and mortality in females.

Nutritional factors

The adverse effects of poor nutrition on susceptibility to certain infectious agents are not now seriously questioned. Experimental evidence in animals has shown repeatedly that inadequate diet may be correlated with increased susceptibility to a variety of bacterial diseases, associated with decreased phagocytic activity and leucopenia. In the case of viruses, which are intracellular parasites, malnutrition might have an effect on virus production, but the usual outcome is enhanced disease due to impaired immune responses, especially the cytotoxic responses.

Mechanisms of innate immunity

Mechanical barriers and surface secretions

The intact skin and mucous membranes of the body afford a high degree of protection against pathogens. In conditions where the skin is damaged, such as in burns patients and after traumatic injury or surgery, infections can be a serious problem. The skin is a resistant barrier because of its outer horny layer consisting mainly of keratin, which is indigestible by most micro-organisms, and thus shields the living cells of the epidermis from micro-organisms and their toxins. The relatively dry condition of the skin and the high concentration of salt in drying sweat are inhibitory or lethal to many micro-organisms.

The sebaceous secretions and sweat of the skin contain bactericidal and fungicidal fatty acids, and these constitute an effective protective mechanism against many potential pathogens. The protective ability of these secretions varies at different stages of life, and some fungal 'ringworm' infections of children disappear at puberty with the marked increase of sebaceous secretions.

The sticky mucus covering the respiratory tract acts as a trapping mechanism for inhaled particles. The action of cilia sweeps the secretions, containing the foreign material, towards the oropharynx so that it is swallowed; in the stomach the acidic secretions destroy most of the micro-organisms present. Nasal secretions and saliva contain mucopolysaccharides capable of blocking some viruses.

The washing action of tears and flushing of urine are effective in stopping invasion by micro-organisms. The commensal micro-organisms that make up the natural bacterial flora covering epithelial surfaces are protective in a number of ways:

- their very presence uses up a niche that cannot be used by a pathogen
- they compete for nutrients
- they produce by-products that can inhibit the growth of other organisms.

It is important not to disturb the relationship between the host and its indigenous flora.

Commensal organisms from the gut or bacteria normally present on the skin can cause problems if they gain access to an area that they do not normally populate. An example of this is urinary tract infections resulting from the introduction of *Escherichia coli*, a gut commensal, by means of a urinary catheter. Commensal organisms that are provided with the circumstances by which to cause infections are called *opportunistic pathogens*. Infections with these opportunists are quite widespread, often appearing as a result of medical or surgical treatment that breaches the innate defences or reduces the host's ability to respond.

Humoral defence mechanisms

A number of microbicidal substances are present in the tissue and body fluids. Some of these molecules are produced constitutively, e.g. lysozyme, and others are produced in response to infection, e.g. acute-phase proteins and interferon. These molecules all show the characteristics of innate immunity – there is no specific recognition of the micro-organism and the response is not enhanced on re-exposure to the same antigen.

Lysozyme. This is a basic protein of low molecular weight found in relatively high concentrations in neutrophils as well as in most tissue fluids, except cerebrospinal fluid, sweat and urine. It functions as a mucolytic enzyme, splitting sugars off the structural peptidoglycan of the cell wall of many Gram-positive bacteria and thus causing their lysis. It seems likely that lysozyme may also play a role in the intracellular destruction of some Gram-negative bacteria. In many pathogenic bacteria the peptidoglycan of the cell wall appears to be protected from the access of lysozyme by other wall components, e.g. lipopolysaccharide. The action of other enzymes from phagocytes or of complement may be needed to remove this protection and expose the peptidoglycan to the action of lysozyme.

Basic polypeptides. A variety of basic proteins, derived from tissues and blood cells, have some antibacterial properties. This group includes the basic proteins called spermine and spermidine, which can kill tubercle bacilli and some staphylococci. Other toxic compounds are the arginine- and lysine-containing proteins protamine and histone. The bactericidal activity of basic polypeptides probably depends on their ability to react non-specifically with acid polysaccharides at the bacterial cell surface.

Acute-phase proteins. The concentration of acute-phase proteins rises dramatically during an infection. Microbial products such as endotoxin can stimulate macrophages to release IL-1, which stimulates the liver to produce increased amounts of various acute-phase proteins, the concentrations of which can rise over 1000-fold. One of the best-characterized acute-phase proteins is *C-reactive protein*, which binds to phosphorylcholine residues in the cell wall of certain micro-organisms. This complex is very effective at activating the classical complement pathway. Also included in this group of molecules are α_1-antitrypsin, α_2-macroglobulin, fibrinogen and serum amyloid A protein, all of which act to limit the spread of the infectious agent or stimulate the host response.

Interferon. The observation that cell cultures infected with one virus resist infection by a second virus, i.e. viral interference, led to the identification of the family of antiviral agents known as *interferons*. A number of molecules have been identified; α- and β-interferons are part of innate immunity, and γ-interferon is produced by T cells as part of the acquired immune response (see Chapter 12).

Complement

The existence of a heat-labile serum component with the ability to lyse red blood cells and destroy Gram-negative bacteria has been known since the 1930s. The chemical complexity of the phenomenon was not appreciated by early workers, who ascribed the activity to a single component, called complement. Complement is in fact composed of a large number of different serum proteins present in low concentration in normal serum. These molecules are present in an inactive form but can be activated to form an enzyme cascade, i.e. the product of the first reaction is the catalyst of the next and so on.

There are about 30 proteins involved in the complement system, some of which are enzymes, some are control molecules and others are structural proteins with no enzymatic activity. A number of the molecules involved are split into two components (a and b fragments) by the product of the previous step. There are two pathways of complement activation, the alternative and classical, that lead to the same physiological consequences, namely:

- opsonization
- cellular activation
- lysis.

The two pathways use different initiation processes. Component C3 forms the connection between the two pathways, and the binding of this molecule to a surface is the key process in complement activation.

Classical pathway. The classical pathway of activation leading to the cleavage of C3 is initiated by the binding of two or more of the globular domains of the C1q component of C1 to its ligand: immune complexes containing IgG or IgM and certain micro-organisms and their products. This causes a conformational change in the C1 complex that leads to the auto-activation of C1r. The enzyme C1r then converts C1s into an active serine esterase that acts on the thioester-containing molecule C4 to produce C4a and a reactive C4b (Fig. 11.2). C4a is released and some of the C4b becomes attached to a surface. The rest is inactivated by reacting with water. C2 binds to the surface-bound C4b, becomes a substrate

for the activated C1 complex and is split into C2a and C2b. The C2b is released, leaving C4b2a – the classical pathway C3 convertase. This active enzyme then generates C3a and the unstable C3b from C3. A small amount of the C3b generated will bind to the activating surface and act as a focus for further complement activation. The activation of the classical pathway is regulated by C1 inhibitor and by a number of molecules that limit the production of the 'C3 convertase'.

The so-called *lectin pathway* is initiated by mannose binding lectin attaching to the surface of a micro-organism. This leads to the production of C4b2a and the generation of C3b on the activating surface.

Alternative pathway. Intrinsically, C3 undergoes a low level of hydrolysis of an internal thioester bond to generate C3b. This molecule complexes, in the presence of Mg^{2+} ions, with factor B, which is then acted on by factor D to produce C3bBb. This is a 'C3 convertase' that is capable of splitting more C3 to C3b, some of which will become membrane-bound.

The initial binding of C3b generated by either the classical or alternative pathway leads to an amplification loop that results in the binding of many more C3b molecules to the same surface. Factor B binds to the surface-bound C3b to form C3bB, the substrate for factor D – a serine esterase – that is present in very low concentrations in an already active form. The cleavage of factor B results in the formation of the C3 convertase, C3bBb, which dissociates rapidly unless it is stabilized by the binding of properdin (P) – forming the complex C3bBbP. This convertase can cleave many more C3 molecules, some of which become surface-bound. This amplification loop is a positive feedback system that will cycle until all the C3 is used up unless it is regulated carefully.

Regulation. The nature of the surface to which the C3b is bound regulates the outcome. Self-cell membranes contain a number of regulatory molecules that promote the binding of factor H rather than factor B to C3b. This results in the inhibition of the activation process. On non-self structures the C3b is protected since regulatory proteins are not present, and factor B has a higher affinity for C3b than factor H at these sites.

Thus the surface of many micro-organisms can stabilize the C3bBb by protecting it from factor H. In addition, another molecule, properdin, stabilizes the complex. The deposition of a few molecules of C3b onto these surfaces is followed by the formation of the relatively stable C3bBbP complex. This C3 convertase will lead to more C3b deposition. Immune complexes composed of certain immunoglobulins, e.g. IgA and IgE, also function as protected sites for C3b and activate complement by the alternative pathway. Poor activation surfaces will be made more susceptible to

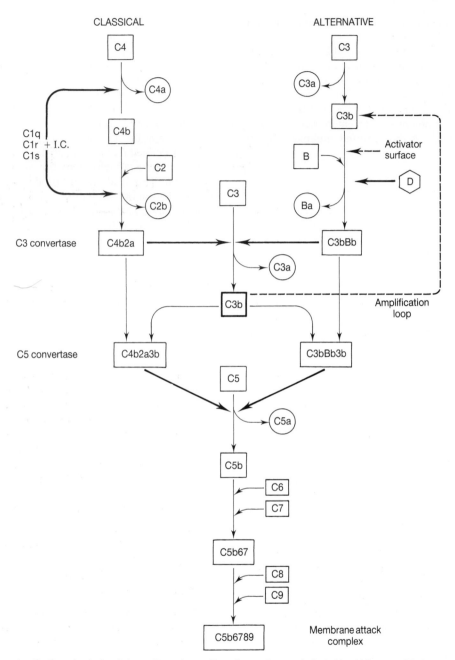

Fig. 11.2 Complement activation: classical and alternative pathways. Enzymic reactions are indicated by thick arrows. I.C., immune complex.

deposition by the presence of antibody that generates C3b by the classical pathway.

Membrane attack complex. The next step after the formation of C3b is the cleavage of C5 (Fig. 11.3). The 'C5 convertases' are generated from C4b2a of the classical pathway and C3bBb of the alternative pathway by the addition of another C3b molecule. These membrane-bound trimolecular complexes selectively bind C5 and

cleave it to give fluid phase C5a and membrane-bound C5b. The formation of the rest of the membrane attack complex is non-enzymatic. C6 binds to C5b, and this joint complex is released from the C5 convertase. The formation of C5b67 generates a hydrophobic complex that inserts into the lipid bilayer in the vicinity of the initial activation site. Usually this will be on the same cell surface as the initial trigger, but occasionally other cells

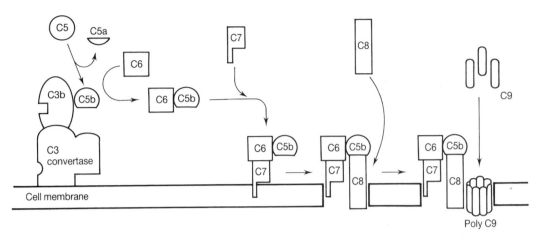

Fig. 11.3 Membrane attack complex.

may be involved. Therefore, 'bystander' lysis can take place, giving rise to damage to surrounding tissue. There are a number of proteins present in body fluids to limit this potentially dangerous process by binding to fluid phase C5b67. C8 and C9 bind to the membrane-inserted complex in sequence, resulting in the formation of a lytic polymeric complex containing up to 20 C9 monomers. A small amount of lysis can occur when C8 binds to C5b67, but it is the polymerized C9 that causes the most damage.

Functions. The activation of complement by either pathway gives rise to C3b and the generation of a number of factors that can aid in the elimination of foreign material.

The complete insertion of the membrane attack complex into a cell will lead to membrane damage and lysis, probably by osmotic swelling. Some thin-walled pathogens, such as trypanosomes and malaria parasites, are killed by complement-mediated lysis. Some Gram-negative bacteria can be killed by complement in conjunction with lysozyme. However, complement-mediated lysis is of limited importance as a bactericidal mechanism when compared to phagocyte destruction of bacteria. Inherited deficiencies of the terminal components are associated with infection by gonococci and meningococci, which can survive inside neutrophils and for which complement-mediated killing is important.

Phagocytic cells have receptors for C3b and iC3b that facilitate the adherence of complement-coated particles. Therefore, complement is an *opsonin*, and in certain circumstances this attachment may lead to phagocytosis.

Two of the molecules released during the complement cascade, C3a and C5a, have potent biological activities. These molecules, known as *anaphylatoxins*, trigger mast cells and basophils to release mediators of inflammation (see below). They also stimulate neutrophils to produce reactive oxygen intermediates, while C5a on its own is a chemoattractant and acts directly on vascular endothelium to cause vasodilatation and increased vascular permeability.

Cells

Phagocytes. Micro-organisms entering the tissue fluids or bloodstream are very rapidly engulfed by *neutrophils* and *mononuclear phagocytes*. In the blood the latter are known as *monocytes* while in the tissues they differentiate into *macrophages*. In connective tissue they are known as *histiocytes*, in kidney as *mesangial cells*, in bone as *osteoclasts*, in brain as *microglia* and in the spleen, lymph node and thymus as the *sinus-lining macrophages*.

The essential features of these cells are that they:

- are actively phagocytic
- contain digestive enzymes to degrade ingested material
- are an important link between the innate and acquired immune mechanisms.

Part of their role in regard to acquired immunity is that they can process and present antigens and produce molecules that stimulate lymphocyte differentiation into effector cells.

The role of the phagocyte in innate immunity is to engulf particles (phagocytosis) or soluble material (pinocytosis), and digest them intracellularly within specialized vacuoles. The macrophages present in the walls of capillaries and vascular sinuses in spleen, liver, lungs and bone marrow serve a very important role in clearing the bloodstream of foreign particulate material such as bacteria. So efficient is this process that the finding of a few micro-organisms in the bloodstream usually indicates that there is a continuing release of micro-organisms from an active focus such as an abscess or the heart valve vegetations found in bacterial endocarditis.

The ability of macrophages to ingest and destroy micro-organisms can be impaired or enhanced by depression or stimulation of the phagocyte system. Some micro-organisms, such as mycobacteria and brucellae, can resist intracellular digestion by normal macrophages, though they may be digested by 'activated' ones.

Chemotaxis. For phagocytic cells to be effective they must be attracted to the site of infection. Once they have passed through the capillary walls they move through the tissues in response to a concentration gradient of molecules produced at the site of damage. These chemotactic factors include:

- products of injured tissue
- factors from the blood (C5a)
- substances produced by neutrophils and mast cells (leukotrienes and histamine)
- bacterial products (formyl-methionine peptides).

Neutrophils respond first and move faster than monocytes.

Phagocytosis. Phagocytosis involves:

- recognition and binding
- ingestion
- digestion.

It may occur in the absence of antibody, especially on surfaces such as those of the lung alveoli and when inert particles are involved. Cell membranes carry a net negative charge that keeps them apart and stops autophagocytosis. The hydrophilic nature of certain bacterial cell wall components stops them passing through the hydrophobic membrane. To overcome these difficulties the phagocytes have receptors on their surface that mediate the attachment of particles that have been coated with the correct ligand. Phagocytes have receptors for the Fc portion of certain immunoglobulin isotypes and for some components of the complement cascade. The presence of these molecules or *opsonins* on the particle surface markedly enhances the ingestion process and, in some cases, digestion. Whether mediated by specific receptors or not, the foreign particle is surrounded by the cell membrane, which then invaginates and produces an *endosome* or *phagosome* within the cell (Fig. 11.4).

The microbicidal machinery of the phagocyte is contained within organelles known as *lysosomes*. This compartmentalization of potentially toxic molecules is necessary to protect the cell from self-destruction and produce an environment where the molecules can function efficiently. The phagosome and lysosome fuse to form a *phagolysosome* in which the ingested material is killed and digested by various enzyme systems.

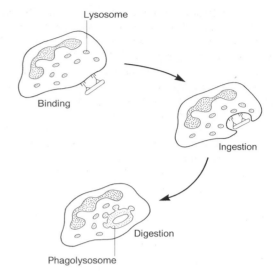

Fig. 11.4 Stages in phagocytosis.

Ingestion is accompanied by enhanced glycolysis and an increase in the synthesis of proteins and membrane phospholipids. After phagocytosis there is a respiratory burst consisting of a steep rise in oxygen consumption. This is accompanied by an increase in the activity of a number of enzymes and leads to the reduction of molecular oxygen to various highly reactive intermediates, e.g. the superoxide anion (O_2^-), hydrogen peroxide (H_2O_2), singlet oxygen ($O^{\cdot}$) and the hydroxyl radical ($OH^{\cdot}$). All these chemical species have microbicidal activity and are termed oxygen-dependent killing mechanisms. The superoxide anion is a free radical produced by the one-electron reduction of molecular oxygen; it is very reactive and highly damaging to animal cells, as well as to micro-organisms. It is also the substrate for superoxide dismutase that generates hydrogen peroxide for subsequent use in microbial killing. Myeloperoxidase uses hydrogen peroxide and halide ions, such as iodide or chloride, to produce at least two bactericidal systems. In one, halogenation (incorporation of iodine or chlorine) of the bacterial cell wall leads to death of the organism. In the second mechanism, myeloperoxidase and hydrogen peroxide damage the cell wall by converting amino acids into aldehydes that have antimicrobial activity.

Within phagocytes there are several oxygen-independent mechanisms that can destroy ingested material. Some of these enzymes can damage membranes. For example, *lysozyme* and *elastase* attack peptidoglycan of the bacterial cell wall, and then hydrolases are responsible for the complete digestion of the killed organism. The cationic proteins of lysosomes bind to and damage bacterial cell walls and enveloped viruses, such as herpes simplex virus. The iron-binding protein *lactofer-*

rin has antimicrobial properties. It complexes with iron, rendering it unavailable to bacteria that require iron for growth. The high acidity within phagolysosomes (pH 3.5–4.0) may have bactericidal effects: it probably results from lactic acid production in glycolysis. In addition, many lysosomal enzymes, such as acid hydrolases, have acid pH optima. There are significant differences between macrophages and neutrophils in the killing of micro-organisms. Although macrophage lysosomes contain a variety of enzymes, including lysozyme, they lack cationic proteins and lactoferrin. Tissue macrophages do not have myeloperoxidase but probably use catalase to generate the hydrogen peroxide system. Normal macrophages are less efficient killers of certain pathogens, such as fungi, than neutrophils. The microbicidal activity of macrophages can, however, be greatly improved after contact with products of lymphocytes, known as lymphokines.

Once killed, most micro-organisms are digested and solubilized by lysosomal enzymes. The degradation products are then released to the exterior.

Natural killer cells. NK cells recognize changes on virus-infected cells and destroy them by an extracellular killing mechanism. After binding to the target cell, by an as yet undefined mechanism, the NK cell produces molecules that damage the membrane of the infected cell, leading to its destruction.

Natural killing is a function of several different cell types. This activity is performed by cells described as large granular lymphocytes and also by cells with T cell markers, macrophage markers and others that do not have the characteristics of any of the main cells of the immune system. Natural killing is present without prior exposure to the infectious agent and shows all the characteristics of an innate defence mechanism. NK cells have also been implicated in host defence against cancers. They are thought to recognize changes in the cell membranes of transformed cells in a mechanism similar to that used to combat virus infection. Natural killing is enhanced by interferons that appear to stimulate the production of NK cells and also increase the rate at which they kill the target cells.

Eosinophils. Eosinophils are polymorphonuclear leucocytes with a characteristic bilobed nucleus and cytoplasmic granules. They are present in the blood of normal individuals at very low levels (<1%), but their numbers increase in patients with parasitic infections and allergies. They are not efficient phagocytic cells but their granules contain molecules that are toxic to parasites. Large parasites such as helminths cannot be internalized by phagocytes and therefore must be killed extracellularly. Eosinophil granules contain an array of enzymes and toxic molecules that are active against parasitic worms. The release of these molecules must be

controlled so that tissue damage is avoided. The eosinophils have specific receptors, including Fc and complement receptors, which bind the labelled target, i.e. antibody or complement-coated parasites. The granule contents are then released into the space between the cell and the parasite, thus targeting the toxic molecules onto the parasite membrane.

Temperature

The temperature dependence of many micro-organisms is well known, and it is therefore apparent that temperature is an important factor in determining the innate immunity of an animal to some infectious agents. It seems likely that the pyrexia that follows so many different types of infection can function as a protective response against the infecting micro-organism. The febrile response in many cases is controlled by IL-1 produced by macrophages as part of the immune response.

Inflammation

A number of the above factors are responsible for the process of *inflammation*. This is the reaction of the body to injury, such as invasion by an infectious agent, exposure to a noxious chemical or physical trauma. The signs of inflammation are redness, heat, swelling, pain and loss of function. The molecular and cellular events that occur during an inflammatory reaction are:

- vasodilatation
- increased vascular permeability
- cellular infiltration.

These changes are brought about mainly by chemical mediators (Table 11.3), which are widely distributed in a sequestered or inactive form throughout the body and are released or activated locally at the site of inflammation. After release they tend to be rapidly inactivated to ensure control of the inflammatory process.

There is increased blood supply to the affected area due to the action of vasoactive amines such as histamine and 5-hydroxytryptamine and other mediators stored within mast cells. These molecules are released:

- as a consequence of the production of the anaphylatoxins (C3a and C5a) that trigger specific receptors on mast cells
- following interaction of antigen with IgE on the surface of mast cells
- by direct physical damage to the cells.

Other mediators, such as bradykinins and prostaglandins, are produced locally or released by platelets. The vasodilatation causes increased blood supply to the area, giving rise to redness and heat. The result is an

Table 11.3 Mediators of inflammation

Mediator	Main source	Function
Histamine[a]	Mast cells, basophils	Vasodilatation, increased vascular permeability, contraction of smooth muscle
Kinins (e.g. bradykinin)	Plasma	Vasodilatation, increased vascular permeability, contraction of smooth muscle, pain
Prostaglandins	Neutrophils, eosinophils, monocytes, platelets	Vasodilatation, increased vascular permeability, pain
Leukotrienes	Neutrophils, mast cells, basophils	Vasodilatation, increased vascular permeability, contraction of smooth muscle, induce cell adherence and chemotaxis
Complement components (e.g. C3a, C5a)	Plasma	Cause mast cells to release mediator C5a is chemotactic factor
Plasmin	Plasma	Breaks down fibrin, kinin formation
Cytokines	Lymphocytes, macrophages	Chemotactic factors, colony-stimulation factors, macrophage activation

[a] In rodents, 5-hydroxytryptamine (serotonin) is present in mast cells and basophils.

increase in the supply of the molecules and cells that can combat the agent responsible for the initial trigger.

The same molecules, vasoactive amines, prostaglandins and kinins, increase vascular permeability, allowing plasma and plasma proteins to traverse the endothelial lining. The plasma proteins will include immunoglobulins and molecules of the clotting and complement cascades. This leaking of fluid will cause swelling (oedema) that will in turn lead to increased tissue tension and pain. Some of the molecules themselves, e.g. prostaglandins and histamine, stimulate the pain responses directly. The inflammatory exudate has several important functions. Bacteria often produce tissue-damaging toxins that will be diluted by the exudate. Clotting factors present result in the deposition of fibrin, creating a physical obstruction to the spread of bacteria. The exudate is drained continuously by the lymphatic vessels, and antigens, such as bacteria and their toxins, are carried to the draining lymph node where immune responses can be generated.

Chemotactic factors produced, including C5a, histamine, leukotrienes and molecules specific for certain cell types, will attract phagocytic cells to the site. The increased vascular permeability will allow easier access for neutrophils and monocytes and the vasodilatation means that more cells are in the vicinity. The neutrophils will arrive first and begin to destroy or remove the offending agent. Most will be successful but a few will die, releasing their tissue-damaging contents to increase

the inflammatory process. Mononuclear phagocytes will arrive on the scene to finish off the removal of the residual debris and stimulate tissue repair.

When the swelling is severe there may be loss of function to the affected area. If the offending agent is quickly removed then the tissue will soon be repaired. The inflammatory process continues until the conditions responsible for its initiation are resolved. In most circumstances this occurs fairly rapidly with an acute inflammatory reaction lasting a matter of hours or days. If, however, the causative agent is not easily removed or is reintroduced continuously, then chronic inflammation will ensue with the possibility of tissue destruction and complete loss of function.

ACQUIRED IMMUNITY

Micro-organisms that overcome or circumvent the innate non-specific defence mechanisms or are administered deliberately, i.e. active immunization, come up against the host's second line of defence – *acquired immunity*. To give expression to this acquired form of immunity it is necessary that the antigens of the invading micro-organism should come into contact with cells of the immune system (macrophages and lymphocytes) and so initiate an immune response specific for the foreign material. The cells that respond are precommitted, because of their surface receptors, to respond to a particular epitope on the antigen. This response takes two forms, *humoral* and *cell-mediated*, which usually develop in parallel. The part played by each will depend on a number of factors, including the nature of the antigen, the route of entry and the individual who is infected.

Humoral immunity depends on the appearance in the blood of antibodies produced by plasma cells.

The term 'cell-mediated immunity' was originally coined to describe localized reactions to organisms mediated by T lymphocytes and phagocytes rather than by antibody. It is now used to describe any response in which antibody plays a subordinate role. Cell-mediated immunity depends mainly on the development of T cells that are specifically responsive to the inducing agent and is generally active against intracellular organisms.

Specific immunity may be acquired in two main ways:

- it may be induced by overt clinical infection or inapparent clinical infection
- deliberate artificial immunization.

This is *active acquired immunity*, and contrasts with *passive acquired immunity*, which is the transfer of pre-formed antibodies to a non-immune individual by means of blood, serum components or lymphoid cells.

Actively acquired immunity is long-lasting although it may be circumvented by antigenic change in the infecting micro-organism. Passively acquired immunity provides only temporary protection. Passive immunity may be transferred to the fetus by the passage of maternal antibodies across the placenta.

Tissues involved in immune reactions

For the generation of an immune response, antigen must interact with and activate a number of different cells. In addition, these cells must interact with each other. The cells involved in immune responses are organized into tissues and organs in order that these complex cellular interactions can occur most effectively. These structures are collectively referred to as the *lymphoid system*, which comprises lymphocytes, epithelial and stromal cells arranged into discrete capsulated organs or accumulations of diffuse lymphoid tissue. Lymphoid organs contain lymphocytes at various stages of development and are classified into primary and secondary lymphoid organs.

The primary lymphoid organs are the major sites of lymphopoiesis. Here, lymphoid progenitor cells develop into mature lymphocytes by a process of proliferation and differentiation. In mammals, T lymphocytes develop in the thymus, and B lymphocytes in the bone marrow and fetal liver. It is within the primary lymphoid organs that the lymphocytes acquire their repertoire of specific

antigen receptors in order to cope with the antigenic challenges that the individual receives during its life. It is also within these tissues that self-reactive lymphocytes are eliminated to protect against autoimmune disease.

The secondary lymphoid organs create the environment in which lymphocytes can interact with each other and with antigen and then disseminate the effector cells and molecules generated. Secondary lymphoid organs include lymph nodes, spleen and mucosal-associated lymphoid tissue, e.g. tonsils and Peyer's patches of the gut. These organs have a characteristic structure that relates to the function they carry out, with areas composed mainly of B cells or T cells.

Development of the immune system

In humans, lymphoid tissue appears first in the thymus at about 8 weeks of gestation. Peyer's patches are distinguishable by the fifth month, and immunoglobulin-secreting cells appear in the spleen and lymph nodes at about 20 weeks. From this period onwards, IgM and IgD are synthesized by the fetus (Fig. 11.5). At birth the infant has a blood concentration of IgG comparable to that of the maternal circulation, having received IgG but not IgM via the placenta. The rate of synthesis of IgM in the infant increases rapidly within the first few days of life but does

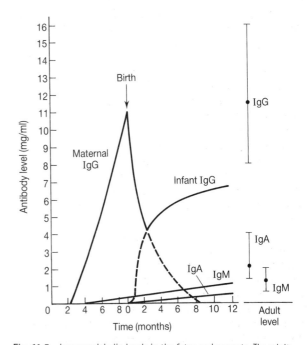

Fig. 11.5 Immunoglobulin levels in the fetus and neonate. The adult levels of the major isotypes are shown as normal ranges with mean serum levels (•).

not reach adult levels until about a year. Serum IgG does not reach adult levels until after the second year, and IgA takes even longer. There is an actual drop in the level of IgG from birth due to the decay of maternal antibody, with the lowest levels of total IgG at around 3 months of age. This corresponds to an age of marked susceptibility to a number of infections. Cell-mediated immunity can be stimulated at birth, but these reactions may not be as powerful as in the adult.

Lymphocyte trafficking

Lymphocytes differentiate and mature in the primary lymphoid organs and then enter the blood lymphocyte pool. B cells are produced in the bone marrow and mature there before proceeding via the circulation to the secondary lymphoid organs. T cell precursors leave the bone marrow and mature in the thymus before migrating to the secondary lymphoid organs. Once in the secondary lymphoid tissues the lymphocytes do not remain there but move from one lymphoid organ to another through the blood and lymphatics (Fig. 11.6). One of the main advantages of this *lymphocyte recirculation* is that during the course of a natural infection the continual trafficking of lymphocytes enables very many different lymphocytes to have access to the antigen.

Only a very small number of the lymphocytes will recognize a particular antigen. Pathogens can enter the body by many routes but must be carried from the site

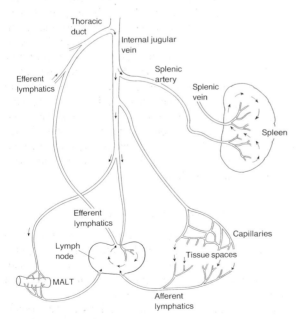

Fig. 11.6 Lymphocyte recirculation. MALT, mucosal-associated lymphoid tissue.

of infection to the secondary lymphoid tissues where they are localized and concentrated on the dendritic processes of macrophages or on the surface of antigen-presenting cells. If the infection is in the tissues, antigen is carried in the lymphatics to the draining lymph node. Under normal conditions there is a continuous active flow of lymphocytes through lymph nodes, but when antigen and antigen-reactive cells enter there is a temporary shutdown of the exit. Thus, antigen-specific cells are preferentially retained in the node draining the source of the antigen. This is partly responsible for the swollen glands (lymph nodes) that can sometimes be found during an infection. Antigens that enter through a mucosal surface are collected into the mucosal-associated lymphoid tissues such as the tonsils and Peyer's patches. Blood-borne antigens are trapped in the spleen. The passage of lymphocytes through an area where antigen has been localized facilitates the induction of an immune response. Lymphocytes with appropriate receptors bind to the antigen and become activated. Once activated the lymphocytes mature into effector cells. In the case of B lymphocytes they become plasma cells and secrete antibody. T lymphocytes will leave the secondary lymphoid tissue and return to the site of infection to destroy the infectious agent.

There is now evidence for non-random migration of lymphocytes to particular lymphoid compartments. For example, lymphocytes that home to the gut are selectively transported across endothelial cells of venules in the intestine. It appears that lymphocytes have specific molecules on their surface that preferentially interact with endothelial cells in different anatomical sites. A lymphocyte that was initially stimulated by antigen in a Peyer's patch will migrate to the draining lymph node, respond, and memory cells will be produced. It is important that these memory cells migrate back to the area where the same pathogen might be encountered again. Therefore, they are found preferentially in the mucosal-associated lymphoid tissue.

Clonal selection

During their development in the primary lymphoid tissues both T and B lymphocytes acquire specific cell surface receptors that commit them to a single antigenic specificity. For T cells this receptor will remain the same for its life, but the surface immunoglobulin on B cells can be modified due to somatic mutations. In the B cell this is mirrored in the modification of the antibody the cell produces on exposure to its specific antigen. The lymphocytes are activated when they bind specific antigen and then proliferate, differentiate and mature into effector cells.

The lymphocytes reactive to any particular antigen are only a small proportion of the total pool. Therefore, antigen binds to the small number of cells that can recognize it and *selects* them to proliferate and mature so that sufficient cells are formed to mount an adequate immune response. A cell that responds to an antigenic trigger and proliferates will give rise to cells with a genetically identical make up, i.e. *clones*. Therefore, this phenomenon is known as *clonal selection*.

Lymphocyte receptors, generated in the primary lymphoid tissues, are created in a random fashion, so there is no reason why some could not recognize 'self' molecules. It is obviously an important attribute of the immune system that it is able to discriminate between 'self' and 'non-self'. During development, any lymphocyte with a receptor that binds strongly to self molecules is eliminated.

Cellular activation

When an individual is exposed to foreign material, selected lymphocytes respond. B lymphocytes proliferate and differentiate into antibody-producing plasma cells and memory cells. T lymphocytes are stimulated to become effector cells that can directly eliminate the foreign material or produce molecules that help other cells destroy the pathogen. The type (immunity or tolerance) and magnitude of the response, if generated, will depend on a number of factors, including the nature, dose and route of entry of the antigen and the individual's genetic make up and previous exposure to the antigen.

The first stage in the production of effector cells and molecules is the activation of the resting cells. This involves various cellular interactions with maturation of the response, leading to a co-ordinated, efficient production of effector T cells, immunoglobulin and memory cells.

Cross-linking of the B cell antigen receptor, surface immunoglobulin, is the initial trigger for activation. When this happens, a number of biochemical changes are instigated. These changes probably act through protein kinases that cause the synthesis of RNA and ultimately immunoglobulin production. In a number of cases this is all that is required to stimulate antibody production. However, for the majority of antigens this initial cross-linking is not enough, and molecules produced by T cells are also required.

Thymus-independent antigens. A number of antigens will stimulate specific immunoglobulin production directly. These T-independent antigens are of two types: *mitogens* and certain large molecules.

Mitogens are substances that cause cells, particularly lymphocytes, to undergo cell division, i.e. proliferation. Certain glycoproteins, called lectins, have mitogenic activity. These molecules have specificity for sugars and bind to the cell surface and will activate all responsive cells. The response to the mitogens will therefore be polyclonal since lymphocytes of many different specificities will be activated. However, at low concentrations these mitogens do not cause polyclonal activation but can lead to the stimulation of specific B cells. Lipopolysaccharide is an example of a B cell mitogen.

Some large molecules with regularly repeating epitopes, e.g. polymers of D-amino acids and simple sugars such as pneumococcal polysaccharide and dextran, can interact directly with the B cell surface immunoglobulin. They may also be held on the surface of specialized macrophages in secondary lymphoid tissues and the B cells interact with them there. The multiple repeats of the epitope interact with a large number of surface immunoglobulin molecules and the signal that is generated is sufficient to stimulate antibody production.

The immune response generated to these antigens tends to be similar on each exposure, i.e. IgM is the main antibody, and the response shows little memory. This suggests that class switch and memory production require additional factors, i.e. products of T lymphocytes.

Thymus-dependent antigens. Many antigens do not stimulate antibody production without the help of T lymphocytes. These antigens first bind to the B cell, which must then be exposed to T cell-derived lymphokines, i.e. helper factors, before antibody can be produced. For the second activation signal, i.e. help, to be effectively targeted at the B cell the T and B cells must be in direct contact. For this to happen the B and T cell epitopes must be physically linked. However, T cells only recognize antigen that has been processed and is presented in association with products of the major histocompatibility complex (MHC), so it is impossible for native antigen to form a bridge between surface immunoglobulin and the T cell receptor. The B cell binds to its epitope on free antigen, but there is no site on this molecule to which the T cell can bind since it requires antigen associated with MHC products. The answer to this problem can be seen when the requirements for antigen presentation in T cell recognition are considered.

Antigen processing and presentation

The development of an antibody response to a T-dependent antigen requires that the antigen becomes associated with MHC class II molecules, i.e. *processed*, and expressed on the cell surface, i.e. *presented*, in a form that helper T cells can recognize.

All cells express MHC class I molecules, but class II molecules are confined to cells of the immune system – the antigen-presenting cells. These cells present antigen

Table 11.4 Antigen-presenting cells in the lymph nodes

Area	Antigen-presenting cell	Antigen
Subcapsular marginal sinus	Marginal zone macrophage	T-independent antigens
Follicles and B cell areas	Follicular dendritic cells	Antigen–antibody complexes
Medulla	Classical macrophages	Most antigens
T cell areas	Interdigitating dendritic cells	Most antigens

to MHC class II-restricted T cells (the CD4-positive (CD4+) population) and therefore play a key role in the induction and development of immune responses. Within lymph nodes, different antigen-presenting cells are found in each of the main areas (Table 11.4).

There are a large number of antigen-presenting cells in the body, most of which constitutively express MHC class II molecules. Other cells, such as T lymphocytes and endothelium, can be induced to express MHC class II molecules by suitable stimuli such as lymphokines. The relative importance of each type depends on whether a primary or secondary response is being stimulated and on the location. The most studied antigen-presenting cells are the macrophages and dendritic cells. However, it is now apparent that in certain situations B cells may be important antigen-presenting cells. The relative importance of B cells becomes greatest during secondary responses, especially if the antigen concentration is low. Here the B cells can specifically engulf antigen via their surface immunoglobulin. In a primary response, specific B cells are at a low frequency and their receptors are of low affinity; in this situation macrophages and dendritic cells are probably most important.

The key feature of all antigen-presenting cells is that they can ingest antigen, degrade it and present it, in the context of MHC class II molecules, to T cells. The antigen is taken into the antigen-presenting cells and enters the endocytic pathway. Before it is completely destroyed, peptide fragments are taken to a structure called the compartment for peptide loading (CPL). MHC class II molecules are synthesized within the endoplasmic reticulum and are also transported to the CPL, where they associate with the processed antigen. The MHC class II molecule with the bound peptide is then transported to the cell surface.

T cell activation

The activation of resting CD4+ T cells requires two signals. The first is antigen in association with MHC class II molecules and the second is the *co-stimulatory signal*. The generation of the first of these signals has just been discussed, i.e. antigen presentation. The second signal is delivered by the same antigen-presenting cell

that gave the first signal. The co-stimulatory signal is mediated by the interaction of a molecule on the antigen-presenting cell engaging with its receptor on the T cell. The best characterized pairing is B7 on the antigen-presenting cell, and CD28 on the T cell.

When both these signals are generated, biochemical changes occur within the T cell, leading to RNA and protein synthesis. The responsive cells progress through the cell cycle from the G_0 to the G_1 phase. The cells start to express IL-2 receptors and produce IL-2, a T cell growth factor that causes the expansion of the responsive T cell population. IL-2 was originally thought to be the only T cell growth factor, but it is now known that IL-4 and IL-1 will support T cell growth although they are not as potent. After about 2 days, IL-2 synthesis stops, while IL-2 receptors remain for up to a week if the cell is not reactivated. Therefore, there is a built-in limitation on T cell growth and clonal expansion. When stimulated, T cells secrete IL-2, which interacts with IL-2 receptors to mediate growth. This can be in an 'autocrine' fashion if the same cell that released the IL-2 is stimulated. If the responding cell is in the vicinity of the producer then the stimulation is in a 'paracrine' manner. IL-2 is not present at detectable levels in the blood, therefore there is no 'endocrine' activity involved, i.e. action at a distant site. The end result is the production of a large number of activated CD4+ T lymphocytes.

The other main type of T lymphocyte is the CD8+ T cell. Antigen recognition by these cells is restricted by MHC class I molecules. Again, these cells require two signals to be activated – antigen fragment in association with MHC class I is the first signal, and the co-stimulatory signal the second signal. A cell that 'sees' both these signals responds by clonal expansion and differentiation into a fully active effector T cell.

B cell activation

Mitogens and T-independent antigens have an inherent ability to drive B cells into division and differentiation. T-dependent responses rely on T cells and their products to control the antibody class, affinity and memory. The first cells to be activated are CD4+ T cells that recognize the antigen in association with MHC class II molecules (see above). These cells respond to the signal of the antigen fragment–MHC complex, and produce a variety of lymphokines that act on B cells.

As far as B cell development is concerned, the antigen-stimulated cells develop under the influence of IL-4 (previously known as B cell stimulation factor) that is produced by closely adherent T cells. IL-5 and IL-6 then bring the cells to a state of full activation with terminal differentiation into an immunoglobulin-producing plasma cell. All this will happen within a germinal centre of a lymph node secondary follicle that has evolved to facilitate the necessary cellular and molecular interactions.

Therefore, for both B and T cell activation two stimuli are required.

- The recognition of antigen makes sure that only those cells that will be effective against the foreign material are recruited.
- The provision of the co-stimulatory signal has evolved to control the process and aid discrimination of 'self' and 'non-self'.

Humoral immunity

Synthesis of antibody

On exposure to antigen, antibody production follows a characteristic pattern (Fig. 11.7). There is a lag phase during which antibody cannot be detected. This is the time taken for the interactions described above to take place and antibody to reach a level that can be measured. Then there is an exponential rise in the antibody level or titre. This log phase is followed by a plateau with a constant level of antibody when the amount produced equals the amount removed. The amount of antibody then declines due to the clearing of antigen–antibody complexes and the natural catabolism of the immunoglobulin.

If the response is to a T-dependent antigen then the B cells can switch to the production of another isotype,

e.g. in a primary response IgM gives way to IgG production. This process is under the control of T cells, since the class of antibody produced will depend on signals from the T cell. At some point, again under the control of T cells, a proportion of the antigen-reactive cells will develop into memory cells. These cells will react if the epitope is encountered again.

There are a number of differences in the reaction profile on second and subsequent exposures to an antigen compared to the primary response (Fig. 11.8). There is a shortened lag and an extended plateau and decline. The level and affinity of antibody produced are much increased, and it is mostly of the IgG isotype. Some IgM will be generated, but it will follow the same pattern as in the primary response.

When first introduced the antigen selects the cells that can react with it. However, before antibody is produced the B cell must differentiate into a plasma cell, involving the interactions already described. The B cells that are stimulated in the primary response synthesize IgM. With time, class switch will occur in some of the B cells, leading to the production of other isotypes. Somatic mutations will occur, giving rise to *affinity maturation* through selection of cells bearing high-affinity receptors as the amount of antigen in the system falls. Memory cells will also be produced. An equilibrium is reached where there is a balance between the amount of antibody synthesized and the amount used. Various mechanisms then come into play to turn off the response when it is no longer needed (see below). The simplest is the removal of the stimulant, i.e. antigen. So the production of antibody is stopped and there is a natural decline in antibody levels.

On subsequent exposure the responding cells, i.e. memory cells, are at a different level of activation and are present at an increased frequency. Therefore, there is a shorter lag before antibody can be detected: the main isotype is IgG. The level of antibody produced is 10 or more times greater than during the primary response. The antibody is present for an extended period and has a

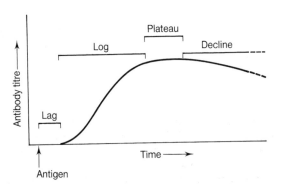

Fig. 11.7 Pattern of antibody production following antigen exposure.

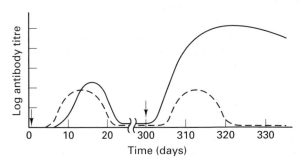

Fig. 11.8 Primary and secondary antibody response. The level of serum IgM (- - -) and IgG (—) detected with time after primary immunization (day 0) and challenge (day 300) with the same antigen.

higher affinity for antigen due to affinity maturation. As is seen in Fig. 11.8 some IgM is also produced during a secondary response. This immunoglobulin is produced by the activation of B cells that were not present in the lymphocyte pool on the previous exposure but have developed since. The development of these cells follows the characteristics of a primary response, and they will give rise to a secondary response if the antigen is encountered again.

Monoclonal antibodies

When an antigen is introduced into the lymphoid system of a mouse, all the B cells that recognize epitopes on the antigen will be stimulated to produce antibody. The serum of the immunized animal is known as a polyclonal antiserum since it is the product of many clonally derived B cells. Even if highly purified antigen is used, the antiserum produced will contain a number of antibodies that react to the antigen and others that interact with antigens that the animal encountered naturally during this time. It is extremely difficult to purify the antibodies of interest from this complex mixture, but it is possible to fuse single plasma cells with a myeloma (a tumour) cell line to form a hybridoma that will grow in tissue culture. These cells will all be identical and therefore secrete the same antibody, a *monoclonal antibody*.

Human monoclonal antibodies are potentially of value in patient treatment. As starting material, peripheral blood or secondary lymphoid tissue such as tonsils have been used. It is impossible for ethical reasons to expose human subjects to most of the antigenic material that would be required to induce useful antibodies. Therefore, cells are only available from patients with certain diseases, such as tumours, infections and auto-immune diseases, or from individuals who have received immunizations.

All the molecules in a monoclonal antibody preparation will have the same isotype, specificity and affinity, in contrast to the polyclonal antiserum produced by the inoculation of antigen into an experimental animal. In addition, the same polyclonal antiserum can never be reproduced, not even when using the same animal. However, monoclonal antibodies are defined reagents that can be produced indefinitely and on a large scale. They provide a standard material that can be used in studies ranging from the identification and enumeration of different cell types to blood typing and diagnosis of disease. They are also increasingly used in attempts to treat and prevent disease.

Cell-mediated immunity

Specific cell-mediated responses are mediated by two different types of T lymphocyte. T cells that have the CD8 molecule on their surface recognize antigen frag-

ments in association with MHC class I molecules on a target cell and cause cell lysis. MHC class II-restricted recognition is seen with T cells that have the CD4 marker. These cells secrete lymphokines when stimulated by the antigen–MHC class II complex. CD4+ T cells are involved in two main activities:

1. Cell-mediated reactions, as the lymphokines can aid in the elimination of foreign material by recruiting and activating other leucocytes and promoting an inflammatory response.
2. The generation and control of an immune response, as some of the lymphokines produced are growth and differentiation factors for T and B cells.

The other cell types, NK cells and phagocytes, which can participate in cell-mediated defence mechanisms have been described.

Cell-mediated cytotoxicity

Certain subpopulations of lymphoid and myeloid cells can destroy target cells to which they are closely bound. The stages and processes involved are similar for the different cell types although the molecules that mediate the recognition of the target by the effector differ.

Cytotoxic T lymphocytes. Cytotoxic T cells (T_c cells) are small T lymphocytes that are derived from stem cells in the bone marrow. These cells mature in the thymus. Most cells that mediate MHC-restricted cytotoxicity are CD8+ and, therefore, recognize antigen in association with MHC class I antigens. Some are CD4+ and, therefore, MHC class II-restricted.

MHC-unrestricted cytotoxic cells. A number of partially overlapping cell populations are able to carry out MHC-unrestricted killing. These include NK cells, lymphokine-activated killer (LAK) cells and killer (K) cells.

Most cells that have the capacity to perform natural killing have the morphology of large granular lymphocytes and have a broad target range. The receptor on the NK cell and the structures that they recognize on the target have not been fully characterized. NK cells have been shown to produce a number of cytokines, including γ-interferon.

Several types of cells are able to destroy foreign material by antibody-dependent cell-mediated cytotoxicity. The cells that carry out this activity have a receptor for the Fc portion of immunoglobulin and are, therefore, able to bind to antibody-coated targets.

Lytic mechanism. Three distinct phases have been described in cell-mediated cytotoxicity (Fig. 11.9):

- binding to target
- rearrangement of cytoplasmic granules and the release of their contents
- target cell death.

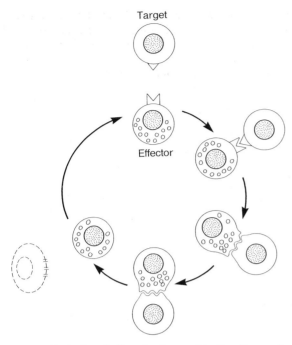

Target

Effector

Fig. 11.9 Mechanism of cell-mediated cytotoxicity. The effector cell has a receptor that is able to bind to a target cell that possesses the appropriate ligand (Δ).

Once the effector–target conjugate is formed the cytoplasmic granules appear to become rearranged and concentrated at the side of the cell adjacent to the target. The granule contents are then released into the space between the two cells. There are at least three different types of molecule stored within the granules that can cause cell death. T cells and NK cells contain perforin, which is a monomeric protein related to the complement component C9. In the presence of Ca^{2+} ions the monomers bind to the target cell membrane and polymerize to form a transmembrane pore. This upsets the osmotic balance of the cell and leads to cell death. The granules also contain at least two serine esterases that may play a role in destroying the target cell. Several other toxic molecules are produced by cytotoxic cells, including tumour necrosis factor (TNFα), lymphotoxin (TNFβ), γ-interferon and NK cytotoxic factor. The process is unidirectional with only the target cell being destroyed. The effector cell can then move on and eliminate another target cell.

Lymphokine production

The other arm of cell-mediated immunity is dependent on the production of lymphokines from antigen-activated T lymphocytes. These molecules, produced in an antigen-specific fashion, can act in an antigen-non-specific manner to recruit, activate and regulate effector cells with the potential to combat infectious agents.

The first documented reference to the production of lymphokines is credited to Robert Koch in 1880. Injection of purified antigen (tuberculin) into the skin of immune individuals produced a reaction that peaked within 24–72 h. The response was characterized by reddening and swelling and was accompanied by the accumulation of lymphocytes, monocytes and basophils. Because of the time course of the reaction this response has become known as *delayed-type hypersensitivity* (DTH) and the cells responsible were called delayed-type hypersensitivity T lymphocytes (T_{DTH} or T_D cells). These cells are identical to the helper T (T_H) cell subset as far as antigen recognition is concerned. CD4+ T cells, usually still referred to as T_H cells, are therefore capable of mediating both helper activities and so-called delayed hypersensitivity reactions by producing lymphokines. Although the term 'delayed hypersensitivity' suggests a disease process, the production of lymphokines has a physiological function, and only in some situations do pathological consequences occur.

Cytokines are biologically active molecules released by specific cells that elicit a particular response from other cells on which they act. A number of these regulatory molecules produced by lymphocytes (lymphokines) and monocytes (monokines) are shown in Table 11.5. The responses caused by these substances are varied and interrelated. In general, cytokines control growth, mobility and differentiation of lymphocytes, but they also exert a similar effect on other leucocytes and some non-immune cells.

The exact signals and mechanisms controlling the activation of T cells and the release of lymphokines are not known. The balance between the different lymphokines produced will determine the response generated. CD4+ T cells can be divided into two main types depending on the profile of lymphokines they secrete. The T_H2 subset produces IL-4 and IL-5, which act on responsive B cells with antibody production as the main feature of the response. The T_H1 subset secretes mainly IL-2 and γ-interferon. The production of IL-2 stimulates T cell growth while γ-interferon will have multiple effects, including macrophage activation.

Role of macrophages

Macrophages are able to carry out a remarkable array of different functions (Fig. 11.10). They play a key role in several aspects of cell-mediated immunity, being involved at the initiation of the response, as antigen-presenting cells, and as effector cells having microbicidal and tumoricidal activities. They also produce a number of cytokines (or more precisely monokines)

Table 11.5 Examples of some of the cytokines that are of importance in the immune system. Many of the molecules detailed below act synergistically to produce their biological effects

Cytokine	Source	Target	Main effects
IL-1	Macrophages Endothelial cells Some epithelial cells	T lymphocytes Tissue cells	Fever Inflammation T cell activation Macrophage activation Stimulate acute phase protein production
IL-2	T lymphocytes	T lymphocytes NK cells B lymphocytes	Proliferation
IL-4	T_H2 cells Mast cells	B lymphocytes T lymphocytes Mast cells	Stimulates proliferation, differentiation and class switch in B cells Differentiation and proliferation of T_H2 cells Mast cell growth
IL-8	Macrophages Endothelial cells	Neutrophils	Chemotaxis
IL-13	T_H2 cells	Macrophages	Inhibits macrophage activation and activities
TNF	Macrophages T lymphocytes	Macrophages Tissue cells	Fever Inflammation Macrophage activation Stimulates acute phase protein production Kills certain tumour cells
Type I IFN (α and β)	Virally infected cells	Tissue cells	Antiviral effect Induction of MHC class I Antiproliferative effects Activation of NK cells
IFN-γ	T lymphocytes (T_H1 and TC) NK cells	Leucocytes and tissue cells	Macrophage activation Induction of MHC class I and II Antibody class switch Antiviral effect
GM-CSF	T lymphocytes Macrophages Endothelial cells Fibroblasts	Immature and committed progenitor cells in bone marrow	Stimulate division and differentiation Macrophage activation

IL, interleukin; TNF, tumour necrosis factor; IFN, interferon; GM-CSF, granulocyte–macrophage colony-stimulating factor; NK, natural killer; MHC, major histocompatibility complex.

that function as regulatory molecules. These monokines contribute to inflammation and fever and affect the functioning of other cells. Macrophages can also produce various enzymes and factors that are involved in reorganization and repair following tissue damage. However, since they contain many important biological molecules they themselves can cause damage if these enzymes and factors are released inappropriately.

Many of these activities are enhanced in macrophages that have been '*activated*' by exposure to lymphokines, such as γ-interferon produced by T cells. Macrophage activation is a complex process that probably occurs in stages with different effector functions being expressed at different stages. Macrophages from different sites in the body show different characteristics, i.e. they are very heterogeneous, and will have different activation requirements.

γ-Interferon is a powerful macrophage-activating molecule, which increases the uptake of antigens by an enhanced expression of Fc and complement receptors; the activities of intracellular enzymes involved in killing are also elevated. Since γ-interferon causes an increase in MHC class II expression there will be an enhanced presentation of antigen to CD4$^+$ T cells. This will lead to

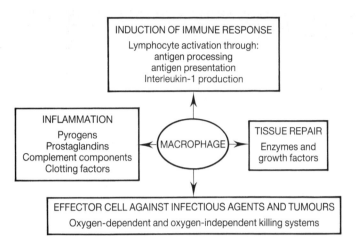

Fig. 11.10 The central role of macrophages.

the production of more lymphokines and more effective elimination of the offending material.

CD4$^+$ T cells secrete the lymphokines that activate macrophages. Therefore, the presentation of antigen by an antigen-presenting cell will lead to the production of lymphokines by T$_H$1 cells *specific* for the antigen involved. The lymphokines produced will then activate *any* responsive macrophage in the vicinity of the responding cells. The activation process appears to depend on the presence of a number of lymphokines that act synergistically to induce activation. For example, pure IL-2, IL-4 or γ-interferon is unable to induce resistance to infection, but if γ-interferon is combined with any of the others then resistance is observed.

Macrophages and monocytes themselves are capable of producing a number of important cytokines. These monokines include:

- IL-1
- IL-6
- various colony-stimulating factors and tumour necrosis factor.

Tumour necrosis factor and IL-1 acting independently and together have effects on many leucocytes and tissues. Tumour necrosis factor is responsible for the tumoricidal activity of macrophages but is also implicated in the elimination of certain bacteria and parasites. It has a synergistic effect with γ-interferon on resistance to a number of viral infections.

Generation of immune responses

As discussed previously, the generation of humoral and cell-mediated responses requires the recognition of antigen, by the responding cell, as the first signal and a co-stimulation second signal. T$_H$ cells, as has been emphasized, only recognize antigen fragments in association with MHC class II molecules. The distribution of MHC class II molecules is limited, in normal situations, to certain cells of the immune system – the antigen-presenting cells. In certain circumstances non-lymphoid cells can present antigens if they are induced to express MHC class II molecules. To stimulate a T$_H$ cell the antigen must be taken into the cell and re-expressed on the surface in association with MHC class II molecules. Since the T cell antigen receptor recognizes antigen fragments bound to the MHC molecules, the antigen-presenting cell must also be able to process the antigen. MHC class I- and class II-restricted recognition by CD8$^+$ and CD4$^+$ T cells requires antigen processing. The pathways that lead to association of an antigen fragment with a particular restriction element are not fully understood.

Immune responses are generated in secondary lymphoid tissues, such as lymph nodes. Since a number of cells and molecules must all interact, the architecture of the secondary lymphoid tissue has evolved for the efficient induction of an immune response. In a secondary immune response the cells involved are at a different stage of activation, i.e. they are memory cells having already been exposed to antigen. Therefore, the growth factor signals may not be so critical but antigen in association with MHC class II molecules is still required. In this situation B cells are important as antigen-presenting cells.

CD8$^+$ T cells, as we have seen, recognize antigen fragments associated with MHC class I molecules. All cells have MHC class I molecules on their surface and would therefore be expected to be capable of presenting antigen fragments to cytotoxic T cells that are in the most part MHC class I-restricted. The antigen fragments derived from endogenously synthesized molecules, e.g. from a virus, are produced at a site distinct from the endocytic vesicles where exogenous antigens are processed.

At or around the site of protein synthesis, endogenously produced antigen fragments become associated with the newly produced MHC class I molecules. The MHC class II molecule picks up internalized antigen within the compartment for peptide loading (CPL), as it moves to the cell surface. In this compartment, antigen fragments cannot bind to the MHC class I molecules because these molecules have already associated with endogenously produced antigenic fragments within the endoplasmic reticulum and never go to the CPL. Thus the site where the antigen is processed determines whether it will associate with MHC class I or class II molecules. This separation of processing pathways explains why CD4$^+$ and CD8$^+$ T cells are involved in the destruction of exogenous and endogenous antigens, respectively.

If a particular antigen does not become associated with either MHC class I or II molecules then no T-dependent immune response will be directed against that antigen. Since MHC class II molecules are involved in the initiation of immune responses by presenting antigen fragments to T_H cells, they can control whether a response takes place or not. It has been clearly shown that the level of an immune response to a particular antigen is controlled by the MHC class II molecules. The genes that code for these molecules, i.e. MHC class II genes, have therefore been referred to as *immune response genes* (*Ir* genes).

It should be obvious that if an antigen cannot associate with the MHC class II molecules of an individual then no immune response will be generated. Since the MHC molecules are polymorphic, the cells of some individuals will present, and therefore respond to, certain antigen fragments while cells from other individuals will not. Fortunately, more than one antigenic fragment can be generated from each pathogen, otherwise individuals who did not respond to the particular sequence would be vulnerable to that micro-organism. In addition, individuals have at least six different MHC class II genes and therefore an increased chance that some fragments will bind to at least one of their MHC class II molecules. Variations in the levels and specificity of response will occur in individuals who have different MHC class II molecules and have therefore produced different MHC–antigen complexes on their cells.

Ir gene effects can also be controlled at the level of the T cell receptor. If an individual does not have a T cell with a receptor that recognizes a particular antigen–MHC complex then no response will be generated. The T cell receptor repertoire is generated in the thymus where the genes of the immature T cells are rearranged to give rise to a functioning receptor. T cells that cross-react too strongly with self molecules are deleted, as are cells whose receptors do not interact with self MHC molecules. Therefore, T cells that interact weakly with MHC molecules are selected to mature and leave the thymus. When these cells later come across an antigen–MHC complex the presence of antigen strengthens the weak T cell receptor–MHC interaction, leading to a stimulatory signal being transmitted to the T cell. If for some reason T cells that respond to a particular MHC–antigen configuration have been deleted, suppressed or not formed then no immune response will be generated to that antigen. There is what is known as a 'hole' in the T cell repertoire.

Control of immune responses

An antigen can induce two types of response, immunity or tolerance. Tolerance is the acquisition of non-reactivity towards a particular antigen. The generation of immunity or tolerance depends largely on the way the immune system first encounters the antigen. Once the immune system has been stimulated the cells involved proliferate and produce a response that will eliminate the offending agent. It is then important to dampen down the reacting cells and various feedback mechanisms operate to bring this about.

Role of antigen

The primary regulator of an immune response is the antigen itself. This makes sense since it is important to initiate a response when antigen enters the host and once it has been eliminated it is wasteful and in some cases dangerous to continue to produce effector mechanisms.

Role of antibody

Many biological systems are controlled by the product inhibiting the reaction once a certain level is reached. This type of negative feedback is seen with antibody, which may act by blocking the epitopes on the antigen so that it can no longer stimulate the cell through its receptor.

As antibody levels rise there is competition between free antibody and the B cell receptor. Consequently, only those B cells that have a receptor with a high affinity for antigen will be stimulated and therefore produce high-affinity antibody. For this reason antibody feedback is thought to be an important driving force in affinity maturation.

Regulatory T cells

T_H cells control the generation of effector cells by producing helper factors. However, the factors that stimulate the expansion of B and T cell numbers do not work indefinitely. Maturation factors are also produced that control terminal differentiation into effector cells. Under the influence of these latter lymphokines the action of the proliferation factors is inhibited mainly by making the effector cell unresponsive to their effects.

Other T lymphocytes have been described that provide negative signals to the immune system. Suppressor T cells (T_s cells) limit the development of antibody-producing cells and effector T cells. The activity of suppressor cells can involve both the production of soluble factors and direct cell–cell interactions.

Tolerance

Two forms of tolerance can be identified – *natural* tolerance and *acquired* tolerance. The non-response to self molecules is due to natural tolerance. If this tolerance breaks down and the body responds to self molecules then an auto-immune disease will develop. Natural tolerance appears during fetal development when the immune system is being formed. In experimental animals the introduction of foreign material at the time of birth leads to tolerance. Acquired tolerance arises when a potential immunogen induces a state of unresponsiveness to itself. This has consequences for host defences since the presence of a tolerogenic epitope on a pathogen may compromise the ability of the body to resist infection.

An antigen can induce different effects on the two arms of the immune system. During an infection the host will be exposed to a variety of antigenic determinants on a micro-organism. These epitopes will be present at differing concentrations and possibly at different times during the infection. The epitopes can act as either immunogens or tolerogens. Therefore, it is possible that the antibody response to a particular antigen may be quite pronounced while the cell-mediated response might be lacking, or vice versa. Alternatively, both arms of the immune response may be stimulated or tolerized.

Generally, high doses of antigen tolerize B cells, while minute doses given repeatedly tolerize T cells. For acquired tolerance to be maintained the tolerogen must persist or be repeatedly administered. This is probably necessary because of the continuous production of new T and B cells that must be made tolerant.

Several mechanisms play a role in the selective lack of response to specific antigens. Since each lymphocyte has a receptor with a single specificity the elimination of a specific cell will render the individual tolerant to the epitope it recognizes and leave the rest of the repertoire untouched. This mechanism relies on self molecules interacting with the receptor and causing their elimination. It is proposed that during lymphocyte development the cell goes through a phase in which contact with antigen leads to death or permanent inactivation. Immature B cells encountering antigen for the first time are particularly susceptible to tolerization in the presence of low doses of antigen. The requirement for two signals in the stimulation of B cells and the generation of effector T cells can give rise to tolerance. Both cell types require stimulation via the antigen receptor and 'help' from a specific T cell. If the helper factors are not produced then the responding cells will be functionally deleted. Therefore, the elimination of self-reactive T cells in the thymus during T cell maturation is an important step in maintaining a state of tolerance. Tolerance can also be induced by active suppression. Some T cells are capable of inducing unresponsiveness by acting directly on B cells or other T cells. These T_s cells can be antigen-specific and probably produce signals that actively suppress cells capable of responding to a particular antigen.

It was originally thought that unresponsiveness to self was controlled by the elimination of all self-reactive cells before they matured. This cannot be true since self-reactive B cells are found in normal adult animals. It is thought that these B cells are controlled by a lack of T cell help, i.e. T_H cells have been eliminated. It is thought that T_s cells play a subordinate role acting as a back-up mechanism.

Immunodeficiency

The immunologically competent cells of the lymphoid tissues derived from, renewed by and influenced by the activities of the thymus, bone marrow and other lymphoid tissues can be the subject of disease processes. The deficiency states seen are due either to defects in one of the components of the system itself, or are secondary to some other disease process affecting the normal functioning of some part of the lymphoid tissues. Deficiency of one or more of the defence mechanisms can be inherited, developmental or acquired. The types of infections and diseases seen in patients with immunodeficiencies relate to the role the affected component plays in the normal situation. An individual whose immune system has been depressed in any of these ways is said to be immunocompromised. The *compromised host* is prone to infectious diseases that the normal individual would easily eradicate or not succumb to in the first place. Some examples of predisposing factors are given in Table 11.6.

Table 11.6 The compromised host

Predisposing factor	Effect on immune system	Type of infection
Immunosuppression for transplant or cancer	Diminished cell-mediated and humoral immunity	Lung infections, bacteraemia, fungal infections, urinary tract infections
Viral immunosuppression, e.g. measles, human immunodeficiency virus, Epstein–Barr virus	Impaired function of infected cells	Secondary bacterial infections, opportunistic pathogens
Tumour of immune cells	Replacement of cells of the immune system	Bacteraemia, pneumonia, urinary tract infections
Malnutrition	Lymphoid hypoplasia Decreased lymphocytes and phagocyte activity	Measles, tuberculosis, respiratory infections, gastrointestinal infections
Breakdown of tissue barriers, e.g. surgery, burns, catheterization	Breach innate defence mechanisms	Bacterial infections Opportunistic pathogens
Inhalation of particles due to employment or smoking	Damage to cilia, destruction of alveolar macrophages	Chronic respiratory infections, hypersensitivity reactions

Defective innate defence mechanisms

Defects in phagocyte function take two forms.

1. Where there is a quantitative deficiency of neutrophils which may be congenital (e.g. infantile agranulocytosis) or acquired as a result of replacement of bone marrow by tumour cells or the toxic effects of drugs or chemicals.
2. Where there is a qualitative deficiency in the functioning of neutrophils which, while ingesting bacteria normally, fail, because of an enzymatic defect, to digest them.

Characteristic of these diseases is a susceptibility to bacterial and fungal, but not viral or protozoan, infections. Among the enzyme deficiency disorders are *chronic granulomatous disease* and the *Chédiak–Higashi syndrome.*

The complement system can also suffer from certain defects in function leading to increased susceptibility to infection. The most severe abnormalities of host defences occur, as would be expected, if there is a defect in the functioning of C3. Severe deficiency or absence of C3 is associated with increased susceptibility to infection, particularly septicaemia, pneumonia, meningitis, otitis and pharyngitis.

Defective acquired immune defence mechanisms

Primary immunodeficiencies. Primary deficiencies in immunological function can arise through failure of any of the developmental processes from stem cell to functional end cell. A complete lack of all leucocytes is seen in *reticular dysgenesis* due to a defect in the development of bone marrow stem cells in the fetus. A baby born with this defect usually dies within the first year of life from recurrent, intractable infections. Defects in the development of the common lymphoid stem cell give rise to severe combined immunodeficiency. Both T and B lymphocytes fail to develop but functional phagocytes are present.

There are several types of B cell defect that give rise to hypogammaglobulinaemias, i.e. low levels of γ-globulins (antibodies) in the blood. Deficiency of immunoglobulin synthesis is almost complete in X-linked infantile hypogammaglobulinaemia (*Bruton's disease*). Male infants suffer from severe, chronic bacterial infections after maternal antibody has disappeared. There is an absence, or deficiency, of all five classes of serum immunoglobulins. Therefore, the defect is thought to be caused by the absence of B cell precursors or their arrest at a pre-B cell stage. In these patients cell-mediated immune mechanisms function normally and they seem to be able to handle viral infections relatively well.

Partial defects in immunoglobulin synthesis have been described affecting one or more of the immunoglobulin classes. In the *Wiskott–Aldrich syndrome* that is inherited as an X-linked recessive character there are low IgM levels but IgA and IgE levels are elevated. Patients are susceptible to pyogenic infections, along with recurrent bleeding and eczema. The bleeding is due to reduced platelet production (thrombocytopenia), and the allergy-related eczema is linked to the elevated IgE levels. In patients with *dysgammaglobulinaemia* there is a deficiency in only one antibody class. Some patients have reduced levels of IgA whereas the other isotypes are normal. These patients have an increased incidence of infections in the upper and lower respiratory tracts where IgA is normally protective.

Individuals with T cell defects tend to have more severe and persistent infections than those with antibody deficiencies. A lack of T lymphocytes is often associated with abnormal antibody levels since T_H cells are involved in the generation and control of humoral immunity. Patients with T cell defects suffer from viral, intracellular bacterial, fungal and protozoan infections rather than acute bacterial infections. In the *DiGeorge syndrome* (congenital thymic aplasia) the patient is born with little or no thymus. Individuals who survive develop recurrent and chronic infections, including pneumonia, diarrhoea and yeast infections once passive maternal immunity wanes.

Secondary immunodeficiencies. Acquired deficiencies can occur secondarily to a number of disease states or after exposure to drugs and chemicals.

Deficiency of immunoglobulins can be brought about by excessive loss of protein through diseased kidneys or via the intestine in protein-losing enteropathy. Malnutrition and iron deficiency can lead to depressed immune responsiveness, particularly in cell-mediated immunity. Medical and surgical treatments such as irradiation, cytotoxic drugs and steroids often have undesirable effects on the immune system. Viral infections are often immunosuppressive. For example, measles, human immunodeficiency and other viruses infect cells of the immune system.

In contrast to the deficiency states just described, raised immunoglobulin levels are found in certain disorders of plasma cells due to malignant proliferation of a particular clone or group of plasma cells. In these conditions, such as chronic lymphocytic leukaemia and multiple myeloma, malignant clones will each produce one particular type of antibody. There is usually a decreased synthesis of normal immunoglobulins and an associated deficiency in the immune response to acute bacterial infections. These B-lymphoproliferative disorders contrast with the situation in *Hodgkin's disease*, a reticular cell neoplasm, where the patients show defective cell-mediated immunity and are susceptible to viruses and intracellular bacteria.

Hypersensitivity

Immunity was first recognized as a resistant state that followed infection. However, some forms of immune reaction, rather than providing exemption or safety, can produce severe and occasionally fatal results. These are known as *hypersensitivity reactions* and result from an excessive or inappropriate response to an antigenic stimulus. The mechanisms underlying these deleterious reactions are those that normally eradicate foreign material but for various reasons the response leads to a disease state. When considering each of the four hypersensitivity states it is important to remember this fact and consider the underlying defence mechanism and how it has given rise to the observed immunopathology.

Various classifications of hypersensitivity reactions have been proposed, and probably the most widely accepted is that of Coombs and Gell. This recognizes four types of hypersensitivity that will be considered in turn.

Type I: anaphylactic

If a guinea-pig is injected with a small dose of an antigen such as egg albumin, no adverse effects are noted. If a second injection of the same antigen is given intravenously after an interval of about 2 weeks a condition known as *anaphylactic shock* is likely to develop. The animal becomes restless, starts chewing and rubbing its nose, begins to wheeze and may develop convulsions and die. The initial injection of antigen is termed the sensitizing dose while the second injection causes anaphylactic shock. Such a reaction is seen in humans after a bee sting or injection of penicillin in sensitized individuals. Localized reactions are seen in patients with hay fever and asthma. In all these situations the host responds to the first injection by producing IgE, and it is the level of IgE produced to a particular antigen that will determine whether an anaphylactic reaction will occur on re-exposure to the same antigen. Asthma results from a similar response in the respiratory tract.

The biologically active molecules that are responsible for the manifestations of type I hypersensitivity are stored within mast cell and basophil granules or are synthesized after cell triggering. The signal for the release or production of these molecules is the cross-linking of surface-bound IgE by antigen. The release of these molecules, vasoactive amines and chemotactic factors, is responsible for the symptoms of type I hypersensitivity. IgE has been implicated in the control of parasitic worms, and the importance of this is discussed in Chapter 13.

Type II: cytotoxic

Type II reactions are initiated by the binding of an antibody to an antigenic component on a cell surface. The antibody is directed against an epitope that can be a self molecule or a drug or microbial product passively adsorbed onto a cell surface. The cell that is covered with antibody is then destroyed by the immune system. A variety of infectious diseases caused by salmonella organisms and mycobacteria are associated with haemolytic anaemia. There is evidence, particularly in studies on salmonella infections, that the haemolysis is due to an immune reaction against a lipopolysaccharide bacterial endotoxin that becomes coated onto the erythrocytes of the patient.

Type III: immune complex

As discussed previously, when a soluble antigen combines with antibody the size and physical form of the immune complex formed will depend on the relative proportions of the participating molecules and will be affected by the class of antibody. Monocytes and macrophages are very efficient at binding and removing large complexes. These same cell types can also eliminate the smaller complexes made in antibody excess but are relatively inefficient at removing those formed in antigen excess. Type III hypersensitivity reactions appear if there is a defect in the systems involving phagocytes and complement that remove immune complexes or if the system is overloaded and the complexes are deposited in tissues. This latter situation occurs when antigens are never completely eliminated, as with persistent infection with an organism, auto-immunity and repeated contact with environmental factors.

The tissue damage that results from the deposition of immune complexes is caused by the activation of complement, platelets and phagocytes; in essence, an acute inflammatory response. In general, the degree and site of damage depend on the ratio of antigen to antibody. At equivalence or slight excess of either component the complexes precipitate at the site of antigen injection or production and a mild, local type III hypersensitivity reaction occurs, e.g. the *Arthus reaction*. In contrast, the complexes formed in large antigen excess become soluble and circulate, causing more serious systemic reactions, i.e. *serum sickness*, or eventually deposit in organs, such as skin, kidneys and joints. The type of disease and its time course will depend on the immune status of the individual.

The local release of antigens from an infectious organism can cause a type III reaction. A number of parasitic worms, although undesirable, cause little or no damage. However, if the worm is killed it can become lodged in the lymphatics, and the inflammatory response initiated by antigen–antibody complexes causes a blockage of lymph flow. This leads to the condition of elephantiasis in which enormous swellings can occur. In some cases of tuberculosis, sarcoidosis, leprosy and streptococcal infections, vascular inflammatory lesions are seen mainly in the legs. These are variously referred to as *erythema nodosum, nodular vasculitis* and *erythema induratum*, and may be due to the deposition of immune complexes and the development of an Arthus reaction.

In systemic disease the clinical manifestations depend upon where the immune complexes form or lodge – skin, joints, kidney and heart being particularly affected.

Drugs such as penicillin and sulphonamides can cause type III reactions. The most susceptible patients will develop rashes (urticarial, morbilliform or scarlatiniform), pyrexia, arthralgia, lymphadenopathy and perhaps nephritis some 8–12 days after being given the drug. It is likely that similar events occur in many bacterial and viral infections (see Chapters 14 and 12, respectively).

Type IV: cell-mediated or delayed

This form of hypersensitivity can be defined as a specifically provoked, slowly evolving (24–48 h), mixed cellular reaction involving lymphocytes and macrophages. The reaction is not brought about by circulating antibody but by sensitized lymphoid cells. This type of response is seen in a number of allergic reactions to bacteria, viruses and fungi, in contact dermatitis and in graft rejection. The classical example of this type of reaction is the tuberculin response that is seen following an intradermal injection of a purified protein derivative (PPD) from tubercle bacilli in immune individuals. An indurated inflammatory reaction in the skin appears about 24 h later and persists for a few weeks. In humans the injection site is infiltrated with large numbers of mononuclear cells, mainly lymphocytes, with about 10–20% macrophages. Most of these cells are in or around small blood vessels. The type IV hypersensitivity state arises when an inappropriate or exaggerated cell-mediated response occurs.

Cell-mediated hypersensitivity reactions are seen in a number of chronic infectious diseases due to mycobacteria, protozoa and fungi. Because the host is unable to eliminate the micro-organism the antigens persist and give rise to a chronic antigenic stimulus. Thus, continual release of lymphokines from sensitized T cells results in the accumulation of large numbers of activated macrophages that can become epitheloid cells. These cells can fuse together to form giant cells. Macrophages will express antigen fragments on their surface in association with MHC class I and II molecules and will therefore be the targets of T_c cells and stimulate more lymphokine production. This whole process leads to tissue damage with the formation of a chronic granuloma and resultant cell death.

Penicillin sensitization is a common clinical complication following the topical application of the antibiotic in ointments or creams. This and other substances that cause contact sensitivity are not themselves antigenic and only become so in combination with proteins in the skin. The Langerhans cells of the epidermis are efficient antigen-presenting cells favouring the development of a T cell response. These cells pick up the newly formed antigen in the skin and transport it to the draining lymph node where a T cell response is stimulated. Here, the specific T cells will be stimulated to mature and will then return to the site of entry of the offending material and release their lymphokines. In a normal situation these would help to eliminate a pathogen but in this case the continual or subsequent exposure to the foreign material leads to an inappropriate response. The reaction site is characterized by a mononuclear cell infiltrate peaking at 48 h. The clinical symptoms in these contact dermatitis lesions include redness, swelling, vesicles, scaling and exudation of fluid, i.e. eczema.

Auto–immunity

A fundamental characteristic of the immune system of an animal is that it does not, under normal circumstances, react against its own body constituents. Mechanisms, as we have seen, exist that allow the immune system to tolerate self and destroy non-self. Occasionally these mechanisms break down and auto-antibodies are produced.

Genetic factors appear to play a role in the development of auto-immune diseases and there is a strong association between several auto-immune diseases and particular HLA (human leucocyte group A) specificities, suggesting that *Ir* gene effects may be involved.

There are a number of examples where potential auto-antigenic determinants are present in exogenous material. These preparations may provide a new carrier, i.e. a T cell-stimulating determinant that provokes auto-antibody formation. The encephalitis sometimes seen after rabies vaccination with the older vaccines is thought to result from a response directed against the brain that is stimulated by heterologous brain tissues present in the vaccine.

Micro-organisms are a source of cross-reacting antigens sharing antigenic determinants with tissue components. These may provide an important way of inducing auto-immunity. The group A streptococci, which are closely associated with rheumatic fever, share an antigen with the human heart. Heart lesions are a common finding in rheumatic fever, and anti-heart antibody is found in just over 50% of patients with this condition. Nephritogenic strains of type 12 group A streptococci carry surface antigens similar to those found in human glomeruli, and infection by these organisms has been associated with the development of acute nephritis. Some of the immunopathology seen in Chagas' disease has been attributed to a cross-reaction between *Trypanosoma cruzi* and cardiac muscle.

Auto-immunity can be induced by bypassing T cells. Self-reactive cells can be directly stimulated by polyclonal activators that directly activate B cells. A number of micro-organisms or their products are potent polyclonal activators; however, the response that is generated tends to be IgM and to wane when the pathogen is eliminated. Bacterial endotoxin, the lipopolysaccharide of Gram-negative bacteria, provides a non-specific inductive signal to B cells, bypassing the need for T cell help. A variety of antibodies are present in infectious mononucleosis, including auto-antibodies, as a result of the polyclonal activation of B cells by Epstein–Barr virus.

RECOMMENDED READING

Abbas A K, Janeway C A 2000 Immunology: improving on nature in the twenty-first century. *Cell* 100: 129–138
Abbas A K, Lichtman A H, Pober J S 2000 *Cellular and Molecular Immunology*, 4th edn. Saunders, Philadelphia
Janeway C A, Travers P, Walport M, Capra J D 2001 *Immunobiology; the Immune System in Health and Disease*, 5th edn. Current Biology, London
Weir D M, Stewart J 1997 *Immunology*, 8th edn. Churchill Livingstone, Edinburgh

Internet sites

www.cellsalive.com/
squier.ucsd.edu/research/sb/ve/immunology/
www.copewithcytokines.de/

12

Immunity in viral infections

J. Stewart

The host response to an invading virus will depend upon the characteristics of the infectious agent and where it is encountered. In many cases viral infections are subclinical, i.e. symptomless. A vast array of host defence mechanisms work in a concerted way to protect the individual from viruses and to eliminate them if an infection occurs. In several instances, virus-induced immune responses may have immunopathological consequences.

THE RESPONSE TO VIRAL INFECTIONS

Interferons

At the time of their discovery in 1957 the term *interferon* identified a factor produced by cells in response to viral infection that protected other cells of the same species from attack by a wide range of viruses. It is now clear that this activity is mediated by members of a family of regulatory proteins.

In humans, as in a number of other species, there are three main types of interferon:

- α-interferon (IFN-α), produced mainly by peripheral blood mononuclear cells
- β-interferon (IFN-β), produced predominantly by fibroblasts
- γ-interferon (IFN-γ), a lymphokine produced in response to a specific antigenic signal.

There is only one gene for IFN-β and one for IFN-γ but there are at least 18 different IFN-α genes coding for 14 functional proteins. All the IFN-α genes are closely related and clustered on chromosome 9, close to the IFN-β gene; the IFN-γ gene is on chromosome 12. The production of interferons is under strict inductional control. IFN-α and IFN-β are produced in response to the presence of viruses and certain intracellular bacteria. Double-stranded RNA may be the important inducer. IFN-γ, which has an extensive role in the control of immune responses, is produced by antigen-activated T lymphocytes and natural killer (NK) cells (see pp. 137–139).

To exert their biological effects these molecules must interact with cell surface receptors. IFN-α and IFN-β share a common receptor while IFN-γ binds to its own specific receptor. After binding to the cell surface receptors, interferons act by rapidly and transiently inducing or up-regulating some cellular genes and down-regulating others. The overall effect is to inhibit viral replication and activate host defence mechanisms.

The antiviral activity is mediated by the interferon released from a virus-infected cell binding to a neighbouring cell and inducing the synthesis of antiviral proteins (Fig. 12.1). Interferons are extremely potent in this function, acting at femtomolar (10^{-15} M) concentrations. They can inhibit many stages of the virus life cycle – attachment and uncoating, early viral transcription, viral translation, protein synthesis and budding. Many new proteins can be detected in cells exposed to interferon, but major roles have been proposed for two enzymes that inhibit protein synthesis: 2′,5′-oligoadenylate synthetase (2,5-A synthetase) and a protein kinase. The activity of both these enzymes is dependent on double-stranded RNA provided by viral intermediates in the cell. The protein kinase is responsible for phosphorylation of histones and the protein synthesis initiation factor eIF$_2$. This leads to the inhibition of protein synthesis within interferon-stimulated cells due to inhibition of ribosome assembly. The 2,5-A synthetase is strongly induced in human cells by all three types of interferon and forms 2′,5′-linked oligonucleotides of adenosine from ATP. These oligonucleotides activate a latent cellular endonuclease that degrades both messenger and ribosomal RNA with a resultant inhibition of protein synthesis. The requirement for the presence of double-stranded RNA for the full expression of these responses will safeguard uninfected cells from the damaging effects of the enzymes. Apart from these well characterized changes, many other changes occur in cells treated with interferons. Some viral proteins can inhibit the interferon response.

Some effects of interferon are viral-specific. The Mx protein induced in mice by IFN-α/β is specifically

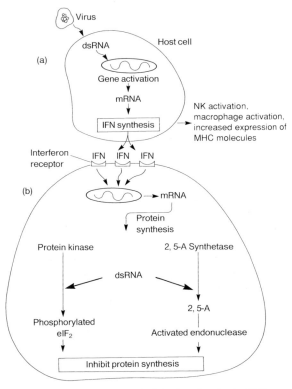

Fig. 12.1 Proposed mechanisms of **a** induction of synthesis of IFN-α and IFN-β and **b** production of resistance to virus infection. dsRNA, double-stranded RNA; mRNA, messenger RNA; 2,5-A, 2',5'-oligoadenylate; MHC, major histocompatibility complex; NK, natural killer cells.

involved in the resistance to influenza virus infection. There is a related protein in human cells, and it is possible that some of the other interferon-induced proteins may confer resistance to specific virus types. Resistance of IFN-γ-treated cells to the parasite *Toxoplasma gondii* is associated with induction of the enzyme indolamine dioxygenase, which catabolizes the essential amino acid tryptophan. However, interferons have effects on host cell growth and differentiation. Interferons, particularly IFN-α and IFN-β, are potent inhibitors of normal and malignant cell growth. A number of clinical trials have shown that IFN-α is active against some human cancers, especially those of haemopoietic origin.

Interferons are able to modify immune responses by:

- altering expression of cell surface molecules
- altering the production and secretion of cellular proteins
- enhancing or inhibiting effector cell functions.

One of the main ways in which interferons control immune responses is by the induction or enhancement of major histocompatibility complex (MHC)-encoded molecules.

Class I MHC genes are up-regulated by all types of interferon, as is the production of β_2-microglobulin. IFN-γ induces and increases the expression of MHC class II antigens. In addition, interferons can induce or enhance the expression of Fc receptors and receptors for a number of cytokines. These activities will increase the efficiency of antigen recognition and lead to a more effective immune response.

Interferons have also been implicated in the control of B cell responses. When added in vitro or in vivo they can suppress or enhance primary or secondary antibody responses, depending on the dose and time of addition. The regulatory effects seem to be on the B cells themselves, on increased antigen presentation and through an effect on regulatory T cells.

A number of immune effector cells act by killing infected target cells. The cytotoxicity of macrophages, neutrophils, T cells and natural killer (NK) cells is enhanced by interferons. IFN-γ produced by T lymphocytes is capable of activating macrophages to kill intracellular bacteria. This lymphokine has all the activities of the molecule that used to be known as macrophage-activating factor (MAF). NK cells are able to destroy a range of syngeneic, allogeneic and xenogeneic cells in an MHC-unrestricted fashion (see below). All three types of interferon increase NK cell activity in vitro and in vivo, not only by recruiting pre-NK cells to become actively lytic but also by increasing the spectrum of cells lysed. The mechanisms by which interferons make cells cytotoxic are not clear but it is of interest that interferons can stimulate the production of cytotoxins such as TNF.

TNF has also been reported to have several antiviral activities similar to IFN-γ, but working through a different pathway. However, if both TNF and IFN-γ are added together then a synergistic effect is seen. If TNF is added to cells after viral infection, it can lead to their destruction even though the cells are normally resistant to TNF. This effect is also synergistic with IFN-γ. Certain viruses have been shown to trigger the release of TNF from mononuclear cells, and it seems likely that this cytokine is an important host response to viral infections.

Certain cell-mediated reactions are also part of the innate defences against viral infections. The structures recognized by NK cells are not known, but changes in the level of expression of MHC class I molecules on the infected cells are important. A number of viruses, especially those causing latent infections, evade immune recognition by interfering with the MHC class I processing pathway. Cells infected with these viruses do not display MHC class I molecules on their surface and are therefore not recognized by cytotoxic T cells. However, the infected cells are recognized by NK cells. The formation of a close conjugate between the NK cell and the target induces the effector cell to produce molecules that lead to the death of the infected cell by apoptosis. Antibodies that recognize NK cells have been used to deplete these cells in mice. It was found that the treated mice were more susceptible to murine cytomegalovirus than were normal mice. Natural killing may form a first-line defence against viral attack, most importantly by herpesviruses, before the acquired immune response is generated. Natural killing is increased by interferons, both the number of effector cells and their killing potential, and, therefore, these two innate defence mechanisms appear to work together to protect the host from viral infections.

The interferon response is rapid and will help to protect the host until acquired responses develop. Interferons induce a febrile response and this may also be important in inhibiting viral growth in some infections with viruses that have low ceiling temperatures for growth.

Acquired immunity

The response to viral antigens is almost entirely T cell-dependent. Immunodeficiencies involving T cells are always characterized by markedly enhanced susceptibility to viral infections. However, this tells us little about the effector mechanisms involved as T cells are required for both antibody production and cytotoxic reactions.

The viral epitopes to which the immune system responds have been studied to give an insight into the mechanisms involved in the host response to these pathogens and also to aid in the development of better vaccines. The recognition of viral antigens is similar to that for all foreign material. B cells and immunoglobulin are able to combine with exposed epitopes while processed viral fragments presented in the context of MHC molecules are recognized by T cells.

Antigen-specific B cells can act as antigen-presenting cells and therefore generate an immune response. B cells will present antigen to T cells and in return will be stimulated by growth and differentiation molecules. Intramolecular help may explain hapten-carrier effects. The uptake of an intact virion will mean that the B cell will be able to present peptides derived from internal proteins to T cells (Fig. 12.2). Thus, a B cell specific for a surface antigen can receive help from a T cell specific for another molecule as long as it is present within the same particle, i.e. intrastructural help.

In most cases, exogenous virus proteins, i.e. those derived from an extracellular virus and taken into a cell, will be presented in the context of MHC class II molecules and stimulate T_H cells. Cells that are supporting viral replication express virus-derived peptides in association with MHC class I molecules, i.e. the endogenous pathway. The fact that some endogenous

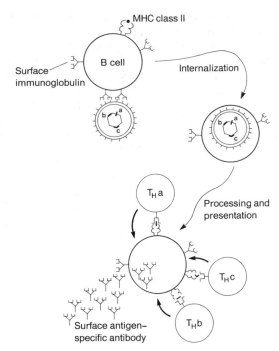

Fig. 12.2 Intrastructural T cell help. A B cell that is specific for a surface component of a virus binds the virus through its receptor, surface immunoglobulin. The virus contains three potential T cell epitopes (a, b and c) within its nucleocapsid. The entire virus can be internalized, and all viral polypeptides will be processed and fragments will be re-expressed in association with MHC class II molecules (presentation) on the B cell surface.

produced viral proteins are presented in the context of MHC class II molecules suggests that there can be some overlap between the MHC class I and class II pathways.

Humoral immunity

There are several ways in which antibody against viral components can protect the host. Antibodies cannot enter cells, and therefore are ineffective against latent viruses and those that spread directly from cell to cell. They will, however, bind to extracellular viral epitopes. These epitopes can be on intact virions or on the surface of infected cells. The binding of antibody to free virus can inhibit a number of processes essential to virus replication. Antibodies can block binding to the host cell membrane, and thus stop attachment and penetration. The immunoglobulins IgG and IgM have this important function in serum and body fluids, and IgA can neutralize viruses by a similar mechanism on mucosal surfaces. Antibody can also work at stages after penetration. Uncoating, with its release of viral nucleic acid into the cytoplasm, can be inhibited if the virion is covered by antibody.

Antibody can also cause aggregation of virus particles, thus limiting the spread of the infectious particles and forming a complex that is readily phagocytosed. Complement can aid in the neutralization process by opsonizing the virus or directly lysing enveloped viruses. In certain cases complement alone can inactivate viruses. Some retroviruses have a protein that can act as a receptor for C1q, and other viruses have been reported to activate the alternative pathway. In some infections, viral proteins remain on the surface of the cell after entry or become associated with the cell membrane during replication. Antibodies against these molecules can cause cell lysis by the classical pathway but an intact alternative pathway is necessary to amplify the initial triggering by the antibody-dependent pathway. In certain situations antibody-mediated reactions are not always of benefit (see below). Antibodies are also capable of modulating or stripping viral antigens from the cell surface, allowing the infected cell to avoid destruction by other effector mechanisms.

Viral infections, particularly those caused by enteroviruses, are frequent and severe when humoral immunity is impaired, as in certain inherited immuno-deficiency states. In Bruton-type deficiencies, polio-myelitis may develop after vaccination with the live virus vaccine; meningoencephalitis caused by echovirus and coxsackievirus may also be seen. In many situations, viruses seem to be able to escape the humoral defence mechanisms. Some viruses become latent, e.g. herpesviruses, and are reactivated despite the presence of circulating antibody, as they can pass directly from cell to cell. Other escape mechanisms include antigenic variation in which the antigenic structure of the virus (e.g. influenza type A) changes so that antibodies formed to the previous strain are no longer effective.

In viral infections the efficiency of antibody depends largely on whether the virus passes through the bloodstream outside host cells to reach its target organ. Poliovirus crosses the intestinal wall, enters the bloodstream to cause a cell-free viraemia and passes to the spinal cord and brain where it replicates. Small amounts of antibody in the blood can neutralize the virus before it reaches its target cells in the nervous system.

In comparison, in viral diseases such as influenza and the common cold, the viruses do not pass through the bloodstream. These infections have a short incubation period, their target organ being at the site of entry into the body, namely the respiratory mucous membranes. In this type of infection a high level of antibody in the blood will be relatively ineffective in comparison with its effect on blood-borne viruses. In this case the antibody must be present in the mucous secretions at the time of infection. There are very low levels of IgG or IgM in secretions but IgA has been shown to be respon-sible for most of the neutralizing activity present in nasal secretions against rhinoviruses and other respiratory tract viruses.

One consequence of this is that conventional immunization methods using killed virus or viral subunits, which produce high levels of circulating antibody, are unlikely to be effective against viruses that attack the mucous membranes. Some considerable effort is being directed at developing methods for stimulating local production of IgA in the mucous membranes themselves. Live virus vaccines are effective in this respect, and the intranasal administration of a live-attenuated influenza virus vaccine is an attempt to overcome this problem. The high degree of immunity provided by the oral polio vaccine is due in part to locally produced antibody in the gut neutralizing the virus before it attaches to cell receptors to cause infection. The presence of IgA against polio has been demonstrated in faeces, in duodenal fluid and in saliva. Recent evidence suggests that parenteral administration of a killed virus may give rise to a secretory IgA response if the individual has been previously exposed to the virus or has received an oral-attenuated vaccine. So there appears to be a link between the systemic immune system and local mucosal immunity.

Humoral immunity does play a major protective role in polio and a number of other viral infections, and is probably the predominant form of immunity responsible for protection from reinfection. Passively administered antibody can protect humans against several infections, including measles, hepatitis A and B and chickenpox, if given before or very soon after exposure. Immunity to many viral infections is life-long. This may occur because antibodies are boosted by occasional re-exposure to the virus.

Cell-mediated immunity

The destruction of virus-infected cells is an important mechanism in the eradication of virus from the host. Antibody can neutralize free virions but once these agents enter cells other strategies are employed. The destruction of an infected cell before progeny particles are released is an effective way of terminating a viral infection. For this process to occur the immune system must recognize the infected cell and various types of effector cell have evolved to mediate these processes.

As viral proteins are synthesized within the cell some of these molecules are processed into small peptides. These endogenously produced antigen fragments become associated with MHC class I molecules, and this complex is then transported to the cell surface where it acts as the recognition unit for cytotoxic T (T_C) lymphocytes. Most T_C cells have a receptor that binds to fragments of the virus sitting in the cleft of an MHC class I molecule. This T cell will also have the CD8 molecule on its surface. Some T_C cells are restricted in their recognition of antigen by MHC class II molecules and therefore have the CD4 molecule. Once these T_C cells have bound to the infected cell they release molecules that induce apoptosis.

Many viruses, such as poliovirus and papillomavirus, replicate and produce fully infectious particles inside the cell. These viruses are liberated from the infected cell as it disintegrates. However, other viruses do not wait for the cell to die but are released by a process of budding through the cell membrane. During their replication, virus-encoded molecules, i.e. viral antigens, are inserted into the host cell membrane, and the nucleocapsid becomes associated with these molecules. The virus particle finally acquires an envelope as it is released. Such viruses include herpesviruses, alphaviruses, flaviviruses, retroviruses, hepadnaviruses and orthomyxoviruses and paramyxoviruses. Viral antigens often appear on the cell surface very early in the replicative cycle, many hours before progeny virus is liberated. In cells infected with herpes simplex virus as many as five different viral glycoproteins appear on the cell surface. In other virus infections, such as those caused by poxviruses and papovaviruses, the viral particles are not released by budding, but viral antigens appear on the cell surface. These molecules, including those which are not incorporated into the released virion, can therefore act as signals indicating the presence of virus within a cell. If antibody binds to these cell surface viral antigens then the infected cell can be destroyed by antibody-dependent cell-mediated cytotoxicity. The effector cells have an Fc receptor that recognizes the Fc portion of immunoglobulin bound to viral antigens present on the infected cell surface. This interaction brings the two cells close together, and toxic molecules are released onto the target cell membrane causing cell death.

CD4[+] and CD8[+] T cells can produce various lymphokines when stimulated by antigen. These will include molecules that are active in the elimination of virus, e.g. IFN-γ and TNF and others that generally increase the effectiveness of the immune system by attracting cells to the site of infection, stimulating the production of more cells and supporting their growth. Macrophages will be activated, and this will lead to enhanced microbicidal activities and the production of monokines.

Induction of an immune response

The precise nature of the acquired immune reactions that are generated in response to infection will depend to a great extent on the site of infection, type of virus, previous exposure to the agent and the genetic make-up of the host. Both humoral and cell-mediated responses will be produced to all infections. The importance of genetic factors is illustrated by the severe *X-linked recessive lymphoproliferative syndrome* in which fatal infectious mononucleosis results from the unrestricted replication of Epstein–Barr virus as affected males have reduced numbers of normal lymphocytes.

The virus or viral components entering the peripheral tissues or being produced there will be carried to the draining lymph node either free in the lymph or in cells such as Langerhans cells. Once in the secondary lymphoid tissues the free virus is taken up by macrophages, processed and viral peptides associate with MHC class II molecules and are transported to the cell surface. Langerhans cells that enter the lymph node become interdigitating cells and present viral peptides, associated with MHC class II molecules, on their surface. A T_H cell will bind to the peptide–MHC class II complex and expand clonally and produce helper factors. The proportions of the different lymphokines produced will determine the type and level of the response generated. B cells will enter the node, and those that bind antigen will be stimulated into antibody production. Other T cells will enter the lymph node. If these cells have a receptor that interacts with an antigen fragment–MHC class I complex then they will respond to the growth factors present in the node and proliferate and mature into effector T_C cells. After a time, the products of the immune response will leave the node to circulate round the body and localize at the site of infection. As the response progresses the pathogen will be eliminated, the tissue repaired and memory cells generated. Finally, when all the antigen is eliminated the immune response will be terminated. In some instances virus-induced immune responses may have immunopathical consequences.

IMMUNOPATHOLOGY

Viruses have evolved a multitude of mechanisms for exploiting weaknesses in the host immune system and avoiding, and sometimes actually subverting, immune mechanisms. Some viruses are so successful in avoiding host defences that they persist in the host indefinitely, sometimes in a latent form without producing disease.

One of the most important strategies developed by viruses is to infect cells of the immune system itself. The effect of this is often to disable the normal functioning of the cell type that has been infected. Many common human viruses, including rubella, mumps, measles and herpesviruses, infect cells of the immune system, as does the human immunodeficiency virus (HIV). The consequences of viral infection of cells of the immune system have been categorized in two ways:

1. Infections that cause temporary immune deficiency to unrelated antigens and sometimes to the antigens of the infecting virus. It is known that infection with influenza, rubella, measles and cytomegalovirus predisposes to bacterial and other infections. This is sometimes associated with depressed immunoglobulin synthesis and interference with the antimicrobial functions of phagocytes.
2. Permanent depression of immunity to unrelated antigens and occasionally to antigens of the infecting virus. The acquired immune deficiency syndrome is an example of such a disease where the patient becomes susceptible to otherwise harmless protozoa, bacteria, viruses and fungi.

Viruses have also developed other mechanisms to avoid the immune system. These include:

- antigenic variation
- release of antigens
- the production of antigens at sites that are inaccessible to the immune system.

Viruses that cannot enter and replicate within phagocytic cells will be destroyed if they are engulfed by a neutrophil or macrophage. Since neutrophils are short-lived cells they do not usually give rise to progeny virus. On the other hand, monocytes and macrophages are long-lived cells and can be responsible for disseminating a virus throughout the body. Viruses that do replicate within macrophages must escape from the phagosome very rapidly before it fuses with the lysosome. Reovirus infection of macrophages is actually helped by the lysosomal enzymes which initiate 'uncoating' of the virus and therefore enhance viral replication.

A virus will remain relatively safe from immune destruction if it remains within the cell and allows only very low or no viral antigen expression on the infected cell membrane. This is what happens in latent infections where herpes simplex or varicella-zoster virus is present in the dorsal root ganglion.

Antibody can actually remove viral antigens from cell membranes, as cross-linking of antigens on the cell surface can lead to their internalization by capping. Here the antigens complexed with the antibody are drawn to one pole of the cell and are internalized or shed into the surrounding tissue. Capping occurs on brain cells infected with measles virus in subacute sclerosing panencephalitis. Viruses that move from cell to cell without entering the extracellular fluids will also escape the action of antibodies, as will those passed from cell to cell by cell division.

A number of infections continually shed virus into external secretions, such as saliva, milk or urine. As long as the infected cell only forms virus on the luminal surface of the mucosa then cells of the immune system and antibody will be unable to destroy the infected cell. IgA present in the secretions may neutralize the virus, but this class of antibody does not activate complement efficiently so the cell will not be lysed. A similar situation applies to epidermal infections with wart virus. The infected cell is keratinized and about to be released from the surface of the body before any virus or viral antigens are produced. The infected cell is therefore isolated from the host's immune cells.

During the course of an infection various antibodies will be formed against different epitopes on a virus. These antibodies will be of differing affinities and also stimulate different effector functions. Antibodies against some of the epitopes will neutralize the virus, but other antibodies will be against unimportant epitopes or be of an ineffective isotype, which may fail to neutralize the virus and may actually aid in its infectivity by allowing uptake of virus–antibody complexes via Fc receptors or cause tissue damage through immune complex disease. Soluble antigens liberated from infected cells could 'mop-up' free antibody so that it can no longer interact and destroy extracellular virus. Whether the small particles present in the serum of patients and carriers with hepatitis B virus infections function in this way is not known, although patients in the prodromal phase may suffer from rash, myalgia and arthralgia. Polyarteritis nodosa and glomerulonephritis can also occur, all suggestive of immune complex formation.

Susceptibility to infection is generally greater in the very young and very old because of a weaker immune response. However, the immunopathology tends to be less severe. In the very young, infections can spread rapidly and prove fatal without the clinical and pathological changes seen in adults. Latent infections are kept under control by the immune system, and in older people the infections show an increased incidence of activation, e.g. zoster or shingles. Immunological immaturity makes the neonate highly susceptible to many viral infections. Maternal-derived antibody provides passive protection for 3–6 months, after which time the infant is at risk of infection: respiratory and alimentary tract infections are frequent.

Physical and physiological differences may also contribute to age-related disease susceptibility. Respiratory infections in old age are probably a bigger problem than in young adults because of weaker respiratory muscles and a poorer cough reflex. In the young the airways are narrower and more easily blocked by secretions and exudate. Infants, because of their low body weight, show signs of distress from loss of fluid and electrolytes, so that fever, vomiting and diarrhoea tend to be very serious at this time of life. Often the reasons for the differences between infants and adults are not known.

Respiratory syncytial virus causes severe illness in the early months of life with croup, bronchiolitis and bronchopneumonia, despite the presence of maternal IgG. In adults the virus usually causes a mild upper respiratory tract infection.

Certain viral infections produce a milder disease in children than in adults, e.g. varicella, mumps, poliomyelitis and Epstein–Barr virus infections. Varicella often causes pneumonia in adults, and mumps may involve the testes and ovaries after puberty, giving rise to orchitis and oophoritis. Epstein–Barr virus is excreted in saliva, and in developing countries most individuals are infected early in life, usually asymptomatically. In developed countries where the childhood infection is less common, first infection can be delayed to adolescence or early adulthood, when salivary exposure occurs during kissing. In this age group, Epstein–Barr virus infection gives rise to glandular fever. It is not clear why these infections are more severe in adults, but it may be linked to the more powerful immune defences giving rise to immunopathological sequelae in adults.

There are also age-related differences in the incidence of infections. It is not surprising that most infections are commonest in childhood when the individual will be exposed to the micro-organisms for the first time.

Antigenic variation

A micro-organism can avoid the acquired immune response by periodically changing the structure of molecules that are recognized by the host immune system. The immune system will select the variants by not being able to mount an immune response against them before they are shed. The micro-organism will only be able to change a component in a way that does not alter the functioning of the molecule. The molecules involved can be active enzymes, recognition molecules or structural proteins. HIV shows considerable variation in parts of the envelope glycoprotein within a given individual.

The significance of antigenic variation is well illustrated by influenza viruses. Here changes in the surface glycoproteins are linked to the occurrence of epidemics of infection (see Chapter 49).

With influenza virus the infection is localized to the respiratory tract where the principal protection against reinfection will be secretory IgA. The virus-specific IgA still present at the mucosal surface a few years after infection can protect against the original infecting virus but may be insufficient to deal with an antigenic variant despite antigenic overlap. Thus, in effect, IgA levels become a selective pressure, which will allow infection by the mutant, and antigenic drift occurs. The very short incubation period (1–3 days) is more rapid than the sec-

ondary antibody response so that the IgA levels cannot be boosted in time to abort infection.

Antigenic variation is likely to be an important viral adaptation for overcoming host immunity in long-lived species such as humans where there is a need for multiple re-infection of the same individual if the virus is to survive and the virus is unable to become latent. In shorter-lived animals such as mice and rabbits a susceptible population appears quickly enough to maintain the infectious cycle.

Persistence of virus

Certain viruses give rise to a persistent infection, which is held in check as long as the immune system remains intact.

Chickenpox is a persistent infection characterized by latency in that there is apparent recovery from the original infection but the virus can reappear later in life when a localized eruption, shingles, results. Other herpesviruses, cytomegalovirus and Epstein–Barr virus also persist after infection. If the carrier's immune system remains intact, there will be no evidence of disease. However, cytomegalovirus causes many problems in immunosuppressed patients. The polyomavirus, JC, usually causes asymptomatic infections, but, in the immunosuppressed, it has been found in areas of destruction in the central nervous system: the disease is progressive multifocal leucoencephalopathy.

In other persistent infections, the immune system contributes to the pathology of the disease, often over a period of years. Thus, in subacute sclerosing panencephalitis, persistence of measles virus in neurones triggers their destruction by the host's immune system. Similarly, the chronic active hepatitis seen in those carriers of hepatitis B who continue to produce virions appears to be caused by a T_C cell response to viral antigens present in the hepatocyte membrane. In both examples, several years may elapse before symptoms appear.

VACCINES

Natural infection with a virus is an extremely effective means of giving life-long immunity from the disease. In most cases, where there is one virus type, this means that second attacks are extremely rare. The memory of the immune system ensures that for these infections a secondary response can be generated before the virus has time to cause the disease. The level of immunity needed to protect an individual will depend on the incubation period of the virus and its life cycle. For viruses with very short incubation periods a high level of protective immunity must be present before exposure to the infective agent. In the case of a virus with a long incubation period (10–20 days) then the immune system has time to generate a protective response.

It is also important to consider the type of immune response that will be protective against different viruses. If antibody gives protection then steps must be taken to ensure that the material to be used for immunization contains the correct epitopes. A denatured antigen will not generate antibodies that can combine with the native virus. Sometimes the chemical treatment of the antigen may destroy important components. Thus the original killed measles virus vaccine did not contain the fusion protein. As a result, vaccinees suffered enhanced disease when exposed to the virus as viral replication and spread could occur in the presence of antibody to the other viral proteins. If T cell immunity is important then the vaccine must be in a form that will give rise to peptides in the correct compartment of the cell to produce antigen fragments in association with MHC-encoded products. It will have to associate with the MHC class II molecules to generate help and MHC class I molecules to stimulate effector cell formation. For antibody production, T cell help will also be required. Therefore, for an antibody response, a killed vaccine may be sufficient but, when T cell immunity is required, a live-attenuated vaccine will be needed.

Vaccination has been responsible for the elimination of smallpox and reducing the incidence of other viral diseases. It should be possible to control many viral diseases but with some the problem is more difficult. New technologies and a better understanding of the immune system are helping with this task.

RECOMMENDED READING

Alcami A, Koszinowski U H 2000 Viral mechanisms of immune evasion. *Immunology Today* 21: 447–455

Biron C A 1999 Initial and innate responses to viral infections – pattern setting in immunity or disease. *Current Opinion in Microbiology* 2: 374–381

Mims C, Nash A, Stephen J 2000 *Mims' Pathogenesis of infectious Disease*, 5th edn. Academic Press: London

Stark G R, Kerr I M, Williams B R G, Silverman R H, Schreiber R D 1998 How cells respond to interferons. *Annual Review of Biochemistry* 67: 227–264

Internet site

www.virology.net/garryfavwebindex.html

13

Parasitic infections: pathogenesis and immunity

J. Stewart

By convention the term 'parasitic diseases' refers to those caused by protozoa, worms (helminths) and arthropods (insects and arachnids). Such parasites affect many hundreds of millions of people in tropical parts of the world and are responsible for many severe and debilitating diseases (see Chapters 61–63).

These infections are associated with a broad spectrum of effects. Some are due to the parasites themselves and others are a consequence of the host response to the invader. The nature and extent of the pathological effects are dependent upon the site and mode of infection and also on the level of the parasite burden.

Development of protective immunity to such parasites is more complicated than to bacteria and viruses because of the complicated life cycles of the parasites involved.

PATHOGENIC MECHANISMS

As with other infectious agents the site occupied by a parasite is important. A host will survive with a large number of lung flukes, *Paragonimus* spp., in the lungs, but infection in the brain may cause far more serious effects. The severity of disease depends not only on the degree of infection but also on the physiological state of the host. A lowering of general health, due to malnutrition for example, will predispose to more serious consequences following infection by parasites.

Mechanical tissue damage

Physical obstruction of anatomical sites leading to loss of function can be a major component of the diseases caused by parasites. The intestinal lumen can be blocked by worms such as *Ascaris* spp. or tapeworms, and filarial parasites (*Wuchereria* and *Brugia* spp.) can obstruct the flow of lymph through lymphatics.

Intestinal infection with the tapeworm *Taenia solium* is usually of little consequence, but the eggs may develop into larvae (cysticerci) in humans, causing cysticercosis. The cysticerci can be found in muscle, liver, eye or, most dangerously, in the brain. Hydatid cysts, the larval stage of the dog tapeworm (*Echinococcus granulosus*) in humans, may reach volumes of 1–2 litres, and such masses can cause severe damage to an infected organ.

Physiological effects

Large numbers of *Giardia* spp. covering the walls of the small intestine can lead to malabsorption, especially of fats. Competition by parasites for essential nutrients leads to host deprivation. Thus, depletion of vitamin B_{12} by the tapeworm *Diphyllobothrium latum* sometimes leads to pernicious anaemia. Other forms of anaemia result from blood loss, especially in hookworm infection, and from red blood cell destruction in malaria.

Some parasites produce metabolites that may have profound effects on the host. *Trypanosoma cruzi* secretes a neurotoxin that affects the autonomic nervous system. Malaria parasites are thought to produce a metabolite with vasoconstrictor activity.

Tissue damage

The presence of parasites can result in the release of proteolytic enzymes that damage host tissues. Ulceration of the intestinal wall occurs in amoebic dysentery, and trophozoites (the active, motile forms of a protozoan parasite) can penetrate deep into the wall of the intestine to reach the blood and hence the liver, lungs and brain where secondary amoebic abscesses may occur. The skin damage caused by skin-penetrating helminths, such as *Strongyloides* spp. and hookworms, can also permit entry of other infectious agents.

The host reaction to parasites and their products can evoke immunological reactions that may lead to secondary damage to host tissues. This is seen in schistosomiasis where the host response to parasite eggs in tissues leads to the formation of a granuloma with subsequent tissue destruction through fibrosis. Other types of hypersensitivity reactions can be generated in various parasite infections (see below).

IMMUNE DEFENCE MECHANISMS

The large size of parasites means that they will display more antigens than bacteria or viruses to the immune system. When the parasite has a complicated life cycle some of these antigens may be specific to a particular stage of development. Parasites have evolved to be closely adapted to the host, and most parasitic infections are chronic and show a degree of host specificity. For example, the malaria parasites of humans, birds and rodents are confined to their own particular species. An exception to this is *Trichinella spiralis*, which is able to infect many animal species.

In the natural host there is no single defence mechanism that acts in isolation against a particular parasite. In turn the parasite will have evolved a number of strategies to evade elimination. In general terms, cell-mediated immune mechanisms are more effective against intracellular protozoa while antibody, with the aid of certain effector cells, is involved in the destruction of extracellular targets. Again, because of the life cycles of some parasites, either cell-mediated or humoral immunity may be of greater importance at different states of their development.

Innate defences

Several of the innate or natural defence mechanisms that are active against bacteria and viruses are also effective against parasitic infections. The physical barrier of the skin protects against many parasites but it is ineffective against those that are transmitted by a blood-feeding insect. In addition, other parasites, such as schistosomes, have evolved mechanisms for actively penetrating intact skin. Certain individuals are genetically less susceptible to certain parasites. Thus, individuals with the sickle cell trait have a genetic defect in their haemoglobin that causes a mechanical distortion in their erythrocytes. This somehow leads to the destruction of intracellular malaria parasites. The Duffy blood groups antigen is the attachment site for one of the plasmodium parasites. Individuals who lack this determinant are therefore protected from malaria caused by *Plasmodium vivax*.

Several other non-specific host defence mechanisms are involved in the control of parasitic infections. These include direct cellular responses by monocytes, macrophages and granulocytes, and by natural killer cells. The by-products of acquired immune reactions will enhance the antiparasitic activity of these cells. For example, certain protozoan parasites infect macrophages. In particular, *Leishmania* spp. are obligate parasites of mononuclear phagocytes, and are completely dependent upon macrophages, where they survive in the phagolysosome. The parasite appears to be able to survive within non-stimulated resident macrophages whereas they are destroyed in activated macrophages.

Complement, through activation by the alternative pathway, is active against a number of parasites, including adult worms and active larvae of *T. spiralis* and schistosomula of *Schistosoma mansoni*. The spleen is thought to be active in the elimination of intracellular parasites as its filtering of infected erythrocytes is thought to remove intracellular plasmodium.

Macrophages

Macrophages play an important role in the elimination and control of parasitic protozoa and worms. They secrete monokines, such as interleukin-1, tumour necrosis factor and colony-stimulating factors that affect not only T cells and antibody production but also granulocytes. However, other monokines, e.g. prostaglandins, are immunosuppressive. Macrophages are also phagocytic cells and function as such in the elimination of parasites. In the same way as in the eradication of other infectious agents, opsonins will greatly enhance this process. Once internalized, the parasite will be killed, by oxygen-dependent and -independent mechanisms, and digested. Many of the molecules produced by macrophages are cytotoxic, and when produced in close proximity to a parasite will kill it. Specific antibody, IgG and IgE, can mediate the attachment of the macrophage to the surface of parasites that are too large to internalize but are vulnerable to antibody-dependent cell-mediated cytotoxicity. Acting as antigen-presenting cells, they can aid elimination by helping in the initiation of an immune response.

In addition to lymphokines some products of parasites themselves, such as those produced by *Tryp. brucei* and the malaria parasite, can cause macrophage activation. These may be direct effects or result from the production of monokines such as tumour necrosis factor.

In some parasitic infections the immune system is unable to eradicate the offending organism. The body reacts by trying to isolate the parasite within a granuloma. In this situation there is chronic stimulation of those T cells specific for antigens on the parasite. The continual release of lymphokines leads to macrophage accumulation, release of fibrogenic factors, stimulation of granuloma formation and, ultimately, fibrosis. Granuloma formation around schistosome eggs can occur in the liver, and this response is thought to benefit the host by isolating host cells from the toxic substances produced by the eggs. It can, however, lead to pathological consequences if the damage to the liver leads to loss of liver function.

Granulocytes

Neutrophils and eosinophils are thought to play a role in the elimination of protozoa and worms. The smaller parasites can be phagocytosed and destroyed by both oxygen-dependent and -independent processes. The phagocytic capacity of neutrophils is superior to that of eosinophils. Both cell types possess receptors for the Fc portion of immunoglobulin and for various complement components, so the presence of opsonins increases phagocytosis. Extracellular destruction of large parasites can occur by antibody-dependent cell-mediated cytotoxicity.

Neutrophils are attracted to sites of inflammation and will clear the offending parasite. They have been reported to be more effective than eosinophils at eliminating several species of nematode, including *T. spiralis*, although the relative importance of the two cell types may depend on the class of antibody present.

Eosinophilia and high levels of IgE are characteristics of many parasitic worm infections. It has been suggested that eosinophils are especially active against helminths, and IgE-dependent degranulation of mast cells has evolved to attract these cells to the site where the parasite is localized. The eosinophilia is T cell-dependent and the lymphokines that induce the production of the cells also cause an increase in their activation state. These effector cells are attracted to the site by chemotactic factors produced by mast cells (see below). Once at the site they degranulate in response to perturbation of their cell membrane induced by antibodies and complement bound to the surface of the parasite. The toxic molecules are therefore released onto the surface of the target and cause its destruction.

Mast cells

The mediators stored and produced by mast cells play an important role in eliminating worm infections. Parasite antigens cause the release of mediators from mast cells; these molecules induce a local inflammatory response. Chemotactic factors are produced and attract eosinophils and neutrophils. Thus the IgE-dependent release of mast cell products helps in the expulsion of the worm. The number of mucosal mast cells rises during a parasitic worm infestation due to a T cell-dependent process.

Platelets

Platelet activation results in the release of molecules that are toxic to various parasites, including schistosoma, *Toxoplasma gondii* and *Tryp. cruzi*. The release process does not require antibody, although IgE-dependent cytotoxicity is possible, but seems to involve acute-phase proteins. The cytotoxic potential of platelets is enhanced by various cytokines, including γ-interferon and tumour necrosis factor.

Acquired immunity

An individual with a parasitic infection will mount a specific response against the invading parasite. These immune reactions will generate antibody and effector T cells directed against specific parasite antigens. Memory B and T cells will also be produced. For a number of reasons described later, much acquired immunity is ineffective in protecting the host against recurrent infection. However, in certain cases, such as amoebiasis and toxoplasmosis, immunity to re-infection is fairly complete. In schistosomiasis, the presence of surviving adult forms protects against further infections. However, this may be an effect of the parasite and not of the host.

Antibody

The specific immune response to parasites leads to the production of antibody. Infection by protozoan parasites is associated with the production of the immunoglobulins IgG and IgM. With helminths there is, in addition, the synthesis of substantial amounts of IgE. IgA is produced in response to intestinal protozoa, such as *Entamoeba* and *Giardia* spp.

In addition to these specific T-dependent responses a non-specific hypergammaglobulinaemia is present in many parasitic infections. Much of this non-specific antibody is the result of polyclonal B cell activation by released parasite antigens acting as mitogens. This response is ineffective at counteracting the parasite and can enhance the pathogenicity by causing the production of auto-antibodies, and may actually lead to a diminished specific response due to B cell exhaustion. It has also been reported that some parasite molecules are T cell mitogens. This could lead to the generation of autoreactive T cells or activation of suppressor responses.

There are a number of mechanisms by which specific antibody can provide protection against and control parasitic infections (Table 13.1). As with viral infections, antibody is only effective against extracellular parasites and where parasite antigens are displayed on the surface of infected cells. Antibody can neutralize parasites by combining with various surface molecules, blocking or interfering with their function. The binding of antibody to an attachment site will stop infection of a new host cell. The agglutination of blood parasites by IgM may occur, leading to the prevention of spread, as in the acute phase of infection with *Tryp. cruzi*. Toxins and enzymes produced by certain parasites add to their

Table 13.1 Humoral defence mechanisms against parasite infections

Mechanism	Effect	Parasite
Neutralization	Blocks attachment to host cell	Protozoa
	Acts to inhibit evasion mechanisms of intracellular organisms	Protozoa
	Binding to toxins or enzymes	Protozoa and worms
Physical interference	Obstructs orifices of parasite	Worms
	Agglutination	Protozoa
Opsonization	Increases clearance by phagocytes	Protozoa
Cytotoxicity	Complement-mediated lysis	Protozoa and worms
	Antibody-dependent cell-mediated cytotoxicity	Protozoa and worms

pathogenicity and antibodies that inhibit these molecules will protect the host from damage and also affect the infection process directly. Intracellular parasites have evolved a number of mechanisms to allow them to survive in this environment. Antibodies against the molecules that aid the parasite in these activities, e.g. to escape from endosomes or inhibit lysosomal fusion, will lead to removal of the intruder by the phagocyte. Parasitic worms are multicellular organisms with defined anatomical features that are responsible for functions such as feeding and reproduction. Antibodies that block particular orifices, e.g. oral and genital, will interfere with critical physiological functions and could cause starvation or curtail reproduction.

Antibodies can bind to the surface of parasites and cause direct damage, or by interacting with complement lead to cell lysis. Antibody also acts as an opsonin and hence increases uptake by phagocytic cells. In this context, complement activation will lead to enhanced ingestion due to complement receptors. Macrophage activation leads to the expression of increased Fc and complement receptors, so phagocytosis will be enhanced in the presence of macrophage-activating factors. Phagocytes play an important role in the control of infections by *Plasmodium* spp. and *Tryp. brucei*.

Antibody-dependent cell-mediated cytotoxicity has been shown to play a part in infections caused by a number of parasites, including *Tryp. cruzi, T. spiralis, S. mansoni* and filarial worms. The effector cells, macrophages, monocytes, neutrophils, eosinophils and natural killer cells bind to the antibody-coated parasites by their Fc and complement receptors. Close apposition of the effector cell and the target are necessary because the toxic molecules produced are non-specific and could damage host cells. A major basic protein from eosinophils damages the tegument of schistosomes and other worms, causing their death. It appears that different cell types and immunoglobulin isotypes are active against different developmental stages of parasites.

Eosinophils are more effective at killing newborn larvae of *T. spiralis* than other cells, whereas macrophages are very effective against microfilariae.

T cells

The importance of T cells in counteracting protozoan infections has been shown using nude (athymic) or T cell-depleted mice, which have a reduced capacity to control trypanosomal and malarial infections. The transfer of spleen cells, especially T cells, from immune animals gives protection against most parasitic infections. The type of T cell that is effective depends on the parasite. CD4+ T cells transfer protection against *Leishmania major* and *L. tropica*, and may be necessary for the elimination of other parasites. The intracellular parasite of cattle, *Theileria parvum*, is destroyed by cytotoxic T (T_c) cells.

CD4+ T cells may act by providing help in antibody production, but they also secrete various lymphokines that interact with other effector cells. CD8+ cells may be cytotoxic in certain situations, but these cells also produce a variety of lymphokines. Interleukin-2 production has been shown to be deficient during parasitic infections, such as malaria and trypanosomiasis. Administration of interleukin-2 to mice infected with *Tryp. cruzi* reduces parasitaemia and increases survival.

Colony-stimulating factors, e.g. interleukin-3 and granulocyte/monocyte colony-stimulating factor, are also produced by activated T cells. These molecules act on myeloid progenitors in the bone marrow, causing increased production of neutrophils, eosinophils and monocytes. They also increase the activity of these cells; the monocytosis and splenomegaly in malaria are caused by these T cell-derived molecules. The accumulation of macrophages in the liver as granulomata in schistosomiasis and the eosinophilia that is characteristic of worm infestations are also T cell-dependent phenomena.

In certain cases the production of lymphokines may have adverse effects. Leishmania infect macrophages and the release of molecules that stimulate the production of more host cells may potentiate the infection.

γ-Interferon does not inhibit or kill parasites directly, although multiplication of the liver stages of the malaria parasite is inhibited by γ-interferon, possibly through interaction with its receptor on the surface of hepatocytes. γ-Interferon is a potent macrophage activation factor and is probably involved in the resistance and elimination of intracellular parasites, such as *Toxoplasma gondii* and *Leishmania* spp. Activated macrophages are more effective killers and can destroy intracellular parasites before they establish themselves within the cell.

EVASION MECHANISMS

All animal pathogens, including parasitic protozoa and worms, have evolved effective mechanisms to avoid elimination by the host defence systems (Table 13.2).

Seclusion

Many parasites inhabit cells or anatomical sites that are inaccessible to host defence mechanisms. Those that attempt to survive within cells avoid the effects of antibody but must possess mechanisms to avoid destruction if the cell involved is capable of destroying them. *Plasmodium* spp. inhabit erythrocytes while toxoplasmas are less selective and will infect non-phagocytic cells as well as phagocytes. A number of different ways of avoiding destruction in macrophages have evolved. *Leishmania donovani* amastigotes are able to survive and metabolize in the acidic environment (pH 4–5) found in phagolysosomes, while *Toxoplasma gondii* is able to inhibit the fusion of lysosomes with the parasite-containing phagosome.

L. major has a similar escape mechanism by attaching to a phagocyte complement receptor (CR1) that does not

trigger the respiratory burst. The activation of the complement system by protozoan parasites seems to be a common mechanism to achieve attachment to target cells. *Tryp. cruzi* trypomastigotes can infect T cells of both the CD4 and CD8 subsets, and may be similar to retroviruses in using receptor molecules on the T cell surface for penetration.

The effectiveness of macrophages in the elimination of *Tryp. cruzi* depends upon the stage of development of the parasite. Trypomastigotes are able to escape from the phagocytic vacuole and survive in the cytoplasm whereas epimastigotes do not escape and are killed. Macrophages are also the preferred habitat of *Leishmania* spp., which multiply in the phagolysosome where they are resistant to digestion.

In an immune host these evasion mechanisms are less effective because of the presence of antibody and lymphokines. The ability to resist complement destruction also appears to be important. For example, *L. tropica* is easily killed by complement and causes only a localized self-healing lesion in the skin whereas a disseminating, often fatal, disease is seen with *L. donovani*, which is 10 times more resistant to complement killing. Large parasites such as helminths cannot infect individual cells; however, they can still achieve anatomical seclusion. *T. spiralis* larvae avoid the immune system by encysting in muscle; intestinal nematodes live in the lumen of the intestine.

Evasion

Parasites may avoid recognition by:

- antigenic variation
- acquiring host-derived molecules.

African trypanosomes have the capacity to express more than 100 different surface glycoproteins. By producing novel antigens throughout their lives, these parasites continuously evade the immune system. By the time the host has mounted a response against each new antigen the parasite has changed again. Plasmodia pass through

Table 13.2 Parasite escape mechanisms	
Intracellular habitat	Malaria parasites, trypanosomes and *Leishmania* spp.
Encystment	*Toxoplasma gondii* and *Trypanosoma cruzi*
Resistance to microbicidal products of phagocytes	*Leishmania donovani*
Masking of antigens	Schistosomes
Variation of antigen	Trypanosomes and malaria parasites
Suppression of immune response	Most parasites, e.g. malaria parasites, *Trichinella spiralis* and *Schistosoma mansoni*
Interference by antigens	Trypanosomes
Polyclonal activation	Trypanosomes
Sharing of antigens between parasite and host – molecular mimicry	Schistosomes
Continuous turnover and release of surface antigens of parasite	Schistosomes

several discrete developmental stages, each with its own particular antigens. A similar situation is seen in certain helminths such as *T. spiralis*. As a result, each new stage of the life cycle will be seen by the host as a 'new' infective challenge.

A number of parasites are known to adsorb host-derived molecules onto their surface. This is thought to mask their own antigens and enable them to evade immunological attack.

Parasitic protozoa and worms also use devices to avoid immune destruction. Certain parasites retain a surface coat, or glycocalyx, that blocks direct exposure of its surface antigens.

Immunosuppression

Parasites are not always able to evade detection and many have evolved mechanisms to suppress or divert immune reactions. Some parasites produce or generate molecules that act against cells of the immune system. Thus, the larvae of *T. spiralis* produce a molecule that is cytotoxic towards lymphocytes, and schistosomes can cleave a peptide from IgG, thereby decreasing its effectiveness. During many parasitic infections a large amount of antigenic material is released into the body fluids, and this may inhibit the response to or divert the response away from the parasite. High antigen concentrations can lead to tolerance by clonal exhaustion or clonal deletion. The immune complexes formed can also inhibit antibody production by negative feedback via Fc receptors on plasma cells. Many of these released molecules are polyclonal activators of T and B cells. This leads to the production of non-specific antibody, impairment of B cell function and immunosuppression. It has also been proposed that many parasites can cause unresponsiveness by activating immune suppressor mechanisms.

In many cases the immunosuppression has been attributed to macrophage dysfunction associated with antigen overload or the presence of intracellular parasites. In addition to the non-specific immunosuppression there can be parasite-specific effects. Mice infected by *Leishmania* spp. show antigen-specific depression of lymphokine production. Since this genus inhabits macrophages and is partly controlled by activation of these cells by lymphokines the effect is a diminished response against the pathogen.

Schistosomes have a receptor for part of the antibody molecule. They also release several proteases that cleave antibody molecules and release products that prevent macrophage activation. A schistosome-derived inhibitory factor suppresses T cell activity and is believed to allow other parasites to survive the effects of T cells and may explain the inefficiency of cytotoxic T cells in damaging the parasite.

When tested in a lymphocyte proliferation assay, peripheral blood lymphocytes of patients infected with *Plasmodium falciparum* are unresponsive to antigen prepared from the parasite, and in nearly 40% of the patients this persists for more than 4 weeks. Patients infected with *P. falciparum* show a suppression of lymphocyte reactivity that is not related to the degree of parasitaemia or severity of the clinical illness. The depressed lymphocyte reactivity is associated with a loss of both CD4$^+$ and CD8$^+$ lymphocytes from the peripheral blood. Once the parasite is cleared the response returns to normal. An even more sophisticated strategy has been evolved by *Leishmania mexicana* and *L. donovani*, which use interleukin-2 to stimulate their own growth. Mammalian epidermal growth factor has also been shown to stimulate the growth of certain trypanosomes in vitro.

IMMUNOPATHOLOGY

The immune response to parasites is aimed at eliminating the organisms, but many of the host reactions have pathological effects.

The IgE produced in parasitic worm infections can have severe effects on the host if it stimulates excessive mast cell degranulation, i.e. type I hypersensitivity. Anaphylactic shock can occur if a cyst ruptures and releases vast amounts of antigenic material into the circulation of a sensitized individual. Asthma-like symptoms occur in *Toxocara canis* infections when larvae of worms migrate through the lungs.

The polyclonal B cell activation seen with many parasitic infections can give rise to auto-antibodies. In trypanosomiasis and malaria antibodies against red blood cells, lymphocytes and DNA have been detected. Host antigens incorporated into the parasite, as an immune evasion mechanism, may stimulate auto-antibody production by giving rise to T cell help and overcoming tolerance. In Chagas' disease about 20% of individuals develop progressive cardiomyopathy and neuropathy of the digestive tract that is believed to be auto-immune in nature. These effects are thought to result from cross-reactivity between antibody or T cells responsive to *Tryp. cruzi* and nerve ganglia.

Immune complex-mediated disease occurs in malaria, trypanosomiasis, schistosomiasis and onchocerciasis. The deposition of immune complexes in the kidney is responsible for the nephrotic syndrome of quartan malaria.

Enlargement of the spleen and liver in malaria, trypanosomiasis and visceral leishmaniasis is associated with increases in the number of macrophages and lymphocytes in these organs. The liver, renal and cardiopulmonary pathology of schistosomiasis is related to cell-mediated responses to the worm eggs. Symptoms similar to those seen in endotoxaemia induced by Gram-negative bacteria are found in the acute stages of malaria.

The non-specific immunosuppression discussed above may explain why individuals with parasite infections are especially susceptible to bacterial and viral infections.

VACCINATION

No effective vaccine for humans has so far been developed against parasitic protozoa and worms, mainly because of the complex parasite life cycles and their sophisticated adaptive responses. Since protection in many cases depends on both antibody and cell-mediated reactions a vaccine must induce long-lived B and T cell immunity. In addition, since the recognition by T cells is genetically restricted, the vaccine preparation must stimulate T cells from most haplotypes and preferably without suppressor epitopes. Because of the immunopathology seen in many parasite infections, antigens that induce a potentially damaging response must be avoided.

A much better understanding of the biological mechanisms underlying the natural history of parasitic diseases is required before it will be possible to control these globally important diseases.

RECOMMENDED READING

Mims C, Nash A, Stephen J 2000 *Mims' Pathogenesis of infectious Disease*, 5th edn. Academic Press, London
Taussig M J 1996 *Processes in Pathology and Microbiology*, 2nd edn. Blackwell Scientific, Oxford
Wakelin D 1996 *Immunity to Parasites*, 2nd edn. Cambridge University Press, Cambridge

Internet site

www.dpd.cdc.gov/dpdx/HTML/Para_Health.htm

14

Immunity in bacterial infections

J. Stewart

Modern medical science has managed to subdue many of the classical infectious diseases, but has helped to create new ones which result from interference with normal host defence mechanisms, consequent upon medical and surgical procedures such as chemotherapy, catheterization, immunosuppression and irradiation. Infections that develop in this way are known as *iatrogenic* (physician-induced) diseases.

It is important to differentiate infection from disease. A host may be infected with a particular micro-organism and be unaware of its presence. If the microbe reproduces itself to such an extent that toxic products or sheer numbers of organisms begin to harm the host then a disease process has developed. Potentially pathogenic bacteria such as pneumococci, streptococci and salmonellae are found in the nose, throat or bowel; this is known as the carrier state and is a source of infection to other individuals. These bacteria may also cause disease in the carrier if they enter a vulnerable tissue.

HOST DEFENCES

Very few organisms can penetrate intact skin, and the various other innate defence mechanisms are extremely efficient at keeping bacteria at bay. When bacteria do gain access to the tissues the ability of the host to limit damage and eliminate the microbe will depend on the generation of an effective immune response against microbial antigens. In most cases the host defences will be directed against external components and secreted molecules. Bacteria are surrounded by a cytoplasmic membrane and a peptidoglycan cell wall. Associated with these basic structures there can be a variety of other components such as proteins, capsules, lipopolysaccharide or teichoic acids. There are also structures involved in motility or adherence to the cells of the host (see Chapter 2). These are some of the components to which the immune system directs its response. In general, peptidoglycan is attacked by lysosomal enzymes, and the outer lipid layer of Gram-negative

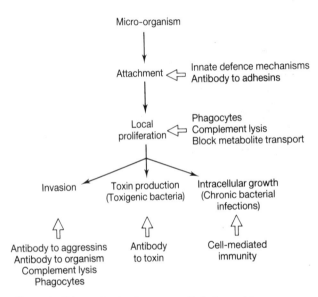

Fig. 14.1 Scheme showing the progress of infection and the immunological defence mechanisms.

bacteria by cationic proteins and complement. Specific antibodies can bind to flagella or fimbriae, affecting their ability to function properly and can inactivate various bacterial enzymes and toxins. Antibodies therefore interfere with many important bacterial processes but, ultimately, phagocytes are needed to destroy and remove the bacteria (Fig. 14.1). In some situations cell-mediated responses are required.

Inflammation

Having successfully avoided the innate immune mechanisms that protect the individual (mechanical barriers, antibacterial substances and phagocytosis; described in Chapter 11), a bacterium starts to proliferate in the tissues, and its toxic products trigger an inflammatory reaction. The resulting increase in vascular permeability leads to an exudation of serum proteins, including complement components, antibodies and clotting factors, as well as phagocytic cells. The phagocytes are attracted to the site of inflammation by chemotactic factors. Anaphylatoxins generated by complement activation further increase vascular permeability and encourage exudation of fluid and cells at the site of inflammation. Many of these mediators also cause vasodilatation, thereby increasing blood flow to the area.

Many types of micro-organisms, e.g. staphylococci and streptococci, are effectively dealt with by the phagocytes. The intensity and duration of the inflammatory process that is stimulated depends on the degree of success with which the micro-organism initially establishes itself. This, in turn, depends on the extent of the injury, the amount of associated tissue damage and the number and type of micro-organisms introduced. A localized abscess may arise at the site of infection.

If bacteria are not eliminated at the site of entry and continue to proliferate, they will pass via the tissue fluids and lymphatics to the draining lymph node, where a specific acquired immune response will be generated. The antibody and effector cells generated will leave the node to return to the area of infection to eliminate the bacteria. Some capsulate micro-organisms, such as pneumococci, are able to resist phagocytosis and are not dealt with effectively until large amounts of antibody are made. These 'mop up' the released capsular polysaccharide, and phagocytosis occurs. Other micro-organisms produce exotoxins, and effective immunity to exotoxins requires the development of specific antibodies against the toxin, i.e. *antitoxin*.

The types of infection described above are usually referred to as *acute* infections, and contrast with the protracted or *chronic* infections that are usually induced by bacteria that are adapted to survive within the cells of the host. Included amongst these are tuberculosis and leprosy, brucella infections and listeriosis. In these infections, cell-mediated immunity plays a predominant part in the final elimination of the micro-organism.

Humoral immunity

The attachment of a micro-organism to an epithelial surface is a prerequisite for the development of an infectious process (see p. 85). A first line of attack by antibody could be to inhibit colonization by stopping attachment.

The immunoglobulin IgA can stop colonization of the mucosal surface if it interferes with the attachment molecules (*adhesins*) present on the bacterial surface. IgA does not activate complement very efficiently; therefore, an inflammatory reaction is not stimulated. Damage to the gut wall during an inflammatory reaction would allow the entry of many potential pathogens into vulnerable tissues.

Many micro-organisms owe their pathogenic abilities to the production of *exotoxins*. Amongst diseases dependent on this type of mechanism are diphtheria, cholera, tetanus and botulism. Antibodies acquired by either immunization or previous infection or given passively as antiserum are able to *neutralize* bacterial toxins.

Many bacterial exotoxins are enzymes, and protective antibody can prevent interaction of the enzyme with its substrate. The antibody can bind directly to the active site of the enzyme or to adjacent residues and inhibit by steric hindrance. Antibody may also act by stopping activation of a zymogen into an active enzyme, interfere with the interaction between the toxin and its target cell or bind to a site on the molecule, causing a conformational change that destroys the enzymatic activity.

The direct binding of antibody to a bacterium can interfere with its normal functioning in numerous ways. Antibody can kill bacteria on its own or in conjunction with host factors and cells. To survive and multiply, bacteria must ingest nutrients and ions mainly by specific transport systems. Antibodies that affect the activity of specific transport systems will deprive the bacteria of their energy supply and other essential chemicals. Some bacteria are invasive, moving into the tissues aided by enzymes that they produce. Invasion can also be inhibited by antibody that attaches to the flagella of the micro-organism in such a way as to affect their motility. Antibodies can agglutinate bacteria, and formation of the aggregate will impede the spread of the organism. In addition, the formation of an immune complex of bacteria and antibody will stimulate phagocytosis and complement activation.

When a particle is coated with antibody a large number of Fc portions are exposed to the outside. This increases the chance that the particle will be held in contact with the phagocyte long enough to stimulate phagocytosis. The interaction of multiple ligands will increase the overall affinity of the binding, and if antibody and complement components are present on the same particle the binding will be even stronger.

The bacteria are internalized and attacked by the oxygen-dependent and oxygen-independent killing mechanisms within the phagocyte. Phagocytes are also responsible for the removal and digestion of bacteria that have been killed extracellularly. Bacteria are susceptible to the lytic action of complement, which may be activated by bacterial components. The presence of antibody on the bacterial cell surface will further stimulate the activation of complement. In certain circumstances, antibodies in conjunction with other bactericidal molecules lead to more efficient bacterial destruction. Gram-negative organisms are normally resistant to the action of lysozyme, probably due to the lipopolysaccharide component of the cell. The action of antibody and complement is thought to expose the underlying cell wall, which is then attacked by the lysozyme.

Cell-mediated immunity

Ultimately, all bacteria will be engulfed by a phagocyte, either to be killed or removed after extracellular killing. The host defence mechanisms of macrophages and monocytes can be enhanced by various activating stimuli, including such microbial products as muramyl dipeptide and trehalose dimycolate. The chemotactic formyl-methionyl peptides have been shown to increase the activities of various macrophage functions. The linkage of chemotaxis to activation has the advantage that the cell that is being attracted to the site of tissue injury will be better equipped to deal with the insult. Endotoxins present in the cell wall of Gram-negative bacteria and various carbohydrate polymers, such as β-glucans, are potent macrophage activators.

The immune system is also active in the production of macrophage-activating factors. In particular, lymphokines, produced by T lymphocytes, are often required to potentiate bacterial clearance both by attracting phagocytes to the site of infection and by activating them. The most important activator is γ-interferon, although tumour necrosis factor and colony-stimulating factors have also been implicated (see Chapter 11). All T lymphocytes produce some lymphokines when stimulated, and the balance of the different factors produced dictates the effect on surrounding cells. The overall effect of the lymphokines is to increase the effectiveness of host defence mechanisms, but if these molecules are produced in excess or to an inappropriate signal then a type IV hypersensitivity reaction can occur.

EVASION

Once a micro-organism becomes established in the tissues, having escaped the innate defence mechanisms, it can often make use of a number of evasion strategies that protect it from the immune reactions of the host. Pathogenic bacteria produce a rather ill defined group of bacterial products called *aggressins* and *impedins*, possession of which is associated with virulence (see Chapter 8). If antibody to such substances is present, the pathogenicity of the micro-organism is likely to be reduced.

Intracellular bacteria

Bacteria that can survive and replicate within phagocytic cells are at an advantage as they are protected from host defence mechanisms. Some micro-organisms reside intracellularly only transiently while others spend most, if not all, their life inside cells. An intracellular lifestyle demands potent evasion mechanisms to survive this hostile environment. Some bacteria, such as *Mycobacterium leprae*, have become so accustomed to their intracellular environment that they can no longer live in the extracellular space.

Listeria monocytogenes, the causative agent of listeriosis, can survive and multiply in normal macrophages, but it is killed within macrophages activated by lymphokines released from T lymphocytes. Listeriosis is most commonly seen in immunocompromised patients, pregnant women and neonates in whom a lack of adequate T cell-derived macrophage-activating factors is probably the critical factor. *Salmonella* spp. and *Brucella* spp. can also survive intracellularly. Unlike *L. monocytogenes* they owe their resistance to a glycolipid capsule that is resistant to destruction.

Mycobacteria have a waxy cell wall that is very hydrophobic. This external surface is very resistant to lysosomal enzymes and persists for a long time even when the bacteria have been killed. In addition, these micro-organisms have evolved other strategies to evade destruction. *Mycobacterium tuberculosis* secretes molecules that inhibit lysosome/phagosome fusion, while *M. leprae* can escape from the phagosome and grow in the cytoplasm. The cell wall of both these bacteria contains lipoarabinomannan that blocks the effects of γ-interferon on macrophages.

T lymphocytes represent the major host defence against intracellular pathogens. In many cases the bacteria themselves do not directly harm the host but the pathogenesis is caused by the immune response. After invasion of the host, intracellular bacteria will be taken up by macrophages, evade intracellular killing and multiply. During intracellular replication some microbial molecules will be processed and presented on the surface of the infected cell in association with major histocompatibility complex (MHC) gene products. The exact nature of the microbial molecules and the processing mechanism are not known. The processing appears to produce mainly antigen fragments in association with MHC class II molecules. This complex on the cell surface will be recognized by specific CD4+ T cells, which will be stimulated to release lymphokines. These molecules will in turn activate the macrophage so that the intracellular bacteria are killed.

It has also been proposed that peptides derived from the bacteria can become associated with MHC class I molecules. This complex will lead to the destruction of the infected cell by CD8+ T cells. These cells also produce lymphokines that can aid in the elimination of the infection. The lymphokines produced will attract blood monocytes to the site and activate them. If these newly recruited cells take up the released mycobacteria they will be more likely to destroy them since they will be in an activated state. The accumulation of macrophages will also cause the formation of a granuloma, which will prevent dissemination of the bacteria to other sites in the body. As conditions for the survival of the pathogens become less suitable they stop replicating and die. Some intracellular bacteria infect cells that are unable to destroy them. In this situation a more aggressive immune response may be needed to remove the pathogen and this can cause pathogenic damage unless kept under control (see below).

IMMUNOPATHOLOGY

The immune response to an organism will lead to some tissue damage through inflammation, lymph node swelling and cell infiltration. Sometimes the damage caused by the immune system is very severe, leading to serious disease and death. Rheumatic fever can follow group A streptococcal infections of the throat and is believed to be due to antibodies formed against a streptococcal cell wall component cross-reacting with cardiac muscle or heart valve. Myocarditis develops a few weeks after the throat infection and can be restimulated if the patient is re-infected with different streptococci.

Immune complex disease (type III hypersensitivity) is frequently associated with bacterial infections. Infective endocarditis caused by staphylococci and streptococci is associated with circulating complexes of antibody and bacterial antigen. Detection of these complexes can be helpful in diagnosis, but they can lead to joint and kidney lesions, vasculitis and skin rashes. Immune complexes may play a role in the pathogenesis of leprosy, typhoid fever and gonorrhoea.

Effects of endotoxin

Endotoxin interacts with cells and molecules of inflammation, immunity and haemostasis.

- Fever is induced by interleukin-1, produced by the liver in response to endotoxin, acting on the temperature-regulating hypothalamus.
- The action of lipopolysaccharide on platelets and activation of Hageman's factor causes disseminated intravascular coagulation with ensuing ischaemic tissue damage to various organs.
- Septic shock occurs during severe infections with Gram-negative organisms when bacteria or lipopolysaccharide enter the bloodstream.

Endotoxin acts on neutrophils, platelets and complement to produce, both directly and through mast cell degranulation, vasoactive amines that cause hypotension. The mortality is very high.

Endotoxin causes macrophages to produce large quantities of potent cytokines such as interleukin-1, tumour necrosis factor and colony-stimulating factors. It also causes polyclonal activation of B cells and can stimulate natural killer cells and other cell types to produce γ-interferon. A substantial part of the pathogenesis of endotoxin shock is probably due to the production of these molecules by cells of the immune system. In small amounts, endotoxin may actually be beneficial to the host but when present in excess the results can be disastrous.

Mycobacterial disease

Activated macrophages secrete a variety of biologically active molecules, including:

- proteases
- tumour necrosis factor
- reactive oxygen intermediates that are harmful to the surrounding tissue.

Tissue destruction will be an inevitable side-effect of this important mechanism of resistance. In the acute phase of a response this is likely to be tolerated; however, in the case of resistant organisms such as mycobacteria the process may become chronic and the tissue destruction extensive. Mycobacterial components are still able to stimulate a response after the bacterium has been killed since they persist for a long time, adding to the tissue damage.

Recent evidence suggests that lysis of infected cells may also occur. At first sight this may appear beneficial. Such a direct effect may be particularly relevant in the case of obligate intracellular pathogens like *M. leprae*. Release into the hypoxic centre of a productive granuloma may also be fatal for *M. tuberculosis*, which is highly sensitive to low oxygen pressures. The same cytolytic event may also result in microbial discharge from the granuloma into surrounding capillaries or alveoli and hence facilitate dissemination to other parts of the body or to other individuals. Lysis of infected cells causes tissue destruction, the severity of the effects depending on the importance of the tissue involved. *M. leprae* infects the Schwann cell, an irreplaceable component of the peripheral nervous system. Although the presence of *M. leprae* does not appear to affect the host cell to any extent, the presence of activated macrophages releasing toxic molecules or direct lysis by cytotoxic cells constitutes a major pathological mechanism in leprosy.

If the leprosy bacillus is released from a lysed non-phagocytic cell to be engulfed by an activated macrophage then the bacterium will be eliminated. Therefore, macrophage activation and target cell lysis can be beneficial as well as detrimental to the host.

The cell-mediated response that has the potential to eliminate these infections will give rise to type IV hypersensitivity reactions if the antigen is not efficiently removed. Chronic production of lymphokines will cause granuloma formation that with time can lead to fibrosis and loss of organ function. This type of response is particularly prevalent in patients with tuberculosis.

RECOMMENDED READING

Kaufmann S H E 1993 Immunity to intracellular bacteria *Annual Review of Immunology* 11:129–163
Mims C, Nash A, Stephen J 2000 *Mims' Pathogenesis of Infectious Disease*. 5th edn. Academic Press, London
Patrick S, Larkin M J 1995 *Immunological and Molecular Aspects of Bacterial Virulence*. Wiley, Chichester

Internet sites

www.bioscience.drexel.edu/immunology/presentations/group2/webpage/bacterial.html
infections.bayer.com/immune_system_bacteria/immune_system_bacteria_en.html

PART 3
BACTERIAL PATHOGENS AND ASSOCIATED DISEASES

15

Staphylococcus

Skin infections; osteomyelitis; food poisoning; foreign body infections

H. Humphreys

Sir Alexander Ogston, a Scottish surgeon, first showed in 1880 that a number of pyogenic diseases in humans were associated with a cluster-forming micro-organism. He introduced the name 'staphylococcus' (Greek: *staphyle* = bunch of grapes; *kokkos* = grain or berry) now used as the genus name for a group of facultatively anaerobic, catalase-positive, Gram-positive cocci. The major pathogen within the genus, *Staphylococcus aureus*, causes a wide range of major and minor infections in man and animals (Table 15.1) and is characterized by its ability to clot blood plasma by action of the enzyme *coagulase*. There are at least 30 other species of staphylococci, all of which lack this enzyme. The coagulase-negative staphylococci are skin commensals that can cause opportunistic infections associated with prostheses or foreign bodies, catheters and implants (usually *Staph. epidermidis*), and urinary tract infections (*Staph. saprophyticus*). It is not usually necessary to identify coagulase-negative staphylococci to the species level routinely, apart from confirming the identity of *Staph. saprophyticus* as a cause of urinary infection in young women.

Staphylococci are resistant to dry conditions and high salt concentrations, and are well suited to their ecological niche, which is the skin. They may also be found as part of the normal flora of other sites such as the upper respiratory tract. Staphylococci are commonly present on animals; mastitis caused by *Staph. aureus* is a common and costly complication of milking. Contamination of food can result in staphylococcal food poisoning.

STAPHYLOCOCCUS AUREUS

Description

Staph. aureus is a Gram-positive coccus about 1 μm in diameter. The cocci are mainly arranged in grape-like clusters (Fig. 15.1), but some, especially when examined in pathological specimens, may occur as single cells or pairs of cells. The organisms are non-sporing, non-motile and usually non-capsulate. When grown on many types of agar for 24 h at 37°C, individual colonies are circular, 2–3 mm in diameter with a smooth, shiny surface; colonies appear opaque and are often pigmented (golden-yellow, fawn or cream),

Table 15.1	Infections caused by *Staph. aureus*
Pyogenic infections	**Toxin-mediated infections**
Boils, carbuncles	Scalded skin syndrome
Wound infection	Pemphigus neonatorum
Abscesses	Toxic shock syndrome
Impetigo	Food poisoning
Mastitis	
Bacteraemia	
Osteomyelitis	
Pneumonia	
Endocarditis	

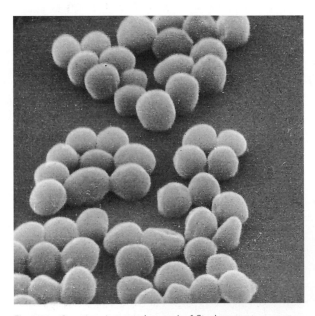

Fig. 15.1 Scanning electron micrograph of *Staph. aureus.*

though a few strains are unpigmented. Staphylococci are salt-tolerant and can be selectively isolated from materials such as faeces and food by use of media containing 7–10% sodium chloride. The main distinctive diagnostic features of *Staph. aureus* are:

- Production of an extracellular enzyme, coagulase, which converts plasma fibrinogen into fibrin, aided by an activator present in plasma. This test is done by adding a drop of fresh young broth culture into a tube containing 0.5 ml of citrated human or rabbit plasma diluted 1 in 10. A positive result is seen within a few hours as a distinct clot.
- Production of thermostable *nucleases* that break down DNA. This activity is detected by the ability of a boiled broth culture to degrade DNA in an agar diffusion test.
- Production of a surface-associated protein known as *clumping factor* or *bound coagulase* that reacts with fibrinogen. Clumping factor is easily detected within a few seconds by adding undiluted plasma to a saline suspension of the organism on a microscope slide.

Various commercial systems are available that rapidly identify coagulase-positive and coagulase-negative species. They are particularly useful for screening large numbers of strains obtained from environmental and food samples.

Pathogenesis

Staph. aureus is present in the nose of 30% of healthy people and may be found on the skin. It causes infection most commonly at sites of lowered host resistance, e.g. damaged skin or mucous membranes.

Virulence factors

Staph. aureus strains possess a large number of cell-associated and extracellular factors, some of which contribute to the ability of the organism to overcome the body's defences and to invade, survive in and colonize the tissues (Table 15.2). Though the role of each individual factor is not fully understood, it is likely that they are responsible for the establishment of infection, enabling the organism to bind to connective tissue, opposing destruction by the bactericidal activities of humoral factors such as complement and overcoming uptake and intracellular killing by phagocytes.

Animal experiments, with mutants defective in individual virulence factors, support the view that no single virulence factor is pre-eminent in overcoming host resistance and establishing a focus of staphylococcal infection. However, particular exotoxins are responsible for the symptoms of certain syndromes.

Table 15.2 Some virulence factors of *Staph. aureus*

Virulence factor	Activity
Cell wall polymers	
Peptidoglycan	Inhibits inflammatory response; endotoxin-like activity
Teichoic acid	Phage adsorption; reservoir of bound divalent cations
Cell surface proteins	
Protein A	Reacts with Fc region of IgG
Clumping factor	Binds to fibrinogen
Fibronectin-binding protein	Binds to fibronectin
Exoproteins	
α-Lysin	
β-Lysin	Impairment of membrane permeability;
γ-Lysin	cytotoxic effects on phagocytic and tissue cells
δ-Lysin	
Panton–Valentine leucocidin	
Epidermolytic toxins	Cause blistering of skin
Toxic shock syndrome toxin	Induces multisystem effects; superantigen effects
Enterotoxins	Induce vomiting and diarrhoea; superantigen effects
Coagulase	Converts fibrinogen to fibrin in plasma
Staphylokinase	Degrades fibrin
Lipase	Degrades lipid
Deoxyribonuclease	Degrades DNA

Staphylococcal toxins

Enterotoxins. Enterotoxins, types A–E, G, H, I and J, are commonly produced by up to 65% of strains of *Staph. aureus*, sometimes singly and sometimes in combination. These toxic proteins withstand exposure to 100°C for several minutes. When ingested as preformed toxins in contaminated food, microgram amounts of toxin can induce within a few hours the symptoms of staphylococcal food poisoning: nausea, vomiting and diarrhoea.

Toxic shock syndrome toxin (TSST-1). This was discovered in the early 1980s as a result of epidemiological and microbiological investigations in the USA of *toxic shock syndrome*, a multisystem disease caused by staphylococcal TSST-1 or enterotoxin, or both. A link was established with the use of highly absorbent tampons in menstruating women, although non-menstrual cases are now as common. The absence of circulating antibodies to TSST-1 is a factor in the pathogenesis of this syndrome.

TSST-1 and the enterotoxins are now recognized as *superantigens*, i.e. they are potent activators of T lymphocytes resulting in the liberation of cytokines such as tumour necrosis factor, and they bind with high affinity to mononuclear cells. These characteristics partly explain the florid and multisystem nature of the clinical conditions associated with these toxins.

Epidermolytic toxins. Two kinds of epidermolytic toxin (types A and B) are commonly produced by strains, mainly belonging to phage group II (see below), that cause blistering diseases. These toxins induce intra-epidermal blisters at the granular cell layer. Such blisters range in severity from the trivial to the distended blisters of *pemphigus neonatorum*.

The most dramatic manifestation of epidermolytic toxin is the *scalded skin syndrome* where the toxin spreads systemically in individuals who lack neutralizing antitoxin: extensive areas of skin are affected, which, after the development of a painful rash, slough off; the skin surface resembles scalding (Fig. 15.2). Such blistering lesions are seen mainly, but not exclusively, in small children.

Epidemiology

Sources of infection

Infected lesions. Large numbers of staphylococci are disseminated in pus and dried exudate discharged from large infected wounds, burns, secondarily infected skin lesions, and in sputum coughed from the lung of a patient with bronchopneumonia. Direct contact is the most important mode of spread, but air-borne dissemination may also occur. Small discharging lesions on the hands of doctors and nurses are a special danger to their patients. Cross-infection is an important method of spread of staphylococcal disease, particularly in hospitals, and scrupulous hand washing is essential in preventing spread. Food handlers may similarly introduce enterotoxin-producing food poisoning strains into food.

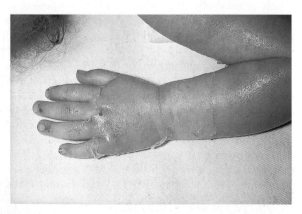

Fig. 15.2 Scalded skin syndrome (toxic epidermal necrolysis). (Photograph courtesy of Dr L G Millard, Queen's Medical Centre, Nottingham).

Healthy carriers. *Staph. aureus* grows harmlessly on the moist skin of the nostrils in many healthy persons, and the perineum is also commonly colonized. Organisms are spread from these sites into the environment by the hands, handkerchiefs, clothing, and dust consisting of skin squames and cloth fibres. Some carriers, called *shedders*, disseminate exceptionally large numbers of staphylococci.

During the first day or two of life most babies become colonized in the nose and skin by staphylococci acquired from their mother, nurse or environment. Nasal carriage in babies, as in older persons, is usually long-lasting. Transmission from babies to nursing mothers, who then develop mastitis, is well described.

Animals. Animals may disseminate *Staph. aureus* and so cause infections in humans, e.g. milk from a dairy cow with mastitis causing staphylococcal food poisoning.

Modes of infection

Acquisition of infection may be either *exogenous* (from an external source) or *endogenous* (from a carriage site, or minor lesion elsewhere in the patient's own body). Staphylococci do not grow outside the body except occasionally in moist nutrient materials such as meat, milk and dirty water, and it is important to remember that the body surfaces of human beings and animals are the main reservoir. Although not spore-forming, they may remain alive in a dormant state for several months when dried in pus, sputum, bed clothes or dust. They are fairly readily killed by heat (e.g. by moist heat at 65°C for 30 min), by exposure to light and by common disinfectants.

Laboratory diagnosis

One or more of the following specimens should be collected to confirm a diagnosis:

- *Pus* from abscesses, wounds, burns, etc., is much preferred to swabs.
- *Sputum* from cases of pneumonia, e.g. postinfluenzal or ventilator-associated pneumonia; bronchoscopic specimens are increasingly used in critically ill patients.
- *Faeces* or *vomit* from patients with suspected food poisoning or the remains of implicated foods.
- *Blood* from patients with suspected bacteraemia, e.g. septic shock, osteomyelitis or endocarditis.
- *Mid-stream urine* from patients with suspected cystitis or pyelonephritis.
- *Anterior nasal* and *perineal swabs* (moistened in saline or sterile water) from suspected carriers; nasal swabs should be rubbed in turn over the anterior walls of both nostrils.

The characteristic clusters of Gram-positive cocci can often be demonstrated by microscopy, and the organisms can be cultured readily on blood agar and most other media. The tube or slide coagulase test is performed to distinguish *Staph. aureus* from coagulase-negative species.

Typing

Most staphylococcal infections are sporadic, but outbreaks occur, especially in hospitals. The identification of an outbreak strain by determining whether all the isolates are of the same type is an important aspect in the investigation of a source, e.g. a heavy shedder in the operating theatre. For many years, strains of *Staph. aureus* have been differentiated into different *phage types* by observation of their pattern of susceptibility to lysis by a standard set of *Staph. aureus* bacteriophages. Virulent phages cause lysis of staphylococci that they can infect, and thus produce a clearing in the lawn of growth. Phage types are designated according to the phages able to cause this effect, and there is international agreement on the interpretation of results. Thus, a strain of type 3B/3C/55 is one that is lysed by phage 3B, phage 3C and phage 55 but not by any of the other phages.

Many strains, especially methicillin-resistant *Staph. aureus* (MRSA), are non-typable with standard and additional or experimental phages. Consequently, phage typing is increasingly being supplemented by genotypic methods such as polymerase chain reaction (PCR) 'fingerprinting', pulsed-field gel electrophoresis, ribotyping, etc. (see Chapter 3). Unfortunately, there are no internationally agreed criteria for assessing the results in the same way as there is for phage typing, but in a local context, it is usually possible to determine the relatedness of strains using a combination of phage typing and genotypic methods.

Treatment

Sensitivity to antibiotics

Staph. aureus and other staphylococci are inherently sensitive to many antimicrobial agents (Table 15.3). Among the most active is benzylpenicillin, but about 90% of strains found in hospitals are now resistant. Resistance to penicillin depends on production of the enzyme penicillinase, a β-lactamase that opens the β-lactam ring. Penicillinase also inactivates most of the other penicillins, but a few, including cloxacillin and flucloxacillin, are stable to the enzyme. Cephalosporins and β-lactamase inhibitors are also stable to penicillinase (see Chapter 5).

Table 15.3 Antibiotics and staphylococci

Active agents	Agents lacking useful activity
Penicillins[a]	Aztreonam
Cephalosporins	Polymyxins
Aminoglycosides[b]	Mecillinam
Tetracyclines	Nitroimidazoles
Macrolides	Quinolones[c]
Lincosamides	
Glycopeptides	
Fluoroquinolones[c]	
Rifampicin[b]	
Fusidic acid[b]	
Trimethoprim	
Chloramphenicol	
Carbapenems	

[a] Resistance common (see text).
[b] Usually used in combination, e.g. with flucloxacillin.
[c] For categorization of quinolones, see Table 5.3 and associated text.

Antibiotic resistance can arise by various mechanisms. MRSA strains are an increasing infection control problem and therapeutic challenge. These strains, which are resistant to all β-lactam agents, and often to other agents such as the aminoglycosides and fluoroquinolones, commonly colonize broken skin, but can cause the full range of staphylococcal infections. The resistance gene *mecA* codes for a unique penicillin-binding protein and is transmitted chromosomally. These are predominantly hospital pathogens in debilitated patients, such as those in intensive care units, where the combination of multiple courses of antibiotics and the use of invasive devices contribute greatly to the risk of acquisition (Fig. 15.3). MRSA is also becoming more common in the community, especially in long-stay institutions. Glycopeptides (vancomycin or teicoplanin) are

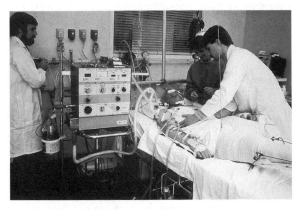

Fig. 15.3 The intensive care unit patient requiring multi-organ support is at particular risk of MRSA.

the agents of choice in the treatment of systemic infection, but these agents are expensive and may be toxic.

Strains of MRSA with reduced susceptibility to glycopeptides have been found in several countries. These bacteria have thickened walls compared to vancomycin-sensitive strains but are difficult to detect by routine methods as the expression of resistance is heterogeneous.

Choice of antibiotic for therapy

Pending receipt of susceptibility test results, the treatment of severe infections suspected to be caused by *Staph. aureus* should be started with flucloxacillin unless MRSA is endemic locally, in which case a glycopeptide such as vancomycin is indicated. If the patient is hypersensitive to penicillin, erythromycin, clindamycin, vancomycin (or teicoplanin) is used. Fusidic acid and rifampicin are not used alone in serious infections since mutation to resistance arises readily.

Infections caused by bacteria exhibiting reduced susceptibility to glycopeptides may be treated (if susceptible) with other anti-staphylococcal agents; in addition, it is often necessary to remove an infected source, such as an intravascular catheter. The efficacy of newer agents such as quinupristin-dalfopristin or linezolid (pp. 52–53) is still being evaluated.

Collections of pus may require surgical drainage, and infected prostheses (e.g. hip joint) or intravascular lines (e.g. Hickmann catheter) usually require removal if antibiotic treatment is to be successful. Life-threatening toxin-mediated disease, such as toxic shock syndrome, requires major medical support such as intravenous fluids to prevent multi-organ failure, often best provided in an intensive care unit.

COAGULASE-NEGATIVE STAPHYLOCOCCI

Coagulase-negative staphylococci comprise a large group of related species, which are commonly found on the surface of healthy persons in whom they are rarely the cause of infection. More than 30 species are recognized, but few are commonly incriminated in human infection. *Staph. epidermidis* accounts for about 75% of all clinical isolates, probably reflecting its preponderance in the normal skin flora. Other species include *Staph. haemolyticus*, *Staph. hominis*, *Staph. capitis* and *Staph. saprophyticus*. The emergence of coagulase-negative staphylococci as major pathogens reflects the increased use of implants such as cerebrospinal fluid shunts, intravascular lines and cannulae, cardiac valves, pace-makers, artificial joints, vascular grafts and urinary catheters, and the increasing numbers of severely debilitated patients in hospitals.

Description

Coagulase-negative staphylococci are morphologically similar to *Staph. aureus*, and the methods for isolation are the same. Colonies are usually non-pigmented (white), and they can be distinguished from *Staph. aureus* by their failure to coagulate plasma and by their lack of clumping factor and deoxyribonuclease. Because *Staph. epidermidis*, which accounts for most isolates, may contaminate clinical specimens, care has to be exercised in assessing its significance, especially from superficial sites. When isolated from sites such as blood or cerebrospinal fluid, further specimens should be obtained to confirm its clinical significance.

Coagulase-negative staphylococci are opportunistic pathogens that cause infection in debilitated or compromised patients such as premature neonates and oncology patients, often by colonizing biomedical devices such as prostheses, implants and intravascular lines. They cause particular problems in:

- cardiac surgery (prosthetic valve endocarditis)
- patients fitted with cerebrospinal fluid shunts (meningitis)
- continuous ambulatory peritoneal dialysis (peritonitis)
- immunocompromised patients (e.g. bacteraemia)
- women during the reproductive years (urinary tract infection with *Staph. saprophyticus*).

Pathogenesis

Production of an exopolysaccharide, allowing adherence and subsequent formation of a multi-layered biofilm, appears to be essential for the pathogenesis of device-related *Staph. epidermidis* infection. A complex array of inter-related chemical messengers controls expression of polysaccharide and drives intercellular adhesion and biofilm formation. Attachment is enhanced by the presence of matrix proteins, such as fibronectin and fibrinogen. The subsequent incorporation of teichoic acid appears to provide the biofilm with stability. There is considerable interest in the development of implantable devices such as prosthetic heart valves or cerebrospinal shunts that are less prone to adherence by *Staph. epidermidis* and subsequent biofilm formation. This may be achieved by altering the structure of the polymer or by incorporating antibacterial agents on the surface of the device.

Treatment

Antibiotic treatment of coagulase-negative staphylococcal infections is complicated because susceptibility is generally unpredictable. Strains resistant to penicillin, methicillin, gentamicin, erythromycin and chloramphenicol are common. If a strain is the cause of systemic infection, then vancomycin or teicoplanin should be used. Rifampicin in combination with a glycopeptide is occasionally useful in treating central nervous system infections. Vancomycin resistance is rare, but one species, *Staph. haemolyticus*, is often resistant to teicoplanin. Uncomplicated urinary tract infection caused by *Staph. saprophyticus* usually responds to trimethoprim or one of the fluoroquinolones such as norfloxacin.

RECOMMENDED READING

Cafferkey M T 1992 Methicillin-resistant *Staphylococcus aureus. Clinical Management and Laboratory Aspects.* Marcel Dekker, New York

Chadwick P R, Wooster S L 2000 Glycopeptide resistance in *Staphylococcus aureus. Journal of Infection* 40: 211–217

Jones D, Board R G, Sussman M 1990 *Staphylococci. Society for Applied Microbiology Symposium Series*, No. 19. Blackwell Scientific, Oxford

Kloos W E, Bannerman T L 1994 Update on clinical significance of coagulase-negative staphylococci. *Clinical Microbiology Reviews* 7: 117–140

Lowy F D 1998 *Staphylococcus aureus* infections. *New England Journal of Medicine* 339: 520–532

Mack D 1999 Molecular mechanisms of *Staphylococcus epidermidis* biofilm formation. *Journal of Hospital Infection* 43: (Supplement) S113–S125

Working Party Report 1998 Revised guidelines for the control of methicillin-resistant *Staphylococcus aureus* infection in hospitals. *Journal of Hospital Infection* 39: 253–290

16

Streptococcus and enterococcus

Pharyngitis; scarlet fever; skin and soft tissue infections; streptococcal toxic shock syndrome; pneumonia; meningitis; urinary tract infections; rheumatic fever; post–streptococcal glomerulonephritis

M. Kilian

Streptococci is the general term for a diverse collection of Gram-positive cocci that typically grow as chains or pairs (from the Greek *streptos*, pliant or chain; and *coccos*, a grain or berry) (Fig. 16.1). Virtually all the streptococci that are important in human medicine and dentistry fall into the genera *Streptococcus* and *Enterococcus*. Occasional opportunistic infections are associated with other genera of streptococci such as *Peptostreptococcus* (p. 340) and *Abiotrophia* ('nutritionally variant streptococci').

Streptococci are generally strong fermenters of carbohydrates, resulting in the production of lactic acid, a property used in the dairy industry. Most are facultative anaerobes, but peptostreptococci are obligate anaerobes. Streptococci do not produce spores and are non-motile. They are catalase-negative.

CLASSIFICATION

The genus *Streptococcus* includes important pathogens and commensals of mucosal membranes of the upper respiratory tract and, for some species, the intestines. The genus *Enterococcus*, which is also an intestinal commensal, is related to the other streptococci, but is classified separately.

The genus *Streptococcus* includes nearly 40 species. With few exceptions, the individual species are exclusively associated, either as pathogens or commensals, with man or a particular animal. The genus consists of six clusters of species (Table 16.1), each of which is characterized by distinct pathogenic potential and other properties.

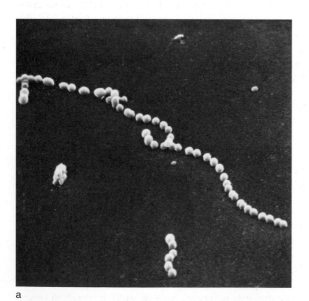

a

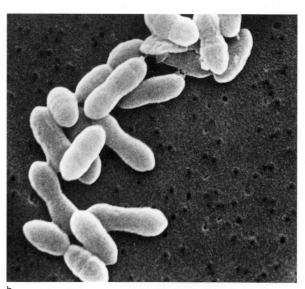

b

Fig. 16.1 Scanning electron micrograph of **a** *Str. pyogenes* showing typical chain formation (2000 × magnification), and **b** *Str. pneumoniae* showing typical diplococcus formation (7000 × magnification). (By courtesy of A P Shelton, Nottingham Public Health Laboratory.)

Table 16.1 *Streptococcus* species of clinical importance

Phylogenetic group	Species	Lancefield group	Type of haemolysis[a]
Pyogenic group	*Str. pyogenes*	A	β
	Str. agalactiae	B	β
	Str. equisimilis	C	β
Mitis group	*Str. pneumoniae*	O	α
	Str. mitis	O	α
	Str. oralis	Not identified	α
	Str. sanguis	H	α
	Str. gordonii	H	α
Anginosus group	*Str. anginosus*	G, F (and A)	α
	Str. intermedius		α
Salivarius group	*Str. salivarius*	K	None
Bovis group	*Str. bovis*	D	α or none
Mutans group	*Str. mutans*	Not designated	None
	Str. sobrinus	Not designated	None

[a] On horse blood agar.

- The *pyogenic* group includes most species that are overt pathogens of man and animals.
- The *mitis* group includes commensals of the human oral cavity and pharynx, although one of the species, *Streptococcus pneumoniae,* is also an important human pathogen.
- The *anginosus* group and the *salivarius* group are part of the commensal microflora of the oral cavity and pharynx.
- The *bovis* group belongs in the colon.
- The *mutans* group of streptococci colonizes exclusively tooth surfaces of man and some animals; some species belonging to this cluster are involved in the development of dental caries.

Virtually all the commensal species, including the enterococci, are opportunistic pathogens, primarily if they gain access to the bloodstream from the oral cavity or from the gut.

Haemolytic activity

Early attempts to distinguish between pathogenic and commensal streptococci recognized different types of haemolysis around colonies on blood agar plates. Colonies of streptococci belonging to the pyogenic group are generally surrounded by a clear zone, usually several millimetres in diameter, caused by lysis of red blood cells in the agar medium induced by bacterial haemolysins. This is called *β-haemolysis* and constitutes the principal

marker for potentially pathogenic streptococci in cultures of throat swabs or other clinical samples.

In contrast, most commensal streptococci give rise to a green discoloration around colonies on blood agar. This phenomenon is termed *α-haemolysis*. The factor causing the green discoloration is not a haemolysin, but hydrogen peroxide, which oxidizes haemoglobin to the green methaemoglobin.

Collectively, commensal streptococci are often called '*viridans streptococci*' which refers to their α-haemolytic property (*viridis* = green). Not quite logically, this term also includes the few streptococci (e.g. the salivarius and mutans groups of streptococci) that induce neither α- nor β-haemolysis. Moreover, in common usage, the term excludes *Str. pneumoniae*, although this species is also α-haemolytic.

Lancefield grouping

An important method of distinguishing between pyogenic streptococci is the serological classification pioneered by the American bacteriologist Rebecca Lancefield, who detected different versions of the major cell wall polysaccharide among the pyogenic streptococci.

This polysaccharide can be extracted from streptococci with hot hydrochloric acid and the different forms can be distinguished by precipitation with specific antibodies raised in rabbits. The polysaccharide is referred to as the group polysaccharide and identifies a number of different groups labelled by capital letters (Lancefield groups A, B, C etc.).

Among the pyogenic streptococci the individual serological groups are, with few exceptions, identical to distinct species (Table 16.1). Subsequently, serological grouping has been applied also to viridans streptococci and to enterococci, and the number of serological groups has been extended to a total of 21 (A–H and K–W). However, this has limited practical significance because there is no direct correlation between individual serogroups of viridans streptococci or enterococci and species.

STREPTOCOCCUS PYOGENES

This species, which consists of Lancefield group A streptococci, is among the most prevalent of human bacterial pathogens. It is exclusively associated with infections in man. It causes a wide range of suppurative infections in the respiratory tract and skin, life-threatening soft tissue infections, and certain types of toxin-associated reactions. Some of these infections may, in addition, result in severe non-suppurative sequelae due to adverse immunological reactions induced by the infecting streptococci.

The spectrum of infections caused by *Str. pyogenes* resembles that of *Staphylococcus aureus*, but the clinical characteristics associated with these two groups of pyogenic cocci are often distinct. Similarities and differences can be explained by the virulence factors expressed by the two species.

Pathogenesis

Virulence factors

Strains of *Str. pyogenes* express a large arsenal of virulence factors and, hence, their pathogenicity and the clinical signs that they induce are very diverse. The virulence factors are involved in adherence, evasion of host immunity and tissue damage (Fig. 16.2). While some factors are expressed by all clinical isolates, others are variably present among *Str. pyogenes* strains. This variation is due to the horizontal transfer of virulence genes among strains, primarily by transduction (see p. 66), and probably explains the temporal variations in the prevalence of severe infections and sequelae. It furthermore explains differences in virulence of individual strains and the different clinical pictures that may be associated with infections due to *Str. pyogenes*. Many of the virulence factors of *Str. pyogenes* are also expressed by some of the other species of pyogenic streptococci. In some species pathogenic for animals the corresponding virulence factors are expressed in a form specifically adapted to interact with their particular host.

Adhesion. Interaction with host fibronectin, a matrix protein on eukaryotic cells, is considered the principal mechanism by which *Str. pyogenes* binds to epithelial cells of the pharynx and skin. The structure that recognizes host fibronectin is located on the F protein, which is one of the many proteins expressed on the surface of *Str. pyogenes* (Fig. 16.2). The interaction between the streptococcal F protein and host cell fibronectin also mediates internalization of the bacteria into host cells.

In addition to the F protein, surface-exposed lipoteichoic acid and M proteins appear to be involved in adherence to mucosal and skin epithelial cells.

M proteins. The ability of *Str. pyogenes* to resist phagocytosis by polymorphonuclear leucocytes is to a

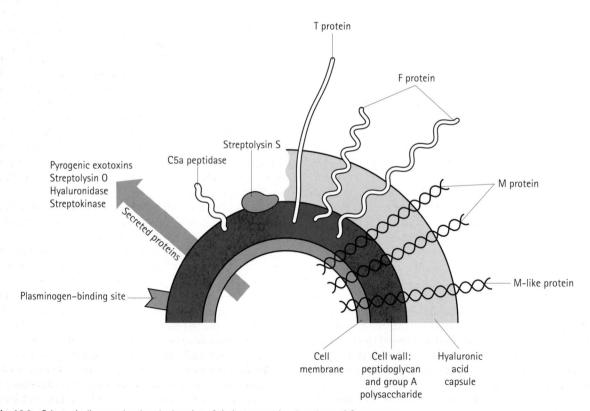

Fig. 16.2 Schematic diagram showing the location of virulence-associated products of *Str. pyogenes*.

high degree due to the cell surface-exposed M protein. The M protein is anchored in the cytoplasmic membrane, spans the entire cell wall, and protrudes from the cell surface as fibrils (Fig. 16.2). Acquired resistance to infection by *Str. pyogenes* is the result of antibodies in secretions and sera to the M protein molecule. However, as a result of genetic polymorphism in the gene encoding the M protein, the most distal part of the protein shows extensive variability among strains. As a consequence, individuals may suffer from recurrent *Str. pyogenes* infections with strains expressing different versions of the M protein. More than 80 different types of M protein have been identified by serological means.

Some strains produce two different M proteins with antiphagocytic activity and some, in addition, a structurally related M-like protein. All these proteins can bind various serum proteins of the host, including fibrinogen, plasminogen, albumin, IgG, IgA, the proteinase inhibitor α2-macroglobulin, and some regulatory factors from the complement system (factor H and C4b-binding protein). As well as masking the bacterial surface with host proteins some of these affinities are probably responsible for the ability of M proteins to resist phagocytosis. Thus, factor H is capable of destabilizing the important opsonin C3b when deposited on the bacterial surface. Likewise, the C4b-binding protein inhibits surface complement deposition by stimulating degradation of both C4b and C3b.

Capsule. Some strains of *Str. pyogenes* form a capsule composed of hyaluronic acid. Such strains grow as mucoid colonies on blood agar and are highly virulent in animal models. While capsule production is rare among isolates from uncomplicated pharyngitis, a significant proportion of isolates from severe infections have a capsule. Like other bacterial capsules it has an antiphagocytic effect. The relative significance of the M protein and the capsule as antiphagocytic factors differs among strains.

The capsule is identical to the hyaluronic acid of the connective tissue of the host and is not immunogenic. The bacteria may, in this way, disguise themselves with an immunological 'self' substance.

C5a peptidase. The C5a peptidase, which is found also in human pathogenic strains of *Str. agalactiae*, is presented on the surface of all strains of *Str. pyogenes*. It specifically cleaves, and thereby inactivates, human C5a, one of the principal chemoattractants of phagocytic cells.

Streptolysins. *Str. pyogenes* produces two distinct haemolysins, termed streptolysins O (oxygen-labile) and S (serum-soluble), both of which lyse erythrocytes, polymorphonuclear leucocytes and platelets by forming pores in their cell membrane.

Streptolysin O belongs to a family of haemolysins found in many pathogenic bacteria. Intravenous injection into experimental animals causes death within seconds, as the result of an acute toxic action on the heart. Streptolysin O may play a role in the pathogenesis of post-streptococcal rheumatic fever. Serum antibodies can be demonstrated after streptococcal infection, particularly after severe infections.

Streptolysin S is responsible for the β-haemolysis around colonies on blood agar plates. It can also induce the release of lysosomal contents with subsequent cell death after engulfment by phagocytes. In contrast to streptolysin O it is not immunogenic.

Pyrogenic exotoxins. Most strains of *Str. pyogenes* produce one or more toxins that are called *pyrogenic exotoxins* because of their ability to induce fever. Three, SPE A, SPE B and SPE C, have been extensively characterized, but there are several others. Purified SPE A causes death when injected into rabbits, and is the most toxic of the three, but SPE B also causes myocardial necrosis and death in experimental animals.

The genes for SPE A and SPE C are transmitted between strains by bacteriophage, and stable production depends on lysogenic conversion in a manner analogous to toxin production by *Corynebacterium diphtheriae* (p. 67). Even among strains that possess the genes the quantity of toxin secreted varies dramatically.

SPE A and SPE C are also called erythrogenic toxins, as they are responsible for the rash observed in patients with scarlatina. They are genetically related to *Staph. aureus* enterotoxins and, like these, have superantigen activity. By cross-linking MHC class II molecules and the Vβ-domain of the antigen receptor on a subset of T lymphocytes, these toxins cause comprehensive (antigen-independent) activation of helper T lymphocytes. The result is substantial release of interleukins IL-1 and IL-2, tumour necrosis factor-α (TNF-α) and interferon-γ. These cytokines may cause a variety of clinical signs, including inflammation, shock and organ failure characteristically seen in patients with severe streptococcal disease.

Unlike SPE A and SPE C, all strains of *Str. pyogenes* produce SPE B, which is a potent cysteine proteinase capable of cleaving many host proteins.

None of the three pyrogenic exotoxins is unambiguously associated with any of the clinical syndromes caused by *Str. pyogenes*. However, most isolates from episodes of severe invasive disease and toxic shock-like syndrome produce SPE A, and the protease SPE B appears to be responsible for the extensive tissue destruction observed in many patients with severe invasive infections, including toxic shock-like syndrome.

Hyaluronidase. *Str. pyogenes* and several other pyogenic streptococci use a secreted hyaluronidase to degrade hyaluronic acid, the ground substance of host connective tissue. This property may facilitate the spread of infection along fascial planes. During infections, particularly those involving the skin, serum antibody titres to hyaluronidase show a significant rise.

Streptokinase. Streptokinase, also known as fibrinolysin, is another spreading factor. It is expressed by all strains of *Str. pyogenes* and co-operates with a surface-expressed plasminogen-binding site on the bacteria. Once host plasminogen is bound to the bacterial surface, it is activated to plasmin by streptokinase. Thus, in contrast to *Staph. aureus*, which aims at hiding behind a wall of coagulated plasma (fibrin), *Str. pyogenes* employs host plasmin to hinder build-up of fibrin barriers. As a result, soft tissue infections due to *Str. pyogenes* are more diffuse, and often rapidly spreading, in contrast to the well localized abscesses that typify staphylococcal infections.

Lipoproteinase. This enzyme is also called *opacity factor*, as it induces opalescence in growth media containing serum. The exact biological significance is not known but there is a strong correlation between the production of this enzyme and particular M types, and it is produced mainly by strains causing skin infections.

Deoxyribonucleases (DNAases). At least four distinct forms of DNAases, designated A, B, C and D, are produced by *Str. pyogenes*. DNAase B is the most common form. The enzymes hydrolyse nucleic acids and may play a role as spreading factors by liquefying viscous exudates.

Clinical features

While a general decrease in the prevalence of serious infections with *Str. pyogenes* has occurred since the mid 19th century, a resurgence in severe streptococcal infections and increased mortality due to streptococcal sepsis has been observed since the early 1980s.

The most common route of entry of *Str. pyogenes* is the upper respiratory tract, which is usually the primary site of infection and also serves as a focus for other types of infections. Spread from person to person is by respiratory droplets or by direct contact with infected wounds or sores on the skin. Not all individuals colonized by *Str. pyogenes* in the upper respiratory tract develop clinical signs of infection.

After an acute upper respiratory tract infection, the convalescent patient may carry the infecting streptococci for some weeks. Only a few healthy adults carry *Str. pyogenes* in the respiratory tract, but the carriage rate in young school children is just over 10%. It may be considerably higher before or during an epidemic.

Non-invasive streptococcal disease

The most common infections caused by *Str. pyogenes* are relatively mild and non-invasive infections of the upper respiratory tract (*pharyngitis*) and skin (*impetigo*). In the USA more than 10 million cases of non-invasive *Str. pyogenes* infection are estimated to occur annually.

Pharyngitis. This is the most common infection caused by *Str. pyogenes*. Clinical signs such as abrupt onset of sore throat, fever, malaise and headache generally develop 2–4 days after exposure to the pathogen. The posterior pharynx is usually diffusely reddened, with enlarged tonsils that may show patches of grey-white exudate on their surface and, sometimes, accumulations of pus in the crypts. The local inflammation results in swelling of cervical lymph nodes. Occasionally, tonsillar abscesses develop; this is a very painful condition and potentially dangerous as the pathogen may spread to neighbouring regions and to the bloodstream.

Despite the significant symptoms and clinical signs, differentiating streptococcal pharyngitis ('*strep throat*') from viral pharyngitis is impossible without microbiological or serological examination. Culture studies have demonstrated that 20–30% of cases of pharyngitis are associated with *Str. pyogenes*.

Occasional cases of streptococcal sore throat are caused by species belonging to Lancefield groups C and G.

Scarlet fever. Pharyngitis caused by certain pyrogenic exotoxin-producing strains of *Str. pyogenes* may be associated with a diffuse erythematous rash of the skin and mucous membranes. The condition is known as *scarlet fever* or *scarlatina*. The rash develops within 1–2 days after the first symptoms of pharyngitis and initially appears on the upper chest and then spreads to the extremities. After an initial phase with a yellowish-white coating the tongue becomes red and denuded ('*strawberry tongue*').

Between 1860 and 1870 the mean annual death rate from scarlet fever in England and Wales was close to 2500 per million of the population. Since then a steady decline in the incidence has been observed. The total number of scarlet fever cases in 1999 in England and Wales was 25 per million — the lowest annual total ever recorded — and death is now extremely rare.

Skin infections. *Str. pyogenes* may cause several types of skin infection, sometimes in association with *Staph. aureus*. The superficial and localized skin infection, known as *impetigo* or *pyoderma*, occurs mainly in children (Fig. 16.3). It primarily affects exposed areas on the face, arms or legs. The skin becomes colonized after contact with an infected person and the bacteria enter the skin through small defects. Initially, clear vesicles develop, which within a few days become pus-filled. Secondary spread is often seen as a result of scratching.

Potentially more severe is the acute skin infection *erysipelas* (*erythros*, red; *pella*, skin). It occurs in the

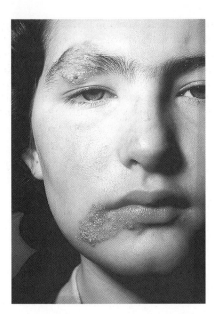

Fig. 16.3 Impetigo. (Photograph courtesy of Dr L G Millard, Queen's Medical Centre, Nottingham.)

superficial layers of the skin (cellulitis) and involves the lymphatics. The infection is characterized by diffuse redness of the skin and the patients experience local pain, enlargement of regional lymph nodes and fever. Untreated, the infection may spread to the bloodstream, and was often fatal before antibiotics became available.

Invasive soft tissue infections

Severe, sometimes life-threatening *Str. pyogenes* infections may occur when the bacteria get into normally sterile parts of the body. The most severe forms of invasive infections are *necrotizing fasciitis*, streptococcal *toxic shock syndrome* and *puerperal fever*, all of which are associated with bacteraemia.

Worldwide, rates of invasive infections increased from the mid 1980s to the early 1990s. In 1999, nearly 10 000 cases of invasive *Str. pyogenes* infection occurred in the USA. Although these infections may occur in previously healthy individuals, patients with chronic illnesses like cancer and diabetes, and those on kidney dialysis or receiving steroids have a higher risk. Even with antibiotic treatment death occurs in 10–13% of all invasive cases: 45% of patients with toxic shock syndrome and 25% of patients with necrotizing fasciitis.

Necrotizing fasciitis. This infection progresses very rapidly, destroying fat and fascia. Although *Str. pyogenes* gains entry to these tissues through the skin after trauma, often of a minor nature, the skin itself may show only minimal signs of infection and may indeed be spared. Systemic shock and general deterioration occur very quickly. The disease affects the fit, young person with no obvious underlying pathology, as well as the immunocompromised.

The clinical diagnosis may be difficult because *Staph. aureus* and anaerobes such as *Clostridium perfringens* can produce a similar clinical picture. Streptococci can be isolated from the blood, blister fluid and from cultures of the infected area.

Streptococcal myositis. This rare infection mimics necrotizing fasciitis clinically, although at operation they look quite different. As a breach of the skin or soft tissue damage is unusual, the source is considered to be the throat, with bacteraemic spread to the muscle. The infection may be precipitated by trauma or muscle strain.

Streptococcal toxic shock syndrome. Patients with invasive and bacteraemic *Str. pyogenes* infections, and in particular necrotizing fasciitis, may develop streptococcal toxic shock syndrome. The disease, which was first described in the late 1980s, is the result of the release of streptococcal toxins to the bloodstream. A striking feature of this acute fulminating disease is severe pain at the site of initial infection, usually the soft tissues. The additional clinical signs resemble those of staphylococcal toxic shock syndrome (p. 169) and include fever, malaise, nausea, vomiting and diarrhoea, dizziness, confusion, and a flat rash over large parts of the body. Without treatment, the disease progresses to shock and general organ failure.

Other suppurative infections. Historically, *Str. pyogenes* has been an important cause of puerperal sepsis. However, after the introduction of antibiotic therapy this and other suppurative infections such as lymphangitis, pneumonia and meningitis are relatively rare.

Bacteraemia. *Str. pyogenes* is the second most common (after *Str. agalactiae*) of the pyogenic streptococci isolated from blood cultures. Bacteraemia is regularly seen in patients with necrotizing fasciitis and toxic shock syndrome, but rarely as a complication to pharyngitis and local skin infections. Once in the blood, *Str. pyogenes* multiplies with incredible speed (doubling time, 18 min), and the mortality rate approaches 40%. The potential complications include acute endocarditis leading to heart failure.

Non-suppurative sequelae

Two serious diseases may develop as sequelae to *Str. pyogenes* infections:

- *Rheumatic fever*, a potential sequela to pharyngitis (including scarlatina).
- *Acute glomerulonephritis*, which is primarily, but not exclusively, associated with skin infections.

Both are caused by immune reactions induced by the streptococcal infection. The first clinical signs appear 1–5 weeks after the infection and at a time when the bacteria may have been eradicated by the immune system or as a result of antibiotic therapy.

Clinical correlations suggest that *psoriasis* may also be triggered by *Str. pyogenes* throat infection. Preliminary evidence supports the hypothesis that some streptococcal superantigens cause disruption of immunological tolerance of a CD8+ T cell subset that recognizes cross-reactive epitopes on M proteins and skin keratin.

Rheumatic fever. This manifests as an inflammation of the joints (arthritis), heart (carditis), central nervous system (chorea), skin (erythema marginatum), and/or subcutaneous nodules. Polyarticular arthritis is the most common manifestation, whereas carditis is the most serious as it leads to permanent damage, particularly of the heart valves.

Rheumatic fever is a major cause of acquired heart disease in young people throughout the world. The incidence of rheumatic heart disease worldwide ranges from 0.5 to 11 per 1000 of the population. New cases are relatively rare in most of Europe, but increased incidences have been observed among the aboriginal populations of Australia and New Zealand, and in Hawaii and Sri Lanka. Outbreaks of rheumatic fever have also been seen in the USA.

The disease is autoimmune in nature and is believed to result from the production of autoreactive (and polyspecific) antibodies and T lymphocytes induced by cross-reactive components of the bacteria and host tissues. Therefore, repeated episodes of *Str. pyogenes* infection increase the severity of the disease. The major antigens involved are myosin, tropomyosin, laminin and keratin in the human tissues and the group A antigen (a polymer of *N*-acetylglucosamine) in the *Str. pyogenes* cell wall in addition to epitopes on some variants of surface M proteins.

Acute post-streptococcal glomerulonephritis. The clinical manifestations include:

- coffee-coloured urine caused by haematuria
- oedema of the face and extremities
- circulatory congestion caused by renal impairment.

Unlike rheumatic disease, outbreaks of post-streptococcal acute glomerulonephritis have continued to decline in most parts of the world. Regions that still exhibit a high incidence of this disease include Africa, the Caribbean, South America, New Zealand and Kuwait.

Post-streptococcal glomerulonephritis is usually referred to as an immune complex-mediated disease. However, the exact pathogenesis is not clear. Several mechanisms have been proposed, including:

- immune complex deposition in the glomeruli
- reaction of antibodies cross-reactive with streptococcal and glomerular antigens
- alterations of glomerular tissues by streptococcal products such as streptokinase
- direct complement activation by streptococcal components that have a direct affinity for glomerular tissues.

Disease is associated with a limited number of M types of *Str. pyogenes,* and there is evidence that particular variants of streptokinase are crucial nephritogenic factors.

Unlike rheumatic fever there is a general absence of individual recurrences which suggests that antibodies to nephritogenic factors protect against disease rather than the opposite.

STREPTOCOCCUS AGALACTIAE

Str. agalactiae belongs to Lancefield group B. Its primary human habitat is the colon. It may be carried in the throat and, importantly, 10–40% of women intermittently carry *Str. agalactiae* in the vagina.

Previously, *Str. agalactiae* was recognized primarily as a cause of bovine mastitis (*agalactia,* want of milk). However, since 1960 it has become the leading cause of neonatal infections in industrialized countries and is also an important cause of morbidity among peripartum women and non-pregnant adults with chronic medical conditions. Among β-haemolytic streptococci, *Str. agalactiae* is the most frequent isolate from blood cultures.

Pathogenesis

Virulence factors

Str. agalactiae produces several virulence factors, including haemolysins, capsule polysaccharide, C5a peptidase (only human pathogenic strains), hyaluronidase (not all strains), and various surface proteins that bind human IgA and serve as adhesins.

Nine different types of the capsular polysaccharide have been identified (Ia, Ib, and II-VIII). The serotype most frequently associated with neonatal infections is type III, whereas infections in adults are more evenly distributed over the different serotypes.

Among the haemolysins produced by *Str. agalactiae*, one, known as the CAMP factor (so-called because it was originally described by Christie, Atkins and Munch-Petersen), plays an important role in the recognition of this species in the laboratory. The CAMP factor lyses sheep or bovine red blood cells pre-treated

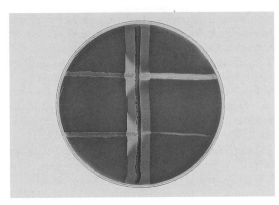

Fig. 16.4 Blood agar culture of strains of *Str. pyogenes* (group A) (upper right), *Str. equisimilis* (group C) (lower right), and *Str. agalactiae* (group B) (upper and lower left) surrounding a vertical streak of *Staph. aureus*. The two *Str. agalactiae* strains show a positive CAMP reaction.

with the β-toxin of *Staph. aureus* (Fig. 16.4). Purified CAMP factor protein is lethal to rabbits when injected intravenously.

Clinical features

Infection in the neonate

Two different entities are recognized:

- *early-onset disease*, most cases of which present at or within 12 h of birth
- *late-onset disease*, presenting more than 7 days and up to 3 months after birth.

Early-onset disease. This results from ascending spread of *Str. agalactiae* from the vagina into the amniotic fluid, which is then aspirated by the infant, and results in septicaemia in the infant or the mother or both. Infants borne by mothers carrying *Str. agalactiae* may also become colonized during passage through the vagina, but early-onset disease is an uncommon outcome (about 1% of cases).

Depending on the site of initial contamination, neonates may be ill at birth or develop acute and fulminating illness a few hours, or a day or two, later. The clinical symptoms include lethargy, cyanosis and apnoea; when septicaemia progresses, shock ensues and death will occur if treatment is not quickly instituted. Meningitis and pulmonary infection may be associated.

Due to improved recognition and prompt treatment of babies with symptoms, the fatality rate has been reduced to less than 10%. However, considerable morbidity persists among some survivors, especially those with meningitis.

Risk factors for neonatal colonization and infection are:

- premature rupture of membranes
- prolonged labour
- premature delivery
- low birth weight
- intrapartum fever.

The immune status of the mother, and hence the level of maternal IgG antibodies in the infant, appears to be more important than the degree of colonization of the mother's genital tract by *Str. agalactiae*.

It is possible that *Str. agalactiae* may itself cause premature rupture of membranes as a result of secretion of proteases and activation of local inflammation.

Late-onset disease. Purulent meningitis is the most common manifestation, but septic arthritis, osteomyelitis, conjunctivitis, sinusitis, otitis media, endocarditis and peritonitis also occur. The incidence of invasive infection is higher among preterm infants than among those born at term.

The pathogenesis is distinct from that of early-onset disease. There is usually no history of obstetric complications and the disease is unrelated to vaginal colonization in the mother. Many cases are acquired in hospital. Ward staff can be carriers of *Str. agalactiae*, and contamination of the baby may occur during nursing procedures, with subsequent baby-to-baby spread. Mastitis in the mother has also been described as a source of infection.

Infections in the adult

Ascending spread of *Str. agalactiae* leading to amniotic infection may result in abortion, chorioamnionitis, postpartum sepsis (endometritis) and other infections (e.g. pneumonia) in the postpartum period in young, previously healthy women.

Str. agalactiae is also a frequent cause of infection in certain risk groups of non-pregnant adults. Disease may manifest as sepsis, pneumonia, soft tissue infections such as cellulitis and arthritis, and urinary tract infections complicated by bacteraemia. The risk factors in these patients are diabetes mellitus, liver cirrhosis, renal failure, stroke and cancer. Older age, independent of underlying medical conditions, increases the risk of invasive *Str. agalactiae* infection.

OTHER PYOGENIC STREPTOCOCCI

Group C and G streptococci

Several species of streptococci that carry the Lancefield group C or group G antigens occasionally cause infections similar to those of *Str. pyogenes*. Most of these species have their primary habitat in horses, cattle and pigs, but some strains have become adapted to the human host and then produce some of the virulence factors primarily associated with *Str. pyogenes*. They can cause epidemic sore throat, especially in communities such as schools, nurseries and institutions often associated with consumption of unpasteurized milk. Group C streptococci have been associated with acute glomerulonephritis but not with rheumatic fever. The most important of the group C streptococci in human medicine is *Str. equisimilis*.

Group R streptococci

Str. suis serotype 2 (group R streptococci) cause septicaemia and meningitis in pigs. They belong to a phylogenetic lineage separate from the other pyogenic streptococci. They occasionally infect people in contact with contaminated pork or infected pigs, and may cause septicaemia, meningitis and respiratory tract infections. Abattoir workers, butchers and, to a lesser extent, housewives are at risk.

STREPTOCOCCUS PNEUMONIAE

Str. pneumoniae, commonly called the pneumococcus, is a member of the oropharyngeal flora of 5–70% of the population, with the highest isolation rate in children during the winter months. In contrast to other streptococci, *Str. pneumoniae* generally occurs as characteristic diplococci (Fig. 16.1). Although genetically closely related to the commensal *Str. mitis* and *Str. oralis*, *Str. pneumoniae* is an important pathogen, which is largely ascribed to its capsular polysaccharide. It primarily causes disease of the middle ear, paranasal sinuses, mastoids and the lung parenchyma but may spread to other sites, such as the joints, peritoneum, endocardium and biliary tract and, in particular, the meninges.

Str. pneumoniae is genetically very flexible because of frequent recombination between individual strains. Gene transfer is by transformation and may result in expression of a different capsular serotype. Experimental transfer of capsule genes in pneumococci was the basis of the original demonstration that DNA contains the genetic information in cells.

Pathogenesis

Virulence factors

Capsule. The capsular polysaccharide is a crucial virulence factor. The capsule is antiphagocytic, inhibiting complement deposition and phagocytosis where type-specific opsonic antibody is absent. A total of 90 different capsular serotypes have been identified.

The serotypes are designated by numbers, and those that are structurally related are grouped together (1, 2, 3, 4, 5, 6A, 6B etc.). The different serotypes differ in virulence. Thus, about 90% of cases of bacteraemic pneumococcal pneumonia and meningitis are caused by some 23 serotypes.

IgA1 protease. Like the two other principal causes of bacterial meningitis (*Neisseria meningitidis* and *Haemophilus influenzae*), pneumococci produce an extracellular protease that specifically cleaves human IgA1 in the hinge region. This protease enables these pathogens to evade the protective functions of the principal immunoglobulin isotype of the upper respiratory tract.

Pneumolysin. Pneumococci produce an intracellular membrane-damaging toxin known as pneumolysin, which is released by autolysis. Pneumolysin inhibits:

- neutrophil chemotaxis
- phagocytosis and the respiratory burst
- lymphocyte proliferation and immunoglobulin synthesis.

In experimental models it induces the features of lobar pneumonia and contributes to the mortality of this disease. Pneumolysin is immunogenic and it might be suitable for a new pneumococcal vaccine.

Autolysin. When activated, the pneumococcal autolysin breaks the peptide cross-linking of the cell wall peptidoglycan, leading to lysis of the bacteria. Autolysis enables the release of pneumolysin and, in addition, large amounts of cell wall fragments. The massive inflammatory response to these peptidoglycan fragments is an important component of the pathogenesis of pneumococcal pneumonia and meningitis.

Clinical features

Predisposing factors

Most *Str. pneumoniae* infections are associated with various predisposing conditions. Although occasional clusterings of pneumococcal infections are recognized, person-to-person spread is uncommon.

Pneumonia results from aspiration of pneumococci contained in upper airway secretions into the lower respiratory tract; for example, when the normal mechanisms of mucous entrapment and expulsion by an intact glottic reflex and mucociliary escalator are impaired. This situation may arise in:

- disturbed consciousness in association with general anaesthesia, convulsions, alcoholism, epilepsy or head trauma

- respiratory viral infections, such as influenza
- chronic bronchitis and other forms of chronic bronchial sepsis.

Other predisposing disease states in which pneumococcal pneumonia may be the terminal event include:

- valvular and ischaemic heart disease
- chronic renal failure
- diabetes mellitus
- bronchogenic and metastatic malignancy
- advancing age.

Immune deficiencies that predispose to pneumococcal infection include:

- hypogammaglobulinaemia
- asplenia or hyposplenism
- malignancies such as multiple myeloma.

In these conditions there is either a relative or absolute deficiency of opsonic antibody activity or an inability to induce a sufficient type-specific antibody response. *Tuftsin*, a naturally occurring tetrapeptide secreted by the spleen, also plays a role in combating pneumococcal sepsis; particularly at risk are those deficient in splenic activity:

- congenital asplenia
- traumatic removal
- functional impairment, e.g. homozygous sickle cell disease.

Human immunodeficiency virus (HIV) infection carries an increased risk of bacterial infections, including those caused by the pneumococcus, particularly in children.

Acute infections of the middle ear and paranasal sinuses occur in otherwise healthy children, but are usually preceded by a viral infection of the upper respiratory tract leading to local inflammation and swelling and obstruction of the flow from these sites.

Pneumonia

Str. pneumoniae is the most frequent cause of pneumonia. The estimated annual incidence is 1–3 per 1000 of the population, with a 5% case fatality rate. Pneumococcal pneumonia follows aspiration with subsequent migration through the bronchial mucosa to involve the peribronchial lymphatics. The inflammatory reaction is primarily focused within the alveolus of a single lobule or lobe, although multilobar disease can also occur. Contiguous spread commonly results in inflammatory involvement of the pleura; this may progress to empyema.

Pericarditis is another uncommon but well recognized complication. Occasionally, lung necrosis and intrapul-monary abscess formation occur with the more virulent pneumococcal serotypes. Bacteraemia may complicate pneumococcal pneumonia in up to 15% of patients. This can result in metastatic involvement of the meninges, joints and, rarely, the endocardium.

Mortality from pneumococcal pneumonia in those admitted to hospital in the UK is approximately 15%. It is increased by age, underlying disease, bloodstream involvement, metastatic infection and certain types of pneumococci with large capsules (e.g. serotype 3).

Otitis media and sinusitis

Middle ear infections (otitis media) affect approximately half of all children between the ages of 6 months and 3 years; approximately one-third of cases are caused by *Str. pneumoniae*. Disease occurs after acquisition of a new strain to which there is no pre-existing immunity. The prevalence is highest among children attending primary school, where there is a constant exchange of pneumococcal strains.

Meningitis

Str. pneumoniae is among the leading causes of bacterial meningitis. It is assumed that invasion arises from the pharynx to the meninges via the bloodstream since bacteraemia usually co-exists. Meningitis may occasionally complicate pneumococcal infection at other sites, such as the lung.

The incidence of pneumococcal meningitis is bimodal and affects children less than 3 years of age and adults of 45 years and above. The fatality rates are 20 and 30%, respectively, which are considerably higher than those associated with other types of bacterial meningitis.

COMMENSAL STREPTOCOCCI

Viridans streptococci

The viridans streptococci, and in particular the species of the mitis and salivarius groups, are dominant members of the resident flora of the oral cavity and pharynx in all age groups. They play an important role by inhibiting the colonization of many pathogens, including pyogenic streptococci. This is achieved by two different mechanisms:

- production of bacteriocins (p. 34)
- production of hydrogen peroxide (also responsible for α-haemolysis).

Most strains secrete bacteriocins. Experimental implantation of strains of *S. salivarius* with strong bacteriocin activity prevents colonization with *Str. pyogenes* in man.

Mitis group. *Str. mitis, Str. oralis, Str. sanguis* and *S. gordonii* colonize tooth surfaces as well as mucosal membranes. Because of their presence in the bacterial deposits (dental plaque) on tooth surfaces, these species may enter the bloodstream during dental procedures such as tooth extraction or vigorous tooth cleaning, particularly if the gingival tissue is inflamed.

In healthy individuals, such bacteria of low virulence are cleared from the circulation within 1 h. However, in patients with various predisposing conditions (Table 16.2), in particular heart valve damage due to post-streptococcal rheumatic fever, the circulating streptococci may settle in a niche protected from phagocytic cells. Local growth on the surface of heart valves eventually causes scarring and functional deficiency. As the disease progresses over several months, it is referred to as *subacute bacterial endocarditis*. It is usually accompanied by intermittent fever. Disruption of bacteria from the cardiac vegetations may cause embolic abscesses in various organs, including the brain. Until endocarditis due to skin staphylococci became more prevalent as a result of intravenous drug abuse, viridans streptococci were the most frequent causes of infective endocarditis.

Str. mitis and *Str. oralis* are increasingly recognized as causes of often fatal septicaemias in immunocompromised patients.

Mutans group. *S. mutans* and *S. sobrinus* exclusively colonize tooth enamel and do not occur until tooth eruption. Their proportions in dental plaque are closely related to sugar consumption, and they are a major cause of dental caries because of their ability to produce large amounts of lactic acid even at pH values below pH 5.0. Like most other plaque streptococci they may cause subacute bacterial endocarditis.

Anginosus group. *S. anginosus, S. intermedius* and several other ill-defined taxa are regular members of the commensal bacteria on tooth surfaces, in particular in the gingival crevices. They are often isolated from abscesses and other opportunistic purulent infections.

Bovis group. *Str. bovis* is found in various animal species, including the human gut. It occasionally causes bacteraemia and subacute endocarditis, and is then often associated with colon carcinoma, which jeopardizes the barrier function of the intestinal wall.

Abiotrophia species

These bacteria were formerly referred to as 'nutritionally variant streptococci'. They grow as satellite colonies around other micro-organisms and in complex media only when supplemented with cysteine. They were previously thought to be mutants of other streptococci, but are genetically quite distinct from members of the genus *Streptococcus*. The three current species are all normal inhabitants of the oral cavity and occasionally cause infective endocarditis.

Enterococcus species

As indicated by the name, members of the genus *Enterococcus* have their natural habitat in the human intestines. The species most commonly associated with human disease are *E. faecalis* and *E. faecium*. The diseases with which they are associated are:

- urinary tract infection
- infective endocarditis
- biliary tract infections
- suppurative abdominal lesions
- peritonitis.

E. faecalis and *E. faecium* are important causes of wound and urinary tract infection in hospital and may cause sporadic outbreaks. Bacteraemia carries a poor prognosis as it often occurs in patients with major underlying pathology and in those who are immunocompromised.

LABORATORY DIAGNOSIS

Collection of specimens

The diagnosis of streptococcal infections is established by demonstrating the presence of the pathogen in throat or skin swabs, pus, blood cultures, cerebrospinal fluid (CSF), expectorates or urine according to the site of infection.

Particular problems are associated with the collection of expectorates for detection of *Str. pneumoniae*. Although it is the commonest cause of community-acquired pneumonia, sputum culture is positive in only about 20% of cases for several reasons:

- There may be difficulty in obtaining an expectorated specimen; postural drainage or inhaled aerosolized saline can encourage its production. Sputum may also

Table 16.2 Factors predisposing to infective endocarditis	
Cardiac factors	Non-cardiac factors
Rheumatic heart disease	Dental manipulations[a]
Atherosclerotic heart disease	Endoscopy
Congenital heart disease	Intravenous drug abuse
Cardiac surgery	Intravenous cannulae and shunts
Prosthetic heart valves	Sepsis
Previous endocarditis	
[a] Procedures in which bleeding occurs.	

be obtained by bronchoscopy in patients who are ventilated.

- Previous antibiotic treatment substantially reduces the chance of isolating the pneumococcus from the sputum.

The adequacy of the sputum sample should be confirmed by microscopy, which should show a predominance of pus cells rather than squamous epithelial cells from the mouth. The specimen is then homogenized with an agent such as *N*-acetylcysteine which permits semi-quantitative culture.

In pneumococcal meningitis the CSF is often macroscopically cloudy. The cell count is usually markedly increased and shows a predominance of polymorphonuclear leucocytes. Typical Gram-positive diplococci can commonly be demonstrated, sometimes in enormous numbers, by Gram stain examination of a CSF deposit. The appearance is often typical, and a presumptive diagnosis can be made to allow appropriate therapy to be started before the identity of the organism is confirmed by culture.

Blood cultures are of value in patients with invasive streptococcal infections. This is also the case in patients with suspected pneumococcal pneumonia, particularly when this is severe, since up to 15% of patients will be bacteraemic.

Other body sites that may merit investigation according to the clinical presentation include joint and peritoneal fluids. Tympanocentesis provides the possibility of establishing the microbial cause of otitis media, but since most of these infections settle spontaneously, or with the assistance of a few days' antibiotic treatment, tympanocentesis is not usually necessary.

Cultivation and identification

Unlike staphylococci, streptococci lack the enzyme catalase, which releases oxygen from hydrogen peroxide. Catalase-negative Gram-positive cocci are therefore likely to be streptococci. The appearance of cocci in obvious chains (Fig. 16.1) is another useful criterion, but the length of the chains varies with the species and the conditions of growth. Optimal chain formation is seen in broth cultures. There may be marked variation in size and shape, particularly in older cultures or in direct smears from purulent exudates.

The primary cultivation medium for streptococci is blood agar, supplemented, whenever enterococci are suspected, with an agar medium (e.g. MacConkey's medium) selective for enterobacteria. Streptococci of aetiological significance will usually predominate in the culture even when the sample is taken from a site with a resident microflora.

The pyogenic streptococci are detected initially by their β-haemolytic activity. The colonies are small (1 mm in diameter) and, in contrast to those of staphylococci, lack pigment. Colonies of pneumococci are α-haemolytic, smooth and may vary in size according to the amount of capsular polysaccharide produced; those of serotypes 3 and 37 are usually larger than the rest and have a watery or mucoid appearance. During prolonged incubation, autolysis of bacteria within the flat pneumococcal colonies results in a typical subsidence of the centre ('*draughtsman colonies*').

Species identification of pyogenic streptococci is largely based on serological detection of group antigens by immune precipitation or co-agglutination techniques. An additional test that is helpful in the presumptive identification of *Str. pyogenes* is the bacitracin sensitivity test. In contrast to most other streptococci, *Str. pyogenes* is uniformly sensitive and large inhibition zones are formed round bacitracin discs on blood agar. Likewise, *Str. agalactiae* can be presumptively identified by the CAMP reaction (Fig. 16.4).

Pneumococci are distinguished from other α-haemolytic streptococci by their characteristic sensitivity to optochin (ethylhydrocupreine). Growth of pneumococci is inhibited around an optochin disc applied to an inoculated blood agar plate. With few exceptions other α-haemolytic streptococci are not inhibited. In doubtful cases the identity of pneumococci is confirmed by demonstrating bile solubility, autolysis or reactivity to a poly-specific antiserum ('omni-serum') against capsular polysaccharides.

Other streptococci are identified by biochemical characteristics, such as the ability to ferment various carbohydrates and hydrolyse amino acids. However, some of the viridans streptococci are notoriously difficult to identify.

Enterococci are unique among the streptococci in their ability to grow on bile-containing media.

Antigen detection

Numerous commercial kits are available for the detection of *Str. pyogenes* directly in throat swabs without cultivation. These diagnostic kits use specific antibodies to detect the group A antigen in the material on the swab. They allow private practitioners to test if a throat infection is caused by *Str. pyogenes*, but the sensitivity and specificity of individual tests vary.

Antibody detection

Detection of antibodies against antigens of *Str. pyogenes* is an important means of establishing the diagnosis of post-streptococcal rheumatic fever and glomerulonephritis. In many cases the initiating infection in the throat or on the skin is no longer present.

Immune responses vary depending on whether the original focus is the throat or skin. Antibodies against streptolysin O (the ASO test) are used to document antecedent streptococcal infection in the throat of patients with clinical signs of rheumatic fever. A significant increase in antibody titre appears 3–4 weeks after the initial exposure to the micro-organism. Detection of increased levels of serum antibodies to streptococcal hyaluronidase and DNAase B is also of diagnostic importance.

ASO estimation is unreliable in pyoderma-associated acute glomerulonephritis. An elevated ASO titre is not observed in these patients, perhaps because lipids present in the skin inactivate the streptolysin O. Detection of antibodies against streptococcal DNAase B is recommended as a diagnostic tool in these patients.

Typing of streptococci

Strains of *Str. pyogenes* can be subdivided into serological types. The most comprehensive typing scheme is based on structural differences in the highly variable surface M protein. Over 80 different M types may be distinguished with type-specific antisera. Some reference laboratories perform M typing by detecting sequence differences in the gene (*emm*) encoding the M protein. An alternative typing scheme is based on the surface protein known as the T antigen.

Apart from serving epidemiological purposes, particular M types are associated with particular types of infections. Thus, certain M types are more commonly associated with skin infections than mucosal infections. Recent increases in the rate and severity of invasive *Str. pyogenes* infections (toxic shock syndrome and necrotizing fasciitis) have been primarily associated with serotypes M-1 and M-3. Rheumatic fever is often, but not exclusively, associated with serotypes M-5 and M-6. Recent outbreaks in the USA were due to M-18.

Pneumococci are typed on the basis of the differences in capsular polysaccharides, of which 90 have been described. The addition of India ink to a suspension of pneumococci will show the presence of the capsule as a clear halo around the organisms. Mixing a suspension of pneumococci with type-specific antisera increases the visibility of the capsule in the microscope, and is the basis of the *quellung reaction* or *capsular swelling test*. Serotyping of pneumococci is mainly carried out in reference laboratories.

TREATMENT

Streptococci are naturally susceptible to penicillin and to a wide range of other antibiotics. However, acquired resistance to other agents has become an increasing problem. Although streptococci are intrinsically resistant to aminoglycosides, these agents interact synergically with penicillins and the combination is often used in the treatment of streptococcal and enterococcal endocarditis.

Penicillin resistance has never been detected in *Str. pyogenes*. As a result, benzylpenicillin (penicillin G) or oral phenoxymethylpenicillin (penicillin V) are the drugs of choice for treatment of infections with *Str. pyogenes*. Antibiotic sensitivity tests are currently unnecessary if that species is identified as the infecting organism. In cases of hypersensitivity to penicillin, erythromycin is usually the second choice, but resistance occurs and is common in some countries.

Treatment for 3–5 days will limit the effect of severe attacks of streptococcal infection and prevent suppurative complications such as otitis media, but the streptococci will be eliminated from the infected area only if treatment is continued for 10 days. Treatment of uncomplicated throat infections with *Str. pyogenes* is not warranted in areas in which post-streptococcal sequelae are rare.

Surgery is essential to remove damaged tissue in case of necrotizing fasciitis, as antibiotic penetration of the infected area is poor. Clindamycin is preferred to penicillin because it inhibits protein synthesis, including production of exotoxin.

Most strains of *S. agalactiae* are susceptible to penicillins, macrolides and glycopeptides.

Resistance to penicillin in pneumococci and viridans streptococci, caused by mutations in the target penicillin-binding proteins, is widespread. These mutations have accumulated in strains of *Str. mitis* and *Str. oralis* and the altered genes have subsequently been transferred by genetic transformation to *Str. pneumoniae*.

Most pneumococcal infections with strains exhibiting intermediate-level resistance to penicillin (minimum inhibitory concentration 0.1–1 mg/l) respond to high dose therapy; an exception is meningitis, because of problems of penetration into the CSF. High-level penicillin resistance (minimum inhibitory concentration above 2 mg/l) was first recognized in 1977 in South Africa, where it was responsible for an epidemic of pneumococcal meningitis unresponsive to penicillin. The incidence of penicillin resistance is quite variable geographically and reflects the local level of usage of antibiotics.

Penicillin resistance in pneumococci and other viridans streptococci is often linked to resistance to several other antibiotics. Resistance to erythromycin, tetracycline and chloramphenicol is not uncommon, and even tolerance to vancomycin has been reported.

The dose of penicillin necessary to treat susceptible pneumococcal infection is largely determined by pharmacological factors at the site of infection. For example, pneumococcal pneumonia will respond to doses of penicillin as low as 0.3 g (0.5 mega-units) twice daily, whereas pneumococcal meningitis requires much higher doses. In patients unable to tolerate penicillin, erythromycin is the most widely used alternative agent for respiratory pneumococcal infections.

Unlike other streptococci, enterococci are intrinsically resistant to cephalosporins. Sensitivity to penicillins and other antibiotics varies widely, and clinical isolates must be tested for their susceptibility. Vancomycin resistance has been observed in enterococci and is a problem in high-dependency areas of some hospitals.

PREVENTION AND CONTROL

Hygienic measures

Skin infections with *Str. pyogenes* are usually associated with poor hygiene, and can to a large extent be prevented by standard hygienic measures. Late-onset neonatal infections with *Str. agalactiae* may also be prevented or significantly reduced by standard aseptic nursing procedures.

Likewise, hygiene is the most important preventive measure in relation to dental caries, which can be largely prevented by regular tooth-brushing with a fluoride-containing dentifrice.

Chemoprophylaxis

Prophylactic use of antibiotics is relevant in some streptococcal infections. As the primary attack of rheumatic fever usually occurs during childhood, long-term penicillin prophylaxis until adulthood is recommended to reduce the risk of further attacks and further heart injury. This is not the case in patients with acute glomerulonephritis because of the lack of recurrences.

Two different approaches are used to prevent early-onset neonatal *Str. agalactiae* infections:

- A risk-based strategy in which women of unknown colonization status receive intrapartum antibiotic prophylaxis in case of: threatened delivery <37 weeks' gestation; premature rupture of the membranes; intrapartum fever; or previous delivery of a child developing neonatal infection.
- A screening-based approach in which all pregnant women at 35–37 weeks' gestation are screened for

S. agalactiae colonization in vaginal and rectal specimens. All identified carriers are offered intrapartum chemoprophylaxis.

Intravenous or intramuscular penicillin is the agent of choice because its antimicrobial spectrum, narrower than that of ampicillin, reduces the likelihood of resistance developing in other bacteria. A cephalosporin is an appropriate alternative for patients with penicillin allergy as increasing proportions of *Str. agalactiae* are resistant to erythromycin and clindamycin.

Patients at risk of developing infective endocarditis (Table 16.2) should be given prophylactic antibiotics in association with dental procedures that lead to bleeding. The current international recommendations are amoxicillin 1 h before dental treatment or, in case of penicillin allergy, clindamycin. If the patient has been on long-term penicillin prophylaxis the oral streptococci are likely to have reduced susceptibility to penicillins, and clindamycin or vancomycin are recommended as the alternative. It is imperative that patients at risk maintain healthy periodontal conditions and that the amount of dental plaque is kept to a minimum.

Vaccines

Pyogenic streptococci

Attempts to develop a vaccine against *Str. pyogenes* infections have been hampered by two problems:

- the considerable antigenic diversity of the M protein and other vaccine candidate antigens
- the potential immunological cross-reactivity of many of the antigens with host tissue components.

Several strategies are currently being tested, including oral vaccination.

A vaccine against neonatal *Str. agalactiae* infection based on protein-conjugated type III capsular polysaccharide is being tested for use primarily in women of reproductive age. However, additional serotypes are increasingly prevalent.

Pneumococci

Before the widespread availability of effective antimicrobial drugs the treatment of pneumococcal infections was based on the use of type-specific antiserum. This reduced mortality in bacteraemic pneumococcal pneumonia but not to the same extent that penicillin was subsequently shown to achieve. However, it indicated that type-specific antibody had a role in the control of pneumococcal disease and led to a variety of prototype vaccines. The vaccine that has been in use for many years contains a mixture of 23 polysaccharide serotypes chosen according to the prevalence of serotypes responsible for bacteraemic pneumococcal infection. It offers protection against 90% of isolates.

Like other vaccines based on pure polysaccharides, the immunogenicity of the multivalent vaccine is inadequate in those below 2 years of age and in those immunosuppressed as a result of malignancy, steroid therapy or other chronic disease. To overcome this problem, new pneumococcal vaccines containing capsular polysaccharide coupled to a carrier protein are becoming available. These vaccines increase the immunogenicity of the polysaccharide by rendering the response dependent on T lymphocyte help. The current conjugate vaccine only includes seven of the capsular polysaccharides, but vaccines with more comprehensive coverage are anticipated. Some countries contemplate inclusion of the new vaccine in the childhood vaccination programme.

The recommended indications for vaccine use in the UK are shown in Table 16.3. In some countries, including the USA, where the vaccine has been used most widely, it is also recommended for those over 65 years of age, with or without previous ill health, although there have been difficulties in establishing scientifically the efficacy in this group.

Immunization is particularly recommended for those with congenital or surgical asplenia and those with hereditary haemoglobinopathies such as sickle cell disease, since in these patients pneumococcal infection can be fulminant. Vaccine efficacy is not complete and many clinicians also prescribe oral phenoxymethylpenicillin as long-term chemoprophylaxis in this high-risk group.

Table 16.3 Recommended indications for the use of pneumococcal vaccine in the UK (for use in children over 2 years and adults)

Asplenia or severe dysfunction of the spleen
Homozygous sickle cell disease and coeliac disease
Chronic renal disease or nephrotic syndrome
Immunodeficiency or immunosuppression caused by disease or treatment, including HIV infection at all stages
Chronic heart disease
Chronic lung disease
Chronic liver disease, including cirrhosis
Diabetes mellitus

RECOMMENDED READING

Cunningham M W 2000 Pathogenesis of group A streptococcal infections. *Clinical Microbiology Reviews* 13:470–511

Douglas C W I, Heath J, Hampton K K, Preston F E 1993 Identity of viridans streptococci isolated from cases of infective endocarditis. *Journal of Medical Microbiology* 39: 179–182

Fraser J, Arcus V, Kong P, Baker E, Proft T 2000 Superantigens – powerful modifiers of the immune system. *Molecular Medicine Today* 6:125–132

Johnson A P, Speller D C E, George R C et al. 1996 Prevalence of antibiotic resistance and serotypes in pneumococci in England and Wales: results of observational surveys in 1990 and 1995. *British Medical Journal* 312: 1454–1456

Kilian M 1998 *Streptococcus* and *Lactobacillus*. In Balows A and Duerden BI (eds) *Topley and Wilson's Microbiology and Microbial Infections*, 9th edition, Volume 2. Arnold, London, pp. 633–667

Marsh P D, Martin M W 1999 *Oral Microbiology*, 3rd edn. Wright, Oxford

Schrag S J, Zywicki S, Farley M M et al. 2000 Group B streptococcal disease in the era of intrapartum antibiotic prophylaxis. *New England Journal of Medicine* 342:15–20

Schuchat A 1999 Group B streptococcus. *Lancet* 353:51–56

Stevens D L, Kaplan E L (ed) 2000 *Streptococcal Infections. Clinical Aspects, Microbiology, and Molecular Pathogenesis*. Oxford University Press, Oxford

Tomasz A 2000 *Streptococcus pneumoniae. Molecular Biology and Mechanisms of Disease*. Mary Ann Liebert, Inc., Larchmont, NY

Internet site

Centers for Disease Control and Prevention:
www.cdc.gov/ncidod/dbmd/diseaseinfo/

17

Coryneform bacteria, listeria and erysipelothrix

Diphtheria; listeriosis; erysipeloid

J. McLauchlin and P. Riegel

CORYNEFORM BACTERIA

The term *coryneform* is used to describe aerobic, non-sporing and irregularly shaped Gram-positive rods. According to this broad definition, they include bacteria of the genus *Corynebacterium* with a typically club-shape morphology (Greek κορσυνη = club), environmental bacteria such as *Rhodococcus*, *Gordonia* and *Brevibacterium* species, and preferentially anaerobic bacteria of the genera *Actinomyces* (Chapter 20), *Arcanobacterium* and *Propionibacterium*, which exhibit some branched forms.

CORYNEBACTERIUM DIPHTHERIAE

The major disease caused by *C. diphtheriae* is *diphtheria*, an infection of the local tissue of the upper respiratory tract with the production of a toxin that causes systemic effects, notably in the heart and peripheral nerves. Diphtheria has virtually disappeared in developed countries following mass immunization, but is still endemic in many regions of the world. Skin infections are prevalent in some countries. Non-toxigenic strains have been associated with endocarditis, meningitis, cerebral abscess and osteo-arthritis throughout the world.

Description

C. diphtheriae, like other members of the genus, are non-motile, non-spore forming, straight or slightly curved rods with tapered ends. They are Gram-positive, but are easily decolorized, particularly in older cultures. Cells often contain metachromatic granules (polymetaphosphate), which stain bluish-purple with methylene blue. Snapping division produces groups of cells in angular and palisade arrangements that create a 'Chinese character' effect.

C. diphtheriae is aerobic and facultatively anaerobic, growing best on a blood- or serum-containing medium at 35–37°C with or without CO_2 enrichment. On agar medium containing tellurite, colonies of *C. diphtheriae* are characteristically black or grey after 24–48 h.

Biotypes of *C. diphtheriae* named *gravis*, *intermedius* or *mitis* are genomically similar variants exhibiting distinct biochemical features and cultural morphology. Bacilli of the *gravis* biotype are usually short, whereas biotype *mitis* are long and pleomorphic; biotype *intermedius* ranges from very long to short rods. In broth medium, *C. diphtheriae* biotype *gravis* forms a pellicle and a granular deposit whereas *C. diphtheriae* biotype *mitis* produces a diffuse turbidity. The biotype *intermedius* forms no pellicle, but a fine granular deposit can be observed.

Pathogenesis

To cause disease *C. diphtheriae* must:

- invade, colonize and proliferate in local tissues
- be lysogenized by a specific β-phage, enabling it to produce toxin.

In the upper respiratory tract, diphtheria bacilli elicit an inflammatory exudate and cause necrosis of the cells of the faucial mucosa (Fig. 17.1). The diphtheria toxin possibly assists colonization of the throat or skin by killing epithelial cells or neutrophils.

The organisms do not penetrate deeply into the mucosal tissue and bacteraemia does not usually occur. The exotoxin is produced locally and is spread by the bloodstream to distant organs, with a special affinity for heart muscle, the peripheral nervous system and the adrenal glands.

C. diphtheriae can colonize the throats of people who have been immunized against diphtheria or who have become immune as a result of natural exposure, but usually no pseudomembrane develops.

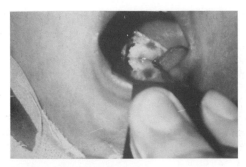

Fig. 17.1 Diphtheritic membrane on throat.

The diphtheria toxin is a heat-stable polypeptide, composed of two fragments: A (active) and B (binding). The toxin binds to a specific receptor on susceptible cells and enters by receptor-mediated endocytosis. The A subunit is cleaved and released from the B subunit as it inserts and passes through the membrane into the cytoplasm. Fragment A catalyses the transfer of ADP-ribose from nicotinamide adenine dinucleotide (NAD) to the eukaryotic elongation factor 2, which inhibits the function of the latter in protein synthesis. Inhibition of protein synthesis is probably responsible for both the necrotic and neurotoxic effects of the toxin. Production of toxin by lysogenized *C. diphtheriae* is enhanced considerably when the bacteria are grown in low iron conditions. Other factors such as osmolarity, amino acid concentrations and pH have a role.

The *Schick test*, an intradermal injection of stabilized diphtheria toxin, was formerly used to determine individual susceptibility to the toxin. A localized erythema and, sometimes, severe local reactions reaching maximum size and intensity in 2–4 days, indicate that there is little or no neutralizing antitoxin in the tissue, and that the individual is susceptible to diphtheria. Absence of a reaction indicates immunity. Tissue culture neutralization tests, enzyme-linked immunosorbent assay (ELISA) and passive haemagglutination assay to measure serum antitoxin levels are now preferred. For epidemiological purposes the minimum protective level is considered to be 0.01 International Units of diphtheria antitoxin per millilitre in a serum sample. A level of 0.1 IU/ml is desirable for individual protection.

Nontoxigenic strains of *C. diphtheriae* may cause pharyngitis and cutaneous abscesses. Systemic disease, including endocarditis, septic arthritis and osteomyelitis, has also been reported. The virulence factors of these strains remain unknown. Conversion of a nontoxigenic strain to a toxigenic strain by phage infection can occur in human populations.

Clinical features

The incubation period of diphtheria is 2–5 days, with a range of 1–10 days. At first, patients present with malaise, sore throat and moderate fever. A thick, adherent green *pseudomembrane* is present on one or both tonsils or adjacent pharynx. In nasopharyngeal infection, the pseudomembrane may involve nasal mucosa, the pharyngeal wall and the soft palate. In this form, oedema involving the cervical lymph glands may occur in the anterior tissues of the neck, a condition known as *bullneck diphtheria*.

Laryngeal involvement leads to obstruction of the larynx and lower airways. Organisms multiply within the membranes and toxaemia is prominent. The patient is gravely ill, with a weak pulse, restlessness and confusion. Intoxication takes the form of myocarditis and peripheral neuritis, and may be associated with thrombocytopenia. Visual disturbance, difficulty in swallowing and paralysis of the arms and legs also occur but usually resolve spontaneously. Complete heart block may result from myocarditis. Death is most commonly due to congestive heart failure and cardiac arrhythmias.

Cutaneous diphtheria mostly occurs in tropical countries. The lesion is usually characterized by an ulcer covered by a necrotic pseudomembrane and may involve any area of the skin. Although the organism usually produces toxin, systemic toxic manifestations are uncommon.

Diagnosis

The diagnosis is made on clinical grounds, supported by a history of diphtheria among contacts, lack of prior immunization or travel in countries where diphtheria is endemic.

The role of the laboratory is to confirm the diagnosis by recovery of *C. diphtheriae* in culture followed by appropriate tests for detection of toxin production. The clinician should inform the laboratory of the presumptive diagnosis of diphtheria because isolation of *C. diphtheriae* requires special media.

Direct microscopy of a smear is unreliable since *C. diphtheriae* is morphologically similar to other coryneforms. The recommended media include blood agar and a selective medium containing tellurite. Identification is based on carbohydrate fermentation reactions and enzymatic activities. Commercial kits such as the API Coryne strip provide a reliable identification.

Toxigenicity testing is essential. Production of diphtheria toxin is demonstrated by the agar immunoprecipitation test (*Elek test*; Fig. 17.2) or by the tissue culture

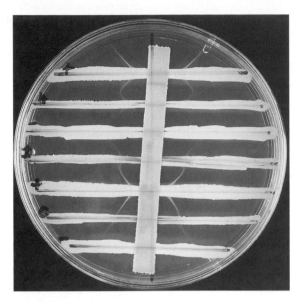

Fig. 17.2 Elek plate for the detection of *C. diphtheriae* toxin production. Cultures are streaked horizontally, then overlayed by an antitoxin-impregnated strip. Toxin and antitoxin diffuse into the culture during incubation and precipitin lines develop where toxin and antitoxin are present in a critical ratio. Positive reactions in test cultures are indicated by precipitin lines that arc with those produced by positive controls. The *C. diphtheriae* cultures are (top to bottom): National Collection of Type Cultures (NCTC) strain 10648 (positive control); test culture (positive); NCTC 10356 (negative control); NCTC 3984 (weak positive control); NCTC 10648 (positive control); test culture (negative); NCTC 10356 (negative control). Photograph courtesy of Dr A. Efstratiou, Central Public Health Laboratory, London.

cytotoxicity assay, which has replaced the virulence test in guinea-pigs. The toxin gene can be detected by the polymerase chain reaction (PCR). This test shows excellent correlation with guinea-pig virulence, though there is the rare possibility of a false-positive PCR assay if the strain harbouring the *tox* gene is unable to express it. The detection of the *tox* gene by PCR directly from clinical specimens is feasible. All biotypes are potentially toxigenic.

Measurement of antibodies to diphtheria toxin in serum collected before administration of antitoxin may support the diagnosis when cultures are negative.

Treatment

If diphtheria is strongly suspected on clinical grounds, treatment should not await laboratory confirmation, which may take several days. Diphtheria antitoxin (hyperimmune horse serum) is given, since antibiotics have no effect on preformed toxin which rapidly diffuses from the local lesions and soon becomes irre-

versibly bound to tissue cells. Because antitoxin neutralizes only circulating toxin it should be administered promptly.

Treatment with parenteral penicillin or oral erythromycin eradicates the organism and terminates toxin production. *C. diphtheriae* is universally sensitive to penicillins but some strains are resistant to erythromycin, tetracyclines and rifampicin. Erythromycin may be preferred to penicillin for elimination of the bacilli from the throat, particularly in treatment of persistent carriers.

Patients should be placed in strict isolation, nursed by staff whose immunization history is documented and have daily platelet counts and electrocardiograms.

Epidemiology

Diphtheria has virtually disappeared in developed countries following mass immunization in the 1940s, but is still endemic in many regions of the world. About 50 000 cases of diphtheria occurred in the newly independent states of the former Soviet union during 1990–1996, leading to infection in short-term visitors from Western Europe. Other countries that have experienced outbreaks of diphtheria in recent years include China, Ecuador, Algeria, South-east Asia and the Eastern Mediterranean. There were 124 cases of diphtheria, with eight deaths in the UK between 1970 and 1994, since when no deaths have been reported. In the USA, only 45 cases were reported during 1980–1995. Non-toxigenic strains able to cause mild disease continue to circulate throughout the world.

Infection is confined to man and usually involves contact with a diphtheria case or a carrier. The most important mode of spread is person-to-person transmission by aerosolized droplets when an infected person coughs, sneezes or talks, or by direct contact with skin lesions. Most clinical infections are probably contracted from carriers rather than symptomatic patients. Prolonged close contact with an infected person and intimate contact increases the likelihood of transmission.

Acquired immunity to diphtheria is due primarily to toxin-neutralizing antibody (antitoxin). Passive immunity in utero is acquired transplacentally and can last for 1 or 2 years after birth. Active immunity can probably be produced by a mild or inapparent infection in infants who retain some maternal immunity. Unimmunized children under 15 years old are most likely to contract diphtheria. The disease is also found among adults whose immunization was neglected. Mortality is highest among young children and in people aged over 40 years. Skin infections caused by *C. diphtheriae* may result in early development of natural immunity against the disease.

C. diphtheriae persists longer in skin lesions than in the tonsils or nose, and cutaneous diphtheria appears to be more contagious than respiratory diphtheria. Untreated people who are infected with the diphtheria bacillus can be contagious for up to 2 weeks, but seldom for more than 4 weeks. If treated with appropriate antibiotics, the contagious period can be limited to less than 4 days. *C. diphtheriae* can survive in the environment in dust and on dry fomites for several months, and transmission via fomites has been documented. Animal-to-human transmission and food-borne transmission by consumption of contamination foods such as raw milk have been described, but are very rare.

Control

High population immunity achieved through mass immunization (at least 95% coverage in children and at least 90% coverage in adults) is the most effective measure to control epidemic diphtheria. Immunization with diphtheria toxoid was first introduced in 1923. Large-scale immunization programmes introduced in the 1940s reduced the incidence of diphtheria dramatically, although the disease was not completely eradicated. Immunization schedules are discussed in Chapter 69.

Prevention of secondary cases by the rapid investigation of close contacts is essential. These investigations should include ascertainment of the immunization histories of all home and school contacts. Primary courses of immunization or a booster are given if necessary.

OTHER MEDICALLY IMPORTANT CORYNEBACTERIA

The non-diphtheria corynebacteria ('*diphtheroids*') are diverse and comprise strictly aerobic bacteria usually isolated from the environment, as well as facultative or preferentially anaerobic bacteria which are commensals of the skin and mucous membranes. The principal species involved and the main clinical syndromes associated with infection are shown in Table 17.1.

Corynebacterium ulcerans

Like *C. diphtheriae* and *C. pseudotuberculosis*, *C. ulcerans* can produce diphtheria toxin. It has been isolated from raw milk and can cause mastitis in cattle. In man, *C. ulcerans* is almost exclusively seen in cases of exudative pharyngitis, but occasional soft tissue infections occur. Some strains cause disease indistinguishable from diphtheria. Infection usually takes the form of acute pharyngitis with pseudomembranes, and cardiac or neurological complications can occur. Therapy involves administration of appropriate antibiotics such as penicillins or erythromycin and administration of diphtheria antitoxin in the case of diphtheria-like disease.

Table 17.1 Habitat and disease associations of corynebacteria

Organism	Major habitat	Disease association
C. diphtheriae	Throat, skin	Diphtheria (toxigenic strains), wound infections, bacteraemia, endocarditis
C. ulcerans	Human throat and skin; animals; raw milk	Man: diphtheria (toxigenic strains), pharyngitis and wound infection; cattle: mastitis
C. pseudotuberculosis	Sheep, horses, goats	Man: lymphadenitis; animals: abscesses and abortion
C. jeikeium	Skin	Bacteraemia, endocarditis; infection of foreign bodies and CSF shunts
C. urealyticum	Skin, urinary tract	Urinary tract infection, pyelonephritis, endocarditis
C. amycolatum	Man and animals	Man: bacteraemia, endocarditis, peritonitis and wound infection; cattle: mastitis
C. glucuronolyticum	Urinary tract of man and animals	Urogenital tract infection
C. minutissimum	Skin, urinary tract	Erythrasma, bacteraemia
C. striatum	Respiratory tract, skin	Respiratory tract infection, wound infection, bacteraemia
C. pseudodiphtheriticum	Respiratory tract	Respiratory tract infection, endocarditis
Arcanobacterium haemolyticum	Throat	Pharyngitis, skin ulcers, endocarditis
Rhodococcus equi	Animals, soil	Pulmonary infection and soft tissue infection

Corynebacterium pseudotuberculosis

C. pseudotuberculosis is primarily an animal pathogen and rarely infects man. It causes caseous lymphadenitis in sheep and goats and abscesses or ulcerative lymphangitis in horses. Human infections mainly occur in patients with animal contact. Infection usually presents as a subacute or chronic granulomatous lymphadenitis involving the axillary or cervical nodes, but pneumonias have been described. Some strains are lysogenized by bacteriophages of *C. diphtheriae* and thus produce diphtheria toxin, but no clinical cases of diphtheria-like disease have been attributed to *C. pseudotuberculosis* infection. Treatment requires prolonged antibiotic therapy with erythromycin, penicillins or tetracycline, and surgical drainage or excision.

Corynebacterium jeikeium

C. jeikeium (formerly CDC coryneform group JK) is part of the normal skin flora, particularly in inguinal, axillary and rectal areas. Colonization by antibiotic-resistant strains is unusual in healthy individuals, but is common in hospital patients, particularly neutropenic patients and those receiving antibiotics. Most infections are associated with skin damaged by wounds or invasive devices. Such infections include:

- prosthetic valve endocarditis
- bacteraemia associated with infected long-term intravenous cannulae
- peritonitis in patients on peritoneal dialysis
- septicaemia and local infection following insertion of an epicardial pacemaker
- central nervous system (CNS) infection in patients with ventriculoperitoneal or atrial shunts for hydrocephalus.

Most infections occur in patients in hospital for prolonged periods and who have received broad-spectrum antimicrobial therapy. Spread is through environmental contamination, the hands of ward staff or auto-infection.

Treatment

Most isolates of *C. jeikeium* recovered from infections are highly resistant to penicillins and cephalosporins in vitro. Even with susceptible isolates, penicillin is incompletely bactericidal, but aminoglycoside-sensitive strains can be successfully eradicated with combined penicillin and aminoglycoside therapy. Systemic amoxicillin, gentamicin, rifampicin or ciprofloxacin can be used if the isolate is susceptible. Resistance to aminoglycosides and macrolides has been reported in more than 60% of isolates and resistance to fluoroquinolones is variable.

Glycopeptides are the drugs of choice for treating serious infections. *C. jeikeium* is sensitive to glycopeptides and these antibiotics are bactericidal. Combinations of vancomycin with gentamicin have been used to treat infective endocarditis. Peritonitis secondary to peritoneal dialysis and meningitis related to shunts can be treated with intraperitoneal or intrathecal vancomycin, respectively.

Corynebacterium urealyticum

C. urealyticum (formerly CDC coryneform group D-2) is a frequent skin colonizer, mainly in hospital patients. The groin is the most frequent skin site of colonization, followed by the abdominal wall and axilla. This microorganism is associated with urinary tract infections, particularly with alkaline-encrusted cystitis related to its strong urease production. Infection is a consequence of bacterial selection attributable to the use of broad-spectrum antibiotics for patients with underlying conditions that predispose to urinary tract infection. *C. urealyticum* may cause pyelonephritis and is an infrequent cause of endocarditis, osteomyelitis or soft tissue infection.

Like *C. jeikeium*, *C. urealyticum* is usually highly resistant to most antimicrobial agents, except glycopeptides. Vancomycin, tetracyclines, erythromycin and norfloxacin have proven effective in treatment. Encrusted cystitis requires endoscopic resection of incrustations in addition to antimicrobial treatment.

Corynebacterium amycolatum

C. amycolatum is a human skin commensal exhibiting characteristics similar to those of other corynebacteria, except for the lack of cell wall mycolic acids. Its biochemical characteristics are variable and it is often misidentified. *C. amycolatum* can be recovered from many body sites. Strains isolated from hospital patients may be multiresistant to antibiotics except glycopeptides. *C. amycolatum* has been reported as causing bacteraemia, endocarditis, peritonitis and wound infection.

Corynebacterium glucuronolyticum

C. glucuronolyticum (syn. *C. seminale*) has been isolated from male patients with genito-urinary tract infections, particularly prostatitis and urethritis. It is the commonest corynebacterium isolated from semen specimens. It exhibits strong β-glucuronidase activity and some strains produce urease. It is usually sensitive to antibiotics, but tetracyclines and macrolides are the most effective in vitro.

Corynebacterium minutissimum

C. minutissimum is believed to be the causative agent of erythrasma, a relatively common and localized infection of the stratum corneum which produces reddish-brown scaly patches in intertriginous sites. Lesions usually involve the groin, toeweb and axillae, which fluoresce coral red when examined by Wood's light. The organism can be cultured from skin scrapings but the diagnosis is usually based on clinical aspects and the characteristic fluorescence. Some more serious infections have been described, including bacteraemia and breast abscess. It is likely that some infections attributed to *C. minutissimum* may have been caused by *C. amycolatum*.

C. minutissimum is sensitive to penicillins; susceptibility to erythromycin is variable.

Corynebacterium striatum

This species is part of the normal flora of the human anterior nares and skin. It is a rare cause of pulmonary infection, particularly in patients with chronic obstructive airway disease or those who are intubated. Nosocomial transmission to mechanically ventilated patients in an intensive care unit has been documented. It has also been isolated from blood, catheter tips, wounds, leg ulcers, peritoneal fluid, urine, semen, vaginal exudate and placental tissues. *C. striatum* is sensitive to penicillins and glycopeptides; susceptibility to aminoglycosides, ciprofloxacin, erythromycin and rifampicin is variable. Many isolates are resistant to broad-spectrum cephalosporins.

Corynebacterium pseudodiphtheriticum

C. pseudodiphtheriticum is a commensal of the human nasopharynx. It is occasionally associated with respiratory tract infections, including tracheobronchitis, necrotizing tracheitis, pneumonia and lung abscess. Most isolates come from patients with endotracheal tubes or chronic obstructive pulmonary disease. It has also been reported to cause endocarditis in patients with prosthetic valves or pre-existing valvular damage. *C. pseudodiphtheriticum* is usually susceptible to most antibiotics except erythromycin.

Arcanobacterium haemolyticum

A. haemolyticum is a catalase-negative, facultatively anaerobic bacterium which is phylogenetically related to *Actinomyces* spp. (see Chapter 20). It causes pharyngitis and chronic skin ulcers. Most patients are young adults who present with sore throat; some have membranous exudates and peritonsillar abscesses, and infection cannot be differentiated from streptococcal pharyngitis on clinical findings alone. The relative frequency of pharyngitis due to *A. haemolyticum* is about 2% in symptomatic patients 15–25 years old, whereas this is rarely found in healthy individuals.

A. haemolyticum is often isolated in association with non-pyogenic streptococci, including the *Streptococcus anginosus* group. A scarlatiniform rash occurs in half the patients with pharyngitis, perhaps caused by a toxin genetically related to the erythrogenic toxin of *Str. pyogenes*. *A. haemolyticum* has occasionally been isolated from cases of cellulitis, osteomyelitis, brain abscesses and endocarditis. This species produces at least two extracellular toxins, phospholipase D and a haemolysin. Erythromycin or other macrolides seem to be effective in treatment. *A. haemolyticum* is also sensitive to penicillin, but treatment failure has been documented.

Rhodococcus equi

R. equi is pathogenic for horses, swine and cattle. It can be found in soil near livestock. It is a rare cause of severe pulmonary infections in patients with the acquired immune deficiency syndrome, neoplastic diseases or renal transplants. Most infections develop insidiously, with fever and respiratory symptoms difficult to distinguish from mycobacterial infection. Infections are often recurrent and refractory to treatment, and may be associated with pleural effusion and bacteraemia. The diagnosis is usually established from bronchoscopy specimens, pleural fluid cultures or blood cultures.

R. equi is usually sensitive to tetracyclines, macrolides, rifampicin, imipenem and vancomycin, but resistance to penicillins has been reported. Treatment includes surgical drainage when feasible and prolonged therapy with an antibiotic combination such as erythromycin and rifampicin or imipenem and vancomycin, established by in-vitro tests.

Other coryneform bacteria

There have been profound changes in the classification and identification of these organisms resulting in the description of new genera and species. For some of them, strong site and disease association have appeared.

- *C. macginleyi* strains have been isolated from the eye, often in association with infections.
- *C. accolens* is usually recovered from respiratory specimens.
- *C. afermentans* ssp. *lipophilum* and CDC coryneform groups G and F-1 may be isolated from a variety of sources, including blood, wound, semen and urine.

- *C. bovis* is commonly isolated from bovine mastitis, but is unlikely to be encountered in human infections.
- *C. argentoratense*, *C. propinquum*, *C. matruchotii* and *C. durum* have been isolated from the throat, but no pathogenic role has been demonstrated.
- *C. xerosis* has been confused with *C. amycolatum* and is very rare.
- *Turicella otitidis* and *C. auris* have been isolated from ears of healthy patients and from patients with ear infections.
- *Rothia dentocariosa* is commonly isolated from respiratory tract specimens and has been associated with endocarditis and brain abscess.
- *Arthrobacter cumminsii* and *A. woluwensis* have been recovered from elderly patients with urinary tract infections.

LISTERIA

Organisms of the genus *Listeria* are non-sporing Gram-positive bacilli. The genus contains six species, but almost all cases of human listeriosis are caused by *L. monocytogenes*. The disease chiefly affects pregnant women, unborn or newly delivered infants, the immunosuppressed and elderly. It is predominantly transmitted by the consumption of contaminated food. *L. ivanovii* is associated with about 10% of infections in livestock animals. This species and *L. seeligeri* have been associated with a very small number of human infections.

Listeria spp. grow well on a wide variety of non-selective laboratory media and some species, including *L. monocytogenes*, exhibit β-haemolysis on blood agar. The bacilli are non-motile at 37°C, but exhibit characteristic 'tumbling' motility when tested at 25°C.

LISTERIA MONOCYTOGENES

Description

L. monocytogenes is very similar to other species, but can be differentiated by biochemical tests. Thirteen serotypes (serovars) are recognized and can be further characterized by phenotypic (bacteriophage typing; multilocus enzyme electrophoresis) or genotypic (plasmid profiling; random amplified polymorphic DNA analysis; pulsed-field gel electrophoresis; amplified fragment length polymorphism typing; direct DNA sequencing) methods.

Most cases of human listeriosis are caused by serovars 4b, 1/2a and 1/2b. Large food-borne outbreaks have predominantly been caused by serovar 4b stains.

The properties of the organism favour food as an agent in transmission of listeriosis. It grows in a wide range of foods having relatively high water activities (A_w >0.95) and over a wide range of temperatures (0–45°C). Growth at refrigeration temperatures is relatively slow, with a maximum doubling time of about 1–2 days at 4°C. Multiplication in food is restricted to the pH range 5–9. *L. monocytogenes* is not sufficiently heat-resistant to survive pasteurization of milk.

Pathogenesis

L. monocytogenes is an intracellular parasite, and it is in this environment that the pathogen gains protection and evades some of the host's defences. However, the host has a number of strategies to deal with such parasites. Non-specific mechanisms of resistance are important as first lines of defence once the mucous membranes are breached. Lysozyme can lyse some strains of listeria, and human neutrophils and non-activated macrophages can phagocytose and kill the bacteria. Protective immunity in man probably depends on T lymphocytes, with antibodies playing little or no role.

L. monocytogenes enters phagocytic and non-phagocytic cells and a listerial surface protein, *internalin* (reminiscent of the M protein of *Str. pyogenes*) is involved with the initial stages of invasion on all cell types. After internalization, *L. monocytogenes* becomes encapsulated in a membrane-bound compartment. In the phagocyte, most cells in the phagocytic vacuole are probably killed. However, those surviving in the phagocytic vacuole, and those in the membrane-bound compartment of non-professional phagocytes, mediate the dissolution of the vacuole membrane by means of a haemolysin (listeriolysin O), and also, possibly, the action of a phospholipase C.

In the host cell cytoplasm, where growth occurs, the organism becomes surrounded by polymerized host cell actin. The ability to polymerize actin by a listeria cell surface protein subverts the host cell's cytoskeleton and confers intracellular motility to the bacterium. The resulting 'comet tail' like structure pushes the bacterium into an adjacent mammalian cell, where it again becomes encapsulated in a vacuole. A listerial lecithinase is involved with dissolution of these membranes; the haemolysin may also contribute in this process. Intracellular growth and movement in the newly invaded cell is then repeated. Similar sets of virulence genes are present in *L. ivanovii* and *L. seeligeri*.

Clinical aspects of infection

L. monocytogenes principally causes intra-uterine infection, meningitis and septicaemia. The incubation period varies widely between individuals from 1 to 90 days, with an average for intra-uterine infection of around 30 days.

Infection in pregnancy and the neonate

Listeriosis in pregnancy is classified by fetal gestation at onset, as this correlates best with the clinical features, microbiology and prognosis. Neonatal infection is divided into early (<2 days old), intermediate (3–5 days old) and late (>5 days old)-onset disease.

Maternal listeriosis occurs throughout gestation, but before 20 weeks of pregnancy is rare. The mother is usually previously well with a normal pregnancy. Pregnant women often have very mild symptoms (chills, fever, back pain, sore throat and headache, sometimes with conjunctivitis, diarrhoea or drowsiness) but may be asymptomatic until the delivery of an infected infant. Symptomatic women may have positive blood cultures.

Cultures from high vaginal swabs (HVSs), stool and midstream urine samples, together with pre- or post-natal antibody tests, are of little help in diagnosis. With the onset of fever, fetal movements are reduced, and premature labour occurs within about 1 week. There may be a transient fever during labour, and the amniotic fluid is often discoloured or stained with meconium. Culture of the amniotic fluid, placenta or HVS after

delivery invariably yields a heavy growth of *L. monocytogenes*. Fever resolves soon after birth, and the HVS is usually culture-negative after about 1 month. While the outcome of infection for the mother is usually benign, the outcome for the infant is more variable. Abortion, stillbirth and early-onset neonatal disease are common, depending on the gestation at infection. However, maternal infection without infection of the offspring can occur and even progress to placental infection without ill effects for the fetus.

Repeated pregnancy-associated infections are exceedingly rare, and an association between listeria carriage and habitual abortion has not been substantiated.

Early neonatal listeriosis is predominantly a septicaemic illness, contracted in utero. In contrast, late neonatal infection is predominantly meningitic and may be associated with hospital cross-infection. The main characteristics of these two forms are summarized in Table 17.2. Early-onset disease represents a spectrum of mild to severe infection which can be correlated with the microbiological findings. Those neonates who die of infection usually do so within a few days of birth and have pneumonia, hepatosplenomegaly, petechiae, abscesses in the liver or brain, peritonitis and enterocolitis.

Late-onset disease is the third commonest form of meningitis in neonates. The CSF protein content is

Table 17.2 Characteristics of neonatal infection with *L. monocytogenes*

	Type of infection	
	Early	Late
Onset after delivery	<2 days	>5 days
Maternal factors[a]	Common	Rare
Source of infection	Intrauterine infection haematogenously acquired from mother	Hospital-acquired from early-onset case, post-natal environment or (?) maternally acquired during delivery
Signs/symptoms	Disseminated infection Cardiopulmonary distress CNS signs Vomiting and diarrhoea Hepatosplenomegaly Skin rash	Meningitis Irritability Poor appetite Fever
Laboratory findings	Leucocytosis or leucopenia Thrombocytopenia Mottling on chest radiograph Increased fibrinogen	Leucocytosis; occasional radiographic changes CSF: total protein and white cell count raised; glucose level lowered
Sites of isolation	Blood, superficial sites and amniotic fluid; less commonly gastric aspirate, CSF and HVS	Commonly CSF; rarely blood
Mortality	30–60%	10–12%

[a] Obstetric problems; low birth weight; maternal fever; abnormal amniotic fluid. CSF, cerebrospinal fluid; HVS, high vaginal swabs.

almost always raised and the glucose level reduced. The total number of white cells is increased but the counts are variable; neutrophils usually predominate, but lymphocytes or monocytes may be the main cell type. In about 50% of Gram films, bacteria, which may resemble rods or cocci, are seen.

Adult and juvenile infection

Listeriosis in children older than 1 month is very rare, except in those with underlying disease. In adults and juveniles the main syndromes are CNS infection, septicaemia and endocarditis. Most cases occur in immunosuppressed patients receiving steroid or cytotoxic therapy or with malignant neoplasms. However, about one-third of patients with meningitis and around 10% with primary bacteraemia are immunocompetent.

Meningitis

The clinical presentation is the same in all groups, but progression is more rapid in immunocompromised subjects. A peripheral blood leucocytosis occurs, and the CSF white blood cell count is raised. The CSF glucose level is low and the protein level is raised; a very high protein concentration may be a poor prognostic indicator. Gram stains of the CSF are often negative, and the clinical features of infection are such that it is not possible to tell listerial meningitis from meningococcal or pneumococcal infection. However, *L. monocytogenes* is isolated from blood cultures in most cases.

In the rare cases of encephalitis, cerebritis or cerebral abscesses the CSF may be normal, but often the white blood cell count is mildly raised and the protein level slightly elevated with a low glucose concentration. The Gram film and culture are usually negative. Blood cultures are the main source of the organism in many of these patients.

Bacteraemia and endocarditis

Primary bacteraemia is more common in men than in women, and occurs most often in patients with haematological malignancy or renal transplants. A few patients develop CNS infection, which has a poor prognosis. Infective endocarditis is twice as common in men as in women. The main predisposing factors are prosthetic valves or damaged natural valves, but some patients belong to other risk groups.

Gastroenteritis

Several food-borne outbreaks of acute gastroenteritis with fever have been described. The foods associated with these outbreaks have been diverse, but heavily contaminated by the bacterium. Symptoms develop in 1–2 days. Large numbers of *L. monocytogenes* are present in the stool, and a few cases develop serious systemic infection. The ability to cause gastroenteritis may be specific to certain strains.

Other infections

Rarer manifestations of listeriosis include arthritis, hepatitis, endophthalmitis, cutaneous lesions and peritonitis in patients on continuous ambulatory peritoneal dialysis. Pneumonia occurs in renal transplant recipients and other groups of patients.

Epidemiology

Incidence

Most western countries report infection rates of 1–10 cases per million of the population per year. Pregnancy and neonatal disease account for 10–20% of cases. Among these, 15–25% of infections lead to abortion and stillbirth, while about 70% are neonatal infections. In about 5% of maternal infections bacteraemia occurs and the fetus is not affected.

The incidence of infection increases with age so that the mean age of adult infections is over 55 years. Men are more commonly infected than women over the age of 40 years, and since women are infected in the childbearing years the overall sex distribution is more or less equal. Immunosuppression is a major risk factor for both the epidemic and sporadic forms of listeriosis and probably accounts for the increasing incidence with age. Human immunodeficiency virus disease is a predisposing factor in some areas. The peak incidence of human disease occurs in July, August or September. Most patients live in urban areas and usually have no exposure to animals.

L. monocytogenes, like other *Listeria* species, has been isolated from numerous sites, including soil, sewage, water and decaying plant material, where it can survive for more than 2 years. Although the true home of listeria is probably in the environment, they are also found in excreta of apparently healthy animals, including man. Up to 5% of healthy adults may have the organism in their faeces. Faecal carriage in man probably reflects consumption of contaminated foods and is likely to be transitory.

Numerous types of raw, processed, cooked and ready-to-eat foods contain *L. monocytogenes*, usually at levels below 10 organisms per gram. The unusual tolerance of the bacterium to sodium chloride and sodium nitrite, and the ability to multiply (albeit slowly) at refrigeration temperatures makes *L. monocytogenes* of particular concern as a post-processing contaminant in long shelf-life refrigerated foods. Even when present at high levels in foods, spoilage or taints are not generally produced. The widespread distribution of *L. monocytogenes* and the ability to survive on dry and moist surfaces favours post-processing contamination of foods from both raw product and factory sites.

Transmission

Most cases are sporadic and in only a few is a route of infection identified. The consumption of contaminated foods is the principal route of transmission. Microbiological and epidemiological evidence supports an association with many food types (dairy, meat, vegetable, fish and shellfish) in both sporadic and epidemic listeriosis. Foods associated with transmission often show common features:

- the ability to support the multiplication of *L. monocytogenes* (relatively high water activity and near-neutral pH)
- relatively heavy contamination ($>10^3$ organisms per gram) with the implicated strain
- processed with an extended (refrigerated) shelf-life
- consumed without further cooking.

Outbreaks of human listeriosis involving >100 individuals have occurred, some lasting for several years. This is likely to represent a long-term colonization of a single site in the food manufacturing environment as well as the long incubation periods shown by some patients. Sites of contamination within food processing facilities involved in human infection have included wooden manufacturing equipment, wooden and metallic shelving, porous conveyor belts, cool-room condensates and floor drains. *L. monocytogenes* survives well in moist environments with organic material, and it is from such sites that contamination of food occurs during processing.

Listeriosis transmitted by direct contact with the environment, infected animals or animal material is relatively rare. Papular or pustular cutaneous lesions have been described, usually on the upper arms or wrists, in farmers or veterinarians 1–4 days after attending bovine abortions. Infection is invariably mild and usually resolves without antimicrobial therapy, although serious systemic involvement has been described. Conjunctivitis in poultry workers has also been reported.

Hospital cross-infection between newborn infants occurs. Typically, an apparently healthy baby (rarely more than one) develops late-onset listeriosis 5–12 days after delivery in a hospital in which an infant with congenital listeriosis was born shortly before. The same strain of *L. monocytogenes* is isolated from both infants and the mother of the early-onset case, but not from the mother of the late-onset case. The cases are usually delivered or nursed in the same or adjacent rooms, and consequently staff and equipment are common to both. There is little evidence of cross-infection or person-to-person transmission outside the neonatal period.

Treatment

L. monocytogenes is susceptible to a wide range of antibiotics in vitro, including ampicillin, penicillin, vancomycin, tetracyclines, chloramphenicol, aminoglycosides and co-trimoxazole. There is little agreement about the best treatment, but many patients have been successfully treated with ampicillin or penicillin with or without an aminoglycoside.

Ampicillin and penicillin are probably equivalent agents for the treatment of meningitis. Co-trimoxazole is an excellent alternative. Aminoglycosides interact synergistically with penicillin or ampicillin and improve mortality rates in experimental animals, but no such evidence exists for human infection. Chloramphenicol, when used alone, is less effective than penicillin or ampicillin and may result in relapses. The combination of chloramphenicol with penicillin or ampicillin has resulted in increased mortality. Cephalosporins are ineffective.

The combination of ampicillin and an aminoglycoside is used most commonly in other forms of neonatal and adult listeriosis. Vancomycin is a useful alternative in bacteraemia.

No significant change in the antimicrobial susceptibility of *L. monocytogenes* has been recognized over the past 30 years, and resistance to any of the agents recommended for therapy is unlikely.

Prognosis

The mortality rate in late neonatal disease is about 10%. In contrast, mortality in early disease is 30–60%, and about 20–40% of survivors develop sequelae such as lung disease, hydrocephalus or other neurological defects. Early use of appropriate antibiotics during pregnancy may improve neonatal survival.

The mortality in adult infection is about 20–50% in CNS infection, 5–20% in primary bacteraemia and 50% in infective endocarditis. About 25–75% of patients surviving CNS infection suffer sequelae such as hemiplegia and other neurological defects.

ERYSIPELOTHRIX

Erysipelothrix is a genus of aerobic, non-sporing, non-motile Gram-positive bacilli. The genus comprises at least two species: *E. rhusiopathiae* and *E. tonsillarum*. *E. rhusiopathiae* causes economically important disease in domestic animals, notably pigs. Human infections are rare, but include a form of cellulitis (*erysipeloid*), which occasionally becomes diffuse and may lead to septi-caemia and endocarditis. Infection is most often associated with close animal contact.

The bacilli are short (1–2 μm), but may produce long filamentous forms resembling lactobacilli. Growth is improved by incubation in 5–10% carbon dioxide. Colonies on blood agar are α-haemolytic.

Penicillin and other β-lactam antibiotics are effective. Erythromycin and clindamycin offer suitable alternatives, but *E. rhusiopathiae* is resistant to vancomycin.

RECOMMENDED READING

Begg N 1994 *Manual for the Management and Control of Diphtheria in the European Region.* WHO Copenhagen, ICP/EPI 038(B)

Brooke C J, Riley T V 1999 *Erysipelothrix rhusiopathiae*: biology, epidemiology and clinical manifestations of an occupational pathogen. *Journal of Medical Microbiology* 48: 789–799

Coyle M B, Lipsky B A 1990 Coryneform bacteria in infectious diseases: clinical and laboratory aspects. *Clinical Microbiology Reviews* 3: 227–246

Efstratiou A, George R C 1996 Microbiology and epidemiology of diphtheria. *Reviews in Medical Microbiology* 7: 31–42

Funke G, von Graevenitz A, Clarridge J E, Bernard K A 1997 Clinical microbiology of coryneform bacteria. *Clinical Microbiology Reviews* 10: 125–159

Hof H, Nichterlein T, Kretschmar M 1997 Management of listeriosis. *Clinical Microbiology Reviews* 10: 345–357

Low J C, Donachie W 1997 A review of *Listeria monocytogenes* and listeriosis. *Veterinary Journal* 153: 9–29

McLauchlin J 1997 The pathogenicity of *Listeria monocytogenes*: a public health perspective. *Reviews in Medical Microbiology* 8: 1–14

McLauchlin J 1997 The identification of *Listeria* species. *International Journal of Food Microbiology* 38:77–81

Robson J M, McDougall R, van der Valk S, Waite E D, Sullivan J J 1998 *Erysipelothrix rhusiopathiae*: an uncommon but ever present zoonosis. *Pathology* 30: 391–394

Schlech W F 1997 *Listeria* gastroenteritis: old syndrome, new pathogen. *New England Journal of Medicine* 336:130–132

18

Mycobacterium

Tuberculosis; leprosy

J. M. Grange

The name of the genus, *Mycobacterium* (fungus-bacterium), is an allusion to the mould-like pellicles formed when members of this genus are grown in liquid media. This hydrophobic property is due to their possession of thick, complex, lipid-rich, waxy cell walls. A further important characteristic, also due to their waxy cell walls, is *acid-fastness*, or resistance to decolorization by a dilute mineral acid (or alcohol) after staining with hot carbol fuchsin or other arylmethane dyes.

There are over 80 named species of mycobacteria, which are divisible into two major groups, the slow and rapid growers, although the growth rate of the latter is slow relative to that of most other bacteria. The leprosy bacillus, *Mycobacterium leprae*, which has never convincingly been grown in vitro, and members of the *Mycobacterium tuberculosis* complex are obligate pathogens. The other species are environmental saprophytes, some of which can cause opportunist disease (see Chapter 19).

MYCOBACTERIUM TUBERCULOSIS COMPLEX

The term *M. tuberculosis complex* refers to a group of very closely related species, which, on genetic analysis, are variants of a single species. All of them cause *tuberculosis*, a chronic granulomatous disease affecting man and many other mammals. The complex includes:

- *M. tuberculosis*, which causes most human tuberculosis.
- *M. canetti*, a very rare variant of *M. tuberculosis* with smooth colonies.
- *M. bovis*, which is the principal cause of tuberculosis in cattle and many other mammals.
- a caprine (goat) variant of *M. bovis,* which has caused a few cases of tuberculosis in veterinary surgeons.
- *M. microti* which is a pathogen of voles and other small mammals, but not of man, and is very rarely encountered.

- *M. africanum*, which appears to be intermediate in form between the human and bovine types. It causes human tuberculosis and is mainly found in Equatorial Africa.

DESCRIPTION

Members of the *M. tuberculosis* complex (*tubercle bacilli*) are non-motile, non-sporing, non-capsulate, straight or slightly curved rods about $3 \times 0.3\ \mu$m in size. In sputum and other clinical specimens they may occur singly or in small clumps, and in liquid cultures they often grow as twisted rope-like colonies termed *serpentine cords* (Fig. 18.1).

Tubercle bacilli are able to grow on a wide range of enriched culture media, but Löwenstein–Jensen (LJ)

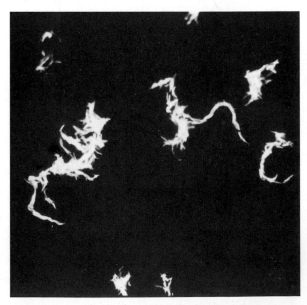

Fig. 18.1 Microcolony of *M. tuberculosis* showing 'serpentine cord' formation.

medium is the most widely used in clinical practice. This is an egg–glycerol-based medium to which malachite green dye is added to inhibit the growth of some contaminating bacteria and to provide a contrasting colour against which colonies of mycobacteria are easily seen. Agar-based media or broths enriched with bovine serum albumin are also used, particularly in automated culture systems.

Human tubercle bacilli produce visible growth on LJ medium in about 2 weeks, although on primary isolation from clinical material colonies may take up to 8 weeks to appear. Colonies are of an off-white (buff) colour and (except for the very rarely encountered *M. canetti* which has smooth colonies) often have a dry breadcrumb-like appearance. Growth is characteristically heaped up and luxuriant or 'eugonic' in contrast to the small, flat 'dysgonic' colonies of bovine tubercle bacilli, which grow much better on media containing sodium pyruvate in place of glycerol.

The optimal growth temperature of tubercle bacilli is 35–37°C, but they fail to grow at 25°C or 41°C. Most other mycobacteria grow at one or other, or both, of these temperatures.

All mycobacteria are obligate aerobes, but *M. bovis* grows better in conditions of reduced oxygen tension. Thus, when incorporated in soft agar media, *M. tuberculosis* grows on the surface while *M. bovis* grows as a band a few millimetres below the surface. This provides a useful differentiating test. Various other differential characteristics of human tubercle bacilli are shown in Table 18.1.

Tubercle bacilli survive in milk and in other organic materials and on pasture land so long as they are not exposed to ultraviolet light, to which they are very sensitive. They are also heat-sensitive, and are destroyed by pasteurization. Mycobacteria are susceptible to alcohol, formaldehyde and glutaraldehyde and, to a lesser extent, to hypochlorites and phenolic disinfectants. They are considerably more resistant than other bacteria to acids, alkalis and quaternary ammonium compounds.

PATHOGENESIS

The tubercle bacillus owes its virulence to its ability to survive within the macrophage rather than to the production of a toxic substance. The mechanism of virulence is poorly understood and is almost certainly multifactorial. The immune response to the bacillus is of the cell-mediated type, which, if mediated by Th1 T helper cells, leads to protective immunity, but the presence of Th2 cells facilitates tissue-destroying hypersensitivity reactions and progression of the disease process. The nature of the immune responses following infection changes with time so that human tuberculosis is divisible into primary and post-primary forms with quite different pathological features.

Primary tuberculosis

The site of the initial infection is usually the lung, following the inhalation of bacilli. These bacilli are engulfed by alveolar macrophages in which they replicate to form the initial lesion or *Ghon focus*. Some bacilli are carried in phagocytic cells to the hilar lymph nodes where additional foci of infection develop. The Ghon focus, together with the enlarged hilar lymph nodes, form the *primary complex*. In addition, bacilli are seeded by further lymphatic and haematogenous dissemination in many organs and tissues, including other parts of the lung. When the bacilli enter the mouth, as when drinking milk containing *M. bovis*, the primary complexes involve the tonsil and cervical nodes (*scrofula*; Fig. 18.2) or the intestine, often the ileocaecal region, and the mesenteric lymph nodes. Likewise, the primary focus may be in the skin, with involvement of the regional lymph nodes. This form of tuberculosis was an occupational disease of anatomists and pathologists and was termed *prosector's wart*.

Within about 10 days of infection, clones of antigen-specific T lymphocytes are produced. These release cytokines, notably interferon-γ, which activate

Table 18.1	Some differential characteristics of tubercle bacilli causing human disease				
Species	Atmospheric preference	Nitratase	TCH	Pyrazinamide
M. tuberculosis[a]	Aerobic	Positive	Resistant[b]	Sensitive
M. bovis	Micro-aerophilic	Negative	Sensitive	Resistant
M. bovis BCG	Aerobic	Negative	Sensitive	Resistant
M. africanum	Micro-aerophilic	Variable	Sensitive	Sensitive

[a] Includes the rare *M. canetti* variant.
[b] Strains from south India may be sensitive.
TCH, thiophen-2-carboxylic acid hydrazide.

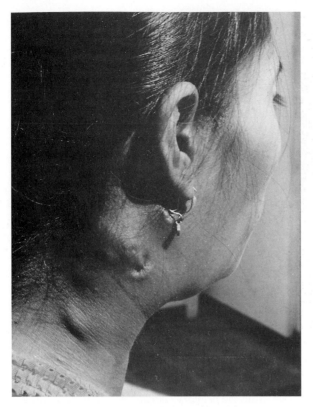

Fig. 18.2 Tuberculous cervical lymphadenitis (scrofula) with sinus formation in an Indonesian woman.

macrophages and cause them to form a compact cluster, or granuloma, around the foci of infection. These activated macrophages are termed *epithelioid cells* from their microscopical resemblance to epithelial cells. Some of them fuse to form multinucleate giant cells. The centre of the granuloma contains a mixture of necrotic tissue and dead macrophages, which, from its cheese-like appearance and consistency, is referred to as *caseation*.

Activated human macrophages inhibit the replication of the tubercle bacilli, but there is no clear evidence that they can actually kill them. Being metabolically very

active, the macrophages in the granuloma consume oxygen, and the resulting anoxia and acidosis in the centre of the lesion probably kills most of the bacilli. Granuloma formation is usually sufficient to limit the primary infection: the lesions become quiescent and surrounding fibroblasts produce dense scar tissue, which may become calcified. Not all bacilli are destroyed: some remain in a poorly understood dormant form which, when reactivated, causes post-primary disease. Programmed cell death (apoptosis) of bacteria-laden cells by cytotoxic T cells and natural killer (NK) cells may also contribute to protective immunity.

In a minority of cases one of the infective foci progresses and gives rise to the serious manifestations of primary disease, including progressive primary lesions (particularly in infants; Table 18.2), meningitis, pleurisy and disease of the kidneys, spine (*Pott's disease*) and other bones and joints. If a focus ruptures into a blood vessel, bacilli are disseminated throughout the body with the formation of numerous granulomata (Fig. 18.3). This, from the millet seed-like appearance of the lesions, is known as *miliary tuberculosis*.

Tuberculin reactivity

About 6–8 weeks after the initial infection, the phenomenon of tuberculin conversion occurs. This altered reactivity was discovered by Robert Koch while attempting to develop a remedy for tuberculosis. When tuberculous guinea-pigs were injected intradermally with living tubercle bacilli, the skin around the injection site became necrotic within a day or two and was sloughed off, together with the bacilli. Koch then found that the same reaction occurred when he injected *old tuberculin* – a heat-concentrated filtrate of a broth in which tubercle bacilli had been grown. This reaction became known as the *Koch phenomenon*, and its characteristic feature is extensive tissue necrosis.

Although Koch's tuberculin proved unsuccessful as a therapeutic agent, it formed the basis of the widely used tuberculin test (see below).

Table 18.2	Stages of primary tuberculosis in childhood		
Stage	Time (from onset)	Characteristics	
1	3–8 weeks	Primary complex develops and tuberculin conversion occurs	
2	2–6 months	Progressive healing of primary complex Possibility of pleural effusion	
3	6–12 months	Possibility of miliary or meningeal tuberculosis	
4	1–3 years	Possibility of bone or joint tuberculosis	
5	3–5 years or more	Possibility of genito-urinary or chronic skin tuberculosis	

Adapted from Miller F J W 1982 *Tuberculosis in Children*. Churchill Livingstone, Edinburgh.

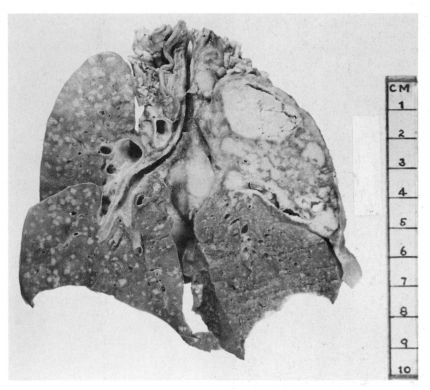

Fig. 18.3 Progressive primary tuberculous lesion in the right upper lobe of the lung and numerous miliary lesions in other parts of the lung in a child aged 6 months.

Post-primary tuberculosis

In many individuals, the primary complex resolves and the only evidence of infection is a conversion to tuberculin reactivity. After an interval of months, years or decades, reactivation of dormant foci of tubercle bacilli or exogenous re-infection may lead to post-primary tuberculosis, which differs in several respects from primary disease (Table 18.3). Endogenous reactivation may occur spontaneously or after an intercurrent illness or other condition that lowers the host's immune responsiveness (see below). For unknown reasons reactivation or re-infection tuberculosis often occurs in the upper lobes of the lungs. The same process of granuloma formation occurs, but the necrotic element of the reaction causes tissue destruction and the formation of large areas of caseation termed *tuberculomas*. Proteases liberated by activated macrophages cause softening and liquefaction of the caseous material, and an excess of tumour necrosis factor (cachectin) and other immunological mediators cause the wasting and fevers characteristic of the disease.

The interior of the tuberculoma is acidic and anoxic and contains few viable tubercle bacilli. Eventually, however, the expanding lesion erodes through the wall of a bronchus, the liquefied contents are discharged and

Table 18.3 Main differences between primary and post-primary tuberculosis in non-immunocompromised patients

Characteristics	Primary	Post-primary
Local lesion	Small	Large
Lymphatic involvement	Yes	Minimal
Cavity formation	Rare	Frequent
Tuberculin reactivity	Negative (initially)	Positive
Infectivity[a]	Uncommon	Usual
Site	Any part of lung	Apical region
Local spread	Uncommon	Frequent

[a] Pulmonary cases.

a well-aerated cavity is formed (Fig. 18.4). The atmosphere of the lung, with a high carbon dioxide level, is ideal for supporting the growth of the bacilli, and huge numbers of these are found in the cavity walls. For this reason, closure of the cavities by collapsing the lung, either by artificial pneumothorax or by excising large portions of the chest wall, was a standard treatment for tuberculosis in the pre-chemotherapy era.

Once the cavity is formed, large numbers of bacilli gain access to the sputum, and the patient becomes an open or infectious case. This is a good example of the

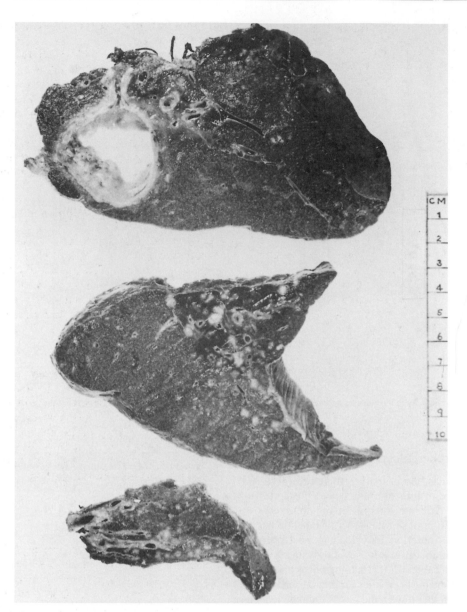

Fig. 18.4 Large tuberculous cavity in the lung of a man aged 24 years. Other parts of the lung show secondary lesions due to endobronchial spread of disease.

transmissibility of a pathogen being dependent upon the host's immune response to infection. Surprisingly, about 20% of cases of open cavitating tuberculosis resolve without treatment.

In post-primary tuberculosis, dissemination of bacilli to lymph nodes and other organs is unusual. Instead, spread of infection occurs through the bronchial tree so that secondary lesions develop in the lower lobes of the lung (Fig. 18.4). Likewise, secondary lesions may occur in the trachea, larynx and mouth, and swallowed bacilli cause intestinal lesions; secondary lesions may also develop in the bladder and epididymis in cases of renal tuberculosis. Post-primary cutaneous tuberculosis (*lupus vulgaris*) usually affects the face and neck. Untreated, it is a chronic condition leading to gross scarring and deformity. Some cases are secondary to sinus formation between tuberculous lymph nodes and the skin (*scrofuloderma*). Most cases of lupus vulgaris were caused by *M. bovis* and this condition is now rarely seen in developed countries.

Immunocompromised individuals

Reactivation tuberculosis is particularly likely to occur in immunocompromised individuals, including the elderly and transplant recipients; it often occurs early in the course of human immunodeficiency virus (HIV) infection. Tuberculosis acts synergistically with HIV to lower the patient's immunity and it is an AIDS-defining condition. As a result, even if tuberculosis is treated effectively in HIV-positive patients, the mortality rate due to other AIDS-related conditions is high, with many dying within 2 years. Cavity formation is unusual in the more profoundly immunocompromised patients, emphasizing the importance of the immune response in this pathological process. Instead, diffuse infiltrates develop in any part of the lung. In contrast to post-primary disease in non-immunocompromised individuals, lymphatic and haematogenous dissemination are common. Sometimes there are numerous minute lesions teeming with tubercle bacilli throughout the body – a rapidly fatal condition termed *cryptic disseminated tuberculosis*. The interval between infection and development of disease is considerably shortened in immunocompromised persons.

The tuberculin test

Although Robert Koch's attempts to use old tuberculin as a remedy for tuberculosis failed, an Austrian physician, Clemens von Pirquet, used the Koch phenomenon as an indication of bacterial 'allergy' resulting from previous infection. Individuals with active tuberculosis were usually tuberculin-positive, but many of those with disseminated and rapidly progressive disease were negative. This led to the widespread but erroneous belief that tuberculin reactivity is an indicator of immunity to tuberculosis.

Old tuberculin caused non-specific reactions, and it has been replaced by *purified protein derivative* (PPD). This is given by:

- intracutaneous injection (*Mantoux* method)
- a spring-loaded gun which fires six prongs into the skin through a drop of PPD (*Heaf* method)
- single-test disposable devices with PPD dried onto prongs (*tine tests*).

The biological activity of tuberculin is compared with international standards and activity expressed in international units (IU). In the UK, solutions of PPD for Mantoux testing are supplied as dilutions of 1 in 10 000, 1 in 1000 and 1 in 100, which correspond to 1, 10 and 100 IU in the injected dose of 0.1 ml. The standard test dose is 10 IU but those suspected of having tuberculosis, and who are therefore likely to react strongly, may first be tested with 1 IU. Undiluted PPD is supplied for use with the Heaf gun.

The tuberculin test is widely used as a diagnostic test, although its usefulness is limited by its failure to distinguish active disease from quiescent infections and past BCG (bacille Calmette-Guérin; see p. 209) vaccination. In addition, exposure to various mycobacteria in the environment may induce low levels of tuberculin reactivity. In the USA, where BCG is not used, more diagnostic reliance is placed on the tuberculin test. The test is used in epidemiological studies as outlined below.

LABORATORY DIAGNOSIS

The definitive diagnosis of tuberculosis is based on the detection of acid-fast bacilli in clinical specimens by microscopy, cultural techniques or by the polymerase chain reaction (PCR) and its various derivatives. Numerous attempts have been made to develop serological tests for the disease with little success.

Specimens

The most usual specimen for diagnosis of pulmonary tuberculosis is sputum but, if none is produced, bronchial washings, brushings or biopsies and early-morning gastric aspirates (to harvest any bacilli swallowed overnight) may be examined. Tissue biopsies are homogenized by grinding for microscopy and culture. Cerebrospinal fluid (CSF), pleural fluid, urine and other fluids are centrifuged and the deposits are examined.

Microscopy

Use is made of the acid-fast property of mycobacteria to detect them in sputum and other clinical material. In the Ziehl–Neelsen (ZN) staining technique, heat-fixed smears of the specimens are flooded with a solution of carbol fuchsin (a mixture of basic fuchsin and phenol) and heated until steam rises. After washing with water, the slide is flooded with a dilute mineral acid (e.g. 3% hydrochloric acid) and, after further washing, a green or blue counterstain is applied. Red bacilli are seen against the contrasting background colour. In some methods, the acid is diluted in 95% ethanol rather than water. This gives a cleaner background but, contrary to a common belief, it does not enable tubercle bacilli to be distinguished from other mycobacteria. Fluorescence microscopy, based on the same principle of acid-fastness, is increasingly used and is much less tiring to the microscopist. Modifications of the various staining techniques are used to examine tissue sections.

Cultural methods

As sputum and certain other specimens frequently contain many bacteria and fungi that would rapidly overgrow any mycobacteria on the culture media, these must be destroyed. Decontamination methods make use of the relatively high resistance of mycobacteria to acids, alkalis and certain disinfectants. In the widely used *Petroff method*, sputum is mixed well with 4% sodium hydroxide for 15–30 min, neutralized with potassium dihydrogen orthophosphate and centrifuged. The deposit is used to inoculate LJ or similar media. Specimens such as CSF and tissue biopsies, which are unlikely to be contaminated, are inoculated directly onto culture media. As an alternative to chemical decontamination, mixtures of antibiotics that kill fungi and all bacteria other than mycobacteria may be added to the culture media. These are used principally in the automated culture systems described below.

Inoculated media are incubated at 35–37°C and inspected weekly for at least 8 weeks. Cultures of material from skin lesions should also be incubated at 33°C. Any bacterial growth is stained by the ZN method and, if acid-fast, it is subcultured for further identification.

A more rapid bacteriological diagnosis is achievable by use of commercially available automated systems. Systems that detect colour changes in dyes induced by the release of carbon dioxide, or the unquenching of fluorescent dyes on the consumption of oxygen by metabolizing bacilli, have replaced the earlier radiometric method.

The first step in identification is to determine whether an isolate is a member of the *M. tuberculosis* complex. These organisms:

- grow slowly
- do not produce yellow pigment
- fail to grow at 25 and 41°C
- do not grow on egg media containing *p*-nitrobenzoic acid (500 mg/l).

Strains differing in any of these properties belong to other species.

Nucleic acid technology

Nucleic acid probes for the identification of the *M. tuberculosis* complex and, specifically, *M. tuberculosis*, and also for certain other species are commercially available. They are not sensitive enough to detect mycobacteria in clinical specimens and are used to identify mycobacteria cultivated by conventional techniques.

Amplification of specific nucleic acid sequences in specimens is achievable by PCR and related techniques, some of which are commercially available. Problems of

Table 18.4 Examples of the interpretation of drug sensitivity testing by the resistance ratio method

Strain	Increasing drug concentration (mg/l)						Resistance ratio	Result
	1	2	4	8	16	32		
Controls	+	+	–	–	–	–	–	–
Test 1	+	(+)	–	–	–	–	1	Sensitive
Test 2	+	+	–	–	–	–	1	Sensitive
Test 3	+	+	+	–	–	–	2	Sensitive
Test 4	+	+	+	+	(+)	–	4	Resistant
Test 5	+	+	+	+	+	–	8	Resistant
Test 6	+	+	+	+	+	+	>8	Resistant

+, confluent growth or innumerable discrete colonies; (+), 20–100 colonies; –, less than 20 colonies.

low sensitivity, 'false-positive' reactions and cross-contamination have largely been overcome by the introduction of closed-system, isothermal techniques for amplification of species-specific 16S ribosomal RNA.

Most members of the *M. tuberculosis* complex contain 1–20 copies of the insertion sequence IS6110, which has been used to develop DNA 'fingerprinting' (p. 68) methods for epidemiological purposes. Alternatively, detection of spacer oligonucleotides, short DNA sequences found around the sites of the insertion sequences, is useful for typing isolates ('spoligotyping').

Drug susceptibility testing

Several methods have been described:

- The resistance-ratio method in which test strains and susceptible controls are inoculated on sets of LJ medium containing doubling dilutions of drug. The results are expressed as the ratio of the drug concentration inhibiting the test strain to that inhibiting the control strains. Susceptible strains have ratios of 1 or 2, while higher ratios indicate resistance (Table 18.4).
- Radiometric or non-radiometric automated systems, which provide results more quickly.
- Nucleic acid technology, which is even more rapid. Kits able to detect about 95% of mutations to rifampicin resistance caused by mutations in the *rpoB* gene are commercially available.

TREATMENT

The antituberculosis drugs are divisible into three groups (Table 18.5).

Table 18.5 Antituberculosis drugs (in vivo)

Sterilizing	Bactericidal	Bacteristatic
Rifampicin	Isoniazid	Ethionamide
Pyrazinamide	Streptomycin	Prothionamide
	Ethambutol[a]	Thiacetazone
	Quinolones	p-Aminosalicylic acid
	Macrolides	Cycloserine

[a] In early stages of therapy.

- Bactericidal drugs that effectively sterilize tuberculous lesions.
- Bactericidal drugs that only kill tubercle bacilli in certain situations. Streptomycin is ineffective against bacilli within macrophages and acidic inflammatory tissue, and isoniazid kills bacilli only if they are replicating.
- Bacteristatic drugs, which are of limited usefulness and are not included in standard drug regimens.

Mutation to drug resistance occurs at a rate of about one mutation every 10^8 cell divisions. Successful therapy requires the prevention of the emergence of drug-resistant strains by the simultaneous use of at least two drugs to which the organism is sensitive.

The earlier 2-year regimen of streptomycin, isoniazid and p-aminosalicylic acid has been replaced by much more acceptable orally administered regimens based on an initial intensive 2-month phase and a 4–6-month continuation phase depending on the World Health Organization (WHO) treatment category (Table 18.6).

Most patients are in category I when diagnosed and the most widely used regimen therefore consists of an intensive phase of rifampicin, isoniazid, pyrazinamide and ethambutol for 2 months, followed by the first two drugs for a total of 6 months. Ideally, the drugs are given daily, but to ensure compliance by supervising the administration of the drugs, they may be given thrice weekly during the continuation phase or throughout.

The response to therapy of drug-susceptible tuberculosis is divisible into three phases:

- During the first week or two, the large numbers of actively replicating bacilli in cavity walls are killed, principally by isoniazid, but also by rifampicin and ethambutol. The patient rapidly ceases to be infectious, and hospitalization with barrier nursing is now rarely necessary.
- In the following few weeks the less active bacilli within macrophages, caseous material and dense, acidic, inflammatory lesions are killed by rifampicin and pyrazinamide.
- In the continuation phase any remaining dormant bacilli are killed by rifampicin during their short bursts of metabolic activity. Any rifampicin-resistant mutants that start to replicate are killed by isoniazid.

Short-course regimens are usually well tolerated by the patient. Isoniazid, rifampicin and pyrazinamide are all potentially hepatotoxic, and rifampicin may cause an influenza-like syndrome, which, paradoxically, is more likely to occur when the drug is given intermittently. Rifampicin antagonizes the action of oral contraceptives – an important point to be considered when treating

Table 18.6 WHO treatment categories and recommended short-course drug regimens

Treatment category	Definition	Initial phase[a]	Continuation phase
I	New sputum smear-positive; smear-negative with extensive lung involvement; severe non-pulmonary disease	HRZE or HRZS	4 months' HR or 4 months' H_3E_3 or 6 months' HE
II	Sputum smear-positive after relapse, treatment failure or interruption of treatment	HRZE or HRZES	5 months' HRE 5 months' $H_3R_3E_3$
III	New smear-negative (other than Category I) and less severe non-pulmonary disease.	HRZ	4 months' HR or 4 months' H_3E_3 or 6 months' HE
IV	Chronic cases[b]	Advice on use of second-line drugs required from specialized centres	

H, isoniazid; R, rifampicin; Z, pyrazinamide; E, ethambutol; S, streptomycin.
[a] Daily or thrice weekly for 2 months.
[b] Smear positive after supervised re-treatment.
The subscript numeral 3 indicates thrice-weekly doses.

young women. There is also mutual antagonism between rifampicin and the antiretroviral drugs used for HIV infection (pp. 57 and 533–534). Substituting rifabutin for rifampicin reduces this problem. Isoniazid may cause mild psychiatric disturbances and peripheral neuropathy, particularly in alcoholics, but these usually respond to treatment with pyridoxine (vitamin B_6). Ethambutol is toxic for the eye and, although this is rare with standard dosages, care is required and the patient should be informed of this possibility.

The emergence of drug-resistant strains (acquired resistance) during adequately supervised short-course chemotherapy is uncommon – most relapses are due to drug-sensitive bacilli. Multidrug-resistant strains are defined as those resistant to isoniazid and rifampicin; they are sometimes also resistant to other drugs and pose serious problems. The regimens for multidrug-resistant tuberculosis are based on in-vitro drug susceptibility tests; useful agents include the newer fluoroquinolones and macrolides and amoxicillin with a β-lactamase inhibitor such as sulbactam. The mortality rate is high, but with a high level of care this can be reduced to around 15% although HIV seropositivity is a poor prognostic factor.

EPIDEMIOLOGY

Human tuberculosis is principally transmitted by inhalation of bacilli in moist droplets coughed out by individuals with open pulmonary tuberculosis. Dried bacilli in dust appear to be less of a health hazard. Sputum of those patients positive on microscopy contains at least 5000 tubercle bacilli per millilitre and these patients are considerably more infectious than those negative on microscopy. Most transmission of the disease occurs within households or other environments where individuals are close together for long periods.

For epidemiological purposes, the incidence of infection by the tubercle bacillus in a community is calculated from the number of tuberculin-positive individuals in different age groups, provided that they have not received BCG vaccination. The annual infection rate gives an indirect measure of the number of open or infectious individuals in the community. Although subject to many variables, a 1% annual infection rate indicates that there are around 50 infectious cases in every 100 000 members of the community. The prevalence of tuberculosis in a region is not the same as the annual infection rate because only a minority of infected individuals develop overt disease and they often become ill several years after their initial infection.

Determinations of the incidence of tuberculosis worldwide are notoriously difficult. According to WHO estimates:

- one-third of the world's population has been infected
- about 100 million individuals are infected annually and 8–10 million develop overt disease
- 4–5 million become open or infectious and around 3 million die.

In the industrially developed nations, tuberculosis is uncommon, with an annual infection rate of 0.3–0.1% or less, but the previous decline has halted and in several countries there has been an increase in notifications since around 1990. In the developing countries the annual infection rates are usually between 2 and 5%.

Owing to the impact of the HIV/AIDS pandemic the incidence of tuberculosis is increasing in some countries and predictions of future trends are very worrying.

- In 1999, 10% of all cases of tuberculosis were HIV-related, rising to over 20% in Africa and to 60% in some regions of southern Africa.
- In the same year, around 3 million people died of AIDS and tuberculosis was the cause of death in 30%.
- A person dually infected by the tubercle bacillus and HIV has an 8% chance of developing active tuberculosis annually. The risk of developing tuberculosis after infection or re-infection is very much higher, approaching 100%, in patients with AIDS.
- The interval between infection and overt disease is considerably shortened, resulting in explosive mini-epidemics in institutions where HIV-positive persons congregate. Some such mini-epidemics have involved multidrug-resistant strains, notably in the USA.

Bovine tuberculosis is spread from animal to animal, and sometimes to human attendants, in moist cough spray. About 1% of infected cows develop lesions in the udder, and bacilli are excreted in the milk, which can then infect people who drink it. Heat treatment, or pasteurization, prevents milk-borne disease. In most developed countries, bovine tuberculosis has been drastically reduced by regular tuberculin testing of herds and the slaughter of reactors. In such countries, human disease due to *M. bovis* is very rare and is usually the result of reactivation of old lesions. Person-to-person spread of *M. bovis* leading to active disease is very uncommon although a few instances of such spread to HIV-positive persons have been reported.

The total eradication of bovine tuberculosis has been prevented by infection of cattle from wild animals, notably badgers in the UK and possums in New Zealand, and also occasionally from farm workers with open tuberculosis due to *M. bovis*.

CONTROL

Human tuberculosis is preventable:

- by the early detection and effective therapy of the open or infectious individuals in a community
- by lowering the chance of infection by reducing overcrowding
- to a limited extent, by vaccination.

Active case finding involves a deliberate search, often on a house-to-house basis or in workplaces, for suspects with a chronic cough of a month or more in duration. Merely waiting for patients with symptoms to seek medical attention is much less effective, even when supported by education programmes. Regular chest examination by mass miniature radiography detects fewer than 15% of individuals with tuberculosis and is no longer used routinely except in certain high-risk situations.

The most important factors affecting the incidence of tuberculosis are socio-economic ones, particularly those leading to a reduction of overcrowding in homes and workplaces. In the developing countries it is estimated that each patient with open tuberculosis infects about 20 contacts annually, while in Europe the corresponding figure is two or three.

Vaccination

Bacille Calmette-Guérin (BCG) is a living attenuated vaccine derived from a strain of *M. bovis* by repeated subculture between the years 1908 and 1920. This species was selected rather than *M. tuberculosis* on the dubious assumption that it was of limited virulence in man. The vaccine was originally given orally to neonates but is now given by intracutaneous injection.

The protective efficacy of BCG varies enormously from country to country. In the UK, administration of BCG to schoolchildren affords 78% protection, but a major trial in south India involving individuals of all ages found no protection (Table 18.7). This difference appears to be the result of prior exposure of the population to environmental mycobacteria which, in some regions, confer some protection, but in others induce inappropriate immune reactions that antagonize protection. For this reason, vaccination given neonatally, before environmental sensitization occurs, is now gaining popularity.

When BCG vaccination is introduced into a region it has an immediate impact on the incidence of the serious but non-infectious forms of childhood tuberculosis such as meningitis, but it has little impact on the annual

Table 18.7 Variations in the protective efficacy of BCG vaccinations in nine major trials

Country or population	Age range of vaccinees (years)	Protection (%)
North American Indian	0–20	80
UK	14–15	78
Chicago, USA	Neonates	75
Puerto Rico	1–18	31
South India (Bangalore)	All ages	30
Georgia and Alabama, USA	>5	14
Georgia, USA	6–17	0
Illinois, USA	Young adults	0
South India (Chingleput)	All ages	0[a]

[a] Some protection demonstrated in those vaccinated neonatally on 15-year follow-up.

infection rate in the community as the smear-positive source cases arise mostly from among the older, unvaccinated, tuberculin-positive members of the community. Vaccination has therefore not proved to be an effective control measure.

Being a living vaccine, serious infections and even disseminated disease may occur in immunocompromised persons. BCG should never therefore be given to persons known to be HIV-positive.

Prophylactic chemotherapy

In true prophylactic chemotherapy, drugs are administered to uninfected individuals who are in unavoidable contact with a patient with open tuberculosis. The main example is a baby born to a mother with the disease. More usually, it refers to therapy, principally with isoniazid alone, given to individuals who have been infected but show no signs of active disease. In the UK, such therapy may be given to unvaccinated children who have converted to tuberculin positivity after exposure to a source case. The use of prophylactic chemotherapy in older tuberculin reactors is controversial and virtually restricted to countries such as the USA where BCG vaccination is no longer given.

Isoniazid or short (2–4-month) regimens of rifampicin with isoniazid or pyrazinamide give short- or medium-term protection to tuberculin-positive HIV-positive persons. Dually infected persons who are tuberculin-negative, indicative of poor immune responsiveness, are much less protected and thus the WHO recommends prophylactic therapy only for tuberculin reactors.

MYCOBACTERIUM LEPRAE

Leprosy is a particularly tragic affliction as the nature of the infection often causes severe disfigurement and deformity which, throughout history, have led to the social ostracism or total banishment of its victims. The prevalence of leprosy is uncertain. The number of registered patients on treatment declined from over 10 million in 1982 to 1.2 million in 1999, but this may be because of changes in case definition and the much shorter duration of therapy. The annual detection rate of new cases has not shown such a steep decline – indeed, there was a peak of around 800 000 cases in 1998 – but this may reflect a higher case detection rate. About 2–3 million patients have been bacteriologically cured, but have residual deformities requiring life-long care.

Once of worldwide distribution, the disease was reported in 91 mainly tropical countries in the year 2000, with 70% of cases occurring in just three countries: India, Indonesia and Myanmar (Burma). The disease was long endemic in the British Isles, and Robert the Bruce of Scotland was one of its victims. The last British leprosy patient to acquire the disease in this country died in the Shetland islands in 1798. In Norway the disease persisted into the 20th century; the causative organism was first described in that country by Armauer Hansen in 1873.

Leprosy is often cited as a disease of great antiquity but, in fact, literary and skeletal evidence of this very characteristic disease go back no further than 500 BC. Biblical leprosy was almost certainly not the same as the disease that now bears this name.

DESCRIPTION

M. leprae has never convincingly been cultivated in vitro, and this has been a major limiting factor in the study of leprosy. In the 1970s it was found that armadillos infected with *M. leprae* often developed extensive disease, with up to 10^{10} bacilli in each gram of diseased tissue. This animal has therefore provided sufficient bacilli for a number of studies and for the production of a skin test reagent, leprosin-A. Limited replication, yielding 10^6 bacilli after 6–8 months, also occurs in the mouse footpad, and this has been used for testing the sensitivity of bacilli to antileprosy drugs.

Leprosy bacilli resemble tubercle bacilli in their general morphology, but they are not so strongly acid-fast. In clinical material from lepromatous patients they are typically found within macrophages in dense clumps. Studies of the metabolism, biochemical properties and antigenic composition of *M. leprae* are difficult. However, a genomic library has been prepared, providing a potentially unlimited source of recombinant protein antigens for immunological studies. A characteristic surface lipid, peptidoglycolipid 1 (PGL-1), has been extracted from *M. leprae*, and its unique carbohydrate antigenic determinant has been synthesized.

PATHOGENESIS

The principal target cell for the leprosy bacillus is the Schwann cell. The resulting nerve damage is responsible for the main clinical features of leprosy: anaesthesia and muscle paralysis. Repeated injury to, and infections of, the anaesthetic extremities leads to their gradual destruction (Fig. 18.5). Infiltration of the skin and cutaneous nerves by bacilli leads to the formation of visible lesions, often with pigmentary changes.

The first sign of leprosy is a non-specific or indeterminate skin lesion, which often heals spontaneously. If the disease progresses, its clinical manifestation is determined by the specific immune responsiveness of the patient to the bacillus, and there is a distinct immunological spectrum (Table 18.8).

- Hyper-reactive *tuberculoid* (TT) leprosy, with small numbers of localized skin lesions containing so few

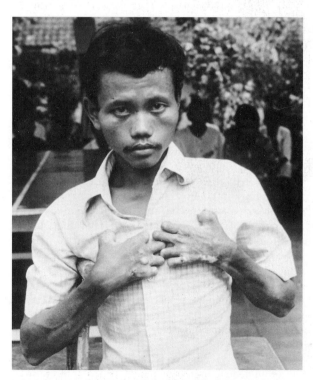

Fig. 18.5 Borderline tuberculoid leprosy. Trophic changes in the hands secondary to nerve damage and anaesthesia. Compare the normal face with Figure 18.6.

Table 18.8 Characteristics of the five points on the spectrum of leprosy

	TT	BT	BB	BL	LL
Bacilli seen in skin	−	+/−	+	++	+++
Bacilli in nasal secretions	−	−	−	+	+++
Granuloma formation	+++	++	+	−	−
Reaction to lepromin	+++	+	+/−	−	−
Antibodies to *M. leprae*	+/−	+/−	+	++	+++
Main phagocytic cell	Mature epithelioid	Immature epithelioid	Immature epithelioid	Macrophage	Macrophage
In-vitro correlates of CMI	+++	++	+	+/−	−
Type 1 reactions	−	+	+	+	−
Type 2 reactions	−	−	−	+/−	++

CMI, cell-mediated immunity; see text for other abbreviations.

bacilli that they are not seen on microscopy and an inappropriately intense granulomatous response that often damages major nerve trunks.

• Anergic *lepromatous* (LL) leprosy, in which the skin lesions are numerous or confluent and contain huge numbers of bacilli, usually seen as clusters or globi within monocytes; cooler parts of the body, such as the ear lobes, are particularly heavily infiltrated by bacilli (Fig. 18.6). There is no histological evidence of an immune response.

• An intermediate form classified as borderline tuberculoid (BT), mid-borderline (BB) or borderline lepromatous (BL).

Destruction of the nasal bones may lead to collapse of the nose (Fig. 18.7). In addition, large numbers of

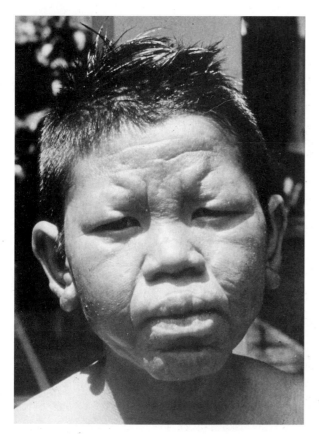

Fig. 18.6 Lepromatous leprosy. Nodular swelling of face, enlargement of ear lobes and loss of eyebrows.

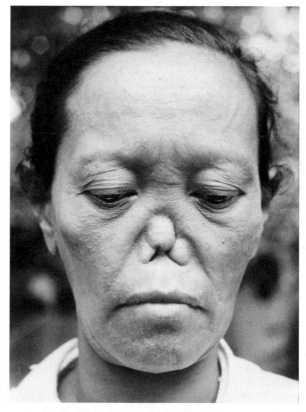

Fig. 18.7 Treated lepromatous leprosy. The nodularity of the skin has resolved on treatment but the absence of eyebrows and the nasal collapse remain.

Table 18.9   Main characteristics of the reactions in leprosy

Characteristics	Type 1 (reversal reaction)	Type 2 (erythema nodosum leprosum)
Immunological basis	Cell-mediated	Vasculitis with antigen–antibody complex deposition
Type of patient	BT, BB, BL	BL, LL
Systemic disturbance	No (or mild)	Yes
Haematological changes	No	Yes
Proteinuria	No	Frequently
Relation to therapy	Usually within first 6 months	Rare during first 6 months

See text for explanation of abbreviations.

leprosy bacilli are discharged in nasal secretions in multibacillary disease. The eye is frequently damaged by direct bacillary invasion, uveitis or corneal infection secondary to paralysis of the eyelids. Blindness is a common and tragic complication of untreated leprosy.

Additional tissue damage in leprosy is caused by immune reactions that are caused by delayed hypersensitivity (Jopling type 1 reactions) or to a vasculitis associated with the deposition of antigen–antibody complexes (Jopling type 2 reactions, *erythema nodosum leprosum*) (Table 18.9). The former, which occurs in borderline cases (BT, BB and BL), may rapidly cause severe and permanent nerve damage, and requires urgent treatment with anti-inflammatory agents and, sometimes, surgical decompression of a greatly swollen nerve.

LABORATORY DIAGNOSIS

The clinical diagnosis may be confirmed by histological examination of skin biopsies and by the detection of acid-fast bacilli in nasal discharges, scrapings from the nasal mucosa and *slit-skin smears*. The latter are prepared by making superficial incisions in the skin, scraping out some tissue fluid and cells, and making smears on glass slides. Smears are obtained from obvious lesions, the ear lobes and apparently unaffected skin. Secretions and skin smears are stained by the ZN method, and the number of bacilli seen in each high-power field is recorded as the *bacillary index* (BI):

1+	1–10 bacilli per 100 fields
2+	1–10 bacilli per 10 fields
3+	1–10 bacilli per field
4+	10–100 bacilli per field
5+	100–1000 bacilli per field
6+	>1000 bacilli per field.

Patients with clinically active leprosy, but in whom no bacilli are seen on slit-skin smear examination, are termed *paucibacillary* (PB) and those who are positive at any site are termed *multibacillary* (MB). This is an important distinction for the selection of treatment (see below).

It is widely assumed, but unproven, that leprosy bacilli that stain strongly and evenly are viable while those that stain weakly and irregularly are dead. The percentage of the former gives the *morphological index*, which declines during chemotherapy. An increase in the morphological index is a useful indication of non-compliance of the patient and the emergence of drug resistance. The PCR is increasingly used to detect *M. leprae* in clinical specimens.

TREATMENT

Monotherapy with dapsone (4,4′-diaminodiphenyl sulphone; DDS) has been abandoned in favour of multidrug therapy based on dapsone, rifampicin and clofazimine. The regimen is determined by whether the patient has paucibacillary or multibacillary disease (Table 18.10).

Table 18.10   WHO recommendations for multidrug therapy

Type of leprosy	Drug	Dose	Frequency	Total duration
Paucibacillary	Rifampicin	600 mg	Monthly, supervised	6 months
	Dapsone	100 mg	Daily, unsupervised	
Multibacillary	Rifampicin	600 mg	Monthly, supervised	2 years or more
	Dapsone	100 mg	Daily, unsupervised	
	Clofazimine	{300 mg	Monthly, supervised	
		{+50 mg	Daily, unsupervised	

Clofazimine causes skin discoloration, particularly in fair-skinned people. If this causes the patient to refuse the drug, prothionamide, ofloxacin or minocycline may be used instead.

The treatment of leprosy demands far more than the administration of antimicrobial agents. It is often necessary to:

- correct deformities
- prevent blindness and further damage to anaesthetic extremities
- treat reactions with anti-inflammatory drugs
- attend to the patient's social, psychological and spiritual welfare.

EPIDEMIOLOGY

Until recently, leprosy was thought to be restricted to man, but the disease has been reported in chimpanzees and sooty mangabey monkeys in Africa and in free-living armadillos in Louisiana, USA. It was also thought that leprosy was transmitted by skin-to-skin contact but it now appears more likely that the bacilli are disseminated from the nasal secretions of patients with lepromatous leprosy. In addition, the blood of patients with lepromatous leprosy contains enough bacilli to render transmission by blood-sucking insects a definite, though unproven, possibility.

As in the case of tuberculosis, transmission of bacilli from patients with multibacillary leprosy to their contacts occurs readily, but only a minority of those infected develop overt disease. The infectivity of patients with paucibacillary leprosy is much lower. Leprosy often commences during childhood or early adult life but, as the incubation period is usually 3–5 years, it is rare in children aged less than 5 years.

Epidemiological studies on the prevalence and transmission of leprosy have been aided by skin test reagents, of which there are two types:

- *lepromins*, which are prepared from boiled bacilli-rich lepromatous lesions
- *leprosins*, which are ultrasonicates of tissue-free bacilli extracted from lesions (the suffixes -H and -A are used to denote human and armadillo origins, respectively).

These reagents elicit two types of reaction:

- The *Fernandez reaction* is analogous to tuberculin reactivity and appears in sensitized subjects 48 h after skin testing. It is best seen with leprosins.
- The *Mitsuda reaction* is a granulomatous swelling which appears about 3 weeks after testing with lepromin. This reaction is indicative of the host's ability to give a granulomatous response to antigens of *M. leprae*, and is positive at or near the TT pole.

Skin testing is of limited diagnostic value, but is useful in epidemiological studies to establish the extent of infection in contacts and in the community, and in classifying patients according to the immunological spectrum.

CONTROL

The most effective control measure in leprosy, as in tuberculosis, is the detection and treatment of infectious cases. This requires that patients should attend for therapy as soon as signs of the disease appear. Unfortunately, owing to the stigma associated with the disease, many patients delay seeking treatment until they have infected many contacts and have developed irreversible disfigurement and handicap.

No living attenuated vaccines have been prepared for *M. leprae*, but BCG vaccine seems to protect against leprosy in those regions where it protects against tuberculosis, strongly suggesting that protection is induced by common mycobacterial antigens.

RECOMMENDED READING

Collins C H, Grange J M, Yates M D 1997 *Tuberculosis Bacteriology: Organization and Practice*, 2nd edn. Butterworth-Heinemann, London
Davies P D O (ed.) 1998 *Clinical Tuberculosis*. 2nd edn. Chapman and Hall, London
Friedland J S 1999 Tuberculosis. In Armstrong D, Cohen J (eds) *Infectious Diseases*. Mosby, London, pp. 2.30.1-16
Grange J M 1996 *Mycobacteria and Human Disease*, 2nd edn. Arnold, London
Porter J D H, Grange J M (eds) 1999 *Tuberculosis. An interdisciplinary Perspective*. Imperial College Press, London
Ridley D S 1988 *Pathogenesis of Leprosy and Related Diseases*. Wright, London
World Health Organization 1997 *Treatment of Tuberculosis. Guidelines for National Programmes* and *Guidelines for the Management of Drug-Resistant Tuberculosis*. World Health Organization, Geneva
Zumla A, Ustianowski A, Lucas S, Munthali L 1999 Leprosy. In: James D G, Zumla A (eds) *The Granulomatous Disorders*. Cambridge University Press, Cambridge, pp 173–188

CD ROMs

Wellcome Trust 1999 *Tuberculosis* (Topics in International Health). CAB International, Wallingford
Wellcome Trust 1999 *Leprosy* (Topics in International Health). CAB International, Wallingford

Internet sites

Tuberculosis

World Health Organization: www.who.int/gtb
Montefiore Medical Center, New York: www.tuberculosis.net
New Jersey Medical School: www.umdnj.edu/~ntbcweb
Division of Tuberculosis Elimination, CDC Atlanta: www.cdc/gov/nchstp/tb
International Union Against Tuberculosis and Lung Disease: www.iuatld.org

TB Focus: www.pol-it.org/cmol/TBFocus.htm
Public Health Laboratory Service: www.phls.org.uk/facts/TB

Leprosy

World Health Organization: www.who.int/lep
International Federation of Antileprosy Associations: www.ilep.org.uk
Forum on Leprosy: www.webspawner.com/users/leprosy

19

Environmental mycobacteria

Opportunist disease

J. M. Grange

In addition to the tubercle and leprosy bacilli there are over 80 species of mycobacteria that normally exist as saprophytes of soil and water. Termed environmental (or non-tuberculous) mycobacteria, some species occasionally cause opportunist disease in animals and man. Although such opportunist pathogens were described towards the end of the 19th century, their classification remained in a state of chaos for over 50 years and they were often called *anonymous mycobacteria*. Order began to replace chaos in 1959 when a botanist, Ernest Runyon, described four groups of mycobacteria associated with human disease according to their production of yellow or orange pigment and their rate of growth:

- *Photochromogens*, which are colourless when incubated in the dark, but develop a bright yellow or orange coloration if young cultures are exposed to a light source for an hour or more and then re-incubated. The caps of the culture bottles must be loosened during exposure to light, as oxygen is essential for pigment formation.
- *Scotochromogens*, which produce pigmented colonies even when grown in the dark.
- *Non-chromogens*, which are unpigmented.
- *Rapid growers*, which may be photochromogens, scotochromogens or non-chromogens; they produce visible growth on Löwenstein–Jensen medium within 1 week on subculture, though growth on primary culture of clinical material often takes considerably longer.

DESCRIPTION

Photochromogens

This group contains the following species:

- *Mycobacterium kansasii*, which grows well at 37°C and is principally isolated from cases of pulmonary disease. On microscopy, it often appears elongated and distinctly beaded.

- *M. simiae*, which, like *M. kansasii*, grows at 37°C and is occasionally involved in pulmonary disease.
- *M. marinum* (previously termed the fish tubercle bacillus) the cause of a warty skin infection known as *swimming pool granuloma*. It grows poorly, if at all at 37°C, and cultures from skin lesions should be incubated at 33°C. Microscopically, it resembles *M. kansasii*.

Scotochromogens

Most slowly growing scotochromogens isolated from sputum or urine are of no clinical significance.

- *M. gordonae* (formerly *M. aquae*), frequently found in water and a common contaminant of clinical material, is a rare cause of pulmonary disease.
- *M. scrofulaceum* is principally associated with scrofula or cervical lymphadenitis, but also causes pulmonary disease.
- *M. szulgai*, an uncommon cause of pulmonary disease and bursitis, is a scotochromogen when incubated at 37°C but a photochromogen at 25°C.

Non-chromogens

The most prevalent and important opportunistic pathogens of man are:

- *M. avium* (the avian tubercle bacillus)
- the closely related *M. intracellulare*, formerly known as the Battey bacillus.

These two species are usually grouped together as the *M. avium* complex. Most clinical isolates are smooth and easy to emulsify; 28 serotypes are delineated by agglutination by specific antisera, although untypable strains are not uncommon. Organisms of the *M. avium* complex cause tuberculosis in birds and lymphadenitis in pigs as well as occasional disease in various other wild and domestic animals. In man, they are responsible for lymphadenitis, pulmonary lesions and disseminated disease, notably in patients with the acquired immune deficiency syndrome (AIDS). Most isolates from AIDS patients are of serotypes 1, 4 and 8 which, on DNA analysis, show homology with *M. avium* rather than *M. intracellulare*.

Other non-chromogens include:

- *M. ulcerans*, a very slowly growing species that will grow in vitro only at 31–34°C. Colonies are non-pigmented or a pale lemon-yellow colour. *M. ulcerans* is the cause of *Buruli ulcer*; unlike other mycobacterial pathogens it produces a toxin that causes tissue necrosis and is involved in the pathogenesis of disease.
- *M. shinshuense*, a very rare cause of skin ulcers in Japan and China, which is a variant of *M. ulcerans*.
- *M. paratuberculosis*, the cause of chronic hypertrophic enteritis or *Johne's disease* of cattle. There have been claims, which remain to be substantiated, that it is a cause of Crohn's disease in man. It produces little or no mycobactin, a lipid-soluble iron-binding compound essential for growth, and this substance must be added to media used for cultivation.
- *M. xenopi*, which was originally isolated from a xenopus toad; it is a thermophile that grows well at 45°C. It is principally responsible for pulmonary lesions in man. Most reported cases have been from London and south-east England and northern France. Two phylogenetically similar species, *M. celatum* and *M. branderi*, have been described.
- *M. malmoense* is a cause of pulmonary disease and lymphadenitis. It grows very slowly, often taking as long as 10 weeks to appear on primary culture, and is therefore likely to be missed if cultures are discarded earlier. For unknown reasons, isolation of this pathogen is increasing in several European countries. In some regions, notably northern England, it has become one of the most frequently isolated of the environmental mycobacteria from cases of pulmonary disease.
- *M. sylvaticum*, the cause of tuberculosis in wood pigeons. Like *M. paratuberculosis* it needs mycobactin for growth.
- *M. lepraemurium*, the cause of a leprosy-like disease of rats, mice and cats.
- *M. terrae*, the radish bacillus, *M. nonchromogenicum* and *M. triviale*, which are sometimes grouped as the *M. terrae* complex.
- *M. haemophilum*, characterized by its growth requirement for haem or other sources of iron, is a rare cause of granulomatous or ulcerative skin lesions in xenograft recipients and other immunocompromised individuals, and lymphadenitis in otherwise healthy children.

- *M. genevense*, a very slow growing organism occasionally isolated from AIDS patients with disseminated mycobacterial disease and from pet birds.

Rapid growers

Only two of the rapidly growing species are well recognized human pathogens:

- *M. chelonae* (the turtle tubercle bacillus), some isolates of which are sometimes classified as *M. abscessus*.
- *M. fortuitum* (the frog tubercle bacillus), some isolates of which are sometimes classified as *M. peregrinum*.

Both species are non-chromogenic. They occasionally cause pulmonary or disseminated disease but are principally responsible for post-injection abscesses and wound infections, including corneal ulcers.

Most of the many other rapidly growing species are pigmented. Disease due to these is exceedingly rare, but they frequently contaminate clinical specimens. They are found on the genitalia, and gain access to urine samples, although, contrary to a common belief, *M. smegmatis* is rarely found in this site. *M. flavescens*, which grows more slowly than other members of this group and is therefore sometimes classified as a slow grower, is an occasional cause of post-injection abscesses.

PATHOGENESIS

Compared with tubercle bacilli, environmental mycobacteria are of low virulence and, although man is frequently infected, overt disease is very uncommon except in those who are profoundly immunosuppressed. Four main types of opportunist mycobacterial disease have been described in man (Table 19.1):

- localized lymphadenitis
- skin lesions following traumatic inoculation of bacteria
- tuberculosis-like pulmonary lesions
- disseminated disease.

Lymphadenitis

This is caused by a number of different species, which vary in relative frequency from region to region. The *M. avium* complex is the predominant cause worldwide. Some reports claim a high incidence of *M. scrofulaceum*, but these strains were probably misidentified members of the *M. avium* complex. In most cases a single node, usually tonsillar, is involved, and most patients are children aged less than 5 years. Unless contra-indicated by

Table 19.1 Principal types of opportunist mycobacterial disease in man and the usual causative agents

Disease	Usual causative agent
Lymphadenopathy	M. avium complex
	M. scrofulaceum
Skin lesions	
Post-trauma abscesses	M. chelonae
	M. fortuitum
	M. terrae
Swimming pool granuloma	M. marinum
Buruli ulcer	M. ulcerans
Pulmonary disease	M. avium complex
	M. kansasii
	M. xenopi
	M. malmoense
Disseminated disease	
AIDS-related	M. avium complex
	M. genevense
Non-AIDS-related	M. avium complex
	M. chelonae

the risk of nerve damage, excision of the node, usually performed for diagnostic purposes, is almost always curative. The incidence of this disease has increased in England since 1990, but it is not clear whether this is a real increase or merely due to a greater diagnostic awareness of mycobacterial disease. Lymphadenitis occasionally occurs as part of a more disseminated infection, particularly in individuals with AIDS.

Skin lesions

Three main types have been described: post-injection (and post-traumatic) abscesses, swimming pool granuloma and Buruli ulcer.

Post-injection abscesses

These are usually caused by the rapidly growing pathogens *M. chelonae* and *M. fortuitum*. Abscesses occur sporadically, particularly in the tropics, or in small epidemics when batches of injectable materials are contaminated by these bacteria. Abscesses develop within a week or so, or up to a year or more after the injection. They are painful, may become quite large – up to 8 or 10 cm in diameter – and may persist for many months. Treatment is by drainage with curettage or total excision. Chemotherapy is not required unless there is local spread of disease or multiple abscesses, as may occur in insulin-dependent diabetics.

More serious lesions, also usually due to *M. chelonae* and *M. fortuitum*, have followed surgery, usually those

procedures involving insertion of prostheses such as heart valves, and corneal infections have followed ocular injuries. Infections by *M. terrae* have occurred in farmers and others who have been injured while working with soil.

Swimming pool granuloma

This is also known as *fish tank granuloma* and *fish fancier's finger*, and is caused by *M. marinum*. Those affected are mostly users of swimming pools, keepers of tropical fish and others involved in aquatic hobbies. The bacilli enter scratches and abrasions and cause warty lesions similar to those seen in skin tuberculosis. The lesions, which usually occur on the knees and elbows of swimmers and on the hands of aquarium keepers, are usually localized, but secondary lesions sometimes appear along the line of the dermal lymphatics. This is termed *sporotrichoid spread* as a similar phenomenon occurs in the fungus infection sporotrichosis (p. 579). The disease is usually self-limiting although chemotherapy with minocycline, co-trimoxazole or rifampicin with ethambutol hastens its resolution.

Buruli ulcer

This disease, caused by *M. ulcerans*, was first described in Australia, but the name is derived from the Buruli district of Uganda where a large outbreak was extensively investigated. Buruli ulcer occurs in several tropical countries, notably Nigeria, Ghana, Zaire, Mexico, Malaysia and Papua New Guinea, and is limited to certain localities, characteristically low-lying marshy areas subject to periodic flooding. *M. shinshuense*, a very rare cause of similar lesions in Japan and China, is a variant of *M. ulcerans*. Although never isolated in culture from the environment, there is strong evidence that *M. ulcerans* is a free-living species that is introduced into the human dermis by minor injuries, particularly by spiky grasses. In recent years the number and severity of cases has increased in western equatorial Africa. This does not appear to be related to infection with the human immunodeficiency virus (HIV) and the cause remains uncertain.

The first manifestation of the disease is a hard cutaneous nodule, which is often itchy. This enlarges and develops central softening and fluctuation owing to necrosis of the underlying adipose subcutaneous tissues caused by a toxin. The overlying skin becomes anoxic and breaks down, the liquefied necrotic contents of the lesion are discharged and one or more ulcers with deeply undermined edges are thereby formed (Fig. 19.1). At this stage the lesion is teeming with acid-fast bacilli, there is no histological evidence of an active cell-mediated

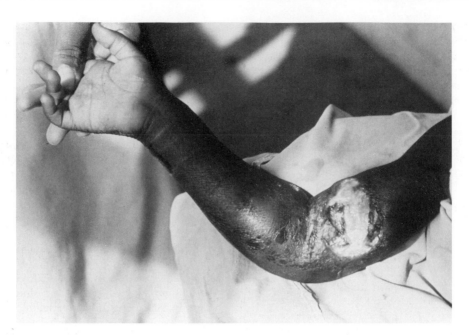

Fig. 19.1 Buruli ulcer. Undermined ulcer overlying the biceps and swelling of the surrounding tissues. (By courtesy of Dr Alan Knell, Wellcome Tropical Institute.)

immune response and the patient does not react to burulin, a skin test reagent prepared from *M. ulcerans*. During this anergic stage the lesion may progressively extend to an enormous size, sometimes involving an entire limb or a major part of the trunk.

For unknown reasons, the anergic phase may give way to an immunoreactive phase when a granulomatous response develops in the lesion, the acid-fast bacilli disappear and the patient reacts to burulin. Healing then occurs but the patient is often left with considerable disfigurement and disability caused by extensive scarring and contractures.

The early, pre-ulcerative, lesions are easily treatable by excision and primary closure by suture. Ulcerated lesions require excision and skin grafting. In the anergic phase, the excision must be extensive enough to remove all disease to avoid recurrences. Therapy with various chemotherapeutic regimens has been attempted but with unconvincing results.

Pulmonary disease

This is most frequently seen in middle-aged or elderly men with lung damage caused by smoking or exposure to industrial dusts. It also occurs in individuals with congenital or acquired immune deficiencies, malignant disease and cystic fibrosis, but a substantial minority of cases occur in persons with no apparent underlying localized or generalized disorder. The disease may be caused by many species, but the most frequent are the *M. avium* complex and *M. kansasii*. Other causative organisms in the UK are *M. xenopi* and *M. malmoense*, with the former being more common in the south of the country and the latter in the north.

Disseminated disease

In the 1980s and early 1990s, up to a half of all persons dying of AIDS in the USA had disseminated mycobacterial disease, almost always due to the *M. avium* complex. This AIDS-related disease was also common in Europe, although it was uncommon in Africa. The introduction of highly active antiretroviral therapy (pp. 533–534) in the developed nations has led to a substantial decline in the incidence of this disease.

The source of the causative organisms is uncertain: some workers consider that disease is due to reactivation of dormant foci of infection acquired in childhood whereas others argue that they result from recent infection from the environment; these explanations are not mutually exclusive. For unknown reasons, the serotypes of the *M. avium* complex causing HIV-related disease are more restricted than those causing non-HIV-related disease and are those corresponding to *M. avium* rather than *M. intracellulare*. Acid-fast bacilli are readily isolated from bone marrow aspirates, intestinal biopsies, blood and faeces. A few cases of AIDS-related disseminated disease have been caused by other species, including *M. genavense*.

Disseminated disease occasionally occurs in individuals with other congenital or acquired causes of immunosuppression, including renal transplantation. Again, the *M. avium* complex is the usual cause, but disseminated *M. chelonae* infections have occurred in recipients of renal transplants and in other immunocompromised patients (Fig. 19.2).

Chronic, localized non-pulmonary lesions, usually in the kidney or bone, caused by various species and with no evident predisposing cause have been described, but they are extremely uncommon.

LABORATORY DIAGNOSIS

Most environmental mycobacteria can be detected microscopically and cultured on media suitable for *M. tuberculosis* (pp. 200–201). However, great care must be taken to differentiate true disease from transient colonization or superinfection. In particular, there are no clinical or radiological characteristics that reliably differentiate pulmonary disease caused by opportunist mycobacteria from tuberculosis, and the diagnosis is therefore made by isolation and identification of the pathogen. As a general rule, a diagnosis of opportunist mycobacterial disease may be made when a heavy growth of the pathogen is repeatedly isolated from the sputum of a patient with compatible clinical and radiological features and in whom other causes of these features have been carefully excluded.

Identification is usually undertaken by specialist reference laboratories. There is no universally recognized identification scheme, although reliance is usually placed on cultural characteristics (rate and temperature of growth and pigmentation), various biochemical reactions and resistance to antimicrobial agents. Many reference centres now use nucleic acid-based methods to identify known species and delineate new ones. The most discriminative methods are based on the detection of sequence differences in 16S ribosomal RNA.

TREATMENT

Most environmental mycobacteria are resistant to many antituberculosis drugs in vitro although infections often respond to various combinations of these drugs. Regimens containing five or six antituberculosis drugs have been used for pulmonary disease caused by the *M. avium* complex, *M. kansasii*, *M. xenopi* and *M. malmoense*, but equal success has been obtained with three drugs – rifampicin, isoniazid and ethambutol – provided that all three are given for up to 18 months. Treatment is, however, unsuccessful in a substantial minority of cases, and localized lesions are surgically excised when possible. Limited experience indicates that the newer macrolides and fluoroquinolones are efficacious.

Pulmonary and non-pulmonary disease due to the rapidly growing species *M. chelonae* and *M. fortuitum* have been treated successfully by various combinations

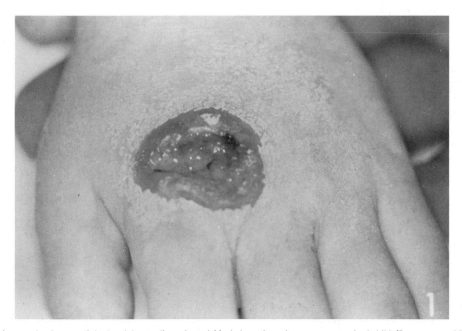

Fig. 19.2 Skin ulcer on the dorsum of the hand due to disseminated *M. chelonae* in an immunocompromised child. (By courtesy of Dr Kurt Schopfer.)

of erythromycin, newer macrolides, sulphonamides, trimethoprim, amikacin, gentamicin, imipenem, extended-spectrum cephalosporins and fluoroquinolones, according to the results of in-vitro susceptibility tests. Despite in-vitro susceptibility, some infections, notably keratitis due to *M. chelonae*, frequently relapse and require surgical intervention.

Various multidrug regimens for AIDS-associated disease caused by the *M. avium* complex have been described. A widely used regimen contains a macrolide (clarithromycin or azithromycin), rifabutin and ethambutol. Amikacin is added if oral regimens are ineffective. Prophylactic therapy is controversial and, with the advent of effective antiretroviral treatment, rarely used.

EPIDEMIOLOGY

Mycobacteria are widely distributed in the environment and are particularly abundant in wet soil, marshland, streams, rivers and estuaries. Some species, such as *M. terrae*, are found in soil while others, including *M. marinum* and *M. gordonae*, prefer free water. Some potential pathogens, notably the *M. avium* complex, *M. kansasii* and *M. xenopi*, are able to colonize pipedwater supplies. Human beings are therefore regularly exposed to mycobacteria as a result of drinking, washing, showering and inhalation of natural aerosols. Such repeated subclinical infection may induce sensitization to tuberculin and other mycobacterial skin-testing reagents. There is also evidence that contact with environmental mycobacteria profoundly affects the subsequent ability of BCG (bacille Calmette-Guérin) vaccine to induce protective immunity, thereby explaining the great regional differences in the efficacy of this vaccine (p. 209).

In countries in which tuberculosis is uncommon, opportunist mycobacterial infections are relatively common. In south-east England, about 5% of mycobacterial disease is due to environmental species; the proportion is much higher in some parts of the USA. In addition, the absolute incidence is increasing as a result of the growing number of immunocompromised individuals, notably patients with AIDS.

A number of 'epidemics' of falsely diagnosed mycobacterial pulmonary disease and urinary tract infection have resulted from the collection of sputum and urine specimens in containers rinsed out with water from taps colonized by mycobacteria. Inadequate cleaning of endoscopes has also led to mycobacterial contamination of clinical specimens and diagnostic confusion. Likewise, false-positive sputum smear examinations for acid-fast bacilli have occurred when staining reagents were prepared from contaminated water.

CONTROL

The incidence and type of disease in any region are determined by the species and numbers of mycobacteria in the environment and the opportunities for human transmission. Unlike tuberculosis, person-to-person transmission of opportunist mycobacterial disease rarely, if ever, occurs. Thus the incidence of such disease is independent of that of tuberculosis and unaffected by public health measures designed to control the latter.

RECOMMENDED READING

Grange J M 1996 *Mycobacteria and Human Disease*, 2nd edn. Arnold, London

Pitchenik A E, Fertel D 1992 Medical management of AIDS patients: tuberculosis and nontuberculous mycobacterial disease. *Medical Clinics of North America* 76: 121–171

Ratledge C, Stanford J L, Grange J M (eds) 1989 *The Biology of the Mycobacteria, Clinical Aspects of Mycobacterial Disease*. Academic Press, London, Vol. 3, Chapters 3, 10 and 11

Salfinger M, Pfyffer G E 1994 The new diagnostic mycobacteriology laboratory. *European Journal of Clinical Microbiology and Infectious Diseases* 13: 961–979

Subcommittee of the Joint Tuberculosis Committee of the British Thoracic Society 2000 Management of opportunist mycobacterial infections. *Thorax* 55: 210–218

Wansbrough-Jones M H 1999 Non-tuberculous or atypical mycobacteria. In: James DG, Zumla A (eds) *The Granulomatous Disorders*. Cambridge University Press, Cambridge, pp 189–204

20

Actinomyces, nocardia and tropheryma

Actinomycosis; nocardiasis; Whipple's disease

J. M. Grange

Gram-positive bacteria with branching filaments that sometimes develop into mycelia are included in the rather loosely defined order Actinomycetales. Although mostly soil saprophytes, four genera, *Actinomyces, Nocardia, Propionibacterium* and *Bifidobacterium* (the latter two are briefly considered in Chapter 36) occasionally cause chronic granulomatous infections in animals and man. *Tropheryma whippelii* is a newly recognized species thought to be an actinomycete on the basis of nucleic acid studies. Another genus, *Streptomyces*, is an extremely rare cause of disease, but is the source of several antibiotics. Repeated inhalation of thermophilic actinomycetes, notably *Faenia rectivirgula* and *Thermoactinomyces* species, causes *extrinsic allergic alveolitis (farmer's lung, mushroom worker's lung, bagassosis)* in those who are occupationally exposed to mouldy vegetable matter.

ACTINOMYCES

DESCRIPTION

Actinomyces are branching Gram-positive bacilli. They are facultative anaerobes, but often fail to grow aerobically on primary culture. They grow best under anaerobic or micro-aerophilic conditions with the addition of 5–10% carbon dioxide. Almost all species are commensals of the mouth and have a narrow temperature range of growth of around 35–37°C. They are responsible for the disease known as *actinomycosis*, which, in man, is usually caused by *Actinomyces israelii*, which accounts for three-quarters of the cases. Less common causes include *A. gerencseriae, A. naeslundii, A. odontolyticus, A. viscosus, A. meyeri, Propionibacterium propionicum* and members of the genus *Bifidobacterium*.

Concomitant bacteria, notably a small Gram-negative rod, *Actinobacillus actinomycetemcomitans*, but also *Haemophilus* species, fusiforms and anaerobic streptococci, are sometimes found in actinomycotic lesions, but their contribution to the pathogenesis of the disease, if any, is unknown. *Act. actinomycetemcomitans* is a rare cause of endocarditis.

PATHOGENESIS

Actinomycosis is a chronic disease characterized by multiple abscesses and granulomata, tissue destruction, extensive fibrosis and the formation of sinuses. Within diseased tissues the actinomycetes form large masses of mycelia embedded in an amorphous protein–polysaccharide matrix and surrounded by a zone of Gram-negative, weakly acid-fast, club-like structures (Fig. 20.1). These clubs were once thought to consist, at least in part, of material derived from host tissue, but it now appears that they are formed entirely from the bacteria. The mycelial masses may be visible to the naked eye and, as they are often light yellow in colour, they are

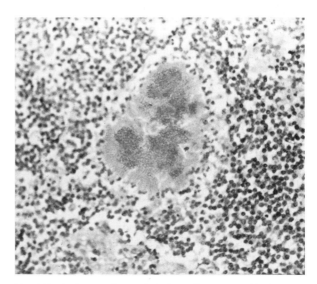

Fig. 20.1 Actinomycotic granule in tissue. (By courtesy of Professor R. J. Hay.)

called *sulphur granules*. In older lesions the sulphur granules may be dark brown and very hard because of the deposition of calcium phosphate in the matrix.

Human actinomycosis may take several forms:

- Around 98% of cases of occur in the cervicofacial region; the jaw is often involved. The disease is endogenous in origin: dental caries is a predisposing factor, and infection may follow tooth extractions or other dental procedures. Men are affected more frequently than women, and in some regions the disease is more common in rural agricultural workers than in town dwellers, probably owing to lower standards of dental care in the former.
- Thoracic actinomycosis commences in the lung, probably as a result of aspiration of actinomyces from the mouth. Sinuses often appear on the chest wall, and the ribs and spine may be eroded.
- Abdominal cases commence in the appendix or, less frequently, in colonic diverticula.
- Pelvic actinomycosis occasionally occurs in women fitted with plastic intra-uterine contraceptive devices.
- 'Punch actinomycosis' is a rare infection of the hand acquired by injury of the knuckles on an adversary's teeth.

The lymphatics are not usually involved in actinomycosis, but haematogenous spread to the liver, brain and other internal organs occasionally occurs. Involvement of bone is much less common in man than in animals and is usually the result of direct extension of adjacent soft tissue lesions.

LABORATORY DIAGNOSIS

Specimens should be obtained directly from lesions by open biopsy, needle aspiration or, in the case of pulmonary lesions, by fibre-optic bronchoscopy. Examination of sputum is of no value as it frequently contains oral actinomycetes. Material from suspected cases is shaken with sterile water in a tube. Sulphur granules settle to the bottom and may be removed with a Pasteur pipette. Granules crushed between two glass slides are stained by the Gram and Ziehl–Neelsen (modified by using 1% sulphuric acid for decolorization) methods, which reveal the Gram-positive mycelia and the zone of radiating acid-fast clubs. Sulphur granules and mycelia in tissue sections are identifiable by use of fluorescein-conjugated specific antisera.

For culture, washed and crushed granules are used to inoculate suitable media, which include blood or brain–heart infusion agar, glucose broth and enriched thioglycollate broth. Cultures are incubated aerobically and anaerobically for up to 10 days. After several days on agar media, *A. israelii* may form so-called *spider colonies* that resemble molar teeth. The identity may be confirmed by biochemical tests, staining with specific fluorescent antisera or by gas chromatography of metabolic products of carbohydrate fermentation.

TREATMENT

Actinomyces are sensitive to many antibiotics, but the penetration of drugs into the densely fibrotic diseased tissue is poor. Thus, large doses are required for prolonged periods, and recurrence of disease is not uncommon. Surgical debridement reduces scarring and deformity, hastens healing and lowers the incidence of recurrences. Penicillins are frequently used. As lesions are often concomitantly infected with β-lactamase-producing bacteria, the preferred treatment for cervico-facial disease is a 2-week course of co-amoxiclav (p. 49). Thoracic disease requires treatment for up to 4 weeks and, in severe cases, the addition of 2 g of ampicillin thrice daily. Tetracyclines are used if the patient is allergic to penicillin. Additional drugs, including aminoglycosides, clindamycin and metronidazole, may be required if concomitant organisms are present.

NOCARDIA

DESCRIPTION

The nocardiae are branched, strictly aerobic, Gram-positive bacteria, which are closely related to the rapidly growing mycobacteria. Like the latter, but unlike actinomyces, they are environmental saprophytes with a broad temperature range of growth. The properties of nocardiae and actinomycetes are compared in Table 20.1. Most species are acid-fast when decolorized with 1% sulphuric acid; some bacteriologists prefer to place the few that are not acid-fast in the separate genus *Actinomadura*.

Many species of nocardiae are found in the environment, notably in soil, but opportunist disease in man is

Table 20.1 Differences between the genera *Actinomyces* and *Nocardia*

Actinomyces spp.	*Nocardia* spp.
Facultative anaerobes	Strict aerobes
Grow at 35–37°C	Wide temperature range of growth
Oral commensals	Environmental saprophytes
Non-acid-fast mycelia	Usually weakly acid-fast
Endogenous cause of disease	Exogenous cause of disease

almost always caused by *Nocardia asteroides*, so named because of its star-shaped colonies, *N. brasiliensis*, *N. farcinica*, *N. otitidis caviarum*, *N. nova* and *N. transvalensis*.

Bovine farcy, a lymphocutaneous disease of cattle in Africa, formerly thought to be nocardial, is now known to be caused by *Mycobacterium farcinogenes* and *M. senegalense*. Other nocardia-like organisms that are very rare causes of human disease are included in the separate genera *Gordona*, *Oerskovia*, *Rothia* and *Tsukamurella*.

PATHOGENESIS

Nocardiae, principally *N. asteroides*, are uncommon causes of opportunist pulmonary disease that usually, but not always, occurs in immunocompromised individuals, including those receiving corticosteroid therapy, post-transplant immunosuppressive therapy, chemotherapy for cancer and those with the acquired immune deficiency syndrome (AIDS). As a result, the frequency of nocardial disease has increased over the last 20 years.

Pre-existing lung disease, notably alveolar proteinosis, also predisposes to nocardial disease. The infection is exogenous, resulting from inhalation of the bacilli. The clinical and radiological features are highly variable and non-specific, and diagnosis is not easy. In most cases there are multiple confluent abscesses with little or no surrounding fibrous reaction and local spread may result in empyema. In some cases the disease is very chronic while in others it spreads rapidly through the lungs. Secondary abscesses in the brain and, less frequently, in other organs occur in about one-third of patients with pulmonary nocardiasis. Acute dissemination with involvement of many organs occurs in profoundly immunosuppressed persons, notably those with AIDS.

Other conditions associated with nocardiae include:

- Primary post-traumatic or post-inoculation cutaneous infections with involvement of the lymphatics, usually caused by *N. asteroides*.
- Fungating tumour-like masses termed *mycetomata* (Fig. 20.2) resulting from cutaneous infections. The condition is found in the USA and the southern hemisphere, but rarely in Europe; the causative agent is *N. brasiliensis* or, less frequently, *N. caviae*.
- *Madura foot*, a chronic granulomatous infection of the bones and soft tissues of the foot resulting in mycetoma formation and gross deformity. It occurs in Sudan, north Africa and the west coast of India, principally among those who walk barefoot and are therefore prone to contamination of foot injuries by soil-derived organisms. A common causative organism is *Actinomadura (Nocardia) madurae*, but it is also

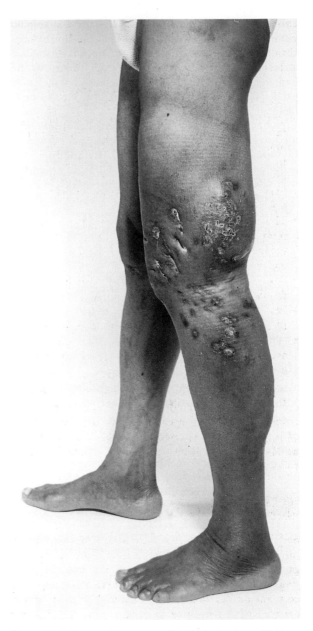

Fig. 20.2 Actinomycotic mycetoma of the thigh, showing multiple fungating nodules and sinuses. (By courtesy of Mr R. D. Rosin.)

caused by other actinomycetes, including *Streptomyces somaliensis*, and by fungi (see p. 578).

LABORATORY DIAGNOSIS

A presumptive diagnosis of pulmonary nocardiasis may be made by a microscopic examination of sputum. In many cases the sputum contains numerous lymphocytes and macrophages, some of which contain pleomorphic Gram-positive and weakly acid-fast bacilli, and occasionally extracellular branching filaments. Nocardiae are not so easily seen in tissue biopsies stained by the Gram or modified Ziehl–Neelsen methods but they may be seen in preparations stained by the Gomori methenamine silver method.

Nocardiae grow on most standard bacteriological media in 2 days to 1 month. Selective growth is favoured by incubation at 45°C. In addition, the technique of *paraffin baiting* may be used: a paraffin wax-coated glass rod is placed in inoculated carbon-free broth. Nocardiae grow on the rod at the air–liquid interface and may be subcultured onto agar media.

Colonies of nocardiae are cream, orange or pink-coloured; their surfaces may develop a dry, chalky appearance and they adhere firmly to the medium. Identification of species is not easy and is usually undertaken in reference laboratories by sequence analysis of the 16S ribosomal RNA (ribotyping).

TREATMENT

The therapy of choice for disease caused by *N. asteroides* and *N. farcinica* is high-dose imipenem with amikacin for 4–6 weeks. Other species may be resistant to one or other of these agents, but they usually respond to treatment with a sulphonamide, with or without trimethoprim, or minocycline for an extended period, often 3 months or more. Mycetomata due to nocardiae are much easier to treat than those caused by fungi. Even long-standing cases with extensive mycetoma formation respond well to chemotherapy.

TROPHERYMA WHIPPELII

Whipple's disease is a multisystem disease with symptoms including diarrhoea and malabsorption, often with arthralgia, fever and, in 10% of cases, central nervous system (CNS) involvement. Gene amplification techniques indicate that a Gram-positive bacillus seen histologically in gut tissue is an actinomycete with a unique 16S ribosomal RNA sequence. The organism, which does not grow on conventional culture media, but replicates in human fibroblast cells, has been named *Tropheryma whippelii*. Diagnosis is usually made by histological examination of intestinal biopsies and by PCR. The usual treatment consists of a 2-week course of streptomycin with either benzylpenicillin or, in the case of CNS involvement, ceftriaxone, followed by co-trimoxazole for 1 year. Relapses involving the CNS have responded to a 1-year course of chloramphenicol.

RECOMMENDED READING

Curry W A 1980 Human nocardosis – a clinical review with selected case reports. *Archives of Internal Medicine* 140: 818–826

Gyles C L 1995 Nocardia; actinomyces; dermatophilus. In: Gyles C L, Thoen C O (eds) *Pathogenesis of Bacterial Infections in Animals*. Iowa State University Press, Ames, pp 124–132

Hay R J 1995 Nocardiasis. In: Weatherall D J, Ledingham J G G, Warrell D A (eds) *Oxford Textbook of Medicine*, 3rd edn. Oxford University Press, Oxford, pp 686–687

Roberts I F, Karim Q N, Rosin R D 1988 Actinomycotic mycetoma of the thigh. *Journal of the Royal Society of Medicine* 82: 552–553

Schaal K P, Lee H-J 1995 Actinomycete infections in humans – a review. *Gene* 115: 201–211

Schaal K P 1998 Actinomycosis, actinobacillosis and related diseases. In: Collier L, Balows A, Sussman M (eds) *Topley and Wilson's Microbiology and Microbial Infections*, 9th edn. Vol. 3. Arnold, London, pp 777–798

Veitch A M, Farthing M J G 1999 Whipple's Disease. In: Armstrong D, Cohen J (eds) *Infectious Diseses*. Mosby, London, pp 2.36.1–4

21

Bacillus

Anthrax; food poisoning

R. C. B. Slack

The genus *Bacillus* originally included all rod-shaped bacteria, but now comprises only large, spore-forming Gram-positive bacilli that form chains and will usually grow both aerobically and anaerobically. They are common environmental organisms and are frequently isolated in laboratories as contaminants of media or specimens. *Bacillus anthracis*, the cause of *anthrax*, is the most important pathogen of the group. Although rare in the industrialized nations, the very name *anthrax* strikes terror in the public, evoking horrors of 'germ warfare'. *B. cereus* may contaminate food, especially rice, in large numbers and is commonly implicated in episodes of food poisoning. Other species of *Bacillus* are less often incriminated as pathogens, usually in the immunocompromised.

Anthrax is a zoonotic disease, primarily recognized in large domesticated animals, which infects man accidentally through contact with infected products. The disease holds a crucial place in the history of medical microbiology:

• Robert Koch's work on anthrax showed that a causative organism could be isolated from the blood of infected animals, artificially grown in pure culture and then used to reproduce the disease in animals. This led to the development of the present-day methods of isolation and identification of bacteria, and to the formulation of *Koch's postulates* (see Chapter 1).

• Louis Pasteur showed that animals could be actively immunized by infecting them with cultures of *B. anthracis* that had been attenuated by growth at 43°C.

Anthrax is a disease in which the infection is transmitted by the spores of the bacillus, which are shed in large numbers in the terminal stages of infection. The disease is therefore unusual in that the infection is spread only from a dying or dead host and that the causative organism may survive for a long time in the environment. More recent work has elucidated the mechanism of virulence of *B. anthracis* and improved protective vaccines have been developed.

BACILLUS ANTHRACIS

Description

B. anthracis is a non-motile straight, sporing bacillus, rectangular in shape and 4–8 by 1–1.5 μm in dimensions, i.e. just smaller in length than the diameter of a red blood corpuscle. The spore is oval, refractile, central in position and of the same diameter as the bacillus. The organism is a strongly Gram-positive aerobe and facultative anaerobe with a temperature range for growth of 12–45°C (optimum, 35°C); it grows on all ordinary media as typical colonies with a wavy margin and small projections, the so-called *medusa head* appearance. Table 21.1 lists some of

Table 21.1 Distinguishing properties of some important *Bacillus* species

Property	B. anthracis	B. cereus	B. subtilis	B. stearothermophilus
Cell size (mm)	Large (6 × 1.5)	Large	Small (3 × 0.6)	Small
Motility	–	+	+	+
Capsule	+	–	–	–
Mouse pathogenicity	+++	+	–	–
Anaerobic growth	+	+	–	+/–
Temperature for optimal growth (°C)	35	30	37	55

the differences between *B. anthracis* and other important members of the genus *Bacillus*.

Spores are never found in the tissues, but appear when the organism is shed or grown on artificial media; they stain only with special spore-staining procedures. The spores are resistant to chemical disinfectants and heat: the spores of many strains will resist dry heat at 140°C for 1–3 h and boiling or steam at 100°C for 5–10 min. However, autoclaving at 121°C (15 lb/in^2 or 1 bar) destroys them in 15 min. The spores are relatively resistant to chemical agents.

Pathogenesis

Clinical infection

Man is relatively resistant to infection with *B. anthracis* and anthrax most commonly arises by inoculation through the skin of material from infected animals or their products. The resulting lesion of cutaneous anthrax is often described as a *malignant pustule* because of its characteristic appearance (Fig. 21.1). Coagulation necrosis of the centre of the pustule results in the formation of a dark-coloured *eschar*, which is later surrounded by a ring of vesicles containing serous fluid and an area of oedema and induration which may become extensive. In patients with severe toxic signs and widespread oedema the prognosis is poor.

Inhalation of spores in dust or wool fibres may result in respiratory anthrax: *wool-sorter's disease*. This condition carries a high mortality due to the intense inflammation, haemorrhage and septicaemia which result from the multiplication of organisms in bronchi and spread to the lungs, lymphatics and bloodstream. The production of toxins and the considerable bacterial load that rapidly occurs in the terminal septicaemic phase produce increased vascular permeability and hypotension similar to endotoxic shock.

The intestinal form of anthrax occurs among pastoralists who may be forced through poverty to eat infected animals that have been found dead. An individual may suffer after a day or so from haemorrhagic diarrhoea, and dies rapidly from septicaemia. Often these episodes occur as small outbreaks in a family or village. Because some individuals may only suffer cutaneous lesions the recognition of the microbial cause of the outbreak is easily made clinically.

Animal infection

All mammals are susceptible, though to a varying degree. Guinea-pigs and mice are highly susceptible to experimental inoculation. If a guinea-pig is injected subcutaneously with pathological material containing the

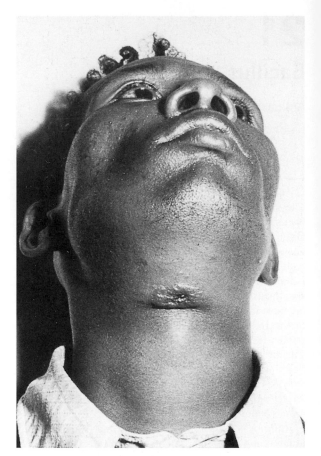

Fig. 21.1 A malignant pustule in a Kenyan farmer. (By courtesy of Professor I. A. Wamola, University of Nairobi Medical School.)

bacilli, or with pure cultures, the animal dies, usually within 2–3 days, showing a marked inflammatory lesion at the site of inoculation and extensive gelatinous oedema in the subcutaneous tissues. Large numbers of the bacilli are present in the local lesion, and are also profusely present in the heart blood and in the capillaries of the internal organs. They are especially numerous in the spleen (Fig. 21.2), which is enlarged and soft, giving rise to the description *splenic fever* in the ox and the German name for the organism – *Milzbrandbazillus* (spleen-destroying bacillus).

The production of anthrax in monkeys and guinea-pigs by inhalation of contaminated aerosols has also been studied experimentally. Spores deposited on the alveolar walls are taken up by phagocytes and carried to the tracheobronchial glands, which become inflamed and enlarged. Infection spreads via the lymphatics to the general circulation. About 20 000 organisms can produce lethal infection if the particle size of the aerosols is less than 5 μm. The smaller particles are

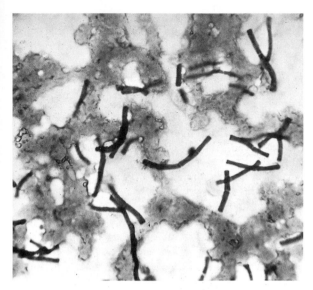

Fig. 21.2 Guinea-pig spleen imprint showing typical anthrax bacilli.

more likely to penetrate in the air-stream to the alveolar walls, but the lethal dose is much higher if the particles are larger. Much of the work on the aerobiology of infection has been conducted in military establishments, and many of the results have not been released in the public domain.

In natural conditions both wild herbivores and domesticated animals are susceptible. The condition is usually septicaemic following ingestion of contaminated pasture. The spores are ingested with coarse vegetation, which probably predisposes to trauma of the intestinal tract. Infection also occurs by inhalation of dust into the respiratory tract and, as in human disease, through skin abrasions leading to malignant pustules.

The spores germinate and the vegetative cells produce toxin, leading to the formation of gelatinous oedema and haemorrhage. In susceptible animals the bacilli resist phagocytosis and reach the lymphatics and the bloodstream. Before death the bacilli multiply freely in the blood and tissues. In resistant animals there is a more profuse leucocyte response with phagocytosis and decapsulation of the organism.

Virulence determinants

The pathogenicity of *B. anthracis* depends on two properties not found in saprophytic *Bacillus* species:

- The capsule, which is unusual in being a polypeptide of D-glutamic acid, and which inhibits opsonophagocytosis.
- The plasmid-encoded toxin complex comprising three proteins, all of which are required for pathogenicity:

the *protective antigen* binds the complex to receptors on the macrophage surface; after proteolysis, *oedema factor* and *lethal factor* are released and, after endocytosis, block the adenyl cyclase pathway within the cell.

The main effect of this toxin complex is to increase vascular permeability, which leads to shock. Knowledge of the biochemistry of these determinants has led to the development of protective antigen vaccines to replace the original non-capsulate avirulent strains.

Laboratory diagnosis

Clinical specimens

The fully developed malignant pustule may be difficult to swab and the central necrotic area gives a poor yield. Fluid aspirated from the surrounding vesicles, when present, is more likely to yield anthrax bacilli. Specimens should be taken before antibiotic therapy has been instituted.

In laboratories unfamiliar with the disease, additional precautions for staff safety need to be organized. However, the relative ease of clinical diagnosis, given the characteristic appearance and occupational exposure, often makes laboratory confirmation superfluous.

Gram's stain may show typical large Gram-positive bacilli, and culture on blood agar yields the large, flat, greyish colonies with the characteristic 'medusa head' appearance. Staining of films from these colonies will show long chains of Gram-positive bacilli, some containing spores. Serological diagnosis by enzyme-linked immunosorbent assay (ELISA) may be of value retrospectively, but is seldom used diagnostically.

Confirmatory tests

Simple biochemical and physiological reactions are used (Table 21.1). Demonstration of non-motility, gelatin liquefaction, growth in straight chains and enhanced growth aerobically, as seen in the characteristic *inverted fir tree* appearance in a gelatin stab, will generally identify *B. anthracis* completely. Toxin production can be demonstrated by immunological or gene probe methods in reference laboratories.

Subcutaneous inoculation of guinea-pigs with a suspension of bacilli was formerly used to confirm that the organism was *B. anthracis*. Death usually ensues within 2–3 days, and post mortem reveals numerous bacteria on cardiac puncture or impression of splenic cells (Fig. 21.2). These specimens, when stained with polychrome methylene blue, show large, blue bacilli surrounded by a red granular-stained capsule (*McFadyean's reaction*). This appearance is given only by *B. anthracis*.

Environmental samples

It is occasionally necessary to isolate *B. anthracis* from potentially contaminated material such as animal hair, hides or soil. This task is particularly difficult because of the large number of non-pathogenic *Bacillus* spp. found in the environment.

Treatment

B. anthracis is susceptible in vitro to a wide range of antimicrobial agents and many have been used successfully in the treatment of anthrax in man. Penicillin remains the drug of choice as β-lactamase-producing strains are rare. In contrast, penicillin resistance is common in other *Bacillus* species. This may be partly due to the fact that *B. anthracis* generally is found in remote areas where antibiotic pressures for selection of resistance are less. Most strains are also sensitive to macrolides, aminoglycosides, tetracyclines and chloramphenicol.

Ciprofloxacin or a similar fluoroquinolone is recommended as prophylaxis or early treatment for those considered at greatest risk of exposure following a large-scale release of anthrax spores in a deliberate attack. This is because it can be easily stockpiled and distributed and it is probable that an aggressor would use a genetically modified penicillin-resistant strain.

The choice of antimicrobial agent is not a limiting factor in the treatment of anthrax; a delay in initiating therapy is the main reason for failure. This is due to late presentation for medical care or, in the case of intestinal or respiratory infection, lack of specific symptoms to establish the diagnosis before an overwhelming septicaemia. In the later stages of disease, general principles applied to the management of any patient in shock are more important than antimicrobial therapy.

It has been common practice to isolate patients with anthrax because of its highly infectious reputation. In fact, human-to-human spread is extremely uncommon and appropriate antibiotics render the patient free from bacilli. In addition, actively multiplying bacteria are not as infectious as spores, which are only found in dead or dying animals.

The use of specific antiserum is not recommended presently although, in the future, immunotherapy may play an important role in the treatment of septicaemic individuals.

Epidemiology and control

Agricultural anthrax

Anthrax is a *zoonosis*: a disease of animals transmissible secondarily to man. The exact incidence in humans and animals is unknown, but many countries in Africa and Asia regularly report cases to the World Health Organization. When the disease is established in livestock and pasture becomes heavily contaminated in a country, an *enzootic* focus is created. Occasionally the disease may erupt into large numbers of domestic animals with associated human cases. In this situation anthrax is *epizootic*. This occurred in the 1980s in Zimbabwe where over 9000 human cases were recorded and countless cattle died. Areas in which anthrax used to be enzootic, such as much of Europe, have been able to control the disease by control of livestock, animal feeds (especially bone meal) and strict regulations on importation of animal hides.

In the UK, the disease is occasionally found in livestock, chiefly cattle, but there were only three confirmed human cases between 1990 and 1999. Sudden death in any herbivore should be treated with suspicion, and a veterinary officer summoned to examine the carcass without a post mortem. A blood slide should be taken for Gram or methylene blue staining. Under the Anthrax Order the animal must remain on the farm and be incinerated on site if found to be positive. Deep burial in quicklime was the alternative method of disposal, but the spores remain viable for many years and may subsequently contaminate pasture and infect grazing animals. Very large numbers of bacilli are present in the terminal stages of disease in animals so that widespread dissemination may occur on death. These highly infectious animals serve as a source of anthrax both by direct spread to another beast and by contamination of the environment.

Heavy contamination of soil exists in enzootic foci in many parts of the world, and spores may be recovered many years after the last known case. Artificial contamination of an uninhabited small island (Gruinard) off the north-west coast of Scotland occurred in 1942–43 as a result of tests of a biological warfare bomb containing live anthrax spores. Subsequent sampling showed wide areas to be contaminated with spores and even by 1979 spores could still be detected in a 3-hectare area of the island. It was calculated that, even if left untouched, it would not be safe to graze sheep on Gruinard for another 70 years. In the 1980s the area was decontaminated by burning the vegetation and spraying with 5% formaldehyde in sea water. By 1987 the ground was declared anthrax-free and, after reseeding, sheep were able to graze safely.

In enzootic areas, disinfection of soil is not a practical control measure, but pastures known to be heavily contaminated should not be used for grazing animals. The organism multiplies when the soil pH is greater than 6 and when early rain has been followed by a long dry spell. Control in animals depends on:

- early diagnosis
- isolation and incineration of infected animals
- the use of vaccines.

Industrial anthrax

In countries in which the disease is relatively rare in animals, contamination with imported materials is the commonest form of infection in man. In general, the infectivity of *B. anthracis* for man is not of a high order, and when a case occurs in a factory spores are often widely distributed in large numbers in the dust and air. Anthrax is a recognized industrial hazard which, in the UK, is notifiable to Consultants in Communicable Disease Control and to the Health and Safety Executive. There is control on the importation of animal hides and hair, which are disinfected if considered infected. Workers at risk of exposure in the leather or wool industries and veterinarians may be offered immunization routinely and antibiotic prophylaxis if exposed to a known risk.

Immunization

Live-attenuated bacilli were first used by Louis Pasteur in May 1881. In spite of great scepticism from professionals about the effectiveness of vaccination outside the laboratory, Pasteur volunteered to make a public demonstration in an area where the disease was common. The Society of Agriculture of Seine-et-Marne took up the challenge, and the experiment took place on a farm in Pouilly-le-Fort. The 25 sheep that were vaccinated with heat-attenuated live bacilli and then inoculated with virulent anthrax material resisted infection whereas 22 of 25 sheep acting as controls succumbed within 48 h. During the next few summer months, thousands of sheep, cattle and horses were vaccinated, and the mortality among domesticated animals fell dramatically. This discovery led to international acclaim for Pasteur and award of the Légion d'Honneur.

Subsequently, the *Sterne strain* of live spore vaccine has been used for animal immunization. Live bacterial vaccines are not considered safe for man. *Alum-precipitated toxoid* has been used to immunize workers at risk of exposure. Frequent booster doses are necessary as immunity, measured by toxin antibodies, declines rapidly. New recombinant protective antigen preparations may give better immunity and fewer adverse reactions.

Concern that 'Gulf War syndrome', an ill-defined illness in military staff, may be a result of anthrax immunization has not been confirmed.

BACILLUS CEREUS

Description

B. cereus is a large Gram-positive bacillus resembling *B. anthracis*, except that it is motile and lacks the glutamic acid capsule. Like other members of the genus it is a saprophyte and frequents soil, water and vegetation. *B. cereus* closely resembles *B. anthracis* in culture, forming large, grey, irregular colonies described as *anthracoid*. Large inocula injected into laboratory animals may cause death but without the haemorrhagic appearance of anthrax, and blood smears do not show the characteristic pink capsule with McFadyean's stain.

Pathogenesis

Spores of *B. cereus* are particularly heat-resistant and most strains produce toxins. The organism is widespread in the environment and is found in most raw foods, especially cereals such as rice. Enormous numbers of organisms (up to 10^{10} per gram) may be found in contaminated food (commonly lightly cooked Chinese dishes), leading to two types of food poisoning:

- Cases in which vomiting, occurring within 6 h of ingestion, is the main symptom. It is caused by preformed toxin, which is a low molecular weight, heat- and acid-stable peptide that can withstand intestinal proteolytic enzymes.
- A diarrhoeal form of food poisoning, occurring 8–24 h after ingestion, similar to enteritis caused by *Escherichia coli* or *Salmonella* serotypes. This is caused by enterotoxins, which, like *Clostridium perfringens* enterotoxin, are heat-labile and formed in the intestine.

B. cereus is also a common cause of post-traumatic ophthalmitis which requires rapid, aggressive management locally.

Laboratory diagnosis

If food is available for testing, and this is often not the case in investigations of gastro-enteritis, laboratory confirmation is easy. High numbers of *B. cereus*, often 10^8 or more per gram, in the absence of other food poisoning bacteria are sufficient to make the diagnosis. Large facultatively anaerobic Gram-positive bacilli that produce anthracoid colonies on blood agar after overnight incubation at 37°C are almost certain to be *B. cereus*. Food reference laboratories are able to confirm identification and type if necessary.

Treatment

Both the emetic and diarrhoeal syndromes are short-lived and no specific treatment is needed. Most sufferers, even those with underlying conditions, seldom come to any harm. Acute symptoms last less than 24 h and recovery on a reduced diet and fluids is rapid.

Control

Disease is easily prevented by proper cooling and storage of food. Ideally, all dishes should be freshly prepared and eaten. Rice, in particular, should not be stored for long periods above 10°C.

OTHER BACILLUS SPECIES

B. subtilis, *B. pumilis* and *B. licheniformis* have been implicated in causing food poisoning similar to that due to *B. cereus*. They do not appear to form toxins, but some strains produce antibacterial peptides, like the antibiotic bacitracin, which may facilitate growth in the intestinal tract. *B. polymyxa* is the source of the antibiotic polymyxin.

B. cereus, *B. subtilis* and, rarely, other members of the genus may be found in wounds and tissues of immunocompromised or burned patients. These opportunist pathogens are also common contaminants of specimens and laboratory media so that the interpretation of significance is sometimes difficult. When found in numbers in otherwise sterile sites, such as blood or cerebrospinal fluid, these otherwise insignificant pathogens require specific treatment. Most strains produce abundant β-lactamase that differs from the enzyme found in staphylococci.

Sterilization test bacilli

B. stearothermophilus was, until the discovery of archaebacteria in hot springs, the most heat-resistant organism known. Spores withstand 121°C for up to 12 min, and this has made the organism ideal for testing autoclaves that run on a time–temperature cycle designed to ensure the destruction of spores. Strips containing *B. stearothermophilus* are included with the material being autoclaved, and are subsequently examined by culture for surviving spores. The organism grows only at raised temperatures, typically between 50 and 60°C; there is hardly any growth below 40°C.

B. globigi, a red-pigmented variant of *B. subtilis*, has been used to test ethylene oxide sterilizers, and *B. pumilis* has been used to test the efficacy of ionizing radiation.

RECOMMENDED READING

Dixon T C, Meselson M, Guillemin J Hanna P C 1999 Anthrax – a review. *New England Journal of Medicine* 341: 815–826

Drobniewski F A 1993 *Bacillus cereus* and related species. *Clinical Microbiology Reviews* 6: 324–338

Farrar W E 1994 Anthrax: Virulence and vaccines. *Annals of Internal Medicine* 121: 379–380

Granum P E 1994 *Bacillus cereus* and its toxins. *Journal of Applied Bacteriology Symposium Supplement* 23: 61S–66S

Nass M 1999 Anthrax vaccine – a review. *Infectious Disease Clinics of North America* 1999: 187–208

Turnbull P C B, Hugh-Jones M E, Cosivi O 1999 World Health Organization activities on anthrax surveillance and control. *Journal of Applied Microbiology* 87: 318–320

Working Group on Civilian Biodefense 1999 Anthrax as a biological weapon. *Journal of the American Medical Association* 281: 1735–1745

22

Clostridium

Gas gangrene; tetanus; food poisoning; pseudomembranous colitis

T. V. Riley

The clostridia are Gram-positive spore-bearing anaerobic bacilli. Most of the species are saprophytes that normally occur in soil, water and decomposing plant and animal matter; they play an important part in natural processes of putrefaction. Some, such as *Clostridium perfringens* and *C. sporogenes*, are commensals of the animal and human gut. On the death of the host, these organisms and other members of the intestinal flora rapidly invade the blood and tissues, and initiate the decomposition of the corpse. A few species are opportunistic pathogens, including:

- *C. perfringens*, *C. septicum* and *C. novyi*, the causes of gas gangrene and other infections
- *C. tetani*, the cause of *tetanus*
- *C. botulinum*, the cause of *botulism*
- *C. difficile*, the cause of pseudomembranous colitis and antibiotic-associated diarrhoea.

A subgroup of *C. perfringens* produces particularly heat-resistant spores and is associated with a form of food poisoning, but classic strains of this species, which are not particularly heat-resistant, can also cause food poisoning.

GENERAL DESCRIPTION

The clostridia are typically large, straight or slightly curved rods with slightly rounded ends. Pleomorphism is common and various forms may be seen in stained smears from cultures or wounds. These include filaments or elongated cells, spindle-shaped forms (*clostridium* is Latin for 'little spindle') and club forms. They are often Gram-variable and may appear to be Gram-negative. All produce spores and these enable the organisms to survive in adverse conditions, e.g. in soil and dust and on skin.

Most species are obligate anaerobes: their spores do not germinate and growth does not normally proceed unless a suitably low redox potential (E_h) exists. However, a few species grow in the presence of trace amounts of air and some actually grow slowly under normal atmospheric conditions.

These organisms are biochemically active, frequently possessing both saccharolytic and proteolytic properties, though in varying degrees. The genus is currently undergoing a major taxonomic revision.

Many clostridia are highly toxigenic. The toxins produced by the organisms of tetanus and botulism attack nervous pathways and are referred to as neurotoxins. The organisms associated with gas gangrene attack soft tissues by producing toxins and aggressins, and they are referred to as histotoxic. *C. difficile* and some strains of *C. perfringens* produce an enterotoxin.

CLOSTRIDIUM PERFRINGENS

This species is commonly implicated in gas gangrene and certain types of food poisoning.

Description

C. perfringens is a relatively large Gram-positive bacillus (about $4–6 \times 1$ µm) with blunt ends. It is capsulate and non-motile. It grows quickly on laboratory media, particularly at high temperatures (approximately 42°C) when the doubling time can be as short as 8 min. It can be identified by the *Nagler reaction*, which exploits the action of its phospholipase on egg yolk medium; colonies are surrounded by zones of turbidity, and the effect is specifically inhibited if *C. perfringens* antiserum containing α-antitoxin is present on the medium. Typical food poisoning strains produce heat-resistant spores that can survive boiling for several hours, whereas the spores of the type A strains that cause gas gangrene are inactivated within a few minutes by boiling.

Gas gangrene

C. perfringens is the commonest cause of gas gangrene, although various other species of clostridia may be

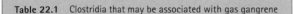

Table 22.1 Clostridia that may be associated with gas gangrene

C. perfringens type A
C. septicum
C. novyi type A
C. histolyticum
C. sordellii

These organisms may occur alone or in combination. Gas gangrene is almost always a polymicrobial infection involving anaerobes and facultative organisms. *C. perfringens* is most commonly involved; other clostridia not listed here are occasionally associated with gas gangrene.

implicated (Table 22.1). The disease is characterized by rapidly spreading oedema, myositis, necrosis of tissues, gas production and profound toxaemia occurring as a complication of wound infection. The diagnosis of gas gangrene is primarily made on clinical grounds with laboratory confirmation.

The main source of the organisms is animal and human excreta, and spores of the causative clostridia are distributed widely. Infection usually results from contamination of a wound with soil, particularly from manured and cultivated land. However, it may be indirectly derived from dirty clothing, street dust, and even the air of an operating theatre if the ventilating system is poorly designed or improperly maintained. The skin often bears spores of *C. perfringens*, especially in areas of the body that may be contaminated with intestinal organisms.

Pathogenesis of gas gangrene

Impairment of the normal blood supply of tissue with a consequent reduction in oxygen tension may allow an anaerobic focus to develop. The patient's condition may deteriorate rapidly with the development of severe shock (Fig. 22.1).

Crushing of tissue and the severing of arteries in accidental injuries, rough handling of tissue and over-zealous clamping during surgery, or shock waves from gunshot injuries may compromise the microcirculation in an extensive area of tissue and prejudice tissue perfusion. The presence of devitalized or dead tissue, blood clot, extravasated fluid, foreign bodies and co-incident pyogenic infection are all factors that promote the occurrence of gas gangrene in a wound. The spores of the clostridia and their vegetative bacilli cannot readily initiate infection in healthy tissues, presumably because the E_h is too high, and the organisms are unable to avoid destruction and clearance by phagocytosis. Predisposing host factors include debility, old age and diabetes.

When clostridial infection has been initiated in a focus of devitalized anaerobic tissue, the organisms

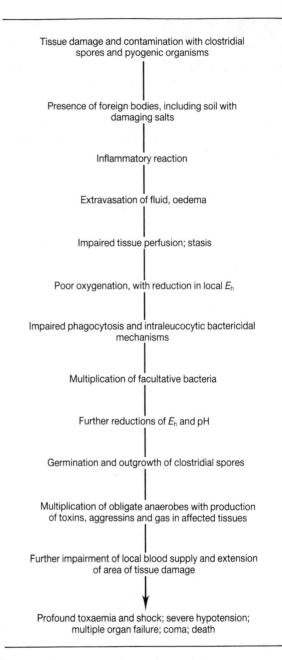

Fig. 22.1 Circumstances and events that may lead to gas gangrene.

multiply rapidly and produce a range of toxins and aggressins. These damage tissue by various necrotizing effects, and some have demonstrable lethal effects. They spread into adjacent viable tissue, particularly muscle, kill it and render it anaerobic and vulnerable to further colonization, with the production of more toxins and aggressins.

- Hyaluronidase produced by *C. perfringens* breaks down intercellular cement substance and promotes the spread of the infection along tissue planes.
- Collagenase and other proteinases break down tissues and virtually liquefy muscles. The whole of a muscle group or segment of a limb may be affected.
- α-toxin, a phospholipase C (lecithinase) is generally considered to be the main cause of the toxaemia associated with gas gangrene, though other clostridial species can produce similar manifestations.

In puerperal infections or in cases of septic abortion, the organisms may gain access from faeces-contaminated perineal skin or contaminated instruments to necrotic or devitalized tissues in the uterus or adnexa. Here they set up a dangerous and often fulminating pelvic infection, possibly with prompt invasion of the bloodstream. There may be intravascular haemolysis and anuria.

C. perfringens may also participate in peritoneal infections occurring as a result of extension of pathogens from the alimentary tract, as in cases of gangrenous appendicitis or intestinal obstruction or mesenteric thrombosis.

If a preparation of adrenaline used for injection is contaminated with clostridial spores, the combination of an infective inoculum with the local ischaemia that follows the injection may be catastrophic. Gas gangrene may be a complication of surgical operations on the lower limb or hip of a patient whose blood supply is inadequate to maintain oxygenation in the postoperative period.

It is important to appreciate that clostridia may be associated with other less severe forms of infection without the toxaemia and aggression of gas gangrene. Moreover, potentially pathogenic anaerobes may be cultivated from a wound that never shows any sign of gas gangrene, and sometimes the laboratory isolation may be attributed to the germination of a few contaminating spores when the specimen is processed. Thus, the onus is on the clinician to relate a laboratory report to the patient's circumstances.

Clinical clues include *crepitus* in the adjacent tissues; this is the sponge-cake consistency caused by small bubbles of gas. In the early stages, the patient has an anxious, frightened appearance. Local pain is increased, and there is swelling of the affected tissues. Toxaemia and shock supervene and the patient's conscious state drifts to drowsiness and into coma. Prompt diagnosis and intensive surgical and antimicrobial treatment greatly influence the patient's chance of survival and may avoid the loss of the affected limb, but all devitalized tissue must be excised (see below).

Laboratory diagnosis

If there are sloughs of necrotic tissue in the wound, small pieces should be transferred aseptically into a sterile screw-capped bottle and examined immediately by microscopy and culture. Specimens of exudate should be taken from the deeper areas of the wound where the infection seems to be most pronounced. Gram smears are prepared. If gas gangrene exists, typical Gram-positive bacilli may predominate, often with other bacteria present in a mixed infection. However, there is usually a pronounced lack of inflammatory cells. Initiation of treatment should not await a full laboratory report and early discussion with the bacteriologist is crucial. A direct smear of a wound exudate is often of great help in providing evidence of the relative numbers of different bacteria that may be participating in a mixed infection or may merely be present as contaminants, but the distinction is not invariably easy and joint discussions are important.

Treatment

Prompt and adequate surgical attention to the wound is of the utmost importance (Fig. 22.2).

- Sutures are removed, necrotic and devitalized tissue is excised with careful debridement.
- Fascial compartments are incised to release tension.
- Any foreign body is found and removed.
- The wound is not resutured but is left open after thorough cleansing and loosely packed.

Antibiotic therapy is started immediately in very high doses. This must account for the likely co-existence of coliform organisms, Gram-positive cocci and faecal anaerobes. Accordingly, penicillin, metronidazole and an aminoglycoside may be given in combination. Alternatively, clindamycin plus an aminoglycoside or a

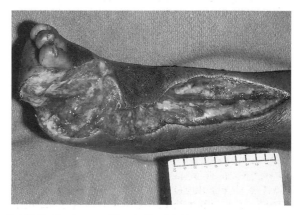

Fig. 22.2 Gas gangrene. Wound after debridement.

broad-spectrum antibiotic such as meropenem or imipenem, may be considered. Much intensive supportive therapy is needed.

Enthusiastic claims have been made for the efficacy of hyperbaric oxygen therapy in gas gangrene; however, clinical trials have given conflicting results. Patients are placed in a special pressurized chamber where they breathe oxygen at 2–3 atm. pressure for periods of 1–2 h twice daily on several successive days. This may limit the amount of radical surgery needed.

A polyvalent antiserum containing *C. perfringens*, *C. septicum* and *C. novyi* antitoxins used to be available, but has now been replaced by intensive antimicrobial therapy.

Prophylaxis

Surgical wounds. *C. perfringens* is normally present in large numbers in human faeces, and its spores occur regularly on the skin, especially of the buttocks and thighs. As clostridial spores are very resistant to most disinfectants, they are likely to survive normal pre-operative skin preparation and persist in the area of the planned incision. The numbers can be reduced by more prolonged skin preparation with the sustained action of an antiseptic such as povidone–iodine for a day or two, and this procedure has a place in orthopaedic surgery.

When inevitable skin contamination is combined with circumstances that predispose to devitalization of tissue and reduced oxygen tension, a patient may be vulnerable to the development of postoperative gas gangrene. These circumstances arise if an elderly patient or a patient with some vascular insufficiency receives major surgery to the hip or lower limb. Peri-operative antimicrobial prophylaxis with penicillin is justified in such cases.

Accidental wounds. The prevention of gas gangrene in accidentally sustained wounds must take account of the endogenous factors noted above and the exogenous sources of clostridial spores and vegetative forms in soil, on contaminated clothing, etc. In addition, there is an increased risk of anaerobic infection developing when foreign bodies such as soil, clothing, metal (nails, wire, bullets, shrapnel) and skin are driven into devitalized tissues. Road accidents and gunshot injuries feature in these considerations. Prompt and adequate surgical attention is of paramount importance but prophylactic administration of benzylpenicillin for patients presenting with serious contaminated wounds is also worthwhile. Many workers prefer to avoid such prophylaxis, provided that they can be absolutely sure that the local state of the wound and the patient's general condition are expertly and frequently monitored throughout the recovery period.

C. perfringens food poisoning

Carrier rates for 'typical food poisoning strains' of *C. perfringens* range from about 2% to more than 30% in different groups that have been surveyed across the world. These bacteria also occur in animals; thus, meat is often contaminated with heat-resistant spores. When meat is cooked in bulk, heat penetration and subsequent cooling is slow unless special precautions are taken. Heat-resistant spores may survive and, during the cooling period, germinate in the anaerobic environment produced by the cooked meat and multiply. Anyone who eats this will consume the equivalent of a cooked meat broth culture of the organism. The organisms are protected from the gastric acid by the protein in the meal and pass in large numbers into the intestine.

Ingestion of large numbers of the viable organisms is necessary for the production of the typical disease syndrome, which is mediated by an enterotoxin that is released when sporulation occurs in the gut. Typical symptoms are abdominal cramps beginning about 8–12 h after ingestion, followed by diarrhoea. Fever and vomiting are not usually encountered and symptoms generally subside within a day or two. No specific treatment is indicated. The carrier state persists for several weeks, but this should not be regarded as an indication for exclusion from any duties, since carriers may be quite numerous in various communities.

The vehicle of infection is usually a precooked meat food that has been allowed to stand at a temperature conducive to the multiplication of *C. perfringens*. While the heat resistance of spores of typical food poisoning strains ensures their survival in cooked foods, and presumably accounts for the association of these strains with most of the reported outbreaks of *C. perfringens* food poisoning, similar trouble can be caused by classical heat-sensitive type A strains if they gain access to food during the cooling period under conditions suitable for their subsequent multiplication.

Laboratory diagnosis

This depends upon the isolation of similar strains of *C. perfringens* at a high enough viable count from the faeces of patients and from those at risk who have eaten the suspected food, and from the food itself. The isolates can be sent to a reference laboratory for special typing to prove their relatedness.

Prevention

The occurrence of this type of food poisoning is an indictment of the catering practices concerned, as food has to be mishandled to allow the chain of events to take place.

Nevertheless, *C. perfringens* is the fourth most common cause of food poisoning after *Campylobacter* species, *Salmonella* serotypes and *Staphylococcus aureus*.

C. perfringens colitis

A sporadic diarrhoeal syndrome, usually occurring in elderly patients during treatment with antibiotics, has been described. The circumstances differ substantially from those of *C. perfringens* food poisoning. An enterotoxin with a cytopathic effect can be detected in the patient's faeces.

Enteritis necroticans (pig-bel)

A subgroup of *C. perfringens* type C produces heat-resistant spores. This organism is the cause of a disease that affects New Guinea natives when they have pork feasts. The method of cooking the pork allows the clostridia to survive. When the contaminated meat is eaten along with a sweet potato vegetable that contains a proteinase inhibitor, a toxin (the β toxin) is able to act on the small intestine to produce a necrotizing enteritis.

CLOSTRIDIUM SEPTICUM

Description

C. septicum is generally about 4–6 × 0.6 μm, but shorter, longer and filamentous forms occur. Spores are readily formed and, as they develop, various shapes arise ranging from swollen Gram-positive 'citron bodies' to obviously sporing forms in which the oval spores may be central or subterminal and are clearly bulging. Older Gram-negative cells may be seen.

The organism is actively motile with numerous peritrichous flagella. It is one of the less exacting anaerobes and grows well at 37°C on ordinary media. It is saccharolytic, and glucose promotes growth.

Surface colonies are irregular, transparent and droplet-like, later becoming greyish and opaque, with projecting radiations that are coarser than those of *C. tetani*.

Pathogenesis

C. septicum is one of the gas gangrene group of clostridia. It also occurs harmlessly in the human intestine, but if the integrity of the gut epithelium is impaired, e.g. by leukaemic infiltration, *C. septicum* bacteraemia may occur. Cyclic or other forms of neutropenia are also associated with spontaneous, non-traumatic gas gangrene that begins with a bacteraemic phase. A rapidly fatal terminal ileal infection and septicaemia in immunocompro-

mised patients, sometimes referred to as *typhlitis*, is most commonly associated with *C. septicum*.

Intramuscular injection of cultures into laboratory animals produces a spreading inflammatory oedema, with slight gas formation in the tissues. Organisms invade the blood and the animal dies within a day or two. Smears from the liver show long filamentous forms and citron bodies. *C. septicum* produces several toxins (α, β, δ and ε). The α-toxin, which has lethal, haemolytic and necrotizing activity, appears to be the most important; this does not have phospholipase C activity and is thus different to the α-toxin of *C. perfringens*.

Epidemiology

The primary habitat of *C. septicum* is either the soil or the animal intestine. Areas with large numbers of spores appear to be associated with a higher incidence of *C. septicum* infections in humans and animals than less heavily infected areas.

CLOSTRIDIUM NOVYI

C. novyi resembles *C. perfringens* in morphology, but is larger, more pleomorphic and a much more strict anaerobe; it is readily killed when vegetative cells are exposed to air. It possesses peritrichous flagella, but its motility is inhibited in the presence of oxygen. The spores are oval, central or subterminal. The organism occurs widely in soil and is associated with disease in man and animals. There are four types – A, B, C and D – distinguished on the basis of permutations of the toxins and other soluble antigens they produce. Only type A strains are of medical interest as they cause some cases of gas gangrene in man. An outbreak of *C. novyi* type A infections in injecting heroin users in the UK killed 35 people.

C. novyi gas gangrene is associated with profound toxaemia. Culture filtrates are highly toxic and possess at least four active substances (α, β, δ and ε toxins) that account for the various haemolytic, necrotizing, lethal, phospholipase and lipase activities of this organism.

CLOSTRIDIUM SPOROGENES

This Gram-positive motile bacillus is very widely distributed in nature, e.g. in soil and in the intestines of animals, and is generally regarded as a harmless saprophyte. Gram-negative forms are frequent in older cultures. Its oval, central or subterminal spores may be highly resistant and the organism is often encountered in mixed cultures in the laboratory, even after preliminary heating of these cultures to select heat-resistant pathogens. Spores may survive boiling for periods ranging from 15 min up to 6 h.

C. sporogenes is frequently isolated from wound exudates in association with accepted pathogens. While its presence may accelerate an established anaerobic infection by enhancing local conditions, it does not by itself cause gas gangrene and cannot be regarded as a pathogen in its own right.

CLOSTRIDIUM TETANI

Description

The organism generally appears by microscopy as a straight, slender rod with rounded ends. Although it is Gram-positive, Gram-negative forms are usually encountered in stained smears. The fully developed terminal spore gives the organism the appearance of a drumstick with a large round end. The tetanus bacillus is an obligate anaerobe, which is motile via numerous peritrichous flagella. It grows well in cooked meat broth and produces a thin spreading film when grown on enriched blood agar. The spores may be highly resistant to adverse conditions, but the degree of resistance varies with the strain. Spores of some strains resist boiling in water for up to 3 h. They may resist dry heat at 160°C for 1 h, and 5% phenol for 2 weeks or more. Iodine (1%) in water is said to kill the spores within a few hours, but this should not significantly influence clinical practice. Glutaraldehyde is one of the few chemical disinfectants that is assuredly sporicidal.

Toxins

C. tetani produces an oxygen-labile haemolysin (tetanolysin), but the organism's neurotoxin (tetanospasmin) is the essential pathogenic product. Strains vary in their toxigenicity; some are highly toxigenic. Most strains produce demonstrable toxin after culture in broth for a few days.

The gene that encodes the neurotoxin is located on a 75-kb plasmid. The toxin is synthesized as a single polypeptide with a molecular weight of 150 000, which undergoes post-translational cleavage into a heavy chain and a light chain linked by a disulphide bond. The estimated lethal dose for a mouse of pure tetanospasmin is 0.0001 μg. It is toxic to man and various animals when injected parenterally, but not by the oral route.

When tetanus occurs naturally, the tetanus bacilli stay at the site of the initial infection and are not generally invasive. Toxin diffuses to affect the relevant level of the spinal cord (local tetanus) and then to affect the entire system (generalized tetanus). These stages,

including the intermediate one of 'ascending tetanus', are demonstrable in experimental animals, but the stages tend to merge in their clinical presentation in man.

The toxin is absorbed from the site of its production in an infective focus, but may be delivered via the blood to all nerves in the body. The heavy chain mediates attachment to gangliosides and the toxin is internalized. It is then moved from the peripheral to the central nervous system by retrograde axonal transport and trans-synaptic spread. The tendency for the first signs of human tetanus to be in the head and neck is attributed to the shorter length of the cranial nerves. In fact, descending involvement of the nervous system is seen as the tetanus toxin takes longer to traverse the longer motor nerves and the toxin also diffuses in the spinal cord.

Once the entire toxin molecule is internalized into presynaptic cells, the light chain is released and affects the membrane of synaptic vesicles. This prevents the release of the neurotransmitter γ-aminobutyric acid. Motor neurons are left under no inhibitory control and undergo sustained excitatory discharge, causing the characteristic motor spasms of tetanus. The toxin exerts its effects on the spinal cord, the brain stem, peripheral nerves, at neuromuscular junctions and directly on muscles.

Occurrence of tetanus bacilli

Tetanus bacilli may be found in the human intestine, but infection seems to be derived primarily from animal faeces and soil. The organism is especially prevalent in manured soil and, for this reason, a wound through skin contaminated with soil or manure deserves special attention. However, tetanus spores occur very widely and are commonly present in gardens, sports fields and roads, in the dust, plaster and air of hospitals and houses, on clothing and on articles of common use.

Spores of C. tetani and other anaerobes may be embedded in surgical catgut and other dressings. This has been the source of infection in some cases in the past; however, the sterility of surgical catgut (prepared from the gut of cattle and sheep) is now rigorously controlled.

Pathogenesis

If washed spores are injected into an animal they fail to germinate and are removed by phagocytosis. Germination and outgrowth of tetanus spores depend upon reduced oxygen tension in devitalized tissue and non-viable material in a wound so that the E_h is significantly lowered. When infection occurs, often assisted by the simultaneous growth of facultatively anaerobic organisms in a mixed inoculum, the tetanus bacillus remains strictly localized, but tetanus toxin is elaborated and diffuses as described earlier.

Conditions that favour the germination of spores and their outgrowth are similar to those that have been discussed earlier in relation to gas gangrene (pp. 231–234).

Cases of tetanus have been reported in which the infection was apparently associated with a superficial abrasion, a contaminated splinter or a minor thorn prick. Indeed, gardening enthusiasts form one of the recognized risk groups.

In some cases the site of infection is assumed to be in the external auditory meatus; thus, *otogenic tetanus* may be attributable to over-zealous cleansing of the meatus with a small stick. In other patients, the site of infection remains undiscovered, and this is referred to as *cryptogenic tetanus*. Tetanus infection may also occur in or near the uterus in cases of septic abortion.

Tetanus neonatorum follows infection of the umbilical wound of newborn infants (see below). Cases of *postoperative tetanus* have been attributed to imperfectly sterilized catgut, dressings or glove powder, and sometimes to dust-borne infection of the wound at operation.

Clinical features of tetanus

The onset of signs and symptoms is gradual, usually starting with some stiffness and perhaps pain in or near a recent wound. In some cases the initial complaint may be of stiffness of the jaw (*lockjaw*). Pain and stiffness in the neck and back may follow. The stiffness spreads to involve all muscle groups; facial spasms produce the 'sardonic grin', and in severe cases spasm of the back muscles produces the opisthotonos (extreme arching of the back) beloved of textbook writers. The period between injury and the first signs is usually about 10–14 days, but there is a considerable range. A severe case with a relatively poor prognosis shows rapid progression from the first signs to the development of generalized spasms. Sweating, tachycardia and arrhythmia, and swings in blood pressure reflect sympathetic stimulation, which is not well understood but creates problems of management.

Treatment

The patient remains conscious and requires skilled sedation and constant nursing. If generalized spasms are worrying, the patient is paralysed and ventilated mechanically until the toxin that has been taken up has decayed; this may take some weeks.

The patient is given 10 000 units of human tetanus immunoglobulin (HTIG) in saline by slow intravenous infusion. Full wound exploration and debridement is arranged, and the wound is cleansed and left open with a loose pack. Penicillin or metronidazole is given for as long as considered necessary to ensure that bacterial growth and toxin production are stopped. The antitoxin and antibiotics are given immediately, and preferably before surgical excision, but delay must be avoided.

Laboratory diagnosis

Gram smears of the wound exudate and any necrotic material may show the typical 'drumstick' bacilli, but this is not invariably so, and it is only presumptive evidence as other organisms that resemble *C. tetani* have terminal spores. Simple light microscopy is often unsuccessful; immunofluorescence microscopy with a specific stain is possible but not generally available.

Direct culture of unheated material on blood agar incubated anaerobically is often the best method of detecting *C. tetani*. There are various other tricks that exploit the organism's motility and fine spreading growth; sometimes these are vitiated by overgrowth with *Proteus* species. Material from the wound or from a mixed sporing subculture may be heated at various temperatures and for various times to exclude non-sporing bacteria; the heated specimens are then seeded onto solid media and incubated anaerobically. Tetanus may be produced in mice by subcutaneous injection of an anaerobic culture prepared from wound material; control mice are protected with tetanus antitoxin.

Epidemiology

Tetanus ranks among the major lethal infections. There are between 800 000 and 1 million deaths annually from tetanus, of which 400 000 are due to neonatal tetanus. The incidence varies enormously from country to country, and it is inversely related to socio-economic development and standards of living, preventive medicine and wound management. There is a direct relationship with fertile soil and a warm climate; thus, people living in the agricultural areas of developing tropical and subtropical countries are exposed to severe challenges associated with poor hygiene, lack of shoes, neglect of wounds and inadequate immunization.

In addition, some local customs promote the occurrence of tetanus:

- treatment of the umbilical cord stump with primitive applications that include animal dung
- tying of the umbilical cord itself with primitive ligatures
- ear-piercing and other operations performed with unsterile instruments.

Fatality rates may exceed 50% and neonatal tetanus carries a very high mortality. Case fatality rates can be greatly reduced to less than 10% by modern methods of treatment in specialist centres. Unfortunately, such expensive skilled help is available for only a small proportion of patients. Under-privileged people in countries with poorly developed or expensive medical services are at greatest risk and are least likely to get sophisticated assistance; 80% of deaths occur in Africa and south-east Asia.

Prevention and control

Prompt and adequate wound toilet and proper surgical debridement of wounds are of paramount importance in the prevention of tetanus. There is an increased risk that tetanus spores may germinate in a wound if cleansing is delayed and if sepsis develops. Clean superficial wounds that receive prompt attention may not require specific protection against tetanus and it is unreasonable to insist that every small prick or abrasion requires protection with antitoxin or antibiotic.

Routine practice should take account of the local incidence of tetanus and the individual circumstances of the case. It is wise to recommend specific prophylaxis for a non-immunized patient with a deep wound, puncture or stab wound, ragged laceration, a wound with much bruising and any devitalized tissue, a wound that is already septic, or a bite wound or other type of wound that is likely to be heavily contaminated. Figure 22.3 shows an approach that reflects current thinking in the UK.

The need for passive immunization is avoided if the patient is known to be properly immunized against tetanus (see Chapter 69).

A patient may be regarded as immune for 6 months after the first two injections, or for 5–10 years after a planned course of three injections (or a subsequent booster injection) of adsorbed tetanus toxoid (p. 275). Tetanus antitoxin should not be given to immune patients, but their active immunity may be enhanced when necessary by giving a dose of tetanus toxoid at the time of injury if the circumstances justify it.

A patient is considered non-immune if there is no history of having had an injection of tetanus toxoid or if only one injection has been given. Take care: a patient may recall having had 'a tetanus shot', but this may have been a previous dose of antitoxin for passive protection (which is transient and cannot be boosted by toxoid). If more than 6 months have elapsed after a course of two injections, or more than 10 years after a full primary course of three injections of adsorbed toxoid (or a booster injection), the patient should be regarded as non-immune. A patient is non-immune if more than 2–3 weeks have elapsed since a previous injection of equine antitoxin, or more than 6–8 weeks in the case of homologous (human) antitoxin. Non-

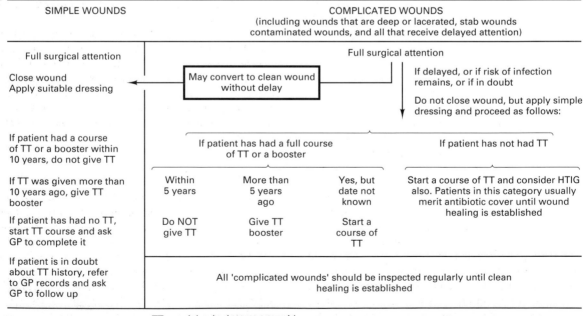

Fig. 22.3 Wound management guidelines, with special reference to the prevention of tetanus.

immunity should be assumed if there is any doubt about the immunization history.

Passive immunization with antitoxin

HTIG (homologous antitoxin) is available for passive protection and now supersedes equine antitoxin (heterologous antitoxin), which has been associated with occasional adverse reactions in the past. However, equine antiserum should not be prematurely discarded in countries that do not yet have HTIG. The prophylactic dose of HTIG is 250–500 units by intramuscular injection.

Combined active–passive immunization

A non-immune patient receiving passive protection with HTIG after injury may be given the first dose of a course of active immunization with adsorbed toxoid at the same time, provided that the injections are given from different syringes and into contralateral sites. The active immunization course must be subsequently completed.

Antibiotic protection

The prophylactic administration of antibiotics to all cases of open wounds is not recommended, but the use of penicillin or clindamycin is justified in some cases when there may be a significant risk of infection. This precaution must not replace prompt and adequate surgical wound toilet.

CLOSTRIDIUM BOTULINUM

Description

C. botulinum is a strictly anaerobic Gram-positive bacillus (about 5×1 μm). It is motile with peritrichous flagella and has spores that are oval and subterminal. It is a widely distributed saprophyte occurring in soil, vegetables, fruits, leaves, silage, manure, the mud of lakes and sea mud. Its optimum growth temperature is about 35°C, but some strains have been shown to grow and produce toxin at temperatures as low as 1–5°C.

The widespread occurrence of C. botulinum in nature, its ability to produce a potent neurotoxin in food, and the resistance of its spores to inactivation combine to make it a formidable pathogen of humans and a range of animals and birds. Spores of some strains withstand boiling in water (100°C) for several hours. They are usually destroyed by moist heat at 120°C within 5 min. Spores of type E strains (see below) are usually much less heat-resistant. Insufficient heating in the process of

preserving foods is an important factor in the causation of botulism, and great care must be taken in canning factories to ensure that adequate heating is achieved in all parts of the can contents. The resistance of the spores to radiation is of special relevance to food processing.

Toxins of C. botulinum

Botulinal toxins are among the most poisonous natural substances known. Seven main types of C. botulinum, designated A–G, produce antigenically distinct toxins with pharmacologically identical actions. All types can cause human disease, but types A, B and E are most common. The importance of this point is that, if antitoxin is given to a patient in an emergency, only the type-specific antitoxin will be effective.

Human botulism

Botulism is a severe, often fatal, form of food poisoning characterized by pronounced neurotoxic effects. The disease has been caused by a wide range of foods, usually preserved hams, large sausages of the German variety, home-preserved meats and vegetables, canned products such as fish, liver paste, and even hazelnut purée and honey. Traditional dishes such as fish or seal's flipper fermented in a barrel buried in the ground cannot be recommended by a bacteriologist! Type E strains are particularly but not invariably associated with a marine source, whereas type A and type B strains are usually associated with soil.

Foods responsible for botulism may not exhibit signs of spoilage. The preformed toxin in the food is absorbed from the intestinal tract. Although it is protein, it is not inactivated by the intestinal proteolytic enzymes. After absorption into the bloodstream, botulinum toxin binds irreversibly to the presynaptic nerve endings of the peripheral nervous system and cranial nerves, where it inhibits acetylcholine release.

Clinical features

The period between ingestion of the toxin and the appearance of signs and symptoms is usually 1–2 days, but it may be much longer. There may be initial nausea and vomiting. The oculomotor muscles are affected and the patient may have diplopia and drooping eyelids with a squint. There may be vertigo and blurred vision.

There is progressive descending motor loss with flaccid paralysis but with no loss of consciousness or sensation, though weakness and sleepiness are often described. The patient is thirsty, with a dry mouth and tongue. There are difficulties in speech and swallowing, with later problems of breathing and despair. There may be abdominal pain and restlessness. Death is due to respiratory or cardiac failure.

Wound botulism

Rare cases of wound infection with *C. botulinum* resulting in the characteristic signs and symptoms of botulism have been recorded.

Infant botulism

The 'floppy child syndrome' describes a young child, usually less than 6 months old, with flaccid paralysis that is ascribed to the growth of *C. botulinum* in the intestine at a stage in development when the colonization resistance of the gut is poor. There are various grades of the syndrome. Some cases have been attributed to the presence of *C. botulinum* spores in honey; when the honey was given as an encouragement to feed, the ingested spores were able to germinate and produce toxin in the infant gut.

Laboratory diagnosis

The organism or its toxin may be detected in the suspected food, and toxin may be demonstrated in the patient's blood by toxin–antitoxin neutralization tests in mice. Samples of faeces or vomit may also yield such evidence. Take care: bear in mind that botulinal toxin is very dangerous – specialist help should be summoned and the laboratory alerted.

Treatment

The priorities are:

- to remove unabsorbed toxin from the stomach and intestinal tract
- to neutralize unfixed toxin by giving polyvalent antitoxin (with due precautions to avoid hypersensitivity reactions to the heterologous antiserum)
- to give relevant intensive care and support.

Control

Home canning of foodstuffs should be avoided, and commercial canning must be strictly controlled. The amateur preservation of meat and vegetables, especially beans, peas and root vegetables, is dangerous in inexperienced hands. Acid fruits may be bottled safely in the home with heating at 100°C, since a low pH is inhibitory to the growth of *C. botulinum*.

A prophylactic dose of polyvalent antitoxin should be given intramuscularly to all persons who have eaten food suspected of causing botulism. Active immunity in man can be produced by injecting three doses of mixed toxoid at intervals of 2 months, but the very low incidence of the disease under normal conditions does not justify this as a routine. Active immunization should be considered for laboratory staff who might have to handle the organism or who might have to handle specimens containing the organism or its toxin.

CLOSTRIDIUM DIFFICILE

Description

C. difficile is a motile Gram-positive rod with oval subterminal spores. It occurs quite commonly in the faeces of neonates, and babies until the age of weaning, but it is not generally regarded as a normal commensal of adults.

The organism produces an enterotoxin (toxin A) and a cytotoxin (toxin B). It is a proven cause of antibiotic-associated diarrhoea, occasionally leading to a life-threatening condition, pseudomembranous colitis (Fig. 22.4). There is almost always a history of prior antibiotic therapy. The lincosamide antibiotics (usually clindamycin) have a particularly high risk. Extended-spectrum cephalosporins are also commonly incriminated and are much more important in terms of quantities used; however, there is virtually no antibiotic that has escaped blame.

Laboratory diagnosis

C. difficile can be isolated from the faeces by enrichment and selective culture procedures. Toxin B can be detected in the patient's faeces by testing extracts against cell monolayers of susceptible cells or both

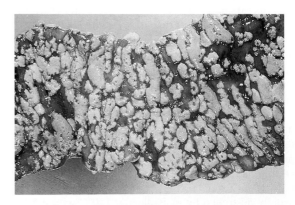

Fig. 22.4 Pseudomembranous colitis.

toxins may be demonstrated by immunological methods, e.g. enzyme-linked immunosorbent assay (ELISA). Toxin A-negative strains of *C. difficile* have been described as a cause of disease and these will not be detected by most current ELISA kits.

Treatment

It is essential to discontinue the antibiotic that is presumed to have precipitated the disease and to suppress the growth and toxin production of *C. difficile* by giving oral metronidazole or vancomycin. Pseudomembranous colitis may be lethal if it is not quickly recognized and treated.

Epidemiology

Evidence usually suggests that the organism is acquired from an exogenous source by a patient whose intestinal colonization resistance has been compromised by antibiotic exposure. Patients with antibiotic-associated diarrhoea tend to spend lengthy periods in hospital. Re-infection occurs in 20–50% of cases as it may take the gut 2–3 months to normalize following perturbation.

Prevention

Clinical awareness is the keynote. *C. difficile* is the most common cause of hospital-acquired diarrhoea. If a patient develops diarrhoea after at least 48 h in hospital, especially while taking antibiotics, the possibility of *C. difficile*-associated diarrhoea must be considered. If several cases occur in a hospital unit, cross-infection should be considered as the hospital environment can become extensively contaminated with *C. difficile* spores. The existing antibiotic policy of the unit should be reviewed.

RECOMMENDED READING

Brazier J S 1995 The laboratory diagnosis of *Clostidium difficile*-associated disease. *Reviews in Medical Microbiology* 6: 236–245

Collee J G, van Heyningen S 1991 Systemic toxigenic diseases (tetanus, botulism). In: Duerden B I, Drasar B S (eds) *Anaerobes in Human Disease*. Arnold, London, pp 372–394

Farrar J J, Yen L M , Cook T, Fairweather N, Binh N, Parry J, Parry C M 2000 Tetanus. *Journal of Neurology, Neurosurgery & Psychiatry* 69: 292–301

Hatheway C L 1990 Toxigenic clostridia. *Clinical Microbiology Reviews* 3: 66–98

Hobbs B C, Roberts D 1993 *Food Poisoning and Food Hygiene*, 6th edn. Arnold, London

Sakurai J 1995 Toxins of *Clostridium perfringens*. *Reviews in Medical Microbiology* 6: 175–185

Shapiro R L, Hatheway C, Swerdlow D L 1998 Botulism in the United States: a clinical and epidemiologic review. *Annals of Internal Medicine* 129: 221–228

23

Neisseria and moraxella

Meningitis; gonorrhoea; respiratory infections

R. C. B. Slack

Neisseriae are Gram-negative diplococci, of which the pathogenic members, the meningococcus and the gonococcus, are characteristically found inside polymorphonuclear pus cells of the inflammatory exudate. Although difficult to differentiate on morphological and cultural characters, these two pathogens are associated with entirely different diseases:

- *Neisseria meningitidis* causes a range of diseases (Table 23.1) embraced by the term *invasive meningococcal disease*. Most common are purulent meningitis (variously called *epidemic cerebrospinal meningitis, cerebrospinal fever* or, because of a purpuric rash which is sometimes present, *spotted fever*) and an acute septicaemic illness with a petechial rash, but without meningitis. About one-third of cases of meningococcal disease present as septicaemia; meningitis accounts for most others.
- *N. gonorrhoeae* causes the sexually transmitted disease *gonorrhoea*, which most commonly presents as a purulent infection of the mucous membrane of the urethra and the cervix uteri in women. In the newborn the gonococcus may give rise to a purulent conjunctivitis, and in young girls a vulvovaginitis.

Disseminated gonococcal infection, which is recognized by a rash and evidence of blood spread, may also occur, more commonly in women.

Other members of the genus are common commensals of the upper respiratory tract, which is also the reservoir of the meningococcus and, occasionally, the gonococcus.

N. lactamica and *N. polysacchareae* are frequently isolated from the nasopharynx. They are of low pathogenicity, but *N. lactamica* is occasionally isolated from blood or cerebrospinal fluid (CSF). Additional commensal species include *N. subflava* (of which there are several biovars), *N. sicca, N. mucosa* and *N. flavescens*. Two others, *N. elongata* and *N. weaveri*, are unusual in being rod-shaped.

Moraxellae are non-fermentative organisms that may be rod-shaped or coccoid. There is still uncertainty as to their taxonomic position. Some strains resemble *Acinetobacter* spp. and other glucose non-fermenters (see p. 287). The most important member of the group, *Moraxella catarrhalis* (*Branhamella catarrhalis*), is a common commensal of the upper respiratory tract, which may give rise to disease, usually as an opportunist pathogen.

Table 23.1 Clinical manifestations of meningococcal infection

Site of infection[a]	Common manifestation	Outcome
Blood	Fulminant septicaemia (Waterhouse–Friderichsen syndrome)	Fatal
Blood	Septicaemia, purpuric rash	} Mortality 14–50%
Blood and CSF	Septicaemia, rash and meningitis	
Blood and CSF	Meningitis with no rash	Mortality 2–6%
Blood	Chronic meningococcal septicaemia (rash, arthralgia, metastatic sepsis)	Recovery with treatment
Blood and site of sepsis	Arthritis, pericarditis, metastatic sepsis, primary peritonitis	Recovery with treatment
Eye	Conjunctivitis, endophthalmitis	Recovery with treatment
Genital tract	Asymptomatic carriage; rarely vulvovaginitis (children), urethritis	Recovery with treatment
Chest	Pneumonia	Recovery with treatment

CSF, cerebrospinal fluid.
[a] In most cases of clinical disease the organism is also carried in the nasopharynx.

NEISSERIA

Description

The two pathogenic neisseriae, *N. meningitidis* and *N. gonorrhoeae*, are very similar in their morphological and cultural characters. They are Gram-negative, oval cocci occurring in pairs with the apposed surfaces flat or even slightly concave (bean-shaped) and with the axis of the pair parallel and not in line as in the pneumococcus. In pus from inflammatory exudates, such as CSF or urethral discharge, many diplococci are found in a small proportion of the polymorphonuclear cells. This is more marked with the gonococcus than with the meningococcus. Extracellular cocci also occur and there may be considerable variation in their size and intensity of staining. In cultures the diplococcal arrangement is less obvious and more coccoid forms may be seen in stained films. Faintly staining involution forms are frequent in older cultures.

Growth requirements

Pathogenic neisseriae are exacting in their growth requirements due, in part, to susceptibility to inhibitory substances in the culture medium. The addition of heated blood or ascitic fluid, or both, to nutrient agar ensures a good growth of colonies from infected material, provided incubation is carried out, preferably at 35–36°C, in a moist atmosphere containing 5–10% carbon dioxide. Growth is rather slow (more so with the gonococcus) but, on a good medium, grey, glistening, slightly convex colonies of 0.5–1.0 mm in diameter appear in 8–24 h. Incubation should, however, be continued for another 24 h, when the colonies will be much larger and the gonococcus in particular tends to have a slightly roughened surface and a crenated margin.

Both meningococci and gonococci may bear fimbriae. The relationship between these and meningococcal disease is uncertain, but gonococcal fimbriae appear to be associated with attachment of the organism to mucosal surfaces and resistance to killing by phagocytic cells:

- the more virulent gonococcal strains (formerly called Kellogg types T1 and T2) bear numerous fimbriae (piliated types P1 and P2)
- the avirulent forms (formerly Kellogg types T3 and T4) are non-fimbriate.

Colonies of meningococci and gonococci react quickly in the test for cytochrome oxidase; non-pathogenic neisseriae react more slowly. Species identification depends on carbohydrate utilization reactions:

- meningococci produce acid from glucose and maltose, although the reactions may be slow and strains may be encountered which ferment only one of these sugars
- gonococci produces acid from glucose only.

Neither species ferments lactose or sucrose. Commercial kits that rapidly detect pre-formed enzymes are commonly used for identification.

Unlike most meningococci and gonococci, non-pathogenic neisseriae grow on ordinary nutrient agar. *N. lactamica* ferments lactose and can be differentiated from the pathogenic neisseriae by its positive reaction in the test for β-galactosidase.

Serological classification

Meningococci are divisible into various serogroups:

- Group A is, in most countries, the serogroup associated with epidemic cerebrospinal meningitis. The ability to cause epidemics seems to be associated with certain genetically defined clones.
- Group B meningococci are seen in both epidemic and outbreak situations.
- Group C strains have been associated with epidemics, but more commonly give rise to local outbreaks.
- Serogroup W135 is occasionally isolated and was associated with a major worldwide outbreak following the pilgrimage to Mecca (the Hajj) in 2000 and 2001.
- A few cases due to serogroups X and Y occur.
- Serogroups Z and 29E (Z′) are killed by normal human serum; they rarely cause disease and then only in patients with underlying disease.
- Capsulate meningococci of serogroups H, I, J, K and L have been described but do not appear to cause disease.

The serogroup of a meningococcus is determined by its lipopolysaccharide (LPS) capsular antigen and can be recognized by a slide agglutination test with absorbed group-specific antisera. Typing, with antisera directed against outer-membrane proteins, and subtyping is used to designate an isolate as, for example, *N. meningitidis* C: 2a: P1.2, P1.5 (serogroup: type: and subtype, respectively) and is usually done in reference laboratories. Further strain characterization is performed by DNA sequence analysis. This is useful in epidemiological studies as some serotypes are also found to be associated with more severe disease or with outbreaks. These are so-called *epidemic strains* of group B and C meningococci and may be a single clone.

Gonococci are antigenically more heterogeneous than meningococci. Strains can be characterized by *auxotyping*, which recognizes requirements for specific nutrients, such as arginine, proline, hypoxanthine and uracil. Panels of monoclonal antibodies that recognize specific proteins are also used to divide strains into various serovars. Epidemiological typing makes use of both methods augmented by nucleic acid methods.

MENINGOCOCCAL INFECTION

Pathogenesis

The natural habitat of the meningococcus is the human nasopharynx. The carrier:case ratio varies in different outbreaks and with the strain and population surveyed.

- Around 5–10% of normal populations are carriers of meningococci, over half of which are non-capsulate strains.
- In communities in which outbreaks of cerebrospinal meningitis are occurring, the carriage rate of the epidemic strain may range from 20% to as high as 90%.
- Some studies have shown that a sharp increase in the carrier rate of group A or other pathogenic groups of meningococci precedes the occurrence of clinical cases.
- There is a significant increase in carriage by University students in their first term when they live in shared accommodation on campus.
- Smokers appear to carry meningococci more often than non-smokers.

   The virulence determinants of invasive meningococci seem to be the LPS capsule (all pathogenic meningococci are capsulate), IgA protease and iron utilization from transferrin.

   The route of spread from the nasopharynx to the meninges is controversial:

- The organism may spread directly through the cribriform plate to the subarachnoid space by the perineural sheaths of the olfactory nerve.
- Much more probably, it passes through the nasopharyngeal mucosa to enter the bloodstream.

   In favour of the latter route are the frequent positive blood cultures in the early stages of infection, the purpuric rash in many cases with the isolation of meningococci from the skin lesions, and the occurrence, particularly during epidemics, of meningococcal septicaemia with rash, but no clinical meningitis.

   Cerebrospinal meningitis occurs among only a limited proportion of the population at risk. The absence of bactericidal antibody in the blood is the factor most closely related to susceptibility to clinical infection. Evidence in support of this relationship is:

- The age distribution of meningococcal disease, which has its highest incidence in infants and young

children 3 months to 3 years of age (Fig. 23.1), among whom humoral meningococcicidal antibodies are rarely found: the analogy with haemophilus meningitis is obvious. Most isolates in this age group are Group B.
- The reciprocal relationship in the appearance of bactericidal antibodies in older children and adults with the decreasing incidence of cerebrospinal meningitis, except when it occurs in outbreaks among young adults brought together for special reasons, e.g. military training, universities and, in earlier days, in ships and gaols. These were more commonly due to Group C before mass vaccination.
- Prospective studies among military recruits which showed that, whereas only 1% of the total population at risk became clinically affected, 38.5% of those lacking specific bactericidal antibody to the meningococcus, and who became infected with the epidemic group C strain, developed meningococcal meningitis.
- Patients convalescent from meningococcal infection develop bactericidal antibody to the infecting strain.

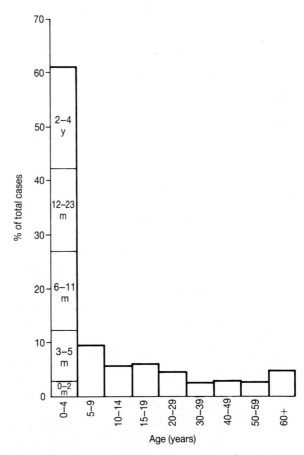

Fig. 23.1   Age distribution of meningococcal infection (England and Wales 1998–9, Public Health Laboratory Service isolates).

It is clear, nevertheless, from the relatively low incidence of meningococcal infections in young children and their absence in the large proportion of adults lacking specific antibody, that in most persons the first infection of the nasopharynx with a meningococcus leads to antibody production without development of clinical disease. It is possible that colonization with *N. lactamica*, which is common in children, may contribute to such antibody production.

Group-specific antibody is protective and this is the basis of the success of vaccination against meningococcal disease. Antibodies to outer-membrane proteins may also protect, but the range of antigens involved in this particular effect and the role of non-specific defence mechanisms in preventing clinical disease are ill-understood. However, the complement system is important, as shown by the recurrent attacks of meningococcal infections in complement-deficient subjects. Other host determinants such as lectin-binding proteins have been identified, but in most cases it is impossible to say why one person suffers invasive disease whereas most individuals remain carriers.

Less common manifestations of meningococcal disease include:

- Purulent conjunctivitis which on rare occasions proceeds to systemic disease.
- Monarticular purulent arthritis without any preceding evidence of septicaemic infection.
- A chronic septicaemic form of disease with both joint and skin involvement.
- Pneumonia, pericarditis and endocarditis, particularly in the elderly.

Laboratory diagnosis

In any suspected meningococcal infection, blood culture must be undertaken; if meningitis is suspected, a lumbar puncture should be performed as soon as possible unless there are signs of raised intracranial pressure. As many patients receive penicillin before admission to hospital, lumbar puncture yields more positive cultures than blood. Where it is available it is preferable to use the polymerase chain reaction (PCR) to detect DNA in blood or CSF.

Typically the CSF contains Gram-negative diplococci which can be recognized by microscopical examination of the stained centrifuged deposit. At a later stage they may be scanty and even apparently absent in films stained by Gram's method.

The CSF is cultured on heated blood (chocolate) agar and on blood agar. In the absence of visible meningococci, glucose broth may be added to the remaining sediment of the centrifuged deposit to facilitate the isolation of very scanty organisms. Cultures are incubated overnight at 37°C in an atmosphere of 5–10% carbon dioxide. Sugar utilization tests or commercial kits are used to identify any Gram-negative diplococci. The oxidase test is performed on colonies on solid medium. Direct slide agglutination with specific antisera may be carried out on suspensions of colonies picked from solid medium.

Non-cultural methods are increasingly used because the rapid institution of chemotherapy reduces the chance of successful culture. Meningococcal capsular polysaccharide may be demonstrated in CSF by counter-current electrophoresis, by latex agglutination and by PCR.

Cultures should be sent, on slopes of chocolate agar, to a reference laboratory for serogrouping and serotyping, procedures that provide important epidemiological information.

Meningococci may be found in genital sites, and it is important to identify these organisms accurately and differentiate them from gonococci.

Treatment

Treatment should begin as soon as meningococcal disease is suspected.

- Intravenous penicillin, cefotaxime or ceftriaxone are the drugs of choice. Although these agents do not cross uninflamed meninges, they readily pass into CSF when inflammation is present.
- Chloramphenicol is effective, but risks of blood dyscrasia have limited its use.
- In the absence of organisms in the Gram-stained CSF deposit, it is wise to give therapy with cefotaxime or ceftriaxone, which cover *Haemophilus influenzae* and *Streptococcus pneumoniae*, the other two principal causes of meningitis in childhood after the neonatal period.
- Meningococci of group A and 'epidemic' strains of group B are commonly resistant to sulphonamides and these drugs are no longer used.

Almost all clinical isolates of meningococci in the UK are presently sensitive to benzylpenicillin. However, meningococci of reduced susceptibility to penicillin have been reported in some countries and are likely to become more common; it is therefore important that accurate sensitivity testing is carried out on all meningococcal isolates from clinical disease.

At the end of a course of therapy with penicillin it is important to give eradicative treatment with rifampicin or ciprofloxacin because penicillin does not eradicate meningococci from the nasopharynx and a patient returning home as a carrier may infect others. This probably does not apply to ceftriaxone or cefotaxime.

The mortality rate in septicaemic illness may range from 14% up to 50% in some outbreaks. The mortality in meningitis is about 2–6%. Bad prognostic signs are:

- The presence of coma on admission to hospital.
- A rapidly coalescing purpuric rash.
- Signs of shock.

Occasionally in the most fulminating forms of septicaemia there may not be time for the rash to develop before death. In such cases meningococci are isolated from the blood in life or post mortem and haemorrhagic adrenals are seen at autopsy, these being characteristic of the *Waterhouse–Friderichsen syndrome*.

Epidemiology

Meningococcal infections occur worldwide and are notifiable in most countries. In the northern hemisphere, they tend to occur during the winter months. About two-thirds of cases occur in the first 5 years of life. The peak prevalence of disease is in the first year of life and there is a smaller peak in adolescence (Fig. 23.1). The incidence is higher in men than women. The prevalence of meningococcal infection fluctuates over time, as does the relative proportion of serogroups (Fig. 23.2).

The incidence of meningococcal infection is increasing. There have been dramatic epidemics due to group A meningococci in many parts of the world; to group C in Brazil and Africa; to group B in Norway; and to W135 following the pilgrimage to Mecca (Hajj).

Outbreaks have occurred frequently among young adult populations recruited for military service, and what might have been limited outbreaks of infection were fanned into great conflagrations of cerebrospinal meningitis in troops in training in both World Wars.

Before the introduction of vaccination, localized outbreaks were common in some US army training camps. Small outbreaks have been seen even in recent times in the UK in schools and universities. Outbreak strains have commonly been group C, although there have been some outbreaks of group B.

Intensive studies have shown that a high proportion of military recruits became nasopharyngeal carriers of meningococci; cases tended to occur as the carriage rate rose, indicating that the critical point at which a patient either becomes ill or immune is at the time of acquiring the organism. Epidemic strains of group A or group B may give rise to a high incidence of disease in susceptible individuals who acquire such a strain. The increase in immunity observed with increasing age is likely to be due to asymptomatic infection with avirulent strains, which are carried by 7–20% of a healthy population, often for many months. Household contacts of a case are 500–800 times more likely to develop meningococcal infection than the general population.

Outbreaks of meningococcal meningitis require at least three factors:

- A population of susceptible individuals who lack bactericidal antibodies to the current strains.
- A high transmission rate from person to person.
- A virulent, capsulate strain of meningococcus.

The factors that determine the virulence and communicability of a meningococcus are still not fully understood, but only capsulate strains are isolated from systemic infections.

Control

Chemoprophylaxis

Outbreaks of disease may be controlled by chemoprophylaxis alone, thus eradicating the organism from carriers, or combined with vaccination. Until the emergence of resistant strains, sulphonamides were effective, but rifampicin is now the preferred drug for children although it is effective in eradicating meningococcal carriage in only 80–90% of the population treated. After prophylaxis, rifampicin-resistant strains may be found in a small number of patients and may, on rare occasions, give rise to disease in contacts. Ciprofloxacin is widely used as a prophylactic for adolescents and adults as a single, oral dose. All household and other intimate (e.g. mouth kissing) contacts of a case should be given chemoprophylaxis as a routine.

Vaccination

Resistance to meningococcal infection is closely associated with the possession of bactericidal antibodies that

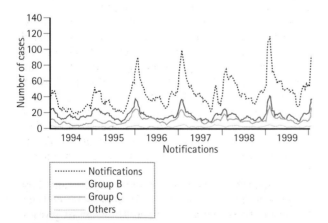

Fig. 23.2 Year (5-week moving average) of cases of meningococcal infection for 1994–99 (England and Wales). (Data from the Communicable Disease Surveillance Centre, Colindale.)

may be maternal in origin or actively produced in response to carriage. Vaccines containing the pure group-specific capsular polysaccharide of meningococci of groups A, C, Y and W135 are available and are good immunogens. However:

- the protection provided is group-specific
- it lasts at most 3 years
- it does not prevent meningococcal carriage
- they are poorly immunogenic in children aged under 2 years.

These shortcomings have limited their use largely for travel to parts of the world in which epidemics due to group A or C meningococci are in progress or are to be expected.

One approach to the management of epidemics of meningococcal infection due to group A or C meningococci has been to vaccinate all the population at risk and to give penicillin to any clinical cases. Any cases that arise before an immune response to the vaccine has commenced are also treated.

The development of protein-conjugated group C vaccines has changed the outlook for prevention (see p. 676). In the UK vaccination has been introduced into the routine programme and it is hoped that clinical infection with group C will be eradicated in those under 18 years, although the effect on carriage is less clear.

Trials are in progress on several vaccines against group B meningococci, but it has been more difficult to find a suitable immunogenic epitope.

GONOCOCCAL INFECTION

The name 'gonorrhoea' derives from the Greek words *gonos* (seed) and *rhoia* (flow) and described a condition in which semen flowed from the male organ without erection. It became apparent that gonorrhoea was associated with sexual promiscuity, one of the diseases celebrated by being named after the Roman goddess of love, Venus. Indeed, gonorrhoea is a classical venereal disease, being almost exclusively spread by sexual contact, having a short incubation period and being relatively easy to diagnose and treat.

Pathogenesis

N. gonorrhoeae is exclusively a human pathogen although chimpanzees have been infected artificially. It is never found as a normal commensal although a proportion of those infected, particularly women, may remain asymptomatic. These individuals may develop systemic or ascending infection at a later stage.

The commonest clinical presentation is acute urethritis in the male a few days after unprotected vaginal or anal sexual intercourse. Dysuria and a purulent penile discharge make most sufferers seek treatment rapidly. A few men have relatively minor symptoms which may disappear rapidly. Truly asymptomatic infection is rare in the active male. However, up to 5% may carry the organism without apparent distress, and this is more common with certain types of gonococci. Rectal and pharyngeal infection is less often symptomatic and may be discovered only after tracing contacts.

In women with vaginal infection, only half may have symptoms of discharge and dysuria. Most seek attention because of their partner's symptoms, as part of contact tracing or screening of high-risk individuals. Asymptomatic carriage in women is common, especially in the endocervical canal. At menstruation or after instrumentation, particularly termination of pregnancy, gonococci ascend to the fallopian tubes to give rise to *acute salpingitis*, which may be followed by *pelvic inflammatory disease* and a high probability of sterility if inadequately treated. Peritoneal spread occasionally occurs and may produce a perihepatic inflammation (*Fitz-Hugh–Curtis syndrome*). Some auxotypes of *N. gonorrhoeae* spread more widely and give rise to disseminated gonococcal infection.

Disseminated infection is seen more commonly in women, who may present with painful joints, fever and a few septic skin lesions on their extremities (Fig. 23.3). The diagnosis of a venereal disease may not be obvious and isolation of gonococci from joint fluid, blood culture and skin aspirates requires particular care. The organisms are invariably present in the cervix, but in many cases antibiotics have been given before the diagnosis is considered. Most strains are highly susceptible to penicillin. Rarely, disseminated gonococcal infection may present as endocarditis or meningitis.

Babies born to infected women may suffer *ophthalmia neonatorum*, in which the eyes are coated with gonococci as the baby passes down the birth canal. A severe purulent eye discharge with peri-orbital oedema occurs within a few days of birth. If untreated, ophthalmia leads rapidly to blindness. It may be prevented in areas of high prevalence by the instillation of 1% aqueous silver nitrate in the eyes of newborn babies. Alternatively, topical erythromycin can be used; this has the advantage of being active against chlamydia and less toxic.

In prepubertal girls, vulvovaginitis may be caused by gonococci. This occurs either in conditions of poor hygiene or by sexual abuse; it should always be investigated carefully and the child put in touch with social services and other professionals capable of dealing with this difficult condition.

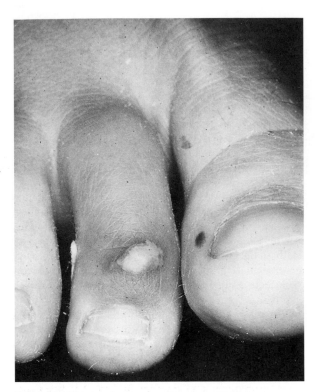

Fig. 23.3 Skin lesions in disseminated gonococcal infection.

Laboratory diagnosis

Cultivation of *N. gonorrhoeae* from sites with scanty commensals, such as the male urethra, rarely presents any problems, and Gram staining of a smear is usually 95% sensitive. *N. gonorrhoeae* is intolerant of drying and temperature changes; it readily undergoes autolysis. It is a fastidious microbe, requiring humidity, 5–7% carbon dioxide and complex media for growth. Ideally, exudate is taken directly from the patient onto appropriate preheated, freshly prepared solid media and immediately placed in a carbon dioxide incubator. This is usually possible only in specialized clinics with sufficient patient numbers to justify the expense. Where there is likely to be any delay, transport media must be used to carry the material on swabs.

Treatment

The susceptibility of isolates of *N. gonorrhoeae* to commonly used antibiotics varies so much that regular testing is essential. Penicillin, especially in slow-release intramuscular forms such as procaine penicillin, remains the preferred therapy. Small decreases in susceptibility occurred in the 1950s and 1960s and were overcome by increasing the size of the single dose. However, by the

1970s the dose of penicillin required to cure simple acute gonorrhoea in men in some parts of the world had reached an impossibly large injection.

Strains of *N. gonorrhoeae* that are completely resistant to penicillins are now common throughout the world, although their prevalence varies from country to country. These strains possess the gene coding for the TEM-type β-lactamase commonly found in *Escherichia coli*.

If penicillin is contra-indicated because of allergy or bacterial resistance there are many alternatives:

- Fluoroquinolones have many advocates although their use is limited in many countries because widespread, inappropriate use has led to a high prevalence of resistance. Failure rates of over 50% have been reported in the Philippines.
- Tetracyclines are effective in most places and also treat concomitant chlamydial infection if given in a sufficiently long course of treatment. Tetracycline resistance in gonococci is increasing in some countries.
- Expanded-spectrum cephalosporins, in particular ceftriaxone, are extremely active, but have to be given by injection and are expensive.
- Co-amoxiclav is suitable for infection with β-lactamase-producing gonococci in a patient not hypersensitive to penicillins; it can be given with a large dose of procaine penicillin to overcome intrinsic penicillin resistance, which is not reversed by clavulanic acid.

Single-dose therapy appears adequate for most cases of acute genital gonorrhoea in men and women. There are obvious advantages to this approach in obtaining complete compliance and stopping the chain of infection. In disseminated gonococcal disease and any complicated infection, treatment for 7–10 days is necessary.

Epidemiology and control

Acute gonorrhoea is usually easily diagnosed and treated, and was well controlled in much of the world until the 1960s. The remarkable changes in travel, migration, sexual licence and availability of oral contraceptives rapidly reversed this process so that there was an increase in gonorrhoea and non-specific genital infection (mainly caused by chlamydiae) every year until scares about the acquired immune deficiency syndrome in the 1980s. Barrier methods of contraception, condoms in particular, greatly reduce the rate of transmission.

The keys to control of gonorrhoea are:

- rapid diagnosis
- use of effective antibiotics
- tracing, examination and treatment of contacts.

Unfortunately, in many places inappropriate self-medication has resulted in widespread antimicrobial resistance. Inability to treat contacts ensures the spread of the disease and re-infections.

MORAXELLA

The genus *Moraxella* is a member of the family Neisseriaceae. The organisms are characterized as asaccharolytic, oxidase-positive, catalase-positive short rods, coccobacilli or, in the case of *M. catarrhalis*, diplococci. They are commensals of mucosal surfaces and occasionally give rise to opportunistic infections. *M. lacunata* is occasionally encountered as a cause of 'angular' blepharoconjunctivitis.

The related genus *Kingella* contains organisms that differ from the moraxellae in being catalase-negative, glucose-fermenting coccobacilli. In common with some other Gram-negative rods, such as *Cardiobacterium hominis*, *Eikenella corrodens* and *Actinobacillus actinomycetemcomitans*, *Kingella* species (usually *K. kingae*) are sometimes found in endocarditis. They have also been implicated in joint infections.

MORAXELLA CATARRHALIS

Pathogenesis

M. catarrhalis is a respiratory tract commensal and, as with other members of the upper respiratory tract flora such as the pneumococcus and *H. influenzae*, it can gain access to the lower respiratory tract in patients with chronic chest disease or compromised host defences. *M. catarrhalis* is commonly isolated from sputum, and a pathogenic role is suspected only if the sputum contains large numbers of pus cells and Gram-negative diplococci, and if culture yields a heavy growth of *M. catarrhalis* in the absence of other recognized respiratory pathogens.

As well as causing chest infection itself, *M. catarrhalis* may also protect other respiratory pathogens from the action of penicillin or ampicillin by producing β-lactamase.

M. catarrhalis has also been incriminated in otitis media and sinusitis, and may be isolated on occasion from blood culture in patients who are immunocompromised.

Laboratory diagnosis

Sputum is examined by Gram film. In true infections large numbers of Gram-negative diplococci may be seen dispersed between the pus cells. Sputum is cultured on media suitable for the isolation of other potential respiratory pathogens (e.g. blood agar and chocolate agar) and incubated in 5% carbon dioxide overnight. In situations in which it is held to be pathogenic, *M. catarrhalis* is predominant in culture.

M. catarrhalis produces rough, circular, convex colonies which can be lifted off intact with a wire loop from agar culture medium. Colonies are oxidase-positive. In common with other moraxellae, they do not ferment sugars and are easily differentiated from neisseriae. Growth on nutrient agar at 22°C has been suggested as a differential characteristic, but clinically significant isolates of *M. catarrhalis* may not grow in these conditions. Tests for deoxyribonuclease and for butyrate esterase are positive. At least 50% of strains produce β-lactamase.

Treatment

M. catarrhalis is sensitive to amoxicillin, combined with clavulanic acid (co-amoxiclav) in the case of β-lactamase-producing strains, and also to cephalosporins, tetracycline, macrolides and fluoroquinolones.

RECOMMENDED READING

Arya O P, Hart C A 1998 *Sexually Transmitted Infections and AIDS in the Tropics*. CABI Publishing, London

Barker R M, Shakespeare R M, Mortimore A J, Allen N A, Solomon C L, Stuart J M 1999 Practical Guidelines for responding to an outbreak of meningococcal disease among University students. *Communicable Disease and Public Health* 2: 168–73

Cartwright K (ed) 1995 *Meningococcal Disease*. Wiley, Chichester

Murphy T R 1996 Branhamella catarrhalis: epidemiology, surface antigenic structure, and immune response. *Microbiological Reviews* 60: 267–279

Nassif X, So M 1995 Interaction of pathogenic neisseria with nonphagocytic cells. *Clinical Microbiology Reviews* 8: 376–388

Oates J K, Csonka G W 1990 Gonorrhoea. In: Csonka GW, Oates J K (eds) *Sexually Transmitted Diseases*. Baillière Tindall, London, pp 209–226

PHLS Meningococcal Infections Working Group and Public Health Medicine Environmental Group 1995 Control of meningococcal disease: guidance for consultants in communicable disease control. *Communicable Disease Report* 5: R189–R195

Rosenstein N E, Perkins B A, Stephens D S, Popovic T, Hughes J M 2001 Meningococcal Disease. *New England Journal of Medicine* 344: 1378–1388

Tunkel A R, Scheld M W 1995 Acute bacterial meningitis. *Lancet* 346: 1675–1680

24

Salmonella

Food poisoning; enteric fever

H. Chart

There are well over 2000 different antigenic types of salmonella. They were originally classified as separate species, but it is now generally accepted that they represent serotypes of a single species, *Salmonella enterica*. Various subspecies are recognized, but most of the serotypes that infect mammals are found in a subspecies also designated *enterica*. The full correct designation is, for example: *S. enterica* subspecies *enterica* serotype Enteritidis, but this is usually abbreviated to *S.* serotype Enteritidis, or simply *S.* Enteritidis.

Many serotypes are host-specific; those causing infections in man may not cause disease in animals and vice versa. Use of the general term 'salmonella' has inadvertently caused confusion in our understanding of the pathogenicity of the various serotypes. This chapter focuses on serotypes of *S. enterica* responsible for human infections unless otherwise stated.

Certain serotypes are a major cause of food-borne infection worldwide. Most infections are relatively benign and restricted to the intestinal tract, causing a short-lived diarrhoea, but some salmonellae cause life-threatening systemic disease. In England and Wales annual isolations of selected serotypes from man almost trebled from 10 251 to 27 000 between 1981 and 1988. This dramatic increase was due largely to the emergence of strains belonging to serotype Enteritidis, which peaked in 1997–98 and continues to be the most frequently isolated serotype. Between 1989 and 1995 the number of infections reported in England and Wales remained steady at about 30 000 infections per year but has more recently fallen by about one-third (Fig. 24.1). However, as in other developed countries, many, perhaps most, infections go unrecognized.

In developing countries in which large-scale farming and processing of food animals has not been established, salmonellae are not as important a cause of community-acquired diarrhoea. However, infections with *S. enterica* serotypes Typhi and Paratyphi, which are mainly encountered as imported infections in developed countries, remain prevalent in other parts of the world.

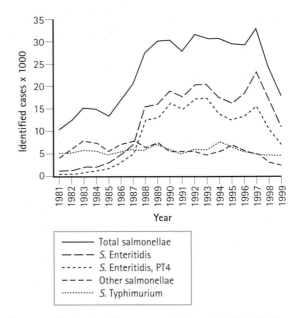

Fig. 24.1 The number of human cases of salmonellosis identified in England and Wales during 1980–99 (Public Health Laboratory Service data).

DESCRIPTION

Salmonellae are typical members of the Enterobacteriaceae: facultatively anaerobic Gram-negative bacilli able to grow on a wide range of relatively simple media and distinguished from other members of the family by their biochemical characteristics and antigenic structure. Their normal habitat is the animal intestine.

Antigens

Typical strains of *S. enterica* express two sets of antigens, which are readily demonstrable by serotyping. Long-chain lipopolysaccharide (LPS) comprises heat-stable polysaccharide commonly known as the *somatic* or *O antigens*. These molecules are located in the outer membrane and are anchored into the cell wall by antigenically conserved lipid A and LPS-core regions. The long-chain LPS molecules exhibit considerable variation in sugar composition and degree of polysaccharide branching, and it is this structural heterogeneity that is responsible for the large number of serotypes of *S. enterica*. Salmonellae are usually highly motile when growing in laboratory media (Fig. 24.2), and flagellar protein subunits contain the epitopes that form the basis of the flagella-based serotyping scheme generally known as the *H antigens*. In most strains of *S. enterica* the flagella exhibit the property of diphasic variation, whereby one of two genetically distinct flagellar structures are expressed. When one flagellar structure is expressed it contains *phase 1* antigens, while when the other set is operative *phase 2* antigens are synthesized.

Certain serotypes of *S. enterica* express a surface polysaccharide, of which the Vi (virulence) antigen of *S*. Typhi is the most important example. Since the polysaccharide may encapsulate the entire bacterium, antibodies designed to recognize the LPS antigens may be prevented from binding, which can occasionally make detection of the O antigens difficult.

The O antigens are numbered with Arabic numerals. The flagellar antigens of phase 1 are designated by lower case letters, and of phase 2 by a mixture of lower case letters and Arabic numerals. The antigenic structure of any serotype of salmonella is expressed as an antigenic formula, which has three parts, describing the O antigens, the phase 1 H antigens and the phase 2 H antigens, in that order. The three parts are separated by colons, and the component antigens in each part by commas.

The original Kauffmann–White scheme, which elegantly catalogued salmonellae (but named them as individual species), placed them into some 30 groups on

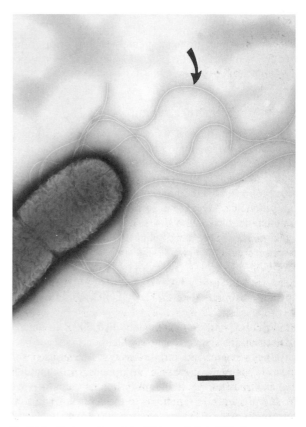

Fig. 24.2 Electron micrograph of *Salmonella* Enteritidis. Arrow indicates the flagella that carry the 'H' antigens (bar = 0.3μm).

the basis of shared O antigens, and further subdivided the groups into clusters with H antigens in common. Some salmonellae, such as *S*. Typhi (9, 12, [Vi]: d-), express only one flagellar phase. Some of the commoner serotypes are shown in Table 24.1.

Table 24.1 The antigenic structure of some representative salmonellae

Serotype	'O' antigens		'H' antigens Phase 1		Phase 2
Typhi	9, 12, [Vi]	:	d	:	–
Paratyphi B	1, 4, 5, 12	:	b	:	1, 2
Typhimurium	1, 4, 5, 12	:	i	:	1, 2
Enteritidis	1, 9, 12	:	g, m	:	1, 7
Virchow	6, 7	:	r	:	1, 2
Kedougou	1, 13, 23	:	i	:	1, w
Hadar	6, 8	:	Z10	:	e, n, x
Heidelberg	1, 4, 5, 12	:	r	:	1, 2
Infantis	6, 7, 14	:	r	:	1, 5
Newport	6, 8, 20	:	e, h	:	1, 2
Panama	1, 9, 12	:	l, v	:	1, 5
Dublin	1, 9, 12	:	g, p	:	–

Phage typing

Phage typing has proved extremely useful for discriminating within strains of *S. enterica* serotypes Typhimurium, Virchow, Enteritidis and Typhi.

Antibiotic resistance typing

Characterization of strains of *S. enterica* has also been facilitated by determining their resistance to a range of antibiotics, including ampicillin, chloramphenicol, gentamicin, kanamycin, streptomycin, sulphonamides, tetracycline and trimethoprim. This has been of particular relevance to certain strains of *S.* Typhimurium (notably definitive type 104) characterized by resistance to ampicillin, chloramphenicol, aminoglycosides and co-trimoxazole.

HOST RANGE AND PATHOGENICITY

Strains of *S. enterica* are widely distributed in nature. All vertebrates appear capable of harbouring these bacteria in their gut, and certain serotypes have also been isolated from a wide range of arthropods, including flies and cockroaches. Most animal infections seem to range from those without symptoms to those resulting in self-limiting gastro-enteritis of variable severity. Some strains, such as those belonging to serotype Typhimurium, show a wide host range, and can be isolated from many different animal species. A small number of strains, the *host-adapted* serotypes, are much more restricted in the species they inhabit, and show a different spectrum of illness.

Host-adapted serotypes

Among the host-adapted serotypes, Typhi and Paratyphi A, B and C are primarily pathogens of humans, and are rarely, if ever, isolated from animals other than man. Paratyphi B, while essentially a human pathogen, is occasionally isolated from cattle, pigs, poultry, exotic reptiles and other animals, although cycles of transmission in these hosts have not been demonstrated.

Human infection with these organisms is characterized by a long incubation period of 10–14 days, followed by a septicaemic illness, *enteric fever*, quite unlike the diarrhoea and vomiting that are characteristic of food poisoning.

Other salmonellae adapted to particular animal hosts include Cholerae-suis (pigs), Dublin (cattle), Gallinarum-pullorum (poultry), Abortus-equi (horses) and Abortus-ovis (sheep). These are all responsible for considerable morbidity, mortality and economic loss among domestic animals. All can cause illness in humans, but only strains of Cholerae-suis and Dublin do so regularly. Strains of *S.* Typhimurium definitive type (DT) 104 isolated from human infection appear to have originated from bovine sources; however, whether these strains can be considered as host-adapted to farm animals remains to be established. The rest of the 2000 or so serotypes of salmonellae show no apparent host preference. The extent to which they cause human infection appears to result from their prevalence in domestic food animals at any particular time and on the opportunity for the contamination of food in which further multiplication can take place. In developed countries most human infections are caused by a relatively small number of locally prevalent serotypes.

PATHOGENESIS

In common with many pathogenic enteric bacteria, strains of *S. enterica* require a range of pathogenic mechanisms to enable them to colonize a host and cause disease. The lack of a good animal model of salmonella pathogenicity has impeded research into how these bacteria cause the symptoms of disease. In general terms, infection is initiated by ingestion of a sufficient number of organisms to colonize the gut, to overcome the host's defences and express the mechanisms resulting in overt disease.

Infective dose

For infections of man, the number of bacteria that must be swallowed in order to cause infection is uncertain and varies with the serotype. The accepted dictum that large inocula of these bacteria are required for induction of human illness is based largely on volunteer studies. In most of these the median infective dose for most serotypes, including Typhi, has varied from 10^6 to 10^9 viable organisms. However, investigation of outbreaks suggests that in natural infection the infective dose might be below 10^3 viable organisms.

Many factors are thought to influence the infective dose. There appears to be considerable strain-to-strain variation in virulence even within a single serotype. Systematic variation in pathogenicity between serotypes is less easy to demonstrate outside the host-adapted strains. The vehicle of ingestion may also influence pathogenesis. Organisms ingested in water and other drinks may be carried through the stomach relatively rapidly, and evade the effect of gastric acid. Similarly, the administration of antacids, or the effects of gastric resection, reduces the infective dose. Bacteria within particles of food would also evade the action of stomach acids.

Host factors

Host factors are also likely to be important, although these may be difficult to separate from other confounding variables. For example, age-specific isolation rates for salmonellae, as for some other gut pathogens, are higher for children less than 1 year of age than for any other age group, but this reflects the fact that a higher proportion of infections are investigated in this age group. This is often misinterpreted as revealing a greater susceptibility.

Initiation of infection

Once salmonellae enter the lumen of the intestine they are able to tolerate the action of digestive bile, but need to be able to compete with the prevailing gut flora, adhere to the gut mucosa and multiply. Certain serotypes, such as *S.* Typhimurium, express type 1 fimbriae, which enable them to adhere to α-mannose-containing molecules on the microvilli of the ileal mucosa; however, surprisingly little is known about the range of fimbriae expressed. Strains of *S.* Enteritidis are thought to express at least three different fimbrial structures, including *S.* Enteritidis fimbriae 14 (SEF 14). Expression of fimbriae is influenced by environmental conditions and, for example, whether SEF 14 is required for colonizing the human gut is not known.

Serotypes such as *S.* Typhimurium and *S.* Enteritidis also express an adhesion mechanism that does not involve fimbriae. Certain strains of enteric bacteria carry DNA sequences that encode several pathogenic mechanisms, termed *pathogenicity islands*. In common with strains of Verocytotoxin-producing *Escherichia coli* belonging to serogroup O157 (see Chapter 26), strains of *S.* Typhimurium and *S.* Enteritidis have pathogenicity islands that encode an adhesion mechanism comprising both a bacterial adhesin and the adhesin receptor which is translocated into the host intestine. This process enables these bacteria to insert their own binding site into the gut, unlike fimbriae, which require host-derived binding sites located in the intestinal wall.

Attachment to the host mucosa is followed by degeneration of the microvilli to form breaches in the cell membrane through which the salmonellae enter the intestinal epithelial cells. For certain strains, further multiplication in these cells and in macrophages of the Peyer's patches follows. Some bacteria penetrate into the submucosa and pass to the local mesenteric lymph nodes. All the clinical manifestations of infection with salmonella, including diarrhoea, begin after ileal penetration. For strains of *S.* Typhi, infection involves the invasion of the bloodstream and various organs.

CLINICAL SYNDROMES

Although salmonellae can cause a wide spectrum of clinical illness there are four major syndromes, each with its own diagnostic and therapeutic problems, which are considered separately. These are enteric fever, gastro-enteritis, bacteraemia with or without metastatic infection, and the asymptomatic carrier state.

Enteric fever

Enteric fever is most usually caused by strains of *S.* Typhi or *S.* Paratyphi A, B or C. The clinical features tend to be more severe with *S.* Typhi (*typhoid fever*). After penetration of the ileal mucosa the organisms pass via the lymphatics to the mesenteric lymph nodes, whence after a period of multiplication they invade the bloodstream via the thoracic duct. The liver, gallbladder, spleen, kidney and bone marrow become infected during this primary bacteraemic phase in the first 7–10 days of the incubation period. After multiplication in these organs, bacilli pass into the blood, causing a second and heavier bacteraemia, the onset of which approximately coincides with that of fever and other signs of clinical illness. From the gallbladder a further invasion of the intestine results. Peyer's patches and other gut lymphoid tissues become involved in an inflammatory reaction and infiltration with mononuclear cells, followed by necrosis, sloughing and the formation of characteristic typhoid ulcers occurs.

Onset

The interval between ingestion of the organisms and the onset of illness varies with the size of the infecting dose. It can be as short as 3 days or as long as 50 days, but is usually about 2 weeks. The onset is usually insidious. Early symptoms are often vague: a dry cough and epistaxis associated with anorexia, a dull continuous headache, abdominal tenderness and discomfort are among the most common symptoms. Diarrhoea is uncommon and early in the illness many patients complain of constipation.

Progression

In the untreated case the temperature shows a step-ladder rise over the first week of the illness, remains high for 7–10 days and then falls by lysis during the third or fourth week. Physical signs include a relative bradycardia at the height of the fever, hepatomegaly, splenomegaly and often a rash of *rose spots*. These are 2–4 mm in diameter, slightly raised discrete irregular blanching pink macules most often found on the front of the chest. They appear in crops of up to a dozen at a time and fade after 3 or 4 days, leaving no scar. They are characteristic of, but not specific for, enteric fever.

Relapse

Apparent recovery can be followed by relapse in 5–10% of untreated cases. Relapse is usually shorter and of milder character than the initial illness, but can be severe and may be fatal. Severe intestinal haemorrhage and intestinal perforation are serious complications that can occur at any stage of the illness.

Morbidity and mortality

Classic typhoid fever is a serious infection which, when untreated, has a mortality approaching 20%. It is notoriously unpredictable in its presentation and course. Mild and asymptomatic infections are not uncommon. In endemic areas, and particularly where it co-exists with schistosomiasis, chronic infection can present with fever of many months' duration, accompanied by chronic bacteraemia. Occasionally, diarrhoea may dominate the picture from the outset, particularly in paratyphoid infections, which sometimes present as typical gastro-enteritis no different from that caused by most *S. enterica* serotypes.

Gastro-enteritis and food poisoning

Acute gastro-enteritis is characterized by vomiting, abdominal pain fever and diarrhoea. It can be caused by ingestion of a wide variety of bacteria or their products, several viruses and a number of vegetable toxins and inorganic chemicals. The term *bacterial food poisoning* is conveniently restricted to cases and epidemics of acute gastro-enteritis that are caused by the ingestion of food contaminated by bacteria or their toxins. It is an important feature of bacterial food poisoning that the bacteria need the opportunity to multiply in the food to reach an infective concentration before being eaten. Infections such as hepatitis A or bacillary dysentery, in which food may be an incidental vector, are not usually considered to be examples of food poisoning. Strains of *S. enterica* commonly cause food poisoning worldwide.

Clinical features

The most common clinical manifestation of infection with non-invasive salmonella serotypes is diarrhoea, often accompanied by headache, malaise and nausea. The incubation period is usually 8–48 h, the onset abrupt and the clinical course short and self-limiting.

Symptoms vary from the passage of two or three loose stools which may be disregarded by the sufferer, to a severe and prostrating illness with the frequent passage of watery, green, offensive stools, fever, shivering, abdominal pain and, in the most severe cases, dehydration leading to hypotension, cramps and renal failure. Vomiting is rarely a prominent feature of the illness.

Severe infections occur most often in the very young and the elderly, although mild, subclinical infections also occur in these age groups. Infections with certain serotypes in those already ill or debilitated for other causes are likely to be more severe and life-threatening. In most cases the acute stage is over within 2 or 3 days, although it may be more prolonged. Persistent or high fever suggests bacteraemia, possibly with metastatic infection.

Bacteraemia and metastatic disease

Bacteraemia is a constant feature of enteric fever caused by strains of *S.* Typhi and *S.* Paratyphi, and can occur as a rare complication of infection with other salmonellae. Transient bacteraemia occurs in up to 4% of cases of acute gastro-enteritis but in most cases the organisms are cleared from the bloodstream without ill effect. Occasionally, dissemination of the bacilli throughout the body results in the establishment of one or more localized foci of persisting infection, especially where pre-existing abnormality makes a tissue or organ vulnerable. Atherosclerotic plaques within large arteries, damaged heart valves, joint prostheses and other implants are all susceptible to metastatic infection. Osteomyelitis is most often found in long bones, costochondral junctions and the spine. Multiple bony sites may be affected, and sickle cell anaemia is an important predisposing factor. Suppurative arthritis can occur either as an extension of contiguous osteomyelitis or as a primary infection.

Meningitis is a particularly serious complication of infection in neonates and very young children. Abscess formation can occur in almost any organ or tissue. Even in the absence of obvious tissue damage the ability of salmonellae to enter and survive within macrophages and other cells, particularly in the liver and biliary tree, but also in bone marrow and the kidney, occasionally leads to persistent infection and the chronic carrier state.

The prolonged carrier state

Most people infected with salmonella continue to excrete the organism in their stools for days or weeks after complete clinical recovery, but eventual clearance of the bacteria from the body is usual. A few patients continue to excrete the salmonellae for prolonged periods. The term *chronic carrier* is reserved for those who excrete salmonellae for a year or more. Chronic carriage can follow symptomatic illness or may be the only manifestation of infection. It can occur with any serotype, but is a particularly important feature of enteric fever; up to 5% of convalescents from typhoid and a smaller number of those who have recovered from paratyphoid fever become chronic carriers, many for a lifetime. The bacilli are most commonly present in the gallbladder, less often in the urinary tract, and are shed in faeces and sometimes in urine. The long duration of the carrier state enables the enteric fever bacilli to survive in the community in non-epidemic times and to persist in small and relatively isolated communities.

Age and sex are important determinants of the frequency of carriage, at least of *S.* Typhi. After enteric fever, less than 1% of patients under 20 years old become carriers, but this proportion rises to more than 10% in patients over 50 years of age. At all ages women become carriers twice as often as men.

Duration of excretion following infection with other salmonellae is less well documented, but over 50% of patients stop excreting the organisms within 5 weeks of infection, and 90% of adults are culture-negative at 9 weeks. The duration of excretion is significantly greater in children under 5 years, but virtually all permanent carriers are adults.

LABORATORY DIAGNOSIS

Selective media, such as desoxycholate-citrate agar or xylose-lysine desoxycholate agar, are used for the isolation of salmonella bacteria from faeces. Fluid enrichment media, such as tetrathionate or selenite broth, are also useful to detect small numbers of salmonellae in faeces or environmental samples. Suspicious colonies from the culture plates are tested directly for the presence of salmonella somatic (O) antigens by slide agglutination and subcultured to peptone water for determination of flagellar (H) antigen structure and for further biochemical analysis. A presumptive diagnosis of salmonellosis can often be made within 24 h of the receipt of a specimen, but confirmation may take another day, and formal identification of the serotype several more days. A negative report must await the result of enrichment cultures, which take at least 48 h.

Enteric fever

Blood culture

The organisms may be recovered from the bloodstream at any stage of the illness, but are most commonly found during the first 7–10 days and during relapses. The organ-isms can also be recovered from the blood clot from a sample taken for serological tests. The clot is digested with streptokinase or minced, and incubated in broth.

Stool and urine culture

Specimens of faeces and urine should also be submitted for examination, but the isolation of salmonella from either of these specimens may merely mean that the patient is a carrier. In typhoid fever, patients' stools may contain salmonella from the second week and urine cultures from the third week of the infection. In paratyphoid B infections the clinical course may be much shorter than in typhoid; diarrhoea may occur early and stool cultures are often positive in the first week of the illness.

Serological tests

Although infections with other invasive serotypes induce specific serum antibodies, serological tests have been applied extensively only in the diagnosis of infection with *S.* Typhi. The Widal agglutination test, formerly used for the detection of specific O, H and Vi antigens, has been largely replaced by sensitive and specific methods such as enzyme-linked immunosorbent assay (ELISA) and immunoblotting. The results of serology should be considered in the light of the level of antibodies to the somatic and flagellar antigens of *S.* Typhi in the healthy population and knowledge of previous vaccination or a history of previous infection.

Cross-reacting antibodies from previous exposure to other salmonellae may confuse the results of serodiagnosis. The O-antigens of *S.* Typhi are also expressed by other serotypes such as *S.* Enteritidis (see Table 24.1). Antibodies specific for group 'd' flagellar antigens can be used to differentiate infections caused by *S.* Typhi from other serotypes that share O antigens.

Use of serology in the search for typhoid carriers, for example in the routine examination of food handlers and waterworks employees, is of doubtful value.

Food poisoning

The laboratory diagnosis of bacterial food poisoning depends on the isolation of the causal organism from samples of faeces or suspected foodstuffs. The more common food poisoning serotypes, such as Enteritidis or Typhimurium, may be characterized more fully by phage typing and antibiotic resistance typing (see above). Strains can be differentiated further by plasmid and pulsed-field gel electrophoresis typing so that the isolates from patients may be matched with those from the infected food and from a suspected animal source. The examination of vomit is rarely of value.

TREATMENT

Enteric fever

The introduction of chloramphenicol in 1948 transformed a life-threatening illness of several weeks' duration and a mortality rate of more than 20% into a short-lasting febrile illness with a mortality below 2%. Many patients can be treated adequately with oral chloramphenicol from the outset. Initial intravenous therapy with the drug may be necessary for the more severely ill patient, who may have anorexia, abdominal distension and, perhaps, vomiting. The intramuscular route gives inadequate blood levels. Treatment should be maintained for 14 days because relapse is more frequent with a shorter course.

The problem of bone marrow toxicity and, in the 1970s, the emergence of plasmid-mediated chloramphenicol resistance in South America and South-East Asia prompted the search for alternative agents. Among these, amoxicillin and co-trimoxazole are as effective as chloramphenicol, and are widely used. Since 1989, however, simultaneous resistance to all three antibiotics has become increasingly common in strains of S. Typhi in several endemic areas, and imported multiresistant typhoid is being encountered worldwide. Ciprofloxacin has emerged as the drug of choice for the treatment of adult typhoid, and is proving equally effective and free from side-effects in children.

Gastro-enteritis

Management of salmonella gastro-enteritis includes replacement of fluids and electrolytes and control of nausea, vomiting and pain. Drugs to control the hyper-motility of the gut are contra-indicated; they may give symptomatic relief for a while, but it is easy to transform a trivial gastro-enteritis into a life-threatening bacteraemia by paralysing the bowel. The role of antibiotics is also limited. Randomized, placebo-controlled, double-blind studies have failed to show any benefit from any antibiotic on the duration and severity of the diarrhoea or the duration of fever; some antibiotics seemed to prolong the carrier state.

Most authorities agree that antibiotics have no part to play in the management in most cases, but when a patient is clearly at increased risk of bacteraemia and generalized invasion, an antibiotic may protect against this serious complication. Such patients include infants under 3 months of age, patients with malignancies, haemoglobinopathies, chronic gastro-intestinal disease such as ulcerative colitis (especially when these need treatment with steroids), and patients who are immuno-suppressed for other reasons. Treatment with an appro-priate agent (see above) should continue until the gastro-enteritis has completely resolved.

Salmonella bacteraemia

Established salmonella bacteraemia requires aggressive antimicrobial treatment with ciprofloxacin, chloramphenicol, co-trimoxazole or high-dose ampicillin. Uncomplicated bacteraemia should be treated for 10–14 days. A careful search for focal metastatic disease should be undertaken, especially when relapse follows cessation of treatment. Surgical drainage of metastatic abscesses may be required, with surgical intervention if heart valves or large vessels are affected.

In salmonella meningitis in infancy, treatment with chloramphenicol or ampicillin may be unsuccessful in up to a third of cases caused by sensitive strains. Since cefo-taxime and ceftriaxone penetrate into the cerebrospinal fluid reasonably well and are highly active against most salmonellae, they offer an effective alternative to the more conventional agents.

Since resistance to any of the drugs used to treat invasive infection may occur, treatment should be supported by susceptibility testing whenever possible.

Chronic asymptomatic carriers

The chronic carrier state presents a particularly difficult therapeutic challenge. The principal site of carriage is the biliary tract, and concomitant biliary disease has significant implications for therapy. When the patient has chronic cholecystitis or gallstones, antibiotics alone are most unlikely to eradicate the infection. Cholecystectomy together with appropriate antibiotic treatment will result in cure in about 90% of cases, but has significant risk, not least from metastatic infection from dissemination of the organisms during surgery.

In the absence of biliary disease, prolonged courses of ampicillin, amoxicillin, co-trimoxazole or ciprofloxacin may cure up to 80% of carriers. However, it is difficult to justify even moderately heroic efforts to cure a condition that has little if any ill effect on the individual and not much direct public health importance. The chronic human carrier is the principal reservoir of enteric fever salmonellae, but even in the developing world direct person-to-person spread by asymptomatic carriers is not common. 'Typhoid Mary', who is reputed to have caused many infections by her cooking, was an exception and must have had peculiar personal habits. Normal personal hygiene, adequate sanitation and a reliable supply of potable water are the real safeguards against enteric fever. Prolonged carriage of other S. enterica serotypes is of even less public health importance, and rarely if ever justifies exclusion from any employment, or intrusive efforts to eradicate the infection.

EPIDEMIOLOGY AND CONTROL

The typhoid and paratyphoid bacilli are essentially human parasites. Man is the reservoir host and most infections can be traced to a human source, or at least to a source of human sewage. All other salmonellae have animal hosts.

Enteric fever

Incidence

In developing countries, *S.* Typhi is common, but data are incomplete. It has been estimated that between 10 and 500 cases of typhoid per 100 000 of the population occur annually throughout the developing world.

In 1938 there were almost 1000 notifications of typhoid fever in England and Wales. Within a decade the incidence had fallen to fewer than 200 cases a year, largely because of the almost universal introduction of chlorination of public water supplies, and improved techniques for the detection of cases and carriers which formed the basis for improved standards of hygiene and sanitation generally. The current incidence throughout most of the developed world is about 0.2 cases per 100 000 of the population. Most contract their infection by travel to endemic areas or by close family contact with excreters. Paratyphoid infections show a similar pattern.

Sanitation

The control of enteric fever is in theory straightforward. Cases occur from the ingestion of food or water contaminated with human sewage carrying typhoid or paratyphoid bacilli. Outbreaks occur when numbers of people are infected from a primary source. This may be a single meal or a briefly contaminated water supply, or may be a water supply or source of food contaminated and available for ingestion over a longer period. Secondary transmission from patients infected by the primary source is rare. Control depends essentially on the wide public availability of wholesome drinking water and the provision of adequate means for the proper disposal of human excreta. Enteric fever is a public health problem only where these provisions do not exist, and where, therefore, the organisms can be spread widely from carriers and from convalescent and sick persons, possibly helped by cultural factors such as food habits, occupation and personal behaviour. In such communities the selection of control measures

may be difficult, and provision of adequate sanitation and pure water may need to be supplemented by prophylactic immunization.

Vaccination

Heat-killed, phenol-preserved whole-cell vaccines containing a mixture of cultures of Typhi, Paratyphi A and Paratyphi B (TAB) have been used for many years in countries with a high endemic level of typhoid fever. Such preparations confer considerable, although not absolute, protection against typhoid for about 3 years. There has always been doubt about the value of the paratyphoid components, as well as concern about the unpleasant side-effects associated with the large antigenic load of the triple vaccine, so that monovalent typhoid vaccines are now preferred. Whole-cell vaccines have been largely replaced by capsular (Vi) polysaccharide vaccines. Alternatively, an oral live-attenuated typhoid vaccine is used.

Travellers to endemic areas in which there are high carriage rates and poor standards of hygiene should be offered immunization, especially if they intend to visit rural areas or to live 'rough'. However, the risk to the air traveller with full board at a reputable hotel is so small that typhoid immunization may be unnecessary. The risk of infection in southern Europe does not justify recommending the vaccine to the many millions travelling there on holiday every year, but vaccination is recommended for travel to Eastern Europe, especially for backpacking holidays outside the main tourist areas.

Salmonella food poisoning

No other zoonosis is as complex in its epidemiology and control as salmonellosis. The biology of different *S. enterica* serotypes varies widely and epidemiological patterns differ greatly between geographical areas, depending on climate, population density, land use, farming practices, food-processing technologies and consumer habits.

Sources

The carcasses or products (cooked meats, eggs, milk) of naturally infected domestic animals are the commonest sources of food poisoning. Flesh may be infected when an ill, septicaemic animal is slaughtered, but in most cases the salmonellae important in human infection cause only mild or inapparent infection in their animal hosts, and abattoir and shop cross-contamination with intestinal contents from a carrier animal is a more important hazard. Poultry (particularly hens), ducks and turkeys are the most significant reservoirs of food poisoning salmonellae in the UK. Pigs share the honours with poultry in much of northern Europe, while beef cattle are important sources in the USA. Duck eggs have always been a problem, since they can be infected in the oviduct before the egg is shelled. Hen eggs acquire their shells higher in the oviduct, and are less commonly infected in this way, although they can be contaminated on the outside if laid on soil contaminated by infected hen faeces.

Food contamination

Rats and mice are commonly infected with food poisoning salmonellae and may contaminate human food with their faeces. Food poisoning may occasionally be caused by food contaminated by a human case or carrier. Thus, even if the foodstuff is initially free from salmonellae the chance of contamination 'from the hoof to the home' is high and the more sophisticated the manipulation of the food, the greater the chance of contamination. For example, one egg containing salmonellae, if eaten by an individual, probably will not give rise to an infection. On the other hand, if such an egg is pooled with others free from salmonellae, as in preparing a mayonnaise or a Hollandaise sauce for communal consumption, and if conditions of temperature and time allow multiplication of the salmonellae, there will be the potential for an outbreak of infection among those who eat the contaminated food.

A clean carcass can be contaminated at the abattoir by instruments or by hanging in contact with an infected carcass in the chilling hall or during transportation to the wholesale and retail butchers' premises. The aggregation of calves or pigs in holding pens greatly increases the occurrence of cross-infection before slaughter. Infection in pigs is most often due to the feeding of swill containing infected animal matter, a practice that is difficult to prevent.

There is a close correspondence between the types of salmonellae prevalent in animals, especially pigs and poultry, and the types causing infection in humans. Strains of S. Typhimurium, which are primary pathogens in a wide variety of animals, are common, and S. Enteritidis has become prevalent in the UK as a result of a widespread epidemic of domestic poultry flocks. Strains belonging to serotypes such as Heidelberg, Brandenburg, Panama and Virchow are rarely found in animals and yet may be responsible for widespread human infections. More needs to be learned about the epidemiology of such infections.

Food preparation

Infection of food with salmonellae is not in itself sufficient to cause food poisoning. It is necessary for the infected food to be moist and to be held long enough under conditions which will allow the bacteria to grow, e.g. overnight in a warm kitchen or several days in a cool larder. If the food is then eaten without further cooking, infection may follow. Although cooking of liquid foods will render them safe, cooking of solid foods often fails to do so because of the relatively poor rate of penetration of heat into the food. A cold or chilled joint of meat, a poultry carcass or a large meat pie may be heated in an oven until the surface is well cooked, while the central part is still insufficiently heated to destroy vegetative bacteria.

Outbreaks

Food poisoning incidents occur most dramatically as explosive outbreaks among members of a community sharing communal meals, as in factories, hospitals or schools or at some celebratory feast, although sporadic incidents affecting a single family or a single person are much more common and much more difficult to track to a source. In the UK, salmonellae account for about 75% of the incidents of food poisoning in which a causal agent is identified. However, this may only reflect the fact that salmonellosis is relatively easy to confirm bacteriologically and is therefore more readily recognized than food poisoning caused by other agents, which often escapes diagnosis.

Prevention

The principles of the prevention of salmonella food poisoning can be readily set out. They are:

- the raising of animals free from infection
- the elimination of contamination by rodents at all levels of food production
- the prevention of contamination by human handlers at the wholesale, retail and hotel levels.

The barriers of economic husbandry, out-of-date premises and, perhaps the most important of all, the need for continuing education of food handlers at all levels of production make implementation of these principles difficult. To reduce the incidence of food poisoning, whether due to salmonellae or to other bacteria, two basic precepts must be observed:

- raw foodstuffs of animal origin, which are always potentially contaminated, must never have direct or indirect contact with cooked foods
- foodstuff thought to be contaminated should be treated or held under temperature conditions which prevent the organisms from growing.

Cooked foods should be served and eaten immediately after cooking, and while still hot, or cooled rapidly and held at refrigerator temperature until eaten, so that at least the inoculum eaten by any individual is small. It is often found that the food incriminated in an outbreak had been cooked several hours or even a day or two before and then left at room temperature before being reheated immediately before serving. This procedure ensures that salmonellae which survived the initial cooking or gained access to the food from contaminated kitchen surfaces or implements had excellent opportunities to multiply in the interval before being warmed up for consumption.

As in most other endeavours to control the spread of infection the human element is the weakest link in the chain, so that health education, particularly of food handlers, is a most important and continuing requirement.

RECOMMENDED READING

Baumler A J, Tsolis R M, Heffron F 1997 Fimbrial adhesins of *Salmonella typhimurium:* role in bacterial interactions with epithelial cells *Advances in Experimental Medicine and Biology* 412:149–58

Bumann D, Hueck C, Aebischer T, Meyer T F 2000 Recombinant live *Salmonella* spp. for human vaccination against heterologous pathogens. *FEMS Immunology and Medical Microbiology* 27: 357–64

Chart H, Cheesbrough J S, Waghorn D J 2000 The serodiagnosis of infection with *Salmonella typhi. Journal of Clinical Pathology* 53: 851–53

Hessel L, Debois H, Fletcher M, Dumas R 1999 Experience with *Salmonella typhi* Vi capsular polysaccharide vaccine. *European Journal of Clinical Microbiology and Infectious Diseases.* 18:609–20

Mandel B K 1994 *Salmonella typhi* and other salmonellas. *Gut* 35: 726–728

Rowe B, Ward L R, Threlfall E J 1997 Multidrug-resistant *Salmonella typhi:* a worldwide epidemic. *Clinical Infectious Diseases* 24 Suppl 1:S106–109

Sirard J C, Niedergang F, Kraehenbuhl J P 1999 Live attenuated *Salmonella*: a paradigm of mucosal vaccines. *Immunological Reviews* 171:5–26

Threlfall E J, Ward L R, Skinner J A, Smith H R, Lacey S 1999 Ciprofloxacin-resistant *Salmonella typhi* and treatment failure. *Lancet* 353:1590–1591

WHO 1988 Salmonellosis control: the role of animal and product hygiene. *WHO Technical Report Series*, No. 774. World Health Organization, Geneva

WHO 1994 Control of *Salmonella* infections in animals and prevention of human foodborne *Salmonella* infections. *Bulletin of the World Health Organization* 72: 831–833

Internet sites

Centers for Disease Control and Prevention:
www.cdc.gov/ncidod/dbmd/diseaseinfo/typhoidfever_g.htm
Centers for Disease Control and Prevention:
www.cdc.gov/od/oc/media/fact/salmonel.htm
Public Health Laboratory Service: http://www.phls.co.uk/
The Wonderful World of Diseases: www.diseaseworld.com/typhoid.htm

25

Shigella

Bacillary dysentery

H. Chart

Dysentery, the bloody flux of biblical times, is a clinical entity characterized by the frequent passage of blood-stained mucopurulent stools. Aetiologically it is divisible into two main categories, amoebic and bacillary. Both forms are endemic in most warm-climate countries. Bacillary dysentery, caused by members of the genus *Shigella*, is also prevalent in many countries with temperate climates.

DESCRIPTION

The genus *Shigella* is subdivided on biochemical and serological grounds into four species:

- *Shigella dysenteriae*
- *Sh. flexneri*
- *Sh. boydii*
- *Sh. sonnei*.

They are typical members of the Enterobacteriaceae and are closely related to the genus *Escherichia*. Studies focusing on the ancestral lineage of these bacteria suggest that *Sh. boydii* is only distantly related to other members of the genus *Shigella*, which are more closely related to entero-invasive serotypes of *Esch. coli* (p. 270).

Microscopically, in stained preparations, shigellae are Gram-negative bacilli indistinguishable from other enterobacteria. They are non-motile and non-capsulate. Culturally they are similar to most other enterobacteria. In common with members of the genus *Salmonella* they do not ferment lactose following overnight incubation, although *Sh. sonnei* ferments lactose slowly.

The antigenic structure is complex. Strains of *Sh. dysenteriae* can be subdivided into 13 and *S. boydii* into 18 specific serotypes. A combination of group- and type-specific antigens allows subdivision of *Sh. flexneri* into six serotypes, each of which can be further subdivided. Strains of *Sh. sonnei* are serologically homogeneous, and a variety of other markers such as the ability to produce specific colicines, the carriage of drug-

resistance or other plasmids, or lysogeny by a panel of bacteriophages are used to discriminate between strains for epidemiological purposes.

CLINICAL FEATURES

The incubation period is usually between 2 and 3 days, but may be as short as 12 h. The onset of symptoms is usually sudden, and frequently the initial symptom is abdominal colic. This is followed by the onset of watery diarrhoea, and in all but the mildest cases this is accompanied by fever and malaise. Many episodes resolve at this point, but others progress to abdominal cramps, tenesmus and the frequent passage of small volumes of stool, predominantly consisting of bloody mucus. The symptoms typically last about 4 days, but may continue for 10 days or more.

The severity of the clinical illness is to some extent associated with the species involved. Infection with *Sh. dysenteriae* is usually associated with a severe illness in which prostration is marked and, in young children, may be accompanied by febrile convulsions. Members of the *Sh. flexneri* and *Sh. boydii* groups may also cause severe illness. In contrast dysentery associated with *Sh. sonnei* (*Sonne dysentery*) in an otherwise healthy person may be confined to the passage of a few loose stools with vague abdominal discomfort, and the patient often continues at school or work.

Strains of *Sh. dysenteriae* type 1 have been responsible for many cases of the haemolytic uraemic syndrome accompanying outbreaks of dysentery in several countries. The condition, with its triad of haemolytic anaemia, thrombocytopenia and acute renal failure, can be caused by many pathogens (in particular, *Esch. coli* O157; p. 271). It is associated with complement activation and disseminated intravascular coagulation, and in some parts of the world is one of the commonest forms of acute renal failure in children.

Death from bacillary dysentery is uncommon in the developed world; it occurs mostly at the extremes of life or in individuals who are suffering from some other disease or debilitating condition.

PATHOGENESIS

Shigella spp. are pathogens of man and other primates, and the pathogenesis of infection with these bacteria and entero-invasive *Esch. coli* (EIEC; p. 270) is very similar. The infective dose is small: bacillary dysentery may follow the ingestion of as few as 10 viable bacteria. The site of infection is the M cells in the Peyer's patches of the large intestine. Strains of *Shigella* spp. are non-motile and it is not known how the bacteria reach and adhere to the M cells.

Association with the intestinal mucosa initiates mucosal inflammation leading to apoptosis, which is thought to facilitate the invasion of the M cells, after which the bacteria are phagocytosed. The shigellae multiply within the epithelial cells and spread laterally into adjacent cells and deep into the lamina propria. The infected epithelial cells are killed and the lamina propria and submucosa develop an inflammatory reaction with capillary thrombosis. Patches of necrotic epithelium are sloughed and ulcers form. The cellular response is mainly by polymorphonuclear leucocytes, which can be seen readily on microscopic examination of the stool, together with red cells and sloughed epithelium.

Dysentery bacilli rarely invade other tissues. Transient bacteraemia can occur but septicaemia with metastatic infection is rare.

Pathogenic mechanisms

Strains of *Shigella* spp. have been examined for a range of putative pathogenic mechanisms. Since the infective dose for these organisms is small, shigellae might have innate tolerance to the low pH and bile encountered in the human digestive tract.

Pathogenic strains of shigellae, like entero-invasive *Esch. coli*, carry a plasmid of 100 to 140 MD, which encodes the pathogenic mechanisms involved with eukaryotic cell invasion. Certain plasmid-encoded elements are regulated chromosomally.

Lipopolysaccharide (LPS) has been implicated in causing localized cytokine release, and the resultant inflammatory response and cellular disruption enables these bacteria to enter intestinal cells. Plasmid-encoded proteins are required for bacteria to break free from cellular endosomes and for the migration between epithelial cells. *Sh. flexneri* and *Sh. sonnei* express an aerobactin-mediated high-affinity iron uptake system; however, since *Sh. dysenteriae*-1 does not express this siderophore the role of aerobactin in the pathogenesis of the disease is unclear.

Sh. dysenteriae-1 produces a potent protein toxin (*Shiga toxin*) very similar to VT1 expressed by strains of Verocytotoxigenic *Esch. coli* (VTEC; p. 271); however, in contrast to VTEC, the genes encoding Shiga toxin are located on the chromosome. Expression of Shiga toxin has been shown to be iron-regulated, with toxin production increasing under conditions of iron restriction. Shiga toxin is a subunit toxin comprising an A portion and five B subunits. The A subunit possesses the biological activities of the toxin while the B subunits mediate specific binding and receptor-mediated uptake of the toxin. In common with the Verocytotoxins of *Esch. coli*, Shiga toxin binds to globotriosylceramide (Gb_3) molecules present on the surface of certain eukaryotic cells. During pathogenesis the release of the inflammatory mediators tumour necrosis factor (TNF) and interleukin-1 (IL-1) increase the number of Gb_3 receptors on the surface of eukaryotic cells, increasing the binding of toxin to these cells.

Like Verocytotoxin, Shiga toxin becomes internalized by host cells and remains active within endosomes, eventually reaching the Golgi apparatus. Within the host cell the A subunit divides to form portions A_1 and A_2, and the A_1 portion of the toxin prevents protein synthesis and causes cell death. Haemolytic uraemic syndrome is thought to be caused by the action of Shiga toxin on kidney tissues; however, Shiga toxin has also been shown to have neurotoxic properties and the role of this toxin in the pathogenesis of bacillary dysentery remains to be elucidated fully.

LABORATORY DIAGNOSIS

A specimen of faeces is always preferable to a rectal swab. Rectal swabs do not allow adequate macroscopic and microscopic examination of the stool, and unless properly taken and bearing obvious faecal material may be no more than a swab of peri-anal skin. Moreover, because of drying of the swab, pathogenic species die quite rapidly, and may not survive transport to the laboratory.

The faeces are inoculated on desoxycholate citrate agar or MacConkey agar. Mucus, if present in the specimen, may be used as the inoculum. After overnight incubation, pale non-lactose-fermenting colonies are tested by standard biochemical and sugar utilization tests to differentiate them from other enterobacteria. Identity is confirmed by serological investigation with species-specific rabbit antibodies, and then with type-specific sera unless the strain is *Sh. sonnei*. It is rarely necessary to take strain identification any further except when investigating major outbreaks in endemic areas.

Plasmid pattern analysis and colicine typing may help elucidate patterns of spread of *Sh. sonnei*.

Primers developed to amplify DNA sequences located on the invasive plasmids of shigellae and entero-invasive *Esch. coli* can assist in the identification of strains of *Shigella* spp. Similarly, tests for the production of Shiga toxin can also facilitate the identification of these organisms. Since Shiga toxin and VT1, expressed by certain verocytotoxigenic *Esch. coli*, are similar in structure and mode of action, Shiga toxin can be tested for by Vero and HeLa cell tests (p. 271) and immunoassays designed for Verocytotoxin.

Patients infected with *Sh. dysenteriae*-1 produce serum antibodies to the LPS antigens, but tests for LPS-specific antibodies are not normally available in areas where infection with shigellae is endemic.

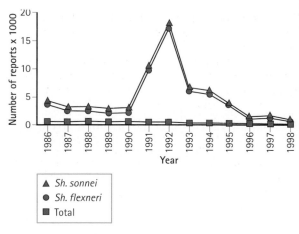

Fig. 25.1 Laboratory reports of shigella, England and Wales 1986–1998

TREATMENT

Most cases of Shigella dysentery, especially those due to *Sh. sonnei*, are mild and do not require antibiotic therapy. Symptomatic treatment with the maintenance of hydration by use of oral rehydration salt solution (see Table 30.2, p. 299) is all that is required. As with salmonella infections, drugs that impair gut motility should be avoided. Treatment with a suitable antibiotic is necessary in the very young, the aged or the debilitated, and in severe infections. Ampicillin, co-trimoxazole, tetracycline or ciprofloxacin is an appropriate choice, provided the drug is shown to be active in vitro; each may be administered orally. There is no evidence that antibiotics reduce the period of excretion of the organisms, and they should not be used in the asymptomatic person, either prophylactically or in attempts to hasten clearance after recovery.

EPIDEMIOLOGY

The 20th century saw a steady and remarkable change in the relative frequency of the different *Shigella* species in the UK and other European countries. Infections due to *Sh. dysenteriae* and *Sh. boydii* are now rare and *Sh. sonnei* has become dominant. In the UK the annual incidence of Sonne dysentery reached a peak in 1956 with over 49 000 notifications. The incidence then declined steadily to an annual average of about 3000 notified cases between 1970 and 1990. However, the number of cases rose sharply in 1991, when there were several widespread community outbreaks, and continued to rise to a peak of 17 000 cases in 1992 (Fig. 25.1), the highest level in the UK for more than 20 years. Infections caused by *Sh. flexneri*

remained at around 700–800 until a decline in 1993. The incidence of *Sh. boydii* is almost ten-fold lower than that of *Sh. flexneri*, while faecal isolations of *Sh. dysenteriae* have remained essentially constant at between 40 and 50 per year.

Similar changes have taken place in the USA, although more slowly. Up to 1968, *Sh. flexneri* and *Sh. sonnei* were equally common, but *Sh. sonnei* now accounts for 65% of cases and *Sh. flexneri* for about 30%. Over the past several decades the other two *Shigella* species have been responsible for less than 5% of notifications, but there has been a recent increase in cases imported from Asia and South America.

In tropical areas of the developing world, shigellosis is endemic; it has been estimated that some 5 million cases require hospital treatment and about 600 000 die every year. Young children are particularly vulnerable.

Sources and spread

Bacillary dysentery is usually spread by the faecal–oral route. The case or carrier, after contaminating his or her hands while cleansing at toilet, touches and thus contaminates the lavatory flush handle, door knobs, washbasin taps, hand towels and other objects which, when handled by another individual, allow transfer of dysentery bacilli to the recipient's hands and thence to the mouth. Such spread is facilitated by separating the washbasin from the lavatory compartment so that the handle of the intervening door acts as an efficient vehicle of infection. The carrier may also touch and thus infect food that is eaten, or eating utensils that are used by another person, who is thereby infected. Dysentery bacilli are also liberated into the air in an aerosol when an infected loose stool is flushed from the toilet, and after settling on the surfaces of toilet seats, furniture and surroundings may survive for some days in a moist atmosphere.

An important feature of the epidemiology of bacillary dysentery in the UK and other countries with good environmental sanitation is that the main patient group involved is school age children and particularly primary school children. Here, unwitting neglect of toilet hygiene by children at school undoubtedly plays a part. The disease is often endemic among adults living in residential institutions where, for one reason or another, high standards of hygiene are difficult to maintain, and has in the past been a scourge in gaols and in armies in the field. The seasonal distribution of bacillary dysentery in the UK is bimodal, with the highest incidence in spring and a second peak in October and November. The incidence is at its lowest in summer, when school children are on holiday. Since this is the period when flying insects are most abundant, this suggests that in this country insects play little, if any, part in transmission. However, in communities without satisfactory methods of sewage disposal, insects can gain access to infected human excreta and transfer shigellae mechanically to foodstuffs. Foods may also be contaminated directly by human cases or carriers.

Occasional epidemics of bacillary dysentery have been traced to water supplies when chlorination of the supply has not been instituted or has been defective. Such waterborne epidemics are usually spectacular in the large numbers of people simultaneously infected and in the speed with which they can be terminated when the water supply is adequately treated. Epidemic infection may also follow the contamination of milk or ice cream.

CONTROL

The mild and often fleeting nature of the clinical illness associated with *Sh. sonnei* infection means that frequently the patient with bacillary dysentery remains ambulant and follows his or her daily labour and leisure pursuits, remaining in circulation as a disperser of the causal organism. The pressure on toilet facilities, particularly in schools, allows hand-to-mouth spread of the bacilli. The provision of washbasins in the same compartment as the toilet pedestal would allow some reduction in spread, especially if flushing mechanisms and washbasin taps could be operated by foot instead of by hand.

Hand washing, although very important, cannot be guaranteed to remove all the dysentery bacilli from the hands. During diarrhoea, faecal soiling of the fingers can be heavy, and hand washing will at best only reduce the numbers of bacteria present. The normal disinfecting effect of the skin fatty acids and competing skin organisms may take up to half an hour to destroy the rest. For this reason it is important that people with symptoms such that they need to go to stool during a normal working shift should stay off work and as far as possible out of circulation until the symptoms have subsided, especially when their work involves preparation of food or direct contact with other people. Asymptomatic carriers are far less important in the spread of this disease, and seldom, if ever, need to be excluded from any employment.

Control of an outbreak

Outbreaks of dysentery in schools and other institutions are notoriously difficult to control. In nursery school outbreaks, infection is usually widespread before the first cases are notified, with considerable environmental contamination. Some children will be incubating the infection; others will have recovered from the diarrhoea but still be excreting the organisms. In this situation the acute case is far more important in the spread of infection than the symptomless excreter. There is little to be gained by trying to ascertain bacteriologically who is infected and who is not once the cause of the outbreak has been established, since there is little reason to exclude an asymptomatic carrier and it is pointless to seek confirmation of a clearly symptomatic case. The practical course is usually to exclude acute cases but to allow children without symptoms to remain at, or return to school.

Having determined the exclusion policy it is important to try to stop hand-to-hand spread among those who remain at school. Supervision of children using the lavatory, supervised hand washing before meals, frequent disinfection of water closets, including seats, lavatory chain and door handles, and the general use of paper towels all play a part. No single measure alone will be sufficient. Staff need support as morale can flag, and they themselves are vulnerable to infection. Outbreaks can persist for weeks despite all measures, and then subside abruptly for little apparent reason.

Similar principles can be applied to outbreaks in residential institutions or a hospital ward. The most important single factor in all these situations is the need for adequate communication. Teachers, nurses, parents and all who are involved in trying to control the outbreak need to have explained to them exactly how the infection spreads, and the reasons for the measures taken or not taken. Finally, the temptation to use antibiotics prophylactically in an attempt to limit the spread must be resisted.

RECOMMENDED READING

Bennish M L, Harris J R, Wojtyniak B J, Struelens M 1990 Death in shigellosis: incidence and risk factors in hospitalized patients. *Journal of Infectious Diseases* 161: 500–506

Dorman C J, Porter M E 1998 The *Shigella* virulence gene regulatory cascade: a paradigm of bacterial gene control mechanisms. *Molecular Microbiology* 29: 677–84

Hale T L, Formal S B 1987 Pathogenesis of shigella infections. *Pathology and Immunopathology Research* 6: 117–127

Lopez E L, Prado-Jimenez V, O'Ryan-Gallardo M, Contrini M M 2000 *Shigella* and Shiga toxin-producing *Escherichia coli* causing bloody diarrhea in Latin America. *Infectious Disease Clinics of North America* 14: 41–65

Nhieu G T, Sansonetti P J 1999 Mechanism of *Shigella* entry into epithelial cells. *Current Opinion in Microbiology* 2: 51–55

Sansonetti P J 1998 Molecular and cellular mechanisms of invasion of the intestinal barrier by enteric pathogens: the paradigm of *Shigella. Folia Microbiologica* 43: 239–246

Sasakawa C 1995 Molecular basis of pathogenicity of *Shigella. Reviews in Medical Microbiology* 6: 257–266

Internet sites

US Food and Drug Administration Center for Food Safety and Applied Nutrition. *Bad Bug Book*: Vm.cfsan.fda.gov/~mow/chap19.html

Public Health Laboratory Service: www.phls.co.uk/

26

Escherichia

Urinary tract infection; travellers' diarrhoea; haemorrhagic colitis; haemolytic uraemic syndrome

H. Chart

Strains of *Escherichia coli* and related Gram-negative 'coliform' bacteria predominate among the aerobic commensal flora in the gut of humans and animals. These bacteria are widespread, and present wherever there is faecal contamination, a phenomenon that can be exploited by public health microbiologists as an indicator of faecal pollution of water sources, drinking water and food. The species encompasses a variety of strains, which may be purely commensal or possess combinations of pathogenic mechanisms that enable them to cause disease in man and other animals.

DESCRIPTION

Strains of *Esch. coli* are usually motile and some, especially those from extra-intestinal infections, may produce a polysaccharide capsule. They grow well on non-selective media, and most strains ferment lactose, producing large, red colonies on MacConkey agar. They grow over a wide range of temperature (15–45°C) and some strains are more heat-resistant than other members of the Enterobacteriaceae and may survive 60°C for 15 min or 55°C for 60 min. Certain strains are haemolytic when grown on media containing suitable erythrocytes.

Esch. coli can be differentiated from other members of the Enterobacteriaceae by the ability to utilize certain sugars and by a range of other biochemical reactions. Many characteristic biochemical reactions, such as indole production and the formation of acid and gas from lactose and other carbohydrates, take place at 44°C as well as at 37°C.

The term *coliform* is commonly used to refer to any member of the Enterobacteriaceae but originally meant 'like *Bacterium* (later *Esch.*) *coli*', and many workers, especially in fields related to public health, prefer to reserve *coliform* to describe genera or species of enterobacteria which normally ferment lactose, using the term *non-lactose fermenter* (NLF) to describe the other bacteria. Neither term has any taxonomic validity.

Studies of DNA–DNA recombination show that strains of *Esch. coli* and *Shigella* spp. form a single genetic species, and it is therefore to be expected that intermediate strains will occur. Certain of these, which are non-motile and anaerogenic, and often ferment lactose late or not at all, have caused difficulties in classification. They were at one time included in the so-called 'Alkalescens-Dispar' group but these strains are now considered to be atypical forms of *Esch. coli*.

Antigenic structure

Serotyping is based on the distribution of lipopolysaccharide (LPS) or somatic (O) antigens, and flagellar (H) and capsular (K) antigens, as detected in agglutination assays with specific rabbit antibodies. Over 170 different O antigens have been described. Serotyping may detect cross-reactions because of shared epitopes on the LPS expressed by strains of *Esch. coli* and organisms belonging to the genera *Brucella, Citrobacter, Providencia, Salmonella, Shigella* and *Yersinia*. In some instances the antigens appearing in the different genera are identical.

More than 50 H antigens have been identified. Most are monophasic but rare diphasic strains have been reported. There are only a few significant cross-reactions between them and with the H antigens of other members of the *Enterobacteriaceae*. Because certain strains of *Esch. coli* cease to express flagella during growth in vitro, strains may need to be grown in semi-solid agar to induce flagella expression.

The term 'K antigen' was first used collectively for surface or capsular antigens that prevent flagellar-specific antibodies from binding to the somatic antigens. In the past these antigens were divided into three classes (L, A and B) according to the effect of heat on the agglutinability, antigenicity and antibody-binding power of bacterial strains that express them. In modern usage, 'K antigen' refers to the acidic polysaccharide capsular antigens, and those of *Esch. coli* may be divided into two groups (groups I and II; Table 26.1) that largely correspond to the former A and L antigens.

Table 26.1 K antigens of *Esch. coli*

Properties	Group I	Group II
Molecular weight	>100 000	<50 000
Acidic component	Hexuronic acid, pyruvate	Glucuronic acid, phosphate, KDO, NeuNAc
Heat stability (100°C, pH 6)	All stable	Mostly labile
O groups	O8, O9	Many
Chromosome site	*His*	*SerA*
Expressed at 17–20°C	Yes	No
Electrophoretic mobility	Low	High

KDO, ketodeoxyoctonate; NeuNAc, *N*-acetylneuraminic acid.

Fimbrial antigens

Like many other members of the Enterobacteriaceae, strains of *Esch. coli* exhibit fimbriae and strains may carry both sex pili and more than one type of fimbrial structure (p. 85). Within a given culture, there may exist individual cells with fimbriae and others with none, and there is reversible variation between the fimbriated and the non-fimbriated phase.

Type 1 fimbriae can mediate adhesion to a wide range of human and animal cells that contain the sugar mannose. Such adhesion might be involved in pathogenicity and there are some examples of this. Filamentous protein structures resembling fimbriae cause mannose-resistant haemagglutination, and there is good evidence to suggest that they play an important part in the pathogenesis of diarrhoeal disease and in urinary tract infection. They include the K88 antigen found in strains causing enteritis of pigs, the K99 antigen found in strains causing enteritis of calves and lambs, and the colonization factor antigens (CFAs) expressed by enterotoxigenic *Esch. coli* (ETEC) causing diarrhoeal disease in humans.

Fimbriae that are of importance in urinary tract infection and cause mannose-resistant haemagglutination are distinguished according to their receptor specificities. These include the P fimbriae that bind specifically to receptors present on the P blood group antigens of human erythrocytes and uro-epithelial cells.

PATHOGENESIS

Strains of *Esch. coli* possess a range of different pathogenic mechanisms. The polysaccharides of the O and K antigens protect the organism from the bactericidal effect of complement and phagocytes in the absence of specific antibodies. However, in the presence of antibody to K antigens alone, or to both O and K antigens, opsonization may occur.

Many strains express haemolysin(s), and in general strains of *Esch. coli* isolated from human extra-intestinal infections are more likely to be haemolytic than strains isolated from the faeces of healthy humans. Haemolysin production is an important pathogenic mechanism for releasing essential ferric ions bound to haemoglobin.

Strains of *Esch. coli* can express siderophores, such as enterobactin, which readily removes iron from mammalian iron transport proteins such as transferrin and lactoferrin (see Chapter 8). Some strains also express another siderophore, aerobactin, which may be plasmid-mediated. The ability of strains of *Esch. coli* to acquire ferric ions is a recognized pathogenic mechanism. Expression of the aerobactin-mediated iron uptake system is a common feature of strains isolated from patients with septicaemia, pyelonephritis and lower urinary tract infection.

CLINICAL SYNDROMES

Urinary tract and septic infections

Esch. coli is the most common cause of acute, uncomplicated urinary tract infection outside hospitals as well as causing much hospital-associated urinary tract sepsis. These bacteria may also cause neonatal meningitis and septicaemia, sepsis in operation wounds and abscesses in a variety of organs.

As many as 80% of *Esch. coli* strains causing neonatal meningitis and 40% of those isolated from infants with septicaemia but without meningitis express a K1 antigen. Strains possessing the K1 or the K5 antigen may be more virulent than those with other K antigens since they share structural identity with host components.

Strains of *Esch. coli* that cause urinary tract infection often originate from the gut of the patient, and the infection is thought to occur in an ascending manner for physiological reasons. There is evidence that the ability of *Esch. coli* to infect the urinary tract is associated with fimbriae that specifically mediate adherence to the uro-epithelial cells.

Epidemiology

Urinary tract infection occurs more frequently in females than in males since the shorter, wider female urethra appears to be less effective in preventing access of the bacteria to the bladder. Sexual intercourse is a predisposing factor. The high incidence in pregnant women can be attributed to impairment of urine flow due partly to hormonal changes and partly to pressure on the urinary tract. Other causes of urinary stagnation that may predispose to urinary tract infection include urethral obstruction, urinary stones, congenital malformations and neurological disorders, all of which occur in both sexes. In men, prostatic enlargement is the most common predisposing factor. Catheterization and cystoscopy may introduce bacteria into the bladder and therefore carry a risk of infection.

Since most urinary tract infections are thought to be caused by organisms originating from the patient's own faecal flora, each infection is generally regarded as sporadic. However, the prevalence of various serotypes of *Esch. coli* in urinary tract infections varies with geographical location, and this fits well with the view that *Esch. coli* which cause such infections are specific pathogens for the urinary tract. Pathogenic strains, possibly transmitted in contaminated foods, are able to colonize the bowel, and in individuals with predisposing factors may cause a urinary tract infection. The prevalence of infections due to a particular strain may therefore increase for a time in a locality.

Laboratory diagnosis

Clinical specimens may be stained by Gram's method for microscopical examination, and are cultured on MacConkey agar or other suitable media. In the case of suspected urinary tract infection, culture is semi-quantitative; in acute *Esch. coli* infections the organism is generally present in pure culture at a count of 10^5 or more per millilitre of urine.

Treatment and control

In the absence of acquired resistance *Esch. coli* is susceptible to many antibacterial agents, including ampicillin, cephalosporins, tetracyclines, quinolones, aminoglycosides, trimethoprim and sulphonamides. Many strains, however, have acquired plasmids conferring resistance to one or more of these drugs, and antimicrobial therapy should be guided by laboratory tests of sensitivity if possible.

Uncomplicated cystitis usually responds to minimal treatment with oral agents such as trimethoprim or nitrofurantoin, but more serious infections require specific antimicrobial therapy based on laboratory results. In particular, bacterial meningitis is a medical emergency and vigorous early treatment with cefotaxime and gentamicin is required.

Urinary catheterization and cystoscopy require rigorous aseptic technique to minimize the introduction of bacteria into the bladder. Bladder irrigation and systemic treatment with antimicrobial agents has been used in catheter-associated infections but such treatment is seldom more than palliative and encourages infections with resistant organisms.

Diarrhoea

Although *Esch. coli* is normally carried in the gut as a harmless commensal, it may cause gastro-intestinal disease ranging in severity from mild, self-limiting diarrhoea to haemorrhagic colitis. Such strains fall into at least five groups, each associated with specific serotypes (Table 26.2) and with different pathogenic mechanisms:

- *Enteropathogenic Esch. coli (EPEC)*, which cause infantile enteritis, especially in tropical countries.
- *Enterotoxigenic Esch. coli (ETEC)*, which are responsible for community-acquired diarrhoeal disease in areas of poor sanitation and are the commonest cause of *travellers' diarrhoea.*
- *Entero-invasive Esch. coli (EIEC)*, which cause an illness resembling shigella dysentery in patients of all ages.
- *Verocytotoxin-producing Esch. coli (VTEC)*, which cause symptoms ranging from mild, watery diarrhoea to severe diarrhoea with large amounts of fresh blood in the stool (*haemorrhagic colitis*). An important complication, especially in children, is the *haemolytic uraemic syndrome.*
- *Entero-aggregative Esch. coli (EAggEC)*, which cause chronic diarrhoeal disease in certain developing countries.

Table 26.2 The major groups of diarrhoea-causing *Esch. coli*

Pathogenic group	Common serogroups
Enteropathogenic *Esch. coli* (EPEC)	O26, O55, O86, O111, O114, O125, O126, O127, O128, O142.
Enterotoxigenic *Esch. coli* (ETEC)	O6, O8, O15, O25, O27, O63, O119, O125, O126, O127, O128, O142
Entero-invasive *Esch. coli* (EIEC)	O78, O115, O148, O153, O159, O167
Verocytotoxin-producing *Esch. coli* (VTEC)	O26, O28ac, O111, O112ac, O124, O136, O143, O144, O152, O157[a], O164
Entero-aggregative *Esch. coli* (EAggEC)	>50 O serogroups

[a] Other serogroups are far less common than O157 in human disease.

Enteropathogenic Esch. coli (EPEC)

Pathogenesis. EPEC strains were originally identified epidemiologically as a cause of diarrhoeal disease in infants; certain strains belonging to characteristically EPEC serogroups, such as O26 and O111, were later shown to express Verocytotoxin. The ability of EPEC strains to cause diarrhoea has been confirmed by oral administration of the organisms to babies and adults.

Colonization of the upper part of the small intestine occurs in infantile enteritis associated with EPEC. Electron microscopy of intestinal biopsy specimens has shown that EPEC become intimately associated with the mucosal surface and partially surrounded by cup-like projections ('pedestals') of the enterocyte surface. In areas of EPEC attachment the brush border microvilli are lost. Adhesion to the gut wall and the subsequent mucosal damage has been termed an 'attaching and effacing' lesion, and the strains exhibiting this phenotype have been termed attaching and effacing *Esch. coli* (AEEC). The genes responsible are located on a 'locus for enterocyte effacement' pathogenicity island located on the *Esch. coli* chromosome. One of the proteins involved, intimin, appears to be the key EPEC adhesin. These EPEC also synthesize a translocated intimin receptor, which is inserted into the host gut wall providing a binding site for intimin. These strains of EPEC use a novel mechanism of adhesion where both the adhesin and its receptor are synthesized by the bacteria.

Epidemiology. Since 1971 few epidemics of EPEC enteritis have been reported in the UK or the USA, but a satisfactory explanation for this has not been put forward. Strains responsible for sporadic cases which continue to occur in the UK, especially in the summer months, possess the same pathogenic mechanisms as those that caused earlier outbreaks.

EPEC enteritis is still common in communities with poor hygiene. In these countries sporadic cases and outbreaks occur very frequently in the general community as well as in institutions. The importance of EPEC as a cause of enteritis in adults is difficult to evaluate since few laboratories look for these organisms in patients over 3 years of age. However, a few outbreaks have been described.

Laboratory diagnosis of EPEC. Stool specimens are plated on media such as MacConkey agar, and bacteria fermenting lactose are examined by slide agglutination with polyvalent rabbit antisera designed to detect the somatic antigens of strains belonging to EPEC-associated serogroups. Bacteria agglutinated by these sera are then identified with monovalent antisera to individual serogroups. Isolates should also be identified as *Esch. coli* since there is widespread sharing of somatic antigens among members of the Enterobacteriaceae.

Tests to determine the ability of strains of EPEC to adhere to cultured HEp-2 (human epithelial) cells, and DNA probes for the detection of the EPEC adherence factor are available in some laboratories.

Enterotoxigenic Esch. coli (ETEC)

Pathogenesis. ETEC produce a heat-stable enterotoxin (ST) or a heat-labile (LT) cholera toxin-like enterotoxin or both. In addition, they usually express fimbriae that are specific for the host animal species and which enable the organisms to adhere to the epithelium of the small intestine. Infection is usually of brief duration, often beginning with the rapid onset of loose stools and accompanied by variable symptoms, including nausea, vomiting and abdominal cramps.

Heat-labile enterotoxin (LT). LT is closely related to the toxin produced by strains of *Vibrio cholerae*. There are two main forms, termed LT-I and LT-II (Table 26.3). Different forms of LT-I associated with human, porcine and chicken infection have been described; similarly, two forms of LT-II (LT-IIa and LT-IIb) have been detected. Although these toxins have a degree of structural variation, they are all subunit protein toxins comprising one A subunit and five B subunits with molecular weights of 26 000–28 000 and 11 500–11 800, respectively. The mechanism by which diarrhoea is caused is identical to that of cholera toxin (p. 297).

Heat-stable enterotoxin (ST). In contrast to LTs, the STs of *Esch. coli* (Table 26.4) have a low molecular weight which is probably responsible for their heat stability and poor antigenicity. There are two major classes, designated ST-I (ST_a) and ST-II (ST_b). Variants of ST-I have been associated with porcine and human infec-

Table 26.3 Differential properties of heat-labile toxins (LT) of *Esch. coli*

	LT-I	LT-II
Cell changes		
CHO cells	+	+
Y1 cells	+	+
Vero cells	+	+
Molecular weight (kDa)		
A subunit	26	28
B subunit	11.5	11.8
Isoelectric point	8.5	6.8[a], 5.4[b]
Genetic location	Plasmid	Chromosome
Action	Binds to gangliosides	Activates cAMP

[a]LT-IIa, [b]LTIIb. CHO, Chinese hamster ovary

Table 26.4 Differential properties of heat-stable toxins (ST) of *Esch. coli*

	ST-I (ST$_a$)	ST-II (ST$_b$)
Molecular weight (kDa)	2	5
Infant mouse test	+	−
Methanol	Soluble	Insoluble
Pig intestinal loop	+	+
Rabbit ileal loop	+	−
Rat gut loop	+	−
Action	Activates cyclic guanosine monophosphate	Unknown (cyclic nucleotides)

tions. ST-I was originally detected by an infant mouse test in which secretion occurs in the intestine within 4 h after intragastric administration; it can now be detected by immuno-assay. This toxin activates guanylate cyclase activity resulting in an increase in the level of cyclic guanosine monophosphate (cGMP). The activity of ST-I is rapid, whereas LTs act after a lag period. The mechanism of secretion caused by ST-I, via cGMP, is not known but calcium may play a role. ST-I is plasmid-encoded, and these plasmids may also encode the genes for LT, adhesive factors and antibiotic resistance.

ST-II is distinguished from ST-I by its biological activity and by its insolubility in methanol. It stimulates fluid accumulation in ligated intestinal loops of piglets but not in the infant mouse test. The mechanism of action is not known but it appears not to act via cAMP or cGMP.

Adhesive factors. Enterotoxin alone is not sufficient to enable *Esch. coli* to cause diarrhoea. The organism must initially be able to adhere to the mucosal surface of the epithelial cells of the small intestine. This adhesion is usually mediated by fimbriae that bind to specific receptors in the intestinal cell membrane. These adhesins have been termed *colonization factors antigens* (CFAs), which can be detected in agglutination or immunodiffusion assays. Heterogeneity among CFAs has been shown by polyacrylamide gel electrophoresis and immunoblotting. The expression of CFAs can also be demonstrated by haemagglutination, by experimental colonization of animal intestines, or by tissue or organ culture methods. CFAs exhibit mannose-resistant haemagglutination. Plasmids that simultaneously carry genes for both CFAs and enterotoxin production have been described.

The first colonization factor to be recognized in *Esch. coli* was a fimbrial antigen, K88, controlled by a transferable plasmid. Loss of the K88 plasmid from a strain of *Esch. coli* known to cause piglet enteritis was accompanied by the loss of its capacity to cause diarrhoea in piglets. This was restored by introducing a K88 plasmid from another strain of *Esch. coli*. There is a gene in pigs which is inherited in a simple Mendelian manner and which determines the presence of receptors for K88 in the pig intestinal epithelium; pigs lacking this receptor are resistant to colonization of the small intestine by *Esch. coli* strains with the K88 antigen.

Several colonization factors have subsequently been discovered in human strains of ETEC and, no doubt, others remain to be discovered. The properties of some of the more important colonization factors are shown in Table 26.5.

Epidemiology. In developing countries ETEC are a major cause of mortality in children under the age of 5 years, and a significant cause of diarrhoea in travellers

Table 27.5 Properties of some important human colonization factors

Colonization factor	Components	MRHA Human	Bovine	Guinea pig	Fimbrial type	Associated toxin	Associated serogroups
CFA I		+	+	−	Rod-like	ST or ST/LT	04, 07, 015, 020, 025, 063, 078, 090, 0104, 0110, 0126, 0128, 0136, 0153, 0159
CFA II	CS1	(+)	+	−	Rod-like	ST/LT	06, 0139
	CS2	−	+	−	Rod-like	ST/LT	06
	CS3	−	+	−	Fibrillar	ST/LT	08, 078, 080, 085, 0115, 0128, 0139, 0168
CFA III		−	−	−	Rod-like	LT	025
CFA IV	CS4	+	+	−	Rod-like	ST/LT	025
	CS5	+	+	+	Helical	ST	06, 029, 092, 0114,
	CS6	−	−	−	None	ST or LT	0115, 0167, 025, 027, 079, 089, 092, 0148, 0153, 0159, 0169

MRHA, mannose-resistant haemagglutinin; CS, coli surface antigen; (+), weak reaction.

visiting countries where ETEC are endemic. There have been several studies of travellers' diarrhoea in Mexico where 'turista' has an attack rate of 29–48%; in African countries ETEC have been found in 31–75% of Peace Corps volunteers with diarrhoea.

The sources and modes of spread of ETEC infection in warm-climate countries are not well understood, but it seems likely that water contaminated by human or animal sewage plays an important part in the spread of infection.

Laboratory diagnosis of ETEC

Detection of LT. Tissue culture assays with monolayers of mouse adrenal cells (Y1), Chinese hamster ovary (CHO) or African green monkey kidney (Vero) cells have been used for detecting LT (Table 26.3). Toxin present in culture supernates has a cytotonic effect on these cells, producing characteristic changes in cell morphology. This is in contrast to the cytotoxic effect of Verocytotoxin (see below).

Several immunological techniques are available for the detection of LT, including enzyme-linked immunosorbent assay (ELISA) and a solid-phase radio-immunoassay (RIA). For the ELISA, plates are coated with ganglioside GM_1 which is used to 'capture' LT present in culture supernates. Bound toxin is then detected with toxin-specific rabbit antibodies. A precipitin test (the *Biken test*) performed directly on bacterial colonies growing on a special agar medium may be suitable for use in field laboratories. Rabbit antibodies specific for LT are incorporated into the agar culture medium. As the bacteria grow and secrete LT, the toxin binds to the anti-LT antibodies, forming a precipitin line. A commercial latex particle agglutination test is also available as a screening test.

Detection of ST. Many enterotoxigenic strains of *Esch. coli* produce ST only and it is essential to include tests for ST production in any survey of enterotoxigenicity. Injection of both LTs and STs into ligated ileal loops of rabbits leads to the accumulation of fluid. The action of ST can be distinguished by its relative stability to heat and by the rapidity of its action. So far it has proved impossible to devise tissue culture tests for ST, and until recently the most widely used method for detecting ST-I was the infant mouse test. The intestines are removed after the injection of culture supernates, and the ratio of gut weight to remaining body weight is used as an objective measure of fluid accumulation.

The non-antigenic nature of ST initially prevented the development of immunological tests. This problem was overcome by preparing antiserum from toxin coupled to a hapten comprising a bovine serum albumin carrier and using the antiserum in a RIA. Subsequently, ELISA tests with monoclonal antibody specific for ST have become available and have largely replaced the infant mouse test.

Genetic probes. Gene probes have been developed for the detection of ETEC with genes encoding STs and LTs.

Entero-invasive Esch. coli (EIEC)

Pathogenesis. EIEC and shigellae (see Chapter 25) both cause disease by invading intestinal epithelia. Infection is by ingestion; only a small number of bacteria need to be swallowed as they are relatively resistant to gastric acid and bile, and pass readily into the large intestine where they multiply in the gut lumen. The bacteria pass through the overlying mucus layer, attach to the intestinal epithelial cells and are carried into the cell by endocytosis into an endocytic vacuole, which then lyses. The ability to cause the vacuole to lyse is an important virulence attribute, as organisms unable to do this cannot spread to neighbouring cells. After lysis of the vacuole the bacteria multiply within the epithelial cell and kill it. Spread to neighbouring cells leads to tissue destruction and consequent inflammation, which is the underlying cause of the symptoms of bacillary dysentery.

Pathogenicity in shigellae and EIEC depends on both chromosomal and plasmid genes. A large plasmid carries genes for the expression of outer membrane proteins that are required for invasion as well as genes that may be necessary for the insertion of these proteins into the cell membrane. Plasmid genes are also required for the ability to escape from the endocytic vacuole and to invade contiguous host cells. Chromosomal genes encoding pathogenic mechanisms include those required for the expression of long-chain LPS and those encoding aerobactin iron-sequestering system.

Epidemiology. The epidemiology and ecology of EIEC have been poorly studied, but there appears to be no evidence of an animal or environmental reservoir. Surveys suggest that they cause about 5% of all diarrhoeas in areas of poor hygiene. In the UK and USA, outbreaks are occasionally described, especially in schools and hospitals for the mentally handicapped. Infections are usually food-borne but there is also evidence of cross-infection. The most common serogroup is O124.

Laboratory diagnosis of EIEC. The original *Serény test* in which the bacteria are tested for the ability to cause conjunctivitis in guinea-pigs has been superseded by tissue culture methods. Monolayers of HEp-2 or HeLa cells are exposed to suspensions of the test organism. After an appropriate infection period the cells are washed with a solution containing gentamicin and lysozyme to remove extracellular organisms. After a further period to allow intracellular growth the cells are examined microscopically for the presence of intracellular organisms.

Verocytotoxigenic Esch. coli (VTEC)

Strains of *Esch. coli* expressing a protein cytotoxic for Vero cells were discovered in 1977. Once epidemiologists were aware of VTEC, the importance of these bacteria in human disease became increasingly apparent and the link with two diseases of previously unknown aetiology, *haemorrhagic colitis* and *haemolytic uraemic syndrome*, was established. Outbreaks were first recognized in the USA in 1982 and strains of VTEC belonging to serogroup O157 emerged as the major cause. Since then, outbreaks and sporadic cases have been reported in several other countries and VTEC belonging to many other serotypes have been described. The ability to cause haemorrhagic colitis has led some workers to refer to these strains as enterohaemorrhagic *Esch. coli*, or EHEC. Since 1995 well publicized major episodes in the USA, Canada, Japan and Scotland have heightened general awareness of the importance of this disease.

Human VTEC infection can be associated with a range of clinical symptoms from mild, non-bloody diarrhoea to the severe manifestations of haemolytic uraemic syndrome; a wide spectrum of illness can occur even within a single outbreak.

Haemorrhagic colitis is a grossly bloody diarrhoea, usually in the absence of pyrexia. It is usually preceded by abdominal pain and watery diarrhoea. Haemolytic uraemic syndrome is characterized by acute renal failure, micro-angiopathic haemolytic anaemia and thrombocytopenia. Haemolytic uraemic syndrome occurs in all age groups, but is more common in infants and young children, and is a major cause of renal failure in childhood. Haemolytic uraemic syndrome is usually associated with a prodromal bloody diarrhoea, but an 'atypical' form occurs without a diarrhoeal phase. It may be accompanied by thrombotic thrombocytopenic purpura in which the clinical features are further complicated by neurological involvement and fever.

VTEC have also been implicated as a cause of disease in animals, particularly calves and pigs.

Pathogenesis – nature and mode of action of Verocytotoxin (VT). The biological properties, physical characteristics and antigenicity of VT are very similar to those of Shiga toxin, produced by strains of *Sh. dysenteriae* type 1 (p. 261). The terms 'Shiga-like toxin' and 'Shiga toxin' have also become widely used. Serological tests have revealed two antigenically distinct forms, termed VT1 and VT2. Antibodies prepared to VT1 neutralize Shiga toxin, while antibodies specific for VT2 do not. Variant forms of VT2 have been described in strains of human and porcine origin. The genes controlling production of these variant toxins are not phage-encoded, and the toxin receptor also differs from that used by VT1 and VT2 (Table 26.6).

Table. 26.6 Differential properties of Verocytotoxins expressed by *Esch. coli*

	VT1	VT2	VT2v[a]
Synonyms	SLT1	SLT2	SLT2v
Cytotoxicity			
Vero cells	+	+	+
HeLa cells	+	+	–
Molecular weight (kDa)			
A subunit	32	35	33
B subunit	7.7	10.7	7.5
Genes phage-encoded	+	+	–

[a] Human and porcine variants.

Like Shiga toxin, VT1 and VT2 comprise A and B subunits. For both toxins the A subunit possesses the biological activities of the toxin while the B subunits mediate specific binding and receptor-mediated uptake of the toxin. VT1 and VT2 bind to globotriosylceramide (Gb_3) molecules present on the surface of certain eukaryotic cells. In contrast VT2 variant toxins bind to globotetraosylceramide (Gb_4). During infection with VTEC the inflammatory mediators tumour necrosis factor (TNF) and interleukin-1 (IL-1), in combination with LPS, increase the number of ceramide receptors on the surface of eukaryotic cells, enhancing the binding of VT to these cells. Infection also results in expression of VT molecules that bind to Gb_3 receptors located in the kidneys, leading to haemolytic uraemic syndrome. Molecules of Gb_3 have been detected on mammalian erythrocytes that have P^k antigens. About 75% of the human population carry this antigen, and it has been suggested that such people might have protection from developing haemolytic uraemic syndrome. Red blood cells expressing P^k antigens bind VT via Gb_3 receptors. The extent to which other mammalian cells bind VT remains to be determined, but since they bind to human platelets via Gb_3, VT receptors may exist on other mammalian tissues.

VT1 and VT2, like Shiga toxin, are cytotoxic for Vero and HeLa cells, although VT2 variant toxins do not bind to HeLa cells since this particular cell line does not express Gb_3 receptors. Enterotoxicity in ligated rabbit gut loops and mouse paralytic lethality can also be used to detect VTs.

VT1 causes a direct, dose-dependent cytotoxic effect on human umbilical cord endothelial cells in culture; actively dividing cells are the most sensitive. Since a micro-angiopathy of the capillaries is a characteristic renal lesion in haemolytic uraemic syndrome this supports the hypothesis that vascular endothelial cells are primary targets for VT.

Once bound to the eukaryotic cell surface, the holo-toxin becomes internalized by host cells and remains active within endosomes. The toxin eventually reaches the Golgi apparatus by mechanisms as yet unknown. At some point within the host cell, the A subunit becomes enzymically 'nicked' to form portions A_1 (28 kDa) and A_2 (4 kDa); the A_1 portion of the toxin prevents protein synthesis and results in cell death.

Strains of O157 VTEC express an attaching and effacing (AE) phenotype and, in common with strains of EPEC, the genes involved are located on a pathogenicity island located on the *Esch. coli* chromosome (see p. 268). Although the mechanisms of bacterial adhesion expressed by O157 VTEC are similar to those of EPEC, antigenic variation in, for example, the respective intimin proteins has been detected.

Epidemiology. Outbreaks of infection with VTEC have occurred in the community, in nursing homes for the elderly and in day care centres for young children. The most severe clinical manifestations are usually seen in the young and the elderly.

Food is an important source. In several outbreaks of haemorrhagic colitis due to O157 VTEC in the USA and Canada the causative organism has been isolated from products as diverse as hamburger meat, unpasteurized apple juice and unpasteurized milk. In the outbreak of infection in Lanarkshire, Scotland, in which a number of elderly people died, cooked meat from an award-winning butcher was implicated, indicating that bacteria have no respect for reputations. Verocytotoxin-producing strains of *Esch. coli* O157.H7 were also isolated from healthy heifers on the farms associated with the milk-borne incidents, and it is now generally accepted that cattle are a major reservoir of *Esch. coli* O157.H7.

Laboratory diagnosis. The proportion of VTEC in the faecal flora may be low, often less than 1%, so that testing of individual colonies from culture plates may not always detect the presence of VTEC. DNA probes for the genes encoding VT1 and VT2 have been developed, and by using these probes in colony hybridization tests several hundred colonies from each faecal specimen can be examined, giving a considerable increase in sensitivity. The polymerase chain reaction (PCR) with VT-specific primers has also been used to detect VTEC.

While 95% of *Esch. coli* ferment sorbitol, O157 VTEC do so only slowly. This property is exploited by replacing the lactose present in MacConkey agar with sorbitol. Most strains of O157 VTEC produce colourless colonies after overnight incubation and these can be tested with an O157 LPS-specific antiserum in a simple agglutination assay. Identification of putative strains of *Esch. coli* O157 must be confirmed by routine bacteriology and serotyping. Toxigenicity is confirmed by gene probes, by PCR, by testing strains for a cytotoxic effect on Vero cells, or by a specific ELISA.

Evidence for VTEC O157 infection has also been obtained by detecting patients' serum and salivary antibodies directed against the O157 LPS antigens.

Entero-aggregative Esch. coli (EAggEC)

EAggEC are characterized by their ability to adhere to particular laboratory-cultured cells, such as HEp-2, in an aggregative or 'stacked brick' pattern. This property is usually encoded on a 60-MDa plasmid. Strains of EAggEC were first reported in 1987 as a cause of chronic diarrhoea in malnourished young children living in Chile, and were reported subsequently in Brazil, India, Mexico and Zaire. EAggEC diarrhoea is comparatively rare in industrialized countries, although occasional outbreaks have occurred in Europe, including the UK, and travellers may become infected following visits to countries in which the strains are endemic.

Pathogenesis. Volunteer studies have failed to identify an infective dose for strains of EAggEC. The characteristic pattern of adhesion to HEp-2 cells may be a putative pathogenic mechanism. Although strains of EAggEC may express fimbriae, adhesion to HEp-2 cells can also occur in the absence of these structures and for certain strains adhesion involves cell-surface charge. The site of adhesion within the human host has not been determined. Strains have been reported to produce an ST-like toxin, but this has not been demonstrated in all EAggEC and the mechanisms by which these strains cause a diarrhoeal illness are only poorly understood. Some isolates express haemolysins, an aero-bactin-mediated high-affinity iron uptake system and a range of haemagglutinins; however, apart from the ability to adhere to HEp-2 cells in the stacked-brick formation, these strains are generally quite distinct.

Epidemiology. Strains of EAggEC belong to very diverse combinations of O and H type, and even within an outbreak of diarrhoeal disease strains with several different serotypes may be isolated. The diversity of serotypes and pathogenic mechanisms observed suggests that the genes encoding the aggregative phenotype may be accepted readily by strains of commensal and potentially pathogenic strains of *Esch. coli*, causing these bacteria to be considered as EAggEC.

Laboratory diagnosis. The only methods currently available for detecting these bacteria are the HEp-2 cell test for determining the aggregative phenotype, and DNA probes. The HEp-2 cell test involves allowing strains of *Esch. coli* to adhere to cell monolayers in vitro and observing the pattern of adhesion by microscopy. Although tissue culture tests are laborious, the pattern of adhesion remains the key assay for detecting EAggEC.

An aggregative adhesion gene probe has proved useful as a comparatively rapid means of screening strains as a prelude to HEp-2 adhesion tests.

Prevention and treatment of Esch. coli enteritis

General measures. As with most diarrhoeal disease, the early correction of fluid and electrolyte imbalance is the most important single factor in preventing the death of the patient in severe infections.

The most effective means of preventing infection is to avoid exposure to the infecting agent. Contaminated food and water are probably the most important vehicles of ETEC infection in developing countries. The provision of safe supplies of water together with education in hygienic practice in the handling and production of food, particularly that given to young children, are essential. Travellers to countries with poor hygiene, especially in the tropics, should select eating places with care and, if possible, should consume only hot food and drinks, or bottled water. Self-peeled fruits are probably safe, but salads should be avoided. Unheated milk should always be considered unsafe.

The spread of infantile enteritis in hospitals and nurseries is mainly from patient to patient, generally on the hands of attendants, or from contaminated infant feeds. It can be prevented only by very strict hygiene. Infected patients, and recently admitted patients suspected of being infected, must be isolated by barrier nursing techniques to prevent faecal spread. In some cases outbreaks can be terminated only by closing the ward or nursery and cleaning thoroughly before re-opening.

VTEC infections are acquired most frequently from meat, unpasteurized milk and direct contact with animals. Food-borne infections should be avoided by normal food hygiene with particular attention to processing and handling cooked meat products separately from raw meat, and the thorough cooking of raw meats, especially if minced.

Vaccination. The most extensive studies of the use of vaccines have so far been in the veterinary field. A potential vaccine for human use has been prepared by cross-linking a synthetically produced ST with the non-toxic B subunit of LT. Tests in the rat showed that the vaccine protects against subsequent challenge with ST or LT or with organisms that produce them. In human volunteers, oral administration causes an increase in antitoxin levels in serum samples and jejunal aspirates. Vaccines for preventing infections with O157 VTEC have been considered, using the O157 LPS antigens as the main vaccine component.

Inhibition of enterotoxin activity. Several substances such as activated charcoal, bismuth subsalicylate and non-steroidal anti-inflammatory drugs inhibit or reverse the secretory effects of enterotoxins in experimental animals and may be of value in the prevention or treatment of diarrhoea. Clinical trials have shown some benefit from such substances but more work needs to be done to establish the optimum conditions for their use.

An experimental silica-based compound has been advocated for treating patients suspected of being infected with VTEC. The compound is designed to bind VT synthesized by bacteria present in the intestine, preventing the toxin entering the patient's tissues.

Antimicrobial prophylaxis. A number of antimicrobial drugs reduce the incidence of diarrhoea in travellers to tropical areas. These include doxycycline, trimethoprim, norfloxacin and other fluoroquinolones. However, the widespread use of antibiotic prophylaxis has been criticized both on the grounds of drug toxicity and because of the possibility that the development and spread of drug resistance might be encouraged among a variety of enteropathogens. Also, certain antimicrobial drugs have been shown to increase expression of VT by strains of VTEC such that administration of antibiotics may be counterproductive.

OTHER ESCHERICHIA SPECIES

Esch. blattae was first described among bacteria isolated from the gut of the cockroach. It differs from *Esch. coli* both in oxidizing gluconate and fermenting malonate, as well as in failing to form indole, acidify mannitol or sorbitol, or produce β-galactosidase. It would probably be better placed in another genus. The species has not been reported from human clinical specimens. *Esch. fergusonii*, *Esch. hermanii* and *Esch. vulneris* have been recovered from various clinical specimens, especially faeces and wounds, but their clinical significance is usually unclear.

RECOMMENDED READING

Chart H 1998 Toxigenic *Escherichia coli. Journal of Applied Microbiology* 84: 77S–86S

Chart H, Jenkins C 1999 The serodiagnosis of infections with Verocytotoxin-producing *Escherichia coli. Journal of Applied Microbiology* 86: 731–740

Echeveria P, Savarino S J, Yamamoto T 1993 *Escherichia coli* diarrhoea. *Baillière's Clinical Gastroenterology* 7: 243–261

Gross R J 1991 The pathogenesis of *Escherichia coli* diarrhoea. *Reviews in Medical Microbiology* 2: 37–44

Johnson J R 1991 Virulence factors in *Escherichia coli* urinary tract infection. *Clinical Microbiology Reviews* 3: 80–128

Kaper J B 1998 EPEC delivers the goods. *Trends in Microbiology* 6: 169–173

Law D, Chart H 1998 A Review: Enteroaggregative *Escherichia coli. Journal of Applied Microbiology* 84: 685–697

Schoolnik G K 1989 How *Escherichia coli* infects the urinary tract. *New England Journal of Medicine* 12: 804–805

Tarr P I 1995 *Escherichia coli* O157:H7 Clinical, diagnostic and epidemiological aspects of human infection. *Clinical Infectious Diseases* 20: 1–10

Internet sites

US Food and Drug Administration Center for Food Safety and Applied Nutrition. *Bad Bug Book*: vm.cfsan.fda.gov/~mow/chap15.html#updates

Public Health Laboratory Service: www.phls.co.uk/

27

Klebsiella, enterobacter, proteus and other enterobacteria

Pneumonia; urinary tract infection; opportunist infection

H. Chart

The genera described in this chapter conform to the general definition of the Enterobacteriaceae in that they are aerobic or facultatively anaerobic, ferment glucose and produce catalase but not oxidase. Together with organisms of the genera *Salmonella* (see Chapter 24), *Shigella* (see Chapter 25), *Escherichia* (see Chapter 26) and *Yersinia* (see Chapter 35), they are commonly referred to as enterobacteria. Species of clinical interest are listed alphabetically in Table 27.1, along with common synonyms.

KLEBSIELLA

CLASSIFICATION

The classification of the genus *Klebsiella* has a complex history that must be considered briefly to avoid confusion. In the past the name *Klebsiella aerogenes* was used for the non-motile, capsulate, gas-producing strains commonly found in human faeces and in water. These probably corresponded to strains described in the 19th century as *Bakterium lactis aerogenes*, referred to later as *Bacterium aerogenes*, and subsequently transferred to the genus *Klebsiella*. Unfortunately, the term '*Bact. aerogenes*' (later *Aerobacter aerogenes*) was also used by water bacteriologists to refer to organisms that were subsequently shown to be motile and are now classified as *Enterobacter* species. In an attempt to resolve the resultant confusion, some taxonomists adopted 'pneumoniae' as the species name for the non-motile aerogenes-like organisms, although it had earlier been used to designate certain biochemically atypical *Klebsiella* strains isolated from the respiratory tract of man and animals. The name *K. pneumoniae* has now been accepted formally, and appears in the Approved Lists of Bacterial Names, while *K. aerogenes* is omitted. In this chapter the name *K. pneumoniae* is therefore used for the species as a whole, but the most frequently encountered, biochemically typical form of

Table 27.1 The principal genera and species of Enterobacteriaceae of clinical interest

Genus	Species	Synonyms
Citrobacter	C. amalonaticus	Levinea amalonatica
	C. freundii	
	C. koseri	C. diversus, L. amalonatica
Edwardsiella	E. tarda	E. anguillimortifera
Enterobacter	Ent. aerogenes	K. mobilis
	Ent. cloacae	
	Ent. agglomerans	Erwinia herbicola
Escherichia[a]		
Hafnia	H. alvei	Ent. alvei, Ent. hafniae
Klebsiella	K. oxytoca	
	K. pneumoniae	
	ssp. aerogenes	K. aerogenes
	ssp. ozaenae	K. ozaenae
	ssp. pneumoniae	K. pneumoniae
	ssp. rhinoscleromatis	K. rhinoscleromatis
Morganella	M. morganii	Pr. morganii
Proteus	Pr. mirabilis	
	Pr. vulgaris	
Providencia	Prov. alcalifaciens	
	Prov. rettgeri	Pr. rettgeri
	Prov. stuartii	
Salmonella[a]		
Serratia	S. liquefaciens	Ent. liquefaciens
	S. marcescens	
	S. odorifera	
Shigella[a]		
Yersinia[a]		

[a] See appropriate chapter.

it is referred to as *K. pneumoniae* ssp. *aerogenes*. The atypical respiratory strains are included in the subspecies *ozaenae*, *pneumoniae* and *rhinoscleromatis*. A further species, *K. oxytoca*, is occasionally encountered in clinical specimens.

DESCRIPTION

Members of the genus *Klebsiella* are straight rods about 1–2 μm long. They can be differentiated by simple biochemical tests and often have a pronounced capsule which can be demonstrated by Gram's stain. Capsular material is produced in greater amounts on media rich in carbohydrate. In these conditions the growth on agar is luxuriant, greyish white and extremely mucoid (Fig. 27.1). The polysaccharides of the different capsular types are all complex acid polysaccharides, which usually contain glucuronic acid and pyruvic acid. They resemble the K antigens of *Escherichia coli* (p. 266).

Klebsiellae are non-motile but most strains express fimbriae. The organisms grow at temperatures between 12 and 43°C (optimum, 37°C) and are killed by moist heat at 55°C for 30 min. They may survive drying for months and, when kept at room temperature, cultures remain viable for many weeks. They are facultatively anaerobic, but growth under strictly anaerobic conditions is poor. There is no haemolysis of horse or sheep red cells.

Antigenic structure

About 80 capsular (K) antigens are presently recognized. Among current UK isolates, types K2, K3 and K21 predominate, and the prevalence of these types

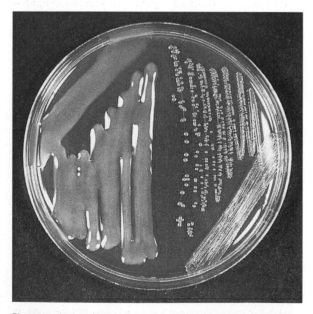

Fig. 27.1 Mucoid (left) and non–mucoid (right) variants of *Klebsiella* species on carbohydrate-rich medium. (By courtesy of George Sharp and Richard Edwards, Nottingham Public Health Laboratory.)

limits the usefulness of capsular serotyping as an epidemiological tool.

In addition to the capsular antigens, five different somatic or O antigens occur in various combinations with the capsular antigens. Four of the five *Klebsiella* O antigens are identical to or related to *Esch. coli* O antigens. It is therefore possible to divide *Klebsiella* strains into a small number of groups which may be further subdivided into capsular types, but this is of little practical value in the classification of the capsulate members of the genus.

There is some association between antigenic structure, biochemical activities and habitat. Members of capsular types 1–6 occur most frequently in the human respiratory tract.

Considerable overlap occurs between *Klebsiella* antigens and those of unrelated organisms. Capsular type 2, for example, is immunologically similar to the type 2 pneumococcus. Capsular antigens are usually detected by means of the capsular 'swelling' reaction, but various other techniques are used, including countercurrent immuno-electrophoresis and enzyme-linked immunosorbent assay (ELISA).

Other typing methods

Many *Klebsiella* strains produce bacteriocins, which appear to be distinct from colicins because they have no action on *Esch. coli*. They have a narrow range of activity on other klebsiellae and epidemiological analysis may be improved by the use of bacteriocins as an adjunct to capsular serotyping. Phage typing has also been used, and biotyping has been recommended instead of serotyping for use in less well equipped laboratories.

Molecular typing methods have also been developed. These include plasmid analysis, DNA profiling by random amplified polymorphic DNA (RAPD) and pulsed-field gel electrophoresis.

PATHOGENESIS

Klebsiellae are a fairly common cause of urinary tract infection and occasionally give rise to cases of severe bronchopneumonia, sometimes with chronic destructive lesions and multiple abscess formation in the lungs (Friedländer's pneumonia). Cases are sporadic and usually occur in members of the general population rather than in hospital patients. In many cases there is also bacteraemia, and the mortality rate is high. This condition is usually but not always associated with members of capsular types 1–5, which are often biochemically atypical.

However, the main importance of klebsiellae as human pathogens is in causing infections in hospital patients; the strains responsible are nearly always biochemically typical members of *K. pneumoniae* spp. *aerogenes*, most of which belong to higher-numbered capsular types. Clinical sepsis develops in surgical wounds and in the urinary tract; a number of patients have bacteraemic infections and some die.

Colonization of the respiratory tract is very common in hospital patients receiving antibiotics, but its clinical significance is often difficult to assess. Some debilitated patients develop bronchopneumonia in which a *Klebsiella* spp. appears to be the primary infecting agent. In the early days of antibiotic usage, klebsiellae were naturally resistant to the available antibiotics and with the passage of time they acquired resistance to the newly developed ones. The emergence of klebsiella as an important cause of infection in hospitals is undoubtedly related to the use of antibiotics.

The *ozaenae* and *rhinoscleromatis* subspecies of *K. pneumoniae* take their names from the diseases with which they are associated. Rhinoscleroma is a chronic upper respiratory tract disease that occurs in a number of countries in eastern Europe and other parts of the world, where it is associated with prolonged exposure to crowded and unhygienic conditions. The lesions occur in the nose, larynx, throat and, to a lesser extent, in the trachea, and consist of granulomatous infiltrations of the submucosa. Ozaena is an uncommon, chronic disease in which there is atrophy of the nasal mucosa, in which *K. pneumoniae* spp. *ozaenae* is of doubtful significance.

Pathogenic mechanisms

Long-chain lipopolysaccharide (LPS) protects strains from the action of serum complement, and polysaccharide capsules are thought to confer protection against phagocytosis. Adhesion to host tissues has been attributed to the expression of a range of fimbrial and non-fimbrial adhesins. In common with other members of the Enterobacteriaceae, klebsiellae express type 1 fimbriae that exhibit mannose-sensitive haemagglutination. Type 3 fimbriae also cause haemagglutination of erythrocytes pre-treated with tannin. Additional fimbrial structures (type 6 and KPF-28) and non-fimbrial adhesins have been described. Adhesin CF29K is a plasmid-encoded protein that enables strains to adhere to cultured human intestinal cell lines.

In common with many enteric bacteria, klebsiellae express an enterobactin-mediated iron-sequestering system which uses ferric-siderophore receptors antigenically related to those expressed by strains of *Esch. coli*. Strains of *Klebsiella* may also express a plasmid-encoded aerobactin-mediated high-affinity iron uptake system. Heat-labile and heat-stable toxins have been described in strains isolated from burns patients; however, the role these toxins play in the pathogenesis of disease remains to be determined.

TREATMENT

Clinical isolates of *Klebsiella* characteristically produce a β-lactamase that renders them resistant to ampicillin, amoxicillin and other penicillins, but combinations of these drugs with β-lactamase inhibitors such as clavulanic acid are usually effective. Klebsiellae are normally susceptible to cephalosporins, especially β-lactamase-stable derivatives such as cefuroxime and cefotaxime, and to fluoroquinolones. Resistance to chloramphenicol and tetracycline varies from strain to strain; they are often sensitive to gentamicin and other aminoglycosides, but transferable enzymic resistance to aminoglycosides and other antimicrobial agents has become common in strains found in some hospitals.

Klebsiella infection of the urine often responds to trimethoprim, nitrofurantoin, co-amoxiclav or oral cephalosporins. Pneumonia and other serious infections require vigorous treatment with an aminoglycoside or a cephalosporin such as cefotaxime.

Vaccines based on *Klebsiella* LPS and capsular polysaccharides have been considered for the prevention of infections with these organisms. The toxic lipid-A component appears to be obstructing the use of LPS vaccines; similarly, capsular vaccines are being hampered by the range of different capsular antigen types expressed by strains of *Klebsiella*.

ENTEROBACTER

DESCRIPTION

Enterobacter species have many features in common with those of the genus *Klebsiella*, but are readily distinguished by their motility, though non-motile variants occasionally occur. Several species are recognized; *Enterobacter aerogenes* and *Ent. cloacae* are much the most important clinically. *Ent. agglomerans*, an anaerogenic, yellow-pigmented organism formerly known as *Erwinia herbicola* is also occasionally encountered.

The colonies of *Enterobacter* strains may be slightly mucoid. In general, their fermentative activity is more limited than that of typical klebsiellae. *Ent. aerogenes* is usually able to express a lysine decarboxylase enzyme, but not arginine decarboxylase, whereas *Ent. cloacae* decarboxylates arginine, but not lysine.

Serotyping and phage typing schemes have been developed to characterize strains of *Enterobacter* spp. associated with hospital infections. Plasmid analysis, multilocus enzyme electrophoresis and amplification of selected DNA sequences by the polymerase chain reaction are also being used.

PATHOGENESIS

The normal habitat of *Enterobacter* spp. is probably soil and water, but the organisms are occasionally found in human faeces and the respiratory tract. Infection of hospital patients occurs, but *Enterobacter* spp. are a much less important cause of hospital infection than *Klebsiella* spp. Most infections are of the urinary tract, although members of the genus are an important cause of bacteraemia in some hospitals.

The pathogenic mechanisms expressed by strains of *Enterobacter* spp. are poorly understood. In common with certain strains of *Klebsiella*, they express type 1 and type 3 fimbriae. Most strains also express an aerobactin-mediated iron uptake system, which is generally associated with extra-intestinal human bacterial pathogens. Strains may produce a haemolysin resembling the α-haemolysin produced by strains of *Esch. coli*. Very rarely strains hybridize with gene probes for Verocytotoxin 1 (p. 272).

An outer membrane protein, termed OmpX, may be a pathogenic factor for strains of *Ent. cloacae*. This protein appears to reduce production of porins, leading to decreased sensitivity to β-lactam antibiotics, and might play a role in host cell invasion.

TREATMENT

Enterobacter strains are nearly always highly resistant to penicillins and to the earlier cephalosporins because they produce a chromosomal β-lactamase with cephalosporinase activity. Many are also resistant to tetracycline, chloramphenicol and to streptomycin, although most are sensitive to other aminoglycosides, including gentamicin, and to fluoroquinolones. Most strains appear susceptible to cefotaxime on primary testing, but they often possess an inducible chromosomal cephalosporinase, which allows the rapid development of resistance during therapy. *Enterobacter* strains differ from *Serratia* strains in being sensitive to the polymyxins.

HAFNIA

DESCRIPTION

Hafnia alvei was formerly placed in the genus *Enterobacter*, but DNA–DNA hybridization studies show that this organism deserves a separate generic status. Three DNA-related groups have been recognized, but at present the genus contains only the one species.

Strains grow well on general laboratory media, but *H. alvei* ferments a much narrower range of sugars than members of the genus *Enterobacter*. It does not express a capsule and does not liquefy gelatin. All *H. alvei* strains are lysed by a single phage, which does not affect other members of the Enterobacteriaceae. There is an antigenic scheme that includes many serotypes.

PATHOGENESIS

Strains are isolated from the faeces of man and other animals and are also found in sewage, soil, water and dairy products. They are occasionally encountered as opportunist pathogens. Some strains carry the genes encoding the ability to cause 'attaching and effacing' lesions of intestinal cells, as described for strains of enteropathogenic *Esch. coli* (EPEC, p. 268).

SERRATIA

DESCRIPTION

Although numerous species of the genus *Serratia* have been described, *S. marcescens* is the one most commonly encountered in clinical specimens. Several others, including *S. liquefaciens* (formerly known as *Ent. liquefaciens*) and *S. odorifera*, are sometimes isolated. They vary considerably in size. Even on the same type of medium a single strain may at one time give rise to coccobacillary morphology and at another to rods indistinguishable from other enterobacteria. Capsules are not normally formed, but capsular material is formed on a well aerated medium poor in nitrogen and phosphate.

Most *Serratia* strains are motile and some strains of *S. marcescens* produce red pigmented colonies on agar. Pigment is formed only in the presence of oxygen and at a suitable temperature, which is not necessarily the same as that for optimal growth. Thus, many strains grow best at 30–37°C but form little or no pigment, whereas at lower temperatures growth is poorer and pigment formation is abundant.

The red pigment, prodigiosin, is soluble in absolute alcohol and other organic solvents but is insoluble in water. It has been separated into three red fractions and one blue fraction with different absorption spectra. Prodigiosin is also formed by certain organisms unrelated to *S. marcescens*, including an actinomycete, and certain Gram-negative rods isolated from sea water.

Typing methods

Several typing methods have been developed, including bacteriocin and phage typing. Strains may also be differentiated by multilocus enzyme electrophoresis and molecular methods such as ribotyping and pulsed-field gel electrophoresis. Plasmid typing has been used, but only a limited proportion of strains carry plasmids.

PATHOGENESIS

S. marcescens is widely distributed in nature, but faecal carriage is uncommon in the general human population. Pigmented strains may cause concern by giving rise to red colours in various foods or by simulating the appearance of blood in the sputum or faeces. Pigmented and non-pigmented strains are found occasionally in the human respiratory tract and in faeces. Most infections occur in hospital patients; they include infections of the urinary and respiratory tracts, meningitis, wound infections, septicaemia and endocarditis. Some strains become endemically established in hospitals and outbreaks of infection are also frequently reported. *Serratia* spp. can multiply at ambient temperatures in fluids containing minimal nutrients and outbreaks have followed the introduction of the organisms directly into the bloodstream in contaminated transfusion fluids. Only a small proportion of the strains responsible for infection are pigmented.

The other *Serratia* species also occur commonly in the natural environment, especially in water; *S. liquefaciens* and *S. odorifera* are occasionally found in clinical specimens.

Pathogenic mechanisms

Serratia spp. may express a range of fimbrial haemagglutinins although the tissue specificity of these adhesins appears to be unknown. Some strains express cell surface components causing these bacteria to be highly hydrophobic, and this may be involved in adhesion to eukaryotic cell surfaces. An iron-regulated haemolysin has been described, but a role for this toxin in the pathogenesis of disease has not been demonstrated. *Serratia*

spp. also express an enterobactin-mediated high affinity iron uptake system and some may acquire ferric ions through an aerobactin-mediated iron uptake system. Extracellular enzymes may be responsible for host tissue damage. Toxins resembling *Esch. coli* Verocytotoxin and heat-labile toxin have been described.

TREATMENT

Serratia strains, like *Enterobacter* strains, are commonly resistant to cephalosporins. Resistance to ampicillin and gentamicin is variable, but many strains destroy these antibiotics enzymically.

An aminoglycoside, such as gentamicin, is usually the most reliable first-line choice. Fluoroquinolones or carbapenems may be useful in recalcitrant cases.

PROTEUS AND RELATED GENERA

CLASSIFICATION

The history of the genera *Proteus*, *Providencia* and *Morganella* is inextricably linked, and they are best considered together. The organism first isolated by Morgan was formerly included in the genus *Proteus*, but genetic evidence and enzyme studies show that a separate genus is justified with a single species, *Morganella morganii*.

There has been similar debate over the taxonomy of the remaining species in this group, with successive proposals to combine and separate the genera *Proteus* and *Providencia*. The organisms once known as biotypes A and B of *Proteus inconstans* are now regarded as separate species of the genus *Providencia*: *Providencia alcalifaciens* and *Prov. stuartii*. As a result of genetic studies, *Proteus rettgeri* has also been transferred to the genus *Providencia* as *Prov. rettgeri*, even though it resembles *Proteus* spp. rather than other organisms of the genus *Providencia* in producing urease. This leaves only *Pr. vulgaris* and *Pr. mirabilis* in the genus *Proteus*.

DESCRIPTION

There is considerable morphological variation, but in agar-grown cultures the microscopical appearance is much like that of other coliform bacteria.

All grow well on laboratory nutrient media. A notable property of *Pr. vulgaris* and *Pr. mirabilis* strains is the ability to swarm on solid media: the bacterial growth spreads progressively from the edge of the colony and eventually covers the whole surface of the medium. This swarming characteristically takes place in a discontinuous manner, with each period of outward progress followed by a stationary period (Fig. 27.2). A number of methods have been devised to inhibit swarming, mainly to avoid interference with the isolation of clinically more important organisms.

The various species are differentiated by standard biochemical tests. *M. morganii* and *Proteus* and *Providencia* species have the almost unique ability to deaminate amino acids oxidatively, which is shown by growing the organism in a medium containing phenylalanine, from which phenylpyruvic acid is formed (the PPA test).

Typing methods

Phage typing, bacteriocin-typing and serotyping schemes have been developed for *Proteus* and *Providencia* species. Swarming *Proteus* strains exhibit the Dienes phenomenon (the mutual inhibition of swarming), and this forms the basis for a precise method of differentiation among such strains. Test organisms are inoculated onto the surface of an agar plate, and those that show no line of demarcation in areas where the swarming growths meet are regarded as identical.

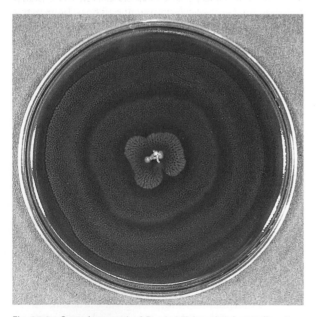

Fig. 27.2 Swarming growth of *Pr. mirabilis* inoculated centrally onto a blood agar plate and incubated overnight at 37°C. (By courtesy of George Sharp and Richard Edwards, Nottingham Public Health Laboratory.)

PATHOGENESIS

Strains of *Pr. mirabilis* are a prominent cause of urinary tract infection in children and in domiciliary practice. Indole-producing strains of *Proteus* and *Providencia* are usually isolated from hospital patients, especially in elderly men following surgery or instrumentation. Septicaemia generally occurs only in patients with serious underlying conditions or as a complication of urinary tract surgery, but outbreaks of septicaemia, often with meningitis, may occur among the newborn in hospitals. A variety of other infections, usually of surgical wounds or bedsores, occur in hospitals and are usually considered to originate from the gut flora.

M. morganii is uncommon in human disease but occasionally causes infections in hospital patients.

Pathogenic mechanisms

These bacteria are characteristically highly motile and chemotaxis may play a part in pathogenesis. Strains of *Proteus* spp. may also express calcium-dependent and calcium-independent haemolysins in addition to a range of proteases such as an IgAase.

Proteus spp. and other urease-producing organisms create alkaline conditions in the urine and may provoke the formation of calculi (stones) in the urinary tract.

TREATMENT

Most strains of *Pr. mirabilis* do not produce β-lactamase; they are consequently moderately sensitive to benzylpenicillin and fully sensitive to ampicillin, and most other β-lactam antibiotics. *Pr. vulgaris* strains are usually resistant to penicillins and many cephalosporins, although they may be sensitive to β-lactamase-stable derivatives such as cefotaxime. All strains are resistant to polymyxins and tetracyclines. *Proteus* and *Providencia* strains are inherently sensitive to aminoglycosides, but resistance, which may be due to enzymic or non-enzymic mechanisms, is now common.

Pr. mirabilis urinary tract infections usually respond to ampicillin or trimethoprim but nitrofurantoin is not effective. Treatment of infection associated with renal stones is often unsuccessful. Serious infection with other *Proteus*, *Providencia* or *Morganella* strains can often be treated with an aminoglycoside or a cephalosporin such as cefotaxime. However, susceptibility is unpredictable and treatment should be guided by laboratory findings.

CITROBACTER

DESCRIPTION

The genus *Citrobacter* was first proposed for a group of lactose-negative or late lactose-fermenting coliform bacteria that share certain somatic antigens with salmonellae and were also known as the Ballerup-Bethesda group. These organisms are now known as *Citrobacter freundii*. Other species included in the genus are *C. koseri* (known as *C. diversus* in the USA) and *C. amalonaticus*. They grow well on ordinary media and are unpigmented. Mucoid forms sometimes occur.

Serotyping schemes have been developed and antigenic diversity in expression of somatic (LPS) antigens is recognized. Antigen–antibody cross-reactions between strains of *Citrobacter* spp. and strains of *Salmonella* and *Esch. coli* have been described. For example, certain strains of *C. freundii* share LPS epitopes with *Esch. coli* expressing O157 antigens.

PATHOGENESIS

Citrobacter spp. are often found in human faeces and may be isolated from a variety of clinical specimens. They do not often give rise to serious infections. *C. koseri* occasionally causes neonatal meningitis; in this condition there is a high mortality and the formation of cerebral abscesses is common.

Pathogenic mechanisms expressed by strains of *Citrobacter* spp. are poorly understood. Strains of *C. koseri* express type 1 (mannose-sensitive) fimbriae

and occasional strains produce a form of *Esch. coli* Verocytotoxin type 2.

TREATMENT

C. freundii is usually sensitive to aminoglycosides, fluoroquinolones and chloramphenicol while sensitivity to ampicillin, tetracycline and cephalosporins varies. Resistance to aminoglycosides occurs frequently among *C. koseri* strains. Choice of treatment should be based on laboratory tests of susceptibility.

EDWARDSIELLA

Edwardsiella tarda was first described under the name *Asakusa* to include a group of enterobacteria that appeared to be quite distinct from all others. It grows well on ordinary media but produces only small colonies of 0.5–1 mm diameter after 24 h.

Edwardsiella strains are frequently isolated from healthy cold-blooded animals and their environment. They are pathogenic for eels, catfish and other animals, sometimes causing economic losses. The occasional human infections probably originate from contact with cold-blooded animals. *E. tarda* mainly causes wound infection, but meningitis and septicaemia have also been reported. It is rarely found in the faeces of healthy people, but a higher isolation rate has been found in patients with diarrhoea, and the role of the species in the aetiology of diarrhoea requires further study. Some strains produce a heat-stable toxin causing fluid accumulation in the infant mouse test developed for detecting *Esch. coli* heat-stable toxin I.

RECOMMENDED READING

Lund B M, Sussman M, Jones D, Stringer M R (eds) 1988 *Enterobacteriaceae in the environment and as pathogens.* Society of Applied Bacteriology Symposium Series, No. 17. Blackwell Scientific, Oxford (published as a supplement to *Journal of Applied Bacteriology* 65)

O'Hara C M, Brenner F W, Miller J M 2000 Classification, identification and clinical significance of *Proteus, Providencia,* and *Morganella. Clinical Microbiology Reviews* 13: 534–546

Podschun R, Ullmann U 1998 *Klebsiella* spp. as nosocomial pathogens: epidemiology, taxonomy, typing methods, and pathogenicity factors. *Clinical Microbiology Reviews* 1998 11: 589–603

Williams P, Tomas J M 1990 The pathogenicity of *Klebsiella pneumoniae. Reviews in Medical Microbiology* 1: 196–204

28

Pseudomonads and non–fermenters

Opportunist infection; cystic fibrosis; melioidosis

J. R. W. Govan

The term *pseudomonads* describes a large group of aerobic, non-fermentative, Gram-negative bacilli belonging to over 100 species that were originally contained within the genus *Pseudomonas*. Most are saprophytes found widely in soil, water and other moist environments. Historically, the genus *Pseudomonas* has been used as a microbial repository for a vast range of species, often with diverse phenotypic characteristics. Molecular analyses of the group have led to revised taxonomic classifications, and many species have been allocated to new genera which include *Burkholderia, Comamonas, Stenotrophomonas, Ralstonia* and *Brevundimonas* (Table 28.1). Some pseudomonads are pathogenic for plants, insects and animals.

Pseudomonas aeruginosa is the species most commonly associated with human disease but *Burkholderia* (previously *Pseudomonas*) *pseudomallei* is an important pathogen in tropical areas of the world. *Burkholderia*

(previously *Pseudomonas) cepacia*, which is now encompassed within the *B. cepacia* complex, has emerged as an important pathogen in immunocompromised patients, particularly in individuals with cystic fibrosis or chronic granulomatous disease. *Stenotrophomonas maltophilia* also infects immunocompromised patients, with a mortality reaching 60% in patients with haematological malignancies.

Several other species are occasionally isolated from human clinical specimens as opportunistic pathogens, including *Ps. putida, Ps. fluorescens, Ps. stutzeri* and a number of other glucose non-fermenters.

There are several reasons for the pre-eminence of *Ps. aeruginosa* as a human pathogen:

- its adaptability
- its innate resistance to many antibiotics and disinfectants
- its armoury of putative virulence factors
- an increasing supply of patients compromised by age, underlying disease or immunosuppressive therapy.

The genome of *Ps. aeruginosa* consists of 6.3 million base pairs – the largest bacterium sequenced to date. This information has already provided insights into the organism's versatility and inherent resistance. The challenge of sequencing the larger genomes of *B. pseudomallei* and *B. cepacia* is under way.

PSEUDOMONAS AERUGINOSA

Description

Ps. aeruginosa is a Gram-negative bacillus, non-sporing, non-capsulate, and usually motile by virtue of one or two polar flagella (see Fig. 2.10, p. 16). It is a strict aerobe but can grow anaerobically if nitrate is available. The organism grows readily on a wide variety of culture media over a wide temperature range and emits a sweet grape-like odour that is easily recognized. Most strains produce diffusible pigments; typically, the colony and surrounding medium is greenish-blue due to

Table 28.1 The principal genera and species of pseudomonads of clinical interest	
Genus	Species
Pseudomonas	*Ps. aeruginosa*
	Ps. fluorescens
	Ps. putida
	Ps. stutzeri
	Ps. mendocina
Burkholderia	*B. pseudomallei*
	B. mallei
	B. cepacia complex[a]
	B. gladioli
Comamonas	*C acidovorans*
	C. testosteroni
Stenotrophomonas	*Sten. maltophilia*
Ralstonia	*R. pickettii*
Brevundimonas	*Brev. diminuta*
[a] See text.	

production of a soluble blue phenazine pigment, *pyocyanin*, and the yellow-green fluorescent pigment *pyoverdin*, which acts as the major siderophore; additional pigments include *pyorubrin* (red) and *melanin* (brown). Some 10–15% of *Ps. aeruginosa* strains readily produce pigment only when grown on pigment-enhancing media. Individual colonies can occur as five distinct types ranging from dwarf colonies to large mucoid colonies; the most common colonial form is relatively large, low-convex with an irregular surface, an edge that is translucent and an oblong shape with the long axis parallel to the line of inoculum.

Ps. aeruginosa differs from members of the Enterobacteriaceae by deriving energy from carbohydrates by an oxidative rather than a fermentative metabolism. It appears inactive in carbohydrate fermentation tests, and only glucose is utilized. However, all strains give a rapid positive oxidase reaction (within 30 seconds) and this is a useful preliminary test for non-pigmented strains.

Typing for epidemiological purposes, or to investigate clonal relationships between isolates, has traditionally relied on phenotypic markers such as serospecificity of the lipopolysaccharide (LPS), susceptibility to phages and the profile of bacteriocin production. Bacteriocin typing is simple to perform and allows characterization of most isolates, including the mucoid and LPS rough phenotypes. For non-mucoid isolates with smooth LPS, simple LPS-based serotyping methods are suitable. The problem of instability in the phenotypic markers used in serotyping or bacteriocin typing has been circumvented by the development of restriction endonuclease typing with pulsed-field gel electrophoresis (see p. 34). This is the most reliable and discriminatory of the present DNA-based typing methods and is considered to be the gold standard.

Pathogenesis

Ps. aeruginosa can infect almost any external site or organ. Most community infections are mild and superficial, but in hospital patients, infections are more common, more severe and more varied.

Community infections

Infections such as otitis externa and varicose ulcers are often chronic, but not disabling. In contrast, corneal infections resulting from contaminated contact lenses or other sources can be rapidly destructive and painful. Recreational and occupational conditions associated with pseudomonas infections include *Jacuzzi rash* or *whirlpool rash* (an acute self-limiting folliculitis) and industrial eye injuries, which may lead to panophthalmitis.

Hospital infections

Infection in hospital patients is usually localized, as in catheter-related urinary tract infection, infected ulcers, bed sores, burns and eye infections. In patients compromised by age, or immunosuppressing diseases such as leukaemia and AIDS, and in those treated with immunosuppressive drugs or corticosteroids, pseudomonas infections frequently become generalized, and the organism may be cultured from the blood or from many organs of the body post mortem. *Ps. aeruginosa* is not a major cause of Gram-negative septicaemia or necrotizing pneumonia but is associated with high mortality when these infections occur in neutropenic patients. Septicaemic infections are characterized by the black necrotic skin lesions known as ecthyma gangrenosum.

Cystic fibrosis

The lungs of children with cystic fibrosis are particularly susceptible to infections caused by *Ps. aeruginosa* and members of what has become known as the *Burkholderia cepacia* complex. In these patients, asymptomatic pulmonary colonization with typical non-mucoid forms of *Ps. aeruginosa* eventually leads to the emergence of mucoid variants (Fig. 28.1); debilitating episodes of pulmonary exacerbation due to mucoid *Ps. aeruginosa* are the major cause of morbidity and mortality in cystic fibrosis.

Virulence factors

Most strains produce two exotoxins, exotoxin A and exo-enzyme S, and a variety of cytotoxic substances including proteases, phospholipases; rhamnolipids and the blue-green pigment pyocyanin; an alginate-like exopolysaccharide is responsible for the mucoid phenotype (Fig. 28.2). The importance of these putative virulence factors depends upon the site and nature of infection:

- proteases play a key role in corneal ulceration
- exotoxin and proteases are important in burn infections
- phospholipases, proteases and alginate are associated with chronic pulmonary colonization
- fluorescein or pyoverdin pigments act as bacterial siderophores.

Production of fluorescein in vivo allows *Ps. aeruginosa* to compete with mammalian iron-binding proteins such as transferrin. In association with pyocyanin, it gives rise to the characteristic blue-green pus of pseudomonas-infected wounds and the old species name *pyocyanea* (Latin = blue pus), as well as the present

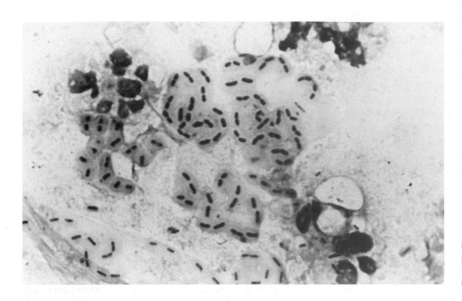

Fig. 28.1 Gram-stained sputum from patient harbouring mucoid *Ps. aeruginosa*. Note spawn-like microcolony and adjacent phagocytes.

aeruginosa (Latin = verdigris; blue-green). The mechanism of action of exotoxin A is similar to that of diphtheria toxin (see Chapter 17) although the molecular receptors are different.

Laboratory diagnosis

Ps. aeruginosa grows on most common culture media, but for specific investigation material should be cultured on a medium that is selective and enhances the production of the characteristic blue-green pigment, pyocyanin. For culture from water or soil, a selective medium containing acetamide as the sole carbon and nitrogen source may be used. Resultant colonies are usually easily identified. About 10% of isolates do not produce detectable pigment even on suitable media; in such cases, a rapid positive oxidase test provides presumptive evidence of the identity. Formal identification can be made with an appropriate multitest system such as API 20NE. Tests for serum antibodies against pseudomonas antigens have no place in diagnosis except in patients with cystic fibrosis or chronic obstructive pulmonary disease, in which increasing antibody levels correlate directly with immune-mediated lung damage.

Treatment

Ps. aeruginosa is normally resistant to many commonly employed antimicrobial agents. Until the 1960s, pseudomonas infections were usually treated with polymyxins, agents that exhibit considerable toxicity. With the development of antipseudomonal β-lactam compounds, including piperacillin, ticarcillin, ceftazidime and

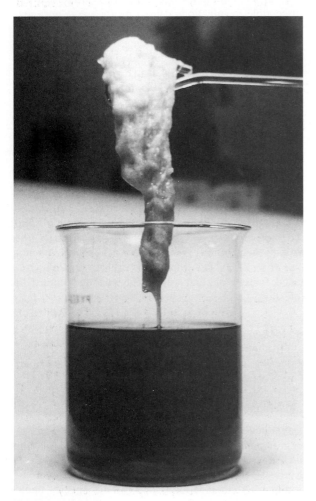

Fig. 28.2 Alcohol extraction of alginate from mucoid *Ps. aeruginosa*.

meropenem, and aminoglycosides such as gentamicin and tobramycin, treatment with a combination of an aminoglycoside and a β-lactam antibiotic was commonly adopted. There is little clinical evidence of the superiority of combined therapy although it has the potential for antibacterial synergy and reduced antibiotic resistance. Monotherapy with broad-spectrum β-lactam agents such as ceftazidime and imipenem is used, but resistance to these agents occurs.

Most antipseudomonal antibiotics have to be given parenterally; in contrast, fluoroquinolones such as ciprofloxacin can be administered orally. Ciprofloxacin exhibits good activity against *Ps. aeruginosa* and penetrates well into most tissues, but resistance may develop. Aerosolized delivery of colistin (polymyxin E) or tobramycin into the lungs appears to be clinically effective in the management of chronic *Ps. aeruginosa* lung infection in individuals with cystic fibrosis.

Passive vaccination may be useful for the treatment of septicaemia and burn infections due to *Ps. aeruginosa*, which are associated with high mortality; active vaccination to prevent pulmonary colonization would be desirable for patients with cystic fibrosis and several conjugate vaccines are in clinical trial.

Epidemiology

Ps. aeruginosa is a hardy saprophyte which can be isolated from a wide variety of environmental sources. Its ability to persist and multiply, particularly in moist environments and on moist equipment (e.g. humidifiers) in hospital wards, bathrooms and kitchens, is of particular importance in cross-infection control. Consumption of salad vegetables contaminated with pseudomonas is a potential risk for immunocompromised patients in intensive care units.

The organism is resistant to, and may multiply in, many of the disinfectants and antiseptics commonly used in hospitals. It can be a troublesome contaminant in pharmaceutical preparations and may cause ophthalmitis following the faulty chemical 'sterilization' of contact lenses.

Most hospital-acquired infections with *Ps. aeruginosa* originate from exogenous sources but some patients suffer endogenous infection, particularly of the urinary tract. Healthy carriers usually harbour strains in the gastro-intestinal tract, but in the open community the carriage rate seldom exceeds 10%. In contrast, acquisition of *Ps. aeruginosa* in a hospital is rapid, and up to 30% of patients may excrete the organisms within 2 days of admission.

Burned patients are especially at risk; the presence of the organism in ward air, dust and in eschar shed from the burns suggests that infection can be air-borne. However, contact spread is probably more important than the air-borne route. Transmission may occur directly via the hands of medical staff, or indirectly via contaminated apparatus. Severely burned patients and those with chest injuries who require artificial ventilation are very susceptible to *Ps. aeruginosa*; pulmonary infection not infrequently precedes septicaemia, which is associated with high mortality. Modern intensive care equipment can be difficult to clean, and there is little doubt that infection can be spread by this source.

Severe eye infections may result from contaminated contact lenses, industrial eye injuries or from introduction of contaminated medicament during ophthalmic procedures. Similarly, in oil exploration, diving operations are occasionally aborted because of outbreaks of troublesome ear infection.

The warm, moist and aerated conditions under which *Ps. aeruginosa* thrives are ideally met in poorly maintained whirlpools or jacuzzis. Ear infections and an irritating folliculitis (jacuzzi rash) may be acquired from such sources.

Epidemics of gastro-intestinal infection can occur in newborn and young infants in maternity units and paediatric wards, and may result from contaminated milk feeds.

Control

Prevention is easier than cure; once *Ps. aeruginosa* has gained access to the hospital environment, or has established infection, it is notoriously difficult to eradicate. Three guidelines to control infection are offered in the knowledge that it is not always easy to put them into practice:

- Patients at a high risk of acquiring infection with *Ps. aeruginosa* (e.g. a patient being evaluated for organ transplantation) should not be admitted to a ward where cases of pseudomonas infection are present.
- Antimicrobial and other therapeutic substances and solutions must be free from *Ps. aeruginosa*. Particular danger exists when multidose ointments, creams or eye drops are used to treat several individuals over a period. Initially, the preparation may be sterile but contamination can easily occur between uses, and *Ps. aeruginosa* can multiply readily at a range of temperatures in many medicaments.
- In hospital units, episodes of cross-infection due to a single strain may occur as sporadic infections in individual patients over a period of months or years. For this reason, if facilities are available, it is advantageous to 'fingerprint' all clinically relevant isolates by a suitable typing system to identify epidemic strains.

BURKHOLDERIA PSEUDOMALLEI

B. pseudomallei is a free-living saprophyte that causes *melioidosis*, a devastating tropical infection of animals and humans that is endemic in eastern Asia and northern Australia. A related organism, *B. mallei*, causes *glanders*, a potentially fatal infectious disease of horses, mules or donkeys. Laboratory-acquired infection with either organism is a serious risk: both species are included in hazard group 3 together with the plague bacillus, *Yersinia pestis*, and must be handled with great care under strictly designated conditions.

B. pseudomallei is easily cultured and produces characteristic wrinkled colonies after several days of growth on nutrient agar; fresh cultures emit a characteristic pungent odour of putrefaction. The organism is oxidase-positive and motile but, unlike some other pseudomonads, does not produce diffusible pigments.

Melioidosis

B. pseudomallei is found in soil and surface water in rice paddies and monsoon drains; isolation rates are highest during the rainy season and in still rather than flowing water. Human infection is mainly acquired cutaneously through skin abrasions or by inhalation of contaminated particles. The clinical manifestations range from a subclinical infection, diagnosed by the presence of specific antibodies, to a benign pulmonary infection that may resemble tuberculosis or fulminating septicaemia with a mortality rate of 80–90%.

In north-eastern Thailand, *B. pseudomallei* is responsible for 20% of all community-acquired septicaemia. Virtually every organ can be affected, and hence melioidosis has been called the 'great imitator' of other infectious diseases. Melioidosis commonly presents as pyrexia and, in endemic areas, serological testing for *B. pseudomallei* is important in the evaluation of pyrexia of unknown origin. The organism can survive intracellularly within the reticulo-endothelial system, and this may account for latency and the emergence of symptoms many years after exposure. Suppurative parotitis is a characteristic presentation of melioidosis in children.

Early diagnosis and appropriate antibiotic therapy are key factors in the successful management of melioidosis. The organism may be observed, usually in very small numbers, as small, bipolar-stained Gram-negative bacilli in exudates, and may be cultured from sputum, urine, pus or blood on selective media. Enzyme-linked immunosorbent assay (ELISA) for detection of bacterial antigen, specific IgG and IgM antibody to *B. pseudomallei*, as well as an indirect haemagglutination test, are useful screening tests in subclinical melioidosis. Polymerase chain reaction (PCR) methods are also available.

Treatment

Intravenous ceftazidime is the treatment of choice for severe melioidosis. In some patients, imipenem has also been shown to be effective when treatment with ceftazidime has proved unsuccessful. Combinations of agents such as tetracycline and chloramphenicol have also been widely used, but prolonged treatment is necessary to avoid relapse. The ability of *B. pseudomallei* to survive and multiply in phagocytes may explain the difficulty of treating melioidosis with antibiotics that are effective against the organism in vitro, and the frequent recurrences seen when the duration of treatment is insufficient.

BURKHOLDERIA CEPACIA

B. cepacia was previously best known as the causative agent of soft rot of onions (*cepia*, Latin = onion). However, in the past two decades it has emerged as a human pathogen causing life-threatening respiratory infection in patients with chronic granulomatous disease or cystic fibrosis. Among the cystic fibrosis population and their carers, anxiety over *B. cepacia* is based on the innate multiresistance of the organism to antibiotics, its transmissibility by social contact and by the risk of *cepacia syndrome*, an acute, fatal necrotizing pneumonia, sometimes accompanied by bacteraemia, which occurs in approximately 20% of colonized patients.

B. cepacia isolates produce few classic virulence determinants; however, pro-inflammatory cytokines such as tumour necrosis factor are stimulated more by LPS from clinical and environmental isolates of *B. cepacia* than by *Ps. aeruginosa* LPS. Laboratory identification is aided by the use of selective media and by multitest identification systems such as API 20NE.

Isolates from human and environmental sources display considerable phenotypic and genomic heterogeneity. Molecular studies show that isolates presumptively identified as *B. cepacia* belong to at least six genomic species, which are referred to as the *B. cepacia* complex.

B. cepacia is probably the most nutritionally adaptable of all pseudomonads and provides a striking example of a soil saprophyte and phytopathogen that has emerged as an important threat to susceptible human hosts. Furthermore, in ironic contrast to its role as a human pathogen, the organism has been developed as a biopesticide for protecting crops against fungal diseases and as a bioremediation agent for breaking down recalcitrant herbicides and pesticides in contaminated soils. Some isolates demonstrate an unusual form of antibiotic resistance by an ability to use penicillin as a sole carbon and energy source.

In vitro, some strains are susceptible to ceftazidime, or the carbapenem, meropenem. However, infections may be particularly intractable. Strict infection control measures, including segregation, are necessary to limit the spread of highly transmissible strains.

GLUCOSE NON-FERMENTERS

The heterogeneous group of aerobic Gram-negative bacilli commonly referred to as *glucose non-fermenters* is taxonomically distinct from the carbohydrate-fermenting Enterobacteriaceae and the oxidative pseudomonads. Their clinical relevance is based on their role as opportunistic pathogens in hospital-acquired infections and their intrinsic resistance to many antimicrobial agents. They grow easily on common culture media, but unequivocal identification may be difficult as most species are relatively inert in the biochemical tests used in identification of Gram-negative bacteria.

Susceptibility to antibiotics of glucose non-fermenters is very variable, and treatment should be based on the results of laboratory tests.

- *Acinetobacter* species are saprophytes found in soil, water and sewage, and occasionally as commensals of moist areas of human skin. The organisms survive well in the hospital environment, and are increasing in importance as opportunist pathogens. Serious infections, including meningitis, pneumonia and septicaemia, are most commonly associated with *Acinetobacter baumannii*. Patients in intensive care units are at particular risk. Isolates are often inherently resistant to many antimicrobial agents, including β-lactam agents (other than carbapenems), aminoglycosides and quinolones.
- *Alcaligenes* and *Achromobacter* species are saprophytes found in moist environments, including those in hospital wards, and are associated with a range of hospital-acquired opportunistic infections, including septicaemia and ear discharges.
- *Eikenella corrodens* is a commensal of mucosal surfaces, which may cause a range of infections, in particular endocarditis, meningitis, pneumonia, and infections of wounds and various soft tissues.
- *Flavobacterium meningosepticum* is a saprophyte whose natural habitat is soil and moist environments, including nebulizers; it may cause opportunistic nosocomial infections, particularly in infants. As the name suggests, this species is associated with meningitis, and has been responsible for high mortality in epidemic outbreaks.

RECOMMENDED READING

Bergogne-Bérézin E, Towner K J 1996 *Acinetobacter* spp. as nosocomial pathogens: microbiological, clinical and epidemiological features. *Clinical Microbiology Reviews* 9: 148–165

Dance D A B 1996 Melioidosis. In: Cook G C ed. *Manson's Tropical Diseases*. WB Saunders pp 925–930

Denton M, Kerr K G 1998 Microbiological and clinical aspects of infection associated with *Stenotrophomonas maltophilia*. *Clinical Microbiology Reviews* 11: 57–80

Gilligan P H 1995 *Pseudomonas* and *Burkholderia*. In: Murray P R, Baron E J, Pfaller M A, Tenover F C, Yolken R H (eds) *Manual of Clinical Microbiology*. American Society for Microbiology, Washington, DC 509–519

Govan J R W, Hughes J, Vandamme P 1996 *Burkholderia cepacia*: medical taxonomic and ecological issues. *Journal of Medical Microbiology* 45: 395–407

LiPuma J J 1998 *Burkholderia cepacia*: management issues and new insights. *Chest Medicine* 19: 473–486

Stover C K, Pham X Q, Erwin S D et al. 2000 Complete genome sequence of *Pseudomonas aeruginosa* PAO1, an opportunistic pathogen. *Nature* 406: 959–964

Internet sites

www.pseudomonas.com
www.go.to/cepacia

29

Campylobacter and helicobacter

Enteritis; gastritis; peptic ulcer

M. B. Skirrow

Campylobacter and *Helicobacter* are members of a group of spirally shaped flagellate bacteria known as rRNA superfamily VI. Both genera contain bacteria of great medical importance. They are specially adapted to colonizing mucous membranes and are able to penetrate mucus with particular facility. In most industrialized countries *Campylobacter jejuni* is the most frequently identified cause of acute infective diarrhoea, and as a result it causes much morbidity and economic loss. The discovery of *Helicobacter pylori* in 1983 has been hailed as the most significant advance in gastroduodenal pathology of the 20th century. Infection of the stomach with this bacterium is essentially the cause of 'idiopathic' peptic ulceration and a significant risk factor for the development of gastric cancer.

CAMPYLOBACTER

Campylobacters were first isolated in 1906 from aborting sheep in the UK. Originally thought to be vibrios, they were later placed in their own genus with *C. fetus* as the type species. *C. fetus* is a major cause of abortion in sheep and cattle worldwide. The discovery that *C. jejuni* and *C. coli* commonly cause acute enteritis in man was not made until the late 1970s. The key to this discovery was the far-sighted application of veterinary microbiological methods to the culture of campylobacters from human faeces by Butzler in Belgium.

Several other species, such as *C. upsaliensis*, *C. lari* and the closely related bacterium *Arcobacter butzleri*, are less commonly associated with diarrhoea, mainly in children in developing countries. *C. fetus* is a rare cause of human fetal infection and abortion, and it occasionally causes bacteraemic infection in patients with immune deficiency. Several other species of campylobacter, notably *C. concisus* and *C. rectus*, are associated with peri-odontal disease.

CAMPYLOBACTER JEJUNI AND C. COLI

Description

C. jejuni and *C. coli* are small, spiral, Gram-negative rods with a single flagellum at one or both poles (Fig. 29.1), which endows the bacteria with exceptionally rapid motility. They are unusually sensitive to oxygen and superoxides, yet oxygen is essential for growth, so micro-aerophilic conditions must be provided for their cultivation. They grow best at 42–43°C. They do not form spores, but undergo coccal transformation under adverse conditions. They are inactive in many conventional biochemical tests, including metabolism of sugars (asaccharolytic), but they are strongly oxidase-positive. Campylobacters are fragile bacteria that are easily destroyed by heat and other physical and chemical agents.

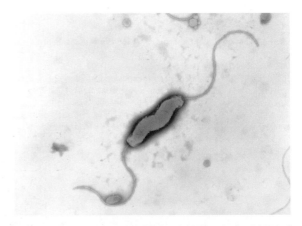

Fig. 29.1 Electron micrograph of *C. jejuni* showing single unsheathed bipolar flagella. X11 500. (Photomicrograph by Dr A. L. Curry and D. M. Jones, Manchester Public Health Laboratory.)

C. jejuni and *C. coli* are closely related, but *C. jejuni* hydrolyses hippurate – the only species of campylobacter to do so. *C. jejuni* accounts for 90–95% of campylobacter infections in most parts of the world.

Antigens and strain typing

C. jejuni and *C. coli* possess two classes of antigen: heat-stable lipopolysaccharide O antigens, and heat-labile surface and flagellar protein antigens. These form the basis of a serotyping system. Serotyping can be used in concert with biotyping or phage typing to give finer discrimination between strains. Genetic 'fingerprinting' methods are gaining favour for epidemiological studies.

Pathogenesis

Infection is acquired by ingestion. In volunteer studies, infection has been established with as few as 500–800 organisms. The jejunum and ileum are the first sites to become colonized, but the infection extends distally to affect the terminal ileum and usually the colon and rectum. The organisms are invasive. In well developed infections, mesenteric lymph nodes are enlarged, fleshy and inflamed, and there may be transient bacteraemia. Histological examination of the mucosa shows an acute neutrophil polymorphonuclear leucocyte response, oedema and sometimes superficial ulceration. These changes are indistinguishable from those seen in salmonella, shigella or yersinia infections.

Immune response

Specific humoral antibodies appear within 10 days of onset, peak in 2–4 weeks, and then rapidly decline. Most of the antibody is in the form of IgG, but healthy persons exposed to repeated infection show a progressive increase in IgA, which provides substantial immunity.

Clinical features

The typical features of campylobacter enteritis are shown in Fig. 29.2. The average incubation period is 3 days, with a range of 1–7 days. The illness may start with abdominal pain and diarrhoea, or there may be an influenza-like prodrome of fever and generalized aching, sometimes with rigors and sweating. Abdominal pain and diarrhoea are the main symptoms. Nausea is common, but vomiting is seldom pronounced. Severe watery diarrhoea may lead to prostration. Leucocytes are almost always present in the faeces, and frank blood may be apparent. Symptoms usually resolve within a few days, but excretion of bacteria may continue for several weeks. Prolonged carriage occurs only in patients with immunodeficiency. Campylobacter enteritis cannot be distinguished clinically from salmonella or shigella infection, but abdominal pain tends to be more severe in campylobacter infection. Indeed, a common reason for patients with campylobacter enteritis to be admitted to hospital is suspected acute appendicitis. Occasionally, illness starts with symptoms of colitis without preceding ileitis, which can make it difficult to distinguish from acute ulcerative colitis.

Complications

There are two conditions that may arise 1–2 weeks after the onset of illness. The first is reactive (aseptic) arthritis, which affects 1–2% of patients. It typically affects the ankles, knees and wrists, and though it may

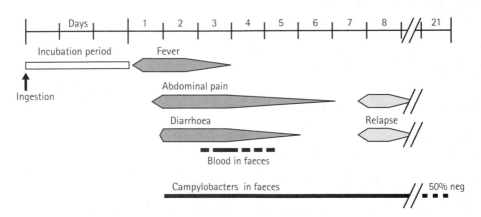

Fig. 29.2 Typical course of untreated campylobacter enteritis of average severity. There is considerable variation among individual patients.

be incapacitating, it is ultimately self-limiting. The second condition is Guillain–Barré syndrome, a form of peripheral polyneuropathy. This is much less frequent, but it may cause serious and potentially fatal paralysis lasting for several months. The problem is thought to be the production of antibodies to certain campylobacter epitopes that cross-react with the myelin in nerve sheaths, thereby producing demyelination.

Laboratory diagnosis

Faecal specimens should be refrigerated pending delivery to the laboratory. Specimens transported by post should be placed in an appropriate transport medium.

Microscopy

The motility and morphology of campylobacters are sufficiently characteristic for a rapid presumptive diagnosis to be made by direct microscopy of fresh faeces, either in wet preparations or stained smears. This is occasionally useful but is not done routinely.

Culture

Isolation of campylobacters from faeces requires some form of selective culture to inhibit competing faecal flora. Charcoal-based blood-free agar containing cefoperazone is widely used. Culture on non-selective media can be achieved by inoculating cellulose acetate membranes (pore size, 0.45–0.65 μm) laid on the surface of the agar; campylobacters are small enough to swim through the membrane, which is removed before incubation. This method has the advantage of detecting fastidious campylobacter species that are sensitive to the antimicrobial agents used in selective media.

Plates are incubated in closed jars with the oxygen tension lowered to 5–15% and carbon dioxide raised to 1–10%. Incubation at 42–43°C gives added selectivity against other faecal flora and more rapid growth of *C. jejuni* and *C. coli*, but it may exclude other species of campylobacter. Plates are incubated for 48 h. Colonies are typically flat and effuse, with a tendency to spread on moist agar.

Serology

Serology can be useful in patients presenting with aseptic arthritis or the Guillain–Barré syndrome after a bout of diarrhoea that was not investigated. Complement fixation test and enzyme-linked immunosorbent assay (ELISA) are group-specific tests that can detect recent infection with *C. jejuni* or *C. coli*.

Epidemiology

Incidence

Campylobacter enteritis is the commonest form of acute infective diarrhoea in most developed countries. In the UK, laboratory reports indicate an annual incidence of about 1 per 1000 of the population, but, as less than 10% of patients are tested, the true figure must be at least 1 per 100. The disease occurs in people of all ages. There is high morbidity in young adults, and an unexplained excess of male patients in this group (male:female ratio 1.7:1).

In developing countries, infection is hyperendemic, and children are repeatedly exposed to infection from an early age. By the time they are 2–3 years old, children have developed substantial immunity that lasts into adulthood. The maintenance of immunity probably depends on continuous exposure to infection.

Sources and transmission

Animals are the main sources of infection. *C. jejuni* and *C. coli* are found in a wide variety of animal hosts, particularly birds, an adaptation that is reflected in their high optimum growth temperature. *C. coli* is particularly associated with pigs. There is a constant shedding of the bacteria from wild birds and other animals into the surface water of lakes, rivers and streams, in which they can survive for many weeks at low temperatures. Farm animals are commonly infected from such sources. *C. jejuni* and *C. coli*, like *C. fetus*, can cause septic abortion in sheep and mild diarrhoea in young animals of several species. Cattle are commonly infected, and raw milk often becomes contaminated. The distribution of raw or inadequately pasteurized milk and untreated water has caused major outbreaks of campylobacter enteritis, some affecting several thousand people.

Poultry and raw meats. *C. jejuni* and *C. coli* colonize domestic poultry with particular ease. At least 60% of chickens sold in shops are contaminated with campylobacters, and broiler chickens are thought to account for about 50% of human infections in industrialized countries. Red meats are less often contaminated.

Properly cooked poultry and meats do not pose a risk; it is what happens to them before they are cooked that can create problems. Cross-contamination from these raw products to other foods, such as bread and salads, probably accounts for most infections. Unlike salmonellae, campylobacters do not multiply in foods, so explosive food poisoning outbreaks are rare. Most infections are sporadic or confined to one household.

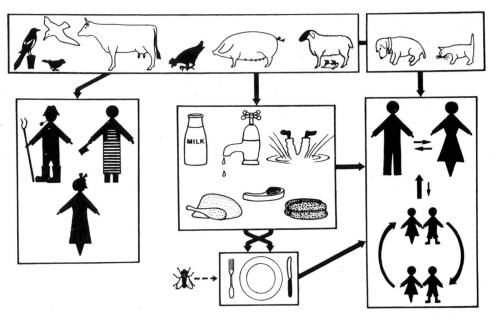

Fig. 29.3 Sources and transmission of *C. jejuni* and *C. coli*. Top boxes: animal reservoirs and sources of infection (the sheep has just given birth to a dead campylobacter-infected lamb). Left-hand box: transmission by direct occupational contact (farmer, butcher, poultry processor). Right-hand box: transmission by direct domestic contact (puppy or kitten with campylobacter diarrhoea; intrafamilial spread mainly from children). Central box: indirect transmission through consumption of untreated water, raw milk, raw or undercooked meat and poultry, food cross-contaminated from raw meats and poultry; possible transmission from flies. (From document VPH/CDD/FOS/84.1 by permission of the World Health Organization, which retains the copyright.)

Other routes of infection. Direct contact with infected animals or their products can also give rise to infection, as shown in Fig. 29.3, which summarizes the principal sources and routes of transmission of campylobacters to man. Spread of infection between humans is of relatively minor importance.

Treatment

Campylobacter enteritis is usually self-limiting and patients seldom require more than fluid and electrolyte replacement. Antimicrobial treatment should be reserved for patients with severe or complicated infections. *C. jejuni* and *C. coli* are moderately resistant to penicillins and most cephalosporins, although several other campylobacter species are sensitive. All species are usually sensitive to erythromycin, which is effective if given early in the disease. Ciprofloxacin and other fluoroquinolones are also effective, but resistance rates are rising.

Campylobacters are highly resistant to trimethoprim, but many strains are sensitive to metronidazole and other nitroimidazoles, an unusual property among bacteria that are not strict anaerobes.

Control

The wide distribution of campylobacters in nature precludes any possibility of reducing the reservoir of infection. Efforts must be directed to interrupting transmission. The purification of water and the heat treatment of milk are obvious and basic measures. The control of infection in broiler chickens merits high priority, but the means to achieve this are beset with difficulty. The terminal γ-irradiation of carcasses eliminates campylobacters and other pathogens, but public acceptability is a problem. Public education on basic hygiene in the handling of raw meats, especially poultry, needs to be strongly promoted.

HELICOBACTER

It is remarkable that *H. pylori*, which colonizes roughly one-half of the world's population, remained undiscovered until 1983. There are various reasons for this, but the turning point came with the introduction of fibre-optic endoscopy and with it the ability to perform biopsy of the gastric mucosa. The discovery was made by Warren and Marshall in Western Australia, and it revolutionized the treatment of duodenal and gastric ulcers; elimination of *H. pylori* produces a lasting cure.

Nearly 20 species are now recognized within the genus *Helicobacter*. Some colonize the stomachs of animals: the monkey, cat, dog, ferret and cheetah each harbour their own species. Others colonize the intestines of a wide range of animals. *H. cinaedi* and *H. fennelliae* are associated with proctitis in homosexual men.

'*H. heilmannii*', which is a larger more tightly spiralled bacterium possessing up to 12 sheathed polar flagella, is also found in the human stomach. It is much less common than *H. pylori*, but it is also associated with gastritis. It has not yet been cultured in vitro, so its name remains provisional. Morphologically indistinguishable organisms have been observed in the stomachs of dogs and cats.

HELICOBACTER PYLORI

Description

H. pylori is a Gram-negative spirally-shaped bacterium, 0.5–0.9 μm wide by 2–4 μm long. Like campylobacters, it is strictly micro-aerophilic and it requires carbon dioxide for growth, but it has a tuft of sheathed unipolar flagella, unlike the unsheathed flagella of campylobacters (Fig. 29.4; cf. Fig. 29.1). It is biochemically inactive in most conventional tests, but it produces an exceptionally powerful urease, almost 100 times more active than that of *Proteus vulgaris*, which is vital to its survival in the stomach (see below). *H. pylori* undergoes coccal transformation even more rapidly than *C. jejuni* when exposed to adverse conditions, and it is even more fragile, a point of importance when referring samples to a laboratory.

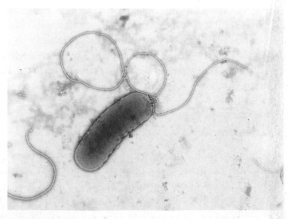

Fig. 29.4 *H. pylori* showing multiple sheathed unipolar flagella. X11 500. (Photomicrograph by Dr A. L. Curry and D. M. Jones, Manchester Public Health Laboratory.)

Antigens and strain typing

Although various antigens are expressed by *H. pylori*, serotyping is of limited practical value. However, its considerable genetic diversity can be exploited by molecular typing based on DNA analysis (see Chapter 3).

Pathogenesis

Site of infection

H. pylori is a highly adapted organism that lives only on gastric mucosa. Colonization ceases abruptly where gastric mucosa ends, e.g. in areas of intestinal metaplasia in the stomach. Conversely, areas of gastric metaplasia elsewhere in the gut, notably the duodenum, may become colonized with *H. pylori*, thus setting the scene for ulceration.

The gastric antrum is the most favoured site, but other parts of the stomach may be colonized, especially in patients taking an acid-lowering drug such as an H_2 antagonist or proton pump inhibitor. The bacteria are present in the mucus overlying the mucosa. Although gastric acid is potentially destructive to *H. pylori*, protection is provided by its powerful urease, which acts on the urea passing through the gastric mucosa to generate ammonia, which neutralizes acid around the bacteria. Colonization often extends into gastric glands, but the mucosa is not invaded by the bacteria (Fig. 29.5). Where they are numerous, the underlying mucosa usually shows a superficial gastritis of the type known as chronic active or type B gastritis (not to be confused with type A atrophic auto-immune gastritis of pernicious anaemia). This is characterized by infiltration with chronic inflammatory cells and polymorphonuclear leucocytes. Mucus-secreting foveolar cells often show damage where the bacteria are numerous.

The course of infection

After an incubation period of a few days, patients suffer a mild attack of acute achlorhydric gastritis with symptoms of abdominal pain, nausea, flatulence and bad breath. Symptoms last for about 2 weeks, but hypochlorhydria may persist for up to a year. Despite a substantial humoral antibody response, infection and chronic gastritis persist indefinitely, but after several decades there may be a progression to atrophic gastritis. Conditions are then inhospitable for *H. pylori*, which disappears or is much reduced in number.

Associated disease

Despite the presence of chronic active gastritis, most infections are symptomless, and endoscopic appearances

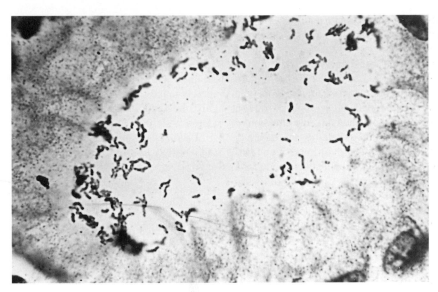

Fig. 29.5 Section of gastric mucosa showing colonization with *H. pylori*. X1400. Warthin–Starry silver stain. (Photomicrograph by Mr G. H. Green, Worcester Royal Infirmary.)

of the stomach are normal. However, a few infected persons develop peptic ulceration. Some cases of non-ulcer dyspepsia are probably caused by *H. pylori*, but there is currently no way of identifying such patients. More importantly, the atrophic gastritis that is the result of longstanding infection is associated with an increased risk of developing gastric cancer. Moreover, a condition known as gastric mucosa-associated lymphoid tissue (MALT) lymphoma is strongly associated with *H. pylori* infection, and complete regression has been observed after elimination of the bacteria.

H. pylori infection has been statistically associated with several conditions outside the digestive tract. Among them are coronary heart disease, iron deficiency anaemia and cot death. Although these are of great potential importance, the links remain unproven because of possible confounding factors.

Peptic ulceration

H. pylori is actively involved in the pathogenesis of what was once regarded as idiopathic peptic ulceration (ulceration not related to non-steroidal anti-inflammatory agents or the Zollinger–Ellison syndrome). Clearly other factors are involved, but the role of *H. pylori* is crucial: infection is virtually a prerequisite for ulceration, and elimination of infection allows healing of ulcers without recurrence, in contrast to short-term treatment with agents that merely suppress gastric acidity. Any recurrence of ulceration is almost always associated with recrudescence of infection.

There are several ways in which *H. pylori* infection might damage the mucosa. One is by the production of virulence factors produced by some *H. pylori* strains, among which are a vacuolating toxin (VacA) and a cyto-toxin-associated gene protein (CagA). The genes controlling the production of VacA and CagA, together with over 40 other genes, are located on a large region of DNA called the *cag* pathogenicity island. Strains possessing this DNA island are more likely to give rise to severe gastritis, peptic ulceration, and gastric cancer than strains without it. The *cagA* gene is a marker for this island, so its detection can help in assessing infected patients. However, bacterial factors are only part of the picture; host factors strongly influence the outcome of infection.

Laboratory diagnosis

Definitive tests for *H. pylori* infection depend on finding the organism in specimens of gastric mucosa obtained by biopsy. In practice, non-invasive tests are used for initial screening.

Non-invasive tests

Serology. Serological tests, mostly based on the ELISA principle, detect antibodies to *H. pylori* or its products and are used routinely to screen patients with dyspepsia. However, they are less useful for screening children and they are unreliable for excluding infection in elderly patients, or as a test for cure in patients who have received treatment (owing to variable persistence of antibody). Rapid bedside tests that use drops of whole blood rather than serum are widely marketed but their accuracy is poor.

Urea breath test. This test detects bacterial urease activity in the stomach by measuring the output of CO_2 resulting from the splitting of urea into CO_2 and ammonia. A capsule of urea labelled with an isotope of carbon (carbon-14 or -13) is fed to the patient, and the emission of the isotope in CO_2 subsequently exhaled in the breath is measured. Patients infected with *H. pylori* give high readings of the isotope. The test has excellent sensitivity and specificity, but there are drawbacks. Carbon-14 is radioactive, albeit weakly, so it is not used in children. Carbon-13 is not radio-active, but a mass spectrometer is needed for its assay, which means that samples must be sent to a specialist laboratory with its attendant costs.

Faecal antigen test. This is a promising new test in which polyclonal antibodies are used to detect *H. pylori* antigens in faeces. It has the potential to supplant serology as a routine screening test.

Polymerase chain reaction (PCR). Various DNA probes have been developed for the direct detection of *H. pylori* by PCR in gastric juice, faeces, dental plaque and water supplies. Some of them have the advantage that they can detect genes expressing antimicrobial resistance and possession of the *cagA* pathogenicity island. Their main drawback is that they are complex to perform and require stringent conditions, so they are unsuitable for general use.

Invasive tests

Collection of specimens. Ideally, patients for endoscopy should not have received antibiotics or proton pump inhibitors for a month before the test. Mucosal biopsy specimens are taken from the gastric antrum within 5 cm of the pylorus, and preferably also from the body of the stomach. For maximum sensitivity, duplicate specimens are taken: one lot for histopathology (placed in fixative); the other lot for culture (placed in the neck of plain bottles made humid by adding a tiny amount of normal saline). Specimens for culture must be processed as soon as possible, certainly on the same day, or else placed in transport medium.

Biopsy urease test. In centres without laboratory facilities, the biopsy urease test is a simple and cheap alternative that can be performed at the bedside. *H. pylori* produces such abundant urease that its action can be detected directly in biopsy specimens. A specimen is placed into a small quantity of urea solution with an indicator that detects alkalinity resulting from the formation of ammonia by urease. Most infected patients (70%) give a positive result within 2 h, 90% after 24 h. Test kits are marketed commercially.

Histopathology and microscopy. Histopathology has the advantage that it provides a permanent record of the nature and grading of a patient's gastritis as well as detecting *H. pylori*. Organisms can be seen in sections stained with haematoxylin and eosin, but more specific stains make the task easier (Fig. 29.5). The bacteria can also be seen in smears of biopsy material stained by Gram's stain.

Culture. Although culture is no more sensitive than the skilled microscopy of histological sections, it has two advantages:

- strains can be tested for antimicrobial resistance
- strains can be typed for epidemiological studies.

Selective agars similar to those used for campylobacters are used for primary isolation. Sensitivity is increased if a non-selective medium is used in parallel. Plates are incubated at 37°C in the same sort of atmosphere as is used for campylobacters. High humidity is essential. Plates are left undisturbed for 3 days and incubated for a week before being discarded as negative. *H. pylori* forms discrete domed colonies, unlike the effuse colonies of *C. jejuni* and *C. coli*.

Epidemiology

Man appears to be the sole reservoir and source of *H. pylori*. How infection is transmitted is unknown, but it is presumed to be by the oral–oral or, possibly, faecal–oral route. Small numbers of *H. pylori* have been detected in dental plaque, saliva and faeces.

Infection rates are strongly related to poor living conditions and overcrowding during childhood. Cross-sectional surveys show that there is a steady rise in seropositivity with increasing age (about 50% infected by the age of 60 years in industrialized countries), but this may simply mean that older people spent their childhood under poorer conditions than younger people (cohort effect) rather than a steady acquisition during life. In developing countries most children become infected by the time they reach puberty. These high rates of infection broadly correlate with high rates of gastric cancer.

Inmates of psychiatric units and orphanages and professional staff carrying out endoscopy examinations show higher than average rates. Nosocomial infection from inadequately disinfected endoscopes has also occurred.

Treatment

The presence of *H. pylori* infection does not necessarily mean that attempts should be made to eliminate it. Two unequivocal indications for treatment are:

- peptic ulcer disease
- gastric MALT lymphoma.

  Possible indications are:

- patients with non-ulcer dyspepsia refractory to conventional treatment
- patients with a family history of gastric carcinoma.

H. pylori is sensitive to most β-lactam antibiotics, macrolides, tetracyclines and nitroimidazoles, but resistant to trimethoprim. It is also sensitive to bismuth compounds (subcitrate, subsalicylate) and partially sensitive to the acid-lowering proton pump inhibitors omeprazole and lansoprazole.

To eradicate *H. pylori* infection, at least two antimicrobial agents must be given in combination with an acid-lowering agent. The reduction of acidity not only enhances antimicrobial action, but it makes the patient feel better and thereby improves compliance. A popular regimen is a 1-week course of the macrolide clarithromycin, plus amoxicillin (or metronidazole) and omeprazole (or lansoprazole). These regimens eliminate *H. pylori* in about 90% of patients. A recrudescence of infection demands a repeat biopsy with culture and sensitivity testing of the infecting strain. High rates of resistance to metronidazole are evident among strains in some regions and resistance to clarithromycin is beginning to appear.

Control

Social deprivation is the dominant factor governing the prevalence of *H. pylori* infection. In western society, social advancement has brought about a reduction of infection, and peptic ulcer disease is on the decline. However, this is far from the case in developing countries, where a cheap and effective vaccine would be valuable, particularly for the prevention of gastric cancer.

RECOMMENDED READING

Altekruse S F, Stern N J, Fields P I, Swerdlow D L 1999 *Campylobacter jejuni* – an emerging foodborne pathogen. *Emerging Infectious Diseases* 5:28–35

Bateson M C 2000 *Helicobacter pylori*. *Postgraduate Medical Journal* 76:141–144

Danesh J, Pounder R E 2000 Eradication of *Helicobacter pylori* and non-ulcer dyspepsia. *Lancet* 355:766–767

McNulty C A M, Wyatt J I 1999 *Helicobacter pylori*. Best Practice No 154. *Journal of Clinical Pathology* 52:338–344

Skirrow M B, Blaser M J 2002 *Campylobacter jejuni*. In: Blaser M J, Smith P D, Ravdin J I et al (eds) *Infections of the Gastrointestinal Tract*, 2nd edn. Raven Press, New York

Stone M A 1999 Transmission of *Helicobacter pylori*. *Postgraduate Medical Journal* 75:198–200

Other resources

Price A, Malfertheiner, Michetti P 1997 *Helicobacter pylori* slide set. Science Press, London

Internet site

Public Health Laboratory Service: www.phls.co.uk

30

Vibrio, mobiluncus, gardnerella and spirillum

Cholera; vaginosis; rat bite fever

H. Chart

VIBRIO

The genus *Vibrio* is the most extensively characterized and medically important group within the family *Vibrionaceae*. The genus includes more than 30 species that are commonly found in aquatic environments. Some cause disease in man as well as in marine vertebrates and invertebrates. The most important pathogens of man are *Vibrio cholerae*, *V. parahaemolyticus* and *V. vulnificus*, but various other species are occasionally implicated as opportunistic pathogens. In the past the importance of vibrios has been associated almost exclusively with the epidemic and pandemic cholera caused by a particular antigenic form of *V. cholerae*.

Until recently it was thought that man was the only natural host of *V. cholerae* and that all infections resulted from direct or indirect contact with human faeces. It is now recognized that *V. cholerae*, like other vibrios, is commonly found as a natural resident of aquatic environments in areas free of cholera, and that its presence is not necessarily associated with faecal contamination. The concept that this organism has only limited potential for survival outside the human intestine has been radically revised.

DESCRIPTION

Vibrios are short, Gram-negative rods, which are often curved and actively motile by a single polar flagellum. Nearly all produce the enzyme oxidase and indole. The genus can be divided into non-halophilic vibrios, including *V. cholerae* and other species that are able to grow in media without added salt, and halophilic species that do not grow in these media (Table 30.1). They grow readily on ordinary media provided that their requirements for electrolytes are met, and grow best when abundant oxygen is present. Most vibrios grow at 30°C but some of the halophilic species grow poorly at 37°C, whereas *V. cholerae*, *V. parahaemolyticus* and *V. alginolyticus* grow at 42°C.

Vibrios are tolerant to alkali but have a low tolerance to acid. Growth is rapid in the pH range 7.4–9.6 while the limits for growth are approximately pH 6.8 and 10.2.

VIBRIO CHOLERAE

Description

The somatic (O) antigen structure is of fundamental importance in the identification of this organism. More than 130 different O serogroups have been described; the causative organism of epidemic cholera (the so-called *cholera vibrio*) is defined by its possession of the O1 antigen, and is known as *V. cholerae* O1. Strains of other serogroups are collectively known as *non-O1 V. cholerae* and correspond to strains known in the past as *non-agglutinable vibrios* or *non-cholera vibrios*. Some of these strains can cause diarrhoea in man. All strains of *V. cholerae* share the same flagellar (H) antigen.

Table 30.1 Salt tolerance of important pathogenic *Vibrio* species				
Salt concentration (%)	*V. cholerae*	*V. parahaemolyticus*	*V. vulnificus*	*V. alginolyticus*
0	+	–	–	–
3	+	+	+	+
6	–	+	+(–)	+
10	–	–	–	+
+, growth; – no growth.				

Strains of *V. cholerae* O1 may be further subdivided on the basis of their O antigens into the subtypes *Inaba* and *Ogawa*. Some strains possess determinants of both of these subtypes and are known as subtype *Hikojima*.

There are two biotypes of *V. cholerae* O1: the *classical* and *El Tor* biotypes. The El Tor variant is distinguished from the classical biotype by the ability to express a haemolysin, and resistance to polymyxin B. The two biotypes can also be recognized by their differential susceptibility to specific phages.

Pathogenesis

Clinical manifestations

Cholera is characterized by the sudden onset of effortless vomiting and profuse watery diarrhoea. Although vomiting is a common feature, the rapid dehydration and hypovolaemic shock, which may cause death in 12–24 h, are related mainly to the profuse, watery, colourless stools with flecks of mucus and a distinctive fishy odour – *rice water stools* – which contain little protein and are very different from the mucopurulent blood-stained stools of bacillary dysentery. Anuria develops, muscle cramps occur and the patient quickly becomes weak and lethargic with loss of skin turgor, low blood pressure and absent or thready pulse. There are, however, all grades of severity, and milder cases cannot be distinguished clinically from other secretory diarrhoeas. Symptomless infections are common.

Pathogenic mechanisms

The sequence of events leading to cholera is confined to the gut. The cholera vibrios are ingested in drink or food and, in natural infections, the dose must often be small. After passing the acid barrier of the stomach the organisms begin to multiply in the alkaline environment of the small intestine.

Once in the small intestine, strains of *V. cholerae* O1 migrate towards epithelial cells, facilitated by active motility and the production of mucinase and other proteolytic enzymes. Once the organism penetrates the mucus layer it adheres to the enterocyte surface. Strains of *V. cholerae* may express a range of haemagglutinins, and lipopolysaccharide has also been implicated in adhesion. Fimbrial expression is co-regulated with the synthesis of cholera toxin.

Adherent bacteria produce a potent enterotoxin known as *cholera toxin*. The toxin consists of five B subunits (molecular weight, 11 600) and a single A subunit (molecular weight, 27 200), and has structural, functional and antigenic similarity to heat-labile toxin expressed by strains of enterotoxigenic *Escherichia coli* (ETEC, p. 268). The A subunit is made up of two peptides (A_1 and A_2) linked by a single disulphide bridge. The B subunit binds to sugar residues of ganglioside GM_1 on the cells lining the villi and crypts of the small intestine. It is thought that insertion of the B subunit into the host cell membrane forms a hydrophilic transmembrane channel through which the toxic A subunit can pass into the cytoplasm. Reduction of the disulphide bond releases the A_1 portion of the molecule, which has enterotoxic activity. The cholera enterotoxin causes the transfer of adenosine diphosphoribose (ADP ribose) from nicotinamide adenine dinucleotide (NAD) to a regulatory protein, which is part of the adenylate cyclase enzyme responsible for the generation of intracellular cyclic adenosine monophosphate (cAMP). The result is irreversible activation of adenylate cyclase and overproduction of cAMP. This in turn causes inhibition of uptake of Na^+ and Cl^- ions by cells lining the villi, together with hypersecretion of Cl^- and HCO_3^- ions. This blocks the uptake of water which normally accompanies Na^+ and Cl^- absorption, and there is a passive net outflow of water across mucosal cells, leading to serious loss of water and electrolytes.

Some strains of *V. cholerae* O1 that cause diarrhoea do not produce cholera toxin. The toxin responsible differs in antigenic nature, receptor site, mode of action and genetic homology from cholera toxin.

Non-O1 V. cholerae

Non-O1 strains of *V. cholerae* cause mild, sometimes bloody diarrhoea, often accompanied by abdominal cramps. Symptoms may occasionally be severe, in which case the disease resembles cholera. Wound infections may occur in patients exposed to aquatic environments, and bacteraemia and meningitis have been reported.

Non-O1 *V. cholerae* strains may elaborate a wide range of virulence factors, including enterotoxins, cytotoxins, haemolysins and colonizing factors. A few strains produce cholera toxin.

Laboratory diagnosis

Stool specimens are inoculated into alkaline peptone water, in which vibrios grow rapidly and accumulate on the surface. After incubation for 3–6 h a loopful from the surface is inoculated on a suitable solid medium such as thiosulphate–citrate–bile salts–sucrose (TCBS agar). On this medium *V. cholerae* strains appear as yellow sucrose-fermenting colonies, which may be tested for the enzyme oxidase and for agglutination with rabbit antibodies specific for the O1 lipopolysaccharide antigens prior to biochemical confirmation.

Cholera toxin is detected by the same tissue culture assays and immunological techniques described for *Esch. coli* heat-labile toxin (p. 270).

Epidemiology

V. cholerae O1

A series of six pandemics of cholera, originating in the Bengal basin, ravaged the world in the 19th and early 20th centuries. Subsequently, cholera was increasingly contained within the endemic foci and surrounding areas of India and Bangladesh until 1961, when a seventh pandemic due to the El Tor biotype of *V. cholerae* O1 spread from Indonesia to the Far East and then swept back through much of southern Asia. Early in the 1970s the pandemic invaded Africa, and in 1991 it reached South America, where the first epidemic in that subcontinent of the 20th century occurred in Peru. By December 1993 more than 820 000 cases of cholera, with almost 7000 deaths, had occurred, and the epidemic had involved all Latin American countries except Uruguay. In the following year the epidemic abated somewhat, with a 46% reduction on the numbers reported in 1993, and the number of cases in the western

hemisphere continues to fall. The progress of the seventh pandemic of cholera from 1959–1994 is shown in Fig. 30.1. The vast majority of cases of cholera now occur in Africa and Asia, where the downward trend seen since 1992 has not been maintained.

The El Tor biotype, originally isolated from pilgrims at the quarantine station known as El Tor, and at first thought to be of doubtful pathogenicity, supplanted the classical biotype in India during the 1960s and spread into Indian states previously free from infection. By 1973 the classical biotype in Bangladesh was also entirely displaced by the El Tor biotype, and it remained in obscurity until October 1979 when five cases were reported. During the 1980s the classical biotype once again replaced the El Tor biotype as the epidemic strain in Bangladesh, but it does not seem to have spread to other countries.

Infection is generally spread by contaminated water or foods such as uncooked seafood or vegetables. The source of the contamination is usually the faeces of carriers or patients with cholera, but contamination can probably sometimes occur from natural aquatic reservoirs. Cholera is characteristically an infection of crowded communities with poor standards of hygiene, often in low-lying areas. Infection tends to persist in

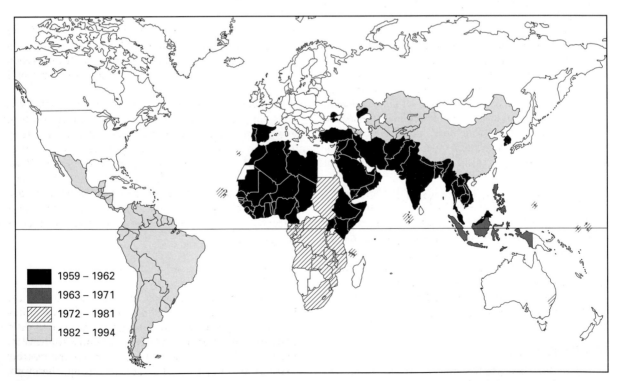

Fig. 30.1 Areas reporting indigenous cholera to the WHO 1959–1994. (After WHO 1991 *Communicable Disease Report* 1: R48–R49 and WHO 1995 *Weekly Epidemiological Record* 70: 202.)

communities with shared communal water supplies such as tanks, ponds, canals or rivers used for bathing, washing and for household use. Outbreaks occur either as explosive epidemics, usually in non-endemic areas, or as protracted epidemic waves in endemic areas. The seasonal incidence is fairly consistent in different endemic regions but the climatic conditions during epidemic waves may be distinctive for each region. For example, in Bangladesh the cholera season (November to February) follows the monsoon rains and ends with the onset of the hot dry months. In Calcutta the main epidemic wave (May to July) rises to its peak in the hot dry season and ends with the onset of the monsoon but extends inland to neighbouring states during the rainy season.

Spread of infection is facilitated by the high ratio of symptomless carriers to clinical cases, which varies from 10:1 to 100:1 depending on living conditions and biotype. Symptomless carriers occur much more frequently in El Tor than in classical infections.

Vibrio cholerae O139

In 1992 cases of cholera indistinguishable from that caused by *V. cholerae* O1 were reported in Madras, India. By mid-January 1993 similar isolates were found in neighbouring Bangladesh, and these rapidly spread north, following the course of the major rivers and raising fears of a new pandemic.

The new strain did not agglutinate with antisera to any of the O serogroups and was assigned to a new serogroup, O139 Bengal. However, it closely resembles *V. cholerae* O1 El Tor biochemically and physiologically, and it may eventually attain the status of a subtype (*Bengal*) of that organism alongside the subtypes *Inaba* and *Ogawa* already recognized. *V. cholerae* O139 may have evolved from *V. cholerae* O1, but with modified lipopolysaccharide structure.

Other non-O1 V. cholerae serogroups

Strains belonging to serogroups other than O1 occur widely in aquatic environments, and many infections are associated with exposure to saline environments or consumption of seafood. They appear to survive and multiply better than *V. cholerae* O1 in a wide range of foods, and it is likely that food-borne outbreaks occur as with other more common enteric pathogens.

Treatment

In cholera absolute priority must be given to the life-saving replacement of fluid and electrolytes. Oral rehydration therapy is often sufficient, but severe cases may

Table 30.2 Formulation of oral rehydration solution recommended by the WHO[a]	
Sodium chloride	3.5 g
Potassium chloride	1.5 g
Sodium citrate	2.9 g
Glucose (anhydrous)	20.0 g

[a] To be dissolved in 1 litre of clean drinking water.

require intravenous rehydration. The World Health Organization (WHO) is promoting the use of oral rehydration therapy in all cases of severe diarrhoea, including that due to *V. cholerae*. The recommended formula is shown in Table 30.2.

Tetracycline, chloramphenicol and co-trimoxazole reduce the period of excretion of *V. cholerae* in the stools of cholera patients. Tetracycline is often given to reduce environmental contamination and to reduce the risk of cross-infection. Tetracycline-resistant strains of *V. cholerae* O1 El Tor began to appear in the 1970s and were soon followed by the appearance of strains resistant to a wide range of antimicrobial agents, including penicillins, streptomycin, chloramphenicol and trimethoprim.

Control

Public health measures used in the control of any disease spread by faecal contamination are of value in the control of cholera. Most important are the provision of safe drinking water supplies and the proper disposal of human faeces.

Knowledge about cholera prevention and control has improved substantially, but the disease still causes fear, especially among travellers to affected areas. They should be reassured; although cholera can be life-threatening it is easily prevented and treated. In 1994, 29 countries that were not affected by endemic cholera reported a total of 283 imported cases, with no deaths. In the context of the millions of people on the move around the world each year this number of cases is insignificant.

Vaccines

The immune response to cholera is directed against the bacterium rather than the toxin. It is specific for a given serotype. Infection with the classical biotype is followed by almost complete immunity for several years, but infection with the El Tor biotype confers little or no immunity. It is not surprising, therefore, that the development of effective vaccines has proved difficult.

Traditional whole-cell vaccines are not very effective and are no longer recommended for travellers. Oral vaccines that combine purified B subunit and killed whole cells are licensed in some countries and appear to be safe and protective. The use of attenuated strains of *Salmonella* bacteria to deliver *V. cholerae* antigens, such as toxin co-regulated pilus proteins, might further improve efficacy.

VIBRIO PARAHAEMOLYTICUS

Description

V. parahaemolyticus was first isolated in 1950 from post-mortem specimens of patients who died during an outbreak of food poisoning due to semi-dried sardines in Japan. It is a halophilic vibrio and will not grow in the absence of sodium chloride (Table 30.1). This property is conveniently demonstrated by inoculating the organism onto cystine-lactose-electrolyte-deficient (CLED) agar, which supports the growth of non-halophilic vibrios but not halophilic species. Strains of *V. parahaemolyticus* from clinical specimens generally form green, non-sucrose-fermenting colonies on TCBS agar, but sucrose-fermenting strains are found in estuarine and coastal waters.

Strains associated with gastro-enteritis usually cause haemolysis of human red cells in Wagatsuma's agar, a special medium containing mannitol. This haemolysis is known as the *Kanagawa phenomenon*.

Pathogenesis

V. parahaemolyticus can cause explosive diarrhoea, but symptoms usually abate after 3 days. Other symptoms include abdominal pain, nausea and vomiting, and there may be blood in the stools. A few extra-intestinal infections have been reported, particularly from wounds.

Kanagawa-positive strains produce a heat-stable cytotoxin and cause diarrhoea in volunteers. In contrast, volunteers have ingested 10^{10} cells of Kanagawa-negative strains without ill effects. Kanagawa-positive strains also adhere to human intestinal cells while Kanagawa-negative strains do not. A heat-labile enterotoxin can be separated from the heat-stable haemolysin and causes morphological changes in tissue culture cells resembling those caused by cholera toxin and the heat-labile enterotoxin of *Esch. coli*.

Most strains from seafood and the environment are Kanagawa-negative although positive colonies can usually be found if a sufficient number are tested. It is likely that a few Kanagawa-positive strains multiply selectively in the human intestine as infection develops and predominate in the stools of patients with diarrhoea.

Laboratory diagnosis

The faeces of patients with a history of recent consumption of seafood may be examined by the methods used for *V. cholerae*. In the examination of seafood and sea or estuarine waters for halophilic species, including *V. parahaemolyticus*, enrichment culture in alkaline peptone water containing 1% sodium chloride is used.

Epidemiology

V. parahaemolyticus is a common cause of diarrhoea in Japan and South-east Asia. It also causes illness associated with seafood in many other countries, including the USA and the UK. The organisms are common in fish and shellfish and in the waters from which they are harvested. Infections occur more frequently in the warmer months when the organisms are most prevalent in the aquatic environment. There is a particular risk associated with the consumption of raw seafood prepared and eaten in Japanese-style restaurants.

Extra-intestinal infections are always associated with exposure to the aquatic environment or handling of contaminated seafood.

Treatment and control

Patients with diarrhoea generally require only fluid replacement therapy. Infection can be avoided by normal food hygiene procedures and by refrigeration of seafood to reduce the possibility of multiplication of *V. parahaemolyticus*.

VIBRIO VULNIFICUS

This halophilic species was first recognized formally in a study in 1976 of a number of halophilic organisms differing from known species.

Pathogenesis

There are three distinct clinical syndromes:

- Rapid onset of fulminating septicaemia followed by the appearance of cutaneous lesions. More than 50% of those with primary septicaemia die. The condition is invariably associated with the consumption of raw shellfish. It is thought that the organisms enter the bloodstream by way of the portal vein or the intestinal lymph system. Elderly males with liver function defects due to alcohol abuse are particularly susceptible, but any deficiency in the immune system may also be a contributing factor.

- A rapidly progressing cellulitis following contamination of a wound sustained during exposure to salt water. Infections of this kind occur in otherwise healthy persons as well as in the debilitated, and are characterized by wound oedema, erythema and necrosis which only occasionally progresses to septicaemia. The infection can be rapidly fatal.
- Acute diarrhoea following the consumption of shellfish. This is less common; victims generally have mildly debilitating underlying conditions. Mortality is rare.

Pathogenicity is associated with the presence of a polysaccharide capsule that probably contributes to the ability to resist phagocytosis and the killing effects of human serum. Strains of *V. vulnificus* lack high-affinity iron uptake systems and are unable to obtain ferric ions bound to human transferrin. Patients with iron overload disorders such as haemochromatosis are highly susceptible; high levels of free serum iron are thought to facilitate the rapid septicaemia observed in patients infected with this organism.

Several toxins may contribute to tissue damage. They include a collagenase and cytolytic and proteolytic substances. A vascular permeability factor has also been described.

Epidemiology

Infections occur most frequently in areas where the water temperature remains high throughout the year, such as the mid-Atlantic and Gulf coast states of the USA. They are much more common during the warmer months of the year when *V. vulnificus* is most abundant. Wound infections are associated with injuries sustained in the aquatic environment while septicaemic infections are associated with the consumption of raw shellfish.

VIBRIO ALGINOLYTICUS

Description

Vibrio alginolyticus is a halophilic organism formerly regarded as biotype 2 of *V. parahaemolyticus*. It fails to grow on CLED agar but grows in the presence of 10% sodium chloride. It forms large, yellow (sucrose-fermenting) colonies on TCBS. There is pronounced swarming on non-selective solid media.

Pathogenesis

It occasionally causes opportunistic self-limiting infections of wounds. Clinical features include mild cellulitis and a seropurulent exudate. The pathogenic mechanism is unknown.

Epidemiology

This organism is widely distributed in sea water and seafood and is probably the most common vibrio found in these sources in the UK. It occurs in large numbers throughout the year. Infections are invariably associated with exposure to sea water.

OTHER VIBRIOS

- *Vibrio damsela* is a halophilic, aerogenic marine vibrio found in tropical and semi-tropical aquatic environments. It is associated with severe infections of wounds acquired in warm coastal areas.
- *Vibrio fluvialis* (previously known as group F vibrios, one biotype of which is now regarded as a separate species, *V. furnissii*) is easily confused with *Aeromonas hydrophila* because of a superficial phenotypic similarity. Patients experience diarrhoea, abdominal pain, fever and dehydration. Strains of *V. fluvialis* can be isolated in low numbers from fish and shellfish, and from sea water in areas where this is warm. It seems likely that infection is from contaminated seafood.
- *Vibrio hollisae* has been associated with bacteraemia and diarrhoea, especially in areas of the USA where the sea water is warm, such as the Gulf of Mexico. Infections are strongly associated with the consumption of raw seafood. Strains of *V. hollisae* exhibit gene sequences homologous with those encoding the thermostable haemolysin of *V. parahaemolyticus*.
- *Vibrio mimicus* occurs in similar environments to *V. cholerae*. Most isolates are from the stools of patients who develop gastro-enteritis after consumption of raw oysters, although a few ear infections have also been reported.

Other aquatic organisms that are probably related to vibrios include *Aeromonas* spp. and *Plesiomonas shigelloides*. *Aeromonas* spp., notably *A. hydrophila*, have been debatably implicated in diarrhoea and occasionally cause more serious infection in compromised individuals. *A. salmonicida* is an economically important pathogen of fish. *P. shigelloides* is an organism of uncertain taxonomic status that sometimes causes water-borne outbreaks of diarrhoea in warm countries.

MOBILUNCUS AND GARDNERELLA

The name *Mobiluncus* was first proposed for a group of curved, motile, Gram-variable, anaerobic bacteria isolated from the vagina of women with bacterial vaginosis. Although the genus was first placed tentatively in the family Bacteroidaceae its taxonomic position is uncertain. Studies of 16S RNA suggest that the genus *Mobiluncus* belongs to the order Actinomycetales, in which it is most closely related to the genus *Actinomyces*.

Gardnerella vaginalis (formerly *Corynebacterium vaginale* or *Haemophilus vaginalis*) is often found in association with *Mobiluncus* spp. in bacterial vaginosis and, for convenience, is included here.

DESCRIPTION

There are two species of *Mobiluncus*: *M. curtisii* and *M. mulieris*. The former is short (mean length 1.5 μm) and Gram-variable while the latter is long (mean length 3.0 μm) and Gram-negative. Both species have multiple flagella originating from the concave aspect of the cells. Cell wall studies show that there is no outer membrane and, although the cell wall is thinner than that of most Gram-positive organisms, it is generally considered that both species are Gram-positive. Two subspecies have been proposed for *M. curtisii*, ssp. *curtisii* and *holmesii*.

G. vaginalis is a micro-aerophilic, pleomorphic, Gram-variable rod of uncertain taxonomic status.

BACTERIAL VAGINOSIS

The clinical condition described as non-specific vaginitis or bacterial vaginosis is characterized by the presence of a thin, homogeneous vaginal discharge with a characteristic 'rotten fish' smell. This becomes more pronounced on alkalization, and can be evoked by placing a drop of potassium hydroxide solution on the fresh exudate on a slide or the speculum used for the vaginal examination. In addition, *clue cells* (epithelial cells covered with bacteria) can be seen in fresh unstained smears, and the vaginal pH is raised above 4.5. The characteristic smell is ascribed to amines produced by one or more of the bacterial species that form the complex microbial flora of the vagina.

Bacterial vaginosis appears to be a polymicrobial infection, with certain organisms playing a key role, especially when they overgrow the lactobacilli of the normal flora. *Mobiluncus* spp. are isolated from less than 50% of women with bacterial vaginosis, but this almost certainly underestimates the prevalence of these fastidious and slow-growing organisms. By use of DNA probes, *Mobiluncus* spp. have been found in the vaginal secretions of over 80% of women with vaginosis, but rarely in women without vaginosis. *Mobiluncus* are frequently found in association with *G. vaginalis* and with other organisms that may also be of aetiological importance. It appears that both the combination of species and their relative numbers are of importance in the development of the syndrome.

Mobiluncus spp. are occasionally isolated from extragenital sites, especially from breast abscesses.

PATHOGENESIS

The mechanisms that allow *Mobiluncus* spp. to cause disease are unknown. They express pili and are able to obtain iron from lactoferrin, but the role of these in the pathogenesis of disease is unknown. It has been possible to infect primates experimentally and animal studies may help elucidate the processes involved in the pathogenesis of vaginitis.

TREATMENT

Mobiluncus spp. and *G. vaginalis* are susceptible to most antimicrobial agents, including benzylpenicillin, clindamycin, erythromycin and nitroimidazoles. *M. mulieris* is more susceptible than *M. curtisii* to metronidazole, but treatment with this drug appears to eliminate all *Mobiluncus* species in patients with vaginosis. Oral or topical (intravaginal) metronidazole or clindamycin have been successfully used for the treatment of bacterial vaginosis.

SPIRILLUM MINUS

The organism commonly known as *Spirillum minus*, one of the causes of rat-bite fever in man, is of uncertain taxonomic position. It was once regarded as a spirochaete but was later placed in the genus *Spirillum*.

DESCRIPTION

S. minus is a short, spiral, Gram-negative organism about 2–5 μm in length and 0.2 μm in diameter. Longer forms up to 10 μm may be observed. The regular short coils have a wavelength of 0.8–1.0 μm. The organisms are very actively motile, showing darting movements like those of a vibrio. The movement is due to polar flagella, which vary in number from one to seven at each pole. The organisms can be demonstrated in fresh specimens by dark-ground illumination or by staining with Leishman's or other stains. Although there have been many unconfirmed claims the organism has not been cultivated on artificial media and many of its properties are therefore unknown.

LABORATORY DIAGNOSIS

In rat-bite fever, *S. minus* may be demonstrated in the local lesion, in the regional lymph glands or in the blood, either by direct microscopical methods or by animal inoculation. Guinea-pigs, white rats and mice are susceptible to infection, and the organism may be detected by microscopy in the peripheral blood following intraperitoneal challenge.

PATHOGENESIS

The clinical syndrome of rat-bite fever begins with an acute onset of fever and chills 1–4 weeks after the animal bite. The bite usually heals before the onset of symptoms but it often re-ulcerates. Local lymphadenopathy and lymphangitis develop with the onset of fever and systemic disease. A generalized rash with large brown to purple macules is usually observed, but some patients present with urticarial lesions. A roseolar rash may spread from the area of the original bite. Fever usually declines within 1 week before returning again after a few days; the fever may then recur in an episodic fashion for months or even years.

Endocarditis, meningitis, hepatitis, nephritis and myocarditis are rare complications. In most untreated cases, symptoms resolve within 2 months, after six to eight episodes of fever, although up to 6.5% of untreated cases may be fatal.

EPIDEMIOLOGY

Strains of *S. minus* occur naturally in wild rats and other rodents, causing bacteraemia. This form of rat-bite fever occurs mainly in Japan and the Far-East and is known as *sodoku*. Cases have been diagnosed, however, in other parts of Asia and in Europe and the USA.

TREATMENT

Infections with *S. minus* respond to treatment with penicillin and tetracyclines. In the rare case of endocarditis the addition of an aminoglycoside may be of value.

RECOMMENDED READING

Catlin B W 1992 *Gardnerella vaginalis*: characteristics, clinical considerations and controversies. *Clinical Microbiology Reviews* 5: 213–237

Jenkins S G 1988 Rat-bite fever. *Clinical Microbiology Newsletter* 10: 57–59

Kaper J B, Morris J G, Levine M M 1995 Cholera. *Clinical Microbiology Reviews* 8: 48–86

Levett P N 1992 Bacterial vaginosis. *Reviews in Medical Microbiology* 3: 15–20

Nair G B, Albert M J, Shimada T, Takeda Y 1996 *Vibrio cholerae* O139 Bengal: the new serogroup causing cholera. *Reviews in Medical Microbiology* 7: 43–51

Powell J L 1999 Vibrio species. *Clinics in Laboratory Medicine* 19:537–552

Rippey S R 1994 Infectious diseases associated with molluscan shellfish consumption. *Clinical Microbiology Reviews* 7: 419–425

Strom M S, Paranjpye R N 2000 Epidemiology and pathogenesis of *Vibrio vulnificus*. *Microbes and Infection* 2:177–188

Toranzo A E, Santos Y, Barja J L 1997 Immunization with bacterial antigens: *Vibrio* infections. *Developments in Biological Standardization* 90:93–105

World Health Organization 2000 Cholera 1999. *Weekly Epidemiological Record* 75: 249–256. Also available at www.who.int/wer

Internet sites

U.S. Food & Drug Administration, Center for Food Safety & Applied Nutrition. *Bad Bug Book*: vm.cfsan.fda.gov/~MOW/chap7.html

University of Wisconsin Department of Bacteriology: www.bact.wisc.edu/Bact330/lecturecholera

31

Haemophilus

Respiratory infections; meningitis; chancroid

M. P. E. Slack

The major pathogen in this group of organisms is *Haemophilus influenzae*, which is associated with a variety of invasive infections such as meningitis, epiglottitis, pneumonia and septic arthritis, and localized disease of the respiratory tract including bronchitis and otitis media. *H. influenzae* biogroup aegyptius (formerly *H. aegyptius*) is a cause of epidemic conjunctivitis and Brazilian purpuric fever. Other haemophili of medical importance include *H. ducreyi*, the causative organism of chancroid, and *H. parainfluenzae*, *H. aphrophilus* and *H. paraphrophilus*, three organisms that are occasionally encountered in patients with infective endocarditis and various other miscellaneous conditions. The generic name (= 'blood-loving') relates to the inability of these organisms to grow on culture media unless whole blood or certain of its constituents are present.

In 1883 Robert Koch described the microscopical appearance of a profusion of minute rods in pus from patients with conjunctivitis while engaged on cholera research in Egypt, and this is thought to be the first documented observation of haemophili. A few years later, during the influenza pandemic of 1889–92, Pfeiffer noted the constant presence of large numbers of small bacilli in the sputum of patients affected with the disease. He established these organisms in stable subculture and in 1893 published a complete account of his work on influenza, arguing that the bacillus was the causative agent of the disease. Considerable controversy surrounded this issue until the matter was resolved in 1933, when Smith, Andrewes and Laidlaw confirmed that the true aetiological agent was a virus. It still remains possible that secondary infection with *H. influenzae* contributed to the high mortality seen in the 1889–92 and 1918–19 pandemics.

In 1995 the entire genome of *H. influenzae* was sequenced, the first bacterium for which this task was achieved.

DESCRIPTION

Morphology

Haemophili are small, pleomorphic Gram-negative rods or coccobacilli. In clinical specimens, *H. influenzae* is most commonly seen as a small, uniform coccobacillus. In some cultures, and occasionally in clinical material, longer, filamentous forms may be seen, often in association with large, spherical or fusiform bodies.

Encapsulation

Some strains of *H. influenzae* produce a capsule, which is demonstrable by capsule stains and a *Quellung* reaction (swelling of the capsule) with type-specific antisera. The capsules are polysaccharide in composition and represent six distinct antigenic types, designated a–f. The most important of these is type b, which is a polymer of ribosyl ribitol phosphate. Strains possessing the type b capsule are associated with most invasive infections. The six capsular types can be identified by a polymerase chain reaction (PCR) method.

Growth on laboratory media

Growth depends on a requirement for two factors, termed *X* and *V*.

- X factor (haemin) is required for the synthesis of cytochrome *c* and other iron-containing respiratory enzymes. Unlike most bacteria, haemin-dependent haemophili cannot synthesize protoporphyrin from δ-aminolaevulinic acid.
- V factor is nicotinamide adenine dinucleotide (NAD), NAD phosphate (NADP) or certain unidentified precursor compounds. It is essential for oxidation–reduction processes in cell metabolism.

Ordinary blood agar contains X and V factors, but growth of *H. influenzae*, which requires both factors, is poor. The major growth restriction is due to the lack of availability of V factor, and enhancement of growth is obtained if the medium is supplemented with NAD. Streaking an organism which excretes an excess of this substance (e.g. *Staphylococcus aureus*) across the surface of the agar will produce growth stimulation in its vicinity (*satellitism*). Utilization of V factor in blood agar is also limited by the presence of serum nicotinamide adenine dinucleotidase (NADase). This can be inactivated by heating blood agar for a few minutes at 70–80°C until it turns brown (*chocolate agar*). This process also liberates extra X and V factors from the lysed red cells into the medium. X factor is heat-stable, but heating of media at 120°C for several minutes destroys V factor.

Transparent media containing blood extracts (e.g. Levinthal agar or Fildes' peptic digest agar) are useful for demonstrating capsulate strains, colonies of which are iridescent when viewed obliquely with transmitted light. Type b capsulate strains can also be detected by the presence of precipitin haloes on transparent media containing hyperimmune *H. influenzae* type b antiserum.

Metabolism

Haemophilus species are aerobic and facultatively anaerobic. Anaerobic growth considerably reduces the haemin requirement of X-dependent species. *H. aphrophilus* has a requirement for carbon dioxide, but this character may be lost on subculture. *H. influenzae* does not require a carbon dioxide-enriched atmosphere, but often grows better in such conditions.

Biochemical reactions

Haemophili are generally catalase-positive and oxidase-positive; they reduce nitrate to nitrite and ferment glucose. Patterns of acid production from other carbohydrates are used to identify the species. *H. influenzae* can be divided into eight biotypes on the basis of indole production, urease activity and ornithine decarboxylase reactions. Biotypes I–III are the most common, and most invasive (type b) organisms are biotype I.

PATHOGENESIS

Normal carriage

H. influenzae is exclusively a human parasite, which resides principally in the upper respiratory tract. Non-capsulate organisms are present in the nasopharynx or throat of 25–80% of healthy people; capsulate strains (about half of which are capsular type b) are present in 5–10%. Immunization of infants with *H. influenzae* type b (Hib) conjugate vaccine significantly reduces pharyngeal carriage of Hib, but has no effect on the carriage of other capsular types or non-capsulate strains.

H. influenzae is associated with two types of infection: invasive infections and non-invasive infections, which are quite distinct in their epidemiological profiles.

Invasive infections

Meningitis is the most common manifestation, but *H. influenzae* also causes epiglottitis, septic arthritis, osteomyelitis, pneumonia and cellulitis (Table 31.1). In some cases the patient develops a bacteraemia without a clearly defined focus of infection. Most bacteraemic infections are caused by Hib.

These infections are unusual in the first 2 months of life, but are otherwise mainly seen in early childhood. Most cases occur in children under 2 years of age, but acute epiglottitis has a peak incidence between 2 and 4 years of age. The introduction of conjugate vaccines effective against Hib in infants (see below) has dramatically reduced the incidence of invasive disease in children in countries using Hib vaccine, and consequently the epidemiology is changing.

The polysaccharide capsule is the major virulence factor for Hib. The rarity of infections in the first 2 months of life correlates with the presence of maternal antibodies to this substance, and the occurrence of infection in early infancy with the absence of antibodies having such specificity. As the prevalence and mean level of capsular antibodies in the population rise, *H. influenzae* type b infections become less common (Fig. 31.1).

Table 31.1 The clinical presentation of 749 cases of invasive *H. influenzae* type b infections

Clinical diagnosis	No. of cases	%
Meningitis	437	56
Epiglottitis	111	14
Bacteraemia	63	8
Cellulitis	54	7
Pneumonia	41	6
Septic arthritis	37	5

Data from Public Health Laboratory Service Regional *H. influenzae* survey 1990–92.

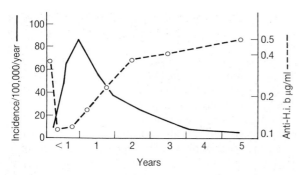

Fig. 31.1 The incidence of *H. influenzae* meningitis (continuous line) during the first 5 years of life and the corresponding mean level of anti-*H. influenzae* type b capsular polysaccharide antibodies (broken line). (From Peltola H, Käyhty H, Sivonen A, Mäkelä H 1977 *Haemophilus influenzae* type b capsular polysaccharide vaccine in children: a double blind field study of 100 000 vaccinees 3 months to 5 years of age in Finland. *Pediatrics* 60: 730–737.)

What determines whether acquisition of type b organisms in a susceptible host will lead to asymptomatic carriage and the stimulation of protective antibodies, or to the induction of invasive disease, is unclear. However, animal experiments suggest that when invasion occurs, the organism penetrates the submucosa of the nasopharynx and establishes systemic infection through the bloodstream.

The type b capsular polysaccharide facilitates all phases of the invasion process. Other virulence factors that may be involved include:

- fimbriae, which assist attachment to epithelial cells
- IgA proteases, which are also involved in colonization
- outer membrane components, including outer membrane proteins and lipopolysaccharide, which may contribute to invasion at several stages.

Initiation of invasive infection may be potentiated by intercurrent viral infection. Host genetic factors and immunosuppression may also play a role. It is unclear whether it is exposure to *H. influenzae* type b, or some other organism (e.g. *Escherichia coli* K100) possessing cross-reacting antigens, which usually stimulates natural protective antibody production.

Non-capsulate *H. influenzae* occasionally cause invasive disease. Meningitis and septicaemia due to non-capsulate *H. influenzae* is sometimes seen in the neonate. Infections with non-capsulate strains are also sometimes seen in adults. Pneumonia and bacteraemia are the commonest manifestations, often in patients with an underlying disease, notably chronic lung disease or malignancy. The highest rates occur in patients aged over 60 years, and the case fatality rate is high.

Invasive infections due to *H. influenzae* of serotypes other than b (principally types e and f) are rare. The spectrum of disease is similar to that seen with type b.

Non-invasive disease

H. influenzae produces a variety of local infections, which are often associated with some underlying physiological or anatomical abnormality. Most are caused by non-capsulate strains. The commonest are:

- otitis media
- sinusitis
- acute exacerbations of chronic obstructive airway disease
- conjunctivitis.

Acute sinusitis and otitis media are usually initiated by viral infections, which predispose to secondary infection with potentially pathogenic components of the local resident microbial flora. The mechanisms may involve:

- obstruction to the outflow of respiratory secretions
- decreased clearance of micro-organisms via the normal mucociliary mechanism
- depression of local immunity.

Acute exacerbations of chronic obstructive airway disease are similarly initiated by acute viral infections. Respiratory viruses compromise an already impaired mucociliary clearance mechanism in patients with chronic lung disease and allow bacterial colonization of the lower respiratory tract. In this situation *H. influenzae* can establish purulent infection and further damages pulmonary function by a direct toxic effect on cilia.

LABORATORY DIAGNOSIS

Direct examination

Gram-stained smears of cerebrospinal fluid, pus, sputum or aspirates from joints, middle ears or sinuses can provide a rapid, presumptive identification. Haemophili tend to stain poorly and dilute carbol fuchsin is a better counterstain than neutral red or safranin.

General considerations

The viability of *H. influenzae* in clinical specimens declines with time, particularly at 4°C. For optimal yield, specimens should be transported to the laboratory and cultured without delay. Chocolate agar is a good, general purpose medium and can be used without further supplementation for specimens obtained from sites that would normally be expected to be sterile. Plates should be incubated in an aerobic atmosphere enriched with 5–10% carbon dioxide.

Sputum

Specimens of expectorated sputum inevitably become contaminated by upper respiratory flora. This will commonly include *H. influenzae*, and the finding of the organism in such specimens cannot be automatically taken to imply involvement in a pathological process. Support for the significance of *H. influenzae* is provided if, in a purulent sample, the organism is present as the predominant isolate, or in a viable count of over 10^6 colony-forming units per millilitre. Addition of bacitracin (10 IU/ml) facilitates the selective isolation of *H. influenzae* from mixed cultures of respiratory organisms. Obtaining bronchial secretions by bronchoalveolar lavage reduces the problem of contamination with commensal organisms.

Throat swabs

The temptation to obtain throat swabs in patients with suspected acute epiglottitis should be resisted, since attempts to obtain the sample may precipitate complete airway obstruction. Blood cultures are usually positive in this condition.

Blood culture

Blood should be drawn for culture from patients with suspected invasive disease. Any good blood culture medium is satisfactory. Visual examination of the bottles cannot be relied upon to indicate positive growth. Bottles must be routinely subcultured onto solid medium, or some other detection system (e.g. fluorescent detection of released carbon dioxide) used.

Identification

H. influenzae colonies have a characteristic seminal odour. Confirmation of the identity depends on demonstrating a requirement for one or both of the growth factors, X and V.

- *H. influenzae* requires both
- *H. parainfluenzae* requires V factor only
- *H. aphrophilus* and *H. ducreyi* require X factor only.

The culture is plated on nutrient agar that is deficient in both X and V factor, and paper discs containing X factor, V factor and X+V factor are placed on the

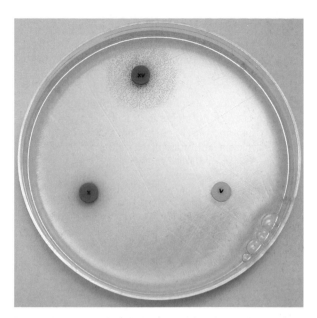

Fig. 31.2 Determination of the growth factor requirement of *H. influenzae*. Growth around the disc containing both X and V factors, but not round discs of the individual factors indicates that the organism is *H. influenzae* (see text).

surface of the agar. After overnight incubation, growth is observed around the discs supplying the necessary growth factors (Fig. 31.2).

The capsular type of *H. influenzae* isolates should be determined by slide agglutination with type-specific antisera, or a PCR-based method.

Antigen detection

The detection of type b polysaccharide antigen in body fluids or pus is a useful and rapid diagnostic aid, particularly in patients who have received antibiotics before specimens are obtained. The most commonly used technique is the demonstration of agglutination of latex particles coated with rabbit antibody to type b antigen.

In the absence of confirmatory cultures, the results should be regarded with caution as some serotypes of *Streptococcus pneumoniae* and *Esch. coli* may share similar antigens.

Molecular techniques

Techniques such as PCR are used to identify *Haemophilus* species in clinical specimens and as confirmatory tests on isolates.

Antibiotic sensitivity tests

Because of the fastidious nature of the organism, accurate determination of the antibiotic susceptibility of *H. influenzae* requires careful standardization of the methodology. Disc tests are less reliable for detecting enzyme-mediated ampicillin (β-lactamase) and chloramphenicol (chloramphenicol acetyl transferase) resistance than microbiological or biochemical techniques that demonstrate antibiotic inactivation.

TREATMENT

H. influenzae is sensitive to a wide range of antibiotics and is usually inhibited by low concentrations of ampicillin (or amoxicillin), chloramphenicol and tetracycline. Early cephalosporins were relatively ineffective against this species, but compounds such as cefuroxime, cefotaxime and ceftriaxone are highly active. Other antibiotics active against *H. influenzae* include co-amoxiclav, ciprofloxacin, azithromycin and clarithromycin.

Ceftriaxone and related cephalosporins such as cefotaxime are the antibiotics of first choice for the treatment of meningitis. They are bactericidal for *H. influenzae*, achieve good concentrations in the meninges and cerebral tissues and have proved highly effective in clinical practice.

Chloramphenicol was formerly the treatment of choice. Resistance may be encountered, but in most parts of the world this remains uncommon. Ampicillin is also effective and was once popular for the primary treatment of bacterial meningitis as it appeared to cover all the pathogens likely to be responsible and avoided the potential toxicity of chloramphenicol. However, resistance to the drug due to the production of a β-lactamase is now encountered in up to 25% of type b strains in the UK. In view of this level of resistance, ampicillin should no longer be used as a single agent in meningitis if *H. influenzae* is a possibility and the results of sensitivity tests are not available.

Antibiotic therapy is only one component of the clinical management of patients with haemophilus meningitis and full supportive care is required to achieve the most favourable outcome. Skilled medical and nursing care is also vital in the management of acute epiglottitis where maintenance of a patent airway is crucial. Ceftriaxone is the antibiotic of choice.

For the treatment of less serious respiratory infections, such as otitis media, sinusitis and acute exacerbations of chronic bronchitis, oral antibiotics such as amoxicillin, co-amoxiclav and clarithromycin are all effective. β-Lactamase-mediated amoxicillin resistance is seen in about 20% of invasive non-capsulate isolates in the UK.

EPIDEMIOLOGY OF INVASIVE DISEASE

H. influenzae is an important cause of serious systemic bacterial disease in children throughout the world. Meningitis is more common in winter months, in families of low socio-economic status and in household contacts of a case. The disease is usually seen in the youngest member of a family and uncommonly in children who have no siblings. Household contacts of patients with invasive disease have an increased risk of acquiring infection if they are less than 5 years of age. The risk for children under 2 years of age is 600–800-fold higher than the age-adjusted risk for the general population.

Outbreaks of infection have been described in close communities, such as nursery schools. Contact with a case in a day care centre or nursery has also been associated with increased attack rates in children under 2 years of age although the calculated risk is lower than that seen in household contacts.

Very high incidence rates have been reported in several distinct populations, e.g. Navajo and Apache Indians and Alaskan Eskimos. By contrast, very low rates have been reported in Hong Kong Chinese. It is possible that socio-economic considerations are important in determining such racial differences, but host genetic factors may also play a role. Immunosuppression, whether iatrogenic or associated with malignancies (especially Hodgkin's disease), asplenia or agammaglobulinaemia, also predispose to invasive disease.

The mortality associated with *H. influenzae* meningitis is around 5%. Neurological sequelae, especially hearing loss, may be present in 10–30% of survivors.

H. influenzae type b conjugate vaccines (see below) have had a dramatic impact on the incidence of Hib invasive disease. Before the introduction of immunization, *H. influenzae* was the leading cause of bacterial meningitis, accounting for about 12 000 cases annually in the USA. Routine immunization with conjugate vaccine has dramatically reduced the incidence of haemophilus meningitis in countries in which it has been adopted. Since 1992, when routine immunization was introduced in the UK, immunization rates have remained high (about 94%) and *H. influenzae* type b disease in children less than 5 years old has declined by 95% (Fig. 31.3).

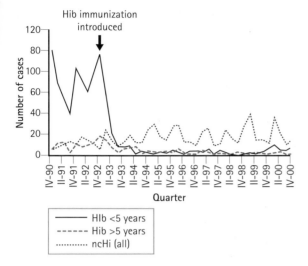

Fig. 31.3 Quarterly incidence of invasive infections caused by *H. influenzae* type b (Hib) and non-capsulate *H. influenzae* (ncHi). (From the Public Health Laboratory Service Regional Survey of invasive *H. influenzae* infections in five regions of England for the period from October 1990 to December 2000.)

CONTROL

Active immunization

The early haemophilus vaccines consisted of purified type b capsular polysaccharide. Unfortunately these proved to be poorly immunogenic in children less than 2 years old – the group most at risk of haemophilus meningitis – and in patients with immunodeficiency. Conjugate vaccines in which the polysaccharide is covalently coupled to various proteins (e.g. tetanus toxoid, a non-toxic variant of diphtheria toxin, *Neisseria meningitidis* outer membrane protein, and diphtheria toxoid) produce a lasting anamnestic response, which is not age-related and may be effective in high-risk patients who respond poorly to polysaccharide vaccine alone. In the UK, *H. influenzae* type b vaccine is routinely offered to infants at 2, 3 and 4 months of age, concurrently with diphtheria, tetanus and pertussis (DTP) immunization (see Chapter 69). There is no booster dose in the second year of life.

Prophylaxis

Rifampicin (20 mg/kg, up to a maximum of 600 mg) given orally once daily for 4 days eradicates carriage of *H. influenzae*. The drug has been used to prevent sec-

ondary infection in household and nursery contacts, but conclusive evidence of efficacy is not available.

- Unvaccinated siblings who are more than 4 and less than 10 years old should be immunized with conjugate vaccine.
- Unvaccinated siblings younger than 4 years old should be given both chemoprophylaxis and vaccine.
- Children less than 4 years of age with invasive *H. influenzae* type b disease should also be offered both vaccine and chemoprophylaxis to eliminate nasopharyngeal carriage as the disease sometimes fails to induce immunity in the very young.

The widespread use of conjugate vaccine may soon render chemoprophylaxis unnecessary.

HAEMOPHILI OTHER THAN H. INFLUENZAE

H. influenzae biogroup aegyptius

This organism, formerly known as the *Koch–Weeks bacillus* and *H. aegyptius*, is now thought to be a subgroup of *H. influenzae*. It is indistinguishable from *H. influenzae* biotype III in routine tests, but can be identified by a PCR method. It causes a purulent conjunctivitis and *Brazilian purpuric fever*, a clinical syndrome that was first recognized in Brazil in 1984, in which conjunctivitis proceeds to an overwhelming septicaemia resembling fulminating meningococcal infection. Ampicillin in combination with chloramphenicol has been successful when treatment has been started sufficiently early.

H. ducreyi

This organism is responsible for a sexually transmitted disease, *chancroid*, which is most prevalent in tropical regions, particularly Africa and South-East Asia. Patients present with painful penile ulcers (*soft sore* or *soft chancre*) and inguinal lymphadenitis. Typical small Gram-negative bacilli can be seen in material from the ulcers or in pus from lymph node aspirates. It is likely that the lesions of chancroid have facilitated the transmission of human immunodeficiency virus (HIV) in some tropical countries.

Chancroid may be treated with azithromycin, erythromycin, ciprofloxacin or ceftriaxone. Resistance to sulphonamides, trimethoprim and tetracyclines has reduced the usefulness of these agents. Strains with intermediate resistance to ciprofloxacin or erythromycin have been reported. Treatment failures are much more likely in patients with concurrent HIV infection.

An unrelated Gram-negative rod, *Calymmatobacterium granulomatis*, causes a somewhat similar sexually transmitted disease, *granuloma inguinale*, in parts of the tropics. Intracellular organisms, known as *Donovan bodies* (not to be confused with the Leishman–Donovan bodies of leishmaniasis), can be demonstrated in the stained smears from the lesions. Tetracyclines are usually used in treatment.

Other haemophili

Various other species of *Haemophilus*, notably *H. parainfluenzae*, *H. aphrophilus* and *H. paraphrophilus*, are occasionally implicated in human disease, notably infective endocarditis, but also including dental infections, lung abscess and brain abscess. Endocarditis is usually treated successfully with a combination of ampicillin and gentamicin.

RECOMMENDED READING

Alphen van L, van Ham S M 1994 Adherence and invasion of *Haemophilus influenzae*. *Reviews in Medical Microbiology* 5: 245–255

Jordens J Z, Slack M P E 1995 *Haemophilus influenzae*: then and now. *European Journal of Clinical Microbiology* 14: 935–948

Sahm D F, Jones M E, Hicket M L *et al.* 2000 Resistance surveillance of *Streptococcus pneumoniae, Haemophilus influenzae* and *Moraxella catarrhalis* isolated in Asia and Europe, 1997–1998. *Journal of Antimicrobial Chemotherapy* 45: 457–466

Slack M P E, Azzopardi H J, Hargreaves R M, Ramsay M E 1998 Enhanced surveillance of invasive *Haemophilus influenzae* disease in England, 1990 to 1996; impact of conjugate vaccines. *Paediatric Infectious Disease Journal* 17:S204–207

Swaminathan B, Mayer L W, Bibb W F *et al.* The Brazilian Purpuric Fever Study Group 1989 Microbiology of Brazilian Purpuric fever and diagnostic tests. *Journal of Clinical Microbiology* 17: 605–608

Wenger J D 1994 Impact of *Haemophilus influenzae* type b vaccines on the epidemiology of bacterial meningitis. *Infectious Agents and Disease* 2: 324–333

Internet sites

Clinical Effectiveness Group (Association for Genitourinary Medicine and the Medical Society for the study of Venereal Diseases) 2001. National Guideline for the management of chancroid: www.mssvd.org.uk/PDF/CEG/S43chancroid.PDF

MMWR 1986 International notes Brazilian Purpuric fever: *Haemophilus aegyptius* bacteraemia complicating purulent conjunctivitis. *Morbidity and Mortality Weekly Report* 35:553–554: www.cdc.gov/mmwr/preview/mmwrhtml/00000789.htm

Musher D M *Haemophilus* species: gsbs.utmb.edu/microbook/ch030.htm

Pan-American Health Organization 1999. *Haemophilus influenzae*: epidemiology and prevention: 165.158.1.110/english/hvp/hvp_hib_epidprev.htm

Todar K 1999 Bacteriology Lecture Topics: *Haemophilus influenzae*: www.bact.wisc.edu/Bact330/lectureHflu

32

Bordetella

Whooping cough

N. W. Preston and R. C. Matthews

The genus *Bordetella* constitutes one of the groups of very thin ovoid or rod-shaped Gram-negative bacilli, often described as parvobacteria. The genus contains two notable human pathogens, *Bordetella pertussis* and *B. parapertussis*, which cause one of the most frequent and serious bacterial respiratory infections of childhood in communities not protected effectively by vaccination.

DESCRIPTION

Bordetellae used to be classified in the genus *Haemophilus*. However, growth is not dependent on either of the nutritional factors X and V (see p. 307), and *B. parapertussis* and *B. bronchiseptica* do not require blood for their growth. The three species resemble each other in being small Gram-negative bacilli, in causing infection of the respiratory tract, and in sharing some surface antigens.

Bordetella pertussis

This is the most fastidious of the bordetellae. It produces toxic products which must be absorbed by a culture medium containing charcoal, or starch, or a high concentration of blood as in the original Bordet–Gengou medium. Because agglutination forms an important part of identification, a smooth growth is essential, and this is best provided by charcoal–blood agar. *B. pertussis* is a strict aerobe, with an optimal growth temperature of 35–36°C. Even under these conditions it usually takes 3 days before colonies are visible to the naked eye.

Typical colonies are shiny, greyish white, convex and with a butyrous consistency. By slide agglutination, they react strongly with homologous (pertussis) antiserum, and weakly or not at all with parapertussis antiserum, depending on the specificity of the reagent. Subculture reveals no growth on nutrient agar.

The organism produces three major agglutinogens (1, 2 and 3), which can be detected by the use of absorbed single-agglutinin sera. Factor 1 is common to all strains; the three serotypes pathogenic to humans (type 1,2, type 1,3, type 1,2,3) also possess factor 2 or factor 3 or both factors, and these type-specific agglutinogens have a role in immunity to infection.

Bordetella parapertussis

This organism is readily distinguished from *B. pertussis* by its ability to grow on nutrient agar, with the production of a brown diffusible pigment after 2 days (Table 32.1). It also grows more rapidly than *B. pertussis* on charcoal–blood agar, and is agglutinated more strongly by parapertussis than by pertussis antiserum.

It usually causes less severe illness than *B. pertussis*, and is uncommon in most countries, though occasionally it has been responsible for outbreaks of whooping cough, as in the former Czechoslovakia.

Bordetella bronchiseptica

Colonies of this species are visible on nutrient agar after overnight incubation; it differs from the other species by also being motile and by producing an obvious alkaline reaction in the Hugh and Leifson medium that is used to differentiate oxidative from fermentative action on sugars. It is therefore placed by some taxonomists in the genus *Alcaligenes*; however, it is readily distinguished

Table 32.1 Differential properties of *B. pertussis* and *B. parapertussis*

Property	B. pertussis	B. parapertussis
Duration of incubation to yield visible colonies	3 days	2 days
Growth on nutrient agar	None	Good
Pigment diffusing in medium	None	Brown
Slide agglutination with:		
Pertussis antiserum	Strong	Weak
Parapertussis antiserum	Weak	Strong

from the intestinal commensal *Alcaligenes faecalis* by its rapid hydrolysis of urea.

Although rarely encountered in human infection, *B. bronchiseptica* is a common respiratory pathogen of animals, especially laboratory stocks of rodents. Because it shares antigens with other bordetellae, animals must be checked for freedom from bordetella antibody before they are used in the preparation of specific antisera. For this reason, sheep or donkeys have sometimes been used in preference to rodents.

PATHOGENESIS

Whooping cough is a non-invasive infection of the respiratory mucosa, with humans as the only natural hosts. In a typical case, an incubation period of 1–2 weeks is followed by a 'catarrhal' phase with a simple cough but no distinctive features. Within about a week, this leads into the 'paroxysmal' phase, with increasing severity and frequency of paroxysmal cough, which may last for many weeks and be followed by an equally prolonged 'convalescent' phase.

In the initial preventable stage of the infection there is colonization of the ciliated epithelium of the bronchi and trachea with vast numbers of bacteria whose agglutinogens play a vital and type-specific role in attachment. *B. pertussis* produces a tracheal cytotoxin which paralyses the cilia, and leads to paroxysms of coughing as an alternative means of removing the increased mucus. Another bacterial product, called pertussis toxin, is responsible for the characteristic lymphocytosis in uncomplicated whooping cough. A subsequent increase in the number of neutrophils, together with fever, suggests bronchopneumonia or other secondary infection, maybe with pyogenic cocci. Blockage of airways may cause areas of lung collapse, and anoxia may lead to convulsions, though with modern intensive care the disease is rarely fatal.

Clinical features

Per–tussis (severe cough) has been recognized as a clinical entity for several centuries. Typically, the child suffers many bouts of paroxysmal coughing each day; during these, with no pause for air intake, the tongue is protruded fully, fluids stream from the eyes, nose and mouth, and the face becomes cyanotic; when death seems imminent, a final cough clears the secretions and, with a massive inspiratory effort, air is sucked through the narrowed glottis, producing a long high-pitched whoop — hence the term *whooping cough*. Such attacks often terminate with vomiting. Between them the patient does not usually appear ill.

If a characteristic attack is witnessed, a diagnosis of pertussis is usually made on clinical grounds alone. However, the illness is often mild and atypical, especially in:

- older children and adults
- younger children who have been incompletely immunized
- very young infants partially protected by maternal antibody.

In these cases, the laboratory has a vital role in diagnosis, because similar coughing may be caused by a variety of viruses and such illness is generally mild and of short duration. Here, the term *pseudo-whooping cough* has been applied aptly. False diagnosis may create a popular impression of pertussis as a trivial disease; it is recommended that, in the absence of positive bacterial culture, whooping cough should not be diagnosed for paroxysmal coughing lasting less than 3 weeks. With genuine pertussis, the illness is likely to persist for months rather than weeks. Furthermore, because pertussis vaccine cannot be expected to protect against viral infection, estimates of vaccine efficacy require an accurate diagnosis. Thus, a study in the UK by the Public Health Laboratory Service found an efficacy of 93% against pertussis confirmed by bacterial culture, compared with only 82% for cases diagnosed solely on clinical criteria.

In developing countries, whooping cough is still a major cause of death; however, in developed countries, concern is focused on a very prolonged and frightening illness with possible respiratory and neurological sequelae, on the anxiety and exhaustion of parents, and on the heavy use of hospital and community medical resources.

Experimental infection in animals

Some, though not all, of the features of human disease have been produced in animals. Thus, marmosets and rabbits develop catarrh during prolonged colonization of the respiratory tract; they produce a similar range of agglutinin responses to vaccination, and this immunity shows evidence of serotype specificity.

However, the mouse, which has long been used in the evaluation of pertussis vaccine potency, does not show these features. It can be infected and even killed by degraded organisms of serotype 1, which have lost the type-specific agglutinogens (2 and 3) that are necessary for human infection. It also reveals additional properties of pertussis toxin that are not seen in humans: histamine sensitization, and islets activation (including hyperinsulinaemia and hypoglycaemia). Furthermore, pertussis toxin and other components of the organism – filamentous haemagglutinin and pertactin – are virulence factors in the mouse, but their role in human infection is uncertain. It is therefore necessary to interpret with caution experimental evidence from mice or other small rodents.

LABORATORY DIAGNOSIS

Bacterial culture

Because atypical clinical cases occur frequently, laboratory confirmation of the diagnosis is often essential. Bacterial culture has the highest specificity of the tests available. In the absence of really effective therapy, accuracy in the diagnosis is more important than speed. Bacterial culture has the additional advantage that the isolate can be serotyped and genotyped, and thus provide valuable epidemiological information.

So rarely has a positive culture been obtained from a healthy person, other than one incubating the disease, that a false-positive result can be discounted. Moreover, with good technique of swabbing and culture, the organism can be recovered up to 3 months from the onset of illness when coughing persists. This casts doubt on the widespread belief that the bacterium is eliminated in a few weeks, and has implications for the transmission of infection.

Though the disease is mainly in the lower respiratory tract, the organism can be recovered readily from the nasopharynx. 'Cough plates' and postnasal swabs are unsatisfactory because of overgrowth by commensal bacteria. A pernasal swab acquires fewer commensals, and these can be suppressed by penicillin (0.25 unit/ml = 0.15 mg/l) or cephalexin (30 mg/l) in the charcoal–blood agar plate; higher concentrations may suppress bordetellae. Pernasal swabs on flexible wire are available commercially; the tip is directed downwards and towards the midline, passing gently along the floor of the nose for about 5 cm (depending on the patient's age) until stopped by the posterior wall of the nasopharynx. Practice in swabbing is necessary, initially with a co-operative adult! If old enough, patients should be warned to expect a tickling sensation but no pain; and a child's head should be held steady. Ideally, a segment of the culture plate should be inoculated immediately after withdrawal of the swab. The use of transport medium reduces the isolation rate. A single swab may yield a negative culture, but isolation rates of up to 80% may be achieved by taking specimens on several successive days.

In the laboratory, the inoculum is spread to give separate colonies, and the plate is incubated for at least 7 days before being discarded as negative. Because of the prolonged incubation, the medium should have a depth of 6–7 mm (40 ml in a 9-cm dish) and a bowl of water may be placed in the incubator to reduce drying of the culture. Cephalexin tends to give 'rough' growth, which may have to be subcultured on cephalexin-free medium for reliable serological identification.

Detection of bacterial antigens or DNA

Bordetella antigens may be detected in serum and urine in tests with specific antiserum. Alternatively, bacteria in nasopharyngeal secretions are labelled with fluorescein-conjugated antiserum and examined by ultraviolet microscopy. This method has the theoretical advantage, compared with culture, of detecting dead bordetellae. However, false-negative results are likely unless the patient's own antibody is removed from the bacteria by enzyme before application of the fluorescent reagent. Moreover, false-positive results may occur because of serological cross-reactions with organisms such as staphylococci, yeasts, haemophili and moraxellae, some of which resemble bordetellae microscopically. Bordetella antiserum should be absorbed with these organisms, but appropriate reagents are not readily available. Reports on the high specificity of this test lack conviction in the absence of reliable evidence on the true diagnosis.

There have been numerous studies of the polymerase chain reaction (PCR) in the detection of bordetella DNA in nasopharyngeal specimens, by the use of various primers. However, the method is relatively expensive and technically demanding compared with culture; as yet, there is a lack of consensus on its diagnostic reliability, with the need to detect both *B. pertussis* and *B. parapertussis*, and then to distinguish between them. Moreover, to be of epidemiological value, these methods would need modification to enable them to identify the serotype of the infecting strain of *B. pertussis*.

Detection of bordetella antibody

Sera and nasopharyngeal secretions can usefully be examined for antibody. However, a negative result does not exclude pertussis because the serological response is often slow and weak, especially in very young children. More importantly, a positive result needs careful interpretation because antigens are shared with other organisms (see above). Even with insensitive tests, such as agglutination, pertussis antibodies are readily detected in the sera of healthy persons. More sensitive techniques, such as enzyme-linked immunosorbent assay (ELISA), are liable to increase the number of false-positive results, and thereby give spurious respectability to a diagnosis that should rightly be 'pseudo-whooping cough'. The need at present in serological diagnosis is not for greater sensitivity but for greater specificity. Even then, the detected antibody may be an 'anamnestic' response to previous pertussis infection or vaccination, provoked non-specifically by a current, antigenically unrelated, illness.

Nevertheless, bacterial agglutination may be a useful guide in the serodiagnosis of pertussis, provided that sera are absorbed with type 1 organisms and titrated for the more specific agglutinins 2 and 3, and that paired sera are taken about 3 weeks apart to detect a greater than four-fold rise in titre. This requires a serum sample of at least 0.5 ml on each occasion.

Differential blood count

Although lymphocytosis is a characteristic response to pertussis infection, many cases of true pertussis do not develop a significant increase in circulating lymphocytes; conversely, there are so many other causes of lymphocytosis that a positive result lacks diagnostic specificity.

TREATMENT

Antimicrobial drugs

Most antibiotics have little or no clinical effect when the infection is well established, even though the organism may be sensitive in vitro.

The drug of choice is erythromycin (or one of the newer macrolides such as clarithromycin), which may reduce the severity of the illness if given before the paroxysmal stage. If given for at least 14 days it sometimes eliminates the organism and so reduces the exposure of contacts. However, positive cultures are frequently obtained after short periods of erythromycin therapy.

Erythromycin may also be given to protect non-vaccinated infants, though it seems unrealistic to expect this treatment to be maintained throughout the several months that the older sibling (or adult) may remain infectious.

Appropriate antibiotics should, of course, be administered to patients who show signs of secondary bacterial infection.

Other measures

Cough suppressants and corticosteroids may control the paroxysms, but may be harmful by encouraging retention of secretions. Cyanosis and anoxia can be reduced by avoiding sudden noises, excitement or excessive medical examination, which tend to precipitate paroxysms. Mucus and vomit should be removed to prevent their inhalation.

Treatment with pertussis immunoglobulin has been tried, but with limited success, probably because such materials have never been checked for the presence of all three agglutinins.

Because of the dearth of effective therapy for whooping cough, the widespread use of pertussis vaccine is of supreme importance (see below).

EPIDEMIOLOGY

Source and transmission of infection

Most new cases arise from patients (usually children, occasionally adults) with typical symptoms, presumably because the paroxysmal cough provides an efficient means of droplet dissemination. Atypical cases have only a minor role in transmission; long-term asymptomatic carriage is unknown. The degree of contact is important: 80–90% of non-immune siblings exposed in the household become infected, compared with less than 50% of non-immune child contacts at school. Antibiotic therapy may reduce transmission, but is not completely effective.

Incidence and mortality

Pertussis infection occurs worldwide, affects all ages, and is a major cause of death in malnourished populations. In the developed countries, mortality has gradually declined with a combination of improved socio-economic conditions, availability of intensive care in hospitals, and antibiotic therapy to combat secondary infection. However, the latter constitute an unnecessary use of medical resources on a disease that is eminently preventable by vaccination.

The disease is most severe and the morbidity rate highest in the first 2 years of life; most fatal cases are in infants under 1 year old. Even very young babies are not immune: maternal antibody does pass to the fetus, but it rarely contains all three agglutinins, and protection is incomplete.

Although one attack usually confers long-lasting immunity, infection with a different serotype of the organism can occur subsequently.

The disease occurs in epidemic waves at about 4-year intervals – the time needed to build up a new susceptible population after the 'herd' immunity produced by an epidemic. Figure 32.1 illustrates the pattern for England and Wales, where whooping cough has been a notifiable disease since 1940. The maintenance of a 4-year cycle presumably results from the interaction of various factors, such as the degree of artificial immunity produced by high vaccination rates, and the levels of natural immunity that follow either large epidemics or a high background incidence of endemic pertussis in interepidemic intervals.

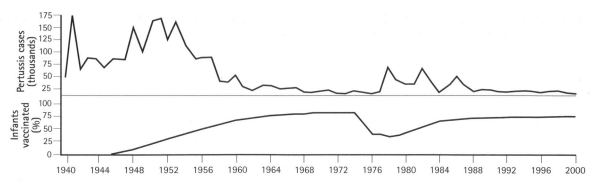

Fig. 32.1 Whooping cough in England and Wales since 1940.

Figure 32.1 also illustrates how variations in the rates of uptake of pertussis vaccine have affected the incidence of whooping cough more than the steady improvement in the general health of the population that continued throughout the period. After the gradual introduction of pertussis vaccination during the 1950s, there was a steady reduction in the size of epidemics until the 1970s. Unfounded fear of brain damage caused a loss of faith in the vaccine, and three large epidemics occurred before the slow restoration of confidence in the vaccine began to take effect.

Prevalence of serotypes

The three serotypes of *B. pertussis* pathogenic for humans are liable to spontaneous reversible variation, as shown by the arrows in Table 32.2. Fimbriae are readily demonstrable on strains possessing agglutinogen 2, aiding colonization of the respiratory mucosa; serotypes 1,2 and 1,2,3 predominate amongst the strains isolated from patients in non-vaccinated communities.

In the 1960s, many countries used type 1,2 vaccine, and these two serotypes were suppressed. However, type 1,3 organisms, which have a weak factor 1 component, became predominant in these countries and caused infection even in vaccinated children before the vaccine was modified in the late 1960s by addition of agglutinogen 3. Similarly, countries which used a vaccine deficient in agglutinogen 2, or in both agglutinogens 2 and 3, saw a predominance of type 1,2 infection, even in vaccinated children.

To be effective, it seems, a vaccine must contain all three agglutinogens, as recommended by the World Health Organization. However, because the agglutinin 3 response is usually the weakest (when type 1,2,3 vaccine is used), type 1,3 organisms are the last to be eliminated from a community with an effective vaccination programme.

Genotypes

It is not possible to trace the spread of infection by serotyping isolates because there are only three

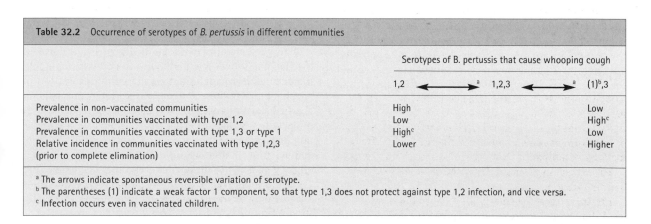

Table 32.2 Occurrence of serotypes of *B. pertussis* in different communities

	Serotypes of B. pertussis that cause whooping cough		
	1,2 ←——→[a]	1,2,3 ←——→[a]	(1)[b],3
Prevalence in non-vaccinated communities	High		Low
Prevalence in communities vaccinated with type 1,2	Low		High[c]
Prevalence in communities vaccinated with type 1,3 or type 1	High[c]		Low
Relative incidence in communities vaccinated with type 1,2,3 (prior to complete elimination)	Lower		Higher

[a] The arrows indicate spontaneous reversible variation of serotype.
[b] The parentheses (1) indicate a weak factor 1 component, so that type 1,3 does not protect against type 1,2 infection, and vice versa.
[c] Infection occurs even in vaccinated children.

serotypes and they undergo spontaneous variation. In contrast, more than 40 genotypes have been demonstrated in macrorestriction profiles by pulsed-field gel electrophoresis of DNA digests. Isolates within a household have been shown to belong to the same genotype, but the technique is probably too expensive and time-consuming for routine use.

CONTROL

Treatment and quarantine

Antibiotics and immunoglobulins currently available are not very effective for the treatment of patients or the protection of contacts. Because patients typically disseminate the organism for many weeks or months, and because children are infectious even before the most characteristic symptoms develop, control of the disease by quarantine is unrealistic.

Vaccination

Vaccination is safe and more than 90% effective and is strongly recommended. The vaccines in general use are suspensions of whole bacterial cells, killed by heat or chemicals, which are administered by deep intramuscular injection. Adsorption of the bacteria on to an adjuvant, such as aluminium hydroxide, enhances the immune response (particularly important with factor 3) and also causes fewer adverse reactions (Table 32.3).

Three conditions are essential for good protection:

- presence of all three agglutinogens in the vaccine
- use of adsorbed vaccine (i.e. with adjuvant)
- a minimum of three doses, at monthly intervals.

Since there is little passive protection from the mother, and since effective active immunity cannot be achieved until after the third injection of vaccine, the first dose is given as soon as a good response can be obtained. In many countries, therefore, the first injection is recommended at 3 months of age. In the UK and some other countries, concern for the vulnerability of the young infant has prompted a start at 2 months, although the immune response is somewhat weaker and there have been doubts about the effectiveness of this

early start. For these and other aspects of vaccination, see also Chapter 69.

Safety of pertussis vaccine

Minor adverse reactions occur in about one-half of vaccinated children, and can be considered as part of the normal immune response. Parents should therefore be warned to expect possible erythema and local swelling, slight feverishness and crying. Of much more concern are possible neurological sequelae, but the National Childhood Encephalopathy Study in the UK and several other studies have shown that pertussis vaccination seems merely to trigger the manifestation of neurological disorders that would occur in any case, and there is no firm evidence that the vaccine causes serious long-term adverse side-effects.

Contra-indications to pertussis vaccination

Severe adverse reaction to a previous dose has been considered the only firm contra-indication. A current feverish illness (not merely snuffles) is cause for postponement until the child is well. Parental concern over a possible neurological contra-indication is due reason for consultation with a paediatrician. Allergy is not a contra-indication, neither is age – children who missed vaccination in infancy may receive the normal three-dose course. Vaccination is also sometimes advised for adults, e.g. nurses and doctors in appropriate hospitals.

Acellular pertussis vaccine

Although doubts about the efficacy and safety of whole-cell pertussis vaccine have largely passed, the urge to identify the essential protective components persists. Trials in different countries (including one with type 1,2 prevalence and another with type 1,3 prevalence), and with vaccines containing various components, may reveal a correlation between protection of children and the response to individual pertussis antigens and type-specific agglutinogens.

A large-scale trial with good diagnostic criteria in Sweden has shown that antibodies to pertussis toxin and filamentous haemagglutinin do not confer protection in the child, though these antigens have been incorporated in nearly all acellular vaccines because they provide mouse-protection (see above). This trial did indicate a correlation between agglutinin titres and protection of children, and it showed that whole-cell vaccine had a higher efficacy than any of the acellular vaccines that were used.

Furthermore, an eventually satisfactory acellular vaccine may be too expensive for routine use, especially for developing countries where the need is greatest.

Table 32.3 Plain and adsorbed pertussis vaccine		
Vaccine	Immune response	Adverse reactions
Plain	Weaker	More
Adsorbed (onto adjuvant)	Stronger	Less

Eradication

Vaccination aims at a herd immunity, which breaks the cycle of transmission because the organism dies before finding a new susceptible host (see Chapter 69).

In several countries, good whole-cell vaccine is available. Eradication is possible but even if high levels of vaccination of infants are maintained it will be some years before adequate herd immunity is achieved within the child population.

RECOMMENDED READING

Cherry J D, Brunell P A, Golden G S, Karzon D T 1988 Report of the Task Force on Pertussis and Pertussis Immunization – 1988. *Pediatrics* 81: 939–984

Editorial 1992 Pertussis: adults, infants, and herds. *Lancet* 339: 526–527

Jenkinson D 1995 Natural course of 500 consecutive cases of whooping cough: a general practice population study. *British Medical Journal* 310: 299–302

Khattak M N, Matthews R C 1993 Genetic relatedness of *Bordetella* species as determined by macrorestriction digests resolved by pulsed-field gel electrophoresis. *International Journal of Systematic Bacteriology* 43: 659–664

Preston N W 1993 Eradication by vaccination: the memorial to smallpox could be surrounded by others. *Progress in Drug Research* 41: 151–189

Preston N W 2000 Pertussis (whooping-cough): the road to eradication is well sign-posted but erratically trodden. *Infectious Diseases Review* 2: 5–11

Preston N W, Matthews R C 1995 Immunological and bacteriological distinction between parapertussis and pertussis. *Lancet* 345: 463–464

Preston N W, Matthews R C 1998 Acellular pertussis vaccines: progress but déjà vu. *Lancet* 351: 1811–1812

Thomas M G, Lambert H P 1987 From whom do children catch pertussis? *British Medical Journal* 295: 751–752

Wardlaw A C, Parton R (eds) 1988 *Pathogenesis and Immunity in Pertussis*. Wiley, Chichester

33

Legionella

Legionnaires' disease; Pontiac fever

J. Hood and G. F. S. Edwards

The Legionellaceae are Gram-negative rods whose natural habitat is water. There are 41 genetically defined species, much the most important of which is *Legionella pneumophila*. This species can be subdivided on the basis of DNA relationships into three subspecies:

- *L. pneumophila* ssp. *pneumophila* and *L. pneumophila* ssp. *fraseri*, which have been described in human disease.
- *L. pneumophila* ssp. *pascullei*, which has so far been isolated only from the environment.

Eighteen *Legionella* species have been associated with human disease (Table 33.1) but most infections are caused by just one of the many serogroups of *L. pneumophila*: serogroup 1. Other serogroups and species such as *L. micdadei*, *L. bozemanii* and *L. longbeachae* account for a few cases; other legionellae are rare causes of infection. Man does not normally carry legionellae.

Table 33.1 *Legionella* species associated with human disease

Species	Number of serogroups	Autofluorescence under ultraviolet light
L. anisa	1	+
L. birminghamensis	1	–
L. bozemanii	2	–
L. cincinnatiensis	1	–
L. dumoffii	1	+
L. feeleii	2	–
L. gormanii	1	+
L. hackeliae	2	–
L. jordanis	1	–
L. lansingensis	1	–
L. longbeachae	2	–
L. maceachernii	1	–
L. micdadei	1	–
L. parisiensis	1	+
L. pneumophila	16	–
L. sainthelensi	2	–
L. tucsonensis	1	+
L. wadsworthii	1	–

+, Blue-white fluorescence; –, no autofluorescence.

Infection is usually acquired accidentally and the disease is not transmissible from person to person.

Legionellae give rise to two main clinical syndromes:

- *Legionnaires' disease*, a pneumonia that may progress rapidly unless treated with appropriate antibiotic therapy. In previously healthy subjects the mortality is about 10%, but in nosocomial infection the rate may be much higher.
- *Pontiac fever*, a brief febrile influenza-like illness that may be slow to resolve fully, but does not cause death.

Legionellae have rarely been associated with other infections such as prosthetic valve endocarditis or wound infection, but these are usually nosocomial infections.

DESCRIPTION

In biological material (e.g. sputum, lung or in water deposits) legionellae are short rods or coccobacilli, but in culture they become longer and are sometimes filamentous. Although they are weakly Gram-negative, they are difficult to visualize in biological material by Gram's stain, but may be stained non-specifically using a silver impregnation method. Specific fluorescent antibody stains are used diagnostically. The organisms may be numerous, particularly in patients who are infected in hospital or who are immunosuppressed, but are often present only in very small numbers in the scanty sputum that is characteristic of Legionnaires' disease. They have not been demonstrated in patients with Pontiac fever.

Legionellae are exacting in their growth requirements and grow best on buffered charcoal yeast-extract agar (BCYE), which contains iron plus cysteine as an essential growth factor. Some legionellae grow better in the presence of 2.5–5% carbon dioxide at 35–36°C. Colonies do not appear until after incubation for 48 h. Usually they appear by 5 days, but species other than *L. pneumophila* may take up to 10 days. Colonies have a 'cut-glass' appearance on examination under the plate microscope. Colonies of some *Legionella* species show blue-white (or red – not yet seen in species isolated from man) autofluorescence on illumination with long-wave ultraviolet light (Table 33.1). Species and serogroups within species have specific heat-stable lipopolysaccharide antigens, and further identification depends on serological examination, usually by the fluorescent antibody test or by slide agglutination with specific antisera. Species may be differentiated further on the basis of serology into serotypes within serogroups, but this applies, at the present time, almost entirely to *L. pneumophila* serogroup1. Subtyping is usually by the use of monoclonal antibodies in an immunofluorescence test. Similarities or differences between strains of the same serogroup may be revealed by genetic studies and this may be useful in the investigation of possible outbreaks.

PATHOGENESIS

Legionnaires' disease

Infection is almost always due to *L. pneumophila* serogroup1. The illness is characterized by:

- an incubation period of 2–10 days
- high fever
- respiratory distress
- confusion, hallucinations and, occasionally, focal neurological signs.

Once infection is established the patient develops pneumonic consolidation with an outpouring of proteinaceous fibrinous exudate, containing macrophages and polymorphs, into the alveoli. Despite the outpouring of cells, patients usually produce little sputum. Infection may extend to involve two or more lobes of the lung and renal impairment leading to renal failure may occur. The severity of the disease may range from a rapidly progressing fatal pneumonia to a relatively mild pneumonic illness. The mechanism of the distant toxic effects of the infection on the nervous system is unknown.

Patients who are debilitated, e.g. by immunosuppression or surgery, are more prone to infections and these are usually more severe than those encountered as sporadic community cases. Smoking is a predisposing factor. The deterioration in body defences associated with ageing is also important: the disease is most common in those over the age of 40 years with a peak in the 60–70-year age group. The only generally accepted mode of infection is inhalation of an aerosol of fine water droplets containing the organism though some believe that aspiration of water containing legionellae can also lead to infection. There is presently no evidence that ingestion plays a part in pathogenesis, although the demonstration of *L. pneumophila* in bowel contents raises this as a possibility.

Animal models provide some insight into the train of events in the lungs. Guinea-pigs infected by inhalation of an aerosol containing legionellae develop a lobular pneumonia which rapidly becomes confluent. Instillation of a protease produced by *L. pneumophila* into the lungs of guinea-pigs produces a pneumonia which appears to be the same as that caused by inhalation of intact bacteria.

At the cellular level, legionellae are engulfed by monocytes and can survive therein as intracellular parasites. The duration of intracellular parasitization is unknown but the persistent excretion of group-specific legionella antigen in the urine of some patients, as opposed to its more transient appearance in most cases of legionella pneumonia, suggests that in some patients intracellular parasitism may be prolonged. There is however, no evidence of a chronic carrier state or chronic infection.

Pontiac fever

The pathogenesis of this non-pneumonic, non-lethal form of legionella infection is not understood. Living legionellae have been isolated from sources of infection associated with outbreaks of Pontiac fever, and legionella antigen has been demonstrated in the urine of some cases, indicating that appreciable quantities of legionellae have been involved in the infection.

LABORATORY DIAGNOSIS

The tests used are listed in Table 33.2. As in any case of pneumonia, respiratory secretions (sputum, bronchial aspirate or washings), as well as pleural fluid, lung biopsy or autopsy material, should be examined by microscopy and culture. Gram-stained films are of little

Table 33.2 Diagnostic tests for legionella infection

Nature of test	Test	Appropriate specimen
Detection of whole organism	Culture FAT Gene probes	Sputum or other pathological material
Detection of soluble antigen	ELISA	Urine
Detection of antibody	FAT RMAT ELISA	Serum

FAT, fluorescent antibody test; ELISA, enzyme-linked immunosorbent assay; RMAT, rapid micro-agglutination test.

value except to demonstrate the presence of other pathogens and organisms that may interfere with the isolation of legionellae. Legionellae have occasionally been isolated from blood culture, but this is not a rewarding routine procedure.

The preferred diagnostic method is immunofluorescent staining with specific monoclonal or polyclonal antisera. Legionellae are usually hard to find in the scanty sputum produced by patients. Specific cultures are made on BCYE medium with and without antibiotics added to suppress other respiratory tract flora. Potentially contaminated material such as sputum or post-mortem material may also be heated at 50°C for 30 min in order to diminish growth by other less heat-stable respiratory tract organisms which have an inhibitory effect on growth of legionellae in culture. In heavy infections, legionellae may appear on BCYE media, but not on standard media, after incubation for 48 h at 36°C in air, preferably enriched with 2.5% carbon dioxide. Some of the less common legionellae may take longer to grow and cultures should not be discarded until after 10–14 days of incubation. Colonies having a 'cut-glass' appearance by plate microscopy or those fluorescing blue-white under ultraviolet light are Gram-stained, and single colonies are subcultured onto blood agar or cysteine-deficient medium to show that they will *not* grow on these media. Cultures are identified by use of specific antisera in an immuno-fluorescence test.

Antigen tests

The examination of urine for legionella antigen by enzyme-linked immunosorbent assay (ELISA) is a rapid and specific method of identifying *L. pneumophila* as the likely cause of a pneumonia.

Serology

Although antibodies take at least 8 days to develop after the onset of infection, some cases may not reach hospital until this period has elapsed so that it is worthwhile to examine serum for antibodies to *L. pneumophila* on admission to hospital. Further sera should be taken at intervals to show the development of antibodies or a rise in antibody titre. Antibodies usually develop after 8–10 days of illness and then increase in titre, but some patients may not produce antibody for some weeks or, rarely, for several months.

- A four-fold or greater rise in antibody titre in a typical clinical case indicates infection with legionella.
- A single titre of 256 or more is presumptive of infection.

In some cases proven by culture, lower titres may be found, especially when death occurs early in the illness. Antibody may persist for months or years and can be a source of confusion, as may cross-reacting antibody produced by some patients with *Campylobacter* infection. At present the only fully validated antibody test is that for infection by *L. pneumophila* serogroup1, although patients proven by bacterial culture to be infected by other legionellae produce antibodies to the infecting strain.

TREATMENT

High-dose intravenous erythromycin is the standard therapy in legionella pneumonia. Azithromycin exhibits better activity than erythromycin in vitro and penetrates well into cells and lung tissue. It may emerge as the drug of choice if its clinical efficacy is confirmed.

In severe cases a macrolide may be supported by rifampicin and, possibly, by the addition of ciprofloxacin, although evidence for the value of this agent is not well documented.

Susceptibility testing of clinical isolates is rarely justified: it is technically demanding and, as person-to-person transmission of infection is extremely rare, antibiotic use is unlikely to contribute to the development of resistance in other patients.

EPIDEMIOLOGY

In 1976 an outbreak of 182 cases of pneumonia, mainly affecting members of the American Legion, occurred at a convention in Philadelphia. This form of pneumonia became known as *Legionnaires' disease*, and the bacterium associated with it as *L. pneumophila*. Since that time, legionella pneumonia has been recognized as the only acute *bacterial* pneumonia that may occur in outbreak form. This is due to the dissemination of the bacteria in aerosols which may travel as much as 1–2 km from the source.

Infected aerosols are usually generated from warm water sources, typically:

- the ponds in cooling towers of refrigeration plants in air-conditioning systems
- domestic hot water systems in hotels and hospitals
- warm water in nebulizers and oxygen line humidifiers
- whirlpool spa baths and showers.

Legionellae are engulfed by, and survive within, free-living amoebae, and the bacteria may be protected from drying and disinfectants when present in the cysts formed by such amoebae. Community outbreaks may occur on a fairly large scale and the source of infection in such outbreaks is invariably a cooling tower in which the bacteria are harboured in the water of the pond associated with the apparatus. Smaller outbreaks have been associated with domestic water supplies in hospitals, spas and hotels and also with whirlpool spas. So-called sporadic cases may, on careful epidemiological examination, prove to be associated with cooling towers. About a third of cases in the UK acquire their infection abroad, usually from domestic water supplies in hotels, and apparently sporadic cases account for many others.

Legionnaires' disease accounts for a small but significant number of pneumonias admitted to hospital. The disease is more prevalent in the late summer and autumn. This may be due to an increase in bacterial numbers in warm water both in natural sources and cooling towers.

The route and source of infection of Pontiac fever are the same as in Legionnaires' disease. It may affect all age groups, including children. The attack rate is high with almost all of those exposed to the infection source being affected whereas, in Legionnaires' disease, the attack rate is low.

CONTROL

There is no vaccine. Nevertheless, unlike most forms of bacterial pneumonia, the disease may be prevented by the eradication of *Legionella* species in the various kinds of water source that may give rise to aerosol production. It is therefore important that any outbreak, or even one case occurring in hospital, is investigated to try to identify possible sources of an infectious aerosol so that it can be eradicated. Information about cases must be notified to epidemiological centres so that any association between cases may be established; once the source is identified, legionellae can be eradicated from water in several ways:

- heat
- disinfection with chlorine or other biocides, including chlorine dioxide
- copper–silver ionization.

Water systems in hotels and hospitals should be managed so that hot water is heated to above 60°C before distribution and does not lie stagnant and cooling in the pipes. As legionellae do not multiply in cold water, cold water supplies should be kept below 20°C; it should not be allowed to stagnate, as it may warm up and allow the multiplication of legionellae. It may be necessary in some infected water systems to dose continuously with a suitable biocide (see above) to maintain suppression of growth. Cooling towers should be disinfected with chlorine or other biocides in a way that ensures that the growth of legionellae and possible supporting organisms, such as algae or amoebae, is suppressed.

RECOMMENDED READING

Bartlett C L R, Macrae A D, Macfarlane J T 1986 *Legionella Infections*. Edward Arnold, London

Fallon R J 1996 Legionellaceae. In: Collee J G, Fraser A G, Marmion B P, Simmons A (eds) *Mackie and McCartney Practical Medical Microbiology*, 14th edn. Churchill Livingstone, Edinburgh, pp 489–499

Harrison T G, Taylor A G (eds) 1988 *A Laboratory Manual of Legionella*. Wiley, Chichester

Joseph C A, Watson J M, Harrison T G, Bartlett C L R 1994 Nosocomial Legionnaires' disease in England and Wales 1980–92. *Epidemiology and Infection* 112: 329–345

Stout J E, Yu V L 1997 Legionellosis. *New England Journal of Medicine* 337: 682–687

Winn W C 1988 Legionnaires' disease: historical perspective. *Clinical Microbiology Reviews* 1: 60–81

34

Brucella, bartonella and streptobacillus

Brucellosis; Oroya fever; trench fever; cat scratch disease; bacillary angiomatosis; rat–bite fever

M. J. Corbel

BRUCELLA

The genus *Brucella* comprises a group of Gram-negative coccobacilli that can infect a wide range of mammals ranging from rodents to killer whales. They are of particular zoonotic and economic importance as a cause of highly transmissible disease in cattle, sheep, goats and pigs. Infection in pregnant animals often leads to abortion, and involvement of the mammary glands may cause the organisms to be excreted in milk for months or even years. Human infections arise through direct contact with infected animals, including handling of infected carcasses; indirectly from a contaminated environment; or through consumption of infected dairy produce or meat.

Brucellosis is a typical zoonosis, and human-to-human infection does not play a significant role in transmission. Infection may remain latent or subclinical or it may give rise to symptoms of varying intensity and duration. Brucellosis can present as an acute or subacute pyrexial illness which may persist for months or develop into focal infection that can involve almost any organ system. The characteristic intermittent waves of elevated temperature that gave the name *undulant fever* to the human disease are now usually seen only in long-standing untreated cases.

DESCRIPTION

Classification

The *Brucella* genus comprises a group of closely related bacteria that probably represent variants of a single species. For convenience these have been classified into nomen species that differ from one another in their preferred animal host, in genetic arrangement, phage sensitivity pattern and oxidation of certain amino acids and carbohydrates. The main human pathogens are *Brucella abortus, B. melitensis, B. suis* and *B. canis.* The first three may be further subdivided into biovars associated

with various animal hosts. *B. abortus* has a preference for cattle and other Bovidae, *B. melitensis* for sheep and goats. The first three biovars of *B. suis* preferentially infect pigs whereas the fourth and fifth biovars have reindeer or caribou and rodents, respectively, as natural hosts. The biovars differ in their sensitivity to dyes, in production of hydrogen sulphide and in agglutination by sera monospecific for A and M epitopes.

Other nomen species that have not been shown to infect man include *B. ovis* and *B. neotomae*, which preferentially infect sheep and desert wood rats, respectively. Strains distinct from all these types have been isolated from seals, dolphins, porpoises and killer whales. They seem to represent at least three new nomen species and appear to be pathogenic for man.

Morphology

Organisms of the genus *Brucella* appear as cocci, coccobacilli and short bacilli, 0.5–0.7 μm wide by 0.6–1.5 μm long. They occur singly, in groups or short chains. They are Gram-negative, non-motile, non-capsulate and non-sporing.

Cultural characteristics

Brucella spp. are aerobic. However, *B. ovis* and many strains of *B. abortus*, when first cultured, are unable to grow without the addition of 5–10% carbon dioxide. All strains grow best at 37°C in a medium enriched with animal serum and glucose.

On clear solid medium the colonies may take several days to appear. With the exceptions of *B. canis* and *B. ovis* strains, which are permanently rough, they are normally smooth, moist, convex, transparent and glistening ('honey droplet'). However, the organisms can mutate, especially in liquid media, forming rough colonies on subculture. There is a corresponding loss in virulence and an antigenic change, so that they are no longer readily agglutinated by homologous antisera prepared against normal smooth strains. Identification can be made by the polymerase chain reaction (PCR) with appropriate primers or by a combination of biochemical, cultural, phage typing and serological tests. Rapid gallery tests may misidentify *Brucella* and are not recommended.

Sensitivity and survival

Brucellae may be killed at a temperature of 60°C for 10 min, but dense suspensions, such as laboratory cultures, can require more drastic heat treatment to ensure their inactivation. Infected milk is rendered safe by efficient pasteurization. Brucellae are very sensitive to direct sunlight and moderately sensitive to acid, so that they tend to die out in sour milk and in cheese that has undergone lactic acid fermentation. The organisms can survive in soil, manure and dust for weeks or months, and remain viable in dead fetal material for even longer. They have been isolated from butter, cheese and ice-cream prepared from infected milk. They may survive in carcass meat, pork and ham for several weeks under refrigeration. Pickling and smoking reduce survival. They are susceptible to common disinfectants if used at appropriate concentration and temperature. They are sensitive in vitro to a wide range of antibiotics, only a few of which are effective therapeutically.

Antigenic structure

In all smooth strains the dominant surface antigen is a lipopolysaccharide (LPS) O chain, which, depending on the three-dimensional structure, forms A, M or C epitopes. These are common to all smooth species, but the distribution of A and M depends on biovar. Rough strains do not produce the O chain but have a common R epitope. The LPS has endotoxin activity and elicits antibody-mediated protection. More complete immunity is dependent on cell-mediated, particularly cytotoxic, responses elicited by ribosomal and other proteins.

PATHOGENESIS

The incubation period is usually about 10–30 days, but infection may persist for several months without causing any symptoms. *B. melitensis* and *B. suis* tend to cause more severe disease than *B. abortus* or *B. canis*. Infection by any species may give rise to a variety of symptoms and, without the fluctuating temperature to act as a guide, diagnosis may be difficult.

Brucellae can enter the body through skin abrasions, through mucosal surfaces of the alimentary or respiratory tracts and sometimes through the conjunctivae, to reach the bloodstream by way of regional lymphatics. The organisms are facultative intracellular parasites and subsequently localize in various parts of the reticulo-endothelial system with the formation of abscesses or granulomatous lesions, resulting in complications that may involve any part of the body. Brucellae surviving within cells may cause relapses of acute disease, or a chronic syndrome may develop that is associated with continued illness and vague symptoms of malaise, low-grade fever, lassitude, insomnia, irritability and joint pain. Such 'chronic brucellosis' may follow an acute attack or develop insidiously over several years without previous acute manifestations. It rarely responds to antibiotic therapy and is probably a post-infectious response similar to the 'myalgic-encephalomyelitis syndrome'.

The signs and symptoms of brucellosis are not specific. Pointers to the diagnosis are a history of occupational exposure or recent travel to endemic areas with consumption of milk products.

LABORATORY DIAGNOSIS

Brucellosis is confirmed in man by isolating the organisms from blood or other tissue samples and by serological and other tests. In animals culture may be attempted from abortion material, placenta, milk, semen or from samples of lymphoid tissue, mammary gland, uterus or testis collected post mortem.

Brucellae are easily transmitted by aerosols, by ingestion and percutaneous inoculation. Cultures must be handled under containment conditions appropriate to Class 3 pathogens.

Blood culture

When brucellosis is suspected, blood culture should be attempted repeatedly, not only during the febrile phase. Because the organisms may be scanty, at least 10 ml of blood should be withdrawn on each occasion, 5 ml being added to each of two blood culture bottles containing glucose–serum broth. One of these bottles should be incubated in an atmosphere containing 10% carbon dioxide. Preliminary lysis and centrifugation of the blood improves the isolation rate. Other materials such as bone marrow, solid tissue samples or exudates are also suitable for culture.

Subculture should be made on to serum–dextrose agar every few days; alternatively, a two-phase Castaneda culture system, in which the broth is periodically allowed to flow over agar contained within the blood culture bottle, may be used. Blood cultures should be retained for 6–8 weeks before being discarded as negative. Automated blood culture systems may also be used.

B. melitensis and B. suis are more frequently isolated from blood than are B. abortus or B. canis.

Serological tests

In the absence of positive cultures, the diagnosis of brucellosis usually depends on serological tests, the results of which tend to vary with the stage of the infection (Table 34.1).

Standard agglutination test

This test usually becomes positive 7–10 days after onset of symptoms. During the acute stage of the disease, levels of agglutinins associated with both IgM and IgG immunoglobulins continue to rise. Since high-titre sera may not cause agglutination in low dilution (the *prozone* effect), a range of serum dilutions from 1 in 10 to over 1 in 1000 should be made.

Rose Bengal plate test

This is a rapid slide agglutination test with a buffered stained antigen. It is widely used as a screening test in farm animals, but also gives good results in human brucellosis. It is not affected by prozones or immunoglobulin switching.

Mercaptoethanol test

Low-titre agglutinins due to residual IgM may persist for many months or even years after the infection has cleared. The mercaptoethanol test is carried out simultaneously and in the same manner as the standard agglutination test except that the saline diluent contains 0.05 M 2-mercaptoethanol. The agglutinating ability of IgM, and sometimes IgA, is destroyed by 2-mercaptoethanol, and therefore agglutination in this test is indicative of the continuing presence of IgG and the likelihood of persisting infection.

Complement fixation test

As the disease progresses from the acute to the chronic phase and the organisms become localized intracellularly in various parts of the body, the IgM antibodies decrease; the agglutination titre falls and may become undetectable even while the patient is still ill. The absence of agglutination therefore does not rule out the possibility of infection. IgG and IgA antibodies that remain present in the serum and are no longer capable of agglutinating may be detected by complement fixation or ELISA tests.

In latent or chronic infection, the complement fixation test is likely to be positive whereas in cases of past infection it is negative.

Enzyme-linked immunosorbent assay (ELISA)

The ELISA for IgG and IgA antibodies shows a good correlation with active disease, especially in long-standing infection. It has largely replaced the anti-human globulin (Coombs') test formerly used for detecting non-agglutinating (IgG) antibodies.

In some rural communities the sera from a proportion of the normal population agglutinate brucellae in low dilutions because of previous subclinical infection.

The sera of persons who have been immunized against cholera and of those who have antibodies to *Francisella tularensis* may give false-positive reactions in the agglutination test against brucellae. More extensive false-positive cross-reactions are produced by infection with *Yersinia enterocolitica* O9, and to a lesser extent *Salmonella* O30 and *Escherichia coli* O157. Western blotting against whole cell protein extracts may be useful for differentiation.

Polymerase chain reaction (PCR)

The PCR with primers specific for the *omp2, omp25* and *rrs-rrl* genes can detect *Brucella* specifically and also give an indication of species and biovar. Promising results have been obtained in clinical studies.

Table 34.1 Results of serological tests used in the diagnosis of brucellosis

Type of brucellosis	Agglutination test	Mercaptoethanol test	Complement fixation test	ELISA
Acute	+	+ or −	+	+
Chronic	(−)	+	+	+
Past infection	(−)	−	−	(−)

(−), weak or negative. ELISA, enzyme-linked immunosorbent assay.

Brucellin skin test

This test, similar to the tuberculin test (p. 205), is no longer recommended as it does not differentiate active from past or subclinical infection. Moreover, intradermal antigen preparations are not readily available and some interfere with the serological response to infection.

TREATMENT

Brucella infections respond to a combination of streptomycin or gentamicin and tetracycline or to rifampicin and doxycycline. Tetracycline alone is often adequate in mild cases. Treatment should be continued for at least 6 weeks. Co-trimoxazole and rifampicin can be used in children. In endocarditis and neurobrucellosis a combination of a tetracycline, aminoglycoside and rifampicin is recommended. Serum antibody titres usually decline sharply after effective treatment. The chronic post-infectious form without localizing lesions responds poorly to treatment.

EPIDEMIOLOGY

B. abortus has been eradicated from cattle in most developed countries. Formerly common in dairy farmers, veterinarians and abattoir workers, it is now a rare cause of human disease. In the UK nearly all human cases are acquired abroad; most are caused by *B. melitensis*, which is still prevalent in Mediterranean countries, the Middle East, central and southern Asia and parts of Africa and South America

Human brucellosis due to *B. suis* is largely an occupational disease arising from contact with infected pigs or pig meat. It was once common in the USA, chiefly among those who handled raw meat shortly after slaughter. It occurs in feral pigs in Australia and the USA and is a hazard to hunters. It is widespread in domesticated pigs in various African, Asian and South American countries; biovar 4 is found only in the Arctic regions of North America and Russia. In some European countries, hares may act as reservoir hosts of *B. suis* biovar 2 which rarely causes human disease.

CONTROL

The live-attenuated *B. abortus* strain S19 vaccine has been used to protect cattle from abortion and so reduce spread of the disease. It can interfere with subsequent diagnostic serology and is now being replaced by the rough strain *B. abortus* RB51, which gives comparable protection, but does not induce interfering antibodies and is less hazardous to man.

The live-attenuated smooth strain *B. melitensis* Rev I is used to protect sheep and goats from *B. melitensis* infection. Vaccination of pigs is not widely practised but the attenuated *B. suis* strain 2 has been used in China.

Human vaccination is not recommended because effective and non-reactogenic vaccines are not currently available.

Pasteurization eliminates the risk of brucellosis from the consumption of infected milk or milk products. However, there remains the possibility of infection due to contact with infected animals or their tissues. Veterinary surgeons, farmers and laboratory workers are particularly at risk.

Eradication depends on the elimination of the infection from domestic animals by a policy of compulsory testing of the animals and slaughtering positive reactors.

BARTONELLA

The genus *Bartonella*, which is genetically related to *Brucella*, comprises over a dozen species of very small Gram-negative bacilli, at least nine of which are responsible for various febrile and localizing diseases in man.

* *Bartonella bacilliformis* is the cause of *Oroya fever* or *Carrion's disease* and *verruga peruana* and is spread by sandflies.
* *Bart. quintana* is the cause of *louse-borne trench fever*.
* *Bart. henselae* and *Bart. clarridgeiae* are the most common causes of *cat scratch disease* and can be transmitted by fleas.

Other *Bartonella* species and subspecies have been identified as pathogens of dogs, mice, voles and other mammals. Some, including *Bart. vinsoni*, *Bart. vinsoni* ssp. *berkhoffii*, *Bart. vinsoni* ssp. *apruensis* and *Bart. elisabethae*, have been identified as causes of fever, bacteraemia and endocarditis in man. *Bart. grahami* has been implicated in ocular disease.

It is becoming apparent that the various species can cause a similar range of syndromes involving many organ systems. As the genus extends, it is likely that other species will be implicated in human disease.

BARTONELLA BACILLIFORMIS

Bart. bacilliformis is responsible for outbreaks of a severe and often fatal disease of man in the mountainous regions of Peru, Colombia and Ecuador. The name Oroya fever was given after an epidemic of the disease in 1870 during the building of a railway between Lima and Oroya, when 7000 labourers died within a few weeks. The infection is spread by sandflies, usually *Lutzomyia verrucarum*.

After recovery from Oroya fever the patient may develop a skin eruption known as verruga peruana. Individuals may act as reservoirs of infection long after recovery from the illness and also after asymptomatic infection, which probably occurs in more than 50% of those exposed. *Bart. bacilliformis* is pathogenic only to humans.

Description

Bart. bacilliformis is a small Gram-negative coccobacillus. The organisms occur singly, in pairs, chains or clumps. In older cultures they tend to be extremely pleomorphic. They are motile through a cluster of about 10 flagella situated at one end of the cell.

It is a strict aerobe and grows best at 25–28°C, pH 7.8, on semisolid agar medium enriched with serum and haemoglobin.

Pathogenicity

After an incubation period of about 20 days, Oroya fever presents as a high fever followed by progressively severe anaemia due to blood cell destruction. There may be enlargement of the spleen and liver and haemorrhages into the lymph nodes.

The case fatality rate in untreated cases may be over 40%, though the overall fatality rate for all forms of the infection is probably only 0.1%. Verruga peruana may occur without the initial attack of Oroya fever or it may develop several weeks after recovery. It consists of a pleomorphic skin eruption of round, elevated, hard nodules that may become secondarily infected, producing ulcers and haemorrhagic lesions. The rash usually appears mainly on the legs, arms and face, although all parts of the body may be affected. The condition may persist for as long as a year, but it is rarely fatal.

Laboratory Diagnosis

In both Oroya fever and verruga peruana, bartonellosis is confirmed by demonstrating the organisms in smears of blood or tissue aspirates stained by Giemsa or immunofluorescent stain. They are seen packing the cytoplasm of the cells and adhering to the cell surfaces.

Culture

Bartonella spp. are dangerous pathogens and should be handled under Class 3 containment conditions. *Bart. bacilliformis* is readily cultured in semisolid nutrient agar supplemented with rabbit serum and haemoglobin, similar to that used for the culture of leptospires. Visible growth may take up to 10 days. Identification can be achieved by PCR or by cultural and serological tests.

Blood culture should be carried out at all stages of infection. It may be difficult to isolate the organisms from the blood when the verruga stage has developed and culture from the skin lesions is rarely satisfactory.

Other tests

PCR with primers for 16S ribosomal RNA sequences provides a rapid means of diagnosis, but is usually available only from reference laboratories. Antibodies to *Bart. bacilliformis* can be detected by indirect haemagglutination, indirect immunofluorescence and ELISA. They are common in inhabitants of endemic areas and are not necessarily diagnostic of active disease.

Treatment

Chloramphenicol is recommended for the treatment of Oroya fever and the frequently associated salmonella infections and can drastically reduce the mortality rate. Newer macrolides such as clarithromycin may be even more effective. Penicillin, streptomycin and tetracycline may also be effective in uncomplicated cases. Blood transfusion may be necessary in severe cases of anaemia.

Control

No vaccines are available. Insecticides are used to eliminate the sandfly vector in likely breeding sites inside and outside houses and surrounding areas. Since the insects bite only at night, individuals may protect themselves by withdrawing from affected areas at nightfall.

BARTONELLA QUINTANA

This organism was formerly classified among the rickettsiae as *Rochalimaea quintana*. However, unlike the rickettsiae these organisms can grow in cell-free media and they tend to be epicellular rather than intracellular parasites of man. Unlike *Bart. bacilliformis* the organism does not possess flagella, although it may exhibit a twitching movement caused by fimbriae.

Bart. quintana was first identified as the cause of the febrile illness known as *trench fever* among the troops in the First World War. It is transmitted by the body louse, *Pediculus humanus*, under unhygienic living conditions and is not uncommon among homeless people in some countries. Trench fever is a bacteraemic condition typically associated with periodic febrile episodes lasting about 5 days. *Bart. quintana* has also been implicated in cases of angiomatosis and endocarditis. The organism may be isolated from the blood of patients by culture on blood agar. *Bart. vinsoni* and its subspecies are similar.

BARTONELLA HENSELAE

Bart. henselae has been isolated from the blood and lymph nodes of patients suffering from *cat scratch disease*, a severe condition of regional lymphadenopathy and fever resulting from the scratch or bite of an infected cat. Cat fleas may be responsible for transmission. *Bart. clarridgeiae*, which can be differentiated from *Bart. henselae* by its flagella, can cause an identical syndrome.

An organism known as *Afipia felis* has also been implicated in a small proportion of cases of cat scratch disease. It is morphologically similar to *Bart. henselae*, but differs biochemically, genetically and in being culturally less fastidious.

Bart. henselae and, less frequently, *Bart. quintana* and other species have been identified in the blood and tissues of individuals suffering from two severe clinical syndromes associated with human immunodeficiency virus (HIV) or other immunosuppressant conditions:

- *Bacillary angiomatosis*, which produces proliferative vascular lesions in the skin, regional lymph nodes and various internal organs.
- *Bacillary peliosis*, which affects the liver and spleen.

Diagnosis

Bart. henselae may be cultured from the pus or lymph node samples of patients with cat scratch disease and from blood, lymphoid tissue, liver and spleen of patients with bacillary angiomatosis or peliosis. In tissue sections the organisms are best demonstrated by silver stain or an immunospecific stain. ELISA, with various protein antigens, is the most useful serological test.

Most *Bartonella* species can be detected and differentiated by PCR methods.

Treatment

Tetracyclines, aminoglycosides, chloramphenicol and clarithromycin are all effective against bartonella infections. Treatment may need to be prolonged for at least 6 weeks.

STREPTOBACILLUS MONILIFORMIS

Streptobacillus moniliformis is one of the causes of *rat bite fever* in man, the other being *Spirillum minus* (p. 302). It is a common commensal occurring in the nasopharynx of rats and other rodents, and sometimes causes epizootic disease in mice and rats, resulting in otitis media, multiple arthritis and swelling of the feet and legs. Laboratory workers who handle rodents are most at risk. Rarely, outbreaks of infection occur as a result of the ingestion of milk or other food contaminated by rats (*Haverhill fever*).

DESCRIPTION

S. moniliformis is Gram-negative, non-motile, non-capsulate and highly pleomorphic. The organisms appear as short bacilli, 1–3 μm in length, forming chains interspersed with long filaments that may show oval or spherical lateral swellings.

It is a facultative anaerobe that benefits from added carbon dioxide and a moist atmosphere. It grows best at 37°C and pH 7.6. Culture media must contain blood, serum or ascitic fluid. Loeffler's serum medium is satisfactory. After incubation for 2 days, discrete, granular, greyish yellow colonies 1–5 mm in diameter are visible on the surface, while minute 'fried egg' colonies appear in the depth of the medium. The latter are L-phase variants that have little or no virulence for laboratory animals. They develop spontaneously and are thought to have a defective mechanism for cell wall formation.

In liquid medium, e.g. serum broth, *S. moniliformis* produces an abundant granular sediment, appearing like cotton wool balls that do not disintegrate on shaking.

Sensitivity

S. moniliformis is destroyed by a temperature of 55°C in 30 min. In culture it survives for only a few days, although in serum broth at 37°C it may remain viable for as long as 1 week. With the exception of the L-forms, *S. moniliformis* is susceptible to penicillin, and both forms are sensitive to streptomycin and tetracycline.

PATHOGENICITY

In man the organism enters the body through wounds caused by rodent bites. It multiplies and invades the lymphatics and the bloodstream, causing a feverish illness with severe toxic symptoms and sometimes complications such as arthritis, endocarditis and pneumonia.

Infection acquired by ingestion of contaminated water, milk or food is known as *Haverhill fever*, a condition characterized by fever, sore throat, polyarthritis and erythema. The duration of the illness varies from a few days to several weeks. Endocarditis, hepatitis and amnionitis may develop as complications. In the pre-antibiotic era a case fatality rate of about 10% was reported. It is much lower nowadays with effective treatment.

LABORATORY DIAGNOSIS

An acute febrile illness associated with arthropathy and a history of contact with rodents may point to the diagnosis.

S. moniliformis can be isolated in culture from the patient's blood during the acute phase of the illness and from the synovial fluid of those who develop arthritis.

Growth occurs in a liquid medium as characteristic 'cotton wool balls'.

Mice are highly susceptible to intraperitoneal inoculation of infected blood or joint fluid, as a result of which they develop either a rapidly fatal generalized condition or a more chronic disease with swelling of the feet and legs.

Specific agglutinins may be detected in the patient's serum as early as 10 days or as late as several weeks after the rat bite. As they can also occur in healthy individuals, at least a four-fold rise in titre is needed for diagnosis. ELISA is the method of choice for detecting antibodies.

TREATMENT

Penicillin or oral tetracycline is usually very effective.

RECOMMENDED READING

Adal K A 1995 Bartonella: new species and new diseases. *Reviews in Medical Microbiology* 6: 155–164

Corbel M J 1998 Brucella. In: Balows A, Duerden B I (eds) *Principles of Bacteriology, Virology and Immunity*, 9th edn, Vol 2. Edward Arnold, London, pp 829–952

Corbel M J, MacMillan A P 1998 *Brucellosis*. In Hausler W J Jr, Sussman M (eds) *Principles of Bacteriology, Virology and Immunity* 9th edn, Vol. 3. Edward Arnold, London, pp 819–847

Jensen W A, Fall M Z, Rooney J, Kordick D L, Breischwerdt E B 2000 Rapid identification and differentiation of *Bartonella* species using a single step PCR assay. *Journal of Clinical Microbiology* 38: 1717–1722

Madkour M M 2001 *Madkour's Brucellosis*. Springer, Berlin

Washburn R G 1995 *Streptobacillus moniliformis* (rat-bite fever). In: Mandell G L, Bennett J E, Dolin R (eds) *Principles and Practice of Infectious Diseases*, 4th edn. Churchill Livingstone, Edinburgh, pp 2084–2086

Welsh D F, Slater L N 1995 *Bartonella*. In: Murray P R, Baron E J, Pfaller M A, Tenover F C, Yolken R H (eds) *Manual of Clinical Microbiology*, 6th edn. ASM Press, Washington, DC, pp 690–695

Wullenweber M 1995 *Streptobacillus moniliformis* – a zoonotic pathogen. Taxonomic considerations, host species, diagnosis, therapy, geographical distribution. *Laboratory Animals* 29: 1–15

35

Yersinia, pasteurella and francisella

Plague; pseudotuberculosis; mesenteric adenitis; pasteurellosis; tularaemia

M. J. Corbel

The organisms within these three genera are animal pathogens that, under certain conditions, are transmissible to man, either directly, or indirectly through food and water or via insect vectors. They are Gram-negative coccobacilli, formerly contained within one genus, *Pasteurella*. Molecular genetics has indicated a completely separate identity for the three genera, each with its own disease manifestations in man and animals.

- *Yersinia* belongs to the Enterobacteriaceae and includes many non-pathogenic species.
- *Pasteurella* is closely related to the *Actinobacillus–Haemophilus* group.
- *Francisella* is distantly related to *Legionella*.

YERSINIA

YERSINIA PESTIS

Yersinia pestis, the *plague bacillus*, is essentially a parasite of rodents. In certain parts of the world, burrowing animals such as ground squirrels, gerbils and voles act as reservoirs of infection that may be transmitted by fleas to susceptible animals such as bandicoots, marmots, squirrels and rats. The animals suffer from outbreaks of plague, and their fleas may transmit the infection to man, giving rise to sporadic disease referred to as *wild* or *sylvatic plague*. Farmers or trappers who come into contact with infected animals are at risk.

More serious for man is *urban plague*, resulting from the spread of infection among rats, especially the black rat, *Rattus rattus*, which used to flourish around human habitation. Outbreaks of human plague, following epidemics in rats, have in the past sometimes developed into pandemics.

Description

Y. pestis is a Gram-negative, non-sporing, non-motile, short coccobacillus. It occurs singly, in pairs or, when in liquid culture, in chains. Pleomorphism is marked, especially in old cultures in which pear-shaped or globular cells, suggestive of yeast cells (*involution forms*) may be seen. In smears from exudates and in cultures grown at 37°C they are frequently capsulate. In smears from tissues stained by methylene blue or Giemsa stain they show characteristic bipolar staining ('*safety pin*' appearance).

Y. pestis grows both aerobically and anaerobically at 0–37°C. It is somewhat sensitive to oxygen, and small inocula may not grow aerobically in ordinary culture media. At the optimum temperature of 27°C, small, slightly viscid, translucent, non-haemolytic colonies develop on blood agar within 24 h. Growth occurs on MacConkey's medium, but tends to autolyse after 2–3 days.

It is killed at 55°C in 5 min and by 0.5% phenol in 15 min. It is sensitive to drying but may remain viable in moist culture for many months, especially at low temperature.

Pathogenesis

The heat-stable somatic antigen complex of *Y. pestis* comprises a rough type lipopolysaccharide (LPS) which has endotoxin activity and is believed to contribute to the terminal toxaemia of plague. The heat-labile Fraction 1 (F1) protein capsular antigen helps the organism to resist phagocytosis and is a protective immunogen. This, and many other proteins associated with pathogenicity, are encoded by three plasmids. The largest of these contains genes activated at low calcium concentration, which express various outer membrane and secreted proteins with a variety of functions, including cell surface adhesion, iron acquisition, inhibition of phagocytosis and intracellular killing. *Y. pestis* also produces a plasminogen activator and fibrinolysin, which are believed to play a critical role in the initial stages of infection. A pathogenicity island also encodes other proteins associated with virulence, including some common to *Y. pseudotuberculosis* and *Y. enterocolitica*.

Traditionally, three severe forms of human plague are described:

- bubonic
- pneumonic
- septicaemic plague.

All of these may occur at different stages in the same patient. The disease may also present as pharyngitis or meningitis.

Bubonic plague

The transfer of *Y. pestis* from rats to man through the bites of infected fleas may occasionally result in a local-ized infection, known as *pestis minor*, with mild consti-tutional symptoms. More often the lymph nodes draining the area of the flea bite become affected, and the resulting adenitis produces intensely painful swellings or *buboes* in the inguinal, axillary or cervical regions, depending on the position of the bite. From these primary buboes the plague bacilli may spread to all parts of the body. Complications such as bronchopneumonia, septicaemia or meningitis may follow. In the absence of adequate antibiotic therapy administered early in the course of the disease, the case fatality rate may exceed 50%.

Pneumonic plague

This can develop in patients presenting with bubonic or septicaemic plague. It may also be acquired as a primary infection by inhalation of droplets infected with *Y. pestis*, usually from an individual with pneumonic disease or as a result of exposure to aerosols generated from cultures. A severe bronchopneumonia develops. The sputum becomes thin and blood-stained. It contains numerous plague bacilli that are demonstrable in stained films or on culture of the sputum. This type of plague is highly contagious and is almost invariably fatal unless treated very early.

Septicaemic plague

This may occur as a primary infection or as a complication of bubonic or pneumonic plague. The plague bacilli spread rapidly throughout the body and the outcome is almost invariably fatal, even in treated cases. Purpura may develop in the skin ('*Black death*') and disseminated intravascular coagulation is usually present. It should be noted that bacteraemia can occur in bubonic or pneumonic plague but is usually intermittent in the early stages.

Laboratory diagnosis

Pneumonic plague is easily acquired in the laboratory by inhalation of aerosols generated from *Y. pestis* cultures. These and clinical specimens suspected of containing the organism should only be handled under containment conditions appropriate for Class 3 pathogens. Laboratory animals used for diagnostic tests must be housed under insect-free containment conditions.

Plague is confirmed by demonstrating the bacilli in fluid from buboes or local skin lesions in the case of bubonic plague, in the sputum in pneumonic plague and in blood films and by blood culture when septicaemic plague is suspected. Blood culture may be intermittently positive in all forms of the disease. Post mortem, the bacilli can usually be isolated from a wide range of tissues, especially spleen, lung and lymph nodes.

Smears of exudate or sputum are stained with methy-lene blue or Giemsa stain. Characteristic bipolar-stained coccobacilli are confirmed as *Y. pestis* by culturing samples on blood agar and incubating at 27°C. If exudate is inoculated subcutaneously into guinea-pigs or white rats, or on to their nasal mucosa, infection follows and the animals die within 2–5 days. The bacilli may then be isolated from the blood or from smears of spleen tissue taken post-mortem.

Characteristic colonies growing on blood agar plates are presumptively identified by various cultural and bio-logical tests, by demonstrating chain formation in broth culture, and by 'stalactite' growth from drops of oil layered on the surface of fluid medium. Demonstration of the F1 capsular antigen by immunospecific staining will confirm the presence of *Y. pestis*.

Serology is most likely to be useful in the convales-cent stage. Tests used to detect antibodies to *Y. pestis* antigens in serum include the complement fixation test, and the haemagglutination test with tanned sheep red cells to which the capsular F1 antigen has been adsorbed. In the latter case a rising titre or a single titre of at least 16 is considered significant. An enzyme-linked immunosorbent assay (ELISA) with F1 antigen is likely to become the method of choice.

A polymerase chain reaction (PCR), with primers based on F1 gene sequences, offers a rapid and less hazardous means of diagnosis than culture.

Treatment

Y. pestis is sensitive to many antibiotics, including aminoglycosides, chloramphenicol, co-trimoxazole and tetracyclines, but not penicillin.

When plague is suspected, patients should be isolated and respiratory precautions observed for at least the first 48 h. Antibiotic therapy should be started without waiting for confirmation of the diagnosis.

Intramuscular streptomycin is highly effective. Chloramphenicol (given intravenously for the first 4 days) is recommended in patients with meningitic symptoms. Tetracycline may be adequate in uncomplicated bubonic plague if given in large doses within 48 h of onset, and continued for 10 days. Experience with other antibiotics is limited, but there are indications that gentamicin and ciprofloxacin are effective.

Although monotherapy is usually adequate, strains carrying antibiotic resistance plasmids have been reported, and combined therapy may be advisable until the sensitivity of the strain is known.

It should be appreciated that plague is a toxigenic infection and that even sterilizing doses of antibiotics will not prevent death once the bacteraemia has exceeded a certain threshold.

Epidemiology

Plague epidemics have probably occurred from the earliest times. The disease was introduced into Europe from Asia in the 13th century and led to the great pandemic known as the Black Death, when about a quarter of the population of Europe succumbed to the disease. It was during a major outbreak of plague in Hong Kong in 1894 that Yersin first described the plague bacillus.

Plague disappeared from Europe in the 17th century, perhaps because the black rat was displaced by the spread of the brown (sewer) rat, *Rattus norvegicus*, which is susceptible to plague, but does not commonly frequent human dwellings. Improvements in housing may also have played an important part in the elimination of plague from Europe.

The bacilli are transmitted from animal to animal and from animal to man by fleas, notably, but not exclusively, *Xenopsylla cheopis*, an ectoparasite of rats. In cool humid weather, fleas multiply and plague spreads readily among susceptible rats. Hot, dry weather, on the other hand, tends to limit the spread of infection because the fleas die out under those conditions.

When a flea feeds on the blood of a sick animal, plague bacilli are sucked into the insect's midgut, where they multiply to such an extent that they may block the proventriculus, a process promoted by secreted proteins. When the animal dies the flea seeks an alternative host, which may be another rodent or man. Because the 'blocked' flea is unable to suck readily, some of the infected blood of the previous host is regurgitated and injected into the bite wound of the new victim.

When the epizootic among rats has reached a stage at which the number of susceptible animals has greatly decreased through death or immunity, it tends to die out, as does any human epidemic associated with it.

Domestic cats may become infected with plague through contact with rodents. The animals may develop atypical disease and then transmit the infection to their owners or to veterinarians by the percutaneous or respiratory routes.

The sputum of persons suffering from pneumonic plague contains large numbers of plague bacilli and under favourable conditions the disease spreads rapidly through the community by droplet infection, independently of rodents or fleas. Epidemics are more likely to occur when overcrowding in insanitary accommodation allows the infected droplets to spread readily from person to person. Cool, humid conditions favour transmission.

Endemic foci of wild rodent plague persist in many rural parts of the world, including North and South America, Africa and many parts of Asia (Fig. 35.1). Constant surveillance must be maintained to prevent its spread to urban populations, especially in areas where living conditions are below standard.

Y. pestis has been employed as a biological warfare agent. Its potential application in bio-terrorism is of major concern.

Control

Bubonic plague

Periodic surveys are advocated in endemic areas to determine the prevalence of rodents and fleas so that control measures can be taken. Rats may be destroyed by rat poison and fleas by the liberal application of insecticide to rat runs.

Other control measures include the construction of rat-proof dwelling houses and buildings such as warehouses in dockland areas. The fumigation of ships and measures to prevent rats gaining access to ships and aircraft help to prevent the spread of plague from one country to another.

Pneumonic plague

Patients suffering from pneumonic plague should be isolated, if possible with full respiratory precautions. Overcrowding of houses and other accommodation should be avoided. Co-trimoxazole or tetracyclines administered to immediate contacts may afford some degree of protection.

Vaccination

Vaccines prepared from killed virulent strains of *Y. pestis* can confer significant protection against bubonic but not pneumonic plague. Live vaccines prepared from avirulent strains are used in some countries, but can cause severe reactions. Neither type can be relied upon to confer long-term immunity, and revaccination is necessary at 6-monthly intervals if exposure

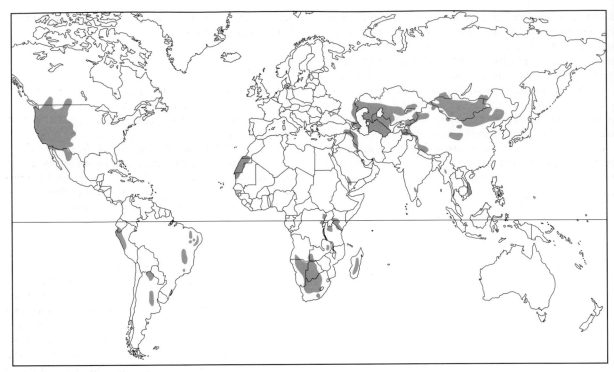

Fig. 35.1 Areas where endemic plague is known to have persisted.

to infection continues. Improved vaccines based on recombinant F1 and V antigens are under development.

YERSINIA PSEUDOTUBERCULOSIS

Y. pseudotuberculosis can cause disease in many species of wild and domesticated animals and birds. Although presentation can vary widely, it typically causes a fatal septicaemia, often accompanied by formation of small whitish nodules in the viscera ('*pseudotuberculosis*').

The infection is indirectly transferable to man, usually through contaminated food or water, resulting in a variety of presentations ranging in severity from subclinical to severe. Gastro-intestinal manifestations are common; acute ileitis and mesenteric lymphadenitis are the most characteristic. Post-infectious immunologically mediated sequelae are not uncommon.

Description

Y. pseudotuberculosis is a small, ovoid Gram-negative bacillus, with a tendency to bipolar staining. Genetically it is very similar to *Y. pestis,* which is probably a rough variant that has acquired additional plasmids encoding virulence factors. Initial growth may be best under anaerobic conditions. Isolation can be improved by

'cold enrichment' in buffered saline incubated at 4°C with periodic subculture for up to 6 weeks.

The organisms may be differentiated from *Y. pestis* by:

- motility when grown at 22°C
- ability to produce urease
- lack of the F1 antigen as shown by immunospecific staining or PCR.

There are eight major O serotypes, several of which can be separated into subtypes based on thermostable LPS somatic antigens. Unlike *Y. pestis* LPS, these are of smooth type and their specificity is determined by the O chain structure. The core regions are common to all serotypes and to *Y. pestis.* Thermolabile flagellar antigens are present in cultures grown at 18–26°C. Many other protein antigens are shared with *Y. pestis* and *Y. enterocolitica.*

Pathogenesis

Like other yersiniae, *Y. pseudotuberculosis* carries a plasmid encoding factors essential for pathogenicity. At least one enterotoxin is also produced as well as *invasin* and iron-regulated proteins encoded by a chromosomal pathogenicity island.

Infection may be subclinical, but occasionally results in a severe typhoid-like illness with fever, purpura and enlargement of the liver and spleen, which is usually fatal. More frequently it causes mesenteric lymphadenitis and terminal ileitis, usually accompanied by fever, diarrhoea and pain simulating acute or subacute appendicitis. All age groups may be attacked but young males aged 5–15 years seem more frequently affected. Recovery is usually uneventful but immunological sequelae such as erythema nodosum or reactive arthritis develop in some patients.

Laboratory diagnosis

Infection in man is confirmed by isolation of the organism in culture from blood, local lesions or mesenteric nodes, particularly the ileocaecal nodes.

Specific serum antibodies are detected and measured by tube or micro-agglutination tests performed during the acute phase of the illness with smooth suspensions of strains of serotypes I–VI grown at 22°C. Haemagglutination of red cells sensitized with LPS, or ELISA can also be used. The agglutinins decline rapidly and reach low levels within 3–5 months.

Treatment

Unlike *Y. pestis*, *Y. pseudotuberculosis* is usually sensitive in vitro to penicillins; it is also usually sensitive to aminoglycosides, chloramphenicol, tetracyclines, co-trimoxazole and quinolones.

Ileitis and mesenteric adenitis are usually self-limiting. Septicaemia demands parenteral treatment with ampicillin, chloramphenicol, gentamicin or tetracycline.

Epidemiology

Many animal species suffer from the infection, but there is little proof of direct transmission to man. Most human infections probably result from the ingestion of contaminated water, vegetables or other food.

About 90% of all human cases in Australia, Europe and North America are attributed to strains of serotype I, followed by serotypes II and III, whereas in Japan serotypes IV and V predominate.

YERSINIA ENTEROCOLITICA

By far the commonest manifestation of *Y. enterocolitica* infection is acute enteritis, which may simulate acute appendicitis. Like many environmental species of *Yersinia*, it may also occasionally cause opportunist infection in compromised patients, sometimes present-

ing as a plague-like syndrome with bubo formation or fulminant septicaemia.

Description

Morphologically and culturally, *Y. enterocolitica* resembles *Y. pestis* and *Y. pseudotuberculosis* but grows more readily; it differs from them antigenically, biochemically and genetically.

At least 54 different O antigens and 19 H factors have been identified, so that a large number of serotypes are recognized. Serotypes 3, 8 and 9 account for most human infections; other serotypes are probably non-pathogenic in immunocompetent individuals.

Pathogenesis

Y. enterocolitica causes mild and occasionally severe enteritis, mesenteric lymphadenitis and terminal ileitis. Septicaemia, which is often fatal, is most common in the elderly or in patients with predisposing conditions such as cirrhosis, iron overload or immunosuppression. Pneumonia and meningitis are rare presentations. Post-infectious complications include erythema nodosum, polyarthritis, Reiter's syndrome and thyroiditis. In young children the infection may produce fever, diarrhoea, abdominal pain and vomiting. The symptoms may last for several weeks.

Laboratory diagnosis

Infection is diagnosed by isolating the organism from blood, lymph nodes or other tissues on blood agar or MacConkey's agar. Isolation from contaminated sources such as faeces is best done by cold enrichment in buffered saline incubated at 4°C for up to 6 weeks, followed by plating on a selective medium. Identity is confirmed by biochemical tests and motility.

The serotype may be determined by slide agglutination with specific rabbit antisera. Serum antibodies are measured by agglutination tests against appropriate O antigens. A significant rise in the titre to 160 or more over a 10-day period indicates acute infection. ELISA may also be used. Cross-reactions occur between serotype O9 and smooth *Brucella* strains because of almost identical O chain structures. These are very difficult to differentiate. PCR may be of value but is difficult to apply to highly contaminated samples such as faeces.

Treatment

Y. enterocolitica is sensitive to many antibiotics, including aminoglycosides, chloramphenicol, co-trimoxazole, quinolones and tetracyclines, but it is resistant to penicillin. Sensitivity to other β-lactam antibiotics is variable.

Uncomplicated gastro-intestinal infection is usually self-limiting and treatment is indicated only in severe cases. Tetracycline is probably the drug of choice. Invasive infections such as septicaemia require intensive parenteral antibiotic treatment.

Epidemiology

Y. enterocolitica has been isolated from caseous abscesses resembling those of pseudotuberculosis, from blood and infected wounds and from the intestinal contents of apparently healthy animals of many species throughout the world. Pigs carry pathogenic serotypes quite frequently, cattle, sheep and goats less so.

Serotypes 3 and 9 account for most human infections in Europe, while serotype 8 is most common in the USA. Human disease usually results from ingestion of contaminated food or from contact with the environment. Raw pork, milk and drinking water have been implicated as sources. Man-to-man transmission also occurs.

Blood transfusion is a significant hazard as the organism can grow in refrigerated contaminated blood donations. Flies are believed to play a role in transmission by contaminating food, and infection has been demonstrated in fleas and lice. However, enteric infection is the usual route of transmission and preventive measures are those appropriate for food-borne disease.

PASTEURELLA

PASTEURELLA MULTOCIDA

Pasteurella multocida (formerly *P. septica*) is a commensal or opportunist pathogen of many species of domestic and wild animals and birds, and is frequently present in the upper respiratory tract. Carriage of the organism is usually asymptomatic but stress may provoke lethal systemic infection. Man occasionally becomes infected, especially following animal bites.

Description

P. multocida organisms are aerobic and facultatively anaerobic coccobacilli, which are appreciably smaller than those of *Yersinia* species, though they are often pleomorphic in culture. They are Gram-negative, non-motile, non-sporing and capsulate in culture at the optimum temperature of 37°C. In smears of blood or tissue stained with

methylene blue they show bipolar staining. *P. multocida* does not grow on MacConkey's medium.

Five capsular antigens A, B, D, E and F (C is not valid) and at least 11 somatic LPS antigens have been identified. The expression of the capsule is affected by cultural conditions and is lost in rough strains, which also fail to express smooth type O antigens.

The organisms are killed in a few minutes at 55°C and by phenol (0.5%) in 15 min. They may survive and remain virulent in dried blood for about 3 weeks, and in culture or infected tissues for many months if kept frozen.

Pathogenesis

P. multocida can be extremely virulent to many species of animals and birds, causing *fowl cholera* and haemorrhagic septicaemia, which are usually fatal. It also causes respiratory infections and contributes to the pathogenesis of atrophic rhinitis in pigs.

The capsule is essential for full virulence, at least in mice and rabbits, and is the major protective antigen. Iridescent smooth strains show the greatest pathogenicity; mucoid strains are of reduced virulence and rough strains are avirulent. A dermonecrotic protein toxin, a cytotoxin and a neuraminidase probably account for many of the local manifestations of infection but the bacteria also contain LPS with endotoxin activity.

Human infections usually present as a local abscess at the site of a cat or dog bite, with cellulitis, adenitis and, sometimes, osteomyelitis. *P. multocida* is also implicated in infections of the respiratory system such as pleurisy, pneumonia, empyema, bronchitis, bronchiectasis and nasal sinusitis.

Rare manifestations of disease include meningitis or cerebral abscess (usually following head injury), endocarditis, pericarditis or septicaemia, and infections of the eye, liver, kidney, intestine and genital tract.

A history of a recent animal bite or of occupational exposure are indicators for suspecting a *Pasteurella* infection. The organisms may also be carried commensally in the respiratory tract and can cause infection after surgical operation or cranial fracture.

Laboratory diagnosis

Swabs from bite wounds, from blood, from cerebrospinal fluid in cases of meningitis and from the secretions in suppurative respiratory tract infections are cultured on blood agar. The organisms are identified by various cultural and biochemical tests. Serology is of no value in diagnosis of acute human infection. PCR is potentially useful but rarely available.

Treatment

Infections usually respond to penicillin. Tetracycline, erythromycin or co-trimoxazole are suitable alternatives. In cases of osteomyelitis following dog or cat bites, antibiotic therapy must be continued for at least 8 weeks.

Epidemiology

P. multocida is carried in the nasopharyngeal region of many species of wild and domestic animals, some of which remain healthy while others suffer septicaemic or respiratory diseases. In human infections following animal bites, the organism passes directly to man in the animal's saliva. Cat bites are particularly hazardous. Man may also become infected through breathing droplets generated by the coughing of animals suffering from respiratory infection. Pig farmers may be particularly at risk.

The disease in farm animals can be prevented by vaccination with preparations derived from killed capsulate bacteria. This is not practicable for human infections because of their rarity.

OTHER PASTEURELLA SPECIES

Pasteurella spp. other than *P. multocida* cause human disease very infrequently.

- *P. caballi* causes respiratory and genital infections in horses and has caused bite wound infections in man.
- *P. dagmatis* has been associated with bite wounds and endocarditis.
- *P. (Mannheimia) haemolytica* causes pneumonia and haemorrhagic septicaemia in sheep, buffalo and cattle, and various diseases in poultry and other domesticated animals. It has been isolated from human cases of endocarditis, septicaemia and wound infection. It differs from *P. multocida* in forming haemolytic colonies on blood agar and by its ability to grow on MacConkey's medium.
- *P. (Actinobacillus) pneumotropica* is frequently isolated from the respiratory tract of laboratory animals. It has occasionally been isolated from human cases of septicaemia, upper respiratory tract infections and from animal bite wounds.
- *P. stomatis* has been isolated from cat bite wounds.
- *P. volantium* has been isolated from the human oropharynx.

FRANCISELLA

FRANCISELLA TULARENSIS

Francisella tularensis produces *tularaemia* in man and certain small mammals, notably rabbits, hares, beavers and various rodent species. It occasionally causes large epizootics in lemmings and other small rodents. It can be transmitted by direct contact, by biting flies, mosquitoes and ticks, by contaminated water or meat, or aerosols.

The closely related *F. novicida* (which is probably a subtype of *F. tularensis*) and *F. philomiragia* have been reported from North America as rare causes of human disease.

Description

When first isolated from infected tissue, *F. tularensis* is a very small, non-motile, non-sporing, capsulate, Gram-negative coccobacillus. In culture it tends to be pleomorphic, and larger, even filamentous, forms are present. It stains poorly with methylene blue but carbol fuchsin (10%) produces characteristic bipolar staining. Two biovars are recognized:

- Jellison type A (formerly *F. tularensis tularensis* or *F. tularensis nearctica*). They are found only in North America, are often transmitted by ticks and are highly pathogenic.
- Jellison type B (formerly *F. tularensis palaearctica* or *F. tularensis holarctica*). They occur in Europe, Asia and North America, are transmitted by mosquitoes rather than ticks, and are much less virulent.

F. tularensis is strictly aerobic. It will not grow on ordinary nutrient media, but grows well on blood agar containing 2.5% glucose and 0.1% cysteine hydrochloride. *F. novicida* and *F. philomiragia* are less fastidious.

F. tularensis is killed by moist heat at 55°C in 10 min, but may remain viable for many years in cultures maintained at 10°C, and for many days in moist soil and in water polluted by infected animals.

Pathogenesis

Little is known about mechanisms of pathogenicity. *F. tularensis* produces a carbohydrate capsule essential for virulence. A smooth type LPS is also present in the outer membrane, but apparently has very low endotoxin activity.

The organism is a facultative intracellular pathogen; in animals suffering from tularaemia the bacteria are present in large numbers within the cells of the liver and spleen, including macrophages.

Most human cases are sporadic, although occasional large outbreaks have been reported. After an acute onset with fever, rigors and headache, the disease develops manifestations that vary according to the route of entry of infection. Thus, following cutaneous inoculation through direct contact with infected animals or a fly or tick bite, a small punched-out skin ulcer develops at the point of entry, accompanied by enlargement of the draining lymph nodes even to the extent of bubo formation (*ulcero-glandular form*). If entry is via the conjunctiva a similar syndrome will develop involving the eye and pre-auricular nodes (*oculo-glandular form*). A glandular form without ulceration also occurs. Inhalation of infected dust or droplets, or ingestion of contaminated meat or water is more likely to lead to pulmonary or typhoidal disease, respectively. Either can be preceded or accompanied by painful pharyngitis. The severity of disease is much greater with type A strains and case fatality rates may exceed 5%. Disease caused by type B strains is much less severe, with very low mortality.

Laboratory diagnosis

F. tularensis is extremely dangerous to handle in the laboratory and Category 3 containment is required for all manipulations and animal work.

Human infections are usually diagnosed by inoculating tissue samples or the discharge from local lesions on to glucose–cysteine blood agar or cystine heart agar and identifying any small mucoid colonies characteristic of *F. tularensis*. Alternatively, the exudate may be inoculated into guinea-pigs or mice and the liver and spleen of the infected animals cultured post mortem. A PCR has been described, but is not widely available.

Serology is most likely to be positive after 3 weeks. Rising titres of agglutinins to *F. tularensis* or individual titres of 160 are diagnostic. Serum from cases of brucellosis may cross-react with *F. tularensis* and vice versa,

usually to relatively low titre. An intradermal delayed hypersensitivity test has been used in the past but the antigen is not readily available.

Treatment

F. tularensis is sensitive to aminoglycosides, chloramphenicol and tetracyclines, but resistant to most β-lactam antibiotics. Streptomycin or gentamicin are the antibiotics of choice in tularaemia and are usually curative. Tetracyclines or chloramphenicol in high dosage are also effective, but relapse may occur with these bacteriostatic agents. Treatment should be continued for at least 10 days.

Epidemiology

Tularaemia has a worldwide distribution, but occurs mainly in the northern hemisphere. Cases have been reported from North America, from several European countries, including Scandinavia, and from Asia. It has not so far been identified in the UK.

The infection, which is a typical zoonosis, is mainly spread by insects or ticks among lagomorphs and rodents. It is transmitted to man through:

- handling of infected animals, e.g. rabbits or hares
- tick, mosquito or fly bites
- inhalation of contaminated dust
- ingestion of contaminated water (as a result of pollution of water with the carcasses or excreta of infected rodents such as water rats or lemmings) or meat.

The organism is highly infectious, with a minimum infectious dose of 1–10 viable bacteria. Laboratory workers are especially at risk through handling infected laboratory animals or cultures of the organism. Man-to-man transmission of infection apparently does not occur. *F. tularensis* has been developed as a biological warfare agent and has potential application in bioterrorism. A vaccine based on the live-attenuated LVS strain confers some protection.

RECOMMENDED READING

Abdel-Haq N M, Asmar B I, Abrahamson W M, Brown W J 2000 *Yersinia enterocolitica* infection in children. *The Pediatric Infectious Disease Journal* 19: 954–958

American Public Health Association 1990 Plague. In: Benenson A S (ed) *Control of Communicable Diseases in Man*, 15th edn. American Public Health Association, Washington, DC, pp 324–329

Bottone E J 1998 Pasteurellosis In: W J Hausler Jr and M Sussman (eds), *Topley and Wilson's Microbiology and Microbial Infections*, Vol. 3 Arnold, London, Ch. 47, pp 931–939

Bottone E J 1999 *Yersinia enterocolitica;* overview and epidemiologic correlates. *Microbes and Infection* 1: 323–333

Butler T 2000 Plague. In: Ledingham J E G and Warrell D A (eds),

Concise Oxford Textbook of Medicine. Oxford University Press, Oxford, Ch. 16.51, pp 1625–1628

Johansson A, Ibrahim A, Goransson I, Eriksson U, Guryeva D, Clarridge J E, Sjostedt A 2000 Evaluation of PCR-based methods for detection of *Francisella* species and subspecies and development of a specific PCR that distinguishes the two major subspecies of *Francisella tularensis. Journal of Clinical Microbiology* 38: 4180–4185

Neubauer H, Sprague L D, Hensel A, Aleksic S, Meyer H 2000 Specific detection of plasmid bearing *Yersinia* isolates. *Clinical Laboratory* 46: 583–587

Smith M D, Thanh N D 1996 Plague. In: Cook G C (ed) *Manson's Tropical Diseases*, 20th edn. W B Saunders, London, pp 918–924

36

Non-sporing anaerobes

Wound infection; periodontal disease; abscess; normal flora

R. P. Allaker and J. M. Hardie

The significance of obligate anaerobes in general, and of non-sporing anaerobes in particular, is increasingly recognized. This heightened awareness of the important role that such organisms play, both as part of the normal microbial flora of the body and in a wide variety of infections, has come about largely through the application of greatly improved laboratory techniques for the isolation and cultivation of anaerobic bacteria, and the pioneering efforts of 'anaerobe enthusiasts' in various parts of the world.

A bewildering range of anaerobes is found in the mouth and oropharynx, gastro-intestinal tract and female genital tract of healthy individuals as part of the commensal flora. These include Gram-positive and Gram-negative cocci, rods and filaments, as well as a number of spiral forms (Table 36.1). Most infections with these organisms are of endogenous origin, except in the case of animal and human bite wounds, where the infecting organisms, usually mixed, are derived from the mouth of the aggressor.

Table 36.1 Anaerobic bacteria found as part of normal flora in man[a]

	Skin	Mouth	Gastro-intestinal tract	Genito-urinary tract
Gram-positive bacilli				
Actinomyces	–	+	+	+
Bifidobacterium	–	+	+	+
Clostridium	–	–	+	+
Eubacterium	–	+	+	+
Lactobacillus	–	+	+	+
Propionibacterium	+	+	+	+
Gram-positive cocci				
Coprococcus	–	–	+	–
Gaffkya	–	–	+	+
Gemmiger	–	–	+	–
Peptococcus	+	–	+	+
Peptostreptococcus	+	+	+	+
Ruminococcus	–	–	+	–
Sarcina	–	–	+	–
Streptococcus	+	+	+	+
Gram-negative bacilli				
Anaerobiospirillum	–	+	+	(?)
Anaerorhabdus	–	–	+	(?)
Bacteroides	–	+	+	+
Bilophila	–	–	+	+
Butyrivibrio	–	–	+	–
Centipeda	–	+	+	(?)
Desulfomonas	–	–	+	–
Fusobacterium	–	+	+	+
Leptotrichia	–	+	+	–
Mitsuokella	–	+	+	(?)
Porphyromonas	–	+	+	+

Table 36.1 (*Continued*)

	Skin	Mouth	Gastro-intestinal tract	Genito-urinary tract
Prevotella	–	+	+	+
Selenomonas	–	+	+	–
Succinimonas	–	–	+	–
Succinivibrio	–	–	+	–
Wolinella	–	+	+	–
Gram–negative cocci				
Acidaminococcus	–	–	+	+
Megasphaera	–	–	+	–
Veillonella	–	+	+	+
Spirochaetes				
Treponema	–	+	+	+
Other spiral forms	–	+	+	+

–, not usually found; +, commonly present; (?), presence uncertain (further data required).
[a] Data from various sources.

The flora of the lower intestinal tract, in particular, harbours vast numbers of anaerobes; quantitative studies on the bacterial flora of human faeces (Table 36.2) reveal a total content of over 10^{10} anaerobes per gram of faeces.

Many of the bacteria isolated from anaerobic infections are opportunistic pathogens. Such organisms are particularly likely to set up infections in damaged and necrotic tissue, when they are translocated to sites other than their normal habitat, or in a host that is compromised or debilitated in a way that leads to impairment of immunological or other defence mechanisms. Anaerobic infections of the head, neck and respiratory tract are often associated with organisms found in the mouth, while infections in the abdominal and pelvic regions are more commonly associated with gut bacteria.

FEATURES OF ANAEROBIC INFECTIONS

Clinical signs

A common, but not invariable, feature is the production of a foul or putrid odour. Foul-smelling pus or discharge should always alert the clinician to the likelihood that anaerobes are present, since no other organisms produce this effect, but the absence of this sign does not necessarily exclude the involvement of anaerobic bacteria. Other clues to the clinical diagnosis are listed in Table 36.3.

Table 36.2 The bacterial flora of faeces of English subjects[a]

Bacterial group	Mean bacterial count[b]
Gram-negative anaerobic rods	9.8
Bifidobacterium spp.	9.8
Clostridium spp.	5.0
Veillonella spp.	4.2
Lactobacillus spp.	6.5
Bacillus spp.	3.7
Enterobacteria	7.9
Streptococcus spp.	7.1
Enterococcus spp.	5.8
Total anaerobes	10.1
Total aerobes	8.0

[a] From Hill M J et al. 1971 Bacteria and aetiology of cancer of large bowel. *Lancet* 1: 95.
[b] Log_{10} viable organisms per gram of faeces.

Table 36.3 Some clinical signs and indicators of non-clostridial anaerobic infections[a]

- Presence of foul-smelling pus, discharge or lesion
- Production of a large amount of pus (abscess formation)
- Proximity of lesion to mucosal surface or portal of entry
- Failure to isolate organisms from pus ('sterile' pus)
- Infection associated with necrotic tissue
- Deep abscesses
- Gas formation in tissues
- Failure to respond to conventional antimicrobial therapy
- Pus which shows red fluorescence under ultraviolet light
- Detection of 'sulphur granules' in pus (actinomycosis)
- Infection of human or animal bite wound
- Gram-negative bacteraemia
- Septic thrombophlebitis

[a] Adapted from Finegold & George (1989).

Polymicrobial flora

Infections involving non-clostridial anaerobes are often polymicrobial. The composition of these mixed infections varies according to the site affected. The complexity may vary from two or three species up to a dozen or more, and may include strict anaerobes, facultatively anaerobic and micro-aerophilic organisms. Such combinations frequently comprise mixtures of Gram-negative rods (such as *Bacteroides*, *Prevotella* and *Fusobacterium* species) and Gram-positive cocci (peptostreptococci or streptococci, or both). In most cases, with the occasional exception of actinomycosis, it is not possible to predict accurately which organisms are present from the clinical presentation, although the detection of red fluorescing pus under ultraviolet light usually indicates the involvement of one of the black-pigmented *Porphyromonas* species.

LABORATORY DIAGNOSIS

When anaerobic infection is suspected, it is important that adequate clinical specimens are collected and transported as soon as possible to the bacteriology laboratory, preferably under reducing conditions. After direct microscopical examination of the material, appropriate culture media should be inoculated for incubation under good anaerobic conditions, either in an anaerobic cabinet or in anaerobic jars. In some laboratories, gas–liquid chromatography is carried out directly on pus and other clinical specimens in order to detect metabolic products, such as butyric and propionic acids, that are characteristic of certain anaerobes. Since many anaerobes are relatively slow-growing, it is essential that cultures are incubated for several days before being discarded. In mixed infections, fast-growing aerobic or facultatively anaerobic organisms are often detected within 24 h, whereas some anaerobes may require incubation for 7–10 days before their colonies can be recognized.

GRAM–NEGATIVE BACILLI

Gram-negative, anaerobic, non-spore-forming, non-motile rods were previously classified within three genera, *Bacteroides*, *Fusobacterium* and *Leptotrichia*, which constituted the family Bacteroidaceae. The assignment of species was based largely on the profile of metabolic end-products produced after growth in a carbohydrate- and protein hydrolysate-rich medium. Thus, *Leptotrichia buccalis* (*Leptotrichia* is a monospecific genus) produces mainly lactic acid, whereas *Fusobacterium* species produce copious amounts of butyric acid and lower levels of acetic and propionic acids. Organisms that possessed other

metabolic end-product patterns were placed in the genus *Bacteroides*, which has now undergone major taxonomic revision.

Morphologically, *Leptotrichia* and some *Fusobacterium* species tend to form long filamentous rods, often with pointed ends. Such filaments are sometimes described as *fusiform* or spindle-shaped. *Bacteroides* species are usually seen as shorter rods or coccobacilli, but may be pleomorphic.

Fusobacterium spp.

Fusobacteria colonize the mucous membranes of humans and animals, and are generally regarded as commensals of the upper respiratory and gastro-intestinal tracts. Species such as *F. nucleatum*, *F. periodonticum* and *F. naviforme* are generally isolated from the oral cavity and are often associated with infections of this and related sites. *F. nucleatum*, the most studied species, is frequently recovered from mixed infections of the head and neck region, including dental abscesses and the central nervous system, and is also quite commonly isolated from transtracheal aspirates and pleural fluid. *F. necrophorum* is an important animal pathogen. It is associated with human necrobacillosis and infections similar to those caused by *F. nucleatum* in man, but is isolated less often.

F. nucleatum now includes the subspecies *nucleatum*, *polymorphum* and *vincentii*; *F. necrophorum* includes the subspecies *funduliforme* and *necrophorum*. *F. nucleatum* subspecies *nucleatum* is an important periodontal pathogen, particularly during the period when quiescent periodontitis becomes active. *F. mortiferum*, *F. necrogenes*, *F. gonidiaformans* and *F. varium* are generally isolated from the gastro-intestinal and urogenital tracts of man and animals. These species, together with *F. nucleatum*, are often associated with mixed intra-abdominal infections, perirectal abscesses, osteomyelitis, decubitus, and other ulcers and various soft tissue infections. *F. ulcerans* was originally isolated from tropical ulcers but may be found in other sites.

Leptotrichia buccalis

This species was originally classified in the genus *Fusobacterium*, and shares a number of properties with the fusobacteria. Although normally considered to be an oral species, it also occurs outside the oral cavity, but has not been widely studied. The association of *L. buccalis* with disease is not clear-cut, although it has been reported in acute necrotizing ulcerative gingivitis (*Vincent's gingivitis*), together with *Treponema*, *Porphyromonas* and *Fusobacterium* species.

Bacteroides, Porphyromonas and Prevotella species

Bacteria once thought of as typical members of the genus *Bacteroides*, especially those isolated from humans, form three broad groups according to whether they are asaccharolytic, moderately saccharolytic or strongly saccharolytic (Table 36.4).

- The asaccharolytic, pigmented species are now classified in the genus *Porphyromonas*, which includes the important periodontal pathogen *P. gingivalis*.
- The moderately saccharolytic species that are inhibited by 20% bile and are largely indigenous to the oral cavity have been assigned to the genus *Prevotella*.
- The genus *Bacteroides* is now restricted to *B. fragilis* and related species that are saccharolytic and grow in 20% bile.

To add to the taxonomic complexity, many other former *Bacteroides* species that are usually isolated from non-human sources have been reclassified in recent years, and several new genus names have been proposed. *B. gracilis* is now considered to belong to the genus *Campylobacter* and the former *B. ochraceus* now belongs to the genus *Capnocytophaga*.

Infections with Bacteroides, Porphyromonas and Prevotella species

Bacteroides species and related Gram-negative rods are, together with anaerobic cocci, the commonest cause of non-clostridial anaerobic infections in man. Organisms of the *B. fragilis* group are particularly significant, since they are the most commonly isolated and tend to be more resistant to antimicrobial agents than most anaerobes.

B. fragilis itself is substantially outnumbered by other *Bacteroides* species in the normal bowel microflora, but it is often associated with intra-abdominal and soft tissue infections below the waist. *B. fragilis* is also the most common anaerobe found in bacteraemia, and has even occasionally been reported from head and neck infections, despite its apparent absence from the normal flora of the mouth. Species of the *B. fragilis* group account for about a quarter of all anaerobes isolated from clinical specimens.

Black-pigmented species, including those from the genera *Porphyromonas* and *Prevotella*, occur in abscesses and soft tissue infections in various parts of the body. They are rarely isolated in pure culture. *P. gingivalis* is associated with chronic adult periodontitis and *P. endodontalis* with dental root canal (endodontic) infections.

GRAM–POSITIVE ANAEROBIC COCCI

Classification and nomenclature of strictly anaerobic Gram-positive cocci (as opposed to facultatively anaerobic, micro-aerophilic or carbon dioxide-dependent cocci, which may also be isolated on primary anaerobic culture plates) are still in need of clarification. Consequently, it is not always easy to identify clinical isolates precisely, and they are often described simply as 'anaerobic cocci'.

Most species known to be clinically significant are regarded as belonging to the genus *Peptostreptococcus* (Table 36.5). Distinguishing between them depends upon a variety of physiological and biochemical tests,

---

Table 36.4 Current taxonomic status of *Bacteroides, Porphyromonas* and *Prevotella* species

Saccharolytic group (*B. fragilis* and related species)
  B. fragilis, B. caccae, B. distasonis, B. eggerthii,
  B. merdae, B. ovatus, B. stercoris, B. thetaiotaomicron,
  B. uniformis, B. vulgatus

Moderately saccharolytic group (*Prevotella* spp.)
  Prev. melaninogenica, Prev. bivia, Prev. buccae,
  Prev. buccalis, Prev. corporis, Prev. denticola,
  Prev. disiens, Prev. enoeca, Prev. heparinolytica, Prev. intermedia,
  Prev. loescheii, Prev. nigrescens, Prev. pallens, Prev. oralis,
  Prev. oris, Prev.oulora, Prev. tannerae, Prev. veroralis,
  Prev. zoogleoformans

Asaccharolytic group (*Porphyromonas* spp.)
  P. asaccharolytica, P. catoniae P. gingivalis, P. endodontalis

Other (uncertain taxonomic status)
  B. ureolyticus, B. splanchnicus, B. forsythus, B. capillosus

---

Table 36.5 Currently recognized species of Gram-positive anaerobic cocci

Peptococcus niger
Peptostreptococcus anaerobius
Peptostr. asaccharolyticus
Peptostr. harei
Peptostr. hydrogenalis
Peptostr. indolicus
Peptostr. ivorii
Peptostr. lacrimalis
Peptostr. lactolyticus
Peptostr. magnus
Peptostr. micros
Peptostr. octavius
Peptostr. prevotii
Peptostr. productus
Peptostr. tetradius
Peptostr. vaginalis

including the analysis of metabolic end-products by gas–liquid chromatography. Many species do not ferment carbohydrate substrates, so that some commonly used identification tests are of little value.

Gram-positive anaerobic cocci comprise part of the normal microbial flora of the mouth, gastro-intestinal tract, genito-urinary tract and skin. They are often isolated from clinical specimens. Other genera, including *Coprococcus*, *Gaffkya*, *Gemmiger*, *Ruminococcus* and *Sarcina*, are found as part of the flora of the bowel (see Table 36.1), but are not usually considered to be significant in infections.

Infections with anaerobic cocci

Anaerobic cocci are isolated from infections in various parts of the body, particularly from abscesses (Table 36.6). They are often found in association with other anaerobes, facultatively anaerobic or aerobic organisms. As with all mixed infections, it is difficult to assess the contribution of each individual organism to the pathogenic process. However, there is sufficient evidence from both clinical and experimental studies to confirm the pathogenic potential of the anaerobic cocci.

GRAM–NEGATIVE ANAEROBIC COCCI

Among genera recorded as part of the normal flora of the gastro-intestinal tract (see Table 36.1) only *Veillonella* is found regularly at other sites. In the mouth, for example, this genus is a regular component of supragingival dental plaque and of the tongue microflora. Veillonellae are able to use some of the lactic acid produced by bacteria such as streptococci and lactobacilli that potentially induce dental caries.

The role of *Veillonella* species and other anaerobic Gram-negative cocci in disease, if any, has not been clearly established, although they may be isolated from a variety of clinical conditions. In general, they are regarded as a minor component of mixed anaerobic

Table 36.6 Types of infection and clinical specimens from which anaerobic Gram-positive cocci are isolated

- Blood cultures
- Central nervous system (including brain abscesses)
- Head and neck infections (including ear)
- Dental abscesses and infected root canals
- Periodontal diseases and infected oral implants
- Human and animal bites
- Pleural infections
- Abdominal infections
- Genito-urinary tract infections
- Decubitus ulcers
- Foot ulcers
- Osteomyelitis

infections, and antimicrobial chemotherapy is not generally directed specifically against them.

NON-SPORING GRAM-POSITIVE RODS

The spore-forming genus *Clostridium* is well known for its involvement in serious infections (see Chapter 22). The role of non-sporing Gram-positive rods, on the other hand, is less well understood, although they are present in significant numbers in the normal flora of the mouth, skin, gastro-intestinal and female genito-urinary tracts, and are isolated from a variety of types of infections. The main genera and some of their characteristics are listed in Table 36.7. As with some other groups of anaerobes, the use of acid end-product analysis by gas–liquid chromatography is an important step in the identification of these bacteria.

Infections with Gram-positive rods

Any of these bacteria can occur as components of mixed anaerobic infections, and *Actinomyces* species can undoubtedly adopt a pathogenic role. Most cases of actinomycosis are caused by *Actinomyces israelii* and are cervicofacial, although the disease can also occur in

Table 36.7 Some characteristics of non-sporing Gram-positive rods

Genus	Sites commonly found	Acid end-products
Propionibacterium	Skin, mouth, gut, vagina	Propionic acid
Bifidobacterium	Gut, mouth, vagina	Acetic and lactic acids
Lactobacillus	Mouth, gut, vagina	Lactic acid (major end-product)
Actinomyces	Mouth, gut, vagina	Succinic, lactic and acetic acids
Eubacterium[a]	Mouth, gut, vagina	Butyric and other acids

[a] Taxonomy in need of revision; probably includes several different genera.

the thorax, abdomen and female genital tract (see Chapter 20). *Actinomyces* species are not themselves strict anaerobes, but *A. israelii* requires good anaerobic conditions for primary isolation, and plates should be incubated for 7–10 days.

Propionibacterium propionicus is morphologically and biochemically very similar to *A. israelii*. It is particularly associated with infection of the tear duct in the condition called *lachrymal canaliculitis*. The significance of other genera in infections is not clear. Some species are found in acne; they are also occasionally isolated in infective endocarditis and in infections associated with implanted prostheses. *Eubacterium* species (possibly mistaken for *Actinomyces* species in some reports) are a large group of up to 45 currently recognized species whose taxonomy is in need of revision. These bacteria may play a role in infections around intra-uterine devices; others may be involved in human periodontal disease, but further studies are required to confirm these observations. Similarly, there is only limited evidence for the pathogenicity of *Bifidobacterium* species, although *Bif. dentium* has been isolated occasionally from pulmonary infections.

SPIRAL-SHAPED, MOTILE ORGANISMS

Several *Treponema* species are found in the mouth and elsewhere in the body (see Table 36.1). They are thought to be an important component of the mixed anaerobic infection associated with acute necrotizing ulcerative gingivitis along with fusobacteria and *Prev. intermedia*, and may also contribute to other forms of periodontal disease. The proportion of motile spiral organisms seen by dark-ground microscopy in samples from the gingival pocket increases markedly when there is evidence of periodontal destruction.

Motile, spiral-shaped Gram-negative anaerobes of the genus *Anaerobiospirillum* have been isolated from patients with diarrhoea and from bacteraemia. Although comparatively rarely isolated from humans, they can cause serious infections. The distribution and normal habitat of this and other morphologically similar organisms are not well understood. In some cases the source of infection may be domestic animals and pets.

TREATMENT

In many infections caused by anaerobes the most important aspect of treatment is surgical. This often involves drainage of pus from abscesses, but may also include debridement, curettage and removal of necrotic tissue. For minor infections surgical drainage alone may be sufficient, but in many cases antimicrobial chemotherapy is also indicated. The main groups of agents used are the penicillins and the nitroimidazoles, particularly metronidazole. Other agents with good anti-anaerobe activity include chloramphenicol, clindamycin and cefoxitin, but resistant strains occur.

Metronidazole is effective against virtually all obligate anaerobes, including *Bacteroides, Porphyromonas, Prevotella* and *Fusobacterium* species, but not against facultatively anaerobic or microaerophilic bacteria such as actinomyces and streptococci. Resistance to metronidazole is still very uncommon.

Most anaerobic species are sensitive to benzylpenicillin, but members of the *B. fragilis* group are usually resistant. Such resistance is associated with β-lactamase production and these organisms are usually susceptible to combinations of penicillins with β-lactamase inhibitors (e.g. co-amoxiclav) and to carbapenems such as imipenem.

RECOMMENDED READING

Allaker R P, Young K A, Langlois T, de Rosayro R, Hardie J M 1997 Dental plaque flora of the dog with reference to fastidious and anaerobic bacteria associated with bites. *Journal of Veterinary Dentistry* 14: 127–130

Bolstad A I, Jensen H B, Bakken V 1996 Taxonomy, biology and periodontal aspects of *Fusobacterium nucleatum*. *Clinical Microbiology Reviews* 9: 55–71

Duerden B I, Drasar B S (eds) 1991 *Anaerobes in Human Disease*. Edward Arnold, London

Finegold S M, George W L (eds) 1989 *Anaerobic Infections in Humans*. Academic Press, San Diego

Johnson C C, Finegold S M 1987 Uncommonly encountered, motile, anaerobic gram-negative bacilli associated with infection. *Reviews of Infectious Disease* 9: 1150–1162

Murdoch D A 1998 Gram-positive anaerobic cocci. *Clinical Microbiology Reviews* 11: 81–120

Shah H N, Gharbia S E 1993 Ecophysiology and taxonomy of Bacteroides and related taxa. *Clinical Infectious Diseases* 16: 160–167

Skinner F A, Carr J G (eds) 1974 *The Normal Microbial Flora of Man*. Academic Press, London

37

Treponema and borrelia

Syphilis; yaws; relapsing fever; Lyme disease

A. Cockayne

Members of the genera *Treponema* and *Borrelia* are spirochaetes belonging to the family Spirochaetaceae.

DESCRIPTION

Spirochaetes are slender unicellular helical or spiral rods (Fig. 37.1) with a number of distinctive ultrastructural features used in the differentiation of the genera

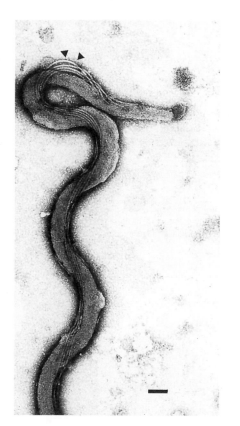

Fig. 37.1 Electron micrograph of *T. pallidum*. The flagella (▼) are inserted at the tip and follow the helical contour of the bacterial cell enclosed within the outer membrane. Bar, 0.1 μm. (Photograph courtesy of Professor C. W. Penn.)

(Fig. 37.2). The cytoplasm is surrounded by a cytoplasmic membrane and a peptidoglycan layer contributes to cell rigidity and shape. In *Treponema* species, fine cytoplasmic filaments are visible in the bacterial cytoplasm (Fig. 37.3), but these are absent in *Borrelia* species. Members of both genera are actively motile; several flagella are attached at each pole of the cell and wrap around the bacterial cell body. In contrast to other motile bacteria, these flagella do not protrude into the surrounding medium but are enclosed within the bacterial outer membrane. Treponemal flagella are complex, comprising a sheath and core (Fig. 37.4), whereas those of *Borrelia* species are simpler and similar to those of other bacteria. The spirochaetal outer membrane is unusually lipid-rich and, at least in some treponemes, appears to be protein-deficient and to lack lipopolysaccharide. This may account for the susceptibility of these organisms to killing by detergents and desiccation.

Although the treponemes are distantly related to Gram-negative bacteria they do not stain by Gram's method, and modified staining procedures are used. Moreover, the pathogenic treponemes cannot be cultivated in laboratory media and are maintained by subculture in susceptible animals. In contrast, borreliae stain Gram-negative, and many pathogenic species can be cultured in vitro in enriched, serum-containing media.

Importance as human pathogens

Human diseases caused by *Treponema* and *Borrelia* species (Table 37.1) include those such as syphilis that have been known for thousands of years, and infections such as Lyme disease, the prevalence and geographical distribution of which are still being evaluated.

Treponemal infections may be spread from person to person by intimate physical contact, contact with infectious body fluids or, in some instances, by fomites. The treponemes infecting man are obligate human parasites, and no other natural hosts are known. In contrast, borreliae are transmitted to man by the bites of infected ticks or lice. The borreliae that cause Lyme disease and endemic

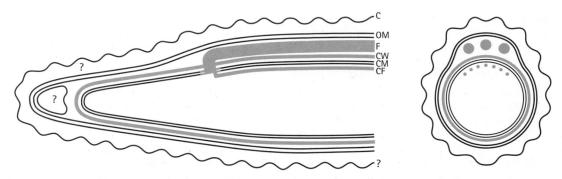

Fig. 37.2 Schematic representation of the structure of *T. pallidum* in longitudinal and cross-section: C, postulated capsular layer; OM, outer membrane; F, flagellum; CW, cell wall peptidoglycan; CM, cytoplasmic membrane; CF, Cytoplasmic filaments (absent in borreliae). Areas of uncertainty, indicated by question marks, concern the existence and form of the capsule, the continuity or otherwise of the outer membrane over the tip of the organism, the nature and form of the tip structure, and the exact juxtaposition of the ends of the cytoplasmic filaments with the bacterial flagellar basal bodies. (After Strugnell et al. 1990 *Critical Reviews in Microbiology* 17: 231–250.)

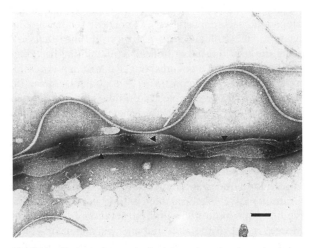

Fig. 37.3 Electron micrograph of a detergent- and protease-treated *T. pallidum* cell showing cytoplasmic filaments (▼) in the bacterial cytoplasm. Bar, 0.1 μm.

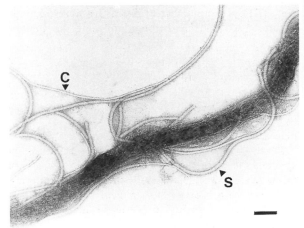

Fig. 37.4 Electron micrograph of a detergent-treated *T. pallidum* cell showing the complex structure of the treponemal flagellum. Both sheathed (S) flagella and the thinner flagellar cores (C) are visible. Bar, 0.1 μm.

Table 37.1 Principal human diseases caused by spirochaetes

Organism	Disease	Distribution	Primary mode of transmission	Animal reservoirs
T. pallidum	Syphilis	Worldwide	Sexual–congenital	None
T. endemicum	Bejel	Arid, subtropical or temperate areas	Mouth-to-mouth via utensils	None
T. carateum	Pinta	Arid, tropical Americas	Skin-to-skin contact	None
B. recurrentis	Epidemic relapsing fever	Central, East Africa; South American Andes	Louse bites	None
Borrelia spp.	Endemic relapsing fever	Worldwide[a]	Tick bites	Yes
B. burgdorferi sensu lato	Lyme disease	Worldwide[a]	Tick bites	Yes

[a] Distribution governed by presence of tick vectors.

relapsing fever also infect many other animal species, which act as reservoirs of infection; man is an unfortunate incidental host in the natural history of these pathogens.

Characteristically, treponemal and borrelial infections occur in several distinct clinical stages. These may be separated by periods of remission, and each stage may have a particular associated pathology. Commonly the causative organism is detectable in early lesions but is much more difficult to identify in later disease. The pathogen spreads from the initial site of infection to many organs via the bloodstream, and in some untreated cases these infections may be progressive, destructive and, in some instances (e.g. tertiary syphilis), may be fatal. In other cases, however, only the early symptoms are apparent and the later pathology is not seen.

Antigenic variation contributes to bacterial virulence for the relapsing fever borreliae but in general the pathogenic mechanisms employed by spirochaetes are poorly understood. No extracellular toxins have yet been identified, and the mechanisms that enable these organisms to persist in tissues despite vigorous immune responses remain unclear. In common with other *Borrelia* spp., *B. burgdorferi* may vary its surface lipoproteins to avoid the immune system. The paucity of exposed, antigenic proteins – so-called '*T. pallidum* rare outer membrane proteins' – on the surface of *T. pallidum* may contribute to immune evasion. It also seems likely that the later manifestations of the treponemal infections may involve auto-immune phenomena.

In addition to the pathogenic species, many other spirochaetes form part of the normal bacterial flora of the mouth, gut and genital tract. Morphological and antigenic similarities between pathogenic and commensal spirochaetes may cause problems in the clinical and serological diagnosis.

TREPONEMA

Treponema species pathogenic for man include:

- the causative agents of venereal *syphilis*
- the non-venereal treponematoses *yaws*, *bejel* and *pinta*.

The spirochaetes causing these different infections are micro-aerobic and morphologically identical – tightly coiled helical rods, 5–15 μm long and 0.1–0.5 μm diameter. They show only subtle antigenic differences and are characterized primarily by the clinical syndromes they cause and minor differences in the pathology induced in experimental animals.

Treponema pallidum ssp. pallidum (T. pallidium)

Treponema pallidum is the causative agent of syphilis,

and was first isolated from syphilitic lesions in 1905. Infection is usually acquired by sexual contact with infected individuals, and is commonest in the most sexually active age group of 15–30-year-olds. *Congenital syphilis* usually occurs following vertical transmission of *T. pallidum* from the infected mother to the fetus in utero, but neonates may also be infected during passage through the infected birth canal at delivery. Infection in utero may have serious consequences for the fetus. Rarely, syphilis has been acquired by transfusion of infected fresh human blood.

Pathogenesis

Untreated syphilis may be a progressive disease with *primary, secondary, latent* and *tertiary* stages. *T. pallidum* enters tissues by penetration of intact mucosae or through abraded skin.

The bacterium rapidly enters the lymphatics, is widely disseminated via the bloodstream and may lodge in any organ. The exact infectious dose for man is not known, but in experimental animals fewer than 10 organisms are sufficient to initiate infection. The bacteria multiply at the initial entry site, and a *chancre*, a lesion characteristic of primary syphilis, forms after an average incubation period of 3 weeks. The chancre is painless and most frequently on the external genitalia, but it may occur on the cervix, peri-anal area, in the mouth or anal canal. Chancres usually occur singly, but in immunocompromised individuals, such as those infected with the human immunodeficiency virus (HIV), multiple or persistent chancres may develop. The chancre usually heals spontaneously within 3–6 weeks, and 2–12 weeks later the symptoms of secondary syphilis develop. These are highly variable and widespread but most commonly involve the skin where macular or pustular lesions develop, particularly on the trunk and extremities. The lesions of secondary syphilis are highly infectious.

These lesions gradually resolve and a period of latent infection is entered, in which no clinical manifestations are evident, but serological evidence of infection persists. Relapse of the lesions of secondary syphilis is common, and latent syphilis is classified as early (high likelihood of relapse) or late (recurrence unlikely). Individuals with late latent syphilis are not generally considered infectious, but may still transmit infection to the fetus during pregnancy and their blood may remain infectious.

Late or tertiary syphilis, which may develop decades after the primary infection, is a slowly progressive, destructive inflammatory disease that may affect any organ. The three most common forms of late syphilis are *neurosyphilis, cardiovascular syphilis* and *gummatous syphilis* – a rare granulomatous lesion of the skeleton, skin or mucocutaneous tissues. Isolation of *T. pallidum* from patients with late syphilis is usually impossible, and much of the observed pathology may be due to auto-immune phenomena.

Treponema pallidum ssp. pertenue (T. pertenue)

T. pertenue is the causative agent of *yaws*, a disease that is endemic among rural populations in tropical and subtropical countries such as Africa, South America, Southeast Asia and Oceania. The number of cases of yaws worldwide was estimated at over 50 million in the 1950s, but eradication programmes sponsored by the World Health Organization reduced the number of cases to less than 2 million in the 1970s. Termination of these programmes has led to a resurgence of pockets of disease, particularly in West Africa.

Infection with *T. pertenue* is non-venereal, and occurs following contact of traumatized skin with exudate from early yaws lesions. Infection is usually acquired before puberty. Primary yaws has an incubation period of 3–5 weeks, and the initial lesions usually occur on the legs. The papular lesions enlarge, erode and usually heal spontaneously within 6 months. Eruption of similar lesions occurs weeks to months later, and relapse is common. Secondary lesions may involve bones, particularly the fingers, long bones and the jaw. Late yaws is characterized by cutaneous plaques and ulcers and thickening of the skin on the palms and soles of the feet. Gummatous lesions may also develop. In contrast to syphilis, neurological and cardiovascular damage does not occur in late yaws. As affected individuals acquire infection early in life, they are essentially non-infectious at childbearing age, and congenital yaws is unknown.

Treponema pallidum ssp. endemicum (T. endemicum)

This organism causes a non-venereal, syphilis-like disease called *endemic syphilis* or *bejel*. Bejel is endemic in Africa, western Asia and Australia, and mainly affects children in rural populations where living conditions and personal hygiene are poor. Transmission is by direct person-to-person contact and by sharing of contaminated eating or drinking utensils.

The initial lesion is usually oral and may not be detected. Secondary lesions include oropharyngeal mucous patches, condyloma lata and periostitis. Late lesions involve gummata in the skin, nasopharynx and bones. As in yaws, the cardiovascular and central nervous systems are not involved, and congenital infection is rare because of the early age of infection.

Treponema carateum

Unlike the other treponematoses, the manifestations of *pinta*, caused by *T. carateum*, are confined to the skin. Although these lesions are non-destructive, they cause disfigurement with associated social problems for infected individuals. Pinta is probably the oldest human treponemal infection, with distribution today being restricted to arid rural inland regions of Mexico, Central America and Colombia.

Spread of infection is by direct contact with infectious lesions. After a 7–21-day incubation period, small, erythematous pruritic primary lesions develop, most commonly on the extremities, face, neck, chest or abdomen. The primary lesions enlarge and coalesce, and once healed may leave areas of hypopigmentation. Disseminated secondary lesions appear 3–12 months later and may become dyschromic. Recurrence of lesions is common up to 10 years after the initial infection. The depigmented lesions are characteristic of the later stages of pinta but do not cause any serious harm.

Other infections

There are several other human infections in which treponemes are implicated. Commonly, the microbial flora associated with these conditions is complex, and the exact role of the spirochaetes in the aetiology of infection remains to be determined. Moreover, the true taxonomic status of some of these organisms is uncertain.

Oral infections

T. denticola, *T. socranskii* and *T. pectinovorum* form part of the normal flora, and numbers of these organisms increase in acute necrotizing ulcerative gingivitis and chronic adult periodontal disease. *T. vincentii* (or Vincent's spirillum) is similarly associated with ulceromembranous gingivitis or pharyngitis, *Vincent's angina*. Several spirochaetes appear to be involved in the aetiology of a similar condition called *trench mouth*.

Gastro-intestinal infections

Several as yet unidentified weakly haemolytic spirochaetes have been implicated in the aetiology of persistent diarrhoea and rectal bleeding in certain human populations. A morphologically similar but genetically distinct organism, *Brachyspira* (formerly *Serpulina*) *hyodysenteriae*, is the cause of swine dysentery.

Skin lesions

Tropical ulcer is a chronic skin condition in which spirochaetes of unknown identity have been implicated, usually in association with fusiform bacteria (p. 339) and other organisms.

LABORATORY DIAGNOSIS

The inability to grow most pathogenic treponemes in vitro, coupled with the transitory nature of many of the lesions, makes diagnosis of treponemal infection impossible by routine bacteriological methods. Although spirochaetes are detectable by microscopy in primary and secondary lesions, diagnosis is based primarily on clinical observations and is confirmed by serological tests. For practical purposes, the serological responses to all these pathogens are identical, and only their use in the serodiagnosis of syphilis will be considered here.

Direct microscopy

Treponemes can be visualized directly in freshly collected exudate from primary or secondary lesions by dark-ground or phase-contrast microscopy. Although this method allows a rapid definitive diagnosis to be made, it may be rather insensitive because primary lesions may contain relatively few bacteria. In addition, care must be taken to differentiate between pathogenic and commensal spirochaetes that may occasionally contaminate such material. More sensitive and specific results may be obtained using fixed material in an immunofluorescence assay with an anti-treponemal antibody.

Serological tests

Infection with *T. pallidum* results in the rapid production of two types of antibodies:

- Specific antibodies directed primarily at polypeptide antigens of the bacterium.
- Non-specific antibodies (reagin antibodies) that react with a non-treponemal antigen called *cardiolipin*.

The mechanism of induction of non-specific antibodies remains unclear. Cardiolipin is a phospholipid extracted from beef heart, and it is possible that a similar substance, present in the treponemal cell or released from host cells damaged by the bacterium, may stimulate antibody production.

Assays for non-specific antibody, because of their low cost and technical simplicity, have routinely been used as screening tests for evidence of syphilis. Since these tests have relatively low specificity, positive results are confirmed by detection of specific anti-*T. pallidum* antibody.

Non-specific serological tests for syphilis

The *Venereal Disease Research Laboratory* (VDRL) test is a non-specific serological test for syphilis which uses a mixture of cardiolipin, cholesterol and lecithin as antigen. IgM or IgG antibody present in positive sera or in cerebrospinal fluid from patients with neurosyphilis causes a suspension of this lipoidal antigen to flocculate, and the result can be rapidly read by eye. This is used as a screening test, and is positive in approximately 70% of primary and 99% of secondary syphilitics, but is negative in individuals with late syphilis. The test can be used quantitatively, and increases in VDRL titre with time may be used to confirm a diagnosis of congenital syphilis.

Since a positive result in the VDRL test usually indicates active infection, it can also be used to monitor the efficacy of antibacterial therapy.

Another non-specific test, the *rapid plasma reagin* (RPR) test, also uses cardiolipin as antigen, but is not suitable for use with cerebrospinal fluid.

Tests for specific antibody

Fluorescent treponemal antibody-absorption (FTA-Abs) test. This is an indirect immunofluorescence assay in which *T. pallidum* is used as an antigen. Acetone-fixed treponemes are incubated with heat-treated sera, and bound antibody is detected with a fluorescein-labelled conjugate and ultraviolet microscopy. The serum is first absorbed with a suspension of a non-pathogenic treponeme, which removes non-specific cross-reactive antibodies that may be directed against commensal spirochaetes. The FTA-Abs test is positive in approximately 80, 100 and 95% of primary, secondary and late syphilitics, respectively, and, unlike the VDRL test, remains positive following successful therapy.

T. pallidum haemagglutination assay (TPHA). In this test, *T. pallidum* antigen is coated onto the surface of red blood cells, and specific antibody in test sera causes haemagglutination. As in the FTA-Abs assay, sera are pre-absorbed with a non-pathogenic treponeme to remove antibody against commensal spirochaetes. The TPHA is less sensitive than the FTA-Abs in primary syphilis (positive in 65%), but both give similar results for secondary and late syphilis; the TPHA also remains positive for life following infection. This assay can be used to detect localized production of anti-treponemal antibodies in cerebrospinal fluid, a marker of neurosyphilis.

Other antibody tests. Production of monoclonal anti-*T. pallidum* antibodies has permitted development of assay systems based on the detection of antibody responses to individual treponemal antigens. Such assays use enzyme-linked immunosorbent assay (ELISA) technology, allowing rapid screening of large numbers of samples with potentially enhanced specificity. Assays that detect either IgM or IgG are available and are increasingly replacing the TPHA and VDRL tests for routine screening. Positive results in ELISA assays should be confirmed by a second specific test such as the TPHA.

Problems in the serological diagnosis of syphilis

Occasionally, both the non-specific and specific tests produce false-positive results. The VDRL assay may give a transient positive result following any strong immunological stimulus such as acute bacterial or viral infection or after immunization. More persistent false-positive results occur in individuals with auto-immune or connective tissue disease, in drug abusers and in individuals with hypergammaglobulinaemia. False-positive results usually become apparent when negative results are found in specific serological tests, but in some cases FTA-Abs results may also be positive or borderline.

Rarely, the FTA-Abs test may be positive and the non-specific VDRL test negative. Lyme disease (see below) induces antibodies that react in the FTA-Abs but not in the VDRL assay. Other spirochaetal diseases such as relapsing fever, yaws, pinta and leptospirosis may give positive results in both specific and non-specific tests. Of particular difficulty is the differential diagnosis of syphilis and yaws in immigrants from areas in which yaws is endemic.

Direct detection of spirochaetal DNA in clinical material by molecular methods, such as the polymerase chain reaction, may have a future role in confirming a diagnosis of syphilis in difficult or atypical cases.

TREATMENT

All the pathogenic treponemes are sensitive to benzylpenicillin, and prolonged high-dose therapy with procaine penicillin has been the traditional method of treatment for primary and secondary syphilis. So far there have been no reports of penicillin resistance. If penicillin allergy is a problem, erythromycin, tetracycline or chloramphenicol may be used. There are reports of treatment failure with erythromycin, and an erythromycin-resistant variant of *T. pallidum* has been isolated. In late syphilis, aqueous benzylpenicillin is used, as this penetrates better into the central nervous system.

In neurosyphilis, successful eradication of the organism may not result in a clinical cure. More aggressive and prolonged antibiotic therapy may be required in HIV patients with syphilis due to impairment of immune function.

Antibiotic therapy of syphilitics, particularly with penicillin, characteristically induces a systemic response called the *Jarisch-Herxheimer reaction*. This is characterized by the rapid onset (within 2 h) of fever, chills, myalgia, tachycardia, hyperventilation, vasodilatation and hypotension. The response is thought to be due to release of an endogenous pyrogen from the spirochaetes.

EPIDEMIOLOGY AND CONTROL

Syphilis

The incidence of all venereal diseases, including syphilis, increased dramatically during the Second World War. The widespread introduction of antibiotic therapy shortly afterwards produced an equally dramatic decrease in the incidence of these diseases, but syphilis remained endemic within the general population.

Until the mid-1980s most cases of syphilis in developed countries occurred in male homosexuals. The advent of HIV and the acquired immune deficiency syndrome (AIDS) in the 1980s reduced the incidence among this group owing to changes in sexual practices. The early 1990s saw a resurgence of syphilis among the heterosexual population in the USA, resulting in an increase in the incidence among women and in the number of cases of congenital syphilis. Subsequent changes in sexual practices among homosexual males have reversed this trend: 50% more cases of primary and secondary syphilis now occur in men than women, while the incidence of congenital syphilis fell from 2000 cases in 1994 to 800 in 1998. Total numbers of cases of syphilis in the USA also fell dramatically from 81 000 to 38 000 over this time period. About 80% of cases of primary and secondary syphilis in the USA now occur in African Americans, probably reflecting differences in poverty levels, access to health care and education facilities among different ethnic groups.

Although the incidence of all forms of syphilis in the UK is currently very low (500–1000 cases reported per year), the disease still has major public health implications. In particular, the possibility of congenital infection and the acquisition of syphilis by blood transfusion necessitate large and costly screening programmes of all pregnant women and blood donations.

Control of syphilis is achieved by treating index cases and any known contacts. Treatment of contacts is important as some may be incubating the infection even if they have no overt signs of disease.

Control of the disease may have additional benefits: primary syphilis increases the risk of HIV infection two- to five-fold, presumably by permitting easier access of the virus through damaged skin or mucosal membranes.

Other treponematoses

The incidence of the other treponematoses is primarily influenced by socio-economic factors. Prevention and control involve treatment of individuals with active or latent disease and contacts, and improvement of living conditions and personal hygiene.

BORRELIA

The two principal human diseases associated with borre- liae are *relapsing fever*, caused by *Borrelia recurrentis* and several other *Borrelia* species, and *Lyme disease* or *Lyme borreliosis*, a multisystem infection caused by *B. burgdorferi* sensu lato. The bacteria causing these infections are morphologically similar helical rods, 8–30 μm long and 0.2–0.5 μm in diameter, with 3–10 loose spirals. Antigenic and genetic differences are used to differentiate the species.

RELAPSING FEVERS

Relapsing fevers are characterized clinically by recurrent periods of fever and spirochaetaemia.

Endemic or *tick-borne relapsing fever* is caused by several *Borrelia* species, including *B. duttoni*, *B. hermsii*, *B. parkeri* and *B. turicatae*, and is transmit- ted to humans by soft-bodied *Ornithodorus* ticks. The natural hosts for these organisms include rodents and other small mammals on which the ticks normally feed. The disease occurs worldwide, reflecting the distribution of the tick vector.

Epidemic or *louse-borne relapsing fever* is caused by *B. recurrentis*, an obligate human pathogen transmitted from person to person by the body louse, *Pediculus humanus*. The incidence is influenced by socio-eco- nomic factors such as lack of personal hygiene, and, his- torically, increases during periods of war, famine and other social upheaval. The disease still occurs in central and eastern Africa and in the South American Andes.

The spirochaetes causing the two forms of relapsing fever differ in their mode of growth in the arthropod vector, and this influences the way human infection is initiated. *B. recurrentis* grows in the haemolymph of the louse but does not invade tissues. As a result the excre- ment of the louse is non-infectious and the bacterium is not transferred transovarially to the progeny. Human infection occurs when bacteria released from crushed lice gain entry to tissues through damaged or intact skin, or mucous membranes. Spirochaetes causing tick-borne relapsing fever invade all the tissues of the tick, includ- ing the salivary glands, genitalia and excretory system. Infection therefore occurs when saliva or excrement is released during feeding. Transovarial transmission to the tick progeny maintains the spirochaete in the tick population.

Pathogenesis of relapsing fever

In both forms of relapsing fever, acute symptoms, including high fever, rigors, headache, myalgia, arthral- gia, photophobia and cough, develop about 1 week after infection. A skin rash may occur, and there is central nervous system involvement in up to 30% of cases. During the acute phase there may be up to 10^5 spirochaetes per cubic millimetre of blood. The primary illness resolves within 3–6 days, and terminates abruptly with hypotension and shock, which may be fatal. Relapse of fever occurs 7–10 days later, and several relapses may take place.

Each episode of spirochaetaemia is terminated by the development of specific anti-spirochaete antibody. Subsequent febrile episodes are caused by borreliae that differ antigenically, particularly in outer membrane protein composition, from those causing earlier attacks. As the cycle of fever and relapse continues, the borreliae tend to revert back to the antigenic types that caused the original spirochaetaemia, and ultimate clearance of the infection appears to be due to antibody-mediated killing.

In general, louse-borne relapsing fever has longer febrile and afebrile periods than tick-borne infection, but fewer relapses. The case fatality rate varies from 4–40% for louse-borne infection and from 2–5% for tick-borne relapsing fever, with myocarditis, cerebral haemorrhage and liver failure the most common causes of death.

Laboratory diagnosis

Definitive diagnosis of relapsing fevers is made by detection of borreliae in peripheral blood samples. Thick or thin blood smears may be stained with Giemsa, or other stains such as acridine orange.

Although antibodies to the borreliae are produced during infection, serological tests are complicated by anti- genic variation and the tendency to relapse. Serological tests for syphilis are positive in 5–10% of cases.

Treatment

Tetracycline, chloramphenicol, penicillin and ery- thromycin have been used successfully. As in the treatment of syphilis, a Jarisch-Herxheimer reaction is produced following administration of antibiotics.

Prevention of infection involves avoidance or eradication of the insect vector. Insecticides can be used to eradicate ticks from human dwellings, but elimination from the environment is not feasible. Prevention of louse-borne infection involves maintenance of good personal hygiene, and delousing if necessary.

LYME DISEASE

Lyme disease, originally called *Lyme arthritis*, was recognized as an infectious condition in 1975, following an epidemiological investigation of a cluster of cases of suspected juvenile rheumatoid arthritis which occurred in Lyme, Connecticut, USA. A common factor in these cases was a previous history of insect bite, and the infectious agent, *B. burgdorferi*, was subsequently isolated from an *Ixodes* tick. Retrospective serological data suggest that Lyme disease was endemic in the USA as early as 1962, and the clinical manifestations of this infection have been known in Europe, including the UK, since the early 1900s. Lyme disease has also been reported in Scandinavia, eastern Europe, China, Japan and Australia.

The natural hosts for *B. burgdorferi* are wild and domesticated animals, including mice and other rodents, deer, sheep, cattle, horses and dogs. The larger animal hosts such as deer are probably more important in maintaining the size of tick populations rather than acting as a major source of *B. burgdorferi*. Infection in these animals may be inapparent, though clinical infection has been observed in cattle, horses and dogs.

B. burgdorferi is transmitted to man by ixodid ticks that become infected while feeding on infected animals. The principal vectors in the USA are *Ixodes dammini* and *I. pacificus*, and in Europe, *I. ricinus*. The life cycle of these ticks involves larval, nymph and adult stages, all of which are capable of transmitting infection, though the nymphal stage is most commonly implicated. In areas endemic for Lyme disease, 2–50% of ticks may carry *B. burgdorferi*. The bacterium grows primarily in the midgut of the tick, and transmission to man occurs during regurgitation of the gut contents during the blood meal. Transmission efficiency appears to be relatively low, but increases with the duration of feeding.

Although there is general similarity, clinical manifestations may differ in the USA and Europe. This variation is due in part to significant differences in the bacterial strains causing infection in the two continents, and has resulted in the division of *B. burgdorferi* into three distinct genospecies:

- *B. burgdorferi* sensu stricto is the principal organism isolated in the USA where Lyme arthritis is a common complication of infection.
- *B. afzeli* and *B. garinii* are more commonly isolated in Europe but not in the USA, and are associated with chronic skin and neurological symptoms of Lyme disease, respectively.

Several other genetically distinct isolates of *B. burgdorferi* have been identified in ticks, but their importance in human infection has yet to be established.

Lyme disease may be a progressive illness, and is divided into three stages:

- *Stage 1* is characterized by a spreading annular rash, *erythema chronicum migrans* (ECM), which occurs at the site of the tick bite 3–22 days after infection. Lesions may contain very small numbers of bacteria, and the disproportionate intensity of the pathology seen may be due to stimulation of cytokine production such as tumour necrosis factor-α, and secondary mediators. The bacterium also disseminates to a variety of other organs. In the USA, secondary lesions similar to those of ECM are common. Malaise, fatigue, headache, rigors and neck stiffness may also be apparent. ECM and secondary lesions fade within 3–4 weeks.
- *Stage 2* develops in some patients after several weeks or months. These patients exhibit cardiac or neurological abnormalities, musculoskeletal symptoms or intermittent arthritis.
- *Stage 3* may ensue months to years later, when patients present with chronic skin, nervous system or joint abnormalities.

Congenital infection may occur with serious, potentially fatal, consequences for the fetus.

Laboratory diagnosis

Once a clinical diagnosis has been made, culture of the spirochaete from suitable biopsy material provides a definitive diagnosis, but this is a lengthy, specialized technique that is not widely available. In addition, the difficulty encountered in detecting the organism in histological sections means that serological tests are routinely used for the confirmation of Lyme disease although polymerase chain reaction (PCR) techniques have been used in some laboratories.

Specific IgM antibodies develop within 3–6 weeks of infection. The earliest response appears to be against the bacterial flagellum and later against outer surface proteins. Subsequently, IgG antibodies are produced, and the highest titre is detectable months or years after infection.

An indirect immunofluorescence test is available, but ELISA is now widely used. Immunoblotting has been proposed as a method of confirming serological diagnosis. Serological diagnosis of early Lyme disease may still pose problems, as in some individuals antibodies to the bacterium are slow to develop and formation of immune complexes may affect the test results. Antibodies that cross-react with *B. burgdorferi* may be produced after infection with other spirochaetes, and sera from Lyme disease patients may give a positive FTA-Abs test, though the VDRL test is negative.

Serological evidence of infection may be detectable in the apparent absence of overt disease. The significance of these findings is unclear but it is possible that such individuals may develop late complications of Lyme disease.

Treatment

Penicillins, the newer macrolides, cephalosporins and tetracyclines have all been used successfully in Lyme disease. Reports suggest that treatment with tetracyclines produces fewer late complications than penicillin therapy. About 15% of patients experience a Jarisch-Herxheimer reaction after antibiotic therapy. Despite antibiotic treatment, some patients suffer from minor late complications of the disease, which may be immunologically mediated or may indicate low-level persistence of the organisms.

Antibiotic therapy may reduce or abolish the antibody response, and this may interfere with the serological confirmation of infection.

Epidemiology and control

The geographical distribution of Lyme disease is governed by that of the tick vector and its associated animal hosts. Forestry workers and farmers are particularly at risk, but infection is also associated with recreational activities. In the UK, Lyme disease occurs in areas that support large populations of wild or domesticated animals on which ixodid ticks feed. Infection may also be acquired after travel to countries where Lyme disease is endemic. It is difficult to assess accurately the true incidence of Lyme disease in the UK since infection may be mild or asymptomatic and consequently not detected. In 1998, 16 800 cases were reported in the USA.

Prevention of infection involves avoidance of endemic areas and education of the public regarding the possible risks of infection in these localities. Eradication of the tick vectors or mammalian hosts from such areas is not feasible. Recombinant vaccines based on the *B. burgdorferi* outer surface proteins OspA and OspC are being tested in human clinical trials and, if successful, could be used to protect residents and visitors in areas in which Lyme disease is endemic.

RECOMMENDED READING

Barbour A G 1990 Antigenic variation of a relapsing fever *Borrelia* species. *Annual Review of Microbiology* 44: 155–171

Egglestone S I, Turner A J 2000 Serological diagnosis of syphilis: PHLS Syphilis Serology Working Group. *Communicable Disease and Public Health* 3: 158–162

Genc M, Ledger W J 2000 Syphilis in pregnancy. *Sexually Transmitted Infections* 76: 73–79

Guy E C 1993 The laboratory diagnosis of Lyme borreliosis. *Reviews in Medical Microbiology* 4: 89–96

Holt S C 1978 Anatomy and chemistry of spirochetes. *Microbiological Reviews* 42: 114–160

Hudson M J 1991 The spirochaetes. In: Duerden B I, Drasar B S (eds) *Anaerobes in Human Disease.* Edward Arnold, London, pp 108–132

Larsen S A, Steiner B M, Rudolph A H 1995 Laboratory diagnosis and interpretation of tests for syphilis. *Clinical Microbiology Reviews* 8: 1–21

O'Connell S 1995 Lyme disease in the United Kingdom. *British Medical Journal* 310: 303–308

Schell R F, Musher D M (eds) 1983 *Pathogenesis and Immunology of Treponemal infections.* Marcel Decker, New York

Shapiro E D, Gerber M A 2000 Lyme Disease. *Clinical Infectious Diseases* 31: 533–542

Szczepanski A, Benach J L 1991 Lyme borreliosis: host responses to *Borrelia burgdorferi. Microbiological Reviews* 55: 21–34

38

Leptospira

Leptospirosis; Weil's disease

T. J. Coleman

The recognition of human leptospirosis as a distinct clinical entity is usually attributed to Adolf Weil of the University of Heidelberg in 1886, although the disease had been described in animals since the mid 19th century. The term *Weil's disease* acknowledges Weil's observations in differentiating what was later proven to be a leptospiral infection from other forms of infective jaundice.

In 1914, Ryokichi Inada and his colleagues in Kyushu, Japan, observed spiral organisms in the livers of guinea-pigs inoculated with blood taken from Japanese miners with infectious jaundice, presumed to be Weil's disease. They named the organisms *Spirochaeta icterohaemorrhagiae*, reflecting their spiral shape and the fact that they caused jaundice (icterus) and haemorrhage. In Europe, similar organisms were demonstrated in some cases of jaundice in German soldiers involved in the First World War. In 1917, another Japanese scientist, Hideyo Noguchi, in a careful study of the structure of the spirochaetes, proposed the genus name *Leptospira*, meaning a 'slender coil'.

Leptospires can be subdivided broadly into two groups:

- those thought to be harmless to animals and man
- those capable of causing the disease, *leptospirosis*.

More than 200 different pathogenic strains, referred to as *serovars*, are currently recognized.

Leptospirosis is a zoonosis and has one of the widest geographical distributions of any zoonotic disease. The highest incidence is in tropical and subtropical parts of the world. Every mammal probably has the potential to become a carrier of some serovar of leptospira. These carriers harbour leptospires in their kidneys and excrete the bacteria into the environment when they urinate. This enables spread among their own kind and to other species, including man, who may directly or indirectly come into contact with their urine.

The disease varies in severity from a mild, self-limiting illness to the fulminating and potentially fatal disease described by Weil. Fortunately, full recovery without long-term morbidity is the most frequent outcome.

DESCRIPTION

Classification

The family Leptospiraceae belongs to the order Spirochaetales and can be subdivided into three morphologically indistinguishable genera: *Leptospira*, *Leptonema* and *Turneria*. Only *Leptospira* spp. are considered to be pathogenic for animals or man.

For practical purposes leptospires can be divided into two species:

- *Leptospira interrogans* comprises the parasitic and pathogenic leptospires.
- *L. biflexa* contains all strains that are found in the environment but cause no disease. Unlike *L. interrogans* they can grow at low ambient temperatures (11–13°C).

L. interrogans is further divided into 23 serogroups, which, in turn, can be split into over 200 serovars based on differences in the outer protein envelope of the bacteria. Similarly, *L. biflexa* can be subdivided into 38 serogroups containing more than 60 serovars.

The accepted nomenclature is generic name followed by species name followed by serovar followed by strain (if appropriate). For example:

- *Leptospira* (generic name) *interrogans* (species name), serovar *icterohaemorrhagiae*
- *Leptospira* (generic name) *interrogans* (species name), serovar *hardjo*, strain hardjoprajitno.

For simplicity the names are often abbreviated to genus and serovar only, so that the examples given are shortened to *L. icterohaemorrhagiae* and *L. hardjo*, respectively.

The organism

Leptospires are about 6–20 μm long, but only about 0.1 μm in diameter, which allows them to pass through filters that retain most other bacteria. They are

Gram-negative, but take up conventional stains poorly. They can be visualized by Giemsa or silver deposition methods or by use of fluorescent antibody. However, they are best viewed by dark-ground or electron microscopy: usually one or both ends appear hooked and they rotate rapidly around their long axis. They have many closely set primary coils that are often difficult to see in living bacteria (Fig. 38.1).

An envelope composed of 3–5 layers of protein, polysaccharide and lipid covers the bacteria and is the main target for the host immune response. Within the outer sheath is the protoplasmic cylinder, bounded by a cell membrane and cell wall (Fig. 38.2). Leptospires have two flagella with their free ends towards the middle of the bacteria. They lie in the periplasmic space between the cell wall and the outer envelope and are wrapped around the cell wall. Each flagellum is attached to a basal body located at either end of the cell. The flagella are similar in structure to those of other bacteria and are responsible for the motility of the leptospires, but the mechanism for their rapid movement is still incompletely understood.

Leptospires are killed rapidly by desiccation, extremes of pH (e.g. gastric acid) and by antibacterial substances that occur naturally in human and bovine milks. They are susceptible to low concentrations of chlorine and are easily killed by temperatures above 40°C. They are killed after about 10 min at 50°C and within 10 s at 60°C.

Metabolism

Leptospires require aerobic or micro-aerophilic conditions for growth. Adequate sources of nitrogen, phosphate, calcium, magnesium and iron (as a haem compound or ferric ions) are essential. They can use fatty acids as their major energy source, but they are unable to synthesize long-chain fatty acids with 15 or more carbon atoms. Members of the interrogans group require the presence of unsaturated fatty acids to utilize saturated fatty acids. Vitamins B_1 (thiamin) and B_{12} (cyanocobalamin) are also required and the addition of biotin is needed for the growth of some strains. These

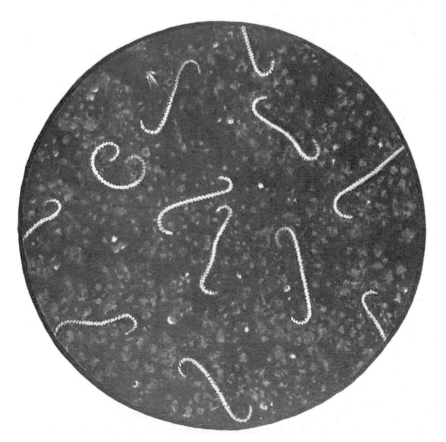

Fig. 38.1 The appearance of living leptospires as seen by dark-ground microscopy. Note the very fine coils and characteristic hooked ends. (From an original painting by Dr Cranston Low, in Low & Dodds 1947 *Atlas of Bacteriology*. Livingstone, Edinburgh.)

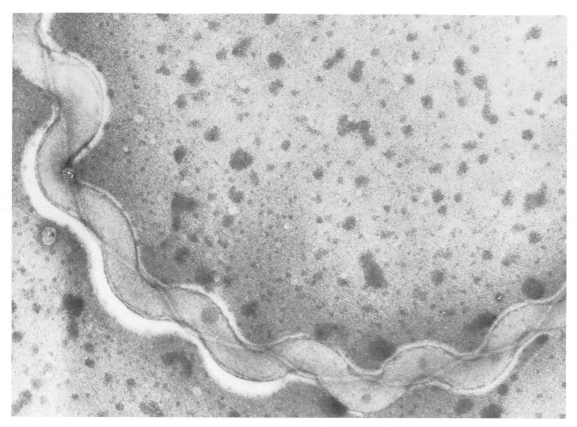

Fig. 38.2 Part of an intact leptospire, showing the protoplasmic cylinder, cell wall, outer envelope and axial filaments (transmission electron micrograph).

components are provided in Ellinghausen–McCullough–Johnson–Harris medium.

Optimal growth of pathogenic species in culture takes place at 28–30°C at pH 7.2–7.6 in media supplemented with 0.1% agar to enhance primary isolation. Growth is often slow, with periods of 3–4 weeks required after inoculation. Since the culture media does not generally contain selective agents, great care must be taken to avoid bacterial or fungal contamination at the time of inoculation of the media and during the prolonged incubation period.

PATHOGENESIS

The pathogenesis of leptospirosis is incompletely understood, but a vasculitis resulting in damage to the endothelial cells of small blood vessels is probably the main underlying pathology.

Infection is acquired by direct or indirect contact with infected urine, tissues or secretions. Ingestion or inhalation of leptospires does not pose a risk and human-to-

human spread is very rare. Leptospires generally gain entry through small areas of damage on the skin or via mucous membranes. It is possible that they may also pass through waterlogged skin, although this is probably not a major route of infection.

The term 'leptospirosis' should be used to describe all infections in both man and animals, regardless of the clinical presentation or strain of *Leptospira* involved. In the past many names (e.g. epidemic pulmonary haemorrhagic fever, cane cutter's disease, Fort Bragg fever, Weil's disease, autumnal fever, etc.) were used to describe the particular clinical presentation or to reflect occupational, geographical, seasonal or other epidemiological features of leptospiral disease. Because of this, the full range of disease presentations was not appreciated and, even now, leptospiral infection may not be suspected unless the patient has the classically severe disease involving the liver and kidneys originally described by Weil. There are no serovar-specific disease patterns although some serovars tend to cause more severe disease than others. There have been reports suggesting that human infection with some serovars can, in rare cases, cause abortion.

Clinical features

Typically, acute symptoms develop 7–12 days after infection although rarely the incubation period can be as short as 2–3 days or as long as 30 days. The infection presents with an influenza-like illness characterized by the sudden onset of headache, muscle pain, especially in the muscles of the lower back and calf, fever and occasionally rigors. Conjunctival suffusion and a skin rash may be seen in some cases.

During a bacteraemic phase lasting 7–8 days after the onset of symptoms, the leptospires spread via the blood to many tissues, including the brain. In severe cases the illness often follows a biphasic course: the bacteraemic phase is followed by an 'immune' phase, with the appearance of antibody and the disappearance of recoverable leptospires from the blood. In this phase patients may show signs of recovery for a couple of days before the fever, rigors, severe headaches and meningism return. Bleeding may occur, together with signs and symptoms of jaundice and renal impairment. Typically, bilirubin concentrations are markedly raised, but other liver function tests are often only moderately elevated.

In severe, fulminating disease the patient may die within the first few days of illness, but with adequate treatment the prognosis is usually good. Many deaths throughout the world are due to the failure to provide adequate supportive management, especially in relation to the maintenance of renal function. Generally, patients are well within 2–6 weeks but some will require up to 3 months to recover fully. In a few patients, symptoms persist for many months but neither long-term carriage of leptospires nor chronic disease has been conclusively demonstrated in man.

After infection, immunity develops against the infecting strain, but may not fully protect against infection with unrelated strains.

LABORATORY DIAGNOSIS

The initial diagnosis must rely on the medical history and clinical findings backed up with details of possible occupational or recreational exposure. The assumption that the laboratory can make the diagnosis as soon as a patient becomes ill is wrong and misleading.

Examination of blood and urine

In theory, leptospirosis can be diagnosed by dark-ground microscopy of blood taken during the first week of illness or, less reliably, in urine during the second week. Dark-ground microscopy of blood is technically demanding since Brownian movement of collagen fibrils, red blood cell membranes and others can resemble viable leptospires. Examination of urine is seldom worthwhile as a method of early diagnosis of infection. Culture of blood may be useful in severe, fulminating disease. Identification of infecting serovars requires specialized techniques that are available only in national reference laboratories.

Serology

In practice the detection of specific antibody is the quickest way to confirm infection in most cases. Antibodies can usually be demonstrated by the sixth day after symptoms have developed although their detection may be delayed if antibiotics have been administered early in the course of the illness.

The microscopic agglutination test (MAT) is generally accepted as the 'gold standard'. In addition to detecting genus-specific antibody, it indicates the likely infecting serogroup or serovar. Doubling dilutions of patient's serum are titrated against pools of reference serovars representing the most common serogroups. The reference antigens may be either live or killed leptospires. Tests with killed leptospires are more sensitive but less specific; they are also safer and have a longer 'shelf-life'. After incubation, tests are read by low power dark-ground microscopy; 50% agglutination of the leptospires by the patient's or control serum represents a positive result.

Other tests give no indication of the infecting serovar. Several enzyme-linked immunosorbent assay (ELISA) kits with good sensitivity and specificity are available. Most detect IgM antibody, which, paradoxically, may remain detectable for several years while IgG antibody may not be identified at all or for only a few months after infection. The complement fixation test is less sensitive and is no longer recommended.

In the MAT, sera collected soon after the onset of symptoms often show cross-reactivity to different serogroups. In contrast, sera obtained during the convalescent phase of the illness generally show a significantly higher titre to the infecting serogroup or serovar.

Reference laboratories can advise on the examination of cerebrospinal fluid or other tissue, including those taken at post mortem.

TREATMENT

Antibiotics have some benefit if started within 4 days of the onset of illness, and preferably within 24–48 h. In severe illness, intravenous benzylpenicillin is the drug of choice. For milder infections a 7–10-day course of oral amoxicillin is appropriate. Patients allergic to penicillins can be treated with erythromycin.

The value of antibiotic treatment is probably overestimated and few trials have been conducted. However, supportive management to maintain tissue and organ function may be life-saving. In particular, the temporary maintenance of renal function by dialysis may be necessary.

EPIDEMIOLOGY

Animals that acquire infection may not develop discernible disease, but become long-term carriers, so-called *maintenance hosts*. Many rodents fall into this category. For example, rats acquiring inapparent infection with *L. icterohaemorrhagiae* may carry the bacteria in the convoluted tubules of the kidney long-term (possibly life-long), resulting in chronic excretion of viable leptospires in their urine. Similarly, cattle are a maintenance host for *L. hardjo*, dogs for *L. canicola*, and pigs for *L. pomona* or *L. bratislava*. The reasons for this tolerance are unclear since infection with other serovars may cause illness of varying severity followed by the transient shedding of the leptospires in the urine for only a few weeks. Moreover, an animal may become a long-term maintenance host for one serovar and yet develop disease and transient carriage after infection with another.

In general, herbivorous animals are more likely to become chronic carriers of infection. The pH of the urine of many carnivores tends to be acidic and this is likely to inflict more damage to any leptospires in the kidneys than the near neutral pH of urine of herbivores.

Changes in industrial, agricultural and social practices may result in the rapid change of both the density and type of animal populations in an area, with subsequent change in the predominant serovars of *Leptospira* causing disease in man and animals. Such a situation occurred with the carriage of *L. hardjo* by cattle in the UK in the late 1960s.

Viable leptospires are present in the semen of infected animals; in rodents a significant increase in the carriage of leptospires is seen after sexual maturity is reached. Spread across the placenta occurs in several animal species, leading to infection and possibly death of the fetus.

Outside the animal host, leptospiral survival is favoured by warm, moist conditions at neutral or slightly alkaline pH. This no doubt contributes to the seasonal pattern of human infections, which peak in the summer months in both hemispheres. Even small reductions below pH 7 markedly reduce their survival. The anaerobic conditions and low pH of raw sewage explains their short survival time compared with aerated sewage. Salt water is also relatively toxic to leptospires. They do not survive well in undiluted cow's milk and therefore drinking unpasteurized milk poses minimal risk. However, they will survive in water at pH 7.0 or damp soil for up to 1 month. If the soil is saturated with urine they may survive for up to 6 months, indicating the potential for long-term exposure to an infection risk even if the reservoir host has been removed for some time.

Epidemiology in the UK

In the UK, dockside fish workers, sewer workers and coal miners accounted for almost half of all reported cases between 1933 and 1948 (Table 38.1). Since 1980 improved health and safety measures adopted in these industries have resulted in a very marked change, and farm workers now represent the group at greatest risk. Most cases are associated with dairy farms. In 'herring-bone' milking parlours the head of the operator is at about the same height as the udder and is, therefore, in danger of direct urine contamination!

Infections related to exposure to surface waters have also shown a significant rise. Here the predominant serovar is *icterohaemorrhagiae*. The increase is almost certainly due to the greater recreational use of surface waters for activities such as canoeing, windsurfing, fishing, pot-holing and the use of rivers for the swimming section of triathlon competitions.

Men and women are equally susceptible, but reported cases in the UK show a marked male preponderance of about 20:1, reflecting differences in occupational and recreational exposure.

Deaths from leptospirosis have declined markedly, although about 4% of patients still succumb each year. This percentage is similar in other developed countries, but in some countries with limited facilities for medical care, death may occur in 25% or more cases.

Table 38.1 Changes in the reported incidence of leptospirosis in various risk groups in the UK

Risk group	Percentage of cases notified in each period	
	1933–1948 (n=891)	1980–1999 (n=898)
Fish worker	24	2
Coal miner	16	–
Sewer worker	9	2
Service personnel	11	<1
Farm worker	5	43
Veterinarian	–	1
Water-related[a]	5	20
Other/not stated	30	32

[a] Accidental or recreational

CONTROL

With over 200 known strains, each able to infect a wide range of animals that may become long-term carriers capable of infecting others, together with the organisms' ability to survive for long periods in the environment, the complete prevention or eradication of leptospirosis is impossible.

Mass immunization of domestic livestock will prevent clinical disease in the animals and reduce the risk of human acquisition of infection. In the UK, immunization and treatment of infected farm and companion animals may have been a significant contributory factor in the reduction in *L. hardjo* infection and the apparent disappearance of the human cases of *L. canicola* infection acquired from dogs.

To be fully effective, a vaccine should not only protect against disease in the animal but also prevent the establishment of the carrier state and the shedding of viable leptospires in the urine. It is also important that the vaccine contains the strains that predominate in the locality since protection will only be optimal against the vaccine components. Current vaccines protect for only 1–2 years and the economics of farming may influence a farmer's decision as to whether or not to immunize his cattle. No human vaccine is licensed for use in the UK.

Awareness of leptospirosis through the education of doctors, employers and the general public has helped develop safer practices or procedures in the workplace and during recreational pursuits. Measures to reduce rodent populations in the vicinity of human activity, such as removing rubbish, especially waste food, and prevention of the access of rats into buildings is most important.

Simple measures will reduce the risks of acquiring infection:

- covering cuts and abrasions with waterproof plasters
- wearing protective footwear before exposure to surface waters
- showering promptly afterwards if immersion takes place.

In parts of the world where the prevalence of human infection in certain groups is high, selective human immunization schemes may be of benefit if a suitable vaccine is available. Antimicrobial prophylaxis with doxycyline may be of value in high-risk exposure situations in which prompt medical help is unavailable.

RECOMMENDED READING

Alston J M, Broom J C 1958 *Leptospirosis in Man and Animals.* Livingstone, Edinburgh

Faine S, Adler B, Bolin C, Perolat P 1999 *Leptospira and Leptospirosis* 2nd edn. MediSci, Melbourne

Kmety E, Dikken H 1993 *Classification of the Species Leptospira interrogans and History of its Serovars.* University Press, Groningen

39

Chlamydia

Genital and ocular infections; infertility; atypical pneumonia

M. E. Ward

Chlamydiae are obligate intracellular bacterial pathogens of eukaryotic cells with a characteristic dimorphic growth cycle quite distinct from that of other bacteria. They are widely distributed in nature and are responsible for a variety of ocular, genito-urinary and respiratory diseases in man. There is some evidence that they may be involved in atherosclerosis and, possibly, other chronic diseases.

DESCRIPTION

Classification

The family Chlamydiaceae was formerly classified into four species, belonging to the single genus *Chlamydia*:

- *Chlamydia trachomatis*, the cause of human oculogenital infections.
- *C. pneumoniae*, the cause of acute respiratory infection.
- *C. psittaci*, the cause of veterinary and zoonotic infections.
- *C. pecorum*, the cause of veterinary infections.

The use of ribosomal sequence data has prompted a revision of this classification. Most importantly, the former *C. psittaci* (long known actually to represent a diverse group of organisms) has become the new genus *Chlamydophila*, which is split into several species; *C. pneumoniae* has been reclassified as *Chlamydophila* (*Ch.*) *pneumoniae*. Although the old system is still widely used, the new classification is adopted here.

Chlamydia species

C. trachomatis is divided into two biovars which reflect fundamental differences in their invasiveness for cell culture, and in their involvement in human disease:

- Those causing *trachoma, inclusion conjunctivitis* (the so-called TRIC agents) and oculogenital infection.

- Those causing a more invasive genital tract infection associated with lymphoid pathology, *lymphogranuloma venereum* (LGV).

A former third biovar, which causes pneumonia in mice, has been reclassified as *C. muridarum*.

Both the trachoma and the LGV biovars can be divided into serotypes (serovars) on the basis of epitopes carried on their major outer membrane protein. There are 14 serovars in the trachoma biovar (with variants within them) which are given the letters A–K, and three serovars, L1, L2 and L3, in the LGV biovar.

- Classic trachoma tends to be caused by serovars A, B, Ba or C.
- Chlamydial genital tract infection or conjunctivitis secondary to genital tract infection in man tends to be caused by serovars D–K.

There are geographic differences in the distribution of these serovars and it is not uncommon for an individual to be simultaneously infected with more than one. There is no apparent difference in virulence among them, but single strains of mixed serovar do arise, presumably due to recombination events within the gene encoding the major outer membrane protein. This occurs in regions of South and East Africa, where there is a high prevalence of genital tract infection. In such areas recombination events may be particularly favoured or recombinants may have a selective advantage in enabling chlamydiae to survive the immune response in persons frequently exposed to infection.

Chlamydophila species

Members of the genus *Chlamydophila* infect both birds and mammals:

- *Ch. psittaci* causes respiratory, gut and systemic infections in birds, particularly in psittacine and ornithine birds (budgerigars, parrots) and may lead to severe and sometimes fatal pneumonia in man (*psittacosis* or *ornithosis*).

- *Ch. pneumoniae*, the former TWAR (Taiwan acute respiratory) agent, is a common cause of mild to severe acute respiratory disease in man.
- *Ch. abortus* causes abortion in sheep, rarely leading to abortion in pregnant women exposed to infected sheep. Sheep and goats often carry a related organism, *Ch. pecorum*, in their guts.
- *Ch. caviae* causes oculogenital infection in guinea-pigs and is an important experimental model of human infection.

Among representatives of related chlamydial families, parachlamydiae commonly occur in symbiotic association with freshwater amoebae and with pathogenic *Acanthamoeba* species. They are sometimes found in nasal swabs, soft contact lenses, humidifier water, etc. *Simkania negevensis* and *Waddlia chondrophila* may be associated with human respiratory tract disease and bovine abortion, respectively.

Morphology

Chlamydiae are small, non-motile bacteria. Although they stain poorly with Gram's stain they have the typical LPS of Gram-negative bacteria. They exhibit a dimorphic growth cycle, in which infection is initiated by environmentally resistant, metabolically inert, infectious structures called *elementary bodies*, while larger, pleomorphic structures, *reticulate bodies*, are responsible for intracellular replication. The species are differentiated on the basis of the following:

- Growth characteristics and host range.
- Characteristic morphology or staining properties of their inclusions. *C. trachomatis* in particular produces inclusions containing a glycogen-like carbohydrate which stains blue with iodine.
- The shape of the elementary bodies.
- DNA and ribosomal RNA sequences.
- The presence of plasmids or bacteriophages or both.
- Serology based on surface antigens, notably the major outer membrane protein.

Elementary bodies

Chlamydial elementary bodies are small, electron-dense structures about 300–350 nm in diameter. They are generally round, though in some strains of *Ch. pneumoniae* they are pear-shaped. The elementary body is the only infectious stage of the chlamydial developmental cycle and is the primary target of efforts to prevent chlamydial infection.

The elementary body may be considered as a tough, rigid, 'spore-like' body whose purpose is to permit survival outside the host cell. In electron micrographs, the most obvious feature is the electron-dense core of DNA, which is tightly compacted onto chlamydial histone protein (Fig. 39.1). Short projections of unknown function radiate from the surface of the elementary body.

The elementary body is thought to be metabolically inert until it attaches to, and is ingested by, a susceptible host cell. Its rigid cell wall contains only small amounts of peptidoglycan and derives its strength mainly from sulphur bridges in the cysteine- and methionine-rich proteins of the outer envelope.

Reticulate bodies

Typically, reticulate bodies have a diameter of around 1 µm or more. They are non-infectious. They are metabolically active, so their cytoplasm is rich in ribosomes, which are required for protein synthesis. Their nucleic acid, unlike the elementary body, is diffuse and fibrillar.

Reticulate bodies, like elementary bodies, are bounded by an inner cytoplasmic membrane and an

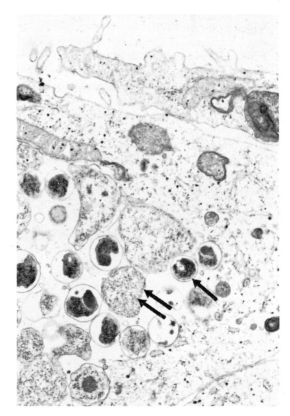

Fig. 39.1 Electron micrograph of a thin section of chlamydial inclusion: ↖, small elementary body; ↖, reticulate body. 15 000. (By courtesy of Dr Douglas R. Anderson, Miami.)

external outer envelope covered with projections and rosettes that are similar to, but more numerous than, those seen on elementary bodies. Reticulate bodies are often packed around the edge of the intracellular inclusion where they grow, in close apposition to the inclusion membrane. The surface projections apparently penetrate the inclusion membrane and they may be part of a bacterial secretion mechanism, injecting chlamydial proteins to subvert the host cell. The reticulate bodies divide by binary fission in typical bacterial fashion. They eventually switch on histone synthesis and differentiate into one or more elementary bodies. A summary of some features of chlamydial elementary and reticulate bodies is shown in Table 39.1.

Nucleic acid

Chlamydiae have one of the smallest genomes among bacteria, with approximately 1.2 Mb of sequence coding for roughly 700 proteins. Gene sequencing has revealed a number of surprising features:

- Genes encoding metabolic pathways for the production of ATP. It had formerly been assumed that high-energy molecules for biosynthesis had to be provided by the host cell.
- Both *C. trachomatis* and *Ch. pneumoniae* have the full complement of molecules required for biosynthesis of peptidoglycan, the site of penicillin action and the main strengthening component of bacterial cell walls.
- The existence of a family of polymorphic membrane proteins, including a cytolysin that may play a key role in pathogenicity.
- A surprisingly large number of chlamydial genes with apparent origins from higher organisms, including animals and plants. This may have implications for understanding the evolution of eukaryotic cells and their organelles.
- The absence of the *FtsZ* gene, previously considered essential for bacterial cell division.

- A family of genes encoding proteins with phospholipase D-like activity and probably concerned with the interaction of chlamydiae with lipid-containing host cell organelles.

Virtually all strains of *C. trachomatis* and several other chlamydiae carry a cryptic plasmid, whose function is unknown. However, as multiple copies of the plasmid are almost always present in *C. trachomatis* it is a particularly useful target for the detection and diagnosis of chlamydial infections by DNA amplification methods. There is no evidence that these plasmids carry antibiotic resistance genes.

Protein

In most chlamydiae the major outer membrane protein is immunodominant at the surface of the elementary bodies, and relatively high amounts of monoclonal antibody to the serovar-specific regions of the protein neutralize chlamydial infection in tissue culture cells. Furthermore, the major outer membrane protein forms a pore in the chlamydial surface, permitting the controlled ingress of molecules. One model of chlamydial infection is that, after entry of the elementary body into the cell, reduction of disulphide bridges permits the entry of nutrients into the elementary body and triggers differentiation.

In *Ch. pneumoniae*, the major outer membrane protein is not immunodominant and it may be overlaid by one of the other membrane proteins that this organism possesses, and which are likely to play an important role in pathogenicity.

Chlamydiae have at least two heat-shock proteins, close relatives of which are found in other bacteria and in man. These proteins rescue and chaperone proteins that have been exposed to stress, and exposure to active oxygen radicals inside cells might be such a stress for chlamydiae. Cross-reactivity of antibodies to human or bacterial heat-shock proteins with the chlamydial protein may interfere with tests such as the micro-

Table 39.1 Comparison of chlamydial elementary bodies and reticulate bodies

Characteristic	Elementary body	Reticulate body
Size	0.2–0.3 μm	1 μm
Morphology	Electron-dense core; rigid	Fragile, pleomorphic
Infectivity to host	Infectious	Non-infectious
RNA:DNA ratio	1:1 (condensed DNA core)	3:1 (increased ribosomes)
Metabolic activity	Relatively inactive	Active, replicating stage
Trypsin digestion	Resistant	Sensitive
Projections and rosettes	Few	More

immunofluorescence test, which measures antibody to whole chlamydiae. It is also possible that auto-immunity caused by the immune response to chlamydial heat-shock protein may contribute to the pathogenesis of chronic chlamydial infection.

Lipopolysaccharide

Chlamydiae have a typical 'rough' Gram-negative LPS which has weak endotoxin activity and which carries a genus-specific antigenic region used for the detection and diagnosis of chlamydial infection.

GROWTH

Laboratory propagation

Chlamydiae are grown in tissue culture cells such as McCoy or HeLa cells. It may be necessary to treat cells with poly-anionic compounds such as DEAD-dextran to reduce the electrostatic barrier to infection before centrifugation of the chlamydiae or clinical specimen onto the cells. The cells are then usually incubated in an anti-metabolite such as cycloheximide to favour chlamydial

competition for host cell amino acid pools. The presence of chlamydial inclusions is determined by microscopy in conjunction with a suitable staining method, preferably fluorescence microscopy with labelled monoclonal antibody.

Growth cycle

The chlamydial growth cycle (Fig. 39.2) is initiated by the attachment of an infectious elementary body to the host cell and entry into the cell, which follows closely. Typically, chlamydiae attach to the host cell near the base of microvilli, from where they are actively enclosed in tight endocytic vesicles. The process of chlamydial entry is relatively efficient, but ill understood. Electron microscopy suggests two possible mechanisms for chlamydial entry:

- A sequential, zipper-like, microfilament-dependent process of phagocytosis requiring direct circumferential contact between bacterial adhesins and unknown host cell receptors.
- Uptake into clathrin-coated vesicles by receptor-mediated endocytosis, a process normally used for the uptake of large molecules into the host cell.

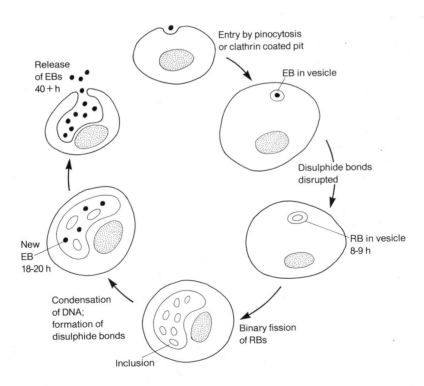

EB = elementary body; RB = reticulate body

Fig. 39.2 The chlamydia growth cycle.

Intrinsic properties of the chlamydial cell wall initially delay normal fusion with lysosomes. Subsequently, the vacuole translocates to the perinuclear region, and chlamydial gene products modify the vacuole so that it intercepts and fuses with a subset of sphingomyelin-containing exocytic vesicles from the host cell Golgi apparatus. The chlamydial vacuole also grows, in part, by acquiring and subsequently modifying glycerophospholipids from the host cell. The result is that chlamydiae have a phospholipid composition that is much closer to the host cell than to other bacteria.

After the differentiation of elementary bodies to reticulate bodies, the latter divide by binary fission within the expanding endosome with a doubling time of about 2 h. After 18–24 h the DNA begins to re-condense, and reticulate bodies are transformed into one or more elementary bodies. The growth cycle is asynchronous, so that reticulate bodies, elementary bodies and various intermediate forms may be found in the same inclusion.

This process of replication, followed by the differentiation of reticulate bodies into elementary bodies, requires amino acids such as cysteine and tryptophan, deprivation of which (for example, as a result of the action of interferon-γ) leads to a reversible cessation of chlamydial growth. This provides an opportunity for persistent quiescent infection, since the amino acid-starved pathogen may lie dormant, transferring with host cell division, until the necessary amino acid becomes available again.

PATHOGENESIS

Comparatively little is known about how chlamydiae produce disease, and what is known relates to *C. trachomatis*. The most severe sequelae of *C. trachomatis* infection (visual loss in trachoma, ectopic pregnancy or infertility in pelvic inflammatory disease) are caused by fibrosis and scarring due to the repair of tissue damaged by chlamydial-induced inflammation. There is little evidence for major differences in the basic virulence of *C. trachomatis* other than the differences between the LGV and trachoma biovars and differences in susceptibility to interferon-γ. The major determinants of severe disease appear to be:

- Socio-environmental factors, particularly in trachoma, affecting the number of infecting organisms, which in turn influences the magnitude of the initial inflammatory response and the likelihood of repeated infection. The more severe the inflammatory response the more likely there is to be significant fibrosis and damage to tissue.
- Host genotypic factors that regulate the immune response and associated repair mechanisms.

- The potential for self-induced (probably cell-mediated) immune damage to the host arising from chlamydial heat-shock proteins or other chlamydial antigens that are similar to, or mimic, host components.
- The ability of chlamydiae to become sequestered at immunologically privileged or inaccessible sites (e.g. coronary arteries for *Ch. pneumoniae*, the joints for reactive arthritis due to *C. trachomatis*).

CLINICAL FEATURES

Ocular infection

Trachoma

Trachoma has been known for thousands of years. Although generally considered a disease of hot climates, it was present in Ireland until 1945 and it is possible that there are still pockets of the disease in Europe. It is caused by several *C. trachomatis* serovars (Table 39.2) that are spread by eye-seeking flies, fingers and contaminated articles. Active trachoma, characterized by the presence of lymphoid follicles on the conjunctiva and intermittent shedding of chlamydiae, is primarily a disease of children.

By contrast, blindness occurs mainly in adults. It is caused by conjunctival scarring leading to distortion of the eyelids (entropion) and abrasion of the cornea by the eye lashes (trichiasis). Adults with trachoma rarely shed viable chlamydiae from their eyes, although it is possible to demonstrate the presence of chlamydial antigen or chlamydial nucleic acid. Ocular damage is probably largely determined by:

- the cell-mediated immune response
- the severity of the original infection in childhood
- the frequency of re-infection
- the prevalence of other agents of bacterial conjunctivitis, such as *Moraxella* spp., which can exacerbate visual loss
- host genotypic factors that influence the balance between protective T-helper 1 and T-helper 2 cell-mediated immune responses.

Trachoma is generally a clinical diagnosis, which has been simplified by a grading scheme introduced by the World Health Organization.

Adult inclusion conjunctivitis

Inclusion conjunctivitis (paratrachoma) occurs worldwide and is most prevalent in sexually active young

Table 39.2 Human infections caused by chlamydiae		
Site of infection	Disease	Organism (serovars)
Eye	Trachoma	*C. trachomatis* (A, B, Ba, C)
	Inclusion conjunctivitis	*C. trachomatis* (D–K)
	Ophthalmia neonatorum	*C. trachomatis* (D–K)
	Contact lens-associated	*Parachlamydia* spp.
Genital tract		
Male	Non-specific urethritis, proctitis, epididymitis	*C. trachomatis* (D–K)
Female	Cervicitis, urethritis, endometritis,	
	salpingitis, PID, perihepatitis, peri-appendicitis, infertility	
	with tubal occlusion	*C. trachomatis* (D–K)
	Abortion, premature birth	*C. trachomatis* (D–K)[a]
	Sheep-related abortion	*Ch. abortus*
Male and female	Lymphogranuloma venereum	*C. trachomatis* (L1–L3)
Respiratory tract	Neonatal atypical pneumonia	*C. trachomatis* (D–K)
	Pharyngitis, bronchitis, pneumonia	*Ch. pneumoniae*
		Simkania negevensis[a]
	Pneumonia	*Ch. abortus*
	Psittacosis, ornithosis	*Ch. psittaci*
Chronic diseases	Atherosclerosis, coronary disease	*Ch. pneumoniae*[a]
	Stroke, multiple sclerosis, sarcoidosis, Alzheimer's disease	*Ch. pneumoniae*[b]

PID, pelvic inflammatory disease
[a] Unproven association
[b] Weak association

people, being spread from genitalia to the eye. In the acute stage it presents as a follicular conjunctivitis, often with a mucopurulent discharge, which persists if untreated. Patients occasionally develop scarring or pannus formation as in trachoma. However, the disease is much milder, is usually self-limiting and rarely causes visual loss, presumably because, unlike trachoma, repeated infection is less common.

Chlamydial ophthalmia neonatorum (inclusion blennorrhoea)

This condition develops in infants around 14 days after birth. Follicles are rarely seen, reflecting the infant's immunological immaturity. The disease presents as a swelling of the eyelids and orbit, hyperaemia and a purulent infiltration of the conjunctiva which does not respond to cleansing of the eye or to chloramphenicol eye ointment.

The organisms are acquired from the mother during birth; about half of infants born through a chlamydia-infected cervix develop ocular infection. These babies often have nasopharyngeal infection also, either from the eyes via the lachrymal ducts, or by direct acquisition at birth. The diagnosis is confirmed by laboratory examination of a conjunctival swab obtained after removing

pus from the eye. A smear stained with *C. trachomatis*-specific fluorescent monoclonal antibody often shows spectacular numbers of chlamydial elementary bodies, looking like the star-spangled sky at night.

If untreated the infection usually resolves, but a substantial proportion of these infants develop chlamydial pneumonia about 6 weeks after birth. This is a mild, atypical pneumonia, with insidious onset and surprisingly marked X-ray changes.

Genital infection

Infection in men

C. trachomatis serovars D–K are responsible for about 30% of cases of non-specific urethritis (NSU) in men. This is one of the commonest sexually transmitted infections worldwide and repeat infections are common.

The infection is often asymptomatic, with infected men serving as a reservoir of infection in the community. In symptomatic patients, varying amounts of mucopurulent discharge are produced. Occasionally this progresses to epididymitis or prostatitis, especially in those aged less than 35 years. It is likely that chronic chlamydial epididymitis may eventually lead to occlusion of the tube and infertility due to azoospermia.

Anal intercourse may cause chlamydial proctitis in either sex. Associated symptoms include rectal pain and bleeding, mucopurulent discharge and diarrhoea.

Infection in women

In symptomatic women, *C. trachomatis* serovars D–K cause mucopurulent cervicitis and urethritis. However, many women harbour the organism asymptomatically in their cervix. Such patients are not only a risk to their sexual partners or offspring, but also to themselves, as ascending infection frequently occurs. This results first in an endometritis, in which chlamydiae survive monthly menstrual shedding of the uterine lining, followed by infection of the Fallopian tubes to cause acute salpingitis. If untreated, this is likely to lead to scarring and tubal occlusion which, if bilateral, leads to infertility. Alternatively, tubal function may be impaired rather than blocked, leading to implantation of the fertilized ovum in the oviduct rather than the womb, resulting in ectopic pregnancy.

Collectively, endometritis and salpingitis are known as *pelvic inflammatory disease*, which, in most developed countries, is largely caused by *C. trachomatis*. Chlamydial pelvic infection may lead to further abdominal involvement and the formation of pelvic adhesions. Perihepatitis (*Fitz-Hugh–Curtis syndrome*) and even peri-appendicitis may result.

Chlamydial pelvic inflammatory disease is a substantial and seldom recognized cause of pelvic pain in young women, leading to greatly increased likelihood of hysterectomy or other surgical interventions. Pain, costly investigations for infertility, and surgery can be avoided by screening young women aged 15–25 years for chlamydial infection. This is particularly important in women seeking a termination of pregnancy or undergoing surgery or instrumentation of the genital tract. Such a strategy presupposes the availability of sensitive tests for the diagnosis of genital chlamydial infection.

Lymphogranuloma venereum

Genital tract infection with *C. trachomatis* serovars L1–L3 may present as lymphogranuloma venereum (LGV). Commonest in the tropics, this condition is occasionally seen in developed countries. It usually begins with a genital ulcer followed by lymphadenopathy of the regional lymph nodes. Buboes are seen in men and, should the infection persist, can spread to the gastro-intestinal and genito-urinary tracts, causing strictures and, in rare cases, penoscrotal elephantiasis.

Infection in pregnancy

Ch. abortus is commonly associated with infectious abortion in sheep. Pregnant women exposed to infection from aborting sheep occasionally suffer miscarriage or intra-uterine death. The organism seems to have a predilection for the placenta, causing placentitis. Patients develop a febrile prodrome a few days to 2 weeks after contact with sheep. There is also a potential hazard to nursing or medical staff dealing with unsuspected cases due to *Ch. abortus* because of the heavy load of the organism in the placenta.

C. trachomatis has also been isolated from abortion products, but its role in abortion, stillbirth, premature birth and premature rupture of the membranes is uncertain.

Respiratory infections

Chlamydophila pneumoniae

This organism causes pneumonia, pharyngitis, bronchitis, otitis and sinusitis with an incubation period of about 21 days. It is suspected to be a significant cause of acute exacerbations of asthma. *Ch. pneumoniae* is one of the commonest causes of community-acquired pneumonia, but is seldom identified as the causal agent because laboratory tests for its diagnosis are not widely used. The organism is a chronic, often insidious, respiratory pathogen to which there appears to be little immunity. Clinical reactivation of existing infection and re-infection are probably common, although the two are difficult to distinguish. Sero-epidemiological studies indicate that some 60–80% of people worldwide become infected with *Ch. pneumoniae* during their life, at an incidence of 1–2 % per year.

Chlamydophila psittaci

Avian strains of *Ch. psittaci* cause psittacosis in man. The disease is more correctly called ornithosis, since infection can be acquired from birds other than psittacines. The incubation period is about 10 days, and the illness ranges from an 'influenza-like' syndrome, with general malaise, fever, anorexia, rigors, sore throat, headache and photophobia, to a severe illness with delirium and pneumonia. The illness may resemble bronchopneumonia, but the bronchioles and larger bronchi are involved as a secondary event and sputum is scanty. The organism is blood-borne through the body, and there may be meningo-encephalitis, arthritis, pericarditis or myocarditis, or a predominantly typhoidal state with enlarged liver and spleen, and even a rash resembling that of enteric fever. Endocarditis resembling that complicating Q fever (p. 376) has been described.

Coronary heart disease

Prospective serological studies initially indicated that *Ch. pneumoniae* was associated with the subsequent development of coronary heart disease, but this association has not been confirmed. However, *Ch. pneumoniae* is shed from the lungs into the bloodstream, and *Ch. pneumoniae* antigen or nucleic acid is commonly found in atherosclerotic plaque. In cell culture *Ch. pneumoniae* can bring about the conversion of macrophages into foam cells, while in experimental animals the organism may exacerbate formation of atheromatous plaque. Taken together, it seems likely that *Ch. pneumoniae*, in association with known risk factors, may be able to exacerbate coronary artery disease, but there is no definitive proof of this. Trials of anti-chlamydial antibiotics in the prevention of coronary heart disease have so far been inconclusive, and the use of antibiotics to prevent coronary artery disease is presently not justified.

Ch. pneumoniae has been suspected of playing a role in other chronic human diseases, including Alzheimer's disease, multiple sclerosis, stroke and sarcoidosis, but the evidence is even more slender than for heart disease.

IMMUNOLOGICAL RESPONSE

Studies in animal models indicate that there are both humoral and cell-mediated immune responses to chlamydial infection.

Initial host response

Chlamydial infection generates a cytokine response by direct infection of the columnar or non-squamous epithelia that they often infect, and by interaction with cells of the immune system, particularly macrophages.

Cytokines generated by direct interaction with epithelial cells help to generate and sustain an inflammatory response. IL-1α is particularly important, stimulating additional production of pro-inflammatory cytokines by adjacent uninfected cells. IL-8 attracts polymorphonuclear leucocytes, which can kill chlamydiae, while IL-6, generated by either epithelial cells or by interaction of chlamydiae with T lymphocytes, is probably important, together with IL-12, for sustaining the protective T-helper 1 cell-mediated immune response.

Tumour necrosis factor-α (TNFα), produced by macrophages in response to chlamydiae, may play an important role in tissue damage. Some virulent strains of *Ch. psittaci* can replicate in macrophages, but it is unclear whether this is significant in the case of *C. trachomatis*. However, it is likely that chlamydial antigens, particularly LPS, persist in macrophages, perhaps acting as a long-term inflammatory stimulus.

Protective immunity

Multiple infections with *C. trachomatis* are common, suggesting that there is little natural immunity to chlamydial infections. Nevertheless, there is evidence that acquired immunity develops:

- Active trachoma is a childhood disease, suggesting that repeated exposure to high levels of re-infection in a hyper-endemic area eventually leads to immunity.
- Genital tract isolation of *C. trachomatis* decreases significantly with age independently of diminished sexual activity, suggesting that exposure leads to moderate protection. Moreover, genital tract infection is relatively uncommon in groups repeatedly exposed to infection, such as commercial sex workers.
- *C. trachomatis* infections are generally limited to the superficial mucosae and shedding tends to resolve if infection is untreated. However, protection appears short-lived.
- Vaccination against trachoma with crude, whole preparations of *C. trachomatis* achieved some short-term protection in volunteers and in field trials. Limited protection has been achieved in experimental animals with various vaccines.

Since they replicate within cells, chlamydiae are, for most of their life cycle, inaccessible to antibody. The simplest model for immunity to chlamydial infections is that neutralizing antibody can protect against initial colonization by blocking attachment and invasion of elementary bodies, but thereafter, cell-mediated immune responses will be necessary to control established infection.

For *C. trachomatis*, the main neutralizing antibody response appears to be directed against the surface exposed epitopes of the major outer membrane protein. Antibody to these epitopes in genital or ocular secretions is probably responsible for the short-term serovar-specific immunity to this organism which was observed in trachoma vaccine field trials and in experimental studies in primates. However, relatively high levels of antibody appear to be needed at mucosal surfaces for effective neutralization. The dilemma for vaccine developers is that this is difficult to achieve.

It is likely that antibody is relatively unimportant compared with cell-mediated immunity for the eradication of established chlamydial infection. Experiments in guinea-pigs infected with *Ch. caviae* and mice infected with *C. muridarum* suggest that, as with other intracellular bacteria, the ability to mount a T-helper 1 response is critical, and interferon-γ is the key protective cytokine. It is possible that the balance of cell-mediated immunity to chlamydiae and chlamydial replication and antigen production may account for the fact that chlamydial infections tend to be chronic, insidious and characterized by occasional periods of intermittent activity and shedding.

INFECTION OF BIRDS AND MAMMALS

Non-human infections are important economically and as a source of human infection. Agricultural economy is affected as outbreaks of ornithosis have been reported in turkeys, geese and ducks. Abortion in ewes can occur in one-third of a previously uninfected flock, and a continuing 1–2% abortion rate is found in infected flocks. The economic loss to the farming industry from *Ch. abortus* ewe abortion is very high. Genital and eye infections of koala bears have been reported in Australia, giving rise to speculation that the species could become endangered due to chlamydial-induced infertility and blindness.

Birds with respiratory and intestinal infections shed the organism in nasal secretions and droppings. The nasal secretions contaminate the feathers, where they dry and produce an infected dust in which the organism can survive for months. There are import controls in many countries to restrict the movement of birds, which are rendered more infectious by travel-induced stress.

The organism has been found in sheep droppings, in the milk, and on the placenta and fleece of sheep. Aerosols can be produced and are a hazard to shepherds, who may develop a respiratory infection, and to pregnant women.

LABORATORY DIAGNOSIS

Cultivation

The classic method for the laboratory diagnosis of *C. trachomatis* infection is the demonstration of characteristic iodine-staining inclusions in McCoy cell tissue culture. However, cell culture is tedious, insensitive, time-consuming and expensive and it necessitates special transit of specimens to the laboratory to ensure chlamydial viability is sustained. It has been almost entirely superseded by diagnostic methods that are not dependent on viability (see below).

Ch. pneumoniae is usually even more difficult to grow but, apart from the availability of a commercial fluorescent monoclonal antibody, there is no commonly accepted laboratory diagnostic method. Many laboratories, recognizing the importance of the organism, have developed their own in-house polymerase chain reaction (PCR) or other nucleic acid-based tests, of variable quality.

Antigen detection

In smears of infected exudate from patients, *C. trachomatis* elementary bodies may be identified with fluorescein-labelled monoclonal antibodies and fluorescence microscopy. This is a sensitive and specific method, but is technically demanding and is appropriate for small numbers of specimens only.

Chlamydial antigen, usually LPS, may also be detected by enzyme immuno-assay, and a number of tests are available commercially. The better methods have excellent specificity, but a sensitivity of only 70–80%. These methods can be automated and are appropriate for screening large numbers of samples. However, positive results need to be confirmed by other tests.

Nucleic acid detection

The best nucleic acid detection tests have sensitivity and specificity approaching 100% and are now the methods of choice for clinical specimens. However, they tend to be expensive and are not widely available. The method usually involves amplification of part of the chlamydial genome or the *C. trachomatis* cryptic plasmid by the PCR or ligase chain reaction. Alternatively, methods for the detection of chlamydial mRNA in infected cells or DNA hybridization may be used.

C. trachomatis DNA can be reliably detected in urine or in vaginal tampons, reducing the need for direct sampling of the female genital tract. However, many of these diagnostic methods were not developed for this kind of sample and it is necessary to include controls to avoid false-negative reactions due to the presence of inhibitors in the specimen.

Serology

The classic micro-immunofluorescence test is based on crude, whole chlamydial antigens, antibody to which may be cross-reactive with other bacterial antigens. This, coupled with the fact that the presence of antibody does not closely coincide with the presence of infection, limits the predictive value of serological tests. Thus, while patients with pelvic inflammatory disease often have high levels of antibody to *C. trachomatis*, the converse is clearly often not true. Similarly, the results of tests for antibody to *Ch. pneumoniae* do not correlate well with the detection of the actual organism by PCR. However, serological tests are useful in the diagnosis of *C. trachomatis* pneumonia in the newborn and can be indicative in the investigation of pyrexia of unknown origin due to *Ch. psittaci*. Serology can be particularly helpful if a rising antibody titre can be demonstrated in acute versus convalescent sera.

TREATMENT

The antibiotic of choice is doxycycline in adults and erythromycin in babies. Penicillin is chlamydiastatic and should not be used. Because chlamydiae have a prolonged replication cycle and may be suppressed, not eradicated, by short courses of antibiotics, treatment must be given for a minimum of 7 days. Many authorities advocate 3 weeks' treatment, especially for ascending and complicated genital infections in women. Azithromycin, which provides sustained tissue levels and is often curative after a single dose, is an important advance, since patients treated with tetracycline often show poor compliance.

In managing ophthalmia neonatorum it is important to remember that the nasopharynx is also infected, so systemic antibiotic, preferably oral erythromycin or azithromycin, should be used. Chloramphenicol eye drops, which have been used to treat neonatal conjunctivitis, are not effective against chlamydiae.

EPIDEMIOLOGY

Both *C. trachomatis* and *Ch. pneumoniae* may cause animal infections, but human infection is almost certainly acquired by person-to-person spread. For *C. trachomatis*, the main route is flies or contaminated secretions (trachoma) or sexual transmission (genital tract infection). Trachoma is a disease of poverty, and improvement in socio-economic conditions has led to a decrease in the incidence of the disease in industrially developed countries. Blindness affects 6–9 million adults, particularly women who care for infected children. Although the incidence of active trachoma in children is decreasing, it is likely that trachoma-induced blindness will increase for some years as populations in the developing world increase their life expectancy.

Ch. pneumoniae is uncommon in childhood, but ultimately most people become infected, with the main route of infection being aerosol droplets. In Scandinavia there have been some spectacular outbreaks of pneumonia caused by this organism in military camps and student populations. There is a large non-human reservoir of infection with *Ch. psittaci* and human infection is acquired incidentally.

CONTROL

Trachoma

Prevention of trachoma relies on:

- Antibiotic prophylaxis with oral azithromycin, which is as effective as tetracycline eye ointment and substantially more convenient.
- Education and face washing campaigns, which are effective but difficult to sustain.

Genital infection

Tracing partners of index cases of *C. trachomatis* genital infection is very important, as it is useless to treat the index case only to leave the patient exposed to a risk of re-infection from an untreated partner. Genital infections can be insidious, not causing clinical signs and symptoms. It is therefore essential that the infected partner should be treated, even if clinically normal. In cases of neonatal infection the mother and her partners should be examined and treated.

Animal contact

The control of importation of psittacine birds has reduced the risk of ornithosis in pet owners and bird fanciers in many countries. Control of *Ch. abortus* infection may mean avoidance of contact with well-known sources of infection, e.g. sheep at lambing, milking and shearing. Pregnant women are particularly at risk from such infection and should avoid contact with sheep during pregnancy.

Immunization

There are no vaccines available against human chlamydial infections, even though it is clear that T-helper 1 cell-mediated immune responses can be protective. A major problem with most of the human infections is that it is unclear how best to sustain immune responses at mucosal surfaces.

RECOMMENDED READING

Barron A L 1988 *Microbiology of Chlamydia*. CRC Press, Boca Raton

Beatty W L, Morrison R P, Byrne G I 1994 Persistent chlamydiae: from cell culture to a paradigm for chlamydia pathogenesis. *Microbiological Reviews* 58: 686–699

Brunham R C, Peeling R W 1994 *Chlamydia trachomatis* antigens: role in immunity and pathogenesis. *Infectious Agents and Disease* 3: 218–233

Danesh J, Whincup P, Walker M, Lennon L, Thomson A, Appleby P, Wong Y, Bernardes-Silva M, Ward M E 2000 *Chlamydia pneumoniae* IgG titres and coronary heart disease: prospective study and meta-analysis. *British Medical Journal* 321: 208–212

Everett K D E, Bush R M 2001 Molecular evolution of the Chlamydiaceae. *International Journal of Systematic and Evolutionary Microbiology* 51: 203–220

Johansson, M, Schon K, Ward M E, Lycke N 1997 Genital tract infection with *Chlamydia trachomatis* fails to induce protective immunity in gamma interferon receptor-deficient mice despite a strong local immunoglobulin A response. *Infection and Immunity* 65: 1032–1044

Stephens R S (ed.) 1999 *Chlamydia: Intracellular Biology, Pathogenesis and Immunity*. American Society of Microbiology, Washington DC

Wong Y, Gallagher P J, Ward M E 1999 *Chlamydia pneumoniae* and atherosclerosis. *Heart* 81: 232–238

Internet sites

University of California at Berkeley: chlamydia-www.berkeley.edu:4231/
www.tigr.org/tigr-scripts/CMR2/GenomePage3.spl?database=ntcp01
Ward M E: www.chlamydiae.com

40

Rickettsia, orientia, ehrlichia and coxiella

Typhus; spotted fevers; scrub typhus; ehrlichioses; Q fever

D. H. Walker and Xue-Jie Yu

Few diseases have had a greater impact on the course of human history than epidemic typhus. Hans Zinsser's classic book *Rats, Lice and History* provides a graphic account of how *Rickettsia prowazekii*, the aetiological agent of this louse-borne disease, has caused millions of deaths and much human suffering in conditions of famine, poverty and war. Epidemic typhus has occurred mainly in poor populations in developing countries as world conditions have improved, but various other rickettsial diseases are still widely distributed. Deteriorating socio-economic conditions in the former USSR and warfare in Africa have led to the re-emergence of louse-borne typhus.

As currently classified, the family Rickettsiaceae includes a diverse group of organisms that share such common features as intracellular growth and transmission by arthropod vectors. Molecular studies reveal that *Rickettsia* species, *Orientia* (formerly *Rickettsia*) *tsutsugamushi* and *Ehrlichia* species evolved from a common ancestor.

Some obligately intracellular Gram-negative bacteria formerly classified with the Rickettsiaceae are no longer considered to be members of the family. *Bartonella* (formerly *Rochalimaea*) *quintana*, the louse-borne aetiological agent of trench fever and bacillary angiomatosis, is a cell-associated bacterium that can be grown in cell-free culture (see Chapter 34). *Coxiella burnetii* is obligately intracellular and can be isolated from arthropods, but does not require an arthropod vector to maintain itself in nature.

RICKETTSIA AND ORIENTIA

DESCRIPTION

The genera *Rickettsia* and *Orientia* include organisms responsible for numerous diseases in many parts of the world (Table 40.1). The pioneering research of Ricketts and others in the early 20th century demonstrated the rickettsial aetiology of Rocky Mountain spotted fever. Several other diseases, including epidemic and murine typhus, were later shown to be rickettsial infections.

Table 40.1 Human diseases caused by *Rickettsia* and *Orientia* species

Species	Disease	Geographical distribution	Mode of transmission	Primary vectors	Main vertebrate hosts
Typhus group					
R. prowazekii	Epidemic typhus	Extant foci in Africa, North and South America	Louse faeces	*Pediculus humanus corporis*	Humans, flying squirrels
R. typhi	Murine typhus	Primarily tropics and subtropics	Flea faeces	*Xenopsylla cheopis* and other fleas	Rodents and other small mammals
Spotted fever group					
R. akari	Rickettsialpox	USA, Ukraine, Croatia, Korea	Bite of mouse mite	*Liponyssoides sanguineus*	House mice; possibly other rodents
R. australis	Queensland tick typhus	Australia	Bite of tick	*Ixodes holocyclus*	Unknown
R. conorii	Boutonneuse fever	Europe, Africa, Middle East, India	Bite of tick	*Rhipicephalus*	Rodents and other small mammals

Table 40.1 (Continued)

Species	Disease	Geographical distribution	Mode of transmission	Primary vectors	Main vertebrate hosts
R. japonica	Japanese spotted fever	Japan	Bite of tick	*Dermacentor, Haemaphysalis, Ixodes*	Unknown
R. rickettsii	Rocky Mountain spotted fever	North and South America	Bite of tick	*Dermacentor, Rhipicephalus sanguineus,* and *Amblyomma cajennense*	Rodents, dogs and other small mammals
R. africae	African tick bite fever	Africa and West Indies	Bite of tick	*Amblyomma hebraeum*	
R. sibirica	North Asian tick typhus	Northern Asia	Bite of tick	*Dermacentor, Haemaphysalis,* etc	Rodents and other small mammals
R. honei	Flinders Island spotted fever	Australia	Bite of tick	Unknown	Unknown
R. felis	Cat flea typhus	North America	Flea Undetermined mechanism	*Ctenocephalides felis*	Opossums
Scrub typhus group *Orientia tsutsugamushi*	Scrub typhus	Asia, Australia, islands of SW Pacific and Indian oceans	Bite of larval mite	*Chiggers* (*Leptotrombidium* species)	Rodents (especially rats)

Hitherto unrecognized spotted fevers caused by *R. japonica, R. africae,* and *R. honei* were discovered in the 1980s and 1990s in Japan, Africa and Australia, indicating that much remains to be learned about these organisms. In addition to species known to be associated with human disease, a number of presumably non-pathogenic rickettsiae have been isolated, primarily from arthropods, including even herbivorous insects, and are poorly understood.

Rickettsia species are small (0.3–0.5 × 0.8–1.0 μm) Gram-negative bacilli. They are obligately intracellular parasites that reside in the cytosol of host cells (Fig. 40.1). All are associated with an arthropod vector. Species that are pathogenic for man parasitize endothelial cells almost exclusively. They are highly specialized and can synthesize adenosine triphosphate (ATP) and proteins. ATP, amino acids and metabolic intermediates are also transported from the cytoplasm of the host cell by specific mechanisms.

The genus *Rickettsia* is currently divided into two antigenically distinct groups: the *typhus group* and the *spotted fever group*, which are very closely related. They have a typical Gram-negative bacterial cell wall, including a bilayered outer membrane that contains the lipopolysaccharide antigens that distinguish the two groups. External to the outer membrane there appears to be a slime layer, probably composed of polysaccharides. Electrophoresis has demonstrated a number of distinct and common proteins in both groups of rickettsiae. The immunodominant rickettsial outer membrane protein A (OmpA) has been studied principally in the spotted fever group rickettsiae. It contains a hydrophilic region of tandem repeat units that determine the diversity of molecular size and antigens largely by the number, order and type of repeat units. OmpB is a typical autotransporter protein and is abundant in both groups of rickettsiae. OmpA and OmpB both contain cross-reactive and species-specific epitopes.

The scrub typhus rickettsiae appear to be fundamentally different and have been classified into a related but distinct genus as *Orientia tsutsugamushi* (Table 40.1). There is no indication of antigenic similarities between *O. tsutsugamushi* and members of the genus *Rickettsia*. The cell wall lacks lipopolysaccharide, peptidoglycan or a slime layer and appears to derive its structural integrity from proteins linked by disulphide bonds. *O. tsutsugamushi* exhibits three or four major antigenic proteins with both strain-specific and cross-reactive epitopes.

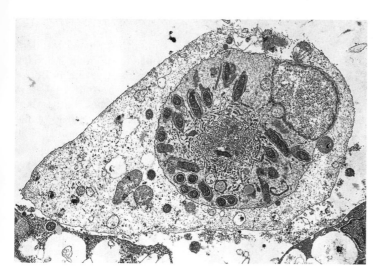

Fig. 40.1 Electron micrograph of a cell infected with *R. rickettsii*, showing dilatation of the endoplasmic reticulum of host cells that occurs as a result of injury associated with infection by spotted fever group rickettsiae.

PATHOGENESIS

Invasion and destruction of target cells

Rickettsiae normally enter the body through the bite or faeces of an infected arthropod vector. They are disseminated through the bloodstream, enter endothelial cells by induced phagocytosis, escape from the phagosome, multiply intracellularly and eventually destroy their host cells. Observations in cell culture systems suggest that spotted fever and typhus group rickettsiae destroy the host cell by different mechanisms. After infection with *R. prowazekii* or *R. typhi*, the rickettsiae continue to multiply until the cell is packed with organisms (Fig. 40.2)

and then bursts, possibly as a result of phospholipase A_2 activity; before lysis, host cells have a normal ultrastructural appearance.

Spotted fever group rickettsiae behave differently; they seldom accumulate in large numbers and do not burst the host cells, but stimulate polymerization of F-actin tails which propel them through the cytoplasm and into filopodia, from which they escape the cell (Fig. 40.3). Infected cells exhibit signs of membrane damage associated with an influx of water, which is sequestered within cisternae of dilated, rough endoplasmic reticulum (see Fig. 40.1). How rickettsiae damage host cell membranes is uncertain, but there is

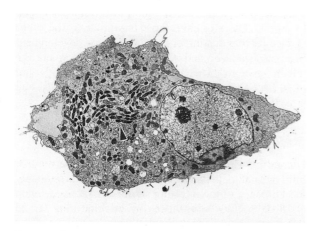

Fig. 40.2 Electron micrograph of a cell infected with *R. prowazekii*. The rickettsiae continue to multiply within the cell until it is completely packed with organisms and bursts. In contrast to cells infected with spotted fever group rickettsiae, the ultrastructural appearance of cells infected with typhus group rickettsiae remains normal until the cell lyses. The region of the cell containing rickettsiae is indicated by the arrow.

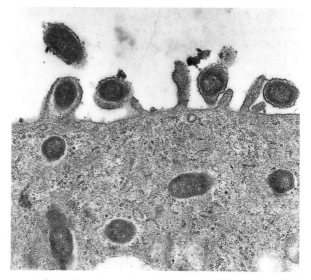

Fig. 40.3 Electron micrograph of *R. conorii* escaping from a host cell. Note the location of the rickettsiae within host cell filopodia.

evidence to suggest a role for free radicals of oxygen, a phospholipase, or a protease.

Scrub typhus rickettsiae also escape from the phagosome, reside free in the cytosol, and are released from host cells soon after infecting them, but little is known about the mechanism(s) by which these organisms damage cells.

Pathological lesions

All members of the genera *Rickettsia* and *Orientia* cause widespread microvascular injury leading to the destruction of infected endothelial cells. The pathological manifestations result more from direct rickettsial injury than by immunopathological mechanisms, mediated via cytokines and cytotoxic T lymphocytes, inflammation, disseminated intravascular coagulation, or endotoxin. Interference with normal circulation and increased vascular permeability following damage of blood vessels can cause life-threatening encephalitis and non-cardiogenic pulmonary oedema.

Clinical aspects of rickettsial diseases

Epidemic typhus

Initial symptoms of the disease are headache and fever 6–15 days after being exposed to *R. prowazekii*. A macular rash, often noted 4–7 days after patients become ill, first appears on the trunk and axillary folds and then spreads to the extremities. In mild cases the rash may begin to fade after 1–2 days, but in more severe cases it may last much longer and become haemorrhagic. Severe cases may also develop pronounced hypotension and renal dysfunction. The mental state of the patient may progress from dullness to stupor and, in very severe cases, even coma. Although the prognosis is grave for comatose patients, prompt treatment may be life-saving.

Individuals who survive a primary infection of louse-borne typhus may develop a relatively milder reactivation of latent infection many years later. This is referred to as recrudescent typhus or *Brill–Zinsser disease*. Such individuals are nevertheless immune to a second louse-borne infection.

Flea-borne fevers

Patients infected with *R. typhi*, the aetiological agent of murine typhus, develop symptoms similar to those of epidemic typhus. Fatal cases are rare but occasionally do occur, particularly in the elderly. Although the disease is much milder than epidemic typhus, it is still severe enough to require several months of convalescence. *R. felis* is transovarially maintained in cat fleas and causes a similar illness.

Tick-borne spotted fever

There are many clinical similarities among the tick-borne rickettsioses of the spotted fever group. Although all can be life-threatening, the most severe is Rocky Mountain spotted fever. Patients become ill within 2 weeks of being bitten by an infected tick. Early symptoms include fever and severe headache, often accompanied by myalgia, anorexia, vomiting, abdominal pain, diarrhoea, photophobia and cough. An eschar frequently occurs at the site of the tick bite in all spotted fever group infections except Rocky Mountain spotted fever. A maculopapular rash usually develops within 3–5 days. The rash of spotted fever usually develops first on the extremities rather than on the trunk. Absence of a rash does not exclude rickettsial infection since a disproportionate number of fatal cases of Rocky Mountain spotted fever are of the 'spotless' variety. Spotted fever group rickettsiae are found within the endothelial cells and less often macrophages of vertebrate hosts, but *R. rickettsii* can also invade vascular smooth muscle.

Vascular damage in severe cases may result in haemorrhagic rash, hypovolaemia, hypotensive shock, non-cardiogenic pulmonary oedema and impairment of central nervous system function. A fulminant form of Rocky Mountain spotted fever sometimes kills the patient within 5 days of the onset of symptoms; this form of the disease is more common in black males who are deficient in glucose-6-phosphate dehydrogenase, and may be related to haemolysis in these patients. Infection confers long-lasting immunity.

Rickettsialpox

Rickettsialpox is a relatively mild infection transmitted by mites. The clinical course is similar to the other spotted fever group infections and includes development of fever, headache and an eschar at the site where the infected mite fed. The rash is initially maculopapular but often becomes vesicular. Fever lasts about a week, and patients usually recover uneventfully.

Scrub typhus

Human infection with scrub typhus rickettsiae may be mild or fatal, depending on host factors and presumably the virulence of the infecting strain. Symptoms develop 6–18 days after being bitten by infected mite larvae (chiggers). An eschar is often apparent at the site of the bite with enlargement of local lymph nodes. Progression of the disease may be accompanied by interstitial pneumonitis, generalized lymphadenopathy, splenomegaly and rash. Death may result from encephalitis, respiratory failure and circulatory failure. Patients who survive generally become afebrile after 2–3 weeks, or sooner if treated. Scrub typhus confers only transient immunity, and re-infection may occur with heterologous or homologous strains.

LABORATORY DIAGNOSIS

Timely and accurate diagnosis of rickettsial disease followed by administration of an appropriate antibiotic may mean the difference between death of the patient and uneventful recovery. The lack of widely available, reliable diagnostic tests that can detect the disease in its early stages remains a problem, particularly as symptoms are often non-specific. The rash may appear at a late stage in the infection and may resemble exanthemata of many other diseases. The presence or significance of an eschar, if present, is also commonly overlooked.

Serological methods

Rickettsial diseases are usually acute and short-lasting. Antibodies appear in the second week of illness, when the patient is usually on the way to recovery. Death may occur before detectable levels of antibody are present. Serology is therefore not suitable for early diagnosis of rickettsial infections and is mainly used to confirm the diagnosis for epidemiologic investigations.

The oldest and most widely used laboratory method is the *Weil-Felix test*, which relies on agglutination of the somatic antigens of non-motile *Proteus* species. Although widely available, this test is not recommended because of unacceptably low levels of sensitivity and specificity.

More reliable diagnostic tests include immunofluorescence and enzyme immuno-assay. These tests are commercially available.

Isolation of rickettsiae

Isolation of the organism provides conclusive proof of rickettsial infection. However, it is seldom attempted because of lack of facilities or expertise and because of the presumed danger to laboratory personnel of handling rickettsiae-infected tissues. Such dangers have been overemphasized in this era of antibiotics, but use of containment facilities is appropriate.

Rickettsiae can be isolated in cell culture, in laboratory animals such as mice or guinea-pigs, or in embryonated chicken eggs. Cell culture yields timely results and is the most widely used method for isolation of rickettsiae from clinical samples. It is possible to detect rickettsiae in cell culture 48–72 h after inoculation by using the shell vial assay.

Detection of rickettsiae in tissue

Skin biopsies from the centre of petechial lesions can be examined for rickettsiae by immunofluorescence or immuno-enzyme methods. This approach is virtually 100% specific and has a sensitivity of 70%. Rickettsiae can be visualized for up to 48 h after the administration of antirickettsial drugs. Formalin-fixed, paraffin-embedded specimens can also be examined for rickettsiae by immunohistological methods. This approach is particularly effective for diagnosing rickettsial infection post mortem. A clever method has been developed for capturing detached, circulating endothelial cells by antibody-coated magnetic beads and immunocytological detection of intracellular rickettsiae.

Polymerase chain reaction (PCR)

Detection of rickettsial DNA by PCR is more rapid than isolation and allows specific identification, but is not yet generally available. Peripheral blood mononuclear cells, skin biopsy and *tache noire* specimens from the site of the bite can be used. Scrub typhus can be diagnosed by PCR amplification of the 56-kDa protein gene of *O. tsutsugamushi*.

PCR amplification of genes encoding 16S rRNA, 17-kDa protein, citrate synthase (*gltA*), OmpA and OmpB has been used for diagnosis of rickettsial infections. All these genes, except *ompA*, are very conserved in the genus *Rickettsia*. A single primer pair that amplifies all or most rickettsiae can be designed from the 16S rRNA, 17-kDa, *gltA* or *ompB* genes. A suitable approach is to use a conserved genus-specific primer pair to amplify a rickettsial gene and then to identify the species by restriction fragment length polymorphism analysis or DNA sequencing.

TREATMENT

Owing to the difficulties of accurate diagnosis and the risks involved in misdiagnosis, empirical therapy is appropriate for patients who have a fever for 3 days or more and a history consistent with the epidemiological and clinical features of rickettsial disease. Tetracyclines are more effective than chloramphenicol. Both are rickettsiostatic and allow the patient's immune system time to respond and control the infection. Sulphonamides should not be administered as they exacerbate rickettsial infections.

Intensive nursing care, management of fluids and electrolytes, replacement of platelets to compensate for those consumed as part of the patient's haemostatic response, and administration of red blood cells to patients who develop anaemia may be needed. Surgery may also be necessary to remove digits and extremities that develop ischaemic necrosis.

EPIDEMIOLOGY

Typhus group infections

Epidemic typhus

R. prowazekii is transmitted from person to person by the body louse, *Pediculus humanus*; the organisms are present in the faeces of infected lice and enter through the bite wound or skin abrasions. *R. prowazekii* causes a fatal infection of the louse, which is therefore incapable of long-term maintenance of the rickettsiae, and humans appear to be reservoirs of epidemic typhus. Patients who suffer a bout of recrudescent typhus (Brill–Zinsser disease) circulate sufficient rickettsiae in their blood to infect approximately 1–5% of lice that feed on them, and this is sufficient to initiate new epidemics of the disease. The importance of non-human reservoirs of the disease is uncertain, but *R. prowazekii* is maintained in an enzootic cycle involving flying squirrels and their own fleas and lice.

Murine typhus

Murine typhus is widely distributed, particularly in tropical and subtropical coastal regions and port facilities where large numbers of rats are found. This disease is maintained in an enzootic cycle involving rats and their fleas, which remain infected for life. Even the inefficient rate of transovarial transmission in fleas may play an important role in maintaining the rickettsiae in nature. Man is infected by the contamination of abraded skin, respiratory tract or conjunctiva with infective flea faeces, in which the rickettsiae can survive for as long as 3 days under optimal conditions of temperature and humidity. The disease is an occupational hazard of working in rat-infested areas such as markets or ports.

Spotted fever group infections

Tick-borne infections

Tick-borne rickettsiae of the spotted fever group are maintained in enzootic cycles involving ticks and their wild animal hosts. Ticks are the primary reservoirs of the rickettsiae, and maintain the organisms by both trans-stadial transmission (larvae to nymph to adult tick) and transovarial or vertical transmission. Some horizontal transmission (tick to rodent to tick) is likely to be essential to the survival of the rickettsiae in nature because the rickettsiae are somewhat pathogenic to ticks.

Man becomes infected following the bite of infected ticks or through contamination of abraded skin or mucous membranes. People place themselves at risk when they enter areas infested with infected ticks. Individuals may also become infected if they are bitten by ticks of domestic dogs or if partially fed ticks rupture during manual deticking of dogs.

Rickettsialpox

R. akari is the only member of the spotted fever group that is transmitted by a mite (*Liponyssoides sanguineus*) rather than ticks. The rickettsiae are maintained in an enzootic cycle that involves house mice (*Mus musculus*) and their mites. As with other spotted fever group infections, the arthropod vector is also the primary reservoir and can maintain the organism by trans-stadial and transovarial transmission. Other rodents and their ectoparasites may be able to maintain the rickettsiae in rural areas, but their importance remains unknown. Rickettsialpox is primarily an urban disease associated with mice-infested buildings.

Scrub typhus

O. tsutsugamushi is transmitted to man by the larval stages of mites of the genus *Leptotrombidium*. The nymphal and adult stages of the mites do not feed on mammals. The parasitic larvae (chiggers) occur in habitats that have been disturbed by the loss or removal of the natural vegetation. The area becomes covered with scrub vegetation, which is the preferred habitat for chiggers and their mammalian hosts, and gives the disease its name. The disease is often localized because of the restricted habitat of the chiggers. Persons entering infected areas are at risk.

CONTROL

It is virtually impossible to eradicate rickettsial infections because of their enzootic nature. Measures aimed at reducing rodent or ectoparasite populations may help to reduce the risk of infection. In addition to delousing infested persons, their clothing and bedding should be decontaminated.

Persons entering areas endemic for spotted fever group infections should wear protective clothing treated with tick repellent. Individuals should also carefully examine themselves for ticks as soon as possible after returning from tick-infested areas. The probability of infection is decreased if the tick is removed soon after it attaches. Transmission may require up to 24 h of feeding, perhaps because starved ticks require a partial blood meal if they are to reactivate the virulence of the rickettsiae.

There is no safe, effective vaccine for any of the rickettsial diseases. The attenuated E strain of *R. prowazekii* induces protective immunity, but is unsuitable for general use because it causes a mild form of typhus in 10–15% of those inoculated and reverts to a virulent state after animal passage. Inactivated vaccines for Rocky Mountain spotted fever may ameliorate the course of the disease, but none prevents illness completely, and all have been removed from the market. Scrub typhus infections also cannot be prevented by administration of vaccines derived from killed rickettsiae. Recombinant vaccines may be more successful, but will have to include those epitopes that are crucial for stimulating cell-mediated immune mechanisms, which are more important than humoral immunity in rickettsial infection.

Prophylactic use of antimicrobial agents is not recommended, since they are only rickettsiostatic and disease develops as soon as the antibiotic regimen is discontinued. Prolonged prophylaxis with weekly doses of doxycycline is effective against scrub typhus, but is probably inappropriate except under exceptional circumstances, e.g. during military operations.

EHRLICHIA

DESCRIPTION

Organisms designated as *Ehrlichia* species (Table 40.2) belong to three genetic clusters that are in the process of reclassification:

- The genus *Ehrlichia* includes the human pathogens, *E. chaffeensis* and *E. ewingii,* and the animal pathogens, *E. canis*, and *E.* (formerly *Cowdria*) *ruminatium.*
- The genus *Neorickettsia* includes organisms with the proposed names *Neorickettsia sennetsu, N. risticii* and *N. helminthoeca.*

- A third genetic cluster contains the human pathogen *Anaplasma phagocytophila* and the animal pathogens, *A. marginale, A. bovis* and *A. platys.*

Long recognized as the aetiological agents of veterinary diseases such as bovine and ovine tick-borne fever in the UK, the first human ehrlichial disease was recognized in 1954 when *N.* (formerly *Ehrlichia*) *sennetsu* was identified as the cause of an illness resembling glandular fever in Japan (*sennetsu* means glandular fever in Japanese). *E. chaffeensis, A. phagocytophila* and *E. ewingii* later emerged as the cause of tick-borne diseases in the USA.

Ehrlichiae are small Gram-negative bacteria. They multiply within membrane-bound cytoplasmic vacuoles, usually in various phagocytes, and form characteristic microcolonies resembling mulberries, termed morulae (Latin *morum* = mulberry) (Fig. 40.4). Electron microscopy reveals two distinct morphological forms, larger reticulate and smaller dense-core cells, both of which divide by binary fission, strong evidence against a

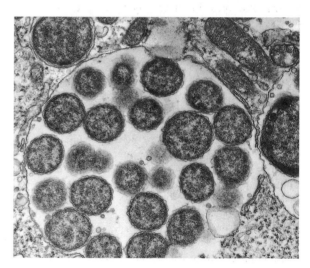

Fig. 40.4 Electron micrograph of *E. chaffeensis* within a cytoplasmic vacuole. (Micrograph by courtesy of Dr Vsevolod L. Popov.)

Table 40.2 Human diseases caused by *Ehrlichia, Anaplasma* and *Neorickettsia* species

Species	Disease	Geographical distribution	Means of transmission	Primary vectors
E. chaffeensis	Monocytic ehrlichiosis	North America, Thailand, Africa	Tick bite	*Amblyomma americanum*
A. phagocytophila	Granulocytic ehrlichiosis	USA, Europe	Tick bite	*Ixodes* species
E. ewingii	Granulocytic ehrlichiosis	USA	Tick bite	*Amblyomma americanum*
N. sennetsu	Sennetsu ehrlichiosis	Japan, Malaysia	Unknown[a]	Unknown

[a] Possibly ingestion of fluke-infested fish.

developmental cycle. Ehrlichiae preferentially metabolize glutamine in the synthesis of ATP.

PATHOGENESIS

Ehrlichia and *Anaplasma* species are transmitted through the bite of ticks. The organisms of *Neorickettsia* are associated with aquatic parasites. *N. sennetsu* is suspected to be ingested with raw fish. The related animal pathogens are either transmitted by ingestion of fish containing certain parasitic flukes that carry *N. helminthoeca* or snails containing the parasite that carries *N.* (formerly *Ehrlichia*) *risticii*.

Few details of the pathogenesis of human infections are known.

- *N. sennetsu* is associated with lymphoid hyperplasia and atypical lymphocytosis.
- Human monocytic ehrlichiosis causes leucopenia, thrombocytopenia, perivascular lymphohistiocytic infiltrates in many organs and non-necrotizing granulomata in bone marrow and liver.
- Human granulocytic ehrlichiosis caused by *A. phagocytophila* is also often associated with leucopenia and thrombocytopenia.

The two latter diseases can be fatal, in some cases owing to opportunistic fungal and viral infections. Ehrlichiae can establish prolonged, even persistent infections in vivo, and some species, including *E. chaffeensis*, can kill heavily infected cells in vitro. The available evidence suggests that cytokine-associated immunopathologic mechanisms are important.

Ehrlichiae enter by phagocytosis and inhibit phagosome–lysosome fusion as well as the signal transduction pathway whereby γ-interferon restricts ehrlichial growth by deprivation of transferrin-associated iron. Antibody to ehrlichiae confers passive protection, and cellular immunity is probably crucial to recovery. Suppression of cellular immunity and neutrophil function by *A. phagocytophila* may predispose to opportunistic infection.

LABORATORY DIAGNOSIS

Ehrlichia and *Anaplasma* grow intracellularly and isolation is extremely difficult. Human infections are diagnosed mainly by demonstrating the development of specific antibodies during convalescence. Indirect immunofluorescence methods use cell culture-propagated organisms. *E. chaffeensis, A. phagocytophilai* and *E. ewingii* are detected diagnostically by PCR with specific primers to amplify the ehrlichial DNA. Human granulocytic ehrlichiosis can often be diagnosed by identification of characteristic morulae in Giemsa-stained peripheral blood neutrophils; *E. chaffeensis* is rarely detected in monocytes in blood smears.

TREATMENT

Doxycycline is very effective in shortening the course of infection and reduces the mortality of human monocytic and granulocytic ehrlichioses.

EPIDEMIOLOGY

Deer and ticks are probably involved in the ecology of both human monocytic and granulocytic ehrlichioses. *Amblyomma americanum* ticks appear to be the major vector of *E. chaffeensis* and *E. ewingii*, and *Ixodes ricinus*-like ticks are probably the vectors of *A. phagocytophila*. Deer, dogs, rodents and domestic ruminants are important reservoirs of various ehrlichiae. Immature ticks obtain ehrlichiae from the blood of infected animals; the organisms are maintained trans-stadially, but not transovarially, and are transmitted during a subsequent blood meal. Human infections have been associated strongly with the season of tick activity and a history of tick bite.

COXIELLA

DESCRIPTION

Query or Q fever was first identified as a distinct clinical entity in 1935 after an outbreak of typhoid-like illness among abattoir workers in Australia. Subsequent studies have shown that this disease is the most widespread of all rickettsial infections with an almost global distribution. The aetiological agent, *C. burnetii*, is an obligately intracellular prokaryote, but genetic analysis suggests it is more closely allied to *Legionella* species.

C. burnetii is a pleomorphic, coccobacillary bacterium. Ultrastructural studies reveal a Gram-negative cell wall. The organisms typically grow within the phagolysosome of macrophages of the vertebrate host (Fig. 40.5). Structurally distinct large and small cell variants of *C. burnetii* have been described, suggesting that it has a developmental cycle. In acidic conditions, similar to those found within a phagolysosome, it actively metabolizes a variety of substrates and can

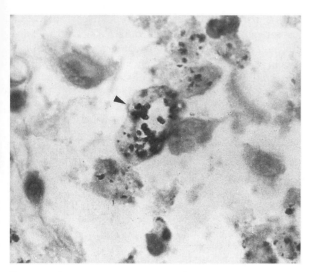

Fig. 40.5 Immunoperoxidase staining of *C. burnetii* in alveolar macrophages in a patient with Q fever. A cell containing many *Coxiella* organisms is indicated by the arrow. (Micrograph by courtesy of Dr J. Stephen Dumler.)

accomplish significant levels of macromolecular synthesis. Prolonged in-vitro cultivation results in a change in antigenic composition, known as phase variation. Phase I organisms are representative of strains isolated from nature, whereas phase II organisms appear in laboratory cultures and are avirulent for laboratory animals. The basis for the phase variation is structural differences in the lipopolysaccharides analogous to the smooth to rough transitions observed in other bacteria. *C. burnetii*, unlike *Rickettsia* species, has been found to contain plasmids.

PATHOGENESIS

Human infection usually follows inhalation of aerosols containing *C. burnetii*. Entry into the lungs results in infection of the alveolar macrophages and a brief rickettsaemia. Many infections are subclinical. The incubation period for the acute form of the disease is usually about 2 weeks but can be longer. In addition to a nonspecific febrile illness, the patient may suffer pneumonitis, hepatic and bone marrow granulomata, meningo-encephalitis and endocarditis. Chronic infections can develop, with the organism persisting in cardiac valves and possibly other foci. Endocarditis is rare, but potentially fatal, and may be accompanied by glomerulonephritis, osteomyelitis or central nervous system involvement. Reactivation of latent *C. burnetii* infections of pregnant women may occur, and the organism is shed with the placenta or abortus.

LABORATORY DIAGNOSIS

Diagnosis relies on the demonstration of specific antibodies in a complement fixation test (CFT) or indirect immunofluorescence assay. Immunofluorescence assay titres peak earlier (4–8 weeks) than those of the CFT (12 weeks) and thus are more sensitive early in the course of the disease. Use of the CFT is also hindered by the anti-complementary activity of some sera.

Isolation of *C. burnetii* from patient specimens is a specialized procedure and is not generally recommended because of the extremely infectious nature of the organism.

TREATMENT

Most *C. burnetii* infections resolve without antibiotic treatment, but administration of doxycycline reduces the duration of fever in the acute infection and is definitely recommended in cases of chronic infection. In Q fever endocarditis, long-term administration of a combination of two drugs among doxycycline, ciprofloxacin and rifampicin has been suggested. Alkalinization of the acidic phagolysosome with chloroquine has been suggested to achieve better bacterial killing.

C. burnetii may be recovered from some patients after months or even years of continuous treatment. In addition to antibiotic therapy, the haemodynamic status should be monitored. Valve replacement may be necessary in some cases of Q fever endocarditis.

EPIDEMIOLOGY

Q fever has been found on all continents except Antarctica, but most cases are reported from the UK and France. Elsewhere, the disease often goes unreported, is misdiagnosed, or causes such mild infections that treatment is not sought. The primary reservoirs of the disease are wild and domestic ungulates, including cattle, sheep, goats, rabbits, cats and dogs. Ticks can maintain *C. burnetii* by trans-stadial and transovarial transmission. Faeces of infected ticks contain very large numbers of *C. burnetii*, but these arthropods are not necessary to maintain the infection in nature.

C. burnetii may be the most infectious of all bacteria. Human infections generally follow inhalation of aerosols or direct contact with the organisms in the milk, urine, faeces or birth products of infected animals. *C. burnetii* can survive on wool for 7–10 months, in skim milk for up to 40 months and in tick faeces for at least 1 year. Most individuals acquire the disease as an occupational hazard. Cases are common among abattoir workers and those associated with livestock rearing or dairy farming. Although Q fever normally occurs as isolated, sporadic cases, a number of well documented outbreaks have been reported.

CONTROL

Elimination of infected reservoir hosts is probably impossible because of chronic infections among the animals and the ability of the organism to survive for long periods in the external environment. Exposure can be reduced by construction of separate facilities for animal parturition, destruction of suspect placental membranes, heat treatment of milk (74°C for 15 s), and efforts to reduce the tick population. Abattoir workers should take care while handling carcasses, especially in the removal and dissection of mammary glands and inner organs. Animal hides should be kept wet until the salting procedure begins. Appropriate containment procedures should be observed in laboratories working with this highly infectious organism.

Vaccines have been developed from formalin-killed whole cells, attenuated *C. burnetii*, and trichloroacetic acid-extracted antigens. Vaccines derived from phase I organisms generate a much greater protective response than similar ones prepared from phase II organisms.

RECOMMENDED READING

Audy J R 1968 *Red Mites and Typhus.* Athlone Press, London

Kass E M, Szaniawski W K, Levy H et al. 1994 Rickettsialpox in a New York City hospital, 1980 to 1989. *New England Journal of Medicine* 331: 1612–1617

Kawamura A, Tanaka H, Tamura A 1995 *Tsutsugamushi Disease.* University of Tokyo Press, Tokyo

McDade J E, Newhouse V F 1986 Natural history of *Rickettsia rickettsii. Annual Review of Microbiology* 40: 287–309

Marrie T J 1990 *Q Fever.* CRC Press, Boca Raton

Maurin M, Raoult D 1999 Q fever. *Clinical Microbiology Reviews* 12: 518–553

Raoult D 1991 Rickettsioses in the Mediterranean – a problem for travellers. *Reviews in Medical Microbiology* 2: 115–120

Raoult D, Brouqui P 1999 *Rickettsial Diseases at the Turn of the Third Millennium.* Elsevier, Amsterdam

Raoult D, Roux V 1997 Rickettsioses as paradigms of new or emerging infectious diseases. *Clinical Microbiology Reviews* 10: 694–719

Walker D H 1998 Emerging human ehrlichioses: recently recognized, widely distributed, life-threatening tick-borne diseases. In: Scheld W M, Armstrong D, Hughes J M (eds) *Emerging Infections I,* 1st edn. ASM Press, Washington DC, 6: 81–91

Winkler H H 1990 *Rickettsia species* (as organisms). *Annual Review of Microbiology* 44: 131–153

41

Mycoplasmas

Atypical pneumonia; genital tract infection

D. Taylor-Robinson

Mycoplasmas are the smallest prokaryotic organisms that can grow in cell-free culture media. They are found in man, animals, plants, insects, soil and sewage. The first to be recognized, *Mycoplasma mycoides* ssp. *mycoides*, was isolated in 1898 from cattle with pleuropneumonia. As other pathogenic and saprophytic isolates accumulated from veterinary and human sources they became known as *pleuropneumonia-like organisms* (PPLO), a term long superseded by mycoplasmas. 'Mycoplasma' (Greek: *mykes* = fungus; *plasma* = something moulded) refers to the filamentous (fungal-like) nature of the organisms of some species and to the plasticity of the outer membrane resulting in pleomorphism.

The term 'mycoplasma(s)' is used often, as here, in a trivial fashion to refer to any member of the class Mollicutes, irrespective of whether they belong to the genus *Mycoplasma*, although the term 'mollicute(s)' is also used.

The class Mollicutes ('soft-skins') contains five families:

- Mycoplasmataceae, which is subdivided into two genera: *Mycoplasma*, of which there are more than 110 named species; and *Ureaplasma*, urea-hydrolysing organisms (trivially termed ureaplasmas), of which there are six species.
- Entomoplasmataceae, which contains the genera *Entomoplasma* and *Mesoplasma* found in insects and plants.
- Spiroplasmataceae, which contains helical, motile organisms (trivially termed spiroplasmas) that cause disease in plants and insects.
- Acholeplasmataceae, which does not depend on sterol for growth, and contains a single genus, *Acholeplasma*, comprising at least 14 species, of which *Acholeplasma laidlawii* was the first to be named.
- Anaeroplasmataceae, which contains strict anaerobes found in the rumen of cattle and sheep.

It has been proposed that several members of the genera *Haemobartonella* and *Eperythrozoon* should be transferred to the genus *Mycoplasma* on the basis of 16S rRNA sequence similarities.

Mycoplasmas are distributed widely in nature, and various species cause economically important infections in cattle, goats, sheep, swine, other mammals, birds and cold-blooded animals (alligators, crocodiles, tortoises) as well as man. In addition, mycoplasmas are of concern to those who use cell cultures because of the problems of contamination.

Ureaplasmas were known originally as *T strains* or *T mycoplasmas*; 'T' for 'tiny' to describe the small size of the colonies in comparison with those produced by other mycoplasmas. Many animals are infected by ureaplasmas. Those of avian, bovine, canine and feline origin are antigenically distinct from the human strains and have been placed in separate species. Ureaplasmas of human origin, formerly classified as *Ureaplasma urealyticum*, which comprises at least 14 serovars, fall into two groups, differentiated in several ways, including genome size. The strains of small genome size are likely to form a new species, *U. parvum*, while those of larger genome size will remain as *U. urealyticum*.

DESCRIPTION

Reproduction

Mycoplasmas multiply by binary fission. However, cytoplasmic division may not always be synchronous with genome replication, resulting in the formation of multinucleate filaments and other shapes. Subsequent division of the cytoplasm by constriction of the membrane at sites between the genomes leads to chains of beads which later fragment to give single cells. Budding occurs when the cytoplasm is not divided equally between the daughter cells. The minimal reproductive unit of mycoplasmas is a roughly spherical cell about 200–250 nm in diameter. It is from organisms of this order of size, whatever the shape, that growth is initiated in cell-free medium; such organisms also make up, with larger forms (0.5–1.0 μm diameter), the substance of the characteristic agar-embedded colonies.

Morphology

Cell morphology varies with mycoplasmal species, environmental conditions and the stage of the growth cycle. Light microscopy reveals pleomorphic organisms, which may range from spherical through coccoid, coccobacillary, ring and dumb-bell forms, to short and long branching (Fig. 41.1), beaded or segmented filaments. The helical shape of spiroplasmas is characteristic but not always seen.

Several mycoplasmas, including *M. pneumoniae, M. genitalium* (Fig. 41.2) and *M. penetrans* of human origin, have specialized structures at one or both ends by which they attach to respiratory or genital tract mucosal surfaces. Sections of the terminal structures of the two former mycoplasmas may exhibit a dense rod-like core when viewed by electron microscopy.

The mycoplasma cell is limited by a membrane, 7.5–10 nm wide, in which two electron-dense layers are separated by a translucent one (Fig. 41.3). Some species have an extramembranous layer, which, in the case of *M. mycoides* ssp. *mycoides*, for example, comprises galactan and has a dense capsular appearance. Some others, for example, *M. gallisepticum* (avian), *M. genitalium, M. pneumoniae, M. pulmonis* (murine) and *Spiroplasma citri*, have surface spikes (sometimes described as a 'nap'), somewhat coarser than those seen on myxoviruses, which may contribute, through adhesin proteins, to attachment to eukaryotic cells. *M. gallisepticum, M. genitalium* and *M. pneumoniae* attach to neuraminic acid receptors. Close adherence enables the mycoplasma to insert nucleases and other enzymes into

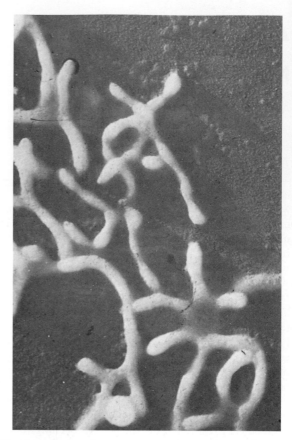

Fig. 41.1 Electron micrograph of *M. mycoides* spp. *mycoides* (bovine origin), gold-shadowed, to show branching filaments. ×28 000. (From Rodwell and Abbot 1961 *Journal of General Microbiology* 25: 201.)

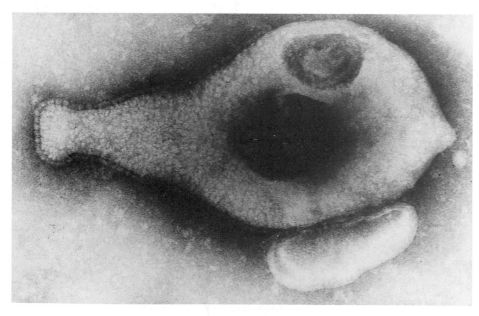

Fig. 41.2 Electron micrograph of *M. genitalium* (human origin), negatively stained, to show flask-shaped appearance and terminal specialized structure covered by extracellular 'nap'. ×120 000. (From Tully et al. 1983 *International Journal of Systematic Bacteriology* 33: 387.)

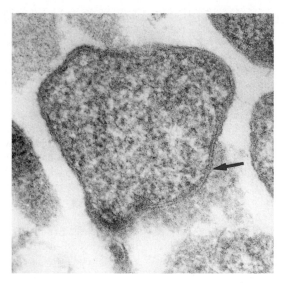

Fig. 41.3 Electron micrograph of *M. pulmonis* (murine origin); thin section illustrating trilaminar membrane (arrow). ×75 000.

The electron-lucent part of the membrane comprises lipids with the long chains of the fatty acids arranged inwards and polar groups to the external and internal parts of the organisms; the electron-dense layers consist of protein and carbohydrate. The mycoplasma membrane is the site of many metabolic reactions involving membrane-bound enzymes and transport mechanisms. Cholesterol, or carotenoid/carotenol, is interspersed between the phospholipid molecules and plays an important part in maintaining membrane integrity in the face of varying external osmotic pressures and in the absence of the rigid cell wall that is found in other bacteria. However, the presence of cholesterol renders the cell membrane susceptible to damage with agents like saponin, digitonin and some polyene antibiotics (e.g. amphotericin B) that complex with sterols. As expected, mycoplasmas are completely resistant to antibiotics that act on bacterial cell wall synthesis and also to lysozyme.

The cytoplasm of mycoplasmas does not contain endoplasmic reticulum but it is packed with ribosomes; nuclear material (unbounded without nucleoli) in fibrillar form (3 nm thick) is centrally placed or dispersed. The ribosomes have a sedimentation coefficient of about 70S and protein synthesis is inhibited by antibiotics such as tetracyclines, aminoglycosides, erythromycin and chloramphenicol.

the cell and to take from it the products of enzyme activity, such as nucleotides. Adherence to erythrocytes (*haemadsorption*), tissue culture cells, spermatozoa and other eukaryotic cells may be demonstrated with certain mycoplasmas (Fig. 41.4).

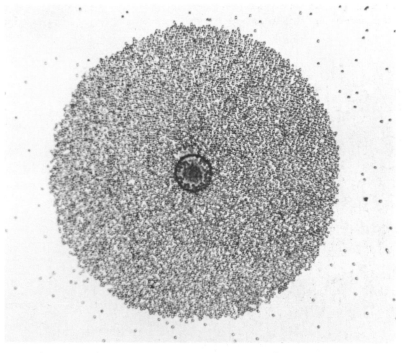

Fig. 41.4 Colony of *M. agalactiae* (caprine origin) showing adherent guinea-pig erythrocytes (phenomenon of haemadsorption).

The genome of *M. genitalium* is the smallest known so far (580 kb) – an important factor in it being the first of any micro-organism to be fully sequenced. It is not much larger than that of a large poxvirus, an indication of the small amount of genetic information needed for a free-living existence and the reason why mycoplasmas have a paucity of biochemical activity and are nutritionally fastidious.

Viruses and plasmids

Fourteen viruses have been identified: six in *Acholeplasma*, four in *Mycoplasma* and four in *Spiroplasma* species. They are rod-shaped (Fig. 41.5) or enveloped spheres that bud from the mycoplasma membrane surface, or are polyhedral with a tail. Those that have been examined in detail contain single- or double-stranded DNA in either a circular or linear form. There is evidence for integration of the viral genome into the mycoplasmal chromosome, especially in spiroplasmas, and this may provide a mechanism for the promotion of genetic diversity. The release of the viruses is continuous and is not accompanied by cell lysis. Plasmids, so far regarded as cryptic, have been detected in *Acholeplasma, Mycoplasma* and, most frequently, *Spiroplasma* species.

Cultivation

Mycoplasmas have limited biosynthetic abilities, so that they need a rich growth medium containing natural animal protein (usually blood serum) and, in most cases, a sterol component. Serum supplies not only cholesterol but also saturated and unsaturated fatty acids for membrane synthesis, components that the organisms cannot synthesize. A widely used isolation medium contains bovine heart infusion (PPLO broth) with fresh yeast extract and horse serum. However, these components vary in their ability to support growth and success may depend on use of different batches of the components, sera from other animal species, or the addition of various supplements.

Cultivation of spiroplasmas is more difficult. The development of a medium designated SP-4 has been helpful in the isolation of spiroplasmas as well as *M. genitalium* and other fastidious mycoplasmas. Although various specific formulations have been described for the isolation of ureaplasmas, most mycoplasmal media are suitable. The sterol-independent organisms also grow readily on these media but serum, which often promotes growth, is not usually essential.

A strategy using Vero cell cultures has been used for isolating *M. genitalium*. The inoculated cell cultures are monitored for mycoplasmal growth by polymerase chain

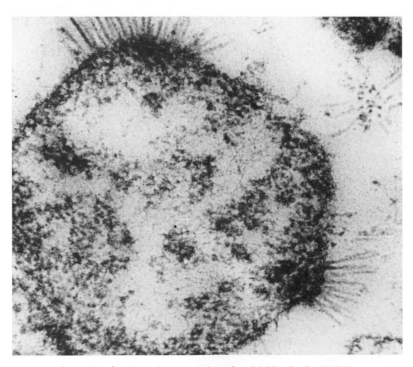

Fig. 41.5 Rod-shaped virus particles (75 × 7.5 nm) radiating from the surface of an *A. laidlawii cell.* ×100 000.

reaction (PCR) technology, followed by subculture to mycoplasmal medium. However, investigators should be cautious about the widespread use of cell cultures (see below).

Most mycoplasmas are facultatively anaerobic but, since organisms from primary tissue specimens frequently grow only under anaerobic conditions, an atmosphere of 95% nitrogen and 5% carbon dioxide is preferred for primary isolation. Continued propagation sometimes requires quite stringent anaerobic conditions and, of course, these are needed for *Anaeroplasma* species. The optimum temperature for most mycoplasmas and ureaplasmas from man or animals is 36–38°C, but is lower for acholeplasmas and spiroplasmas.

Colonial morphology

On agar, mycoplasmas produce colonies that have a 'fried egg' appearance, with an opaque central zone of growth within the agar and a translucent peripheral zone on the surface (Fig. 41.6). The size of the colonies varies widely: colonies of some bovine mycoplasmas and most acholeplasmas may exceed 2 mm in diameter, and are easily visible to the naked eye, whereas those of the ureaplasmas are characteristically small (15–60 μm in diameter) because they usually lack the peripheral zone of growth. Size and appearance also depend on the constituents and degree of hydration of the medium, the agar concentration, atmospheric condition and age of the culture.

Biochemical reactions

Most mycoplasmas use glucose (or other carbohydrates) or arginine as a major source of energy; a few use both, and others do not metabolize either substrate. In most mycoplasmas the respiratory pathways are flavin-terminated so that the haem compounds, cytochromes and catalase, are absent. The unique and distinctive biochemical feature of ureaplasmas is the conversion of urea to ammonia by urease.

Mycoplasma, Ureaplasma, Entomoplasma and *Anaeroplasma* species depend on sterol. They fail to grow in serum-free media and are inhibited by digitonin, distinguishing them from the species that do not require sterol. In addition, most *Mycoplasma* species and ureaplasmas produce hydrogen peroxide, which causes some lysis of guinea-pig or other erythrocytes when these are suspended in agar over developing colonies. *M. pneumoniae* produces clear zones of β-haemolysis. About one-third of all *Mycoplasma* species exhibit haemadsorption (Fig. 41.4).

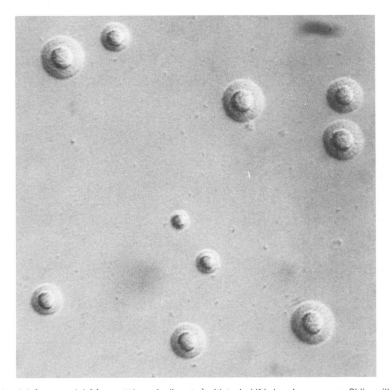

Fig. 41.6   Colonies of *M. hominis* (human origin) (up to 110 μm in diameter) with typical 'fried egg' appearance. Oblique illumination. ×150.

Antigenic properties

DNA analysis has made a fundamental contribution to the taxonomy of mycoplasmas and, in the future, may play an important role in simplifying species classification. For the present, identification and speciation rest largely on the use of specific antisera containing antibodies reflecting the antigenic composition of different mycoplasmas. The Western blot technique is useful in assessing the importance of particular antigens, but gel diffusion and immunoelectrophoresis techniques are important for studying the antigenic structure of mycoplasmas and the relationships between them. For sero-epidemiological studies and for serological diagnosis, more sensitive tests, such as indirect haemagglutination, enzyme-linked immunosorbent assay (ELISA) and micro-immunofluorescence, are used.

The way in which different antigens function is exemplified by considering *M. pneumoniae*. The glucose- and galactose-containing membrane glycolipids of the organism are haptens, which are antigenic only when bound to membrane protein. They induce antibodies that react in complement fixation, metabolism inhibition and growth inhibition tests. Glycolipids with fortuitously similar structure have been found in the human brain. Their cross-reactivity with antibodies to *M. pneumoniae* could account for the neurological manifestations of *M. pneumoniae* infection

(see below). Furthermore, the ability of the organisms to alter the I antigen on erythrocytes sufficiently to stimulate anti-I antibodies (*cold agglutinins*) leads to an auto-immune response and damage to erythrocytes. *M. pneumoniae* has two major surface proteins, including the P1 protein involved in attachment, which are recognized by the host; antibody to them is detected in convalescent sera and in respiratory secretions. Variation in the P1 protein has led to the recognition of two subtypes of strains, which may vary epidemiologically and in pathogenicity.

Variable membrane lipoproteins of several mycoplasmas form an antigenic variation system that provides a means of escaping from the host immune response; the variations are restricted to a small number of protein antigens and do not appear to alter the total cell protein profiles of the organisms.

PATHOGENESIS

Thirteen *Mycoplasma* species, two *Acholeplasma* species and one *Ureaplasma* species presently classified as *U. urealyticum* (see above) have been isolated from man (Table 41.1), mostly from the oropharynx. *M. fermentans*, *M. genitalium*, *M. hominis*, *M. pneumoniae* and *U. urealyticum* unequivocally cause disease or are strongly associated with disease.

Table 41.1 Some properties of mycoplasmas of human origin

| Mycoplasma | Frequency of detection in | | Metabolism of | Preferred pH | Haemadsorption[a] |
	Respiratory tract	Urogenital tract			
M. buccale	Rare	Not reported	Arginine	7.0	−
M. faucium	Rare	Not reported	Arginine	7.0	+
M. fermentans	Common	Rare	Glucose and arginine	7.5	−
M. genitalium	Rare	Rare[b]	Glucose	7.5	+
M. hominis	Rare	Common	Arginine	7.0	−
M. lipophilum	Rare	Not reported	Arginine	7.0	−
A. laidlawii	Very rare	Not reported	Glucose	7.5	−
A. oculi	?	Not reported	Glucose	7.5	−
M. orale	Common	Not reported	Arginine	7.0	+
M. penetrans	Not reported	Rare	Glucose and arginine	7.5	+
M. pirum	Not reported	?	Glucose and arginine	7.5	?
M. pneumoniae	Rare[a]	Very rare	Glucose	7.5	+
M. primatum	Not reported	Rare	Arginine	7.0	−
M. salivarium	Common	Rare	Arginine	7.0	−
M spermatophilum	Not reported	Rare	Arginine	7.0	−
U. urealyticum	Rare	Common	Urea	≤ 6.0	+[c]

[a] Chick red blood cells.
[b] Rare, except in disease.
[c] Serovar 3 only.

Respiratory infections

Mycoplasmal pneumonia

Pneumonias not attributable to any of the common bacterial causes were labelled historically as *primary atypical pneumonias*. In one variety associated with the development of cold agglutinins, a filterable microorganism, first called the *Eaton agent*, was isolated in embryonated eggs. Serious doubts about the possibility of the agent being a virus arose when its growth was found to be inhibited by chlortetracycline and gold salts, and cultivation on cell-free medium in the early 1960s finally clinched its mycoplasmal nature. The organism was subsequently named *M. pneumoniae*, and its importance as a cause of respiratory disease was confirmed by numerous studies based on isolation, serology, volunteer inoculation and vaccine protection.

Epidemiology. Infection occurs worldwide. Although endemic in most areas, there is a preponderance of infection in late summer and early autumn in temperate climates; in some countries, such as the UK, epidemic peaks have been observed about every 4 years. Spread is fostered by close contact, e.g. in a family. Overall, *M. pneumoniae* may cause only about one-sixth of all cases of pneumonia, but in certain populations, such as military recruits, it has been responsible for almost half the cases of pneumonia. Children are infected more often than adults, and the consequence of infection is also influenced by age. Thus, in school-aged children and teenagers, about a quarter of infections culminate in pneumonia, whereas, in young adults, fewer than 10% do so. Thereafter, pneumonia is even less frequent, but severity tends to increase with the age of the patient.

Clinical features. Infections often have an insidious onset, with malaise, myalgia, sore throat or headache overshadowing and preceding chest symptoms by 1–5 days. Cough, which starts around the third day, is characteristically dry, troublesome and sometimes paroxysmal, and becomes a prominent feature. However, patients usually do not appear seriously ill and few warrant admission to hospital. Physical signs, such as rales, become apparent, frequently after radiographic evidence of pneumonia. Most often this amounts to patchy opacities, usually of one of the lower or middle lobes. About 20% of patients suffer bilateral pneumonia, but pleurisy and pleural effusions are unusual. The course of the disease is variable, but cough, abnormal chest signs and radiographic changes may extend over several weeks and relapse is a feature. A prolonged paroxysmal cough simulating the features of whooping cough may occur in children. Very severe infections have been reported in adults, usually in those with immunodeficiency or sickle cell anaemia, although death is rare.

Disease is limited usually to the respiratory tract. Extrapulmonary manifestations include:

- the Stevens–Johnson syndrome and other rashes
- arthralgia
- meningitis or encephalitis (and other neurological sequelae)
- haemolytic anaemia
- myocarditis
- pericarditis.

Haemolytic anaemia with crisis is an auto-immune phenomenon brought about by cold agglutinins (anti-I antibodies). Some of the other complications, such as the neurological ones, may arise in a similar indirect way, although *M. pneumoniae* has been isolated from cerebrospinal fluid.

Respiratory infection in the newborn

M. hominis and ureaplasmas occasionally cause respiratory disease in the newborn, particularly in those of very low birth weight, the infections often being acquired in utero. The likelihood of death or chronic lung disease in infants of less than 1000 g with a ureaplasmal respiratory tract infection within 24 h of birth is double that of uninfected infants of similar birth weight, or heavier infants. However, whether other bacteria that are associated with maternal bacterial vaginosis might also be involved is an unresolved question.

Other respiratory infections

M. hominis has produced sore throats when given orally to adult volunteers; however, it does not seem to cause naturally occurring sore throats in children or adults. *M. fermentans* has been found in the throat and has been associated with adult respiratory distress syndrome with or without systemic disease, and with pneumonia in a few children with community-acquired disease. *M. genitalium* has been isolated, together with *M. pneumoniae*, from the respiratory secretions of a few adults but its role, if any, in respiratory disease seems small.

Urogenital infections

M. fermentans, *M. genitalium*, *M. hominis*, *M. penetrans*, *M. pneumoniae*, *M. primatum*, *M. salivarium*, *M. spermatophilum* and ureaplasmas have been isolated from the urogenital tract; *M. hominis*, *M. genitalium* and ureaplasmas occur most frequently.

Urogenital infections in men

Although *M. hominis* may be isolated from about 20% of patients with non-gonococcal urethritis (NGU), it has not been incriminated as a cause. Furthermore, there is still little evidence to implicate ureaplasmas as a cause of acute NGU, although those of larger genome size might play a part. In contrast, their involvement as a cause of some cases of chronic NGU seems stronger.

M. genitalium has been strongly implicated as a cause of acute and chronic NGU, but there is no evidence that this or other mycoplasmas are a cause of acute or chronic prostatitis.

There is some evidence that ureaplasmas occasionally cause epididymitis, but it is not thought that they cause male infertility; the possible role of *M. genitalium* has not been investigated.

Reproductive tract disease in women

M. hominis organisms and, to a lesser extent, ureaplasmas are found in much larger numbers in the vagina of women who have bacterial vaginosis than in healthy women and, with various other bacteria, may contribute to the development of the condition. These genital mycoplasmas do not cause cervicitis but *M. genitalium* has been associated strongly with the disease.

Bacterial vaginosis, and hence the bacteria associated with it, including *M. hominis,* may lead to pelvic inflammatory disease. *M. hominis* has been isolated from the endometrium and fallopian tubes of about 10% of women with the disease, together with a specific antibody response. This suggests a causal role, but the significance of *M. hominis* is difficult to judge when several other micro-organisms are present. Ureaplasmas have also been isolated directly from affected fallopian tubes, but the absence of antibody responses and failure to produce salpingitis in subhuman primates make them an even less likely cause of disease at this site.

The pathogenic potential of *M. genitalium* seems greater; it has been associated with endometritis and antibody responses in some patients with pelvic inflammatory disease and the production experimentally of salpingitis in subhuman primates suggest that it may have an important role.

The part that *M. hominis* is likely to play in infertility as a result of tubal damage is small and whether ureaplasmas might cause involuntary infertility, or affect sperm, remains speculative. In contrast, serologically, *M. genitalium* has been associated strongly with tubal factor infertility.

Disease associated with pregnancy and the newborn

M. hominis and ureaplasmas have been isolated from the amniotic fluid of women with severe chorio-amnionitis who had preterm labour. Similarly, ureaplasmas have been isolated from spontaneously aborted fetuses and stillborn or premature infants more frequently than from induced abortions or normal full-term infants.

Isolation of ureaplasmas from the internal organs of aborted fetuses, together with some serological responses and an apparent diminished occurrence following antibiotic therapy, support a role for these organisms in abortion. However, bacterial vaginosis is strongly associated with preterm labour and late miscarriage, and, as *M. hominis* and ureaplasmas are part of the extensive microbial flora of bacterial vaginosis, it is possible that they act as part of this flora and not independently. The same may be said about the role of genital mycoplasmas, particularly ureaplasmas, in causing low birth weight in otherwise normal infants. Bacterial vaginosis has been largely ignored in defining the association and a study in which women given erythromycin in the third trimester delivered larger babies than those given a placebo has not been confirmed in later trials. Although there is obvious uncertainty surrounding this issue, premature infants are prone to meningitis caused by *M. hominis* or ureaplasmas within the first few days of life.

After an abortion, *M. hominis* has been isolated, apparently in pure culture, from the blood of about 10% of febrile women; half of them exhibit an antibody response. The organism was not found in the blood of about 5–10% of women who aborted but remained afebrile, but it has been recovered from the blood of about 5–10% of women with postpartum fever. Similar observations have been made for ureaplasmas and it seems that both micro-organisms induce fever by causing endometritis.

Urinary infection and calculi

M. hominis has been isolated from the upper urinary tract of patients with acute pyelonephritis and probably causes about 5% of such cases. Ureaplasmas do not seem to be involved in pyelonephritis. However, the fact that they produce urease, induce crystallization of struvite and calcium phosphates in urine in vitro and produce calculi experimentally in animal models raises the question of whether they cause calculi in the human urinary tract. Ureaplasmas are found more often in the urine and calculi of patients with infective stones than in those with metabolic stones, suggesting that they may have a causal role.

Joint infections

There is evidence that ureaplasmas are involved in the aetiology of sexually acquired reactive arthritis based on synovial fluid mononuclear cell proliferation in response to specific ureaplasmal antigens. They also have a role in arthritis in hypogammaglobulinaemic patients (see below). There are isolated reports of *M. genitalium* in the joints of patients with Reiter's disease and rheumatoid arthritis. *M. fermentans* has been found by a PCR assay in the joints of about 20% of patients with rheumatoid arthritis and in those of patients with other chronic inflammatory rheumatic disorders, but not in the joints of patients with non-inflammatory arthritides.

Infections in immunocompromised patients

M. pneumoniae may cause severe pneumonia in immunodeficient patients and may persist for many months in the respiratory tract of hypogammaglobulinaemic patients, despite apparently adequate treatment. A few of these patients develop suppurative arthritis, and mycoplasmas are responsible for at least two-fifths of the cases. The mycoplasmas involved have been *M. pneumoniae, M. salivarium* (usually regarded as non-pathogenic), *M. hominis* and, particularly, ureaplasmas. In some cases involving ureaplasmas, the arthritis has been associated with subcutaneous abscesses, persistent urethritis and chronic cystitis. Although responding sometimes to tetracyclines, the organisms and disease may persist for many months despite concomitant use of anti-inflammatory and γ-globulin replacement therapy. Administration of specific mycoplasmal antiserum prepared in an animal (e.g. sheep or rabbit) may aid clinical and microbiological recovery.

Septicaemia due to *M. hominis* has occurred after trauma and genito-urinary manipulations, and the mycoplasma has been found in brain abscesses and osteomyelitis. Haematogenous spread leading to septic arthritis, surgical wound infections and peritonitis seems to occur more often after organ transplantation and in other patients on immunosuppressive therapy. Particularly common are sternal wound infections caused by *M. hominis* in heart and lung transplant patients.

It has been suggested that *M. fermentans* infection of peripheral blood monocytes of human immunodeficiency virus (HIV)-positive subjects might lead to more rapid development of the acquired immune deficiency syndrome, and that *M. penetrans* is associated uniquely with HIV-positivity and possibly with Kaposi's sarcoma. Convincing evidence for these propositions has not been forthcoming.

LABORATORY DIAGNOSIS

Mycoplasma pneumonia

Because the clinical manifestations are not sufficiently distinct for definitive diagnosis, laboratory help is required. A non-specific (cold agglutinin) or, usually, a more specific serological test (complement-fixation test or ELISA) is relied upon in routine practice. Cross-reactivity with *M. genitalium* might be a problem with the complement fixation test. Western blotting can be used to check specificity in dubious cases. A four-fold or greater rise in antibody titre in these tests, with a peak at about 3–4 weeks, is indicative of a recent infection.

The cold agglutinin test is less sensitive than the complement fixation test, which enables a rise to be detected in about 80% of cases. Because paired sera are not always available, a single antibody titre of 64–128 or more with either test, in a suggestive clinical setting, should be sufficient to institute therapy.

Attempted isolation of *M. pneumoniae* (and *M. fermentans*) requires the use of mycoplasmal broth supplemented with penicillin and glucose, and with phenol red as a pH indicator. After inoculation with sputum, throat washing, pharyngeal swab, or other specimen, the medium is incubated at 37°C, and a colour change (red to yellow), which may take 3 weeks or longer, indicates fermentation of glucose due to multiplication of the organisms. The broth is then subcultured on agar medium for specific identification of colonies by growth inhibition or immunofluorescence techniques.

Isolation is not often attempted because of the time required. However, the PCR assay is rapid, sensitive and specific. If an isolate is required, a sensible approach is to test specimens by both the PCR assay and culture, and to continue the latter only for those specimens that prove to be PCR-positive.

Urogenital infections

Material from urethral, cervical or vaginal swabs or centrifuged deposit from urine is added to separate vials of liquid mycoplasmal medium containing phenol red and 0.1% glucose, arginine or urea. *M. genitalium* metabolizes glucose and changes the colour of the medium from red to yellow. *M. fermentans* also metabolizes glucose but, in addition, converts arginine to ammonia. The latter conversion is also shown by *M. hominis* and *M. primatum*. The ureaplasmal urease also breaks down urea to ammonia. In each case, the pH of the medium increases, and the colour changes from yellow to red. The colour change produced by ureaplasmas occurs usually within 1–2 days; that caused by *M. hominis* well within a week; *M. genitalium* may take several months or produce no change at all. Subculture to agar medium results usually in the formation of characteristic colonies. On ordinary blood agar, *M. hominis*, but not ureaplasmas, produces non-haemolytic pinpoint colonies.

M. hominis also multiplies in most routine blood culture media; the inhibitory effect of sodium polyanethol sulphonate, included as an anticoagulant, can be overcome by the addition of gelatin (1% w/v).

Serological tests are used for definitive identification. Kits designed to isolate and identify ureaplasmas and *M. hominis* are available commercially and are of particular value if the need to detect these micro-organisms arises infrequently.

DNA primers specific for *M. fermentans, M. genitalium* and *U. urealyticum* have been developed and used for amplification by the PCR. This technique is much more sensitive than culture for detecting the two former mycoplasmas and its use is likely to be the only way of obtaining reliable results.

Genital mycoplasmal infections stimulate antibody responses, but the various techniques to detect them are rarely used diagnostically.

TREATMENT

Mycoplasma pneumonia

M. pneumoniae, like other mycoplasmas, is most sensitive to the tetracyclines in vitro, but is more sensitive to erythromycin than some of the other mycoplasmas of human origin. In clinical practice these antibiotics have proved less effective for treating pneumonia than they have in planned trials, probably because disease is often well established before treatment begins. Nevertheless, it is worthwhile administering a tetracycline to adults and erythromycin to children and pregnant women.

Macrolides, such as clarithromycin and azithromycin and the fluoroquinolones are at least as active in vitro, and quinolones may have some cidal effect. Failure of most antibiotics to kill the organisms, together with the fact that the organisms may become intracellular, probably explains persistence in the respiratory tract long after clinical recovery, as well as clinical relapse in some patients. Furthermore, a functioning immune system is important in eradication, so that in some hypogammaglobulinaemic patients the organisms may persist for months or years.

Antibiotic treatment of *M. pneumoniae* or other mycoplasma-induced infection should start as soon as possible, based on clinical suspicion rather than waiting for laboratory confirmation, and a 3-week course is justified, particularly if supported by serological or other evidence of infection.

Urogenital infections

Treatment must take into account the fact that several different micro-organisms may be involved and that a precise microbiological diagnosis may not be attainable. Patients with NGU should receive one of the tetracyclines, which inhibit chlamydiae, ureaplasmas and *M. genitalium*. However, at least 10% of ureaplasmas are resistant to tetracyclines, and patients who fail to respond to such therapy should then be treated with erythromycin, to which most tetracycline-resistant ureaplasmas are sensitive.

A tetracycline should also be included for the treatment of pelvic inflammatory disease to cover chlamydiae and *M. hominis*. However, since about 20% of *M. hominis* strains are resistant to tetracyclines, other antibiotics such as clindamycin or fluoroquinolones may need to be considered. Azithromycin, which is being used increasingly for chlamydial infections, is also active against a wide range of mycoplasmas, including *M. genitalium* and, to a lesser extent, ureaplasmas.

Fever following abortion or childbirth often settles within a few days, but if it does not, tetracycline therapy should be started, while keeping tetracycline resistance in mind.

MYCOPLASMAS AND CELL CULTURES

Few primary cell cultures become infected with mycoplasmas, but continuous cell lines do so frequently. The mycoplasmas most responsible are *M. arginini, M. fermentans, M. hyorhinis, M. orale, M. salivarium* and *A. laidlawii*. The effects include those caused by mycoplasmal enzymes and toxins, and those resulting from metabolism of cell culture media components or from changes in pH. Despite the presence of up to 10^8 organisms per millilitre of culture fluid, there may be little effect on viral propagation, although it may decrease the yield. Occasionally, the yield may be increased as, for example, with vaccinia virus in *M. hominis*-infected cells.

Culture and an indicator cell system with staining (e.g. Hoechst DNA dye) are used to detect contamination, but these may be superseded by PCR methods. Numerous procedures have been described to eliminate mycoplasmas from cell cultures, but none is consistently successful. Whenever possible it is easier to discard the cultures, replace them with mycoplasma-free cells and adhere to simple guidelines to prevent contamination. If it is imperative to save cells, treatment with an antibiotic that is likely to have mycoplasmacidal activity, such as a fluoroquinolone, identification of the contaminant and use of a specific antiserum, or a combination of these methods is most likely to be successful.

RECOMMENDED READING

Furr P M, Taylor-Robinson D, Webster A D B 1994 Mycoplasmas and ureaplasmas in patients with hypogammaglobulinaemia and their role in arthritis: microbiological observations over 20 years. *Annals of the Rheumatic Diseases* 53: 183–187

Maniloff J, McElhaney R N, Finch L R, Baseman J B (eds) 1992 *Mycoplasmas. Molecular Biology and Pathogenesis.* American Society for Microbiology, Washington DC

Razin S, Tully J G (eds) 1995 *Molecular and Diagnostic Procedures in Mycoplasmology. Molecular Characterization*, Vol. 1. Academic Press, London

Symposium 1993 The changing role of mycoplasmas in respiratory disease and AIDS. *Clinical Infectious Diseases* 17 (Suppl. 1)

Taylor-Robinson D 1995 The history and role of *Mycoplasma genitalium* in sexually transmitted diseases. *Genitourinary Medicine* 71: 1–8

Taylor-Robinson D 1996 Mycoplasmas and their role in human respiratory tract disease. In: Myint S, Taylor-Robinson D (eds) *Viral and Other Infections of the Human Respiratory Tract.* Chapman and Hall, London, p. 319

Taylor-Robinson D 1996 Infection due to species of *Mycoplasma* and *Ureaplasma*: an update. *Clinical Infectious Diseases* 23: 671–684

Taylor-Robinson D, Bebear C 1997 Antibiotic susceptibilities of mycoplasmas and treatment of mycoplasmal infections. *Journal of Antimicrobial Chemotherapy* 40: 622–630

Taylor-Robinson D, Ainsworth J G, McCormack W M 1999 Genital mycoplasmas. In: Holmes K K, Mardh P-A, Sparling P F *et al.* (eds) *Sexually Transmitted Diseases,* 3rd edn. McGraw Hill, New York, p. 533

Taylor-Robinson D, Gilroy C B, Jensen J S 2000 The biology of *Mycoplasma genitalium. Venereology* 13: 119–127

Tully J G, Razin S (eds) 1996 *Molecular and Diagnostic Procedures in Mycoplasmology. Diagnostic Procedures*, Vol. 2. Academic Press, London

Waites K B, Taylor-Robinson D 1999 *Mycoplasma* and *Ureaplasma.* In: Murray P R, Baron E J, Pfaller M A, Tenover F C, Yolken R H (eds) *Manual of Clinical Microbiology,* 7th edn. American Society for Microbiology, Washington DC, p. 782

PART 4
VIRAL PATHOGENS AND ASSOCIATED DISEASES

42

Adenoviruses

Respiratory disease; conjunctivitis; gut infections

J. S. M. Peiris and C. R. Madeley

Adenoviruses have been described as the weeds in the virological garden; always present, not valued for themselves, sometimes decorative and felt to be of only limited interest to serious clinical virologists. As all gardeners will know, a plant is only a weed if it is in the wrong place, and much of the interest in a wild area is provided by 'weeds'. They can also be valued for themselves and, with increasing doubts that viruses are always pathogens, the epidemiology of adenoviruses is becoming of greater interest.

They were named from their original source, *adenoid tissue* removed at operation and cultured as explants in vitro. Cellular outgrowth occurred readily, but this often deteriorated rapidly a week or 10 days later. The cause of the deterioration was found to be *adenovirus(es)* present in the original tissue and which replicated enthusiastically in the new cells growing from the explant.

This discovery initiated much research which established that there were a considerable number of serotypes, or species, and that they were mostly associated with mild *upper respiratory tract infections*. In addition, there were occasional serious (and even fatal) childhood *pneumonias* and infrequent, but readily transmissible, *eye infections*. Some of these infections, mostly in children and not always symptomatic, could persist for weeks or months. The focus of adenovirus research then shifted away from clinical virology with the discovery that some species could cause malignancies in laboratory rodents. As a result, virologists have thoroughly investigated adenovirus structure, replicative mechanisms and oncogenicity during the last 40 years.

Clinical interest revived in the middle 1970s with the discovery of two new serotypes (subsequently numbered types 40 and 41) linked (with several other previously unknown viruses) to that previously elusive entity '*viral gastro-enteritis*'. This revival of clinical interest has been extended by the discovery in rapid succession of six new serotypes (numbered 42–47), most of them in patients with acquired immunodeficiency syndrome (AIDS). While adenoviruses cause serious disease in immunocompromised patients, they may also be present in the stools of congenitally immunodeficient children with little or no associated pathology. This was unexpected, the more so because it is only rarely that adenoviruses have been noted as opportunist invaders of immunosuppressed patients. Why they do not exploit more the vulnerability of these patients is unknown at present. Although they may be present in the stools of congenitally immunodeficient children, adenoviruses rarely damage their human hosts seriously, but their activities and epidemiology should have important lessons for medicine, and investigations into their interactions with our immune mechanisms are overdue. This last point is now very relevant because the use of adenoviruses as vectors in gene therapy is being explored. The apparently low pathogenic potential of adenoviruses has encouraged genetic manipulators to explore their possible use in gene therapy or tumour treatment. Human genes (up to 7 kb in size) have been inserted into replication-crippled adenoviruses and the new gene(s) carried into cells by virus infection in the hope that expression of these genes can correct the defects caused by the absent or defective genes. Alternatively, modified adenoviruses have been used either to target tumour cells (which are often of epithelial origin) to carry lethal mutations into the cell, or to induce the surface expression of target viral antigens which will make the cell vulnerable to normal immune mechanisms.

Both these approaches show some promise, but there remain formidable technical problems to overcome before either gene therapy or oncolysis become useful routinely.

DESCRIPTION

Adenovirus virions provide a very good example of an *icosahedron*. Figure 42.1a shows a group of typical adenovirus particles while Fig. 42.1b, c and d compare a

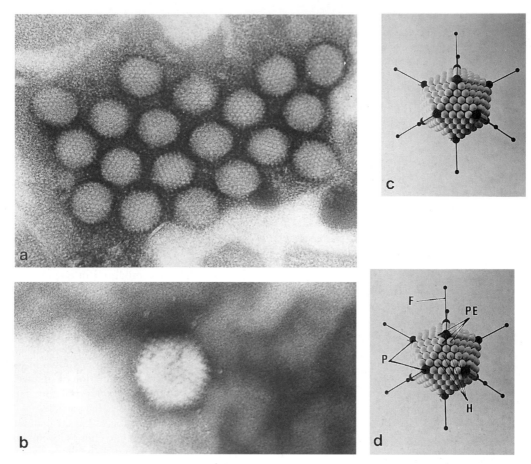

Fig. 42.1 **a** Group of adenovirus particles from a stool extract. These show the typical adenovirus morphology, although apical fibres are not visible. Individual capsomeres are visible as surface 'knobs'. These particles should be compared with the model seen in **c**. Negative contrast, 3%, potassium phosphotungstate, pH7.0 × 160 000. **b** Single adenovirus particle showing some of the apical fibres. This is an unusual finding. Negative contrast, 3% potassium phosphotungstate, pH 7.0 × 280 000. **c** and **d** Photograph of a model with pentons (P), peripentons (PE) and hexons (H) indicated. Note that the fibres are attached to the penton.

single virus particle, as seen in the electron microscope, with a model. The particles in Figure 42.1a lack the fibres projecting from the apices (they are rarely seen in situ in the electron microscope) but otherwise the particles in Figure 42.1a and b resemble the model closely. Indeed, the adenovirus is one of the few viruses of which a convincing model can be made.

The virion is 70–75 nm in size, depending on whether it is measured across the 'flats' or the apices, and there are probably minor variations between preparations and, possibly, serotypes. The surface has 252 visible surface knobs, the capsomers: 12 apical capsomers, each surrounded by five others, are known as *pentons*; 60 peripentons surround the pentons and 180 other capsomers make up the major part of the faces (Fig. 42.1d). Except for the pentons, all the other capsomers are surrounded by six others, and are therefore called *hexons*.

From each penton projects an apical *fibre*. The fibres vary greatly in length between 9 and 31 nm. Collapse of particles on storage or on exposure to some negative stains can release visible fibres in large amounts. Some avian types have double fibres but human strains all have single ones.

Adenoviruses contain a single piece of double-stranded DNA 33–45 kb in size which codes for a considerable number of proteins, with molecular weights between 7500 and 400 000. They include both structural and non-structural proteins. The 10 structural proteins include three polypeptides that make up each hexon, one which forms the penton base and a glycoprotein for the fibre. These five lie on the surface of the particle while the others are internal.

The pentons and fibres bear antigenic determinants that are 'type'-specific, and antibody binding to them results in neutralization of virus infectivity. The hexons also have some type-specific antigenic determinants, but carry group-specific antigens as well. The same group antigens are found on all the mastadenoviruses (see below), the genus to which the medically important human adenoviruses belong. These group-specific antigens provide a basis for tests to detect adenoviruses and antibodies to them (by immunofluorescence, enzyme immuno-assays, complement fixation, etc. – see below).

Classification

The family Adenoviridae comprises two genera:

- *Mastadenovirus*, whose members infect mammalian species, including humans.
- *Aviadenovirus*, whose members infect avian species.

The two genera are completely distinct antigenically. Human adenoviruses are further subdivided into six species (A–F) (Table 42.1), based on DNA homology. By definition, those with more than 50% homology are members of the same species, while those of different species have less than 20% homology.

Within each species, adenovirus serotypes are defined by cross-reactivity in neutralization tests. There are 47 recognized serotypes of human adenoviruses at present, of which types 40–47 have only been recognized within the past 30 years. There may be more types yet to be discovered.

REPLICATION

The virus attaches to susceptible cells by the apical fibres and is then taken into the cell, losing both fibres and pentons in the process. It then passes to the nucleus, losing the peripentons at the nuclear membrane. Inside the nucleus the DNA is released and the process of replication initiated.

The first messenger RNAs (mRNAs) code for non-structural proteins which shut off most host cell activities while switching on the host cell DNA-dependent DNA polymerase, which is required to initiate replication. About 20 of these 'early' proteins are produced, most of which are not incorporated in new particles (i.e. they are non-structural).

Following production of new viral DNA, the remaining genes are transcribed from it to form 'late' proteins. These are produced in quantity in the cytoplasm, are mostly structural and are later transported back to the nucleus where new virus particles are assembled, normally as crystalline arrays. They are assembled on a scaffold protein, initially as empty shells into which the nucleic acid is inserted afterwards. The effects of the shutting down of the host cell metabolism and the accumulation of thousands of new virions results in rupture (lysis) and death of the infected cell with release of the particles.

In cell cultures this process causes the cells to round up, swell and aggregate into clumps resembling bunches of grapes. The cells then disintegrate as they lyse.

Table 42.1 Properties and classification of adenoviruses of species A–F

Species	Serotypes	No. of *Sma*I fragments[b]	Haemagglutination pattern[c]	Oncogenicity in newborn hamsters	Tissues most commonly infected
A	12, 18, 31	4–5	IV	High	Gut (no symptoms)
B	3, 7, 11, 14, 16, 21, 34, 35	8–10	I	Low	Respiratory tract, kidney
C	1, 2, 5, 6	10–12	III	None	Respiratory tract, lymphoid tissue (tonsils and adenoids)
D	8–10, 13, 15, 17, 19, 20, 22–30, 32, 33, 36–39, 42–47	14–18	II	None	Conjunctiva, gut, respiratory tract(?)
E	4	16–19	III	None	Conjunctiva, respiratory tract
F	40, 41	9–12	IV	None	Gut

[a] >50% DNA homology between members.
[b] Restriction endonuclease digestion. Some small fragments probably not included.
[c] I, complete agglutination of monkey erythrocytes; II, complete agglutination of rat erythrocytes; III, partial agglutination of rat erythrocytes; IV, agglutination of rat erythrocytes only after addition of heterotypic serum.
Adapted with permission from Wadell G 2000 In: Zuckerman A J, Banatvala J E (eds) *Principles and Practice of Clinical Virology*, 4th edn. John Wiley and Sons, Chichester

CLINICAL FEATURES

Table 42.2 lists the more common associations of serotypes with disease. However, this does not tell the whole story. On the one hand, the great majority of infections with adenoviruses are probably undiagnosed and the full extent of pathogenesis is under-reported. On the other hand, virus infection and replication are not invariably associated with disease. For example, a wide variety of serotypes are isolated from faeces without evidence of gut pathology, and prolonged tonsillar carriage in children is common. However, some well recognized disease syndromes are caused by adenovirus infections.

Respiratory disease

In childhood

These are usually mild upper respiratory tract infections with fever, a runny nose and a cough. The majority are due to types 1–7, although higher serotypes may be involved sporadically. Types 1, 2, 5 and 6 are more commonly associated with endemic infections while types 3, 4 and 7 are more epidemic. In Newcastle upon Tyne, in the period March 1989 to March 1990, types 1, 2, 5 and 6 accounted for 71 of 103 adenovirus infections (69%), types 3, 4 and 7 for 12 (12%), and other types for 20 (20%). The associated clinical diagnoses included 'upper respiratory tract infection (URTI)', 'increased secretions', 'wheezy', 'cold and cough' and 'failure to thrive'.

These infections are rarely serious but, occasionally and unpredictably, may progress to a pneumonia that is both extensive and frequently fatal. The majority of these pneumonias occur in young children. Unlike other viral respiratory infections, adenoviruses may be associated with raised white cell counts and levels of C-reactive protein, and may be clinically confused with bacterial infections.

In older children and young adults a proportion of these will be labelled as 'colds' but epidemics of adenoviral infection with respiratory symptoms and fever are common in, for example, US military recruit camps, where violent exercise and close proximity combine to make the victims more vulnerable and facilitate spread. These outbreaks can be severe in both numbers and extent of disease; severe enough, in fact, to warrant preparation of a trial vaccine. Eye involvement is a common feature (see below), leading to such outbreaks being called pharyngoconjunctival fever. Types 3 and 7 are more often associated with these outbreaks but other serotypes are found from time to time.

Adenovirus infections are said to mimic whooping cough in some patients, and dual infections with *Bordetella pertussis* have been found. However, there is little doubt that genuine whooping cough is due to the bacterium.

Eye infections

Adenoviruses have been associated with several outbreaks of conjunctivitis in the UK, frequently referred to as 'shipyard eye' because originally it was thought to be caused by steel swarf thrown up from welding and grinding. It was later shown that adenovirus was being transmitted through fluids, eyebaths and other instruments used to treat eye injuries in the shipyard first aid clinic and which had become contaminated by virus

Table 42.2 Disease associated with adenovirus serotypes

Disease	Those at risk	Associated serotypes
Acute febrile pharyngitis		
Endemic	Infants, young children	1, 2, 5, 6
Epidemic	Infants, young children	3, 4, 7
Pharyngoconjunctival fever	Older school-age children	3, 7
Acute respiratory disease	Military recruits	4, 7, 14, 21
Pneumonia	Infants	1, 2, 3, 7
Follicular conjunctivitis	Any age	3, 4, 11
Epidemic keratoconjunctivitis	Adults	8, 19, 37
Haemorrhagic cystitis	Infants, young children	11, 21
Diarrhoea and vomiting	Infants, young children	40, 41
Intussusception	Infants	1, 2, 5
Disseminated infection	Immunocompromised, e.g. AIDS, renal, bone marrow and heart-lung transplant recipients	5, 11, 34, 35, 43–47

Adapted with permission from Wadell G 2000 In: Zuckerman A J, Banatvala J E (eds) *Principles and Practice of Clinical Virology*, 4th edn. John Wiley and Sons, Chichester from the index case. Use of properly sterilized instruments and single-dose preparations of eye ointment have now made this uncommon. Most such outbreaks were due to adenovirus type 8 (although types 19 and 37 may also be involved). This is not one of the easiest types to isolate, and sporadic cases may not be identified as readily as outbreaks, which inevitably attract a more concentrated effort at diagnosis. Eye infections with type 8 do not usually cause systemic symptoms.

Conjunctivitis caused by other serotypes may form part of outbreaks of pharyngoconjunctival fever. It is a follicular conjunctivitis resembling that caused by chlamydiae, from which it should be differentiated, but the associated and usually marked adenovirus respiratory symptoms provide a clue.

Gut infections

The common respiratory serotypes (1–7) are frequently isolated from faeces, and, in young children, the same serotype may be recovered from both ends of the child. Despite some anecdotal reports, there is little evidence to link such isolates with disease of the gut. However, when faecal extracts from children with diarrhoea were examined by electron microscopy, typical adenoviruses were seen in a proportion of cases, often in very large numbers. Surprisingly, these morphologically typical viruses could not readily be isolated in cell culture. It is now clear that these belonged to two hitherto unknown serotypes, 40 and 41. These are associated with a significant proportion of endemic cases of childhood diarrhoea and, in numbers of cases, are second only to rotaviruses. Estimates of the proportion vary between different laboratories but they may contribute up to a third of such cases in which a virus is found. As with other viruses found in diarrhoeal faeces, such adenoviruses may also be present less frequently in the faeces of apparently normal babies, but there is no doubt of their pathogenic potential for the gut. How they differ from the other non-pathogenic types in the gut is not known, nor if they cause respiratory infections.

The role of adenovirus(es) in mesenteric adenitis and intussusception is uncertain. Even when enlarged nodes are identified at laparotomy it is not usual to excise one for diagnosis, and direct evidence is lacking. Finding a coincidental adenovirus in faeces is not proof of involvement, nor is it clear how often adenitis precedes (and possibly initiates) intussusception. Where any such temporal association has been recorded it has involved the common serotypes 1, 2, 5 and 6. Probably the appropriate verdict is the old Scots one of 'not proven'!

Six new serotypes (42–47) have been found, five of them (43–47) in the faeces of patients with AIDS. The sixth was isolated from the faeces of a normal child. Chronic diarrhoea is a feature of AIDS and the role of these adenoviruses, if any, in causing it awaits further investigation. Interestingly, these new serotypes were isolated and identified in cell culture, suggesting they are indeed 'new'. If so, their origin and significance are both unknown.

Other diseases

Infrequently there have been reports of adenovirus (types 11 and 21 mostly) recovered from the urine of children with haemorrhagic cystitis. Finding virus provides a (possible) retrospective cause. Adenoviruses may also be associated with haemorrhagic cystitis, hepatitis (in liver transplant patients) and pneumonitis in immuno-compromised patients. The serotypes involved are often uncommon ones (e.g. types 11, 34, 35). In the newborn, adenoviruses may cause disseminated disease with a 'septic shock' form of presentation.

There are reports in the literature of recovery of adenoviruses from both the male and the female genital tracts. They may be sexually transmitted but are not the cause of a major sexually transmitted disease.

There is no good evidence of adenoviruses being involved in central nervous system disease nor in human tumour production. Experimentally, adenoviruses may induce transformation of hamster cells in culture and such transformed cells will produce tumours in laboratory animals. There is no evidence that this can occur in humans although it has been diligently sought. Under laboratory conditions adenoviruses can also form hybrids with simian virus 40 (SV40), a papovavirus that contaminated early stocks of polio vaccine grown in monkey kidney cells. The hybrids, carrying part of the SV40 genome, are neither pathogenic nor oncogenic in humans.

PATHOGENESIS

Adenoviruses are mostly infectors of mucosal surfaces (respiratory tract, gut and eye) but it is clear that by no means all such infection leads to overt disease. Different serotypes appear to prefer different regions. It is not known what this means at a molecular or cellular level but it may reflect the presence or absence of particular receptors. Infection of an individual cell will cause its death, but several studies have documented prolonged respiratory and gut excretion in healthy children lasting weeks or months. Such respiratory 'carriage' is probably in lymphoid tissue (tonsils and adenoids), and gut carriage may be in the equivalent Peyer's patches, although this has not been documented.

Most infections with adenoviruses, whatever the primary site, probably spread to include the gut. 'Respiratory' strains are frequently recovered from faeces and it seems improbable that this results solely from overflow from the upper respiratory tract. It is much more likely that faecal excretion follows a secondary gut infection, albeit asymptomatic in most cases.

The role of the five newly discovered serotypes (43–47) in patients with AIDS is not known at present. All were recovered from faeces by culture and had not been identified before. They extend the unanswered questions about adenoviruses to include where new types could come from and whether they can arise by mutation and/or recombination.

LABORATORY DIAGNOSIS

Direct demonstration of 'virus'

Electron microscopy

Virus particles may be seen directly in stool extracts by electron microscopy, although this will not identify serotypes. None the less, where virus is seen this will usually be types 40 or 41, particularly where large numbers are present (the level may reach more than 10^{10} particles per gram of faeces). Finding virus in faeces by electron microscopy does not mean that virus must also be present in the nasopharynx or the eye(s).

Virus antigen

The presence of viral antigen in the nasopharynx may be identified by immunofluorescence with group-specific antibodies (polyclonal or monoclonal) directly on aspirates (not swabs), provided they contain respiratory cells. The presence of such infected cells usually indicates a significant infection, in contrast to asymptomatic carriage. Alternatively, viral antigen may be detected by enzyme immuno-assays. However, these detect virus antigen alone without indicating where it was located. Hence they cannot distinguish between a significant presence in respiratory cells (indicating invasion of the mucosal surface) and mostly silent (and clinically insignificant) carriage, probably in the tonsils and adenoids.

Viral DNA

It is also possible to detect viral DNA directly from faeces by polyacrylamide gel electrophoresis. The intact DNA forms a single band found near the top of the gel but its identity as definitely adenovirus in origin can be confirmed only after digestion with restriction endonucleases and repeat electrophoresis. A characteristic 'ladder' of DNA fragments separated by size confirms the diagnosis, distinguishes between types 40 and 41 (and identifies others) and can also indicate subtypes. This approach is particularly useful to identify types 40 and 41, which are difficult or impossible to isolate in cell culture, and for laboratories without access to electron microscopy.

Culture

Virus can be grown in cell culture from respiratory specimens (nasopharyngeal aspirates, and nose and throat swabs), eye swabs, faeces and, occasionally, urine. The speed of isolation can provide a pointer to the significance of the finding. If it takes longer than 12 days it is less likely to be clinically significant, particularly with types 1, 2, 5 and 6.

Isolation of an adenovirus in cell culture from the faeces of patients with diarrhoea is by itself of little significance. As mentioned earlier, diarrhoea-causing adenoviruses are not readily isolated in culture, and cultivable adenoviruses in the stool are not usually those associated with diarrhoea. Nevertheless, the diarrhoea-associated adenoviruses go through partial replication in G293 cells (an adenovirus-transformed human embryo kidney cell line), and the antigens induced in these cells are type-specific. They may be identified by immuno-fluorescence using type-specific antibodies.

Serology

A rise in antibody levels indicates recent infection (though not its site or nature) but absence does not exclude it, especially in babies. Complement fixation is the test most frequently used, and it provides only a group-specific diagnosis. Group- and type-specific enzyme immuno-assays have also been developed but are not used widely. Neutralization tests are both type-specific and more sensitive, but are not available as routine tests; neither is haemagglutination inhibition widely available. However, both tests may be used by reference laboratories or in research.

TREATMENT

There are no antiviral drugs available that are unequivocally effective for the treatment of adenoviral infections. Ribavirin, ganciclovir, vidarabine and cidofavir have all been shown to have antiviral activity in vitro and there are anecdotal reports of their therapeutic use in immunocompromised patients with variable success.

EPIDEMIOLOGY

Adenoviruses are endemic and types 1–7 spread readily between individuals, presumably by droplets. Faecal–oral transmission can also occur and probably does in areas with poverty, poor hygiene and overcrowding. However, it is probable that types 40 and 41, which are widespread causes of diarrhoea even in highly developed countries, also spread via droplets.

Subtyping, which has shown, for example, eight sub-types of adenovirus type 7 (the prototype 7p, and seven variants 7a–7g), has also shown geographical variations in their distribution. Such detailed analysis is not done routinely, however, and no information on subtype distribution of types 40 and 41 is available.

It is probable that only a minority of adenovirus infections are diagnosed virologically. What is known about their epidemiology is therefore only the tip of a considerable iceberg. Using the earlier analogy to weeds, they will always be with us, providing a more luxuriant over-growth from time to time as circumstances allow. It is probable that some individuals are more vulnerable than others to their activity; for example, some young children who develop pneumonia, and, possibly, patients with AIDS. There is a need for more information about these viruses, whose range of activities is wide.

CONTROL

For the same reasons as discussed earlier under treatment, there is little demand for a vaccine. How well it would work can be questioned because circulating antibody may not prevent re-infection, although volunteer studies indicate that re-infection rarely results in disease. Nevertheless, the problems with adenoviruses encountered by US armed forces in recruit camps led them to experiment with a live virus vaccine administered orally in enteric capsules. It provided adequate protection from disease and was licensed for use but only in military personnel. The plethora of serotypes, their widespread presence and their generally benign outcome makes extension to the general public unlikely to be worthwhile.

A careful and rigorous attention to aseptic technique and single-dose vials of materials for use in the eye is the best approach to preventing outbreaks of adenovirus eye infections. As a component of pharyngoconjunctival fever, conjunctivitis is not preventable.

ADENOVIRUS–ASSOCIATED VIRUSES

The adenovirus-associated viruses (AAVs) are members of the parvoviridae. They are about 22 nm in diameter, appear to be more hexagonal than circular in outline and contain insufficient single-stranded DNA to replicate on their own. They form a genus, *dependoviruses*, indicating their dependence on adenoviruses (or herpes simplex virus) to provide the missing functions.

True AAV (also known as adenovirus satellite virus) has not been implicated in clinical disease. However, as with any other virus found in faeces, large numbers of parvovirus-like particles have been seen in extracts of diarrhoeal faeces, sometimes (but not invariably) combined with smaller numbers of adenoviruses. Neither virus grows in cell culture, leaving the significance of these observations obscure (see Chapter 47 on parvoviruses).

RECOMMENDED READING

Alemany R, Balagué C, Curiel D T 2000 Replicative adenoviruses for cancer therapy. *Nature Biotechnology* 18: 723–727

Wadell G 2000 Adenoviruses. In: Zuckerman A J, Banatvala J E, Pattison J R (eds) *Principles and Practice of Clinical Virology*, 4th edn. Wiley, Chichester

43

Herpesviruses

Herpes simplex; varicella and zoster; infectious mononucleosis; B cell lymphomas; cytomegalovirus disease; roseola infantum; Kaposi's sarcoma; herpes B

M. M. Ogilvie

The herpesviruses, a large family infecting many animal species, share a number of features, including their structure and mode of replication and the capacity to establish life-long latent infections from which virus may be reactivated.

Latent infection. This has been defined as 'a type of persistent infection in which the viral genome is present but infectious virus is not produced except during intermittent episodes of reactivation'.

Reactivation. Reactivation from the latent state may be restricted to asymptomatic virus shedding.

Recurrence or recrudescence. These terms are used when reactivated virus produces clinically obvious disease.

At present eight human herpesviruses are recognized, and infection with each of the first seven has been shown to be common in all populations; studies with the eighth suggest it is an uncommon infection in developed countries.

1.	Herpes simplex virus 1	HSV-1
2.	Herpes simplex virus 2	HSV-2
3.	Varicella-zoster virus	VZV
4.	Epstein–Barr virus	EBV
5.	Cytomegalovirus	CMV
6.	Human herpesvirus 6	HHV6
7.	Human herpesvirus 7	HHV7
8.	Human herpesvirus 8	HHV8

The herpes B virus of monkeys can be transmitted to humans accidentally. These viruses, the infections caused by them, and associated diseases will be described here.

DESCRIPTION

Herpesviruses have a characteristic morphology visible in electron microscopical studies (Fig. 43.1). Negative staining reveals the icosahedral protein capsid of

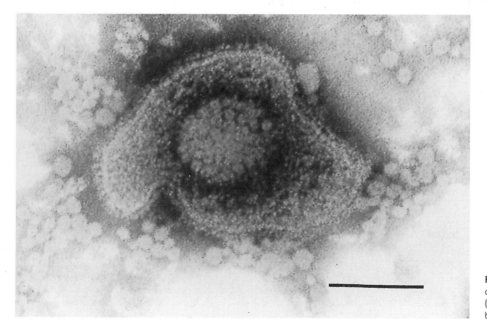

Fig. 43.1 Electron micrograph of HSV. Negative staining (2% PTA). Bar, 100 nm. (Prepared by Dr B. W. McBride.)

average diameter 100 nm, consisting of 162 hollow hexagonal and pentagonal capsomeres, with an electron-dense core containing the DNA genome. Outside the capsid in mature particles is an amorphous proteinaceous layer, the *tegument*, surrounded by a lipid *envelope* derived from cell membranes. Projecting from the trilaminar lipid envelope are *spikes* of viral glycoproteins. Cryo-electron micrographs indicate that the capsid is organized into at least three layers, with viral DNA inserted in the innermost layer. The average enveloped particle diameter is approximately 200 nm.

The genome of herpes virions is linear double-stranded DNA, varying in length from 125 to 245 kbp, with a base content ranging from 42 to 69 G + C mol% for the human herpesviruses. The presence of long and short unique regions bounded by repeated and inverted short segments allows recombination and isomeric forms in some cases (Fig. 43.2). Genes coding for viral glycoproteins, major capsid proteins, enzymes involved in DNA replication and some transcripts associated with latency have been identified. Conserved sequences appear in certain regions, and some genes show homology with regions of human chromosomes. Restriction endonuclease analysis permits epidemiological comparison of strains ('finger-printing') within some herpes species.

Some herpesviruses are predominantly:

- neurotropic (HSV and VZV)
- lymphotropic (EBV, HHV6 and HHV7).

Biological classification

The family Herpesviridae comprises three broad groups (subfamilies):

- Alphaherpesviruses, e.g. HSV, VZV and B virus; rapid growth, latency in sensory ganglia.
- Betaherpesviruses – CMVs; slow growth, restricted host range.

- Gammaherpesviruses, e.g. EBV; growth in lymphoblastoid cells.

Of the newer human herpesviruses, HHV6 and HHV7 have been classified with CMV as betaherpesviruses, and the most recently identified, HHV8, is a gammaherpesvirus like EBV.

The viruses are relatively thermolabile and readily inactivated by lipid solvents such as alcohols and detergents.

Replication

After attachment to receptors, the envelope of herpes virions fuses with the cell membrane. The nucleocapsids cross the cytoplasm to the nuclear membrane; replication of viral DNA and assembly of capsids takes place within the nucleus. With HSV, it is known that tegument protein transactivates expression of the first set of genes. Between 65 and 100 viral proteins are synthesized, in an orderly sequence or cascade.

These proteins are of three types:

1. Immediate early (α) – mainly regulatory functions.
2. Early (β) – includes many enzymes involved in DNA replication.
3. Late (γ) – structural proteins of capsid, glycoproteins.

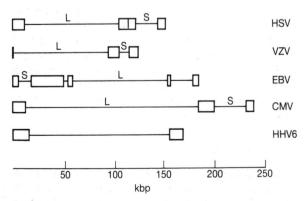

Fig. 43.2 Diagrammatic comparison of herpesvirus DNAs. Lines indicate long (L) or short (S) unique sequences, and repeated regions are boxed.

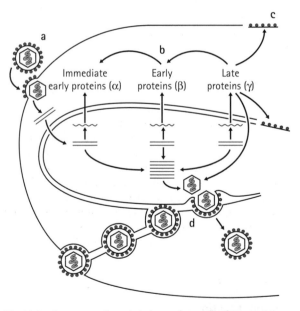

Fig. 43.3 A summary of events in herpesvirus replication; **a**, entry; **b**, viral DNA transcription and replication, showing cascade of proteins synthesized; **c**, glycoprotein expression on cell membranes; **d**, assembly and egress of new virions. (By courtesy of J. P. Vestey, Dermatology, Royal Infirmary, Edinburgh.)

The viral capsid proteins migrate from the cytoplasm to the nucleus where capsid assembly occurs and new viral DNA is inserted and located in the inner shell. Viral glycoproteins are processed in the Golgi complex and are incorporated into cell membranes from which the viral envelope is acquired, usually from the inner layer of the nuclear membrane as the virus buds out from the nucleus (Fig. 43.3). It then passes by way of membranous vacuoles to reach the cell surface. Productively infected cells generally do not survive.

HERPES SIMPLEX VIRUS

HSV is ubiquitous, infecting the majority of the world's population early in life and persisting in a latent form from which reactivation with shedding of infectious virus occurs, thus maintaining the transmission chain.

Description

The virus has the general structure and chemical composition already described. In contrast to other members of the group, HSV can be grown in cells from a wide variety of animals relatively easily, so that far more extensive studies have been undertaken with this virus.

There are two distinct types of HSV, named type 1 (HSV-1) and type 2 (HSV-2). These two types are generally (but not exclusively) associated with different sites of infection in patients (see below); type 1 strains are associated primarily with the mouth, the eye and the central nervous system, while type 2 strains are found most often in the genital tract.

HSV glycoproteins

The envelope of HSV contains several glycoproteins that have been studied in detail both at the structural and functional level. At least 11 glycoproteins are known. Three of the glycoproteins are essential for production of infectious virions: gB and gD, which are involved in adsorption to and penetration into cells, and gH, involved in the release of virus. Some of the glycoproteins have common antigenic determinants shared by HSV-1 and HSV-2 (gB and gD) whilst others have specific determinants for one type only (gG).

Pathogenesis

Primary infection

The typical lesion produced by HSV is the *vesicle*, a ballooning degeneration of intra-epithelial cells. The underlying layer of basal epithelium is usually intact, as

vesicles only occasionally penetrate the subepithelial layer. The base of the vesicle contains multinucleate cells (sometimes called *Tzanck cells*, seen in Giemsa-stained preparations) and infected nuclei contain eosinophilic *inclusion bodies*. The roof of the vesicle breaks down, and an ulcer forms: this happens rapidly on mucous membranes and non-keratinizing epithelia; on the skin the ulcer crusts over, forming a scab, and then heals. A mononuclear reaction is normal, with the vesicle fluid becoming cloudy, and cellular infiltration in the subepithelial tissue. After resorption or loss of the vesicle fluid the damaged epithelium is regenerated. Natural killer cells play a significant role in early defence by recognizing and destroying HSV-infected cells. Synthesis of herpesvirus glycoproteins during the virus growth cycle is followed by the insertion of the glycoproteins into the cell membranes, and some are secreted into extracellular fluid. The infected host responds to all these foreign antigens, producing cytotoxic T cells (CD4$^+$ and CD8$^+$), and helper T lymphocytes (CD4$^+$), which activate primed B cells to produce specific antibodies and are also involved in the induction of delayed hypersensitivity. The different glycoproteins have significant roles in generating these various cell responses; probably all of them induce neutralizing antibody.

During the replication phase at the site of entry in the epithelium, virus particles enter through the sensory nerve endings that penetrate to the parabasal layer of the epithelium, and are transported, probably as nucleocapsids, along the axon to the nerve body (neurone) in the sensory (dorsal root) ganglion by retrograde axonal flow. Virus replication in a neurone ends in neuronal cell death; however, in some ganglion cells a *latent infection* is established in which the neurones survive but continue to harbour the viral genome. Neurones other than those in sensory ganglia can be the site of herpes latency. Whether true latency occurs at epithelial sites is not yet clear; there is some evidence of persistence of virus at peripheral sites, but this may be due to a reactivation with a low level of virus replication.

Antibody does reduce the severity of infections, although it does not prevent recurrences. Neonates receiving maternal antibody transplacentally are protected against the worst effects of neonatal herpes. HSV-2 infection seems to protect against HSV-1, but prior HSV-1 infection only partly modifies HSV-2 disease.

Latent infection

Latent infection of sensory neurones is a feature of the neurotropic herpesviruses HSV and VZV. Most of the information available about the latent state has been obtained from studies of HSV-1 latency. Only a small proportion (about 1%) of cells in the affected ganglion carry the viral genome, which is in a different state to that found in virions. In latency, viral DNA exists as free circular *episomes* – perhaps about 20 copies per infected cell. Very few virus genes are expressed in the latent state; in HSV some viral RNA transcripts (latency-associated transcripts) are found in the nuclei but no virus-coded proteins have been demonstrated in the cells, so these infected neurones are not recognized by the immune system. Latent herpes simplex genomes have been detected in post mortem studies on excised ganglia and other neuronal tissues. HSV-1 is regularly detected in:

- the trigeminal ganglion
- other sensory and autonomic ganglia (e.g. vagus)
- adrenal tissue and in the brain.

HSV-2 latency in the sacral ganglia has been demonstrated. Either type may become latent in other ganglia.

Reactivation and recrudescence

Reactivation processes are still not understood. It is suggested that in some way herpesvirus DNA passes along the nerve axon back to the nerve ending where infection of epithelial cells may occur. Not all re-activation will result in a visible lesion; there may be asymptomatic shedding of virus only detectable by culture.

Whilst some progress has been made in the molecular biology of the latent state in the neurone, the factors influencing the development of recrudescent lesions are not yet clearly identified. An increase of CD8$^+$ suppressor cell activity is common at the time of recurrences. Some mediators, e.g. prostaglandins, and a temporary decrease in immune effector cell function, particularly delayed hypersensitivity, may enhance spread of the virus. Certainly the known triggers for recurrences are accompanied by a local increase in prostaglandin levels and depression of cell-mediated immunity predisposes to herpes recurrence. The mechanism of reactivation is not known, but the event can be accurately predicted in those known to harbour latent virus. Thus, following bone marrow transplant or high-dose chemotherapy, herpes simplex recurs in 80% at a median interval of 18 days in the absence of prophylaxis.

However reactivation is achieved, it is a feature of HSV infection. It occurs naturally, and can be induced by a variety of stimuli such as:

- ultraviolet light (sunlight)
- fever
- trauma
- stress.

The interval between the stimulus and the appearance of a clinically obvious lesion is 2–5 days, as has been regularly demonstrated in patients undergoing neurological interference with their trigeminal ganglion, a common site of herpes latency.

Clinical features

Primary infection. Primary herpetic infection, as the name indicates, is the patient's first experience of HSV and occurs therefore in those with no antibody to the virus. It usually involves the mucous membranes of the mouth, but may include the lips, skin of the face, nose or any other site, including the eye and genital tract.

Recurrence or recrudescence. Symptomatic recurrence is heralded by a *prodrome* in two-thirds of people, who experience pain or paraesthesia (tingling, warmth, itch) at the site, followed by erythema and a papule, usually within 24 h. Progression to a vesicle and ulcer, with subsequent crusting, takes 8–12 days before natural healing. Because of their association with febrile illness the lesions are popularly known as 'cold sores' or 'fever blisters'. The most common site is at the mucocutaneous junction of the lip, seldom inside the mouth. Other sites frequently involved are on the chin and inside the nose. However, recurrent lesions will manifest at any site innervated by the affected neurone, determined by the site of initial infection.

HSV infections may be differentiated according to the immune status of the patient (Table 43.1).

Severe pain, extensive mucosal ulceration and delayed healing are features of recurrent herpes in severely compromised patients. The ulcers provide entry for other infections. Herpes simplex viraemia after reactivation is uncommon, even in the immunocompromised, but can lead to disseminated infection in internal organs. Some sufferers experience *erythema*

Table 43.1 Types of herpes simplex virus (HSV) infection

Type of infection	Immune status of patient
Primary – first HSV infection (any type at any site)	Seronegative
Latent – no symptoms	Seropositive
Recurrent – recrudescence of the latent HSV type(s)	Seropositive
Initial (non-primary) – first episode of the heterologous HSV in a seropositive patient	Seronegative for infecting type; seropositive for latent type
Re-infection (exogenous) – with a strain that differs from the latent HSV type	Seropositive

multiforme following their recurrent herpes. This is associated with reaction to certain herpes antigens, and may take the form of the Stevens–Johnson syndrome. Prophylaxis to prevent the herpes recurring has proved useful.

Oral infection

Classically, the first infection presents as an acute, febrile *gingivostomatitis* in pre-school children. Vesicular lesions ulcerate rapidly and are present in the front of the mouth and on the tongue. Gingivitis is usually present. Vesicles may also develop on the lips and skin around the mouth, and cervical lymphadenopathy occurs. The child is miserable for 7–10 days in an untreated case before the lesions heal. However, the majority of primary infections go unrecognized, the episode being attributed to teething or mistaken for 'thrush' (candida infection). Herpetic stomatitis also occurs in older children and adults acquiring a primary infection. There may be an associated mononucleosis in the older patient; pharyngitis is also notable. Viraemia with dissemination of herpes to internal organs is rare except in pregnancy (primary infection, with hepatitis) or the neonate (see later) or the immunocompromised patient.

Skin infection

Herpetic whitlow.   Hand infections with HSV are not uncommon. Three presentations may be seen:
- The classical primary lesion on the fingers or thumb of the toddler with herpetic stomatitis, due to auto-inoculation.
- Another classical and often primary infection is acquired by accidental inoculation in health care workers. These infections may recur; the majority are HSV-1.
- The commonest hand lesions are, however, recurrent, associated with HSV-2 and genital herpes and seen in young adults. Pain and swelling occur, and the vesicles become pustular, but, if in well-keratinized areas, do not always ulcerate. Associated lymphangitis is common. Primary lesions take up to 21 days to heal, recurrent ones only 10 days.

Eczema herpeticum.   A severe form of cutaneous herpes may occur in children with *atopic eczema* – eczema herpeticum or Kaposi's varicelliform eruption. Vesicles resembling those of chickenpox may appear, mainly on already eczematous areas. Extensive ulceration results in protein loss and dehydration, and viraemia can lead to disseminated disease with severe, even fatal, consequences. A similar picture is occasionally seen in adults with pemphigus who develop herpes simplex. Patients with burns are also at risk. In each instance early recognition and antiviral therapy can be life-saving.

Eye infection

HSV infection of the eye may be initiated during a childhood primary infection or occur from transfer of virus from a cold sore. There may be simply conjunctivitis, or keratoconjunctivitis associated with corneal ulceration. Typically, branching or dendritic corneal ulcers are found, and recur, resulting in corneal scarring and impairment of vision. More extensive ulceration occurs if steroids have been used, but deeper infiltrates are common in long-standing cases and benefit from combined steroid and antiviral therapy. The presence of typical herpes vesicles on eyelid margins is a useful clinical guide but is not always seen. The majority of eye infections are HSV-1, and most patients with recurring eye disease are aged over 50 years. More than half of the corneal grafting performed in the UK is for HSV corneal scarring, but the disease may recur in the graft. Recently, acute retinal necrosis associated with HSV-2 has been recognized.

Central nervous system infection

HSV may reach the brain in several ways. Viraemia has been detected during primary herpetic stomatitis, and infection may be carried within cells into the brain and meninges. Direct infection from the nasal mucosa along the olfactory tract is another possibility, but the most likely route is central spread from trigeminal ganglia.

HSV encephalitis (HSVE).   This is a rare condition, but is the commonest sporadic fatal encephalitis recognized in developed countries. The infection has a high mortality rate and significant morbidity in survivors of the acute necrotizing form. HSVE presents:

- at any time of year
- at any age
- occasionally in the young, but is more frequent in those in the 50–70-year age group
- 70% of cases are in people with serological evidence and often a clinical history of previous herpes simplex.

However, recurrent lesions are seldom apparent at the same time as HSVE. A prodrome of fever and malaise is followed by *headache* and *behavioural change* sometimes associated with a sudden focal episode such as a *seizure*, or *paralysis*; *coma* usually precedes death. The *temporal lobe* is most frequently affected, and virus replication in neurones, followed by the oedema associated with the inflammatory response, accounts for the haemorrhagic necrosis and space-occupying nature of this form of the disease. More *diffuse*, milder disease has been recorded. Brain stem encephalitis is another serious manifestation.

Clinical recognition leading to early specific antiviral therapy will significantly reduce the 70% mortality and serious morbidity of untreated cases, but therapy must be started as soon as possible, before the patient progresses from a drowsy state into coma. Diagnostic confirmation used to be most reliably provided by examination of brain biopsy tissue for virus antigens, virus particles and the characteristic histopathology. Brain biopsy is now seldom performed for suspected HSVE in the UK, but should tissue be available in the course of intracranial pressure monitoring it should be examined. Cerebrospinal fluid (CSF) collected in the acute stages of HSVE should be sent to a laboratory offering HSV DNA amplification by polymerase chain reaction (PCR). This highly sensitive technique is now established in several regional centres, and, unlike previous attempts to find HSV in CSF by culture or antigen detection, can demonstrate the presence of HSV DNA in the majority of cases within the first 10 days of onset. Diagnosis can be confirmed in the convalescent period after therapy by the demonstration of intrathecal synthesis of HSV antibody. For this purpose CSF and peripheral blood taken on the same day are required.

By far the majority of HSVE cases where virus has been identified (outside the neonatal period – see below) have been due to HSV-1. HSV-2 encephalitis does occasionally occur in immunocompromised adults and may be seen more frequently in those infected with the human immunodeficiency virus (HIV).

Genital tract infection

Both types of HSV can infect the genital tract. Although the more common association has been with type 2 strains, type 1 infection is not infrequent, particularly in young women, where it may account for more than half of genital infections. Genital infection may be acquired by auto-inoculation from lesions elsewhere on the body, but most often results from intimate sexual contact, including orogenital contact. The lesions are vesicular at first but rapidly ulcerate.

- In the male, the glans and shaft of the penis are the most frequent sites of infection.
- In the female, the labia and vagina or cervix may be involved.
- In both sexes, lesions may spread to surrounding skin sites.

The incubation period following exposure to virus is 2–20 days, with an average of 7 days. A primary infection is usually the most severe, especially in women. Fever and malaise are accompanied by regional lymphadenopathy, urethritis, and vaginal discharge may be present. The whole episode lasts 3–4 weeks, and high titres of virus are shed. In some cases a lymphocytic meningitis develops, and urinary retention can also be a problem. The latter are manifestations of sacral radiculopathy. Where the infection is an initial (non-primary) genital herpes the attack is generally less severe, but lasts around 2 weeks.

Recurrent genital herpes. This can be as frequent as six or more episodes a year. Although the attacks are milder and shorter (around 7–10 days) than first episodes, the results are socially and psychologically distressing. Some patients experience prodromal symptoms in the distribution of the sacral nerves, but the patient is already infectious by this stage. Virus shedding from the genital tract is often asymptomatic. The patient or general practitioner may not recognize recurrent lesions as herpetic in origin, so that in many instances the risk of transmission to sexual partners is not apparent. HSV-1 genital infection recurs less often than HSV-2, and thus carries a better prognosis. Either type is capable of transmission from mother to infant. Transplacental passage resulting in intra-uterine damage to the fetus has been recorded but is very rare, and is probably limited to cases with substantial maternal viraemia. Ascending infection from the cervix may be more significant, especially when the membranes are ruptured for some time before delivery.

Genital herpes increased in incidence during the 1970s and 1980s. It appears to have decreased now, as reflected in genito-urinary clinic and laboratory reports in the UK. However, the increased role of general practitioner consultations and treatment may be affecting these numbers. Genital herpes can be a significant problem in immunosuppressed patients, and is seen as persistent severe peri-anal lesions with or without proctitis in many HIV-infected male homosexuals. Genital herpetic ulcers are known to increase the risk of transmission of infection with HIV.

Neonatal herpes

A rare but very serious infection, untreated neonatal herpes has a case fatality rate exceeding 60%, with half of the survivors severely damaged. Virus, commonly HSV-2, is acquired by passage through an infected genital tract at birth. The greatest risk, with 50% transmission rate (because there is more virus present and no antibody transfer), occurs with a primary infection in the mother at the time of delivery. With recurrent herpes at term, the transmission rate is only 8% or less. Neonatal infection usually presents about the sixth day post partum. It is important to note that skin lesions may be absent, or few in number, and when they occur, are commonly located on the presenting part, e.g. scalp. Virus dissemination to internal organs is the most serious complication, in which the infant shows signs of general sepsis, including fever, poor feeding and irritability. Pneumonia and jaundice develop, with or without signs of meningitis or encephalitis. Progressive liver failure with coagulopathy leads to death around the sixteenth day in this, the most serious disseminated form. Occasionally, infection is restricted to skin or mucosae, including the conjunctivae, or involves the central nervous system with or without dissemination to internal organs. Early antiviral therapy is the key to survival with minimal morbidity, although local recurrent lesions can be expected, especially at skin sites, in the first year.

The prevention of neonatal herpes is difficult, the vast majority of infections occurring in babies born to women with no past history of genital herpes and in whom the infection at term has either been asymptomatic or has gone unrecognized clinically. Routine preterm screening for virus shedding, particularly as applied to those with a past history, does not predict the babies at risk. Once type-specific antibody tests become available routinely, susceptible women at risk of acquiring HSV-2 from partners could be identified. If any suspicious lesions are seen during labour, swabs for virus culture and a rapid detection test should be taken. Caesarean section is only likely to reduce the risk of infection if performed in the early stages of labour. If the mother is known to have moderate levels of antibody, the baby is unlikely to develop the disease.

Some cases of neonatal herpes are acquired just after birth from contact with sources of HSV other than the mother's genital tract. The clinical presentation is similar, although the virus is likely to be type 1 from oral or skin lesions of attendants or relatives. In the case of suspected neonatal herpes without skin lesions, nasopharyngeal secretions, CSF and blood lymphocytes should be cultured.

Laboratory diagnosis

Virus detection and serological studies both have their place in the diagnosis of infection with HSV. In all instances of acute infection, be it primary or recurrent, virus detection is the method of choice, for antibody responses are naturally later and much less informative. Indeed, in recurrent episodes the antibody titre may not vary. Sensitive assays for IgG antibody, including type-specific antibody, have an important place in prospective testing.

Herpes virus detection

Direct diagnosis of HSV infection is available, and should be sought in cases where there is any doubt as to the clinical diagnosis, or where rapid confirmation is required to support the choice of therapy or other management. Virus isolation is suitable for most common herpes infections, direct diagnosis being reserved for the atypical or serious situations.

Isolation of HSV from an infected patient is now most usually attempted in cultures of human diploid fibroblast cells. Growth is rapid, and within 24 h a cytopathic effect (CPE) may be visible, presenting as rounded, ballooned cells in foci that later expand and eventually involve the whole cell sheet. Virus is released from infected cells into the culture fluid, hence the rapid spread of infection from the initial foci.

Herpes virions may be demonstrated by electron microscopy in vesicle fluid or tissue preparations. Detection of viral antigens in cells (by immunofluorescence, for example) provides a rapid diagnosis on cells scraped from the base of lesions. Unfortunately, in the most serious infections it is often not possible to have easy access to the site of infection. Detection of amplified viral DNA by PCR in CSF or other samples is proving a most sensitive and specific method of diagnosis. The two HSV types can be differentiated either by using type-specific primers in the PCR, or using common primers followed by analysis with restriction enzymes or hybridization probes for each type.

Antibody tests for HSV

Complement fixation tests (CFT) are still useful in the diagnosis of primary infections when a significant change in antibody titre can be expected. The titre of antibody may not be high, especially in genital infection, and the test measures total antibody, not differentiating type-specific antibodies. In the case of herpes encephalitis, a serological diagnosis depends on demonstration of intrathecal synthesis of antibody to HSV. CFT can be used, testing serum and CSF in parallel against HSV antigens and another unrelated antigen. In health there is no antibody detectable by such tests in the CSF. If the serum antibody:CSF antibody ratio is diminished from the normal 200:1 to 40:1 (or less), and the blood–CSF barrier integrity is confirmed by other antibody (or albumin) being excluded from the CSF, intrathecal antibody synthesis is demonstrated. It is also helpful to check for the possible transfer of antibody from blood to CSF by means of an IgG index performed on the same serum and CSF samples by the biochemists or immunologists. Tests on serum alone cannot confirm HSVE.

Enzyme immuno-assays are much more sensitive and specific than CFT. When type-specific antigen preparations based on glycoprotein G are used, type-specific antibody can be detected. Immunoblotting similarly can demonstrate type-specific antibody, and can be used to study changes in the profile of antibodies seen in sequential samples at intervals after infection. Therapy often results in delay in these type-specific antibodies appearing, and late convalescent samples, at 6 weeks, should be included. Previously, type-specific assays were only available on a research basis, although enzyme immuno-assays for total antibody to HSV were supplied commercially. Reliable type-specific antibody assays are now on the market.

Treatment

Specific antiviral therapy has revolutionized the management of HSV infections over the last 20 years. Prior to the development of agents suitable for systemic use, topical application of the relatively non-selective idoxuridine was used successfully in the treatment of eye and skin infections. *Aciclovir* (synonym: *acyclovir*) has a better therapeutic ratio and was proven effective, when used early enough in appropriate dosage, for the whole range of acute HSV infections. Latency is not eradicated by this agent, which inhibits viral DNA synthesis. Prophylactic use of aciclovir is now an established part of the management to prevent reactivation in the immunocompromised, e.g. transplant recipients. Long-term suppressive therapy with aciclovir has been particularly successful in the management of frequently recurring genital herpes and HSV-related erythema multiforme. Patient-initiated early treatment can also abort or modify recurrences.

Aciclovir is the most widely used antiherpes treatment, with an excellent safety record; it is available in preparations for topical, oral and intravenous use. In pregnancy it continues to be monitored for any adverse outcome in the infant. Topical cream or ointment is suitable only for mild epithelial lesions, such as recurrent cold sores or genital herpes or corneal ulcers. Oral or intravenous therapy with aciclovir should be given for:

- Any deeper lesions.
- Disease in immunocompromised hosts.
- Intravenous therapy is required for central nervous system and other systemic infection.
- Any of the serious manifestations.

Dosage varies considerably, depending on the site of infection and whether the aim is suppression of recurrence or therapy of established disease. Because the level of aciclovir achieved in the CSF is only half that in plasma, the dosage for the treatment of encephalitis has to be twice that for other systemic disease. It is important to maintain therapy until clinical signs indicate a favourable response. In serious systemic disease, or in the severely immunocompromised, therapy is continued for 2 weeks or longer.

The poor bio-availability of aciclovir given by mouth has stimulated the development of a prodrug, *valaciclovir*, which is rapidly converted into aciclovir, producing significantly higher plasma levels after oral dosage. Another effective antiherpes agent, *penciclovir*, which is activated and inhibits HSV DNA synthesis in a similar fashion, is given in the form of an oral pro-drug, *famciclovir*. Both of these newer agents are licensed for treatment of genital herpes, and may be administered less frequently than aciclovir.

Resistance to aciclovir does develop in some instances. The commonest forms are HSV strains with deficient or altered thymidine kinase (TK); as a result they cannot phosphorylate aciclovir and the drug is inactive. This has not been a significant clinical problem in general but it must be borne in mind, particularly in severely immunocompromised hosts with the acquired immunodeficiency syndrome (AIDS) or following bone marrow transplant. A few resistant viruses with altered DNA polymerase have also been isolated associated with clinical disease. With widespread use of aciclovir, more resistant strains may be expected to arise, and monitoring of the antiviral sensitivity of herpes isolates will be necessary. Strains resistant to aciclovir are generally also resistant to famciclovir, and may need to be controlled with an agent such as foscarnet that does not require activation by viral TK.

Epidemiology

HSV is probably transferred by *direct contact*. Many children, especially in overcrowded conditions, acquire oral HSV-1 infections in the first years of life. Spread may not occur so readily in better social conditions, with the result that primary infection is delayed to young adulthood. This is the usual time of exposure to genital herpes and, as a result, primary infections may be HSV-2 or HSV-1.

Sensitive immuno-assays and type-specific assays have shown that:

- 60–90% of adults have had HSV-1 infections
- many more adults have had HSV-2 infection than give a history of genital herpes.

However, neonatal herpes is still a rare complication in the UK; the British Paediatric Surveillance Unit reported 37 confirmed neonatal herpes infections over a period of 42 months. Eleven of the infants died within their first month, and several of the survivors suffered adverse sequelae. The rate of cases has increased in some populations as genital herpes has become more common. Herpes encephalitis outside of the neonatal period occurs sporadically at a rate of about 1 per 500 000 of the population per annum.

The role of HSV in human carcinomas, particularly carcinoma of the cervix, is not clear; the ability of the virus to transform cells in vitro is well known, although permissive cells are usually destroyed before any effect can be shown.

Control

Transmission of herpes simplex can be reduced by:

- alleviating overcrowding
- practising simple hygiene
- education regarding the infectious stages
- sexual transmission may be significantly reduced by the use of condoms.

Exposure of the infant at birth can be avoided if delivery by caesarean section is performed in the early stage of labour, but this is only to be recommended when lesions are present in the mother or virus has been demonstrated at that time. Reference has already been made to the use of prophylactic antiviral regimens to control predictable recurrence. Progress in understanding latency and reactivation will provide approaches to preventing re-activation. Protection from ultraviolet light and the use of inhibitors of prostaglandin synthesis may be useful in this context.

Experimental vaccines are under investigation, but none is licensed for use in the UK at present. Research into subunit vaccines based on the viral glycoproteins or other significant viral proteins may lead to an appropriate preparation to elicit the immune responses important in control of herpes simplex.

VARICELLA–ZOSTER VIRUS

Infection with VZV presents in two forms:

- the primary infection *varicella* (or chickenpox) is a generalized eruption
- the reactivated infection *zoster* (or shingles) is localized to one or a few dermatomes.

Description

The viruses isolated from varicella and zoster are identical, and this has now been confirmed by molecular epidemiological studies on viruses isolated from individual patients. The virus has the morphology of all herpesviruses. Seventy genes code for 67 different proteins, including five families of glycoprotein genes. The glycoproteins gE, gB and gH (previously named gpI, gpII and gpIII, respectively) are particularly abundant in infected cells, and are present in the viral envelope (Fig. 43.4).

Virus replication takes place in the nucleus, and histological examination of infected epidermis reveals typical nuclear inclusions and multinucleate giant cells identical to those of herpes simplex. Human fibroblast cell cultures are most often used for isolation, but VZV can grow in a variety of human and simian cell cultures. The enveloped virions released from the nucleus remain closely attached to microvilli along the cell surface, and this 'cell-associated' characteristic, with infection being passed from cell to cell, has limited studies with this virus compared to the lytic HSV. The typical cytopathic effect appears in cell cultures in 3 days to 2 or 3 weeks.

There is only one antigenic type of VZV known, but a limited identification of strains from different geographical sources is possible; vaccine virus can be distinguished from wild-type. Antibodies to the three main glycoproteins all neutralize virus infectivity. One of these glycoproteins, gB, shares 49% amino acid identity with gB of HSV, and this may account for the cross-reactive, anamnestic antibody response that may be detected during infections with either virus.

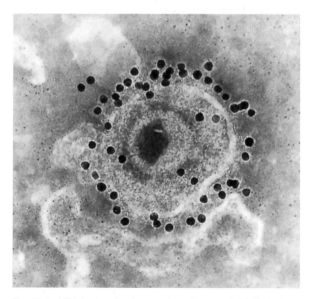

Fig. 43.4 VZV showing the virus envelope glycoprotein I (gE) labelled with monoclonal antibody and goat anti-mouse IgG conjugated with 15 nm colloidal gold. × 150 000. (Micrograph taken by C. Graham, supplied by Dr E. Dermott, Department of Microbiology and Immunobiology, Queen's University, Belfast.)

Pathogenesis

Varicella

This is a disease predominantly of children, characterized by a vesicular skin eruption. Virus is thought to enter through the upper respiratory tract, or conjunctivae, and multiply in local lymph tissue for a few days before entering the blood and being distributed throughout the body. Following replication in reticulo-endothelial sites, a second viraemic stage precedes the appearance of the skin and mucosal lesions. Mucosal lesions are less noticeable and ulcerate early, and the skin rash is readily recognized.

These vesicles lie in the middle of the epidermis, and the fluid contains numerous free virus particles. Within 3 days the fluid becomes cloudy with the influx of leucocytes; fibrin and interferon are also present. These pustules then dry up, scabs form, and they desquamate. It is a noticeable feature that lesions in all stages are present at any time while new ones are appearing. The clearance of virus-infected cells is dependent on functional cell-mediated immune mechanisms, cytotoxic T cells and antibody-dependent cell cytotoxicity in particular. Persons deficient in these responses and in interferon production have prolonged clear-vesicle phases and great difficulty in controlling the infection.

Zoster

The pathogenesis of zoster is not so well established as that of HSV recurrence. Nucleic acid probes have revealed VZV sequences in sensory ganglia, and explant cultures of ganglia produce some VZV proteins, although not fully infectious virus. The latent virus is found in neurones and in satellite cells in sensory ganglia, and more than one region of the genome is transcribed, but the state of the latent VZV is not known. It seems likely that virus reaches the ganglion from the periphery by travelling up nerve axons, as HSV does, but there is also the possibility that during viraemia some virus enters ganglion cells. Another difference from HSV latency lies in the persistent VZV expression that has been detected in some mononuclear cells, which may have a role in VZV disease such as postherpetic neuralgia (see below).

Reactivation of VZV manifested as zoster can occur at any age in a person who has experienced a primary infection that may or may not have been clinically apparent. The rate is much increased in persons aged 60 years or over and, as most primary infection takes place before the age of 20 years, there is usually a latent period of several decades. However, a much shorter latent period is seen in immunocompromised patients, and also in those who acquired primary infection in utero (see below). More than one episode of zoster is uncommon in any individual. The stimulus to reactivation is not known, nor the details, but virus does appear to travel from sensory ganglia to the peripheral site. The zoster is usually limited to one dermatome; in adults, this is most commonly in the thoracic or upper lumbar regions or in the area supplied by the ophthalmic division of the trigeminal nerve. It is thought that this distribution is related to the density of the original varicella rash. There are associations with preceding trauma to the dermatome – injury or injections, for instance, with an interval of 2–3 weeks before the zoster appears. An inquiry usually elicits some such association in immunocompetent hosts. There is an associated suppression of specific cell-mediated responses in acute zoster, but rapid secondary antibody responses are usually found. Reactivation occurs more commonly in T cell immunodeficiency states.

Viraemia may occur in the course of zoster but is unusual, with pre-existing immunity normally being rapidly boosted. In the immunocompromised, however, viraemia leads to dissemination of zoster, either to internal organs or in a generalized manner similar to varicella.

Clinical features

Varicella

The incubation period averages 14–15 days but may range from 10 to 20 days. The patient is infectious for 2 days before and up to 5 days after onset, while new vesicles are appearing.

The rash of varicella is usually centripetal, being most dense on the trunk and head. Initially macular, the rash rapidly evolves through papules to the characteristic clear vesicles ('dew drops').

Presentations vary widely – from the clinically inapparent to only a few scattered lesions, or to a severe febrile illness with a widespread rash, especially in secondary cases in older members of a household. Whilst commonly a relatively mild infection in the young child, the complications of varicella are serious and account for significant morbidity, requiring hospitalization of normal children and adults, unlike the other herpesvirus infections.

Secondary bacterial infection of skin lesions is the commonest complication, mainly in the young child, and it increases the amount of residual scarring. Thrombocytopenic purpura occurs, especially in immunocompromised hosts. A variety of organs may be affected, producing myocarditis, arthritis, glomerulonephritis and appendicitis. The two most frequent problems are related to the lungs and the central nervous system.

Pneumonia.   In varicella, viral pneumonitis is a most serious complication, even in immunologically normal people. It occurs as a subclinical feature evident only by radiography in a proportion of adults, but is increasingly being recognized for the danger it brings, especially to smokers. Cough, dyspnoea, tachypnoea and chest pains begin a few days after the rash. Nodular infiltrates are seen in the lungs on radiography. Specific antiviral therapy is only successful if used early in sufficient dosage, and should be instituted at the first sign of pneumonia in an adult with chickenpox. Early investigations (radiography and gas exchange) are indicated in all smokers with chickenpox. Immuno-compromised patients are even more at risk of varicella pneumonia.

Central nervous system.   Neurological complications include the common but benign cerebellar ataxia syndrome. Acute encephalitis is rare but more serious, and occurs more commonly in immunocompromised patients. This may be confused with postinfectious encephalopathy, which, with other post-infectious manifestations such as transverse myelitis or Guillain–Barré syndrome, is immunologically mediated and not related to viral cytopathogenicity.

Varicella in pregnancy.   Varicella virus can cross the placenta following viraemia in the pregnant woman, and infect the fetus. The infection may be more serious for the mother herself in pregnancy, with pneumonia the major problem. Two types of intra-uterine infection are noted:

1. *The fetal varicella syndrome* is a consequence of fetal infections with VZV in the first half of pregnancy. The birth of infants so infected has been rarely reported but the features include characteristic scarring of the skin, hypoplasia of limbs, and chorioretinitis. The maternal infection is usually varicella but in one case at least it was disseminated herpes zoster. Fetal infection is not inevitable. Silent intra-uterine infection can also occur: no damage is seen, but the baby is born with latent VZV infection, having recovered from infection.

2. *Neonatal (congenital) varicella* occurs when varicella develops within the first 2 weeks of life, following maternal varicella in late pregnancy, depending on the interval between maternal viraemia and delivery of the baby. If the rash in the mother begins 7 days or more prior to delivery, her antibody response will have developed and been transferred across the placenta so that the baby does not develop disease. However, the infant is at serious risk if varicella occurs 6 days or less before delivery (or up to 2 days after); this allows viraemic spread across the placenta, before antibody is made and transferred to the baby. Because the usual respiratory entry route has been bypassed, the incubation period is reduced to 10 days on average. If infection arises, disseminated disease with pneumonitis and encephalitis may be found. The rate of transmission is 1 in 3, but there is no way of knowing which mother will transmit, and in this situation protection of the neonate with passive immunity (see VZIG; p. 411) and early antiviral therapy is indicated.

Zoster

This is the manifestation of reactivated VZV infection. It takes the form of a localized eruption, and is unilateral and typically confined to one dermatome. Prodromal paraesthesia and pain in the area supplied by the affected sensory nerve are common before the skin lesions develop; these are identical to those of varicella except in their distribution. The evolution of the rash is similar, with some new vesicles appearing while the earliest ones are crusting; however, the whole episode in the majority of cases is confined to the affected dermatome and heals in 1–3 weeks. Acute pain is not always a feature, but its presence should alert to the possibility of zoster, and a search for early lesions, perhaps internal, is indicated. Occasionally there are no skin lesions – '*zoster sine herpete*'.

Dissemination of zoster is indicated by lesions appearing in the skin at distant sites or, more seriously, by involvement of internal organs such as the lung and brain. In the immunocompromised this results in severe disease, with occasional fatalities.

Postherpetic neuralgia.   This is the most common complication of zoster, a risk in 50% of patients aged over 60 years, and results in significant morbidity in around 20%. It is defined as intractable pain persisting for 1 month or more after the skin rash. Constant pain at the site, or stabbing pains or paraesthesiae may continue over 1 year or much longer in a number of individuals. This is an exhausting and disabling condition for which no satisfactory cure has been found. The indications are that adequate early antiviral therapy can reduce the incidence.

Ophthalmic zoster.   Involvement of the ophthalmic division of the trigeminal nerve occurs in up to one-quarter of zoster episodes, with ocular complications in more than half the patients. Corneal ulceration, stromal keratitis and anterior uveitis may result in permanent scarring, so this complication may threaten sight when the nasociliary branch is involved. Ocular complications are reduced in patients given oral aciclovir early in ophthalmic zoster. Occasionally acute retinal necrosis is identified.

A contralateral hemiparesis due to granulomatous cerebral angiitis in the weeks following acute ophthalmic zoster is a recognized neurological complication. Other postinfection manifestations are seen, and more acute ones such as the *Ramsay–Hunt syndrome* (facial palsy with aural zoster vesicles) suggest that motor neurones can also be involved. Sympathetic ganglia may also be the site of latency, as indicated by cases where the initial recrudescence has been in gastric mucosa, with subsequent dissemination.

Recurrent and chronic VZV. Immunodeficient patients, most particularly those with CD4+ lymphopenia due to HIV infection, may develop recurrent and chronic infection. New lesions continue to appear, or reappear after aciclovir therapy, often presenting an atypical hyperkeratotic appearance. Aciclovir-resistant VZV has been isolated in this situation.

Laboratory diagnosis

Typical presentations of varicella or zoster seldom need laboratory confirmation; however, atypical presentations merit investigation, especially in the immunocompromised. Vesicular rashes due to enterovirus are sometimes confused with varicella and, in compromised patients, various vesicular lesions may be mistaken for zoster. A common misdiagnosis is the assumption that localized vesicular lesions other than on the face or genitalia are due to zoster. In fact, many are due to herpes simplex recurrences, and this is readily shown by antigen detection and virus isolation.

Virus detection

Early vesicular lesions provide the best diagnostic material. Vesicle fluid can be collected in a capillary tube or aspirated with a fine needle and syringe. Direct examination by electron microscopy will reveal herpes particles; some of the fluid can be diluted in virus transport medium and inoculated into tissue culture for virus isolation, which takes from 5 days to 3 weeks. More rapid detection is possible with centrifugation-enhanced cultures ('shell vials'). If cells swabbed from the base of lesions are available, or biopsy tissue, virus antigens may be sought directly in them, using immunofluorescence tests with monoclonal antibodies. VZV DNA amplification by PCR is also proving valuable for detection of VZV in CSF or aqueous humour. The latter two methods are the ones most used now for rapid diagnosis.

Serological diagnosis

Antibody testing with varicella-zoster antigens is useful in confirming a diagnosis of varicella by demonstration of seroconversion or rising titres of antibody between acute and convalescent serum samples; complement fixation is still a useful test for this purpose. However, the test is not sufficiently sensitive to determine past infection and, to assess immune status, assays need to be based on enzyme or radiolabelled methods, or immunofluorescent staining of varicella-zoster-infected cells. For demonstration of IgM antibody, IgM capture systems have been shown to be useful. IgM to VZV is detectable in both varicella and zoster, appearing early in zoster.

Treatment

Aciclovir given intravenously is effective in the treatment of varicella and zoster in immunocompromised patients. Oral aciclovir can be used to accelerate healing and reduce new lesion formation in zoster in healthy patients if given early enough and may lower the rate of postherpetic neuralgia. VZV is not as sensitive to aciclovir as HSV, with 50% inhibitory dose (ID_{50}) values ranging from 4 to 17 µM aciclovir compared with 0.1–1.6 µM aciclovir for HSV, so a higher dosage is required. For the intravenous preparation this means 10 mg/kg given every 8 h. Oral therapy has to be with the high-dose 800 mg five times a day regimen. Newer preparations such as the oral prodrugs valaciclovir and famciclovir offer the advantage of less frequent dosing. Trials have shown that high-dose oral aciclovir can shorten the course of varicella in healthy children and adults by 1 day if commenced within 24 h of the onset of the rash. The practical difficulties of achieving this rule out routine treatment for all cases of varicella in healthy children, but consideration should be given to treating all adults, and where possible adolescents and family contact cases, who are known to develop more extensive disease. Treatment of VZV infection is given primarily to all 'high-risk of complication' groups:

- neonates (within the first 3 weeks of life)
- immunocompromised patients
- those with ophthalmic zoster
- healthy patients with varicella when there is an additional complicating factor such as smoking or pneumonia.

Epidemiology

Varicella is partly seasonal, being spread mainly by the respiratory route in winter and early spring. Some cases result from contact with zoster and occur sporadically at any season. Varicella is highly infectious to susceptible close contacts, as in a household; a past history of varicella is a good indicator of immunity. The majority of children contract varicella between the ages of 4 and 10 years in western countries, with around 8% of young

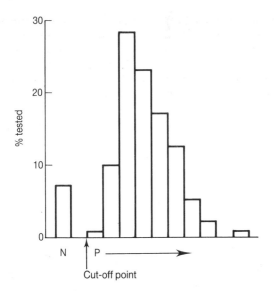

Fig. 43.5 Distribution of antibody (IgG) to VZV in a young adult population (southern England). Percentage confirmed negative (N) was 7.8%; P →, increasing positive result.

adults remaining susceptible (Fig. 43.5). However, a much higher proportion of young adults remain susceptible in subtropical countries. Mortality from varicella is surprisingly high in normal adults, particularly smokers, who develop pneumonia. Zoster is associated with decreased T cell function, and occurs with increased incidence in:

- old age
- the pre-AIDS phase of HIV infection
- organ transplant recipients
- patients on chemotherapy or radiotherapy for lymphoma or leukaemia.

Control

Passive immunization

Passive immunity is partly protective for varicella, as seen in infants with maternal antibody or patients given *varicella-zoster immunoglobulin* (VZIG) within 72 h of exposure. VZIG (in the UK) or another similar high-titre antibody preparation is available for neonates, non-immune pregnant contacts or immunocompromised contacts. As the majority of pregnant contacts will in fact be immune, testing for antibody after exposure may prevent unnecessary use of VZIG. Current preparations will seldom prevent infection, but will modify disease. Recent review of intervention with VZIG in exposed antenatal patients showed that the rate of transmission to the fetus was decreased significantly.

Varicella vaccine

A live-attenuated varicella vaccine has been in use for some years in Japan and some European countries, and was recently approved in the USA for routine childhood immunization. This vaccine, given by intramuscular injection, has been found to be immunogenic in children with leukaemia in remission and in healthy children and adults; vaccinees have resisted infection on close exposure to varicella. Some symptoms are noted around 10 days post vaccine, and vesicles appear at the site of injection in up to 5%. Immunization does not prevent latency developing; however, the incidence of zoster in vaccinees compared to the naturally infected is not increased. Whether vaccination in the elderly will effectively boost immunity to prevent zoster is not yet known. Subunit vaccines would remove the risks of transmission, and latency, inherent in the live vaccine.

EPSTEIN–BARR VIRUS

In 1964 Epstein, Barr and Achong described herpesvirus particles in cells from a common lymphoma in African children studied by Burkitt, who suspected a viral aetiology of the tumour. The link between that new herpesvirus – the *Epstein–Barr virus* – and a variety of lymphoproliferative diseases is now clearer. EBV primary infection is:

- most often asymptomatic and occurs early in childhood
- the classical infectious mononucleosis (*glandular fever*) of adolescents in the developed world.

Humans are the only natural host, but EBV infection can be transmitted to some subhuman primates.

Description

The characteristic morphology seen on electron microscopy placed EBV with the herpesviruses. This virus cannot be grown in human fibroblast or epithelial cell lines and there is no completely productive or permissive system for culture of EBV. This lympho-tropic virus is classified as a gammaherpesvirus, genus lymphocryptovirus.

Replication

The full replication (productive or lytic) cycle of EBV is now known to take place in certain differentiated epithelial cells. EBV receptors (the CD21 molecule) are expressed on mature resting B lymphocytes, and similar receptors are present on cells of stratified squamous epithelium – in the oropharynx, salivary glands and ectocervix for instance. Viral production, however, is restricted to the differentiated cells of the granular layer and above, and virus is shed from the superficial cells. Technical difficulties in growing differentiating epithelia in culture have limited these studies to date, and most work on the lytic cycle of EBV has been done in lymphoblastoid cell lines, in which a proportion of the EBV-infected cells can be induced to produce virions.

The organization of the EBV genome differs from HSV, and some genes are present in one and not the other. Approximately 80 proteins are encoded; some glycoproteins are known, including the major glycoprotein gp350/220, which mediates attachment to CD21, and gp85, which is involved in membrane fusion. The latent (non-productive) state of EBV infection is maintained in a subset of resting memory B lymphocytes, and perhaps in certain epithelial cells. In the B lymphocytes the EBV genome is maintained as multiple full-length copies in the form of circular episomes. Specific EBV early RNA species are found in all cells infected with the virus. A variable number of EBV genes are expressed in the latent state; these are principally genes coding for nuclear antigens (EBNAs) and a gene encoding a latent membrane protein that hardly extends beyond the plasma membrane but may be involved in recognition by immune T cells. It may also have a role in cell transformation.

The EBV nuclear antigen 1 (EBNA 1) is responsible for maintaining the replication of the EBV episome. EBNA 2 is necessary for transformation of B lymphocytes; there are two alleles of this gene, originally designated EBNA 2A and EBNA 2B. There are two EBV strains now termed EBV-1 and EBV-2. The genes of the latent EBV are replicated by host cell DNA polymerase.

The full lytic cycle of EBV replication is accompanied by production of virus structural antigens and assembly of virions. Although EBV does encode a viral thymidine kinase, aciclovir is phosphorylated by cellular TK in cells producing EBV. The viral DNA polymerase is very sensitive to aciclovir triphosphate, and treatment with aciclovir will reduce EBV production but has no effect on latency or the proliferation induced by the virus.

Pathogenesis

Infection of oropharyngeal epithelial cells occurs initially, then infection of B lymphocytes, which disseminate through the circulation, with the potential to enter a productive phase and release virus elsewhere in the body. Most shedding of virus, however, takes place in the oral cavity and this can be detected regularly in the saliva of asymptomatic hosts, increasing in immunosuppressed states. How B cells become infected is not proven, but there are opportunities for close contact between lymphocytes and epithelial cells in the nasopharynx.

A proportion of infected B lymphocytes undergo transformation and continue to proliferate in vitro as a lymphoblastoid cell line (*immortalization*). Activated B lymphocytes secrete immunoglobulin, and EBV is a potent polyclonal activator of antibody production by B cells, independent of any accessory cells. IgM-producing lymphocytes predominate, and IgM antibody is found in high levels, but detectable IgG (especially the IgG3 subclass), IgA and IgD have also been found.

Recovery from primary EBV infection is associated with humoral and cellular responses; any delay in cellular control, or over-vigorous responses, contributes to the disease associated with the infection. Thus, large initial infective doses result in high numbers of circulating infected B lymphocytes, followed by a marked T cell response. The polyclonal activation of B cells results in transient antibodies (predominantly IgM) appearing, both auto and heterophile antibodies. The cellular response is detected as large numbers of 'atypical lymphocytes' in the blood and infiltrating many tissues. These cells have been shown to be mainly cytotoxic/suppressor T cells and NK cells. The suppression is manifested as a general depression of immune responses. The cytotoxic elements carry the ability to kill EBV-infected cells, and this is not entirely human leucocyte antigen (HLA) restricted (Fig. 43.6).

Antibody responses following EBV infection make a characteristic pattern, with the initial IgM response to

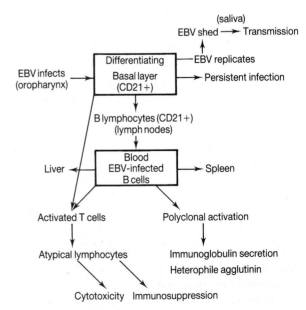

Fig. 43.6 Simplified outline of EBV infection of cells in the oropharynx and interaction with lymphocytes.

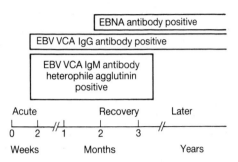

Fig. 43.7 Appearance and duration of diagnostic antibodies following primary EBV infection.

virus capsid antigens persisting for some months. The EBNA complex elicits antibodies in late convalescence only, perhaps after release from B cells lysed by the cytotoxic T cells (Fig. 43.7). Failure to produce antibody to EBNA is a feature of immunodeficiency states. This may be associated with increased levels of antibodies to EBV lytic cycle antigens (early antigen, and viral capsid antigen), reflecting a high virus replication rate. High IgA levels to EBV capsid antigen are found in those at risk of developing nasopharyngeal carcinoma (see later).

Clinical features

Primary infection with EBV is usually mild and unrecognized in the vast majority who acquire it in the first years of life.

Infectious mononucleosis

The disease known as *infectious mononucleosis*, or *glandular fever*, is a primary EBV infection seen pre-dominantly in the 15–25-year age group. The incubation period is 30–50 days, and the onset is abrupt with a sore throat, cervical lymphadenopathy and fever, accompanied by malaise, headache, sweating and gastro-intestinal discomfort. Pharyngitis may be severe, accompanied by a greyish–white membrane and gross tonsillar enlargement. Lymphadenopathy becomes generalized, often with splenic enlargement and tenderness, mild hepatomegaly in some cases and clinical jaundice in 5–10%. Intermittent fevers with drenching sweats occur daily over 2 weeks. A faint transient morbilliform rash may be seen; a maculopapular rash may follow ampicillin administration due to immune complexes with antibody to ampicillin. The illness can last several weeks, and fatigue and lack of concentration are common in the aftermath.

Complications of glandular fever

Complications are rare but some are serious.

- Acute airway obstruction may occur as a result of the lymphoid enlargement and oedema; this merits emergency tracheostomy in some cases, but usually responds well to corticosteroids.
- Splenic rupture is also rare.
- Neurological complications include meningitis, encephalitis and the Guillain–Barré syndrome.

Other EBV-associated disease, tumours and immunodeficiency

EBV is associated with an increasing number of diseases, including malignant tumours, some of which are listed in Table 43.2. The role played by EBV in these is

Table 43.2 Diseases associated with EBV

Disease	Cells infected	Link
Infectious mononucleosis ('glandular fever')	B lymphocytes and nasopharyngeal epithelium	Causal; acute primary infection
Oral hairy leucoplakia (seen in AIDS)	Differentiated epithelium along edge of tongue	Causal; productive recurrence in immunocompromised host
Nasopharyngeal carcinoma (especially in South-East Asia and China)	Undifferentiated nasopharyngeal epithelium (long latent period; 30+ years)	100% EBV-positive cells; co-factor(s) + genetic risk
Burkitt's lymphoma (endemic African form)	Monoclonal B cell tumour (short latent period; 5+ years)	100% EBV-positive; immunocompromised by malaria
Immunoblastic lymphoma (post-transplant/AIDS; X-linked syndrome)	B lymphocytes	70–100% EBV-positive cells; immunodeficiency states genetic defect
Hodgkin's disease	Hodgkin and Reed-Sternberg cells	30–90% EBV-positive cells in subsets of disease
T cell lymphoma	T lymphocytes	30–100% EBV-positive cells in subsets of disease

not clear in all cases. Cellular immunodeficiency states lead to lack of control over the proliferative phase of EBV infection, and a risk of development of lymphomas. In some situations, as in African Burkitt's lymphoma, EBV infection at an early age accompanied by chronic immunosuppression due to endemic malaria proceeds to a highly aggressive tumour.

Laboratory diagnosis

Infectious mononucleosis is accompanied by production of heterophile agglutinins that can be detected by a rapid slide agglutination test or the *Paul-Bunnell* test. Agglutination of horse or sheep red cells by serum absorbed to exclude a natural antibody is the basis of this test. Atypical lymphocytes, accounting for 20% of the lymphocytosis common in this condition, are seen in blood films. Definitive diagnosis requires the demonstration of IgM antibody to the EBV viral capsid antigen, or seroconversion if an earlier serum lacks IgG antibody. These tests, using indirect immunofluorescence or enzyme immuno-assay, are generally available. Other serological tests are applicable in special situations.

EBV virus detection has generally been confined to research laboratories. Saliva or throat washings are suitable specimens. Tissues can be stained for EBNA, or probed for EBV DNA or early RNA species, and these approaches, alongside PCR for EBV, are playing an increasing role in diagnosis of disease in immunodeficiency states, although they are not yet routinely available.

Treatment

Aciclovir therapy does reduce EBV shedding in acute infections, and there may be a place for it in patients suffering from, or at risk of, complications associated with an ongoing viral lytic cycle. Immunotherapy for EBV lymphoproliferative conditions with donor-derived cytotoxic T cells is a possibility in some situations.

Epidemiology

Infection with EBV is transmitted by saliva, and requires intimate oral contact. Transmission has rarely been reported following transfusion of fresh blood to seronegative recipients. Infection is widespread, with most of the population infected from early in life, even in developed countries. Increased numbers of severely immunocompromised hosts are at risk of developing EBV-associated malignant lymphomas, including recipients of solid organ or bone marrow transplants.

Control

A subunit vaccine based on the major membrane glycoprotein gp350/220 is undergoing trials. It has been shown to protect marmosets against tumour-inducing doses of EBV. Screening for IgA to EBV capsid antigen is used in populations at risk of nasopharyngeal cancer to detect preclinical cases.

CYTOMEGALOVIRUS

There are CMVs specific to other animals, and the full name for the virus infecting humans is human cytomegalovirus (HCMV). This will be used only in the descriptions of the features specific to HCMV, otherwise the more usual CMV will be used. The name 'cytomegalovirus' was chosen on account of the swollen state of infected cells as seen in culture and in tissues. Nuclei of productively infected cells contain a large inclusion body, giving a typical 'owl's eye' appearance.

Description

The CMVs have the same general structure as other members of the herpes group.

Human fibroblast cells are required for isolation of HCMV in vitro, but in vivo the virus replicates in epithelial cells in:

- salivary glands
- the kidney
- the respiratory tract.

CMV remains highly cell-associated, and is sensitive to freezing and thawing. Virus shed in urine is stable at 4°C for many days.

Replication

The temporal regulation of viral protein synthesis in the growth cycle is more obvious in laboratory culture of the slower growing CMV than with HSV. Immediate early (non-structural) protein (p72) appears in nuclei within 16 h of inoculation, whilst late (virion-structural) proteins are produced after DNA synthesis, and the typical cytopathic effect is often not recognizable for 5–21 days. Foci of swollen cells slowly expand as infection passes from cell to cell (Fig. 43.8). Passage and storage of virus are best achieved by trypsinization and passage as infected cells.

HCMV does not produce a virus-specified thymidine kinase; the protein kinase product of gene UL97 carries out initial phosphorylation of ganciclovir in CMV-infected cells, and cellular kinases produce the triphosphate, which inhibits CMV DNA polymerase.

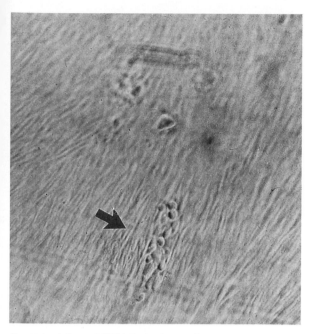

Fig. 43.8 A focus of CMV infection (arrowed) in a tissue culture monolayer of human embryo fibroblasts.

There are several families of glycoproteins in CMV, and these are important antigenic targets. Most neutralizing antibody is directed against gB.

Pathogenesis

Primary infection with CMV may be acquired at any time, possibly from conception onwards.

CMV persists in the host for life. Reactivation is common, and virus is shed in body secretions such as urine, saliva, semen, breast milk and cervical fluid. Mononuclear cells are thought to carry the latent virus genome since viral RNA transcripts of early genes have been detected in them, but the nature and site of latency are not yet clear. Whether any virus persists in epithelial cells is not known.

Recurrent infections may follow reactivation of latent (endogenous) virus, or re-infection with another (exogenous) strain. Isolates can be distinguished by restriction endonuclease analysis. Endothelial giant cells (multinucleate cells) have been found in the circulation during disseminated CMV infection. These cells are fully permissive for CMV replication.

Intra-uterine infection

Maternal viraemia may result in fetal infection in approximately one out of three cases of primary CMV during pregnancy, and this may lead to disease in the fetus. Infection may also be acquired in utero when the mother has a reactivation, but this rarely results in disease. Transplacental infection is probably carried by infected cells, and transmission is associated with a high viraemic load.

Perinatal infection

This is predominantly acquired from infected maternal genital tract secretions or from breast-feeding (3–5% of pregnant women in Europe reactivate CMV). Rarely, perinatal blood transfusion was the source, but as leucodepletion is now common this risk has been reduced.

Postnatal infection

This can be acquired in many ways. Saliva containing CMV is profusely distributed amongst young children, and shared by intimate kissing. Semen can have high titres of virus, and may be a source of sexual transmission or artifical insemination-associated infection. Blood transfusion and donated organs are important sources of CMV. As it is not known which donors are most likely to transmit infection, all antibody-positive ('seropositive') donors are considered potential transmitters as the presence of antibody implies the presence of persistent virus.

Host responses

The host response to primary CMV includes IgM, IgG and T cell responses. Some of the T cell responses may contribute to immunopathology by reacting with HLA molecules induced by CMV. CMV early genes transactivate other viral and cellular genes and this may be an important interaction with HIV, leading to the production of HIV from latently infected cells. Because CMV infects mononuclear cells, there is a degree of immunosuppression associated with the acute infection. Cell-mediated responses are crucial to control of CMV, as shown by the serious consequences of disseminated infections in those deficient in effector cell functions. The incubation period for primary infection is 4–6 weeks; reactivation, after transplantation for instance, appears from 3 weeks onwards.

Clinical features

Congenital CMV infection

This is asymptomatic in 95% of infected babies, but around 15% of these will show sensorineural deafness or intellectual impairment later. Progression of the persistent CMV infection may be involved. All congenitally infected infants excrete abundant virus in urine during the first year. The 5% of symptomatic infants have 'cytomegalic inclusion body disease' with:

- growth retardation
- hepatosplenomegaly
- jaundice
- thrombocytopenia
- central nervous system involvement, a significant problem with CMV; microcephaly, encephalitis and retinitis noted at birth. Some changes may even be detectable on ultrasound scanning in utero.

Mononucleosis

Postnatal infection with CMV is seldom recognized clinically, unless virus is isolated. Respiratory tract infection is common in infancy. A *mononucleosis syndrome* is seen occasionally, especially in young adults or when CMV is acquired from blood transfusion. Hepatitis, fever and atypical lymphocytosis are noted, but pharyngitis and lymphadenopathy are unusual and heterophile agglutinins are not found (see EBV – infectious mononucleosis). This syndrome is also seen in some HIV-infected patients before the development of AIDS, and should prompt HIV-related investigations.

Infection in the compromised patient

Immunocompromised patients may develop symptoms as the result of primary or recurrent CMV infection. Dissemination of the virus in the blood as indicated by a hectic fever is a bad prognostic sign. The complications of CMV infection in cellular immunodeficiency include:

- pneumonitis – has a high mortality in bone marrow allograft recipients
- encephalitis – often fatal
- retinitis – which may occur on its own (10–40% of AIDS patients)
- oesophagitis/colitis – 5–10% of AIDS patients
- hepatitis
- pancreatitis or adrenalitis.

Primary CMV infection in transplant recipients is a significant cause of morbidity and loss of graft. Mortality is high, particularly in allogeneic marrow recipients who develop an immunopathological pneumonitis associated with graft versus host disease. Transplant protocols all include prophylactic or pre-emptive therapy for prevention of CMV disease.

Retinitis due to CMV recurrence is a feature of late-stage AIDS, when the CD4 cell count is less than 50/μl, and early recognition, antiviral treatment and maintenance therapy are important in slowing the progression towards blindness.

Laboratory diagnosis

Detection of CMV is the objective, and, if possible, to show its presence at the site of disease. Samples should include urine, saliva, broncho-alveolar lavage fluid or biopsy tissue if available, and peripheral blood collected in anticoagulant. In the neonate, urine samples taken in the first 2 weeks of life are sufficient for diagnosis of congenital infection.

Virus detection

Rapid diagnostic methods will detect virus DNA in the samples with PCR or a hybridization assay, or CMV early antigen in cell cultures 24 h post inoculation (Fig. 43.9), while conventional culture will be used to isolate virus. High titres of CMV will produce a cytopathic effect very quickly, but most cultures require 2–3 weeks. CMV isolation from urine does not of course prove that the virus is the cause of the disease being investigated. To demonstrate congenital infection, virus must be shown in a sample taken within the first 2 weeks of life as later samples may be due to virus acquired in the postnatal period. Additional confirmation that CMV is related to a disease process comes from showing that the virus is replicating in the affected tissues (perhaps by cytology), and in some cases that a primary infection has occurred. The demonstration of CMV in the circulation is a significant prognostic finding, whether based on detection of DNA (by PCR) or of a late phosphoprotein antigen (pp65), and above a certain level is predictive of clinical disease.

Serology for CMV

This is increasingly important, and sensitive screening tests are widely available. Complement fixation tests are adequate for showing seroconversion after primary infection in competent hosts. To screen for 'seropositive' status a more sensitive assay, such as enzyme immuno-assay for CMV IgG or total antibody or latex agglutination assay, is appropriate. These tests can be done urgently for donor–recipient assessment. CMV IgM is found after primary or secondary infection, but it is not always possible to detect IgM in the neonate or immunocompromised patient.

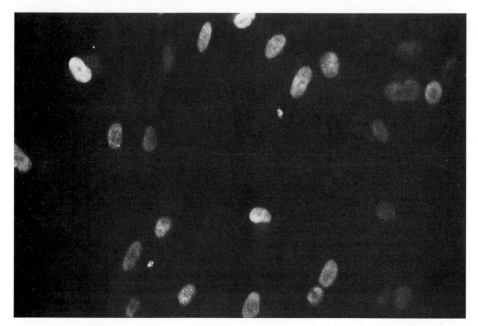

Fig. 43.9 CMV early antigen demonstrated in nuclei of human embryo fibroblasts by immunofluorescence after incubation for 24 h following centrifuge-assisted inoculation.

Treatment

Some antiviral agents for CMV infections are available but serious side-effects limit their use to life- or sight-threatening complications. Ganciclovir is the agent most often used for treatment of serious CMV disease, given intravenously twice a day. Marrow toxicity results in neutropenia, and there is a potential for long-term loss of spermatogenesis. Clinically, treatment has been successful in CMV colitis and encephalitis, and progression of CMV retinitis in AIDS has been controlled with prolonged maintenance therapy, which may now be given orally. Ganciclovir-resistant virus has been found; usually a mutation in the protein kinase gene is responsible. Foscarnet (phosphonoformate) is an alternative agent that does not require phosphorylation. Aciclovir is not effective therapy for CMV, but some benefit from high-dose prophylaxis of CMV in transplant recipients has been noted. More recently, oral ganciclovir has been licensed for prophylaxis in transplant recipients, and an oral prodrug valganciclovir is in trials. Cidofovir is an alternative antiviral agent used locally in the eye for CMV retinitis.

Epidemiology

Primary CMV infection is acquired by 40–60% of persons with limited exposure by mid-adult life, and by over 90% of those with multiple intimate exposures.

Less than 5% of units of blood from seropositive donors result in transmission to seronegative recipients, whilst 80% of kidneys transmit infection from seropositive donors. The full extent of congenital CMV disease is not known, but this infection occurs in approximately three out of 1000 live births in the UK and is thought to be the commonest viral cause of congenital infection.

Control

Some preventive action is undertaken by way of screening organ donors and recipients to avoid, where possible, a seronegative recipient receiving an organ from a seropositive donor. This has been shown to reduce morbidity and mortality significantly in all forms of allogeneic transplant. Blood donor screening to select CMV seronegative units for support of seronegative patients in transplant programmes is important but not always available. The heavy demands for blood do not allow for such a provision generally, but a special case can be made for any seriously compromised host or any very premature baby to receive screened blood (from CMV seronegative donors) or, as is routine now in the UK, leucocyte-depleted blood.

No CMV vaccine is licensed for use. Experimental live-attenuated vaccines have been tried, but hopes rest on subunit vaccines or on a combined approach.

HUMAN HERPESVIRUSES 6 AND 7

Description

The existence of further herpesviruses infecting humans was not suspected until one was first isolated in 1986 from the blood of patients with lymphoproliferative disorders, some of whom had AIDS. Electron microscopy revealed a virus with characteristic herpes group features. DNA sequence studies showed this virus, now officially named human herpesvirus 6 (HHV6), to be distinct from the five known human herpesviruses, but closer to HCMV, with which it has some homology. Two variants have been identified on sequence analysis, HHV6A and HHV6B. Although first isolated from B cells, HHV6 was shown to infect CD4+ T cells preferentially, and HHV6A can be propagated in T cell lines in the laboratory. HHV6B is now known to be the cause of a common disease of infancy called *exanthem subitum* or *roseola infantum*, while variant 6A has no clear disease association.

In 1990 another new human herpesvirus was isolated in similar circumstances, and has been shown to be sufficiently distinct to be called HHV7. Primary infection with HHV7 has been identified in some cases of roseola infantum also. There is a proposal that a new genus *Roseolovirus* be established for these two viruses, which are members of the subfamily betaherpesviruses.

Pathogenesis and clinical features

Roseola infantum (exanthem subitum)

This disease was long considered to be an infection caused by a virus, and transmission by blood was confirmed experimentally years before HHV6 was isolated. The infection is extremely common in the first years of life, presenting between 6 months and 3 years of age with a sudden onset of fever (39.4–39.7°C). The child is not usually ill, remaining alert and playful, with some throat congestion and cervical lymphadenopathy. Sometimes more pronounced respiratory symptoms occur and febrile convulsions have been reported. Fever persists for 3 days, when the temperature suddenly falls; a widespread macular rash appears in around only one-tenth of cases, according to recent studies. HHV6B has been isolated from peripheral blood in the acute febrile phase, in patients who subsequently produced a rash and some who did not. Seroconversion is noted in convalescence, confirming a primary infection with HHV6. Some cases are associated with HHV7 infection, but as yet no other disease association has been found for HHV7.

Complications of primary infection with HHV6 have been noted, particularly neurological ones, and in the rare adult case hepatitis, lymphadenopathy and neurological features have been found. Reactivation in immunocompromised hosts is commonly diagnosed on the basis of serology, and both viruses have been detected by PCR, but the extent of disease in the transplant recipient for instance has still to be established.

Both HHV6 and HHV7 infect T lymphocytes; indeed, HHV7 uses the same receptor (CD4) as HIV. The potential significance of these interactions has still to be established with regard to effects on the progression of AIDS.

Laboratory diagnosis

Isolation of HHV6 or HHV7 involves co-cultivation of peripheral blood lymphocytes with mitogen-activated cord blood lymphocytes. The infected lymphocytes do survive for some time but are not immortalized. Very large refractile multinucleate cells are produced in culture, and many intact enveloped virions are released into the culture medium. These viruses may be isolated from saliva, particularly HHV7. DNA amplification by PCR is also used in diagnosis.

Laboratory diagnosis of HHV6 or HHV7 is currently available only from specialist laboratories. Antibody tests are becoming more widely used. Antibody avidity tests can help to establish whether a primary infection has occurred, and both this method and PCR have proven useful in establishing the correct diagnosis of HHV6-associated roseola infantum in a proportion of suspected cases of infant measles.

Treatment

HHV6 is sensitive to ganciclovir, but not to aciclovir. Treatment is seldom clinically indicated however.

Epidemiology

Antibody analysis to date has been based mainly on immunofluorescence studies with cells infected with either HHV6 or HHV7 as antigen. High antibody titres to HHV6 are found in young children in the first 4 years of life, reflecting recent primary infections in this group. Primary infection, with viraemia and seroconversion, has also been detected in seronegative transplant recipients of liver or kidney from seropositive donors. Possible transmission by blood transfusion has not been excluded. Infection with HHV7 is said to occur a few years later on average. Older persons have lower levels of antibody, but more sensitive enzyme immuno-assay tests reveal almost universal seropositivity. The spectrum of disease associated with these viruses and the extent of asymptomatic shedding remain to be established.

HUMAN HERPESVIRUS 8 (KAPOSI'S SARCOMA-RELATED HERPESVIRUS)

Sequences of DNA representing a completely new human herpesvirus were identified in 1994 in studies of tissue from the epidemic form of Kaposi's sarcoma in patients with AIDS. The DNA fragments unique to the tumour tissue were found to have some homology with the gammaherpesvirus subfamily, including EBV. This is undoubtedly a new virus, officially named HHV8, but also referred to as *Kaposi's sarcoma-associated herpesvirus*, and it is the newest human tumour virus.

Kaposi's sarcoma

Whether the new virus is the cause of Kaposi's sarcoma (KS) is not established yet, but the evidence is that HHV8 is an essential agent but not the only factor. The mucocutaneous neoplasm is the commonest tumour in one group of HIV-infected individuals. The classical form (classic KS) was described as a rare finding in elderly patients of mediterranean descent; a rather more aggressive endemic form is seen in Africa (endemic KS) and in some post-transplant patients, but the aggressive epidemic form (AIDS-KS) has been a feature of HIV-infected, homosexual male patients. A transmissible agent was long suspected on epidemiological grounds, transmitted sexually but rarely by blood, with faecal–oral contact as a risk factor. Endothelial cells of vascular or lymphatic origin are involved; they have a characteristic spindle shape and are arranged in bundles. Although occurring at multiple sites in skin, lymph glands and gastro-intestinal tract, and although these may cause functional problems, the tumour itself does not lead to death. Local radiotherapy and systemic chemotherapy have been used in treatment. Lesions on the exposed parts are blue-pink or red-brown plaques, sometimes raised, and are a cause of considerable concern for the affected individual.

'Body cavity associated lymphomas'

HHV8 genomes have been found in lymphoma cells from AIDS-related B cell lymphomas and similar conditions. These are termed body cavity lymphomas and are found primarily in HIV-infected patients.

Laboratory diagnosis

At present DNA amplification by PCR is the method of detection of HHV8. It has been reported that lytic growth of HHV8 can be induced in latently infected B cell lymphoma lines, and as a result, reagents for antibody testing can be produced. Recombinant proteins are being synthesized. Now that reagents free of EBV are becoming available the epidemiology of infection with this new herpesvirus is being studied. Initial findings indicate that, unlike most of the human herpesviruses, HHV8 infection is not common, at least in developed countries (less than 5% of blood donors in North America and Northern Europe have antibodies). Rates of seropositivity are higher in risk groups for KS, including a high rate in children in some African countries.

CERCOPITHECINE HERPESVIRUS 1 (B VIRUS)

Description

This virus, antigenically related to HSV, commonly infects Old World (Asiatic) macaque monkeys, causing a mild vesicular eruption on the tongue and buccal mucosa analogous to primary herpetic stomatitis in humans. The infection rate in monkeys increases markedly if they are kept in crowded conditions and, whilst relatively benign in the monkey, this virus is highly pathogenic for humans.

Human infection with B virus is rare. It has usually been acquired from a bite or from handling infected animals without appropriate protective wear. In one instance the wife of an infected monkey handler became infected through contact with her husband's vesicles, and B virus has also been transmitted in the laboratory from infected monkey cell cultures. Within 5–20 days of exposure, local inflammation may appear at the site of entry, usually on the skin, accompanied by some itching, numbness and vesicular lesions. Ascending myelitis or acute encephalomyelitis may follow. Delay in specific therapy leads to a high mortality rate and serious neurological sequelae in survivors.

Diagnosis and treatment

Diagnosis is by isolation of the virus from blood, vesicle fluid, conjunctival swabs and CSF. Herpes virions may be detectable on electron microscopy of vesicle fluid. Definitive identification of the virus is available in special reference laboratories, using PCR for DNA, or monoclonal antibodies. Demonstration of specific antibodies is complicated by cross-reacting HSV antibody. B virus is not as sensitive to aciclovir as HSV, requiring concentrations equivalent to those used for VZV. Treatment needs to be given promptly to be effective, and intravenous aciclovir for 14 days or longer is recommended. Ganciclovir should be used when there is evidence of central nervous system involvement. Because of the small number of cases the best therapeutic regimen is not well established.

Prevention of B virus infection

Guidelines have been issued for the protection of those handling monkeys or monkey tissues. These include:

• recommendations for training to prevent exposure

• safe handling and protective wear procedures
• care of wounds
• information as to the risks and nature of the infection.

Prophylaxis in the event of possible exposure involves wound washing, cleansing with 10% iodine in alcohol, and a course of oral aciclovir (high dose, 800 mg five times a day for 3 weeks) with a prolonged observation period as the onset of infection may be delayed.

RECOMMENDED READING

Carrington D, McKendrick M W 1998 Varicella supplement 1998 and consensus guidelines for management. *Journal of Infection* 36 (suppl 1): 1–88

Cinque P, Cleator G M, Weber T et al. 1996 The role of laboratory investigation in the diagnosis and management of patients with suspected herpes encephalitis: a consensus report. *Journal of Neurology, Neurosurgery and Psychiatry* 61: 339–345

Cohen J I 2000 Epstein–Barr virus infection *The New England Journal of Medicine* 343: 481–492

Stanberry L R, Jorgensen D M, Nahmias A J 1997 Herpes simplex viruses 1 and 2. In: Evans A S and Kaslow R A (eds) *Viral Infections of Humans*, 4th edn. Plenum Press, New York

Zuckerman A J, Banatvala J E, Pattison J R (eds) 2000. Section 2 (Herpesviridae) In: *Principles and Practice of Clinical Virology*, 4th edn. Wiley, Chichester
(This has separate chapters on the human herpesviruses, and an overview of the family.)

Internet site

www.virology.net/Big_Virology/BVDNAherpes.html

44

Poxviruses

Smallpox; molluscum contagiosum; parapoxvirus infections

T. H. Pennington

The world's last naturally occurring case of smallpox was recorded in Merca, Southern Somalia, in October 1977. This momentous event marked the end of a long campaign against smallpox, which in its 'modern' phase started with the introduction of vaccination by Edward Jenner at the end of the 18th century. With the eradication of smallpox – which has joined the dodo and the great auk by becoming extinct in the wild at the hand of humans – the importance of poxviruses in medical practice may appear to be much diminished, as the other naturally occurring viruses in this family that infect humans nearly always restrict themselves to causing self-limiting and trivial skin lesions. Smallpox, on the other hand, caused a generalized infection with high mortality, and fell into that small group of viruses (including viral haemorrhagic fevers and, now, human immuno-deficiency virus) which differ from the majority – which usually cause mild or subclinical infections – because their infections are commonly severe and frequently lethal. Notwithstanding their minor role today as human pathogens, poxviruses retain their importance, and their place in this book, for three reasons.

Firstly, the successful smallpox eradication campaign is important in its own right as a major achievement. It is also important because it highlights the principles and problems associated with projects that aim to control infections by eradicating the pathogen. Smallpox was the first disease to fall to this approach and remains the only successful example to date.

Secondly, work on the molecular biology of poxviruses has led to the identification of distinctive properties and the development of techniques and approaches which have made it possible to move significantly towards constructing single-dose vaccines which protect simultaneously against a wide range of diseases. Genes coding for foreign non-poxvirus antigens have been inserted into the poxvirus genome so that the antigens are expressed during virus infection and induce immunity.

Thirdly, no account of virus diseases in general and poxvirus infections in particular is complete without consideration being given to the events which followed the introduction of myxomatosis into Australia, by far the best studied example to date of the evolution of a new virus disease.

DESCRIPTION

Classification

A large number of different viruses belonging to the family Poxviridae have been described. They infect a wide range of vertebrate and invertebrate hosts. The subfamily Chordopoxvirinae contains all the viruses that infect vertebrates; it is divided into six genera, each containing related viruses which generally infect related hosts. Thus, members of the genus *Leporipoxvirus* infect rabbits and squirrels, *Avipoxvirus* members infect birds, *Capripoxvirus* members infect goats and sheep, *Suipoxvirus* members infect swine, and *Parapoxvirus* members infect cattle and sheep. Some viruses, including that of molluscum contagiosum, which infects humans, remain unclassified. By far the most intensively studied poxvirus is vaccinia virus, the Jennerian smallpox vaccine virus. This virus has been placed in the genus *Orthopoxvirus* together with smallpox virus and some viruses which infect cattle and mice.

The virion

Poxviruses are the largest animal viruses. Their virions are big enough to be seen as dots by light microscopy after special staining procedures. They are much more complex than those of any other viruses (Figs 44.1 and 44.2). They are also distinctive in that they do not show any discernible symmetry. The core contains the DNA genome and 15 or more enzymes which make up a transcriptional system whose role is to synthesize biologically active polyadenylated, capped and methylated virus messenger RNA (mRNA) molecules early in infection. The core has a 9-nm thick membrane, with a regular subunit structure. Within the virion, the core

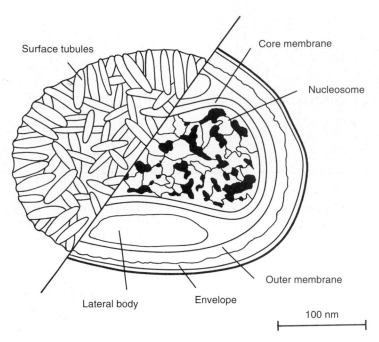

Fig. 44.1 The structure of the vaccinia virion. Right-hand side, section of enveloped virion; left-hand side, surface structure of non-enveloped particle. (From Fenner F et al. 1988 *Smallpox and its Eradication.* World Health Organization, Geneva.)

assumes a dumb-bell shape because of the large lateral bodies. The core and lateral bodies are enclosed in a protein shell about 12 nm thick – the outer membrane – the surface of which consists of irregularly arranged tubules, which in turn consist of a small globular subunit. Virions released naturally from the cell are enclosed within an envelope which contains host cell lipids and several virus-specified polypeptides, including the haemagglutinin; they are infectious. Most virions remain cell-associated and are released by cellular disruption. These particles lack an envelope so that the outer membrane constitutes their surface; they are also infectious. More than 100 different polypeptides have been identified in purified virions.

The genome

Their DNA genomes range in mass from 85 MDa (parapoxviruses) to 185 MDa (avipoxviruses). The vaccinia virus genome has 186 000 base pairs (123 MDa). The poxvirus genome is distinctive in that covalent links join the two DNA strands at both ends of the molecule, the genome thus being a single uninterrupted molecule that is folded to form a linear duplex structure. The occurrence of inverted terminal sequence repetitions is also a characteristic feature, identical sequences being present at each end of the genome.

REPLICATION

Poxviruses are unique among human DNA viruses in that virus RNA and DNA synthesis takes place in the cytoplasm of the infected cell. Because of this they have been intensively studied by workers on gene expression. After entry into the cell the core is uncoated. It starts to synthesize mRNA immediately. About half the genome is transcribed. Genes that are transcribed at this time are called early genes and map throughout the length of the genome. Only a few of their products have been characterized. They include enzymes needed for replication and transcription of viral DNA, such as DNA polymerase. Virus DNA replication starts at about 90 min after infection and goes on for several hours. It takes place in well-defined areas in the cytoplasm called factories. As soon as DNA replication starts, a dramatic change in viral gene expression occurs. Nearly all the genome now becomes available for transcription, and regulatory mechanisms come into play which lead to the synthesis of a new class of gene product, the late polypeptides. Soon after the onset of synthesis of these polypeptides the expression of most of the early genes is turned off. Most virion structural polypeptides are made late. Virion assembly takes place in the cytoplasm and proceeds in a series of steps which include the formation of spherical

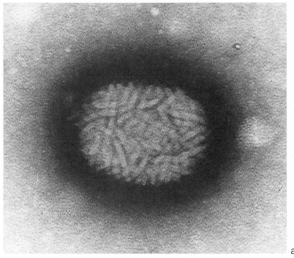

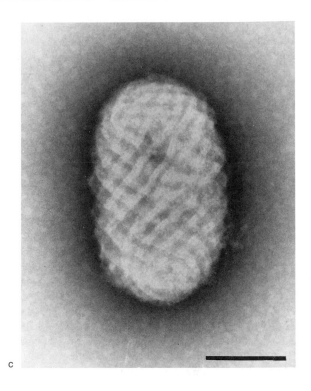

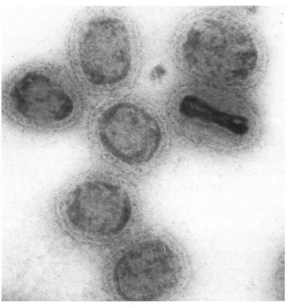

Fig. 44.2 Electron micrographs of poxviruses. **a** Molluscum contagiosum virus (MCV). ×15 000. **b** MCV showing internal structure. ×75 000. (Prepared by N. Atack.) **c** Parapoxvirus: orf. Bar, 100 nm. (By courtesy of Dr D. W. Gregory.)

immature particles. The onset of virus macromolecular synthesis is accompanied by irreversible inhibition of host protein synthesis due to the functional inactivation and degradation of host cytoplasmic RNA molecules. It is probable that this effect on the host, which leads to the death of infected cells, is a major factor in the causation of tissue damage during infection.

CLINICAL FEATURES

Smallpox virus had no animal reservoir and spread from person to person by the respiratory route. After infecting mucosal cells in the upper respiratory tract without pro-

ducing symptoms it spread to the regional lymph nodes and, after a transient viraemia, infected cells throughout the body. Multiplication of virus in these cells led to a second and more intense viraemia which heralded the onset of clinical illness. During the first few days of fever the virus multiplied in skin epithelial cells, leading to the development of focal lesions and the characteristic rash. Macules progressed to papules, vesicles and pustules, leaving permanent pockmarks, particularly on the face. Two kinds of smallpox were common in the first half of the 20th century. These were called:

- variola major, or classical smallpox
- variola minor, or alastrim.

Variola major had case fatality rates varying from 10 to 50% in the unvaccinated. Variola minor caused a much milder disease and had case fatality rates of less than 1%. The viruses are very similar but can be distinguished in the laboratory by restriction enzyme fragment length polymorphisms of their genomes.

CONTROL OF SMALLPOX

Before vaccination

Before the introduction of vaccination, the control of smallpox relied on two approaches, variolation and isolation. Variolators aimed to induce immunity equivalent to that after natural infection. Susceptible individuals were deliberately infected with smallpox pus or scabs by scratching the skin or by nasal insufflation. Although the virus was not attenuated, infections had lower case fatality rates (estimated to be 0.5–2%) and were less likely to cause permanent pockmarks than those acquired naturally. Variolation was first recorded in China nearly 1000 years ago, and was practised in many parts of the world. Variolators were active until very recent times. In Afghanistan, Pakistan and Ethiopia their activities caused problems towards the end of the smallpox eradication programme in the 1970s because they spread virus in a way that evaded the measures erected to control natural virus transmission.

Vaccination

Edward Jenner vaccinated James Phipps with cowpox virus on 14 May 1796 and challenged him by variolation some months later. He repeated this 'trial', as he called it, in other children, and the description of these events in his 'Inquiry' in 1798 led to the rapid worldwide acceptance of vaccination. Introduction of the vaccine virus into the epidermis led to the development of a local lesion and the induction of a strong immunity to infection with smallpox virus that lasted for several years. Although the essentials of *Jennerian vaccination* remained unchanged for the rest of its history, early vaccinators developed their own vaccine viruses, which became known as vaccinia. The origin of these viruses is obscure, and modern vaccinia viruses form a distinct species of orthopoxvirus, related to but very clearly distinct from the viruses of both cowpox and smallpox.

The eradication campaign

Smallpox was brought under control by:

- routine vaccination of children – compulsory in some countries

- outbreak control by isolation and selective vaccination.

This was achieved gradually in Europe, the former USSR, North and Central America, and Japan, and the virus had been eradicated from all these areas by the mid-1950s. In 1959 this achievement prompted the World Health Organization (WHO) to adopt the global eradication of smallpox as a major goal. At this time 60% of the world's population lived in areas where smallpox was endemic. A slow reduction in disease was maintained for the next few years, but epidemics continued to be frequent. Consequently the WHO initiated its Intensified Smallpox Eradication Programme. This started on 1 January 1967 when the disease was reported in 31 countries. It had the goal of eradication within 10 years. The goal was achieved in 10 years, 9 months and 26 days. From a starting point of 10 million to 15 million cases annually (Fig. 44.3) and against a background of civil strife, famine and floods, success came because of a major international collaborative effort – aided by some virus-specific factors (Table 44.1). At the beginning of 1976 smallpox occurred only in Ethiopia (Fig. 44.4). Transmission was interrupted there in August of that year, although an importation of virus into Somalia and adjacent countries had occurred by then. This was the last outbreak. The last case occurred on 26 October 1977. In the final years of the programme its emphasis moved from mass vaccination to a strategy of surveillance and containment. This strategy rapidly interrupted transmission because:

- cases were easy to detect due to the characteristic rash
- patients usually transmitted disease to only a few people – and only to those in close face-to-face contact
- only persons with a rash transmitted infection.

The WHO Global Commission for the Eradication of Smallpox formally certified that smallpox had been eradicated from the world on 9 December 1979. The use of smallpox as a biological weapon has been raised. It could be a severe threat in unprotected populations.

OTHER POXVIRUS INFECTIONS OF HUMANS

Molluscum contagiosum

The lesions of this mild disease are small coppercoloured warty papules that occur on the trunk, buttocks, arms and face. It is spread by direct contact or by fomites. The lesion consists of a mass of hypertrophied epidermis that extends into the dermis and protrudes

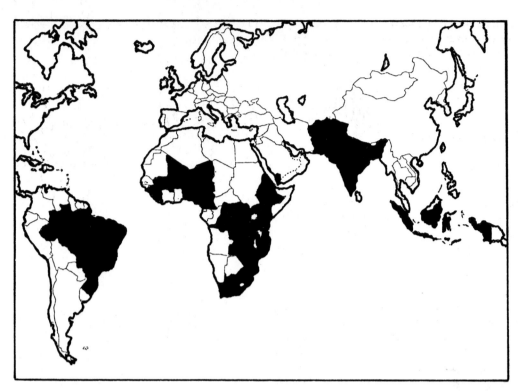

Fig. 44.3 Smallpox in the world, 1967. The map shows the 31 countries with endemic smallpox. (From Fenner et al. (1988) – see Fig. 44.1 for reference.)

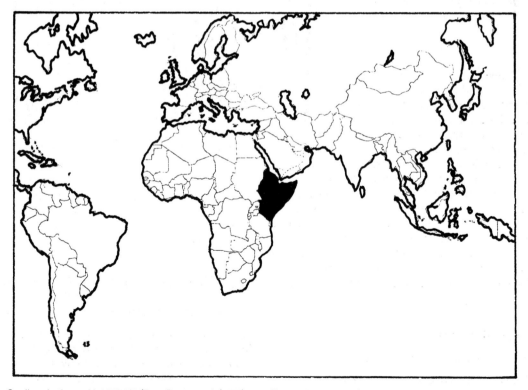

Fig. 44.4 Smallpox in the world, 1976–77. (From Fenner et al. (1988) – see Fig. 44.1 for reference.)

Table 44.1 Features of smallpox that facilitated its eradication

Feature	Importance
Disease severe	Ensured strong public and governmental support for eradication programme
Detection of cases easy because of characteristic rash and subsequent development of facial pockmarks	Facilitated containment of outbreaks and audit of success of programme
Slow spread and poor transmissibility	Facilitated containment of outbreaks by vaccination/isolation
Transmission by subclinical cases not important	Meant that control of spread by isolation of cases was an effective procedure
No carrier state in man	Meant that control of spread by isolation of cases was an effective procedure
No animal reservoir	Meant that control of spread by isolation of cases was an effective procedure
Vaccine technically simple to produce in large amounts, in high quality and at low cost (in skin of ungulates)	Meant that vaccine availability was not an important constraint in the eradication programme
Vaccine delivery simple and optimized by use of re-usable, cheap, specially designed needles to deliver a standard amount of vaccine to scratches in skin	Meant that failure at the point of vaccination was not an important constraint in the eradication programme
Freeze-dried vaccine stocks were heat-stable with very long shelf life in tropics	Meant that vaccine viability under adverse environmental conditions was not an important constraint in the eradication programme

above the skin. In the epithelial cells very large hyaline acidophilic granular masses can be observed. They crowd the host cell nucleus to one side, eventually filling the whole cell. When material from the lesions is crushed, some of the inclusions burst open, and from them large numbers of virions escape. These have the size, internal structure and morphology of vaccinia virus. The infection has been transmitted experimentally to human subjects, but the virus has not been grown in cultured cells. The development of immunity is slow and uncertain. Lesions can persist for as long as 2 years, and re-infection is common.

Monkeypox

This has been occasionally implicated in a smallpox-like condition in equatorial Africa. It may be fatal in unvaccinated individuals, but is less transmissible from person to person than smallpox.

Parapoxvirus infections

The virions of parapoxviruses are characterized by a criss-cross pattern of tubes in the outer membrane (see Fig. 44.2c), and genomes that are considerably smaller – 85 MDa – than those of other poxviruses. They infect ungulates and cause the occupational diseases in humans of *orf* and *milker's nodes*. The lesions of orf (which causes a disease in sheep known as contagious pustular dermatitis) are often large and granulomatous. Erythema multiforme is a relatively frequent complication. The lesions of milker's nodes are highly vascular hemispherical papules and nodules. Both diseases are:

- self-limiting
- commonest on the hands
- contracted by contact with infected sheep (orf) or cows (milker's nodes)
- occupational diseases, mainly seen in farm workers such as shepherds, slaughterhouse workers or butchers.

VACCINIA VIRUS AS A VACCINE VECTOR

The vaccinia virus genome can accommodate sizeable losses of DNA in certain regions, to the extent that as many as 25 000 base pairs can be lost without lethal effect. By replacing this non-essential DNA with foreign genes it has been possible to construct novel *recombinant virus strains,* which express the foreign genes when they infect cells. These genes have been inserted into the vaccinia genome by standard gene manipulation techniques, recombination and transfection.

When a cell is infected with more than one poxvirus strain, recombination can take place between them if they are closely related genetically. Recombination takes place even if one of the poxvirus genomes enters the cell in the form of naked DNA: techniques exist that optimize this process, which is known as *transfection*. Recombination has been used to insert foreign genes into the region of the vaccinia genome that codes for the non-essential enzyme thymidine kinase (TK). A fragment of vaccinia virus DNA containing this gene is taken and by use of gene manipulation techniques the foreign gene is inserted into the TK region, with a vaccinia virus promoter next to it to ensure gene expression. This DNA is then introduced by transfection into cells infected with wild type (TK⁺) vaccinia virus. Recombination takes place at the TK gene, producing viruses whose genomes now contain the foreign gene. Because this is inserted into the TK gene the latter is non-functional (TK⁻). Selection procedures for the absence of TK activity are now applied, aiding the identification of recombinant viruses. Recombinant vaccinia strains containing as many as four foreign genes, coding for combinations of bacterial, viral and protozoal antigens, have been constructed.

The advantages of this ingenious way of developing new vaccines are:

- they are applicable to many different antigens
- the possibility of constructing multivalent vaccines that could give protection against several diseases after a single 'shot'
- stimulates cell-mediated immunity
- the ease of administration
- cheapness of vaccinia as a vaccine.

A strain that expresses the rabies glycoprotein antigen is being used in Europe to protect foxes. Serious disadvantages remain for humans, however. These are primarily those associated with vaccinia virus itself, whose use carried with it a number of serious complications. The most important of these were:

- *progressive vaccinia*, a fatal infection which occurred in immunodeficient individuals
- *eczema vaccinatum*, a serious spreading infection which occurred in eczematous individuals
- *postvaccinal encephalitis*, which, although rare, was severe and occurred in normal healthy individuals.

These disadvantages preclude the use of vaccinia as a vector for foreign antigens in humans, and work is being done on the modification of its virulence to circumvent these problems. So far, studies on virulence genes have shown that poxviruses code for an impressive array of factors interfering with host defences. These include proteins which bind complement components, act as receptors for interleukin-1β, interferon, and tumour necrosis factor, and synthesize steroids.

These factors are all exported from infected cells. Factors that act inside cells include proteins that block the action of interferon, inhibit the post-translational modification of interleukin-1β, and prevent the synthesis of a neutrophil chemotactic factor. It is possible that abrogation of virulence factors such as these may lead to safer vaccines.

MYXOMATOSIS: AN EVOLVING DISEASE

As a rule, virus infections are mild and self-limiting. Viruses are obligate parasites and it is easy to understand that it is not in their interests to cause the extinction or massive reductions in size of host populations. It is reasonable to suppose that the type of disease caused by a virus reflects the outcome of a process in which host and virus have co-evolved to levels of resistance and virulence optimal for the maintenance of their respective population numbers. The high mortality of classical smallpox is considered by some to have been a major factor in the restriction of human population size, and this has been used to support the hypothesis that the association between smallpox and humans has been established – in evolutionary terms – only in recent times, co-evolution of the relationship being a long way from equilibrium. It is impossible to test this hypothesis directly for variola, but the relationship between another poxvirus – myxoma virus – and the rabbit in Australia, has provided a dramatic example. This is the only example of co-evolution where changes in an animal host and virus and the evolution of a disease have been studied in real time.

Myxoma virus is South American. It causes a benign local fibroma in its natural host, the rabbit *Sylvilagus brasiliensis*, but causes *myxomatosis* in the European rabbit, *Oryctolagus cuniculus*. This is a generalized infection with a very high mortality rate. Field trials to test its efficacy as a measure for controlling the European rabbit were carried out in Australia in 1950. The virus escaped and caused enormous epidemics in the years that followed. The original virus caused infections with a case mortality rate greater than 99%, and rabbits survived less than 13 days. Within 3 years virus isolates from epidemics had become much less virulent, causing infections with mortality rates of 70–95% and survival times of 17–28 days. Changes in the resistance of the rabbit also occurred, with mortality rates of infection falling (from 90 to 25% following challenge with strains of virus with modified virulence, for example) and symptomatology becoming less severe. In myxomatosis, natural selection favoured virus strains with intermediate virulence because such strains are transmitted more effectively than highly virulent strains, which kill their hosts too quickly, and non-virulent strains, which are poorly transmitted.

RECOMMENDED READING

Baxby D 1981 *Jenner's Smallpox Vaccine*. Heinemann, London

Fenner F, Ratcliffe F N 1965 *Myxomatosis*. Cambridge University Press, Cambridge

Fenner F, Henderson D A, Arita I, Jezek Z, Ladnyi I D 1988 *Smallpox and its Eradication*. World Health Organization, Geneva

Fields B N, Knipe D M, Howley P M (eds) 1996 *Virology*, 3rd edn. Lippincott–Raven, Philadelphia

Jenner E 1798 *An Inquiry into the Causes and Effects of the Variolae Vaccinae*. Sampson Low, London

45

Papovaviruses

Warts: warts and cancers; progressive multifocal leuco-encephalopathy

H. Cubie

The *pa*pillomavirus, *pol*yomavirus and the *va*cuolating virus of rhesus monkeys (simian virus 40; SV40) are small DNA viruses which are currently classified in two genera (*Papillomavirus* and *Polyomavirus*) of the family Papovaviridae, the name being derived from the first two letters of the names of each of the members. Papovaviruses are all small DNA tumour viruses with icosahedral capsid structure, but the molecular biology and pathogenesis of the two genera differ considerably.

Papillomavirus. Papillomaviruses are widely distributed in nature and are species-specific DNA viruses that infect the squamous epithelia and mucous membranes of vertebrates, including man. They are responsible for many varieties of *warts* and fibropapillomata. Although the lesions are usually benign, their association with tumours of man and other animals is now well documented. The first evidence for oncogenic properties came from the study of the virus types infecting animals. In the 1930s Shope found that the cottontail rabbit papillomavirus caused benign warts with 25% of the lesions undergoing malignant change within a year. Viral DNA remains detectable within the tumours. In domestic rabbits, however, up to 75% of lesions progressed to cancer. Application of tar to the lesions led to more rapid malignant change. Bovine papillomavirus (BPV) causes tumours of the alimentary canal and bladder in cattle fed on a diet containing bracken fern. The tumours are preceded by infection with BPV types 4 and 2, respectively, but the virus is not detected after malignant transformation. These studies show that malignant progression can be influenced by both genetic composition and exposure to chemicals.

Polyomavirus. The name is derived from 'poly' (many) and 'oma' (tumour). The viruses are species-specific, and although tumour induction is well described in experimental animals, there is to date no documented association with any naturally occurring tumour of man. Recognized members of this group include the mouse polyomavirus, SV40 of monkeys and two viruses of man – JC virus (JCV) and BK virus

(BKV), both named after the initials of the people from whom they were first isolated.

HUMAN PAPILLOMAVIRUSES (HPV)

The papillomaviruses are 52–55 nm in diameter and have an icosahedral capsid composed of 72 capsomeres (Fig. 45.1). The genome is a supercoiled double-stranded circle of DNA, with a single coding strand, a molecular weight of approximately 5×10^6 and consisting of about 8000 base pairs.

The existence of different HPV types at different sites was recognized in the late 1960s, with differentiation of cutaneous and genital warts. There are now thought to be over 100 types of HPV, distinguished on the basis of

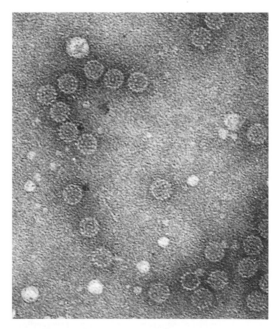

Fig. 45.1 Electron micrograph of wart virus from a plantar wart. PTA stain. ×100 000. (By courtesy of Dr M. M. Ogilvie.)

the homology between their genomes as measured by cross-hybridization between the separated DNA strands. A new type must exhibit less than 50% homology with any other known type. The appearance of the lesions produced and the particular tissue infected is associated with specific virus types.

- Types 1, 2, 3 and 4 commonly infect the keratinized epithelium of the hands and feet.
- Over 30 types infect the mucosal epithelium in the anogenital tract and orolaryngeal cavity, of which HPV types 6, 11, 16, 18, 31, 33 and 45 are the most common.
- Types 2 and 57 can infect both skin and genital mucosa.

Types are categorized as 'low', 'intermediate' or 'high' risk according to the extent of their oncogenic

potential. The tissue tropisms and relatedness of HPVs can be seen in phylogenetic trees produced by computer algorithms of aligned sequences. Cutaneous types form one clear branch of the tree while genital types with greatest malignant potential form a second branch (Fig. 45.2).

Genome organization and replication

While viral DNA can be found in the basal cells of the epithelium, whole virions are found only in the uppermost cell layer in terminally differentiated keratinocytes. This close association of viral replication with tissue differentiation has made the development of tissue culture systems difficult. Understanding of the events in the replication cycle has been largely deduced therefore from knowledge of comparable viruses, with bovine papillomaviruses often being used as model systems to study the biology of HPV.

The genome is divided into an early region with two large (E1 and E2) and several smaller (E4–E7) open reading frames and a late region with two large genes (L1 and L2) which code for the capsid proteins (Fig. 45.3). The E region codes for proteins concerned with DNA replication, transcription and transformation. The E1 and E2 proteins are both essential for replication. The long control region (LCR) is concerned with the control of transcription. Binding of the E2 protein to an enhancer site on the LCR can upregulate transcription of E6 and E7, the genes responsible for transformation.

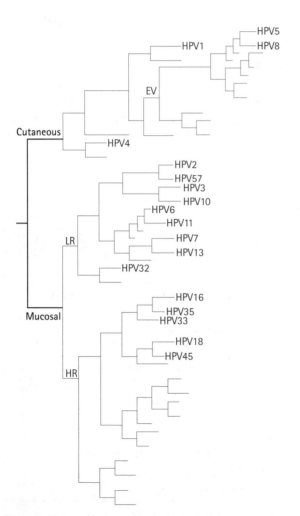

Fig. 45.2 Phylogenetic tree constructed from aligned sequences of part of E6 gene of HPV. LR, HR: low risk, high risk of malignancy (Adapted from van Ranst et al., Current Research in Papillomaviruses, 1996.)

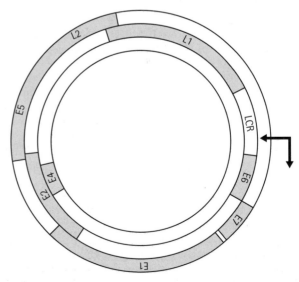

Fig. 45.3 Simplified circular map of HPV 16 genome, identifying early (E) and late (L) open reading frames. Arrow at origin.

Inactivation of E1 leads to integration of viral DNA into the host chromosomes at random sites. E4 causes the collapse of the cellular cytoskeleton, and E5 has transforming activity in some papillomavirus types. The coding sequences are distributed in all three open reading frames with considerable overlap along a single strand of DNA. Complex splicing events allow many different transcripts to be produced, with the resulting proteins having different biological roles. The gene functions are summarized in Table 45.1.

Unravelling the functions of these genes has contributed significantly to our understanding of the pathogenicity of different HPV types and particularly to the transforming ability of the high-risk types. Viral DNA can be found as an episome in productively infected cells but is usually integrated into random sites on a host chromosome in malignant lesions.

Transformation

Transfection of viral DNA into cultured cells has yielded much information on the genes responsible for the tumorigenic potential of HPV. Integration of the viral genome results in disruption of E1 and E2, with subsequent increase in expression of E6 and E7. The immortalizing properties of high-risk HPV types such as HPV 16 and 18 are largely due to expression of E7, but co-operation between E6 and E7 is necessary for efficient transformation. How does this come about?

E7 binds to the tumour suppressor gene product, Rb, which is required for terminal differentiation of keratinocytes. Thus, binding of E7 to Rb permits continued cell growth and viral expression by preventing differentiation. E6 binds to the tumour suppressor gene product p53 and causes its rapid degradation. The function of p53 is to induce cellular arrest to allow repair of DNA damage. Only E6 from high risk HPV types can overcome the growth arrest function of p53. Not all PVs possess an E5 gene so it cannot be vital for transformation. However, in vitro studies with BPV and HPV show several E5 interactions with growth factor receptors, resulting in their sustained activation and a clear contribution to the transformed state. Recent work shows E5 expression to be absent in frank cancers, and further work is required on the role of this protein.

Clinical features and pathogenesis of HPV infections

Cutaneous warts

Cutaneous warts commonly infect the keratinized epithelium of the hands and feet, producing typical warts frequently seen in young children and adolescents. The viruses associated with such lesions are HPV types:

- 1 and 4 (plantar warts)
- 3 and 10 (flat warts)
- 2, 4 and 7 (common warts) (Table 45.2).

Table 45.1 Papillomavirus gene functions

Gene	Function	Comments
LCR (Long control region)	Regulation of gene function and initiator of viral replication	Both positive and negative transcriptional control elements
E1	Episomal maintenance	Frequently disrupted by integration
E2	Regulation of transcription and replication. DNA-binding protein; very similar in BPV and HPV	Regulates transcription and viral replication in association with E1. Frequently disrupted by integration
E4	Virion maturation, disrupts cytoskeleton	
E5	Transforming function – alters signalling from growth factor receptors	Often lost or not expressed after integration. Not found in all papillomaviruses
E6	Transforming function – binds to p53	Co-operates with E7 to increase efficiency of transformation
E7	Major transforming gene – binds to Rb	Transforms cells independently of E6
L1	Production of major capsid proteins	Group- and type-specific determinants
L2	Production of minor capsid proteins	Type-specific determinants

Table 45.2 HPV types associated with specific lesions

Lesion	HPV type
Cutaneous sites	
Deep plantar warts (*verruca plantaris*)	1, 4
Common warts (*verruca vulgaris*)	2, 4, 7
Plane or flat warts	3, 10
Epidermodysplasia verruciformis-like macular lesions	5, 8
Mucocutaneous sites	
Genital warts (*condyloma acuminatum*)	6, 11
Flat condyloma and intra-epithelial neoplasia	16, 18, 31, 33, 45
Laryngeal papillomata	6, 11
Oral papillomata	2, 6, 11, 16, 18, 57
Oral hyperplasia	13, 32

Histologically, the lesions are benign with hypertrophy of all the layers of the dermis and hyperkeratosis of the horny layer (Fig. 45.4). They usually disappear spontaneously but occasionally may be resistant to treatment. Regrowth of the lesions after treatment is thought to be due to persistence of the virus in the skin surrounding the original wart.

Although both humoral immune and cell-mediated immune responses can develop in papilloma infections, regression is usually the result of cellular responses. In patients with primary or secondary cell-mediated

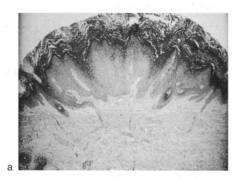

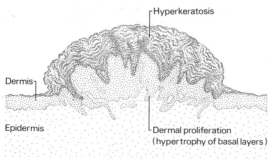

Fig. 45.4 Histology of a wart.

immunodeficiency, there is an increased risk of developing warts which can be extensive, persistent or recurrent and likely to progress. For example, in people suffering from the rare genetic skin disorder *epidermodysplasia verruciformis* (EV) where there is a selective depletion of specific T cell clones, large plane warts associated with virus types such as HPV 5 and 8 develop and persist for life. Similarly, up to 40% of renal allograft recipients will develop cutaneous warts within a year of the graft, rising to more than 90% in those with graft survival greater than 15 years. EV-associated HPV types have recently been detected in a variety of lesions, including a high proportion of psoriatic skin lesions and in non-lesional skin, suggesting that the development of visible lesions is well controlled by the immune system of healthy individuals.

Anogenital warts

These lesions (also known as *condylomata acuminata*) are commonest in sexually active adults. In women they are found:

- on the vulva
- within the vagina
- on the cervix.

Vulvar and vaginal warts are usually plainly visible, but on the cervix they may be indistinguishable from the normal mucosa without the aid of a colposcope to magnify the cervical epithelium. The application of 5% acetic acid causes whitening of epithelium in which there is a high concentration of nuclear material and reveals subclinical lesions as areas of densely white whorled epithelium known as flat or non-condylomatous warts.

Subclinical and latent infections of the genital tract are common. Subclinical lesions may become clinically apparent if the immune response is disturbed, as in pregnancy. Latent virus has been detected in about 12% of women with normal cytology in the superficial cells from cervical scrapes. The prevalence rate is 3–5 times higher in women aged under 35 years than in older women, and HPV16/18 is more commonly found than HPV6/11.

In men the most common sites for lesions are:

- the shaft of the penis
- peri-anal skin
- the anal canal.

Subclinical infection of the genital tract may also occur in men and will be visible colposcopically only if the penis is painted with 5% acetic acid.

HPV types 6 and 11 are commonly found in benign vulval or penile warts. Cervical and anogenital warts may be due to HPV types 16 or 18, both of which are associated with malignant and premalignant lesions of

Hyperkeratosis
Dermis
Epidermis
Dermal proliferation (hypertrophy of basal layers)

the cervix and anogenital tract. Other types frequently found in genital cancers and precursor lesions include types 31, 33 and 45.

Orolaryngeal lesions

Recurrent respiratory papillomatosis. This is a rare condition characterized by the presence of benign squamous papillomata on the mucosa of the respiratory tract, most commonly on the larynx. It has a bimodal age distribution with peaks of incidence in children under 5 years of age and adults after the age of 15 years, and is caused by infection of the respiratory mucosa with HPV types 6 and 11. Children acquire the disease by passage through an infected birth canal, while adults acquire the disease from orogenital contact with an infected sexual partner. The transmission rate is low. The disease presents with hoarseness of voice or, in children, with an abnormal cry. As the lesions grow they may cause stridor and upper airway obstruction which can be life-threatening and require emergency surgery. Recurrence following treatment is common and extension of the disease to the bronchial tree may occur. Malignant conversion of laryngeal papillomas has been described in the past, usually after radiotherapy to treat the initial lesion.

Oral papillomatosis. A variety of papillomata and benign lesions associated with HPV occur on the oral mucosa and tongue. Several HPV types, including types 2, 7, 13 and 32, have been found, the last two in focal epithelial hyperplasia or Heck's disease, which is common in Eskimos. Multiple lesions may develop on the buccal mucosa, a condition known as oral florid papillomatosis. Subclinical lesions can be detected on the oral mucosa of normal adults after the application of acetic acid. The virus types here are those more commonly found in the genital tract, and infection is acquired during orogenital contact with an infected sexual partner.

HPV and cancer

Premalignant lesions of the genital tract

Malignant disease of the cervix is preceded by neoplastic change in the surface epithelium, a condition known as *cervical intra-epithelial neoplasia* (CIN). A similar pattern of events takes place in other sites in the genital tract of both men and women. The initial transforming event takes place in the deepest layer of the epithelium, the germinal layer, and abnormal cells spread through the surface layers. This condition increases in severity from:

- CIN I (low grade squamous intra-epithelial lesions (LSIL in American classification) to
- CIN II and III (high grade or HGSIL), in which abnormal cells including mitotic figures can be found in all layers of the epithelium with loss of stratification and differentiation.

Untreated CIN II/III can progress to invasive cancer in a large percentage of affected individuals while CIN I lesions are less likely to progress. Regression may occur spontaneously at all stages (Fig. 45.5). HPV DNA can be detected in all grades of the premalignant lesions of the female and male genital tract.

- HPV types 6 and 11 are most commonly found in low-grade disease whereas
- HPV types 16 and 18 are more commonly associated with lesions of greater severity and invasive cancer.

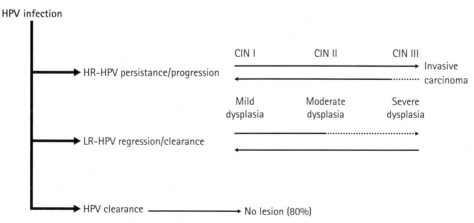

Fig 45.5 HPV infection and pathogenesis of cervical cancer. HR, high risk; LR, low risk; CIN, cervical intra-epithelial neoplasia.

Squamous cell carcinoma

The association of wart viruses with invasive cancers of the skin, larynx and genital tract is well documented. Malignant conversion of skin warts occurs in about one-third of EV patients at a relatively young age on skin exposed to sunlight with HPV type 5 or 8 in over 90% of squamous cancers. Malignant conversion of cutaneous warts in renal allograft recipients has also been documented. Squamous cell carcinoma of the aerodigestive tract has been shown to harbour HPV to varying extents in different studies and in different tumour types. More than 20 HPV types have been found. In tumours of the tonsils HPV 16 and 33 have been particularly noted but the nature of the association is not fully established.

The commonest association with invasive cancer, however, is with tumours of the anogenital tract. About 99% of invasive cervical cancers contain HPV DNA. The proportion of cancers containing different HPV types varies around the world and the incidence shows wide demographic, ethnic and socio-economic variation.

- In Indonesia, for example, HPV18 predominates
- In Europe HPV16 is by far the most common.

HPV18 and the related HPV 45 are more frequently found in the more aggressive adenocarcinomas. In-situ DNA hybridization of tumour biopsies has shown that HPV DNA is unevenly distributed throughout the tumour, suggesting that these cancers are polyclonal in origin.

In most animal cancers associated with papillomavirus there is an identifiable co-factor. In humans, the genetic background of the individual, smoking, seminal fluid factors and immune status all act as co-factors in HPV-associated genital tract malignancies. Thus, CIN is commoner in:

- relatives of affected women than in the population at large
- women who smoke are at increased risk of CIN and cancer of the cervix
- women who are immunosuppressed, whether due to drug treatment (transplant recipients), or secondary to haematological malignancies (leukaemias) or to infection with HIV.

Further risk factors in the development of genital carcinomas include:

- sexual activity
- age at first intercourse (young age favours)
- oral contraceptive use
- occurrence of other sexually transmitted infections.

It is, however, extremely difficult to assess the relative interdependence of all risk factors.

In the development of HPV-related carcinomas at other sites, exposure to ultraviolet or ionizing radiation, smoking, chewing of betel-quid, immunosuppression and genetic make-up are all likely to be important.

Transmission and epidemiology

Clinical studies of the incidence of skin warts show that infection is common in early childhood and is acquired by direct contact with an infected person. HPV is a stable, hardy virus so fomites are also important, as shown by outbreaks of hand warts from the use of gymnastic apparatus and plantar warts acquired from swimming pool surrounds. Mild shearing trauma is necessary to allow the virus to reach the basal layers of the skin.

Transmission of genital warts mainly occurs during sexual activity and there is a strong association between increasing numbers of sexual partners and the prevalence of genital HPV infection. However, there is evidence that genital wart types can also be acquired non-sexually. Vertical transmission of low- and high-risk HPV types from mother to infant at birth and perinatal transmission within the first 6 weeks of life have both been clearly demonstrated. The high rates and persistence of buccal infection with HPV 16 in primary schoolchildren could also be explained by horizontal transmission. Furthermore, genital HPV DNA has been detected in virgins and antibodies to HPV 16 have been demonstrated in up to 10% of young schoolgirls.

Laboratory diagnosis

Morphological identification

HPV infection may be readily diagnosed when there are typical clinical lesions. Subclinical infection requires laboratory confirmation using cytological, histological, immunocytochemical and molecular detection of nucleic acid. HPV infection can be recognized morphologically in cervical smears by the presence of vacuolated cells with atypical enlarged hyperchromatic nuclei described as *koilocytes*. However, koilocytes are not always present, are not sufficiently specific for HPV and cannot differentiate between low and high risk HPV types. Histological examination of a biopsy taken from a lesion identified at colposcopy will show more specific features of HPV infection, including papillomatosis, hyperkeratinization of the surface layer, hypertrophy of the basal layers and disorganization of the epidermal structure.

Molecular methods

It is being recognized increasingly that there is a diagnostic role for specific HPV testing in cervical screening programmes for more effective identification of women with lesions likely to progress to cervical cancer. HPV testing could be used in association with cytology or possibly instead of cytological screening in countries with no cervical screening programmes.

In-situ hybridization on tissue sections or exfoliated cells provides histological information at the same time as HPV detection, but has shown lower sensitivity than methods involving amplification. Hybridization in solution using a cocktail of HR-HPV probes followed by immunochemical signal amplification (Hybrid Capture® assay) has been used in several large cervical screening studies. Amplification of HPV DNA by polymerase chain reaction (PCR) using consensus primers to detect a wide range of HPV types has also been widely used. It is generally agreed that HPV testing is more sensitive than cytology for detection of high-grade CIN, but it has a lower specificity, especially in younger women in whom transient infection is common. Large scale trials are on-going in several countries to evaluate further the effectiveness of HPV testing.

Serology

The lack of native antigen hampered the development of serological assays for many years, but recent production of virus-like particles in eukaryotic expression systems using baculovirus or vaccinia recombinants has allowed the detection of antibodies to specific HPV types. Such assays are more useful for showing evidence of past exposure rather than current infection and are appropriate for epidemiological studies. Studies reporting the detection of antibody to recombinant proteins or synthetic peptides from the E6 or E7 gene in women with high-grade cervical disease suggest there may be a correlation between antibody presence and poor prognosis.

Treatment and control

In most immunocompetent people, warts are a cosmetic nuisance and will eventually disappear spontaneously. Warts may be destroyed by cryotherapy with dry ice or liquid nitrogen but simple topical treatment with salicylic acid at home is often successful. Genital warts are more problematic. They are a common sexually transmitted infection and represent a significant cost to health care resources. In pregnant women, vaginal warts may occasionally grow to such a size that the birth canal is obstructed and surgical removal is required.

Interferon may assist the immune system to eradicate the virus and decrease the likelihood of recurrence. Interferons have been used to treat recurrent CIN or laryngeal warts after reduction of tumour load by laser vaporization or surgery, but it is expensive, lesions recur when the interferon is stopped and side-effects are common. Cytotoxic agents such as podophyllin have been used in specific types of warts, but require close monitoring. Recently the immune modulator imiquimod, which activates monocytes/macrophages and causes direct release of IFN-α, has been shown to be efficacious in clinical trials as a self-applied topical treatment. All of these treatments will remove the lesions but do not always eradicate the virus from surrounding normal epithelium. Incomplete treatment is the commonest cause of recurrence of warts and all of a patient's warts must have disappeared with restoration of normal skin texture before a cure is considered.

Prevention of spread of wart viruses can be achieved by avoiding contact with affected individuals. Thus, the use of condoms will diminish the risk of spread of genital warts. Although HPV DNA has been found on vaginal specula, no woman has been shown to have been infected by this route.

There are a number of vaccines available to prevent the development of papillomas and cancers in cattle and rabbits. These include virus-like particle vaccines consisting of L1 alone or L1 and L2 proteins. In humans, trials using similar prophylactic vaccines to prevent genital infection with HR-HPV are in progress. Therapeutic vaccines containing viral oncoproteins have been used to stimulate cell-mediated immunity and both Phase 1 and Phase 2 trials are currently being carried out to assess their ability to prevent progression to cancer. Results are encouraging but much more work requires to be done.

POLYOMAVIRUSES

The virions are 42–45 nm in size with a 72-capsomere icosahedral capsid. The genome has a molecular weight of 3.4×10^6 and is approximately 5000 bp in length. Like the papillomaviruses, it is a double-stranded supercoiled loop of DNA, but both strands code for virus proteins.

Replication and transformation

The genome of polyomaviruses has an early region which codes for large T and small t antigens. These are the first antigens to appear after infection; they accumulate in the nucleus and stimulate cellular growth and are important for replication. This is followed by a switch to transcription of the late region and production of the structural proteins VP1, VP2 and VP3. The growth cycle in culture is 36–44 h long, and the release of mature virus particles follows lysis of the cell. The structural proteins determine host range and infectivity. BKV can be grown with difficulty in human embryonic kidney cells while JCV, which is not only species but also tissue-specific, replicates only in human embryo glial cell cultures.

The early proteins are associated with immortalization and transformation. Large T antigen binds to both Rb and p53 and prevents the induction of cell death. Only murine and hamster polyomaviruses appear to be oncogenic in their natural hosts. Both BKV and JCV have been shown to be oncogenic for newborn hamsters but have not been found consistently in any human tumours. Nevertheless there are many unanswered questions about the natural history of these viruses.

Clinical features and pathogenesis

BKV has been mainly isolated from immunocompromised individuals, usually from urine or kidney. DNA hybridization studies, however, would suggest that BKV can also be found in tonsils, lung, lymph nodes and spleen. JCV has been isolated principally from the brain, but also from urine and the renal tract of immunocompromised individuals. The genome has been identified in lung, liver, spleen, lymph nodes and leucocytes.

While serological studies suggest infection is common, primary polyomavirus infection is a rare diagnosis and infection is usually asymptomatic. There are a few reports of children with primary BKV infection showing acute respiratory disease or haemorrhagic cystitis. Reactivation, however, is common and can lead to clinical disease, particularly in organ transplant patients, with up to 40% of renal allograft recipients excreting polyomavirus in the early months after transplantation. A similar situation is found after bone marrow transplantation. Reactivations of BKV and JCV infections are quite common in pregnancy, with viruria being detected in 3–7% of women, especially during the second and third trimesters. Although there are no specific associated symptoms, women with persistent viruria have more illnesses and their babies are more often premature or jaundiced, but there is no evidence that polyomaviruses are transmitted transplacentally.

Progressive multifocal leuco-encephalopathy (PML)

This condition was first described in 1958 in patients with *Hodgkin's lymphoma* and *chronic lymphocytic leukaemia*. It is usually a late complication in people immunocompromised due to therapy or disease and is associated with reactivation of JCV in the brain. It is more frequent in later life, but recently cases in younger people have been found, particularly renal allograft recipients and AIDS patients.

PML patients have multiple foci of demyelination, usually in the cerebral hemispheres, but occasionally elsewhere in the central nervous system. A unique combination of pathological changes in PML is identifiable histologically. The peripheral zone surrounding areas of demyelination contains swollen oligodendrocytes, with hyperchromatic nuclei and occasional basophilic inclusions. These cells contain many virions detectable by electron microscopy. Replication of the virus occurs in the nucleus, causing cell destruction and breakdown of the myelin sheath. In the centre of the lesion, oligodendrocytes are absent and in contrast, the astrocytes present look more neoplastic and do not contain virions. Some astrocytes may be transformed but tumour formation is absent. Malignant gliomas are occasionally found near areas of demyelination. JCV is consistently associated with PML but low levels of JCV DNA have been reported in patients without clinical evidence of PML. Whether this indicates a latent state or a preclinical stage of PML is currently unknown.

The clinical features depend on the areas affected. Symptoms include visual, mental and speech impairment, hemiplegia, loss of memory and dementia. Death usually occurs within 6 months of the disease first becoming manifest. Similar symptoms can have other causes and differential diagnosis is essential.

Polyomavirus infection and transplant recipients

In renal transplant recipients, polyomavirus infection appears to be as common as cytomegalovirus infection. Most infections appear to be due to reactivation of BKV, although primary infection with JCV has been recognized with the donor kidney as the likely source of virus. Half of the infections occur between 4 and 8 weeks after transplantation, but subclinical reactivations of virus occurring up to 12 months after transplantation are not uncommon. Polyomavirus infection is associated with a transient decrease in graft function. If this is wrongly interpreted as being a rejection episode and managed by further immunosuppression, complications may occur. Polyomavirus infection of the transplanted ureter results in cell proliferation leading to *ureteric stenosis* and occasionally to obstruction. Both BKV and JCV have been implicated in this condition. Obstruction can occur up to 300 days postoperatively and may not be recognized until nephrectomy or post mortem is performed. In bone marrow transplant recipients, 38% of a study group in the USA were found to be excreting polyomavirus in their urine, with the highest incidence in patients with acute myeloid leukaemia. Excretion of BKV appears much more common than of JCV. Although not associated with graft versus host disease, some patients had a transient post-transplant hepatitis and late-onset BKV viruria has been linked to haemorrhagic cystitis.

Laboratory diagnosis

Isolation of BKV and JCV is too difficult for routine diagnostic use. Detection of virus particles by electron microscopic examination of negatively stained urine deposits or brain homogenates is possible. Viral antigen can be detected using indirect immunofluorescence on exfoliated cells from urine or in acetone-fixed brain smears. Detection of viral DNA by in-situ hybridization is possible, with positive cells showing characteristic morphological changes of swollen oligodendrocytes. PCR to detect JCV DNA in cerebrospinal fluid is more commonly used. When this is combined with intrathecal antibody detection it provides a sensitive non-invasive diagnostic procedure. The most common serological assays to measure antibody to BKV and JCV are haemagglutination inhibition and ELISA. Rising titres and the presence of IgM are diagnostic of recent infection. Failure to detect antibody to JCV nearly always excludes a diagnosis of PML.

Epidemiology

Serological studies in the UK show that BKV infection is a relatively common event in early childhood. By 3 years of age 30% of children have antibody to the virus, and this rises to 90% by the age of 5 years. The pattern of infection is similar in other countries.

Serological evidence suggests that JCV circulates independently of BKV in the community, and acquisition of antibodies is slower and more variable. In the UK, 5% of the pre-school population have antibody, with this proportion rising to 30% by the age of 17 years and to 60% in adults. In Japan, infection is more rapid and widespread, with two-thirds of children seropositive by age 6 years, rising to 90% of adults.

Treatment

There is no established treatment for PML, although many antiviral agents have been tried. Cytarabine may allow some improvement, especially if given intrathecally for a long time. Reducing the level of immunosuppression is likely to be beneficial, but this may not be possible because of the underlying disease.

RECOMMENDED READING

Bunney M H, Benton E C, Cubie H A 1992 *Viral Warts – Biology and Treatment,* 2nd edn. Oxford University Press, Oxford

Knowles W 2000 Human polyomaviruses. In: Zuckerman A J, Banatvala J E, Pattison J R (eds) *Principles and Practice of Clinical Virology,* 4th edn. John Wiley & Sons, Chichester

Lacey C, ed. 1996 *Papillomavirus Reviews: Current Research on Papillomaviruses.* Leeds Medical Information, Leeds

Shah K V, Howley P M 1996 Papillomaviruses. In: Fields B, Kripe D M, Howley P M (eds). *Fields Virology,* 3rd edn. Lippencott Raven, Philadelphia

Zur Hausen H 1998 Papovaviruses. In: Collier L, Balows A, Sussman M (eds). *Topley and Wilson's Microbiology and Microbial Infections,* Vol. 1: Virology, 9th edn. Arnold, London

46

Hepadnaviruses

Hepatitis B infection; deltavirus infection

P. Simmonds and J. F. Peutherer

The family Hepadnaviridae includes the human hepatitis B virus (HBV) and the woodchuck, ground squirrel and Pekin duck viruses; others have been identified, but these are the best known and studied. The viruses show similarities in the structure of their virions and associated particles, the size, nature and replication of the DNA genome and their ability to cause both acute and chronic infections in their natural hosts. HBV is a major cause of chronic liver disease and hepatocellular carcinoma; worldwide it is estimated to cause more than one million deaths each year.

PROPERTIES

Structure

Three different particles can be seen in the blood in HBV infection (Figs 46.1 and 46.2). The predominant form is a

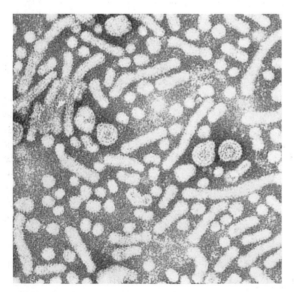

Fig. 46.1 Electron micrograph of the particles in the blood of a patient infected with HBV. ×130 000. (By courtesy of Dr A. Keen, University of Cape Town.)

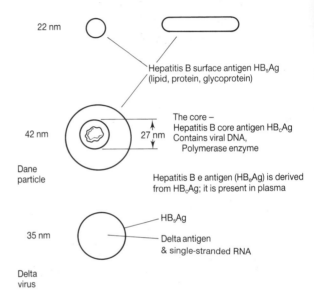

Fig. 46.2 The particles and antigens of HBV and delta virus.

small, spherical particle with a diameter of 22 nm. Filaments are also present with a diameter of about 22 nm. Both types of particle are composed of lipid, protein and carbohydrate; they are not infectious and consist solely of surplus virion envelope. The particles carry the hepatitis B surface antigen (HBsAg). The third type of particle, the virion or *Dane particle*, has a diameter of 42 nm: enclosed within the envelope is the core (27 nm), which contains the viral DNA and polymerase within a shell composed of hepatitis B core antigen (HBcAg). There may be as many as 10^{13} of the small particles and filaments per millilitre. The virions are present in much smaller numbers, usually by a factor of 10 000 or more, and the proportion varies considerably in different stages of the disease. The viral DNA is about 3200 nucleotides long and is circular (Fig. 46.3). The long strand is complete, but there is a gap of variable length of about 1000 nucleotides in the complementary strand: this can be closed via the action of the virion polymerase when virus replication starts.

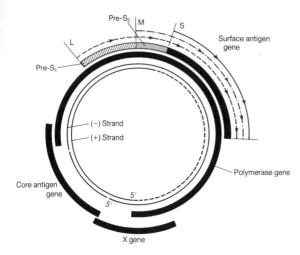

Fig. 46.3 The gene organization of HBV DNA.

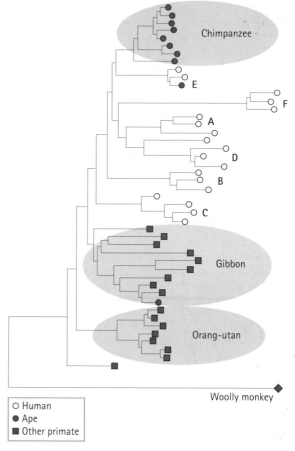

Fig. 46.4 The relatedness of the nucleotide sequences of hepadnavirus genomes from humans and non-human primates.

There are four overlapping genes coding for the core, surface and polymerase proteins and an X protein that may act as an activator of transcription. The hepatitis e antigen (HBeAg) is translated from the HBcAg gene using an upstream initiating codon. The protein is secreted from infected cells into plasma, especially at times when there is active viral replication reflected by the release of Dane particles into the circulation. The surface antigen gene is transcribed to produce three mRNAs, L, M and S. These are translated to give three proteins: each contains the S protein. The product of the M mRNA consists of the S and pre-S_2 proteins. The protein from the L mRNA comprises pre-S_1, preS_2 and S. The L product is present only in the virion, while the M and S proteins are found in each type of particle.

Genetic variation

HBV can be classified into at least six genotypes, A–F, by comparison of their nucleotide sequences (Fig. 46.4). Some genotypes are distributed worldwide, while others have a more restricted geographical distribution; genotype E is found predominantly in sub-Saharan Africa, while genotypes B and C are found in the Far East. In western countries, there are differences in genotype frequencies between risk groups for HBV infection. However, there is no evidence that genotypes of HBV differ from each other in their transmissibility or disease causation, although there are antigenic differences in the HBsAg protein. HBsAg contains a common 'a' antigen, and two sets of mutually exclusive determinants, 'd' or 'y' and 'w 'or 'r', giving the four main types – adw, adr, ayw and ayr, the latter being associated with different HBV genotypes. Fortunately, the invariant 'a' determinant is the main target of the protective antibody

response to infection, and immunity induced by infection or immunization with one HBV genotype will cross-protect against infection with others.

Recently it has been discovered that HBV infection occurs in the wild in a number of non-human primate species, such as chimpanzees, orang-utans and gibbons. Each of these species harbours variants of HBV distinct from those found in humans (Fig. 46.4). Whether primate HBV infection contributes to the pool of human carriers in areas of high endemicity, such as sub-Saharan Africa, is currently unclear. However, in view of the genetic differences between human and non-human genotypes, this seems unlikely, as does the converse possibility that HBV infection of primates resulted from contact with humans.

Stability

It is difficult to assess the stability of HBV due to the lack of a suitable laboratory culture system. Indirect evidence has been obtained from the study of recipients of blood products treated in various ways and chimpanzee inoculation experiments. Thus it was established that:

- heating to 60°C for 10 h inactivates virus by a factor of 100–1000-fold
- treatment with hypochlorite (10 000 ppm available chlorine) or 2% glutaraldehyde for 10 min will inactivate virus 100 000-fold.

Studies based on the survival of HBsAg show that this is much more resistant to destruction.

Replication

Replication of viral nucleic acid starts within the hepatocyte nucleus where viral DNA can be free-, extrachromosomal, or integrated at various sites within the host chromosomes. However, integration is not essential for viral replication. There are some parallels between the hepadnaviruses and the retroviruses, in that:

- both synthesize DNA from an RNA template
- there is amino acid sequence homology between the enzymes involved.

To replicate hepadnavirus DNA, a full-length RNA copy is enclosed in core protein in the hepatocyte nucleus. This is copied to DNA by the polymerase, the RNA is destroyed and the DNA copied to form double-stranded DNA as the virion matures (see Chapter 9).

CLINICAL FEATURES

The possible outcomes of infection with HBV infection are summarized in Fig. 46.5. The incubation period

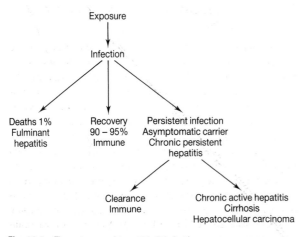

Fig. 46.5 The outcome of hepatitis B infection.

varies widely, from 40 days to 6 months, but is often about 2–3 months. A dose-related effect has been observed as shorter incubation periods have been associated with the inoculation of large doses of virus (as in the transfusion of infected blood). A prodromal illness occurs in some patients, who complain of malaise and anorexia accompanied by weakness and myalgia. Arthralgia also occurs and may be accompanied by an urticarial or maculopapular rash. These features may be related to circulating immune complexes containing HBsAg, which have been implicated in the rarer complications of polyarteritis nodosa and glomerulonephritis. Complexes are usually present in the plasma in cases of fulminant hepatitis B. In an acute case, hepatocellular damage is detectable biochemically before the onset of jaundice and persists after it has resolved. The patient usually begins to feel better when the jaundice appears, accompanied by pale stools and dark urine. Carriers of HBV are initially symptom-free, and many will remain so for many years. As many as 25% of carriers will develop the clinical features of chronic hepatitis and cirrhosis, and eventually hepatocellular carcinoma.

PATHOLOGY

All types of viral hepatitis produce similar changes at the histological level. In the acute stage there are signs of inflammation in the portal triads: the infiltrate is mainly lymphocytic. In the liver parenchyma, single cells show ballooning and form acidophilic (*Councilman*) bodies as they die. In healthy carriers, the inflammatory response is mild, and the affected hepatocytes are pale staining and glassy.

In chronic hepatitis, damage extends out from the portal tracts, giving the piecemeal necrosis appearance. Some lobular inflammation is also seen. As the disease progresses fibrosis develops and, eventually, cirrhosis.

Pathogenesis

Acute disease

HBV replicates in the hepatocytes, reflected in the detection of viral DNA and HBcAg in the nucleus and HBsAg in the cytoplasm and at the hepatocyte membrane.During the incubation period, high levels of virus are present before the host immune response develops and controls the virus. During replication HBcAg and HBeAg are also present at the cytoplasmic membrane. These antigens induce both B and T cell responses; damage to the hepatocyte can result from antibody-dependent, NK and cytotoxic T cell action.

Expression of MHC class I antigens is poor in hepatocytes but can be enhanced as interferons are produced in response to the infection. This in turn leads to increased antigen recognition and lysis of the infected hepatocytes. HBV is non-cytocidal without the assistance of the host's immune system and the disease is usually milder in the immunocompromised. A similar sequence of events occurs in the silent case except that the liver damage is less severe.

Persistence of HBV

Persistence of HBV is indicated by the continued presence of HBsAg and HBV DNA in the blood for more than 6 months. This occurs:

- in 5–10% of adult cases
- in 30% of childhood cases (<6 years)
- in 90% of newborn infections
- more frequently in males
- more often in the immunocompromised.

It is not yet clear what determines that an individual will progress to the carrier state. There may be genetic factors, but it is clear that the absence, or relative inefficiency, of the immune system is important, as shown by the increased likelihood of the carrier state in the very young and the immunocompromised. In the neonate, infection occurs in the presence of maternal IgG anti-HBc and tolerance to HBeAg which can cross the placenta. This will have the effect of masking HBcAg on hepatocyte membranes and thus will prevent its recognition by cytoxic T cells and other immune mechanisms. If there is insufficient anti-HBs, it will be unable to block further infection of cells by circulating virus.

Carriers may continue to replicate virus to high levels (HbeAg-positive; DNA-positive) without evidence of liver damage. This has been called the early replicative phase of chronic infection. It ends with the disappearance of HBeAg and the appearance of anti-HBe. The change happens at a variable time after infection, but each year 5–20% of patients go through this transition, usually associated with a period of liver cell damage. This is often, but not always, accompanied by the disappearance of HBV DNA from the blood, signalling a transition from high to low infectivity carrier status. A carrier may undergo several episodes of hepatitis. Eventually, HBV may disappear in 1–2% of carriers each year.

Chronic liver disease and hepatocellular carcinoma

Chronic liver damage results from continuing, immune-mediated destruction of hepatocytes express-

ing viral antigens. Also, auto-immune reactions may contribute to the damage as immune responses are induced to various liver-specific antigens. There may be a role for the HBeAg-negative mutants that arise during the transition from HbeAg-positive to anti-Hbe-positive.

Hepatocellular carcinoma (HCC) is one of the 10 most frequent tumours in the world, and there is considerable evidence that 80% are caused by chronic infection with HBV. Thus, the highest rates of HCC are found in areas where HBV is highly endemic and where infection occurs at a very early age. This is necessary as there may be an interval of 30–40 years between infection and tumour development, although shorter intervals are seen. Integrated viral DNA can be found in tumour cells but the site differs in different tumours, although the tumour is clonal in origin in each individual. The integrated DNA is extensively rearranged and regions may be deleted. The mechanism of carcinogenesis is not yet clear, although it is usually associated with cirrhosis. As with other tumours, infection with HBV may be only one factor and others, genetic or chemical, may be necessary. The effective administration of HBV vaccine to children in Taiwan has already caused a significant decrease in HCC cases.

The rate of progression to cirrhosis and HCC varies according to:

- the age of infection and stage reached
- the state of the patient's immune system
- geographic factors
- genetic factors.

Several of these may be related, but the relative risk of progression varies from 12–79-fold, with the highest risk of 148-fold seen in Alaska. The risk of developing HCC is 30–98-fold in the Far East.

HBV with mutations in the surface, core and polymerase genes

HBsAg variants were first detected in children born to infected mothers and in patients given a new liver because of chronic HBV disease. In both situations the variants arose during infection in the presence of anti-HBs. The children were exposed to maternal virus during birth and were then given anti-HBs immunoglobulin and active immunization to reduce the risk of infection. This treatment is successful in most cases, but in some, mutant virus appears and allows the virus to escape the neutralizing anti-HBs given to, or induced, in the baby. Escape mutants have been detected in various parts of the world, including Italy, Singapore, Japan, Brunei, USA and China following the start of vaccination campaigns.

In liver transplant recipients, anti-HBs is administered to protect the new liver from infection with virus already present. The variants have been seen to disappear when anti-HBs therapy is stopped. The phenomenon has been found in liver transplant patients in the USA, Germany and UK.

The mutations affect the a determinant of HBsAg, the principal target of anti-HBs. Mutant virus can be transmitted to new hosts; it is associated with the virus-positive carrier state. The widespread occurrence of HBsAg mutants would create considerable problems for vaccination programmes, as well as compromising many existing diagnostic assays for HBsAg that detect epitopes associated with the a determinant. Other isolates with mutations in the pre-S1 and pre-S2 regions have been described. They can replicate and may be the only detectable form of virus in some cases. They appear during the chronic phase of infection.

HBcAg variants are known with mutations in the core promoter or pre-core coding regions of the HBcAg gene. These generally suppress the production of HBeAg, without affecting the synthesis of HBcAg and the assembly of complete virions. They are therefore often found in carriers who are HBeAg-negative, but positive for HBV DNA by polymerase chain reaction (PCR). The mutants are rarely seen in patients with minimal liver disease, but can appear during or after the loss of HBeAg and the development of anti-HBe. The clinical significance and the selection pressures that produce pre-core mutations remain unclear, although there is evidence that *de novo* infection with such mutants may be associated with a higher risk of developing fulminant hepatitis. The loss of HBeAg may affect the outcome of perinatal infections. The transplacental transfer of HBeAg can induce tolerance to HBcAg and hence the baby will not develop an acute hepatitis and clearance of the virus. The baby is very likely to become a long-term carrier. Babies born to HBeAg-negative carrier mothers often develop an acute hepatitis or fulminant hepatitis.

In Greece, 90% of carriers are negative for HBeAg and all carry mutant genomes. Similar variants are found in the Far East and the mediterranean region; such cases are increasingly recognized worldwide.

Polymerase variants can often be detected during therapy with nucleoside analogues and confer drug resistance. Their presence can affect the choice of drugs.

The frequency with which mutations appear in HBV is dependent on the high rate of replication of the virus and its dependence on replicating DNA via RNA and an RNA-dependent DNA polymerase. In highly viraemic carriers as many as 10^{10} mutant genomes may arise each day. Different variants may be present in the blood, liver and peripheral blood mononuclear cells of a carrier. Most mutants are defective, but some may become apparent at certain stages of disease or treatment due to immunological or drug selection pressures and contribute to disease progression or treatment failure.

LABORATORY DIAGNOSIS

The virology laboratory can test for a wide range of HBV antigens and antibodies, using radio-immuno assays and enzyme-linked immunosorbent assays (ELISAs) and for HBV DNA by PCR. The standard screening test is for HBsAg, which, if present in the serum, indicates that the patient is infected with HBV, either as a recent acute infection or as a carrier.

Acute infection

In an acute case (Fig. 46.6), HBsAg is present for some weeks before the onset of symptoms and is at maximum titre at the height of liver damage. In most cases HBsAg cannot be detected beyond 3–4 months. Over this period, HBV DNA can be detected in plasma by PCR, indicating the presence of complete, infectious virus particles. In a few patients, antigenaemia is of short duration and may not be detectable at the onset of symptoms. In such cases the presence of anti-HBc, especially IgM anti-HBc, and anti-HBe, may be the only indications of recent HBV infection. If successive serum samples are examined, the development of anti-HBs will confirm primary infection, although there is considerable variation in the appearance of this antibody.

Typical responses shown by at least three-quarters of cases are outlined in Fig. 46.6. HBeAg is produced when virus is replicating and thus it is usually found soon after HBsAg. IgM anti-HBc is the next response to be detected. HBeAg is correlated strongly with the detection of viral DNA, virions and viral polymerase in the serum. IgM anti-HBc is a transient response and, if present in high titre, indicates a recent acute infection. The response declines with time and is usually absent by 6 months. Tests for HBeAg and anti-HBe during an

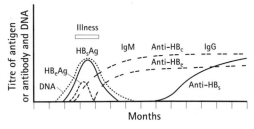

Fig. 46.6 Hepatitis antigens, antibodies and DNA in a patient recovering from acute infection.

acute infection can be helpful in that the disappearance of HBeAg and replacement with anti-HBe indicates that the patient is responding to the infection and will clear HBsAg. Ninety per cent of patients develop anti-HBs; in a few cases it is present at the same time as HBsAg, but usually there is a gap of up to 6 months before anti-HBs is detected. Once present, the patient is immune to further infection with HBV.

Chronic infection

As illustrated (Fig. 46.7), a carrier of HBV is almost always HBeAg-positive and HBV DNA-positive beyond 6 months. During this time, IgM anti-HBc disappears and is replaced with IgG anti-HBc. This is typical of the early replicative phase of chronic infection. It may be succeeded by the loss of HBeAg and the appearance of anti-HBe (Fig. 46.8): the change happens at a variable time. Many patients continue to be positive for HBV DNA.

TREATMENT

Much effort has been focused on the treatment of the chronic carrier with the aims of:

- reducing the possibility of transmission to others
- preventing progression of liver disease and improving liver histology
- preventing the development of HCC.

α-interferon (α-IFN) has been the drug of choice for the treatment of chronic HBV infection. α-IFN inhibits the packaging of RNA in nucleocapsids during virus assembly and thus has a direct antiviral action. It also upregulates expression of HBsAg and other viral pro-

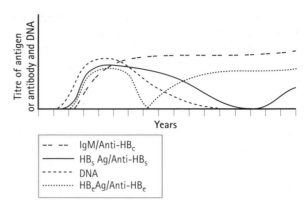

Fig. 46.8   The sequence of laboratory results in a hepatitis B carrier who loses HBeAg.

teins on the surface of the infected cell, and therefore enhances the cytotoxic T cell responses. The standard course of 5 million international units per day for 4 months can achieve a significant reduction in the levels of circulating virus and normalization of alanine aminotransferase (ALT) levels in approximately one-third of those treated. Conversion from HBeAg-positivity to anti-HBe-positive status occurs in approximately 20%, generally followed by the clearance of HBsAg in the following years. Pre-treatment variables favouring response are:

- recent infection
- adult patient
- female
- caucasian
- healthy immune system, anti-HIV-negative
- increased serum ALT
- HBeAg-positive
- low HBV DNA concentration
- hepatitis D virus-negative
- therapy maintained for more than 4 months.

The incidence of the development of cirrhosis of the liver and the development of HCC is lower in those receiving α-interferon therapy. Side-effects are common and include flu-like symptoms, mild exacerbation of hepatitis (often a favourable indication of subsequent response) and granulocytopenia.

More recently, antiviral drugs that inhibit the replication of HBV have been developed. These compounds are nucleoside analogues that, after phosphorylation in the cell, are recognized by the HBV-encoded RNA polymerase/reverse transcriptase. Their incorporation into the synthesized nucleic acid strand usually prevents further addition of nucleotides and therefore terminates replication.

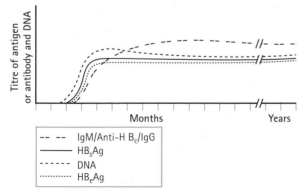

Fig. 46.7   The sequence of laboratory results in a patient who becomes a carrier of HBV.

The most widely used, and currently the only approved nucleoside analogue is lamivudine (2′,3′-dideoxy-3′ thiacytidine[3TC]). It is a potent inhibitor of HBV DNA synthesis and is effective at low concentrations in vitro. At a dose of 100–300 mg daily, lamivudine leads to a marked reduction or elimination of detectable HBV DNA in plasma and normalization of ALT levels in approximately 60–70% of individuals. Over a treatment period of 1 year, about 20% of those who are HBeAg-positive become anti-HBe-positive. Unfortunately, withdrawal of treatment usually leads to the re-appearance of hepatic inflammation and the return of HBV DNA to pre-treatment levels, except in those achieving HBeAg seroconversion. Although toxicity is low, and long term the drug is generally tolerated well, prolonged administration is complicated by the emergence of antiviral resistance, manifested by the re-appearance of HBV DNA in plasma and the development of abnormal ALT levels. Resistance is generally associated with mutations in the catalytic core of the HBV polymerase enzyme (typically a Met->Ile or Val) in the YMDD motif. Antiviral resistance is more frequent in those who are immunosuppressed, a group that includes patients receiving liver transplants.

A number of other nucleoside analogues are currently in phase II or III trials. These include famciclovir, adefovir, entecavir and emtricitabine. These work in a similar way to lamivudine, and can often achieve comparable results in reduction or clearance of HBV DNA and ALT normalization, but all are associated with relapse when treatment is stopped. As antiviral resistance to lamivudine is not associated with resistance to other antivirals such as famciclovir, there is a rationale for the use of combination treatment, as has been pioneered in the therapy of HIV infection.

For end-stage liver disease, liver transplantation is necessary. Attempts have been made to prevent re-infection of the graft with HBV through the administration of anti-HBs immunoglobulin, and more recently this has been combined with a nucleoside analogue such as lamivudine. Used singly, anti-HBs immunoglobulin and lamivudine are rarely effective, but recent studies have indicated that their combined use may prevent HBV recurrence after transplantation, and give improved graft function and significantly improved patient survival.

EPIDEMIOLOGY

HBV is present in the blood and also body fluids such as semen, vaginal secretions and saliva, although the concentration is only about 1 in 1000 of that in blood. Even so, this may still represent a large number of infectious virions. The presence of HBV in blood underlines the original association of infection with blood transfusion or the use of blood products (post-transfusion 'serum' hepatitis) and infections associated with needlestick injuries. Sexual transmission is also recognized, as is that which occurs between family members, siblings, peers and residents in institutions for the learning-impaired. In these circumstances there will be frequent contact with blood and saliva; the virus will gain entry through cuts and abrasions or across mucous membranes. Biting and scratching are also important. Vertical transmission from mother to child is one of the most important routes. Transmission occurs when maternal blood contaminates the mucous membranes of the baby during birth. Transplacental infection is thought to be quite rare.

The prevalence of HBV infection varies widely in different parts of the world:

- *Highest rates*: HBsAg 10–15%; anti-HBs 70–90% in south-east Asia, China, equatorial Africa, Oceania and South America. Vertical and horizontal transmission are both common.
- *Intermediate rates*: HBsAg 5%; anti-HBs 30–40% in Eastern Europe, around Mediterranean, South America and the Middle East.
- *Lowest rates*: HBsAg 0.1–0.5%; anti-HBs not more than 5% in Western Europe, North America and Australia.

Overall, it is estimated that one-third of the world population has been infected with HBV and that there are 300–400 million carriers in the world. In areas of low endemicity the risk of infection varies widely in different groups according to behaviour. Most cases occur in parenteral drug injectors who share scarce needles and syringes, and by sexual transmission by both homosexual and heterosexual intercourse. In about one-third to one-quarter of cases it may be impossible to identify a source. Screening of all blood donations has virtually eliminated transmission by transfusion and blood products. Some groups of patients are at increased risk of infection and of becoming carriers; these include patients on maintenance haemodialysis and in long-stay homes for those with learning difficulties.

Health care personnel and laboratory workers are at risk from patients, although the degree of risk varies with the place and nature of their work, the care with which it is performed and their immune status. Surgery, dental surgery, obstetrics and gynaecology often involve working with sharp instruments, often in restricted spaces. Operators may injure themselves and inoculate patient's blood. The spilling of patient's blood will pose a threat only if there is contamination of unprotected skin, with abrasions, or mucous membranes.

Patients are also at risk from staff, and episodes have been identified in which a surgeon, gynaecologist, dentist or other staff member has transmitted the virus to patients during invasive procedures, especially in difficult operations where the operator's hands are hidden and needles and instruments are guided by touch. Apart from small outbreaks linked to a common source, such as surgery and haemodialysis, epidemics are rare. In the past, before specific tests were available, a few outbreaks were described following the use of blood products prepared in bulk from large numbers of donations. A large number of cases occurred in the US armed forces during the Second World War due to the use of yellow fever vaccine stabilized with infectious human plasma.

CONTROL

Broadly there are two approaches to the prevention of infection with HBV. Firstly, the possibility of transmission can be reduced or removed by modifying risk behaviour. The measures include avoiding unprotected sexual contact by the use of condoms, and sharing needles by injecting drug misusers. Implementation of sensible control of infection policies can reduce the risks considerably to health care workers and patients. It is essential, of course, that blood for transfusion is screened. However, there are limits to these approaches, and immunization, both passive and active, offers many advantages, not least in situations where the prevention of infection is otherwise difficult or impossible.

Passive immunization

Hyperimmune hepatitis B immunoglobulin (HBIG) is prepared from donors with high titres of anti-HBs. Doses of 300–500 IU in 3 ml are given intramuscularly. The use of HBIG is still necessary in the following situations:

- after accidental exposure if not vaccinated, or not responded to vaccine
- to babies born to infected mothers (with active immunization)
- to prevent infection of a new liver transplanted for chronic HBV.

HBIG must be given as soon as possible after an accident and preferably within 48 h; a second dose is given 4 weeks later to those who do not respond to current vaccines. Such a regimen does not give absolute protection, but an efficacy of 76% has been reported. In some such cases, a transient viraemia may occur. If the victim has not been vaccinated, HBIG should be used and a course of active immunization started, injecting the two materials into different body sites. A course of 6-monthly injections of HBIG can reduce the infection rate in babies by 70%, but even greater protection is provided by combining HBIG with active immunization starting at birth. The protective efficacy of this combined treatment is 90%. In transplant recipients, it may be more effective to combine HBIG with lamivudine due to the appearance of HBsAg mutants.

Active immunization

Much effort has been devoted to the development of vaccines for long-term protection against hepatitis B. Current vaccines are produced by cloning the surface antigen gene in yeast cells. The product is particulate and resembles the small particles seen in patients, although it is not glycosylated. The vaccine is administered with alum as adjuvant and injected intramuscularly; care should be taken to avoid injection into fat as this can produce poorer seroconversion rates. For this reason, injection into the deltoid muscle of the upper arm is recommended. The vaccine is free from major side-effects; local swelling and reddening may occur in up to one in five recipients, with a slight fever in only a few cases.

Three doses of vaccine are given at 0, 1 and 6 months. The seroconversion rate is influenced by a number of factors, the most important of which are the age and sex of the vaccinee. Rates in excess of 95% are seen in young women, whereas the rate may drop to 80% in older men. Immunosuppressed patients show even lower rates, e.g. only 50–60% in patients on maintenance dialysis. Because virus challenge doses and the infectivity of sources can vary considerably it is difficult to define a minimum protective level of anti-HBs, but levels should be greater than 100 IU/l. If vaccine is used selectively to protect particular groups in the population, it is reasonable to check the response within a few months of the third dose of vaccine, although this is not appropriate when the vaccine is given as part of a schedule applied to a large part of the population.

The duration of the response to vaccine is variable and dependent on the titre of anti-HBs after completion of the course. In those groups given the vaccine for occupational protection, vaccinees whose anti-HBs titres are in excess of 500 IU/l are likely to maintain adequate levels for at least 4–5 years. If the initial response is between 100 and 500 IU/l, then a boost at 3 years is indicated. If the response is less than 100 IU/l, a booster dose should be given. Low or non-responders need to be identified and told that they are not protected and that they must seek prophylaxis by passive immunization if they suffer accidental exposure. Those who are known to have responded can be given a booster if they are exposed to the virus, although the need for this will depend on the titre of anti-HBs achieved and the time since completion of the course.

Alternative vaccines are under development to improve the seroconversion rate, especially in those who do not respond to current preparations, and the ease of administration by reducing the number of doses needed and by combining with other vaccines. Incorporation of the pre-S1 and pre-S2 proteins is one approach. Alternatives are the use of synthetic peptides and hybrid virus vaccines.

Who should be immunized?

The aim of immunization is to prevent transmission of HBV by the routes described and to eradicate the virus from the population of the world. This will not be achieved quickly or easily. Carriers are an important reservoir and can transmit the virus over many years. Transmission from mother-to-child is an important route and requires intervention at the birth, or within 12 h, to protect the child. As most babies infected at birth will become long-term carriers, it is essential to target this group. Intervention at this early stage is expensive and should be reserved for babies born to carrier mothers identified by antenatal screening. Herd immunity can be provided by incorporation of HBV vaccine into the schedules of routine immunizations. Horizontal transmission occurs at later ages, and this can be tackled by immunization of adolescents before they become sexually active or adopt at-risk life styles. The strategy is:

- antenatal screening to identify infected mothers and protect neonates
- universal infant vaccination
- vaccination of all adolescents.

Vaccine use in this way has been shown to reduce the number of cases of acute hepatitis B and the carrier rate in the population.

In all populations medical staff are at special risk of infection from the nature of their work and should be immunized and their responses checked. This will also protect patients against infection from staff. Until the vaccine has been used routinely in a population for some years, it is sensible to protect other groups at special risk:

- sexual partners of known HBV-positives
- those with frequent unprotected sexual exposure
- parenteral drug misusers (most have been infected by the time identified)
- ambulance, police and fire service staff and military personnel

- patients with learning difficulties living in long-stay homes
- patients needing frequent transfusions and/or blood products
- patients on maintenance dialysis.

The selective use of vaccine in health care staff in the UK has led to a significant reduction in the number of cases of acute infection in this group.

THE DELTA AGENT (HEPATITIS D VIRUS)

The delta (δ) antigen was first identified in Italian patients infected with HBV. Initially, it was thought to be an antigen of HBV, but it is part of another virus that cannot replicate without assistance from HBV (or another hepadnavirus). The virus is a small (35–37 nm) enveloped particle containing a single, small circular molecule of RNA of 1.7 kilobase pairs. The internal protein – the δ antigen – has a molecular weight of 68 000. The envelope of the virus is the same as that of HBV (see Fig. 46.2). The origin of the virus is unknown and it has no homology with HBV. The closest relatives are the satellite viruses of plants.

Analysis of the RNA from different isolates has shown that there are three distinct genotypes.

Clinical features and pathogenesis

HDV can only infect simultaneously with HBV or as a superinfection of a chronic carrier of HBV. The symptoms are similar to those of acute and chronic hepatitis B. The presence of HDV may increase the severity of the clinical features compared to those seen with HBV alone. This is reflected in a 10% risk of fulminant hepatitis with simultaneous HBV and HDV infection, and a 20% risk in superinfections.

In about 10% of cases, co-infection results in a biphasic illness. HDV superinfection can cause an acute hepatitis and may lead to a persistent state. The risk of progression of liver damage is also increased.

Diagnosis

Tests are available for δ antigen and antibody. The sequence of appearance of the various markers in a patient co-infected with HBV and HDV is shown in Fig. 46.9. The initial antibody to HDV is of the IgM class. In cases of superinfection, the test results are as illustrated (Fig. 46.10). During the episode there may be a drop in the HBsAg titre and, although it is usually still detectable, it may disappear temporarily in a few cases. This can cause some confusion if the episode is the first presentation of the patient.

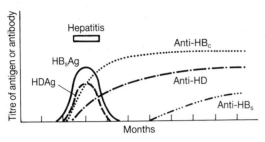

Fig. 46.9 Test results in a patient simultaneously infected with HBV and HDV.

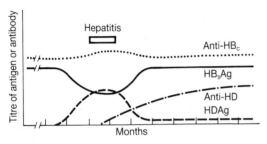

Fig. 46.10 Test results in a hepatitis B carrier superinfected with HDV.

Epidemiology

HDV is not a new virus as there is evidence of infection in the 1930s. It has been estimated that there may be 25 million carriers in the world, but there is considerable geographical variation. The three genotypes are found as follows:

- Type I: Europe, North America, North Africa, Middle East and East Asia

- Type II: Japan, Taiwan and Okinawa
- Type III: North of South America.

In some populations HDV is associated with drug misusers, while in others it is present throughout the population. Sexual transmission is recognized, but is not so easy as via blood as may occur in drug misuse and transfusion. In a number of episodes HDV has spread rapidly among carriers, causing hepatitis, death from fulminant hepatitis and chronic illness.

The incidence of HDV infection in the major risk groups for HBV infection in western countries has declined markedly in the past 10–20 years. Thus, in Italy, the proportion of chronic HBV patients who carry HDV has declined from 23% in 1987 to 8% in 1997, and it is now found mostly in patients aged over 50 years. Over the same period, the proportion of patients with HBV-associated cirrhosis with HDV fell from 30% to 1–3%. Hepatitis B vaccine has been widely used in Italy and this has more than halved the number of acute hepatitis B cases. The disproportionate effect on HDV carriage may be due to the need for dual infection. Thus as HBV infection declines, HDV declines faster as there is less chance of the virus finding a suitable host.

Treatment and control

There is no treatment for HDV infection other than for the co-existing HBV infection. There is some evidence that interferons may induce a temporary drop in δ antigen levels. The same general control measures for HBV are also relevant. HBV vaccine will prevent HDV infection, but there is no means of protecting existing HBV carriers against the consequences of HDV superinfection.

RECOMMENDED READING

Curry M P, Koziel M 2000 The dynamics of the immune response to acute hepatitis B: new lessons using new techniques. *Hepatology* 32: 1177–1179

Fields B N, Knipe D M, Howley P M (eds) 1996 *Virology*, 3rd edn. Lippincott-Raven, Philadelphia

Gunther S, Fischer L, Pult I, Sterneck M, Will H 1999 Naturally occurring variants of hepatitis B virus. *Advances in Virus Research* 52: 25–137

Lee W M 1997 Medical progress: hepatitis B infection. *New England Journal of Medicine* 337: 1733–1745

UK Health Departments 1998 *Guidance for Clinical Health Care Workers: Protection against infection with Blood Borne Viruses.* Recommendations of the Expert Advisory Group, Her Majesty's Stationery Office, London

Zuckerman A J, Banatvala J E, Pattison J R (eds) 2000 *Principles and Practice of Clinical Virology*, 4th edn. Wiley, Chichester

47

Parvoviruses

B19 infection; erythema infectiosum

H. A. Cubie

Parvoviruses have been isolated from a wide range of organisms, from arthropods to humans. The family Parvoviridae is divided into two subfamilies: the Parvovirinae and the Densivirinae. The latter group infects only invertebrates. The Parvovirinae contains three genera: *Parvovirus, Dependovirus* and *Erythrovirus* (Table 47.1).

The *Parvovirus genus* contains the *autonomous* parvoviruses, which are widespread in nature and capable of autonomous replication. They cause a wide variety of diseases in different organs of their natural hosts. The group includes feline and canine parvoviruses (FPV and CPV) which are so important in veterinary medicine that immunization against them is a routine practice in developed countries. Minute virus of mice (MVM) was first discovered in 1966 and, although not very pathogenic, it has served as a model for understanding the function and molecular biology of other members of the genus. It is possible that some of the small round viruses seen in human faeces may be shown to be parvoviruses although none have been recognized as pathogenic in humans. In contrast to parvoviruses, dependoviruses require helper virus functions for replication. They infect a number of species, but the most studied are the human adeno-associated viruses (AAV). Several serotypes have been noted but none have yet been associated with human disease. There is only one parvovirus (B19) known to cause disease in humans and, together with closely related simian viruses, B19 has been placed in a new genus, *Erythrovirus*.

DESCRIPTION

The parvovirus virion (Fig. 47.1) is a relatively simple structure, 20–25 nm in diameter, showing icosahedral symmetry and lacking an envelope. The capsid consists of two proteins, VP1 and VP2, and there are 60 protein subunits, 95% of which are VP2. VP1 and VP2 share significant sequence identity, but VP1 is longer and has a unique region external to the capsid which is accessible to antibody binding. VP1 is necessary for stable conformation and induction of neutralizing antibodies. The virions are extremely resistant to lipid solvents, acid, alkali and high salt concentrations.

Table 47.1 Taxonomic organization of *Parvoviridae*, with particular emphasis on the autonomous parvoviruses, their natural hosts and the diseases they cause

Subfamily	Genus	Virus	Host	Disease
Densovirinae	Three genera	Densonucleosis viruses (DNV)	Arthropods	Many fatal diseases
Parvovirinae	Parvovirus	Minute virus of mice (MVM)	Mice	Subclinical
		Feline parvovirus (FPV)	Cat	Enteritis, leucopenia, cerebellar ataxia
		Canine parvovirus (CPV)	Dog	Enteritis, myocarditis
		Porcine parvovirus (PPV)	Pigs	Reproductive failure
		Aleutian disease virus (ADV)	Mink	Pneumonitis
		Mink enteritis virus (MEV)	Mink	Enteritis
	Dependovirus	Adeno-associated viruses (AAV)	Humans and others	Unknown
	Erythrovirus	B19	Man	Respiratory tract illness, aplastic crisis, Erythema infectiosum/ fifth disease, hydrops fetalis
		Simian parvovirus (SPV)	Monkey	Anaemia

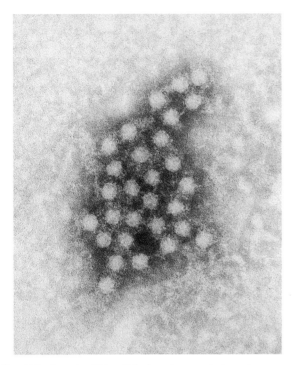

Fig. 47.1 Parvovirus B19 particles in an immune electron microscopy (IEM) preparation of serum of a child with a petechial rash and arthritis ×200 000. (Courtesy of Dr Hazel Appleton, Central Public Health Laboratory, London.)

Specific viral receptors, such as blood group P antigen for B19, explain the narrow host range. Only a very few differences in the coding sequence for capsid proteins between FPV and CPV determine the ability of each to replicate in cats or dogs, respectively. Each species, including humans, is affected by a genetically and antigenically stable virus. Consequently, in normal individ-

uals, infection with B19 virus is followed by life-long immunity.

The genome consists of a single strand of DNA and has a characteristic structure. There is a linear coding region bounded by terminal palindromic sequences which fold to create hairpin loops. Several parvoviruses have been fully sequenced and contain between four and six kilobase pairs. Sequence homology suggests B19, MVM and AAV are equally different from each other. The genome of B19 is 5.6 kilobase pairs in length, making it one of the largest parvovirus genomes. Since both strands are packaged with equal efficiency, B19 DNA spontaneously anneals into a double-stranded form when extracted from virions.

Many animal parvoviruses can be grown in cell culture and the appearance of cytoplasmic vacuolation and intranuclear inclusions is characteristic. Such inclusions can also be seen in B19-infected tissue specimens in human disease (Fig. 47.2) and are caused by the over-production of viral components in infected cells. Propagation of B19 can be achieved in several cells, including bone marrow, fetal liver and some leukaemic cell lines. However, productive infection requires the presence of erythropoietin and only reaches high levels in erythroid progenitor cells.

Replication

Autonomous parvoviruses are so called because they do not require the presence of a helper virus for replication. Nevertheless, they are highly parasitic because of their molecular simplicity and are dependent on cellular factors expressed transiently in the cell during the late S or early G_2 phase of mitosis for virus replication. The necessary factors may only be produced at specific stages of cellular differentiation. Thus, all parvoviruses

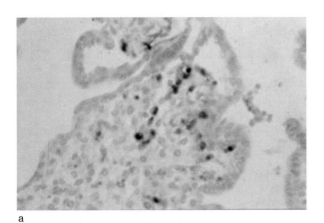

a

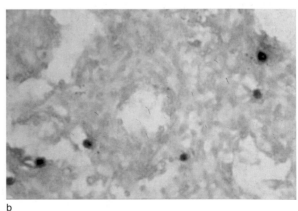

b

Fig. 47.2 In-situ hybridization using a pool of B19 oligonucleotide probes showing enlarged parvovirus B19-infected erythroblast in **a** placenta and in **b** fetal liver from a fatal case of *hydrops fetalis*.

require dividing cells for replication but not all dividing cells are susceptible.

Viral replication and encapsidation takes place within the nucleus. It is initiated from the hairpin loops of the terminal sequences which induce synthesis of the complementary DNA strand. Non-structural proteins play an important role in replication by providing endonuclease and helicase functions. They also inhibit cellular division and initiate the complex transcription processes. DNA replication is by the 'rolling hairpin' model, with DNA replication ceasing as capsid protein accumulates. For B19, about 5000–8000 infectious particles per erythroid cell are produced.

PATHOGENESIS AND CLINICAL FEATURES

All clinical manifestations of parvovirus replication can be attributed to their dependence on cellular helper functions expressed transiently in actively dividing cells. Thus, it is not surprising that disease of the intestine, the haemopoietic system and the fetus feature frequently. Since susceptibility to parvovirus infection is also related to particular stages of differentiation of the cell, very distinct clinical syndromes such as cerebellar ataxia in kittens and aplastic crisis in humans are also features of parvovirus infection.

Animal diseases

In the cat, FPV causes ataxia in kittens if infection occurs in the perinatal period, since the cells of the external granular layer of the cerebellum are dividing rapidly at this stage and become a target for virus-induced damage. As the animals are weaned, the intestinal crypt epithelial cells develop a cell cycle time of 8–12 h, and are thus susceptible to FPV. Consequently, infection at this stage is associated with enteritis. In the dog, the distinct clinical syndrome of perinatal infection by CPV is myocarditis, since in the very young pup there is rapid growth of the myocardium and the mitotic index is high. If infection occurs in older puppies, enteritis is a consistent feature. The white blood cells are also a target for infection by FPV and CPV, and so both kittens and puppies of 2–4 months of age tend to suffer leucopenia and enteritis.

In mink infected with mink enteritis virus (MEV), severe enteritis is the most consistent feature, and there is not a distinct clinical syndrome associated with perinatal infection. However, mink are the natural host of another parvovirus, Aleutian disease virus (ADV). In newborn kits this causes an acute respiratory disease due to infection of type II alveolar cells, which are only susceptible to productive infection in the early stages of life. In later life ADV establishes a persistent infection in the germinal centres of lymph nodes, a plasmacytosis in many organs, hypergammaglobulinaemia and death due to chronic renal failure as a consequence of immune complex glomerulonephritis. This syndrome occurs earlier and more regularly in Aleutian mink because of the linkage of the Aleutian coat colour gene to a gene associated with a lysosomal abnormality leading to failure to destroy immune complexes following phagocytosis.

In rodents, parvoviruses appear to be asymptomatic in their natural hosts, and the same was thought to be true of porcine parvovirus (PPV), a very common infection of pigs. However, the virus was found in tissue, vaginal and seminal samples from pig herds affected by reproductive failure, and it was subsequently shown that infection in early pregnancy leads to transplacental infection, still-birth, mummification or resorption of the piglets.

A new simian parvovirus (SPV) was discovered in cynomolgus monkeys in 1994. The monkeys presented with severe anaemia associated with persistent SPV infection, and it is probable that this was the consequence of immunosuppression due to co-infection with simian retrovirus. SPV is the most closely related type to B19.

Human infections

Dependoviruses

Adeno-associated viruses (AAV) were first discovered in adenovirus stocks, but soon afterwards they were isolated from children with mild disease, usually in association with adenoviruses of different serotypes. It was first thought that only adenoviruses could supply the necessary helper functions but more recently herpesviruses, human papillomaviruses (HPV) and vaccinia have all been shown to be able to provide helper functions for AAV replication.

Antibodies to AAV have been found in 40–80% of humans depending on the test used and population studied. There is as yet no evidence of an association with acute disease. At least four serotypes are known, with types 2 and 3 more common in humans and types 1 and 4 in monkeys. AAV5 was isolated some time ago from a penile condyloma and AAV DNA has been demonstrated in semen. AAV is highly prevalent in the female genital tract, with up to 80% of women tested shown to harbour AAV DNA. Infectious virions have been found in cervical epithelium and HPV was also frequently present. AAV DNA has also been demonstrated in broncho-alveolar lavage samples, again frequently together with HPV DNA. The interaction with the helper virus is beneficial to AAV but usually inhibits the replication of the helper. AAV may therefore be beneficial to the host. However, pregnant women are more often seropositive for AAV than non-pregnant women and women having a miscarriage often have AAV-specific IgM. Transplacental infection with AAV has been demonstrated in mice and occurs naturally with PPV. These interesting results need confirmation and further study.

AAV can become integrated at a specific site on the q-arm of chromosome 19, establishing latency with high frequency and stability for the lifetime of the cell. This makes AAV an important candidate as a gene transfer vector. It provides the smallest well defined delivery system and does not induce a cell-mediated immune response. Since the parental virus does not appear to be associated with significant disease, AAV can readily transduce both dividing and non-dividing cells, with expression of the desired protein on the cell surface. Gene therapy applications already include the delivery of cystic fibrosis transmembrane conductance regulator protein and, for patients with haemophilia B, human factor IX protein.

Erythroviruses

Human parvovirus B19 is found worldwide. It is usually endemic and infections can occur throughout the year.

Volunteer studies

Experimental infection of healthy volunteers has revealed the steps in the pathogenesis of B19 infection (Fig. 47.3). The virus is infectious when given in the form of nasal drops. One week later there is an intense viraemia and virus is excreted in the nasal secretions, but is not found in faeces or urine. The viraemia lasts for only a few days before there is a brisk antibody response, initially of the IgM class but followed rapidly by the appearance of IgG antibody.

Haematological changes take place in the second week after inoculation. Erythroid precursors are absent from the bone marrow of normal individuals 10 days after inoculation, and there is consequent disappearance of reticulocytes from the peripheral blood and a small fall in the haemoglobin level (Fig. 47.2). Lymphocyte, neutrophil and platelet levels sometimes fall transiently, but this is not due to lack of precursors in the bone marrow. Studies with cultured bone marrow cells confirm the in-vivo observations. Haematological changes are the direct result of viral cytopathic effect on erythroid progenitor cells in bone marrow with interruption of erythrocyte production. No effect on the cells of the myeloid series is observed.

The *rash* and *arthralgia* associated with B19 infection occur in infected volunteers during the third week

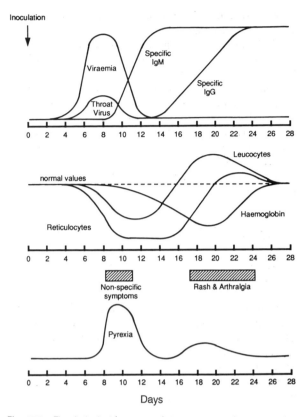

Fig. 47.3 The virological (upper trace), haematological (middle trace) and clinical events (lower trace) following inoculation of B19 virus. (Reproduced with permission of Wiley, Chichester.)

after inoculation. As yet there are no studies of the pathology of either of these features, but since they follow the disappearance of the viraemia and occur at a time when there is an easily detectable immune response it is assumed that the rash and arthralgia are immune-mediated.

The viraemia that is characteristic of B19 infection gives ample opportunity for infection of the placenta and fetus if it occurs during pregnancy. In infected fetuses there appears to be a persistent infection with damage to haematopoietic cells, leading to anaemia, which is one of the factors responsible for *hydrops fetalis*. The other situation in which persistent infection occurs is in the immunosuppressed. The reason is that such individuals produce only small amounts of antibody in response to infection and none of it is capable of neutralizing the virus.

The cell receptor for parvovirus B19 is the P antigen. This is present on red blood cells, erythroid progenitors, vascular endothelium and fetal myocytes. Thus the distribution of the cell receptor is linked to the clinical manifestations of disease. Individuals who lack P antigen (p phenotype) are not susceptible to B19 infection.

Clinical diseases caused by B19

There is a spectrum of clinical consequences of B19 infection (Table 47.2). These depend in part on the natural variation in symptomatology that occurs with common childhood infections and in part on recognizable host factors.

Minor illness. In children, in whom B19 infection is most common, asymptomatic infection accounts for about half of all infections. Non-specific respiratory tract illness is the next most common illness, at least in boys. This can mimic influenza and coincides with the viraemic phase of the infection.

Rash illness. B19 virus causes an erythematous maculopapular rash, which in its most clinically distinct form is called *erythema infectiosum*. It is common in children aged 4–11 years, and is sometimes called *fifth disease* since it was the fifth of six erythematous rash illnesses of childhood in an old classification. Classically, it starts with an intense erythema of the cheeks, hence another of its names – '*slapped-cheek disease*'. The rash then proceeds to involve the trunk and limbs. It lasts only a day or two, although transient recrudescences may occur when the individual is hot. The rash on the limbs tends to have a lacy or reticular appearance. There may be associated lymphadenopathy and joint symptoms.

It is now clear that B19 is a cause of rash illness world-wide, but such illnesses are not always diagnosed clinically as erythema infectiosum. The erythematous rash illness is often very similar to rubella. Erythema of the cheeks is not always prominent and the rash often does not have a lacy appearance. It sometimes occurs on the palms and soles. In the absence of laboratory tests the most frequent clinical diagnoses made are rubella, allergy and 'viral illness', unless there is an outbreak in young children associated with red cheeks, in which case the diagnosis of erythema infectiosum is often made. In a few cases of B19 infection the rash is purpuric in nature. In most of these the platelet count is normal but a transient thrombocytopenia occasionally occurs.

Joint disease. Symptoms and signs of joint involvement occur frequently in B19 infection. Approximately 80% of adult females will report joint symptoms, although the figure is only approximately 10% in childhood cases. Like the rash, the arthropathy of B19 infection is very similar to that seen with rubella, being a symmetrical arthralgia or arthritis involving the small joints of the hands, with wrists, knees and ankles affected in some cases. There is a tendency for the arthropathy to be more severe in children. The symptoms and signs usually resolve within 2 weeks, but in a few cases they will persist for months and very occasionally for years. Some of these patients may be classified clinically as early benign rheumatoid arthritis but they will be found to be rheumatoid factor-negative, and B19 virus is not related to rheumatoid arthritis in any way.

Aplastic crisis. An aplastic crisis is a transient, acute event which complicates chronic haemolytic anaemia. There is a fall in haemoglobin from steady-state values, a disappearance of reticulocytes from the peripheral blood and a virtual absence of red blood cell precursors in the bone marrow at the beginning of the crisis. The cessation of erythropoiesis lasts 5–7 days, and patients present with symptoms of worsening anaemia. Blood transfusion is required in the acute phase, but after a week or so the bone marrow recovers rapidly, there is a reticulocytosis and the haemoglobin concentration returns to steady-state values. The crisis resolves as virus is neutralised by specific antibody production.

Throughout the world B19 infection is responsible for 90% of cases of aplastic crisis. It most commonly occurs

Table 47.2 Spectrum of disease due to B19 related to host factors

Disease	Host	Treatment
Asymptomatic	Normal children and adults	
Respiratory tract illness	Normal children and adults	
Rash illness	Normal children and adults	
Erythema infectiosum/fifth disease/ slapped cheek syndrome	Normal children	
Arthralgia	Normal adults	
Transient aplastic crisis	Patients with increased erythropoiesis	Transfusion
Persistent anaemia	Immunodeficient or compromised patients	Transfusion with intravenous immunoglobulin
Congenital anaemia/hydrops	Fetus <20 weeks	Intra-uterine transfusion

in children with sickle cell anaemia but also in patients with other haemopoietic abnormalities such as hereditary spherocytosis and β-thalassaemia intermedia.

B19 infection in the immunosuppressed. The inability to mount an effective neutralizing antibody response to B19 will result in persistent infection. Such persistent infections have been described in patients with underlying immunodeficiency states, including Nezelof's syndrome, acute lymphatic leukaemia and human immunodeficiency virus (HIV) infection. They have also been noted post-transplant. Sometimes there is evidence of a weak antibody response, particularly of IgM and IgG to VP2 without maturity to the dominant VP1 response. The illness is characterized by either persistent anaemia or a remitting and relapsing anaemia. The bone marrow picture is typical of that seen in aplastic crisis complicating haemolytic anaemia.

B19 in pregnancy. No evidence of B19 infection can be found in sera taken during the first month of life from infants with birth defects and as yet there is no evidence of late developmental abnormalities in children exposed to B19 in utero.

Transplacental infection with B19 can occur during acute maternal infection when the fetus is not protected by passive antibody. Early studies of B19 infection in women known to be pregnant suggested that the spontaneous abortion rate was high. While there is no excess number of abortions following B19 infection in the first trimester of pregnancies, approximately one in 10 of pregnancies complicated by B19 infection end in spontaneous abortion during the second trimester. This is approximately 10 times the incidence in controls.

The severe effects sometimes observed in the fetus are a consequence of the high turnover of red cells and the immaturity of the immune response. The large increase in red cell mass during the second trimester leads to the greater risk at this time and the pregnancy is lost 4–6 weeks after the onset of symptoms of erythema infectiosum in the mother. A more effective fetal immune response to the virus reduces the risk of fetal loss in the third trimester.

Most pregnancies complicated by B19 continue to full-term delivery of normal infants. However, damage without loss sometimes occurs as a consequence of second or third trimester infection. In these cases *fetal hydrops* appears to be a consistent feature. There is a chronic infection in the fetus which leads to anaemia, which is, together with myocarditis, responsible for the hydrops. In these cases maternal B19 infection can range from 2 to 12 weeks prior to the diagnosis of hydrops fetalis. Overall, B19 infection probably accounts for 10% of cases of non-immunological hydrops fetalis.

LABORATORY DIAGNOSIS OF B19 INFECTION

In acquired infection the diagnosis of B19-associated disease follows the classical principles for acute systemic virus infections. The viraemia and throat virus excretion coincide with haematological changes, and detection of virus is a useful diagnostic test in cases of aplastic crisis. Rash and arthralgia occur some days after the end of the short period of circulation and excretion of virus, so in these cases diagnosis by the detection of virus-specific IgM antibody is the best method.

Detection of virus

Serum is the specimen of choice for the detection of virus since it contains the highest concentrations (up to 10^{11} particles per millilitre) of virus and, if virus is not detected in the sample, it can serve as an acute-phase serum for antibody assays. Detection of viral antigen by counterimmuno-electrophoresis with a human convalescent serum as the detector antibody is a simple and rapid technique and detects virus in 30% of sera taken within 3 days of the clinical presentation of aplastic crisis. Enzyme or radio immuno-assays are more sensitive and may also be used. However, detection of the viral genome in serum, blood or bone marrow is often the method of choice these days. Nucleic acid dot blot hybridization will increase detection rates to 60% in samples taken during the acute viraemic phase. A much greater sensitivity is found with polymerase chain reaction-based assays, but this is rarely necessary due to the high DNA copy number in acute infections.

Antibody detection

Most cases have detectable B19-specific IgM within a day or two of the onset of the rash, although in some cases it is necessary to wait for 7 days after the onset to be able to demonstrate such antibody in convincing amounts. Once B19-specific IgM has appeared in the serum it rapidly reaches peak concentrations and persists in decreasing amounts for 2–3 months. High concentrations of IgG antibody are usually found a month or two after infection and in most instances detectable IgG antibody persists for life. Diagnosis of recent infection can also be made by demonstrating seroconversion or increasing amounts of IgG antibody.

The lack of an appropriate cell culture system for B19 meant that serological assays were dependent on scarce supplies of native antigen. Recently recombinant VP1/2 and synthetic peptides have been used in ELISA, but users need to be aware of the great variation in sensitivity and specificity of different tests. IgM capture assays are preferred. Virus-like particles produced by recombinant technology in mammalian or baculovirus systems have provided a new, easy and safe source of viral antigen. Insect cells infected with recombinant baculovirus and expressing B19 virus-like particles are widely used in immunofluorescent assays for both IgG and IgM detection.

Infection in the fetus

The diagnosis of B19 infection in a fetus is complex. Since maternal infection is likely to have occurred some weeks previously, there may be no specific IgM detectable. There is frequently a persistent viraemia, however, and the diagnosis depends upon the detection of virus in fetal specimens, either in fetal blood samples or in fetal tissues taken at autopsy from which DNA has been extracted. B19-infected cells can also be detected by in-situ hybridization on formalin-fixed, paraffin-embedded tissue sections (Fig. 47.2).

EPIDEMIOLOGY

B19 infection has been found in all countries (Europe, North America, Scandinavia, Australia and Japan) in which appropriate diagnostic tests have been applied and it is almost certainly world-wide in distribution. Diseases due to B19 infection cluster in childhood, although some complications such as arthralgia occur more commonly in adult cases. Serological studies indicate that infection is most commonly acquired between 4 and 10 years of age. By the age of 15, approximately 50% of children have detectable B19 antibody, but infection occurs throughout adulthood and up to 90% of elderly people are seropositive. No antigenic strain differentiation has been found, even between isolates from different countries.

B19 virus infections are endemic throughout the year in temperate climates, but there is a seasonal increase in frequency in late winter, spring and early summer months. There are also longer-term cycles of B19 infection with a periodicity of about 4–5 years. The majority of B19 infections are transmitted by close contact by the respiratory route, with a seroconversion rate of 20–30%

for day-care personnel in close contact with infected children. The occurrence of high-titre viraemia enables this infection to be transmitted by blood or blood products. The stability and resistance of erythroviruses has led to transmission of B19 by heat-treated Factor VIII and IX to haemophiliacs.

TREATMENT AND CONTROL

Most cases of B19 infection are mild and self-limiting and specific treatment is not required. However, there are three situations (Table 47.2) in which severe anaemia occurs as a consequence of B19 infection, and in each of these blood transfusion is indicated. In cases of aplastic crisis the transfusion tides patients over the relatively short period of erythroid aplasia before the immune response rapidly clears the virus infection. In the immunosuppressed there is a failure to produce neutralizing antibody so treatment consists of transfusion plus the administration of human normal immunoglobulin for 10 days. This leads to disappearance of the viraemia, sometimes permanently, sometimes only temporarily. The failure of the fetus to eliminate the virus is presumably associated with its inability to mount an immune response. Intra-uterine transfusion has been used to correct the anaemia, and the full-term delivery of normal infants has followed in these cases.

Prevention of disease by isolating susceptible individuals is impractical since infections may be subclinical and symptomatic individuals are infectious before any sign of illness. The rash or arthralgia stages of B19 infection are caused by immune reactions, not viraemia and are therefore not infectious. Theoretically, susceptible individuals with chronic haemolytic anaemia or immunocompromised children could be temporarily protected by the administration of human immunoglobulin but this has not been tried.

There is as yet no vaccine against B19 disease but, by analogy with the animal viruses, such a strategy would be very effective once sufficient quantities of viral antigen capable of stimulating neutralizing antibody are produced. Recombinant B19 virus-like particles can induce neutralizing antibodies and provide a potentially suitable candidate for vaccination of humans.

RECOMMENDED READING

Faisst S 2000 *Parvoviruses, from Molecular Biology to Pathology. Contributions to Microbiology*, Vol. 4. Karger, Basel
Pattison J R 2000 Parvoviruses. In: Zuckerman A J, Banatvala J E, Pattison J R (eds) *Principles and Practice of Clinical Virology*, 4th edn. Wiley, Chichester

Siegl G, Cassinotti P 1998 Parvoviruses. In: Collier L, Balows A, Sussman M (eds) *Topley and Wilson's Microbiology and Microbial Infections*, Vol. 1: Virology. 9th edn. Arnold, London
Young NS 1996 Human Parvoviruses. In: Fields B, Knipe D M, Howley P M (eds). *Virology*, 3rd edn. Lippencott Raven, Philadelphia

48

Picornaviruses

Meningitis; paralysis; rashes; intercostal myositis; myocarditis; infectious hepatitis; common cold

S. M. Burns

The family Picornaviridae comprises small (pico) viruses with a diameter of 27–30 nm and containing single-stranded RNA. It is subdivided into nine genera of which the *Enterovirus, Rhinovirus* and *Hepatovirus* genera are of considerable importance to humans. Viruses in the genus *Enterovirus* infect via the gut, and include the echoviruses, coxsackieviruses and polioviruses. The virus of hepatitis A belongs to the genus *Hepatovirus*. The members of the other genus, *Rhinovirus*, are the most important cause of the common cold. The properties of enteroviruses and rhinoviruses are compared in Table 48.1.

ENTEROVIRUSES

Description

The polioviruses, coxsackieviruses and echoviruses are described as enteroviruses because they are all found in the intestines and are excreted in the faeces. New enteroviruses continue to be isolated, but they are no longer subdivided into the three named groups. Instead they are called enterovirus and are numbered, e.g. enterovirus 71. Hepatitis A, previously classified as enterovirus 72, has now been assigned its own genus, *Hepatovirus*.

Composition. The RNA genome constitutes about one-quarter of the virion. The RNA is single-stranded and of positive sense, and can be translated directly by host ribosomes. The capsid consists of a protein shell arranged in icosahedral symmetry around the RNA molecule, the complete sequence of which is now known for several strains. Four major peptides are recognized in the shell: VP1, VP2, VP3 and VP4, and are formed from a single precursor protein, VP0, by proteolytic cleavage. Specific neutralizing antibodies are considered to be the major mechanism of protection against infection, and a major antigenic site on the VP1 protein of polio type 3 has been identified.

In addition to the properties listed in Table 48.1, the three groups of viruses and those designated enteroviruses 68–71 have a number of features in common:

- They attach to cells in the intestinal tract by specific receptor sites and replicate in cells of the intestinal tract.
- They commonly cause asymptomatic immunizing infections, which protect against future infections with the same virus.
- They can give rise to viraemia.
- They occasionally cause infection of the central nervous system and other target organs.

Table 48.1 Some properties of picornaviruses		
Property	Enteroviruses	Rhinoviruses
Size (nm)	22–30	30
Capsid		
Form	Icosahedral	Icosahedral
Polypeptides	VP1, VP2, VP3, VP4	VP1, VP2, VP3, VP4
RNA type	Single–stranded, positive–sense	Single–stranded, positive–sense
RNA molecular weight	2×10^6–2.6×10^6	2.6×10^6
Acid	Stable (pH 3–9)	Labile (pH 3–5)
Optimal temperature for growth (°C)	37	33–34
Density in caesium chloride (g/ml)	1.34	1.39–1.42

- They are commoner in children than adults.
- In temperate climates they cause infections usually in the summer and autumn.

Reactions to physical and chemical agents. Enteroviruses are among the most stable viruses. They are insensitive to ether and detergents, which destroy enveloped viruses. In faeces, virus can survive for months at 4°C, for years at −20 or −70°C and at room temperature for several weeks, depending on the amount of virus present, the amount of moisture present and other environmental conditions. The virus is readily killed by moist heat at 50–55°C, but less effectively in the presence of organic material.

Virus in foodstuffs may survive exposure to 60°C, and the flash method of pasteurization is necessary to render them safe.

The inactivation of poliovirus is inhibited by magnesium chloride, and this has been incorporated into live polio vaccine as a stabilizer. Drying rapidly inactivates enteroviruses by ultraviolet light, and usually by drying.

Unlike rhinoviruses they are stable to acid pH.

Chemical inactivation. Poliovirus is rapidly inactivated by 0.3% formaldehyde, 0.1 M hydrochloric acid and solutions giving a free residual chlorine concentration of 0.3–0.5 ppm. Higher concentrations are necessary to inactivate virus in the presence of organic matter, e.g. in swimming bath water.

Polioviruses

There are three types of poliovirus, identified by neutralization tests, their RNA molecules differing by 50% in hybridization studies. Two outstanding characteristics of the viruses are their affinity for nervous tissue and the narrow host range, with only humans and primates susceptible. Cynomolgus and rhesus monkeys can be infected by the oral route, and develop paralysis; in chimpanzees the infection is often asymptomatic. Under the influence of cortisone, monkeys become more susceptible to small parenteral doses of the virus.

The prototype strains are:

- Type 1, the Brunhilde and Mahoney strains
- Type 2, which includes the rodent-adapted strains, the Lansing and MEFI strains
- Type 3, the Leon and Saukett strains.

The three types are antigenically distinct, but overlap occurs in neutralization tests. Type 1 is the common epidemic type, type 2 is usually associated with endemic infections, but type 3 has caused recent epidemics. The size, chemical and physical properties, and the resistance of the three types are all identical, and so their anti-genic properties provide one of the main methods of differentiating them.

Echoviruses

Echoviruses were identified by cell culture of faeces of patients suffering from paralytic and non-paralytic illness. There are over 30 serotypes of the *enteric cytopathic human orphan* viruses and, true to their name, there is still no clear association of some types with specific disease. Echoviruses 22 and 23 have a very different RNA sequence and have been classified into a separate genus, *Parechovirus*.

Pathogenicity for animals. None of the main echovirus types produces clinical illness in laboratory animals, although some strains of echovirus 9, which have been adapted to cell culture, can produce myositis in newborn mice (see coxsackievirus infections).

Haemagglutination. Certain types, e.g. 3, 6, 7, 11, 12, 13, 19, 20, 21, 24, 25, 29, 30 and 33, cause haemagglutination of human group O erythrocytes. The virus reacts with a receptor present on group O cells, although not all strains of a particular type may do so. Temperature, pH and the age of the red blood cell donor influence this property.

Antigenic characters. Thirty-three distinct antigenic types have so far been distinguished by neutralization tests in cell cultures. Cross-reactions occur between types 1, 8, 12 and 13 in neutralization tests. Antigenic variation is known to occur in types 4, 6 and 9, and may be a common occurrence under natural conditions. The specificity of strains may be altered by cultivation in the presence of heterologous antiserum.

Coxsackieviruses

This group (of 30 serotypes) was named after the place in New York State where the first member was isolated. Coxsackieviruses are pathogenic for newborn mice and hamsters. Two groups of the viruses were recognized according to the histological nature and the sites of the lesions they produce in mice (Table 48.2):

Table 48.2 Features of coxsackievirus infection in the laboratory

	Types	Growth in MK cell culture	Effect in suckling mice
Coxsackie A virus	1–24[a]	+	Paralysis
Coxsackie B virus	1–6	+	Spasticity

MK, monkey kidney.
[a] Coxsackievirus A23 now classified as echovirus 9.

- *Coxsackie A viruses*. Group A viruses, of which there are 24, cause widespread severe myositis of skeletal muscles and in life the mice appear to have a flaccid paralysis. Usually the signs of infection appear 4 or 5 days after inoculation and progress until the animal dies 4 or 5 days later.
- *Coxsackie B viruses*. Group B viruses, of which there are six, cause widespread lesions in many organs. The myositis produced is characterized by focal lesions and spastic paralysis. The viruses also cause areas of necrosis in the brown fat lobules, meningo-encephalitis and pancreatitis. The incubation period of group B infection in mice is prolonged.

Growth in culture. All group B coxsackieviruses grow readily in monkey kidney cell cultures. Of group A coxsackieviruses, only A7 and A9 grow in monkey kidney cells, and coxsackievirus A21 can be grown in HeLa, HEp2 or human embryonic kidney cell cultures. The viruses that grow in cell culture produce a cytopathic effect similar to polioviruses and echoviruses. Identification of the isolate is made by neutralization tests.

The other type A viruses are isolated by inoculation of suckling mice; thereafter, some can be adapted to cell culture. In monkeys, coxsackie viruses do not usually produce clinical disease, but after inoculation a viraemia develops, and later the virus is excreted for several weeks in the faeces. Types A7 and A14 can cause a mild paralysis in monkeys, with lesions in the central nervous system resembling those of poliomyelitis. Type A7, which has caused paralytic disease in humans, is identical to the Russian AbIV strain, which was at first thought to constitute a fourth type of the poliovirus.

Mouse inoculation is no longer used as a diagnostic test. It has been replaced by RNA detection using the reverse transcription polymerase chain reaction (RTPCR).

Antigenic characters. Thirty antigenic types have been defined by cross-neutralization tests in mice or cell culture, and cross-complement fixation reactions. Twenty-three have the features of group A and six have those of group B. Each of the six group B types is subject to antigenic variation, and sera from convalescent cases may show heterotypic responses. Coxsackievirus A23 has now been reclassified as echovirus 9.

New enteroviruses

Detailed examination of the characteristics of the viruses in cell culture and their ability to infect laboratory animals, which had been the basis of classification into polioviruses, coxsackieviruses or echoviruses, showed that these were not reliable features. Since 1970 new isolates are simply called enterovirus and are given the next available consecutive number. Thus, enterovirus types 68, 69, 70, 71 and 72 are now recognized.

Replication

Knowledge of enterovirus replication is based on studies of poliovirus. The different stages of the cycle are described in Chapter 9. The end of replication is signalled by the lysis of the host cell, with the release of all the new virus particles.

Clinical features and pathogenesis

The enteroviruses are associated with a wide variety of clinical presentations, although the majority of infections are asymptomatic. The sites affected are:

- the central nervous system (meningitis, paralysis)
- the skin (rashes)
- muscle (intercostal myositis, myocarditis).

In neonates infection can be severe, extensive and occasionally fatal. Enteroviruses have been blamed for the development of the chronic fatigue syndrome. Several other viruses have also been implicated and no strong evidence exists to confirm (their role).

Polioviruses

There are three types of poliovirus infection:

1. Asymptomatic infection or a mild, transient 'influenza-like' illness; this is the most likely outcome, with only 1% of infections resulting in recognizable clinical illness. The virus is excreted in the faeces for a limited time, and an immunological response develops which protects against re-infection with the same strain.
2. Infections with the same symptoms as above and evidence of the involvement of the central nervous system with headache, neck stiffness and back pain (meningitis). Rapid and complete recovery in less than 10 days is usual.
3. Paralytic poliomyelitis in which the patient develops paralysis; this is the most dramatic form of the infection but it is very uncommon, occurring in one in 1000 of poliovirus infections in children, although one in 75 adults may be affected. The paralysis is usually flaccid due to destruction of lower motor neurones, although invasion of the brain stem by the virus can lead to inco-ordination of muscle groups and painful spasms. Paralysis occurs early in the illness but the extent is

variable. Often the paralysis is greatest initially; some function may return over the next 6 months. Damage to the nerve cells in the brain stem (bulbar paralysis) can lead to the inability to swallow and breathe.

The time between infection and the development of symptoms is usually 14 days but can range from 3 to 21 days. During this period several factors are known to have an adverse effect on the outcome of infection:

- Severe muscular activity can lead to paralysis of the limbs used, possibly due to increased vascularity, either in the limb or the appropriate area of the spinal cord, allowing increased access of virus to nerve endings.
- Pregnant women in the third trimester of pregnancy can have severe disease, but there is no firm evidence of congenital defects in infants born to mothers with poliomyelitis. Maternal infection acquired late in pregnancy may lead to perinatal infection and disease of the newborn.
- Injection of adjuvant-containing vaccines, and irritant substances such as heavy metals, can result in paralysis occurring in the limbs that received the inoculation. Paralysis develops (incidence one in 37 000 injections) when poliovirus is contracted within 1 month of receiving the inoculation.
- Patients who have had their tonsils removed have a higher chance of developing bulbar poliomyelitis. This has been attributed to the reduction of secretory IgA in the pharynx, and thus reduced neutralization of the virus.

Paralytic poliomyelitis is recognized as a rare complication of oral polio vaccine or following infection from contact with a vaccinee excreting virus.

Non-polio enteroviruses have also been associated with central nervous disease and paralysis (e.g. echovirus 4 and enterovirus 71); as with polio, paralysis is a rare manifestation of infection.

Echoviruses

Most echovirus infections cause few or no clinical symptoms, but some have been associated with clinical syndromes (Table 48.3).

Infection can be widespread in a community, although only a few suffer from clinical illness. Symptoms occur following a short incubation period of 3–5 days (simple fever, upper respiratory symptoms or diarrhoea). Non-specific rashes of fleeting duration have been reported.

The onset of meningitis is abrupt, with severe headache and vomiting. Symptoms are self-limiting, and after a variable convalescent period a full recovery is

Table 48.3 Clinical syndromes associated with echoviruses
Main syndromes
Aseptic meningitis
Paralysis
Rash
Respiratory disease
Other features
Pericarditis and myocarditis
Neonatal infection

made, although rare cases of paralysis have been recorded.

Most of the echovirus types have been associated with sporadic cases of *aseptic meningitis* or one of the other disease patterns already mentioned. A number of types, notably 4, 6, 9, 16, 20, 28 and 30, have considerable epidemic potential, and the clinical features are very varied. As examples, echovirus 9 epidemics have been common in Europe and North America as large outbreaks of a biphasic fever, with a sore throat, rash on face, neck and chest and, less commonly, on the lower trunk and extremities. A minority of patients show clinical signs of meningitis, but many without distinct clinical signs have a pleocytosis in the cerebrospinal fluid.

Echovirus 16 epidemics have been called *Boston fever* after the city where the illness was first reported. Clinically, the infection starts with a sharp fever, abdominal pains and a mild sore throat. After 24–48 h, a pink discrete macular or maculopapular rash, mostly on the face, chest and back appears in children. Echovirus 4, 6 and 30 epidemics have been associated with considerable numbers of cases of meningitis in children and adults. Echoviruses 6, 9 and 11 have caused severe and fatal infections in newborn infants. The virus is probably transmitted during birth or postnatally from the mother or nursery attendants who are asymptomatic. Circulatory collapse, hepatitis and meningo-encephalitis occur in the infant, and infection can spread rapidly to other infants in the nursery or special care baby unit. The type of virus circulating in the community at the time is usually implicated.

Echovirus 18 has been recovered from the faeces of many infants in an outbreak of diarrhoea. The children had no rash and no severe involvement of the central nervous system or meningeal reaction. Several echoviruses, including types 1, 11, 19, 20 and 22, have been isolated from cases of respiratory illnesses in children in whom symptoms include pneumonia, bronchiolitis and upper respiratory tract illness.

Coxsackieviruses

Group A viruses. These viruses give rise to a number of different illnesses (Table 48.4). *Aseptic meningitis*, indistinguishable clinically from that caused by other enteroviruses, is caused by a number of types, e.g. 2, 4, 7, 9 or 23. Type A7 has given rise to epidemics of paralytic disease in Scotland, the former USSR and elsewhere. *Herpangina* is an acute feverish disease, usually in young children, characterized by lesions in the mouth consisting of papules on the anterior pillars of the fauces; these papules become vesicles and finally shallow ulcers with a greyish base and punched-out edge. There are usually small numbers of lesions. A fine macular rash (rubella-like) is a feature of some Coxsackie infections. Outbreaks may be seen in nurseries and schools. *Hand, foot and mouth* disease presents as a painful stomatitis with a vesicular rash on the hands and feet. Typically, it lasts about a week; most cases are seen in the summer in children aged 1–10 years, and cases can occur in clusters, and in families. The viruses usually implicated are types 5 and 16.

Coxsackievirus A21, amongst others, has caused epidemics of colds in camps of military recruits.

Group B viruses. *Epidemic myalgia* or *Bornholm disease*, first described on the Danish Island of Bornholm, is characterized by fever and the sudden onset of agonizing stitch-like pains in the muscles of the chest, epigastrium or hypochondrium. Although the disease is most frequently recognized in its epidemic form, many sporadic cases occur. Pleurisy and pericarditis may complicate epidemic myalgia, although most cases recover within a week.

In newborn infants, severe and often fatal *myocarditis* has been reported, and the virus can be found in high concentrations in the myocardium at autopsy. Epidemics have occurred in nurseries when there is evidence of group B virus activity in a community; the mother is presumed to be the source. The baby is highly suscepti-ble to the virus, like the infant mouse. Myocarditis and pericarditis can occur in children and adults, and virus has been isolated from pericardial fluid.

Coxsackie B viruses are major causes of human *myopericarditis*, but this is a difficult diagnosis to confirm. Although severe in the neonate, it tends to follow a more benign course in the adult. The initial symptoms are often of an upper respiratory or 'influenza-like' illness followed 7–10 days later by clinical heart disease. Chest pain is a feature and electrocardiogram abnormality such as tachycardia and arrhythmias have been found. On clinical examination, murmurs, rubs and, occasionally, pericardial effusions are detected.

Aseptic meningitis, sometimes with paralysis, is a common manifestation of infection due to group B virus. Occasionally a rash is present.

New enteroviruses (Table 48.5)

Enterovirus 68. Has been reported to cause pneumonia.

Enterovirus 69. Not yet associated with significant clinical illness.

Enterovirus 70. In 1969, outbreaks of *acute haemorrhagic conjunctivitis* spread throughout Africa and Asia; more recently the disease has occurred in Mexico. AHC is highly infectious and has a short incubation period of 24–48 h. Attack rates are very high where there is overcrowding and poor sanitation. Although subconjunctival haemorrhage is a complication, most cases recover within 7 days. Neurological complications can occur, including a polio-like paralytic illness.

Enterovirus 71. Like other enteroviruses, enterovirus 71 produces infections that are usually inapparent. It was first recognized in 1969 in California, when it was isolated from the faeces of a 9-month-old infant suffering from encephalitis. Since then it has been isolated from cases showing a spectrum of illness. During an epidemic in Bulgaria in 1975, there was a high incidence of paralytic disease, mostly in children under 5 years of age. A

Table 48.4 Features of coxsackievirus infection in man

Coxsackievirus group	Type	Clinical illness
A	1–24	Aseptic meningitis Febrile illness Herpangina Hand, foot and mouth disease
B	1–6	Neonatal disease Bornholm disease Myocarditis, hepatitis Meningitis

Table 48.5 Illness associated with recently identified enteroviruses

Enterovirus type	Clinical illness
68	Pneumonia and bronchiolitis
69	Isolated from an ill person in Mexico
70	Acute haemorrhagic conjunctivitis
70, 71	Paralysis, meningo-encephalitis
71	Hand, foot and mouth disease
72[a]	Hepatitis A

[a] Reclassified as *Hepatovirus*

large outbreak occurred in Malaysia in 1997 where 2140 children were affected and 27 cases of fatal myocarditis were reported. This was followed by a related large outbreak in Taiwan in 1998.

Pathogenesis

All enterovirus infections follow a similar pattern, as illustrated in Fig. 48.1 for poliovirus, with differences in the target organs, e.g. central nervous system, skin, heart or muscle. Due to the potential severity of infection and the availability of an animal model, most is known about poliomyelitis, although it is reasonable to assume that similar features are seen with all the enteroviruses.

Virus is ingested and multiplies initially in the lymphoid tissue of the tonsil or Peyer's patches in the small intestine and then the local lymph nodes, e.g. cervical or mesenteric. In fatal cases, the Peyer's patches and the mesenteric lymph nodes are found to be greatly swollen and inflamed and to contain large amounts of virus. Virus released from the nodes reaches the blood, and then the central nervous system. The paralytic effect of poliovirus results from infection of motor neurone cells in the anterior horns of the spinal cord or bulbar regions. Localization in the motor neurones is probably due to the presence of receptors for the poliovirus. Once within the brain or cord, spread can occur directly to neighbouring cells or via the cerebrospinal fluid to more remote areas.

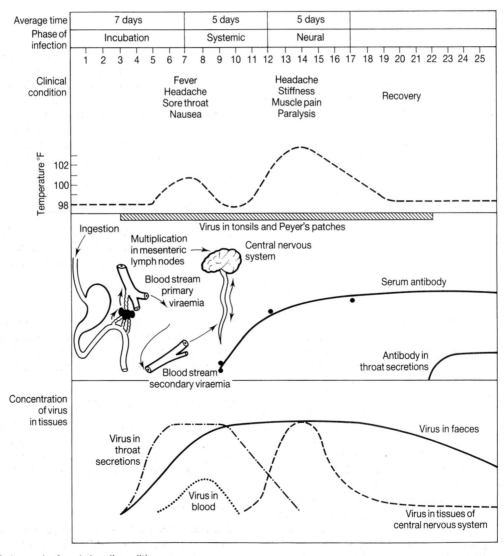

Fig. 48.1 Pathogenesis of paralytic poliomyelitis.

The viraemic phase marks the end of the incubation period, and is manifest in the patient by fever and generalized symptoms; it is followed by a period of about 48 h of relative well-being (the disease is biphasic) while the virus is invading nerve tissue and then, in serious cases, the signs of paralysis appear. Viraemia has been proven to occur after experimental infection of monkeys and has been demonstrated on several occasions in humans. It is probable that the process can be arrested at various stages so that virus may multiply in the intestine without ever reaching the bloodstream. If antibody is present in the blood, virus can be prevented from reaching the central nervous system.

Enteroviruses are lytic, destroying the infected cell within a few hours to days. They are non-enveloped so are unlikely to induce cytotoxic T cell responses. However, cell damage will trigger an inflammatory response; the resultant oedema may affect neurones other than those infected with the virus. As the oedema resolves, function will recover in these cells, thus explaining the apparent improvement in the degree of paralysis in the weeks to months after the acute stage.

Experimentally, it has been shown that the virus can travel along nerves. In most circumstances this is probably not an important route to the central nervous system, but may explain the increased risk of paralysis associated with muscular activity, tonsillectomy and the use of adjuvant vaccines.

Laboratory diagnosis

Culture

Virus isolation was the most useful method for establishing a diagnosis but is gradually being superseded by RTPCR for RNA detection in cerebrospinal fluid (CSF). Examination of CSF is an essential part of the laboratory diagnosis of meningitis. Faecal samples should also be submitted, although isolation can be made from rectal and throat swabs. Since virus excretion can be intermittent, two specimens should be collected on successive days, as early as possible in the illness, ideally within 5 days of the onset.

In culture, virus is detected by the development of a cytopathic effect, usually within a few days; the isolate is identified by neutralization tests with type-specific antiserum. In the UK, poliovirus isolates are likely to be attenuated vaccine strains, which can be differentiated from wild-type virus by several genetic markers.

In paralytic poliomyelitis, the virus can be found in the faeces for a few days preceding the onset of acute symptoms, and is present in over 80% of cases in the faeces during the first 4 days. After 3 weeks some 50% of patients still excrete the virus, and 25% at 5–6 weeks.

Only a few cases continue to excrete the virus after the twelfth week. No permanent carriers are known but prolonged excretion is recognized in immunocompromised hosts. The virus can be isolated from the oropharynx of many cases for a few days before and after the onset of the illness. Isolation from the CSF is seldom successful in cases of paralytic poliomyelitis.

Echoviruses, coxsackie B viruses and coxsackie A9 virus are readily isolated from nose and throat swabs, stools or CSF; they are present in 80% of cases in the faeces for at least 2 weeks after the onset. Identification is by neutralization with reference antiserum.

Isolation of virus from the CSF is a significant finding. However, the relevance of virus isolation from faeces is not always clear, as enteroviruses can be excreted for some time after asymtomatic infection.

Polymerase chain reaction

Identification of conserved sequences within the 5′ non-coding region of the enterovirus genome has resulted in the development of PCR primers that allow the detection of most enteroviruses. Many studies have confirmed that enterovirus RTPCR is more sensitive than culture for the detection of enteroviruses in clinical samples. Such systems can be costly, require sophisticated equipment and do not allow serotype identification.

Serological tests

Although specific IgM and IgG assays for enteroviruses are available their use is limited by the heterotypic and anamnestic responses associated with infections.

Treatment

This is symptomatic. A number of antiviral agents were investigated many years ago for the treatment of paralytic poliomyelitis but they were of no practical value due to the rapid emergence of drug resistance.

Epidemiology and transmission

The only natural source of poliovirus is humans. The virus is spread from person to person, and no intermediate host is known. Echovirus and coxsackievirus have a similar epidemiology; no vaccines are available.

Transmission

All enteroviruses are excreted in large numbers from the gut and are ingested to cause infection. This can be achieved in the following ways:

- By direct transfer on fingers (faecal–oral transfer)
- On eating utensils
- Through contamination of food or drink
- Only rarely by entry through the conjunctiva.

Outbreaks are often seen in closed communities and schools. In the acute phase of infection, virus is present in the throat and, while droplet spread could occur, the faecal–oral route is the usual means of transmission. After the acute phase, it is the only possible route. Cases are most infectious late in the incubation period but infection can be transmitted at any time during virus excretion in the faeces.

Infection rates can equal 100% in closed communities and in households, particularly where children are involved. Social factors, such as standards of hygiene, overcrowding and the age of contacts, are also important. Sewage can contain polioviruses, particularly when there is infection in a community. Enteroviruses can survive for several months in river water, but are unlikely to survive in chlorine-treated water or swimming pools where the recommended level of chlorination (without protein contamination) is achieved. Flies and cockroaches have been found to harbour viruses, but their role in transmission is minimal. Close contact and hygienic standards remain the most important factors.

Prevention and control

After natural infection, immunity is permanent. Virus-neutralizing antibodies are formed early during the disease (often before the seventh day) and persist for several decades. Secretory IgA is produced in the gut. There is some doubt about the duration of immunity to some of the coxsackieviruses.

Immunization

There are two types of polio vaccines:

1. *Inactivated polio vaccine* (Salk vaccine). This was introduced in 1956 for routine immunization. The vaccine contains strains of the three types of virus grown in monkey kidney cell culture and inactivated by exposure to formaldehyde. The batches of vaccine are tested for the presence of residual live poliovirus and must be free of contaminants. Inactivated vaccines are used in Sweden, Finland, Iceland and Holland. With acceptance rates in excess of 90%, these countries have virtually eliminated poliovirus. The circulation of poliovirus in the community has been dramatically reduced despite the fact that inactivated vaccine does not induce much secretory IgA in the alimentary tract. A high rate of immunization is necessary and antibody levels need to be maintained because it has been shown in children that the outcome of

exposure to virus is directly related to the level of antibody at the time of exposure. In an outbreak of poliomyelitis in Finland, the strains of poliovirus type 3 were slightly different from the type 3 poliovirus vaccine strains. Finland has recently introduced a higher potency vaccine that has been shown to produce a good immunological response to all three poliovirus types and it seems likely that this vaccine will give good, long-lasting protection. It was concluded that the outbreak was not due to failure of inactivated vaccine in general but to the poorly immunogenic preparation previously used. The vaccine should be administered by deep subcutaneous or intramuscular injection, and is not associated with local or general reactions. A course of three injections given with intervals of 6–8 weeks between the first and second doses and 4–6 months between the second and third doses produces long-lasting immunity to all three poliovirus types. Inactivated vaccine is recommended for immunocompromised individuals and their contacts and others for whom a live vaccine is contra-indicated.

IPV may be used simultaneously with the triple vaccine for diphtheria, pertussis and tetanus. Booster doses of polio vaccine can be given at the same time as diphtheria/tetanus and also with the combined mumps, measles, rubella (MMR) vaccine.

2. *Live-attenuated polio vaccines* (Sabin vaccine). This replaced the Salk vaccine for routine use in the UK in 1962 and is used extensively in many other countries. It contains live but *attenuated* strains of poliovirus types 1, 2 and 3, grown either in cultures of monkey kidney cells or human diploid cells. The strains, developed by Sabin in 1959, were obtained by growing less virulent polioviruses, which had been isolated in the wild and, after passage, selecting strains that had lost their neurovirulence.

The vaccine is administered orally and parallels natural infection, with stimulation of circulating IgG and local secretory IgA in the pharynx and alimentary tract, thereby producing local resistance to subsequent infection with wild poliomyelitis viruses. Herd immunity is important in preventing the circulation of the wild-type virus and high levels of immunization uptake are necessary. The wide circulation of vaccine virus, which helps to maintain immunity in the community, aids this. However, vaccine strains are not completely stable and studies of sequential isolates of virus from vaccine recipients show that changes can be detected very rapidly. There is therefore the theoretical possibility that vaccine virus, attenuated by serial passage in culture, could revert to neurovirulence with multiple rounds of replication in the vaccinee and after transmission to contacts. Cases of vaccine-associated poliomyelitis have been reported in oral vaccine recipients at a rate of 1 in 2 million doses: it has also been seen in contacts of recipients. It is not possible to predict who will become affected, although the extended replication, which occurs in the immunocompromised, should be avoided, as the rate of vaccine-associated poliomyelitis in such patients is 10 000 times greater than in people with normal immunity. Non-immunized parents and household contacts of children receiving primary immunization should be immunized against poliomyelitis at the same time as the children.

Oral vaccine is recommended for infants from 2 months of age. The primary course consists of three separate doses given at the same time as diphtheria/tetanus/pertussis vaccine (see Chapter 69). Each dose contains all three strains. In infants three drops are dropped from a spoon directly into the mouth, which may be open in response to the simultaneous administration intramuscularly or subcutaneously of diphtheria/tetanus/pertussis vaccine. Breast-feeding does not interfere with the antibody response and should continue. A reinforcing dose is given to children at school entry and prior to leaving, but it is not necessary for adults unless they are at special risk, e.g. through travel or occupational exposure. The effectiveness of live vaccine is shown by the experience in Scotland where the last notified case was in 1994 and was associated with vaccine.

When a case of paralytic poliomyelitis is diagnosed, a dose of oral vaccine should be given to all persons in the immediate neighbourhood of the case who are immunocompetent, whether or not they have a history of previous vaccination against poliomyelitis. This should be followed by completion of the primary course in those not immunized. If the source of the outbreak is uncertain it should be assumed to be a 'wild-type' virus until proven otherwise.

Poliovirus immunization in the tropics. Serological studies in Africa have shown that children will have been infected with two or three types of poliovirus by the age of 5 years. The rate of paralytic disease is low in young children, but significant numbers occur, as the infection is widespread. The disease is known as *infantile paralysis*. Through the expanded programme on immunization the World Health Organisation has increased the rate of immunization chiefly with the use of oral vaccine. Although this is cheaper than inactivated vaccine, it must be stored at 0–4°C and thus requires the existence of an effective cold chain to ensure successful immunization. Apart from inactivation of the vaccine, other explanations for low rates of seroconversion include interference from other enteroviruses, malnutrition and the presence of inhibiting factors in the gastro-intestinal contents.

Global eradication

The World Health Organisation had set a target date of the year 2000 for the global eradication of poliomyelitis.

Although overall the number of cases has fallen by more than 95%, 30 countries in South Asia and West and Central Africa have recent reports of cases. A new deadline has been set of 2005. The eradication is being attempted with annual national immunization days to ensure each child receives an adequate number of doses of oral polio vaccine. Inactivated vaccine has also been shown to provide excellent mucosal protection and with its use countries such as Scandinavia have eliminated wild virus. No decision will be made to discontinue immunization against polio until all countries are free of wild poliovirus infections. In countries where no wild poliovirus infection is reported surveillance systems will need to be in place which are effective at detecting wild poliovirus infections. All cases of paralytic illness should be investigated. Only then will a country be certified poliovirus-free.

Prospects for the future. When the incidence of poliomyelitis falls dramatically, as in the USA for example, the proportion of paralytic cases attributable to vaccine becomes increasingly significant. Recent work has identified the amino acid sequence of antigenic sites, which are important for neutralization of the virus. Information concerning the viral factors necessary for virulence is also available. Therefore, it may be possible to develop modified vaccine viruses, which cannot revert to neurovirulence.

New drugs with some efficacy are under development. Pleconaril is one such drug. It inhibits the uncoating and attachment of virus to cell receptors and shows early promise against enterovirus and rhinovirus.

Hepatovirus (Enterovirus 72/Hepatitis A virus)

Epidemic jaundice has been recognized for centuries; many large epidemics have occurred related to wars, including the Second World War. The virus was first detected by electron microscopical examination of faeces from cases.

Hepatitis A virus (HAV) is the causative agent of *infectious hepatitis*. It is a non-enveloped virus, containing linear, single-stranded RNA. It has similar polypeptides to the four major polypeptides of the Enterovirus family and shares the same properties of resistance to physical and chemical agents. Recently, it has been adapted to cell culture; it will grow only in cells of primate origin.

Clinical features

Although the incidence has fallen in the last decade, hepatitis A is still responsible for almost 60% of acute viral hepatitis in the USA. The illness is usually mild, and occurs after an incubation period of 14–45 days (median,

28 days). There is a prodrome of malaise, muscle pain and headache, and there may be a low-grade fever. The symptoms usually improve and disappear as jaundice develops. Serological tests show that many patients have a subclinical illness, but fulminating hepatitis and liver failure can also occur (overall, less than 0.5%). There are no carriers of the virus. Infection is mildest in young children, often accompanied only by nausea and malaise. Of children under 3 years of age, only 5% develop jaundice, but this rises progressively to more than 50% in adults. The fatality rate also rises with age to 2% in adults. Some patients develop diarrhoea and some appear to have a relapse a few weeks after the onset. Arthritis and aplastic anaemia are rare complications.

Pathogenesis

Like the enteroviruses, HAV probably infects cells in the gut initially and then spreads to the liver via the blood. The histopathology is similar to that of hepatitis B, with peri-portal necrosis and infiltration of mononuclear cells. Viral antigens are seen in the cytoplasm of the hepatocytes. Virus is excreted via the bile into the gut 1–2 weeks before the onset of jaundice, and excretion then declines rapidly over the next 5–7 days. Virus is also present in the urine of clinical and subclinical cases during the same period.

Laboratory diagnosis

Although the virus has been grown in cell culture, it is not possible to do this routinely from the faeces of cases. Diagnosis relies on the demonstration of specific IgM antibody to HAV, which develops very early in the course of infection and is generally present by the time the patient is investigated. It is detectable in the serum for 2–6 months after the onset of symptoms (Fig. 48.2). IgG antibody usually persists for many years and is a useful indicator of immunity.

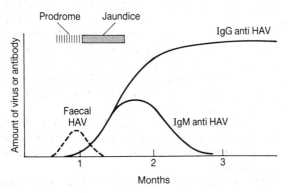

Fig. 48.2 Events in hepatitis A infection.

Epidemiology

Only one major type of HAV has been recognized. Molecular typing is now available to investigate outbreaks and link sporadic cases with common source outbreaks. Serological tests have made it possible to study the rate of infection in different populations throughout the world. Such studies confirm that, as the virus is spread by the faecal–oral route, it is prevalent in countries where sanitation is poor, and children are infected early in childhood. Serological studies also show that, even in developed countries, more than half the population has been infected with HAV. However, with increasing use of vaccine, lower rates are seen. This can result in increased numbers of acute cases in young adults and older patients who may have a history of recent travel to an endemic area.

Outbreaks of HAV infection have been associated with food. Shellfish have often been incriminated, particularly when they are harvested from coastlines adjacent to sewage outlets. The mussel, for example, is a filter feeder and can concentrate the virus. Shellfish are eaten raw or partially cooked, thus protecting the virus. Contaminated raspberries were incriminated in another notorious outbreak in which uncooked frozen raspberries were eaten many months after picking. Infection is assumed to have come from an infected raspberry picker. Because there is only a transient viraemic phase, only a few infections have been recognized after blood transfusion.

Prevention and control

A highly effective and immunogenic vaccine was licensed for use in the UK in 1991. It is a formaldehyde-inactivated vaccine prepared from HAV grown in human diploid cells. A primary course of two doses (or, more recently, a single dose) of vaccine given intramuscularly produces good levels of neutralizing antibody that are likely to persist for at least 10 years. The vaccine is an alternative to human normal immunoglobulin for frequent travellers and those whose occupation takes them to endemic areas abroad. Recent formulations combine hepatitis A and B antigens in the same vaccine.

RHINOVIRUSES

Although other viruses can give a similar illness the viruses of this genus are responsible for the most frequent of all human infections, the 'common cold'. Most people suffer from two to four colds every year and, although the primary infection is not a severe one, the symptoms of secondary bacterial infection often follow and may be more severe than the original cold. Sinusitis and otitis media are quite common. Recently the rhinoviruses have been associated with acute exacerbations of asthma. These viruses are of major economic significance because they cause the loss of many million human-hours of work.

Properties

As the name rhinovirus implies, the genus is associated with the nose. They can be distinguished from the enteroviruses by their acid lability and so do not infect the intestinal tract. There are over 100 serotypes of rhinoviruses; all are fastidious in cell culture. Electron microscopy cannot differentiate them from other family members (Fig. 48.3). Some primates may be susceptible to human viruses, and there are related viruses in cattle, cats and horses. The genomes of some rhinoviruses have 45–60% homology with polioviruses in hybridization tests.

The capsid of rhinoviruses appears to be less rigid than that of the enteroviruses. This loose packing is consistent with its greater buoyant density and sensitivity to acid.

Cultivation

Rhinoviruses show a distinct preference for cells of human origin, especially fetal lung or kidney. They are divided into major (90%) and minor groups (10%) according to their cell receptors.

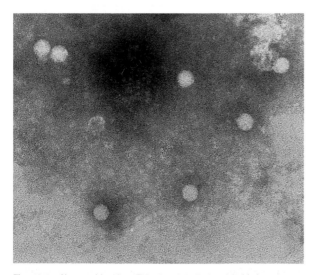

Fig. 48.3 Human rhinovirus. This virus is indistinguishable in appearance from other picornaviruses. Approximate size 25–30 nm. (From Madeley C R, Field A M 1988 *Virus Morphology*, 2nd edn. Churchill Livingstone, Edinburgh.)

Stability

Inactivation of rhinoviruses occurs below pH 6.0 and is more rapid the lower the pH. Complete inactivation occurs at pH 3.0.

Some rhinoviruses may survive heating at 50°C for 1 h. They are relatively stable in the range from 20 to 37°C and can survive on environmental surfaces such as doorknobs for several days. They can be preserved at –70°C.

Rhinoviruses are resistant to 20% ether and 5% chloroform, but are sensitive to aldehydes and hypochlorites.

Replication

Most rhinoviruses attach to the same cell receptors on HeLa cells (90%). The minor group (10%) attaches to a low density lipoprotein receptor and its related protein. The viruses replicate in the cytoplasm of infected cells to give a cytopathic effect (CPE) that coincides with release of the virus in the same way as other picornaviruses. If the infected cultures are incubated at 37°C the yield is reduced to 30–50% of that at 33°C.

Clinical features and pathogenesis

The typical illness is generally referred to as a common cold. The onset, after contact with infection, is usually within 2–3 days, sometimes as long as 7 days. The symptoms are:

- clear watery nasal discharge, which often becomes mucoid or purulent due to secondary bacterial infection
- sneezing and coughing
- sore throat
- headache and malaise.

The symptoms are most severe for 2–3 days when nasal virus titres are maximal and, although recovery is usually complete within a week, symptoms can persist for 2 weeks or longer. The ratio of symptomatic to asymptomatic infection is about 3:1, and the illness is generally worse in cigarette smokers. Rhinoviruses have frequently been isolated from patients during acute exacerbation of chronic obstructive airway disease, and they are the most common viruses to be associated with wheeze in pre-school children.

It should be remembered that all respiratory viruses may cause the symptoms of the common cold and that laboratory diagnosis is necessary to establish the aetiological agent.

Experimental rhinovirus infections in healthy human volunteers and studies on rhinovirus-infected organ cultures have helped to show their pathogenic potential. Humans have proved to be the more sensitive assay as illness can occur when virus cannot be detected by culture in the inoculum. In organ cultures, it has been shown that the virus settles on the ciliated nasal epithelial cells, enters, infects and spreads from cell to cell in the epithelium. The cilia become immobilized, and both cilia and cell degenerate as the virus replicates. Bacterial invasion of the damaged epithelium can then occur. Interferon is usually detectable shortly after the peak of virus shedding and probably plays a part in recovery. When specific antibody is first detected in nasal secretions, virus shedding ceases, suggesting that this may be the main factor leading to recovery. Little is known of the importance of cell-mediated immunity. The symptoms probably relate to the local inflammatory response and interferon release. Rhinoviruses have been recovered in pure culture from sinus fluids collected from patients with acute sinusitis, but secondary bacterial infection is thought to be the usual cause.

Lower respiratory tract infection may occur on some occasions since:

- patients with colds may also have lower respiratory tract symptoms with abnormal lung function
- children who develop colds may develop wheeze
- adults with colds may suffer exacerbation of chronic obstructive airway disease.

Immunity

After the acute illness, neutralizing antibody can be detected both in serum and nasal secretions. It can continue to rise in titre for 4–5 weeks after infection and may persist for up to 4 years, although some infections may provoke only a poor response, leaving the patient susceptible to the same serotype after a few weeks or months. New virus types continue to emerge by a process of immune selection and random mutation.

Laboratory diagnosis

Culture

Nose and throat swabs in virus transport medium are the specimens of choice for the recovery of virus from all age groups. Nasopharyngeal aspirates are excellent specimens from children. Specimens should be taken as early in the illness as possible, preferably within the first 3 days.

Cell cultures of human origin such as MRC5 or WI38 are preferred for the isolation of rhinoviruses. Organ cultures are not used routinely. Cultures are incubated at 33°C and observed microscopically for a CPE.

The majority of isolates are apparent within 2 weeks of inoculation although some may take longer. Identification of an isolate as a rhinovirus may be made by considering the cells in which the CPE develops, the appearance of the CPE and the demonstration of acid lability.

Serology

Serological methods cannot be used in the routine diagnosis of rhinovirus infections because of the multiplicity of serotypes and the lack of a common antigen.

Nucleic acid detection

Culture is slow and cumbersome and serology inadequate, so nucleic acid detection is likely to become a significant tool in diagnosis. However, RNA detection has net yet been optimized and so is not in routine use.

Epidemiology and transmission

Rhinoviruses can be isolated from patients with respiratory illnesses throughout the year but in temperate climates the incidence of colds due to rhinoviruses increases in the autumn and spring and is lowest in the summer months. In the tropics the peak incidence occurs in the rainy season. Deliberate exposure of volunteers to wet and chilling does not cause colds. Rhinoviruses may be transmitted by inhalation of droplets expelled from the nose of a patient and also by hand to surface contact. During the acute phase of the illness high concentrations of virus are present in nasal secretions and may contaminate the fingers, and thereafter the contaminated fingers may touch the eye or nasal mucosa. The incidence of rhinovirus infections is highest in pre-school children and they often introduce colds to the home. People who are in contact with young children are at increased risk of infection.

Colds are mostly trivial and an inconvenience; however, they do cause considerable morbidity and absence from work.

Treatment and control

Although inactivated vaccines can be produced, there remains the considerable problem of deciding on the antigenic composition. Much effort has been devoted to the development of suitable antiviral therapy. Pleconaril is one such drug showing activity against rhinoviruses and enteroviruses (see above). Isolation of the infected person, although perhaps desirable, is not a practical method of preventing the spread of infection. Good infection control practices, including hand washing, will reduce spread of infection in the hospital setting.

RECOMMENDED READING

Andre F E 1990 Inactivated candidate vaccines for hepatitis A. *Progress in Medical Virology* 37: 72–95

Cuthbert J A 2001 Hepatitis A: old and new. *Clinical Microbiology Reviews* 14: 38–58

Grist N R, Bell E J 1984 Paralytic poliomyelitis and non-polio enteroviruses. Studies in Scotland. *Reviews of Infectious Diseases* 6 (Suppl 2): S385–S386

Her Majesty's Stationery Office 1996 *Immunisation against Infectious Disease.* HMSO, London

John T J 2000 The final stages of the eradication of polio. *New England Journal of Medicine* 343(11): 806–807

Roebuck M O 1976 Rhinoviruses in Britain. *Journal of Hygiene* 76: 137–146

Thoren A 1994 PCR for the diagnosis of enteroviral meningitis. *Scandinavian Journal of Infectious Diseases* 26: 249–254

49

Orthomyxoviruses

Influenza

S. Sutherland

The family Orthomyxoviridae comprises four genera: influenza A, B and C viruses and thogotoviruses.

Influenza A viruses can infect a variety of different host species, an ability that is of great importance in determining their ability to cause pandemic infection in humans. Influenza B only infects humans and influenza C, although assumed to be primarily a human infection, has been isolated from pigs in China. The thogotoviruses form a newly discovered fourth genus of the orthomyxovirus family and are found in mosquitoes, ticks and the banded mongoose.

Influenza virus type A was the first to be isolated in 1933, by intranasal inoculation of the ferret. Thereafter, type B was isolated along with type A in cell culture in 1940. One of the most prominent features of the influenza viruses is their ability to change antigenically either gradually (*antigenic drift*) or suddenly (*antigenic shift*). Only influenza A virus has the potential to shift, whereas A, B and C may drift antigenically, although only very minor changes have been demonstrated in influenza C.

THE VIRUSES

The virions are spherical, 80–120 nm in diameter, but may be filamentous, sometimes up to several micrometers in length (Fig. 49.1). They have a helical nucleocapsid comprising eight segments of single-stranded RNA with a total molecular weight of 5×10^6. Also present within the virion is the viral RNA-dependent RNA polymerase: this is essential for infectivity as the virion RNA is of negative sense and therefore has to be transcribed to produce viral messenger RNA (mRNA). The nucleocapsid is surrounded by an M1 protein shell, immediately exterior to which is a lipid envelope derived from the host cell. The M2 protein projects through the envelope to form ion channels, which allow pH changes in the endosome. Two types of spike (Fig. 49.2) project from the envelope, the *haemagglutinin* (H) and the *neuraminidase* (N). The

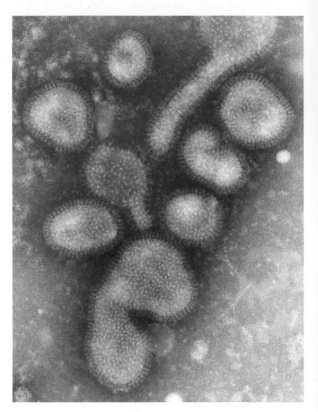

Fig. 49.1 Influenza A/Dunedin/27/83 H,N, virus. Spikes that make up the fringe are also seen in the end-on view, covering the surface of the virus particles and giving them a 'spotty' appearance. Approximate size 80–120 nm. (From Madeley C R and Field A M 1988 *Virus Morphology*, 2nd edn. Churchill Livingstone, Edinburgh.)

haemagglutinin, so called because the virus agglutinates certain species of erythrocyte, is about 10 nm in length, with a molecular weight of 225 000, and consists of trimers of identical glycoprotein subunits, each consisting of two polypeptide chains, HA1 and HA2. The two polypeptides are joined in each subunit by a linkage site that may be a single base, arginine, or multibasic. Cleavage of this link is pH-dependent and

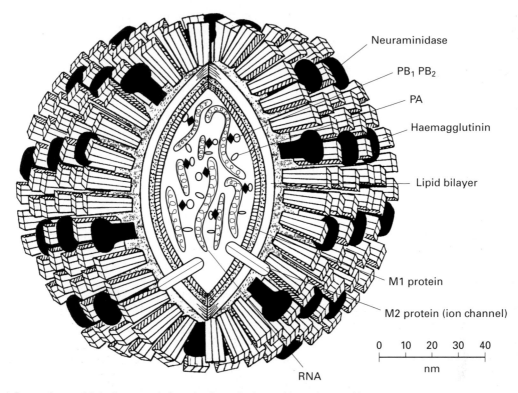

Neuraminidase

PB₁ PB₂

PA

Haemagglutinin

Lipid bilayer

M1 protein

M2 protein (ion channel)

0 10 20 30 40

nm

RNA

Fig. 49.2 Influenza virus particle in diagrammatic form showing projections and internal composition.

allows conformational change that exposes the highly conserved hydrophobic fusion peptide at the N terminal of HA2, necessary for the viral envelope and the endosomal membrane to fuse, thus releasing the nucleocapsid into the host cell cytoplasm. Influenza viruses bind to cells by the haemagglutinin interacting with cell membrane receptors containing *N*-acetylneuraminic acid (sialic acid). The epitopes involved in receptor binding show great variability because of mutations in the RNA causing amino acid substitutions at several sites on the HA1 molecule. These changes can be located in the three-dimensional structure of the molecule and are found only at a few well defined areas close to the attachment site.

Between the H spikes are the mushroom-shaped protrusions of neuraminidase. The head is box-shaped and is assembled from four roughly spherical subunits attached to the stalk containing the hydrophobic region by which it is embedded in the viral envelope. The enzyme catalyses the cleavage of sialic acid and an adjacent sugar residue in glycoproteins found in mucus. This action allows the virus to permeate mucin and escape from these so-called 'non-specific' inhibitors. The neuraminidase also destroys the haemagglutinin receptors on the host cell. Neuraminidase activity is also thought to be important in the final stages of release of new virus particles from infected cells. Sialic acid is always present in newly synthesized virions, and its removal by neuraminidase prevents the new virus particles agglutinating, thus increasing the number of free virus particles and hence spread of the virus from the original site of infection. The viral genes and their functions are shown in Table 49.1.

Nomenclature

The World Health Organization (WHO) system of nomenclature includes the host of origin, geographical origin, strain number and year of isolation; then follows in parentheses the antigenic description of the haemagglutinin and the neuraminidase, e.g. A/swine/Iowa/3/70 (H₁N₁). If isolated from a human host the origin is not given, e.g. A/Scotland/42/89 (H₃N₂). There are 15 different H antigens and nine N antigens. Only H₁–H₃ and N₁–N₂ have been found in epidemic/pandemic viruses from humans, the others being recovered from animals and birds. However, in 1997 an outbreak, with high case mortality, occurred in humans in Hong Kong; the virus was an avian strain, H₅N₁, which appeared to transmit directly from chickens to humans. No human to human spread was demonstrated.

Physical characteristics

The influenza virus withstands slow drying at room temperature on articles such as blankets and glass: it has been demonstrated in dust after an interval as long as 2 weeks. When contained in allantoic fluid or in infected tissues immersed in glycerol saline it will survive for several weeks at 4°C. Virus can survive in cold seawater for a similar period. It can be preserved for long periods at –70°C, and remains viable indefinitely when freeze-dried.

Exposure to heat for 30 min at 56°C is sufficient to inactivate most strains; the few that survive this treatment are killed by exposure to the same temperature for 90 min. The viruses are inactivated by a variety of substances, such as 20% ether in the cold, phenol, formaldehyde, salts of heavy metals, detergents, soaps, halogens and many others.

REPLICATION

Human influenza viruses recognize receptors which contain N-acetylneuraminic acid (sialic acid) attached to the penultimate sugar via an alpha (2,6)-linkage while avian strains prefer receptors with an alpha (2,3)-linkage and in pigs both types are present. After attachment of the viral haemagglutinin to the specific receptors, viruses enter cells by endocytosis. The HA contains a fusion peptide which, at neutral pH, is buried within the spike but at low pH a conformational change occurs which exposes the peptide. Together with several other trimers the fusion peptides form a fusion pore that inserts into the cell lipid layer causing the viral and cell membranes to fuse. This leads to release of the viral ribonucleoprotein (RNP) and associated RNA polymerase into the cell cytoplasm. Transcription of the viral RNA molecules produces 10 mRNA species (Table 49.1) as RNA segments 7 and 8 both have two reading frames. mRNA molecules are processed in the cell nucleus, where poly (A) sequences are removed from host mRNA molecules and added to the viral transcripts. Unlike most other RNA viruses, assembly of the new viral RNP takes place in the nucleus of the host cell.

The viral matrix (M) proteins migrate to the cell membrane and are joined by the H and N glycoproteins. RNP and polymerase locate at the areas of the cell membrane with matrix protein. Release occurs by budding, aided perhaps by the viral neuraminidase. To be infectious the H protein is cleaved into the components HA1 and HA2, which together form the haemagglutinin molecule.

PATHOGENESIS

Pathogenicity of influenza viruses is multifactorial and may involve viral, host and environmental factors. Work with avian strains has identified host receptors and proteases as determinants of tropism and hence of pathogenicity. The sensitivity of strains with monobasic links at the HA1/HA2 junction to the trypsin-like proteases that are active extracellularly tends to limit spread of virus locally in the respiratory tract in humans. Until the H_5N_1 outbreak all human strains were of this type whereas avian strains with multibasic links were associated with systemic spread and were highly pathogenic.

Table 49.1 Influenza virus proteins

Gene segment	Proteins	Molecular weight (×10³)	Location in virion	Function	Comments
1	PB2	0.87	Internal	RNA transcription	Polymerase proteins; highly conserved
2	PB1	0.96			
3	PA	0.85			
4	HA1	47.5	Spikes	Binding to cell receptors envelope fusion to endosome	Glycoprotein; haemagglutinin varies antigenically
	HA2	28.8			
5	NA	48–63	Spikes	Neuraminidase	Glycoprotein enzyme activity
6	NP	50–60	Internal	Subunit of nucleocapsid	Nucleoprotein helical arrangement; type-specific
7	M1	0.28	Beneath lipid bilayer of envelope	Major structural component	Involved in assembly and budding
	M2	11–15	Transmembrane	Ion channel	Changes pH in endosome; blocked by amantadine
8	NS1	0.25	Internal	mRNA transport inhibition; splicing	Non-structural proteins
	NS2	0.13		Unknown	

The NA type may also determine pathogenicity. One NA has been found to bind plasminogen, which could act as a ubiquitous protease even for monobasic strains. Receptor preference will also determine tropism.

Inhaled virus is deposited on the mucous membrane lining the respiratory tract or directly into the alveoli, the level depending on the size of the droplets inhaled. In the former site, it is exposed to mucoproteins containing sialic acid that can bind to the virus, thus blocking its attachment to respiratory tract epithelial cells. However, the action of neuraminidase allows the virus to break this bond. Specific local secretory IgA antibodies, if present from a previous infection, may neutralize the virus before attachment occurs, provided the antibody corresponds to the infecting virus type. If not prevented by one of these mechanisms, virus attaches to the surface of a respiratory epithelial cell and the intracellular replication cycle is initiated.

The major site of infection is the ciliated columnar epithelial cell. The first alteration is the disappearance of the elongated form of these cells, which become round and swollen, the nucleus shrinks, becomes pyknotic and fragments. Vacuolization of the cytoplasm may occur. As the nucleus disintegrates, the cytoplasm shows inclusion bodies, and the cilia are lost.

Release of the virus from the cells allows it to spread via the mucus blanket to other areas of the respiratory tract. The cell damage initiates an acute inflammatory response with oedema and the attraction of phagocytic cells. The earliest response is the synthesis and release of interferons from the infected cells: these can diffuse to and protect both adjacent and more distant cells before the virus arrives. It appears that interferons released in this way cause many of the systemic features of the 'flu-like' syndrome. While viral components are absorbed and trigger the immune system, the virus itself is confined to the epithelium of the respiratory tract. Specific antibody will help to limit the extracellular spread of the virus, while T cell responses are directed against the viral glycoproteins on the surface of infected cells, leading to their destruction by cytotoxic T cells and also by antibody-dependent cell cytotoxicity.

CLINICAL FEATURES

Influenza A

In classical influenza:

- The incubation period is short, 2 days, but it may vary from 1 to 4 days.
- The illness is characterized by a sudden onset of systemic symptoms such as chills, fever, headache, myalgia and anorexia.
- Respiratory symptoms are also common but take second place to the systemic effects, especially early in the illness.

Many patients have both upper and lower respiratory tract infection, often with a troublesome, dry cough. The main physical finding is pyrexia, which rises rapidly to a peak of 38–41°C within 12 h of onset. Fever usually lasts 3 days, but it can be present for 1–5 days. During the second and third days of the illness the systemic effects diminish, and by the fourth day the respiratory symptoms and signs are predominant. In adults, systemic illness without respiratory symptoms is common. Some symptoms are age-specific, e.g. febrile convulsions and otitis media in children and dyspnoea in the elderly. About one-third of patients will suffer only a common cold-like illness, and it has been shown that as many as 20% of cases are subclinical. A long convalescence is common, and cough, lassitude and malaise may last for 1–2 weeks after the disappearance of other manifestations. It should be remembered that many other respiratory viruses can cause typical influenza-like illnesses, although the severity of the systemic symptoms is usually greatest with influenza virus. The similarity to influenza of the prodromal stages of several infections has led to the use of the term 'flu-like' to describe these features.

Influenza B

Symptoms closely resemble those associated with influenza A infections, consisting of a 3-day febrile illness with predominantly systemic symptoms. Overall, the infection is somewhat milder; some studies have shown more involvement of the gastro-intestinal tract, with the coining of the term 'gastric flu'.

Influenza C

Clinically, influenza C causes an afebrile upper respiratory tract infection usually confined to young children: outbreaks are not recognized.

Complications of influenza

- Primary *influenza pneumonia* may occur, especially in young adults during an outbreak, and can be fatal after a very short illness of sometimes less than 1 day. A similar rapid illness can occur in the elderly.
- More commonly a bacterial pneumonia caused by *Staphylococcus aureus* or *Streptococcus pneumoniae* occurs late in the course of the illness, often after a period of improvement, resulting in a classical biphasic fever pattern.

The incidence of chest complications is related to the age of the patient, increasing progressively after the age of 60 years. Severe infections and sudden death can occur, especially if there is some underlying disease, such as cerebrovascular, cardiovascular or chronic respiratory disease.

In the immunocompromised, symptoms may last longer and viral excretion may go on for weeks to months. Excess mortality was reported in pregnant women during the 1918 and 1957 pandemics and even in non-pandemic outbreaks an increase in hospitalization due to cardiorespiratory disease is seen in the second and third trimesters. High case fatality rates were seen in the H_5N_1 human infections in Hong Kong in 1997 when six of 18 laboratory-confirmed cases died.

Immunity

After an attack of influenza the ensuing immunity to the particular subtype of infecting virus is of long duration. It is related to the amount of local antibody (IgA) in the mucous secretions of the respiratory tract together with the specific IgG serum antibody concentration. Immunity to infection, especially with type A, is subtype-specific, giving little or no protection against subtypes possessing immunologically distinct H or N proteins.

LABORATORY DIAGNOSIS

Virus isolation and detection

For primary isolation the most suitable cells are primary monkey kidney or human embryo kidney cells, but since these tissues are scarce most laboratories now use secondary baboon kidney cells or Madin–Darby canine kidney cells. The presence of virus may be detected in baboon kidney cell cultures incubated at 33°C as early as 18 h after inoculation, by haemadsorption with human group O, fowl or guinea-pig red blood cells. Usually, if viable viruses are present in the clinical specimen, isolation is made within 7 days. The virus may then be identified by the fluorescent antibody technique.

Rapid diagnosis

Since the advent of antivirals with activity against influenza viruses, rapid diagnosis has increased in importance, particularly in the hospital or institutional context, such as homes for the elderly, so that attempts can be made to limit the spread of the virus by a combination of patient isolation, vaccination and chemoprophylaxis.

Immunofluorescent detection of influenza antigens in respiratory specimens either directly or following amplification in cell culture for 24 h has speeded up diagnosis considerably. The best specimens are nasal aspirates or nasal washes, but nasal or throat swabs taken vigorously to obtain cells and put in viral transport medium can be satisfactory if taken in the first few days of illness.

It is important in the early stages of an outbreak or in sporadic cases that viruses should be isolated and analysed antigenically for epidemiology and vaccine production. For patient management and control of infection, rapid antigen detection is more useful. Detection of influenza RNA by reverse transcriptase polymerase chain reaction may be more sensitive than antigen detection but is not widely available in diagnostic laboratories.

Serological confirmation of the clinical diagnosis is obtained when a four-fold or greater rise in antibody titre can be shown to any one type of virus. Complement fixation tests (CFTs) are still widely used. This test uses nucleocapsid antigens that are type-specific and can distinguish A from B and C infections. Strain differences can be demonstrated by means of haemagglutination inhibition and neutralization assays or strain-specific CFTs. Single, high CFT titres are difficult to interpret in some patients, especially those with chronic respiratory disease since many may exhibit high titres for many years. In patients who are normally healthy a high titre found during an outbreak can, with some assurance, be related to a recent illness.

EPIDEMIOLOGY

Epidemics, which must have been caused by influenza viruses, have been described for over 2000 years. Typically, there is a sudden appearance of cases of respiratory disease; these occur for several weeks and then suddenly cease. The epidemics occur frequently at irregular intervals and were thought at one time to be under the influence of the stars, hence the term *influenza* (Italian for influence). It is well recognized that epidemics vary in severity. The great pandemic of 1918–19 was particularly severe, killing between 20 million and 40 million people as it spread around the world. It was because of this that a great effort was directed into trying to identify the cause of the illness. Success came in 1933 when Sir Christopher Andrewes and others isolated influenza A virus. Continued isolation studies and analysis of isolates have given an understanding of how the epidemic behaviour relates to changes in the virus. Also, it is possible to deduce which viral antigens circulated before virus isolation was possible by virtue of the phenomenon of *original antigenic sin*. This means that infection with a current virus type stimulates antibody to earlier strains. Thus we can deduce what antigenic components were prevalent back to the end of the 19th century by antibody studies of older people (Fig. 49.3).

The major pandemics are associated with *antigenic shifts* – when the viral H or N, or both, are changed. This is too extensive to be the result of mutation, and analysis of the viral RNA indicates that shift results from the acquisition of a complete new RNA segment 4 and/or 5. In the laboratory it is easy to show that if a cell is infected with two different strains, the progeny will include viruses whose RNA molecules are derived from each parent. Thus, a 'new' virus can result from the process of *reassortment*. All the H and N antigenic subtypes are found in aquatic birds (both seabirds and ducks), but in these the viruses vary little. The genetic reassortment may take place in pigs that have receptors for both human and avian strains, and may act as a mixing vessel from which certain subtypes may transmit to humans.

Until 1977, when H_1N_1 reappeared, it was the rule that when a 'new' virus appeared the 'old' one disappeared, but since that time two subtypes have been circulating concurrently, namely H_3N_2 and H_1N_1. The latter antigens had not been found since the 1950s and since

they were antigenically very similar to viruses from the 1957 pandemic may have reappeared from a frozen source. There is no evidence of latent or persistent infection of humans.

The 1997 Hong Kong outbreak of H_5N_1 virus in humans has added a new dimension to previous thinking about influenza A transmission since this virus seems to have crossed the species barrier from chickens to humans directly. Slaughter of infected chickens ended the outbreak and no cases of human-to-human spread were seen.

Influenza B viruses do not undergo antigenic shift as there is no animal reservoir and, although epidemics do occur at 3–6-year intervals, they never reach pandemic proportions, and their extent is usually limited to small communities such as boarding schools or residences for the elderly. The antigenic changes result from mutation, as do those seen in influenza A after the appearance of 'new' virus strains; the changes are the cause of antigenic drift.

Influenza may occur as:

- pandemics
- epidemics
- sporadically.

A pandemic develops and spreads worldwide, as in 1918, 1957 and 1968 (Fig. 49.3), when a new reassortant virus appears against which there is no immunity in the population. Pandemics have often started in the East, possibly because of the close association of a high-density population with ducks and pigs, and within 2–3 years spread worldwide, involving all age groups. Epidemics result from *antigenic drift* when the virus has drifted so far that the H and N antibodies in the community can no longer prevent large numbers of the population from becoming infected. WHO-designated laboratories monitor influenza A and B throughout the world to check for the appearance of variants. In the UK, influenza activity is monitored in several ways. Spotter general practitioners regularly report the levels of influenza-like illness in their patients. The excess deaths due to respiratory causes rise dramatically over a short period during an influenza epidemic and so are regularly calculated to provide a sensitive measure of increased influenza activity. Laboratories regularly report virus isolations and send isolates to reference laboratories for antigenic analysis.

High rates of infection are found in pre-school children; thereafter the rates are lower even in the elderly. However, elderly patients in residential homes, if not protected, are at particular risk from acute illness and sudden death. Thus, even if the attack rate is low, the case fatality rate is high. Staff, visitors or other patients may introduce the virus.

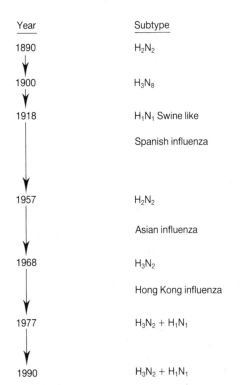

Year	Subtype
1890	H_2N_2
1900	H_3N_8
1918	H_1N_1 Swine like
	Spanish influenza
1957	H_2N_2
	Asian influenza
1968	H_3N_2
	Hong Kong influenza
1977	$H_3N_2 + H_1N_1$
1990	$H_3N_2 + H_1N_1$

Fig. 49.3 Sequential changes in influenza A antigens associated with antigenic shift. Antigenic drift occurs after the appearance of a new subtype.

Influenza virus type C is not associated with epidemics but gives rise only to mild upper respiratory tract infections, especially in young children. Most infections are asymptomatic.

TREATMENT

Oral amantadine hydrochloride was introduced in the early 1980s, followed later by a derivative, rimantadine. These drugs work by blocking the ion channels in the envelope, thus preventing the pH changes that precede the membrane fusion step essential for nucleocapsid release. Unfortunately, these compounds only have activity against influenza virus type A but not B, C or other respiratory viruses. Therefore, it is essential to know which virus is responsible for the illness or outbreak. A clinical diagnosis can be fairly confidently made in a typical case seen during an epidemic due to a known type, but is impossible in sporadic or milder cases. Amantadine is effective when given prophylactically but also therapeutically in patients treated within 24 h of onset of illness. Viruses resistant to amantadine and rimantadine may appear within a few days of drug administration; however, resistant strains show no increased pathogenicity or transmissibility.

More recently two neuraminidase inhibitors, zanamivir and oseltamivir, have received FDA approval for therapeutic use in both influenza A and B infections. They can reduce the duration of symptoms by 1–3 days if given within 36 h of onset of illness. Zanamivir has poor bio-availability and is administered by inhalation of a dry powder twice daily for 5 days. Oseltamivir is given by mouth as a prodrug and has excellent bio-availability. Twice daily dosage for 5–7 days has been used in those with normal renal function though once daily dosage is recommended where renal function is impaired.

Resistance to both these drugs has been demonstrated and may be NA-independent or NA-dependent. Both are effective against amantadine- or rimantadine-resistant strains.

CONTROL

The aim of immunization is to produce haemagglutination inhibiting or neutralizing antibody in all vaccinees. This protects them against infection, but only with strains closely related to those in the vaccine. Vaccine efficacy in the elderly is about 70%, and uptake must be encouraged.

All types of vaccine rely on adequate quantities of virus with the appropriate H and N antigens being produced in the allantoic cavity of embryonated hens' eggs inoculated with seed virus. Reassortment of two strains, one a high-yielding laboratory-adapted strain and the other containing the required H and N antigens, is employed to produce an appropriate inoculum for growth in eggs so that vaccine is prepared as quickly as possible. Separated whole virus particles are inactivated either by formalin or β-propiolactone. Whole virus vaccine should not be given to those who are allergic to egg protein. The H and N antigens may be separated from the whole virus by treatment with detergent, and these subunit or split-virus vaccines are better tolerated, especially in young children. In the UK, influenza vaccines contain three virus strains, two type A and one type B, representing the strains currently circulating in the world. Other types of vaccines have been tried, e.g. live-attenuated vaccines given intranasally. These vaccines have been generally effective in provoking a good local (IgA) antibody response but are not at present widely used. Vaccines containing adjuvants, usually oil-based, have been investigated, but this approach has been abandoned due to the development of very unpleasant local reactions at the site of injection.

RECOMMENDED READING

Andrewes C 1989 *Viruses of Vertebrates*, 5th edn. Baillière Tindall, London
Cox N J, Subbarao K 1999 Influenza. *Lancet* 354:1277–1282
Fields B N, Knipe D M, Howley P M (eds) 1996 *Virology*, 3rd edn. Lippincott-Raven, Philadelphia
Gubareva L V, Kaiser L, Hayden F G 2000 Influenza virus neuraminidase inhibitors. *Lancet* 355: 827–835

Nichol K L, Margolis K L, Wuorenma J, Von Sternberg T 1994 The efficacy and cost effectiveness of vaccination against influenza among elderly persons living in the community. *New England Journal of Medicine* 331: 778–784
Steinhauer D A 1999 Role of hemagglutinin cleavage for the pathogenicity of influenza virus. *Virology* 258: 1–20

50

Paramyxoviruses

Respiratory infections; mumps; measles

J. S. M. Peiris and C. R. Madeley

The paramyxoviruses are a family of enveloped viruses containing single-stranded RNA as a single piece. They resemble the orthomyxoviruses in both morphology and an affinity for sialic acid receptors on mammalian cells, but they are larger and more fragile (Fig. 50.1a).

Within the family Paramyxoviridae there are three genera, each with several members:

- *Paramyxovirus* (para-influenza viruses, mumps virus, Newcastle disease virus (NDV) and simian virus 5 (SV5)).
- *Morbillivirus* (measles virus, canine distemper virus, rinderpest virus, an equine morbillivirus and several strains recently isolated from seals, dolphins and porpoises).
- *Pneumovirus* (respiratory syncytial (RS) virus).

Originally, they were all classified together because they were thought to be similar in structure and function. Neither property is constant throughout the family but there are similarities. For example, para-influenza, mumps and measles viruses are identical as seen in the electron microscope (and as described below), while pneumovirus, although very similar, has slightly longer surface spikes and is more difficult to visualize.

Functionally there are other differences. Para-influenza viruses, NDV and mumps virus have a surface haemagglutinin and neuraminidase, while measles virus has a haemagglutinin but no neuraminidase, and pneumovirus has neither. In addition, measles virus has a haemolysin not possessed by the others, while RS virus has a large surface glycoprotein, G, which has a similar cell-attaching function as a haemagglutinin. Para-influenza, mumps, measles and RS viruses are the common human pathogens.

In the 1990s, two new paramyxoviruses, Hendra and Nipah, were discovered in Australia and South-east Asia; they are animal viruses occasionally transmitted to man. As they are genetically distinct from the other members of this family they will probably be classified as a separate genus. Their full significance as human pathogens is not yet clear.

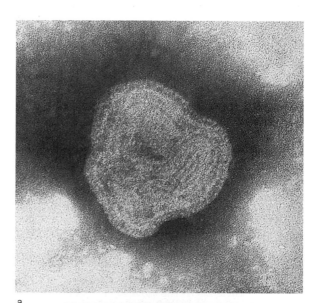

a

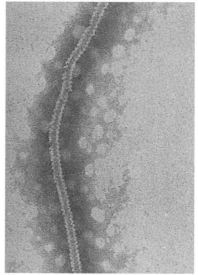

b

Fig. 50.1 **a** Electron micrograph of a typical paramyxovirus. **b** Separate internal helical nucleocapsid. Negative contrast microscopy, ×200 000.

PARA-INFLUENZA VIRUSES

Description

Para-influenza viruses, mumps virus, NDV and SV5 are indistinguishable in the electron microscope. Negatively-stained virions vary in size from 80 to 350 nm; occasionally there are filamentous forms and giant forms up to 800 nm in diameter. The outer surface of the virion is a pleomorphic envelope consisting of a lipoprotein membrane derived from host cell membrane and covered by projections 12–14 nm long and 2–4 nm wide. Although generally similar, orthomyxoviruses and paramyxoviruses are morphologically distinct. Paramyxovirus particles are easily deformed by external forces, may assume a variety of shapes and break up more easily than orthomyxoviruses.

The envelope surface projections are of two kinds:

- The HN, with haemagglutinin (H) and neuraminidase (N) functions, in contrast to orthomyxoviruses, in which these functions are on separate spikes.
- F glycoproteins, which cause cell membranes to fuse, leading to the formation of syncytia – found on all paramyxoviruses.

There are also matrix proteins, M, which line the inner surface of the envelope. All the paramyxoviruses carry an RNA-dependent RNA polymerase within the virion.

Within the enveloped virion is a genome of single-stranded negative-sense RNA complexed with protein to form a helical nucleocapsid. This has a basic length of about 1 μm, and the RNA has a size of 16.5 kilobases, but some particles contain more than one copy. The envelope ruptures readily when the virus is prepared for electron microscopy, releasing the helical nucleoprotein, which has a herring bone or 'zipper'-like appearance (Fig. 50.1b). This is more easily recognized in the electron microscope than the complete particle; it is 15–19 nm wide with a pitch of about 6 nm.

Classification

There are four types of para-influenza viruses (1–4) with antigenically distinct epitopes. Nevertheless, there are conserved antigenic sites on the paramyxovirus envelope proteins, which cause the serological cross-reactions that are found between the para-influenza viruses, mumps virus and SV5. These are particularly close between para-influenza type 1 and a mouse variant (Sendai) that was used for some time as the antigen in complement fixation tests to detect antibody to the former. However, it is apparent that there are other cross-reactions that make the results of serological tests virtually uninterpretable. Responses to previously experienced paramyxoviruses as well as the currently infecting virus are found. This phenomenon of response to 'original antigenic sin' has been seen with other viruses such as influenza and coxsackie B viruses. In addition, type 4 has two subtypes, 4a and 4b, which can be distinguished only by neutralization or haemadsorption inhibition tests.

NDV infects chickens and other domestic birds. Its severity varies considerably from inapparent to fatal. Because some strains can cause major outbreaks with high mortality, an effective live vaccine based on avirulent strains has been developed. NDV is a typical paramyxovirus, and has been shown to be a rare cause of conjunctivitis in humans but only as a result of a laboratory accident. SV5 is often present in normal uninfected monkey kidney cell cultures but does not appear to reduce their sensitivity to other viruses and it does not cause illness in man. Other para-influenza viruses are natural pathogens for cattle and other domestic species; they are not known to infect humans.

Replication

Para-influenza viruses attach via the haemagglutinin to sialic acid-containing receptors on the cell surface. The F protein then fuses the viral envelope with the cell membrane, releasing the nucleocapsid into the cell. The negative-strand genome cannot act as messenger RNA (mRNA) and the RNA-dependent RNA polymerase carried within the virion is required to produce subgenomic-sized mRNA transcripts, which are translated to produce some of the early virus-specific polypeptides. These include a second RNA polymerase which copies the genome into full-length positive complementary strands which are in turn copied back into negative strands for transcription of later mRNA (coding for structural proteins) and for incorporation into new virions.

The viral components are assembled beneath the cell membrane and the surface HN and F proteins are incorporated into a stretch of membrane, converting it to viral envelope. This evaginates and buds off, enclosing a nucleocapsid as it does so to form a new virion. This is probably released from the host cell by the action of the neuraminidase component of the HN spikes. The incorporation of the HN protein into the cell membrane of infected cells allows red blood cells to adhere to their surface – the phenomenon of *haemadsorption*.

Clinical features and pathogenesis

The para-influenza viruses are mostly associated with:

- *Croup*, a harsh brassy cough in children familiar to many mothers as a middle-of-the-night irritant. It is due to a combination of tracheitis and laryngitis.
- Minor upper respiratory tract illness.
- Some cases of *bronchiolitis* and 'failure to thrive'.

They are responsible for 6–9% of respiratory infections for which a virus cause can be identified. The incubation period is from 3 to 6 days, during which the virus spreads locally within the respiratory tract.

Many infections occur in infants in the presence of circulating maternal antibody that does not appear to be protective or to make the illness worse.

Laboratory diagnosis

Rapid diagnosis may be made by immunofluorescent staining of exfoliated respiratory cells separated from well taken nasopharyngeal secretions. Preparation of adequately specific polyclonal sera is time-consuming but practicable, although it may not be possible to separate type 4 positives into subtypes. Preparing satisfactory monoclonal reagents to each type has not proved easy, and available commercial and other kits often offer only a polyvalent one. This reflects the problems of generating and identifying good type-specific monoclonal antibodies against a background of significant antigenic overlap between para-influenza viruses.

Similar antiviral antibodies may also be used in enzyme immuno-assays to identify viral antigen in specimens from the patient. They have the advantage of requiring only antigen to be present in the specimen while other assays require intact infected cells (for immunofluorescence) or infective virus (for culture). However, enzyme immuno-assays give no information on the quality of the specimen nor the extent of infection.

Virus may be isolated in monkey kidney cells. Visible cytopathic effects in the cell sheets are minimal and it will usually be necessary to show infection of the cells by the haemadsorption of 1% guinea-pig or human group O red blood cells. The infecting virus can be typed (or subtyped) by reacting the cell cultures with type-specific antisera before adding the red cells. The appropriate antibody inhibits the haemadsorption. The typing can be confirmed by a neutralization test or by immunofluorescence, but this is not usually necessary.

Serology is not used routinely in diagnosis. Type-specific antibodies may be detected by neutralization or haemadsorption inhibition but these tests are too complex for routine use. Other tests, such as complement fixation, are difficult to interpret because of cross-reactions between para-influenza viruses with mumps virus and, possibly, SV5 (see above).

Epidemiology and transmission

Epidemiologically, para-influenza type 1 infections are more frequent in the winter while type 3 is a summer infection, with small epidemics appearing reliably each year. Type 2 and 4a and 4b infections are more infrequent, in Newcastle upon Tyne at least, although elsewhere in Britain type 2 can be another summer visitor. Type 4 infections are underdiagnosed because of a lack of suitable reagents, but reported figures are too low for epidemiological patterns to be clear. The reasons underlying these individual epidemiological patterns are unknown.

Numerically, para-influenza infections are far fewer than those due to RS virus (q.v.) and most diagnosed infections are in pre-school and primary school children. Fatalities are very rare, and re-infections occur.

The viruses are present in respiratory secretions and are expelled during coughing and sneezing. Infection is acquired by inhalation and by person-to-person contact.

MUMPS

Description

Mumps virus is a typical paramyxovirus, indistinguishable in appearance from para-influenza viruses, measles virus and NDV. A similar herring-bone or zipper-like ribonucleoprotein is frequently seen to leak from the virions in preparations examined by electron microscopy, and may be the only unequivocally virus-like material seen. However, if it is found in CSF it is diagnostic of mumps meningitis because the only other similar virus found in the central nervous system, measles, does not reach levels detectable by electron microscopy in CSF.

The spikes on the envelope carry either a combined haemagglutinin and neuraminidase (HN) or a fusion (F) protein. The envelope also contains a matrix (M) protein. There is only one serotype, although monoclonal antibodies have shown minor variations in the various surface antigenic epitopes.

Replication

This is indistinguishable from that already described for para-influenza viruses. Infected cells show haemadsorption but little obvious damage. New virus is released by budding.

Clinical features and pathogenesis

Mumps is an 'iceberg' disease which, although common as a childhood infection, is often subclinical. Although the salivary glands are often involved, inapparent or minor infections are more common. Difficulty in recovering the virus and ambiguity in serology mean that infections are rarely confirmed by the laboratory. The USA was the first country to propose a vaccine to control mumps, but elsewhere surprise was expressed that anyone should bother. More complete monitoring of its activity suggests otherwise, and it is a full partner in the MMR vaccine (see below), not an afterthought.

Infection is probably by droplet into the respiratory tract. The incubation period is 14–18 days and is followed by a generalized illness with localization in the salivary glands, usually the parotids. The generalized phase is the usual 'flu-like' illness with fever and malaise, followed by developing pain in the parotid glands, which then swell rapidly. Much of the swelling is due to blockage of the efferent duct and the sucking of a lemon in front of a sufferer is a refined form of torture!

Neurological involvement is common in mumps (over 50% of infections), though the majority of cases are not clinically apparent. However, clinical meningitis remains the most common serious complication of mumps, occurring in 1–10% of patients with mumps parotitis. Meningitis (like any other complication of mumps) can occur before, during, after or in the absence of salivary gland involvement. Prior to the widespread use of MMR vaccine, mumps virus and the enteroviruses accounted for most of the cases of aseptic meningitis in the UK. Mumps meningitis is rarely fatal and complete recovery is usual. Meningo-encephalitis has been described, but is much rarer, carries a poorer prognosis and may result in long-term neurological sequelae or in death. Deafness and tinnitus have also been described, but are very rare.

In prepubertal children the acute illness usually subsides in 4–5 days, with complete recovery. The best known complication, in postpubertal males, is *orchitis*. This, though painful and causing softening and atrophy of the affected testicle, is usually unilateral and rarely causes sterility. *Oophoritis* also occurs in girls, and should be distinguished from a ruptured cyst or acute appendicitis. Both orchitis and oophoritis usually develop as the parotitis resolves, and a history of previous parotid pain and swelling will usually provide the clue.

The role of mumps in pancreatitis is difficult to establish. There may be abdominal pain in acute mumps but the levels of serum amylase do not correlate with the clinical picture. High levels may provide supportive evidence but are not diagnostic. Though uncomfortable it is not fatal.

Laboratory diagnosis

Typical mumps does not usually require laboratory confirmation but mild cases with little parotid swelling may not be noticed until complications develop. By this time virus may not be plentiful in the oropharynx. Direct demonstration by immunofluorescence on secretions is very rarely successful, and the diagnosis will depend on growing the virus from throat swabs, from saliva from affected glands or from the CSF. Collection of infected saliva is difficult but throat swabs provide a satisfactory specimen, although the virus may take up to a week to grow. Virus may be present in urine but not reliably so. The detection of ribonucleoprotein helix in CSF by electron microscopy is diagnostic, but the small quantities of fluid usually taken make this impractical.

Growth of virus in cell cultures (usually monkey kidney or HEp2 cells) produces little cytopathic effect, but the virus can be detected by haemadsorption, which can be inhibited by specific antiserum to confirm the presence of mumps virus.

The diagnosis can be made serologically by showing a rise in antibody between acute and convalescent specimens. Complement fixation is the usual test, using soluble (S) and viral (V) antigens. Antibodies to the S antigen are said to develop early, within a week of onset, followed by anti-V antibodies, which persist longer. However, these patterns are not invariable, and only a rise in titre to both antigens can be relied on. A rise to only one antigen in the absence of typical illness will be difficult to interpret and may reflect infection with other paramyxoviruses. Low rises or low static titres in cases of meningitis should also be interpreted with caution – cross-reactions with other paramyxoviruses provide traps for the unwary, and only isolation of the virus provides unequivocal evidence.

Other serological tests have been used, based on enzyme immuno-assays and single radial haemolysis. They have not been used as widely as complement fixation, being more often used in serological surveys or to complement other assays. Neutralization and haemagglutination inhibition tests are more complex to carry out and do not offer any advantages in routine diagnosis.

Epidemiology

Mumps is a worldwide disease, with humans the only known reservoir. Most infections are in children of school age, with those in adults being more severe and more likely to develop complications. Although epidemics occur, mumps is less infectious than measles or chickenpox. Infection appears to confer life-long immunity, and second infections do not occur.

Control

Some, but not very reliable, protection can be given by passive immunization; it may prevent severe orchitis even when given at the stage of parotitis.

Mumps vaccine, based on the *Jeryl Lynn* or *Urabe* strains, has been available as a monovalent vaccine for some time, particularly in the USA, but is now incorporated into a triple vaccine against measles, mumps and rubella (MMR). All three components are live-attenuated viruses, and the mumps component induces good antibody levels, lasting long enough to suggest that the recipients will not become susceptible as adults. A few cases of mild post-vaccine meningitis have been described but have not caused serious concern.

MEASLES

Description

Measles virus, a *morbillivirus*, is morphologically indistinguishable from para-influenza viruses, mumps virus and NDV, although there are important functional differences. The ribonucleoprotein helix is readily released from the virion and may, as with the others, be the only identifiable virus structure seen in the electron microscope. The virion structure includes:

- spikes, carrying a haemagglutinin but not a neuraminidase function
- an F protein that is also a haemolysin
- a matrix protein, M, below the envelope lipid bilayer.

There is only one serotype of measles virus and no subtypes have yet been recognized, although monoclonal antibodies show that there may be differences between wild and cultivated strains.

Human morbilliviruses are related to a number of animal strains. *Canine distemper* and *rinderpest* in cattle are well known relatives, but in the past few years other similar viruses have been isolated from seals (of several species), dolphins and porpoises, and an equine morbillivirus has reappeared which has apparently been transmitted to humans in contact, fatally in one case. All are distinct but can cause serious illness in their natural species though survivors develop solid immunity. There is partial cross-protection in ferrets between measles and canine distemper viruses.

Pathogenesis

Measles is an acute febrile illness, mostly in childhood, after an incubation period of 10–12 days. The onset is 'flu-like', with high fever, cough and conjunctivitis. *Koplik's spots* (red spots with a bluish–white centre on the buccal mucosa) may be present at this stage. After 1–2 days the acute symptoms decline, with the appearance of a widespread maculopapular rash. Viral antigen but not infectious virus may be found in the spots. The rash can be inhibited by local injections of immune serum, but will not appear at all in those who are severely immunocompromised, and this has been thought to point to an immunopathological (T cell-mediated) mechanism.

Over the next 10–14 days, recovery is usually complete as the rash fades, with considerable desquamation. Complications include:

- giant cell pneumonia, more common in adults
- otitis media
- post-measles encephalitis.

The pneumonia is due to direct invasion with virus, but the role of virus in the other two is uncertain. Measles encephalitis can cause severe and permanent mental impairment in those it does not kill. It is rare but disastrous.

The mortality of uncomplicated measles in immunocompetent well nourished children is low but rises rapidly with malnourishment (marked in Africa), in the immunocompromised and, to a much lesser extent, with age. It has also been devastating in isolated populations into whom it was introduced as a 'new' disease.

One further complication of measles is *subacute sclerosing panencephalitis* (SSPE), which occurs in children or early adolescents who have had measles early in life, usually under 2 years of age. It is a progressive and inevitably fatal degenerative disease. Within infected cells is a defective form of measles virus, which, because it is unable to induce the production of a functional M protein, is not released as complete virus from the cells. Patients deteriorate over several years, losing intellectual capacity before motor activities. Oligoclonal antibodies to measles virus proteins appear in the CSF, but the virus cannot be cultivated unless it is 'rescued' by co-cultivating neuronal cells with a susceptible cell type.

The virus has been linked with multiple sclerosis, Paget's disease of bone and Crohn's disease. In each case, tubular structures resembling measles nucleocapsids have been seen by thin section electron microscopy, and immunofluorescence has been used to demonstrate measles 'antigens' in biopsy material. Serum from about 50% of adults aged over 50 years, however, will fix complement with measles antigen although the individuals give no history suggestive of recent measles, and it is possible that auto-antibodies to a measles-like protein can be induced with age. If so, its significance is unknown but would be a factor in assessing measles involvement in older patients with chronic diseases. At present, the evidence linking measles virus in the aetiology of these diseases is less than compelling.

Laboratory diagnosis

Most cases of measles are diagnosed clinically, usually in the patient's home. Direct virological confirmation is often not attempted and is difficult to do in general practice. In hospital and particularly in immunocompromised patients, in whom the disease will often be rashless, the diagnosis may be made rapidly by immunofluorescence on exfoliated respiratory cells in well taken nasopharyngeal secretions. The presence of a large number of giant cells, particularly in patients on cytotoxic drugs, is a bad prognostic sign.

Other immuno-assays have been developed but give no feedback on the extent of the infection. Otherwise the virus may be grown in human fibroblasts, primary monkey cells and vero cells, although it does not grow readily.

Measles induces a good antibody response, and a rise in complement-fixing antibody is diagnostic. However, complement-fixing antibody in older patients is often detected and its significance is unknown. Other tests for antibody have been developed but are not used widely because diagnosis is usually made clinically. As measles vaccine (see below) is used more widely, clinical measles is becoming rarer and the need for laboratory confirmation of probable cases is rising. Antibody tests for measles-specific IgM and IgG on specimens of saliva are now available in some countries and avoid the need for venesection.

Epidemiology

Transmission is person-to-person, probably by respiratory droplets, but the associated conjunctivitis may also be a source. Despite some anecdotal evidence, there is no good evidence that distemper in dogs can be a source of measles in humans.

Measles epidemics occur every 2 years in developed countries in the absence of widespread use of the vaccine. This periodicity will be absent in isolated populations too small to maintain transmission (<400 000), in poverty and overcrowding and following widespread use of vaccine. The disease is ubiquitous throughout the world and, although a candidate for eradication, this may be difficult to achieve.

In tropical areas, particularly Africa, children become infected under the age of 1 year, and the mortality rises in consequence, reaching as high a figure as 42% in children under 4 years of age. Malnutrition is one of the main underlying causes of this excess mortality. The attack rate is also very high in isolated populations that have not experienced the disease for some years. In the Faroes in the 1840s, three-quarters of the population were infected, although the mortality was low. Most of those who were not infected were aged over 65 years, the interval since the last time the disease had been present in the islands, and confirms that infection gives prolonged immunity.

In the USA, where a serious attempt to eradicate measles has been made, the number of cases was reduced from over 500 000 per year to about 2000 (a reduction of over 99%), but outbreaks in immigrants and high-school students have recently emphasized the problems of preventing imported cases and of keeping up a high level of immunization.

Control

The first measles vaccine was a formalin-inactivated one. Although inducing circulating antibody, it was found that vaccinees exposed to natural measles were likely to develop atypical disease. The rash was more peripheral, involving the palms and soles, and pneumonia was common. It was later recognized that the vaccine had failed to induce adequate levels of antibody to the haemolytic F protein, and the immunity induced did not inhibit cell-to-cell spread of the virus. Consequently it was withdrawn and replaced with a live-attenuated vaccine. Early versions of the latter were only partially attenuated and were thought to offer only a choice of when to have measles, but with the added uncertainty over whether the resulting immunity was as long-lasting as that following natural measles. Later versions, containing the *Edmonston B* or *Schwarz* strains, have been better attenuated while giving a seroconversion rate of over 90%. So far (over about 30 years) the immunity induced by the vaccine has persisted and may be life-long.

In the UK, vaccine uptake has been relatively low until recently, when its use was promoted more strongly. A nationwide campaign was promoted in 1994–95 to avert a predicted epidemic. High levels of uptake were achieved, and no epidemic occurred. In contrast, eradication has been attempted in the USA, where evidence of vaccination or clinical disease is a legal requirement for school entry. This has reduced the disease incidence substantially but importation has so far frustrated any hopes of interrupting transmission completely.

Measles vaccine has now been combined with those against mumps and rubella to form the MMR vaccine. This combination of three attenuated viruses has been shown to induce good immunity to all three. Introduced initially in the USA, it is now the preferred vaccine in the UK for administration between 12 and 18 months.

Immunization in the high endemic regions of Africa still presents problems, however. Because many infants are infected before their first birthday, the vaccine has to be given under 6 months to have any effect. Passively transferred maternal antibody often interferes with the immune response to a live vaccine, and such early immunization does not always produce adequate immunity. A second dose at 12–13 months is then probably necessary but adds to the cost and the logistic difficulties. Solutions to both will have to be found before progress is made towards measles eradication in the developing world.

RESPIRATORY SYNCYTIAL VIRUS

Description

Superficially, RS virus resembles other paramyxoviruses, with a similar pleomorphic envelope studded with surface spikes that may be seen more clearly in the electron microscope than those on the para-influenza viruses, mumps and measles. The spikes may also be slightly longer, but neither the complete virus particles nor the nucleoprotein helix (with a diameter of 17 nm) are easy to visualize in the electron microscope. However, individual particles are generally larger than other paramyxoviruses (Fig. 50.2).

RS virus is placed in a separate genus – *Pneumovirus* – because of these minor physical differences and the lack of a haemagglutinin, a haemolysin or a neuraminidase. The nucleic acid is negative-sense single-stranded RNA of 15 kb, coding for both structural and non-structural proteins. RS virus has no haemagglutinin but has a G glycoprotein instead. It is a receptor for cell attachment but not to red blood cells, and differs in chemical composition from the HN protein of other paramyxoviruses. There are fusion (F), matrix (M), polymerase and nucleocapsid proteins. The F protein induces the syncytia in cell cultures from which the virus gets its name, and is probably responsible for both virus penetration and spread in the host. The virus is relatively fragile and may not survive even snap-freezing to –70°C. Specimens for isolation should not be frozen.

For most purposes there is only one serotype, although the advent of monoclonal antibodies has confirmed that there are two subtypes, A and B. In Newcastle upon Tyne, strains of subgroup A have been prevalent every year since 1974, but subgroup B strains have been more erratic and have not been isolated every winter. The reason for this phenomenon is unknown. Analysis of the genome has revealed further minor differences which appear unimportant in diagnosis (i.e. do not represent major antigenic variations) but which have allowed various strain lineages to be recognized. These may reflect selection pressure by immunity but new ones are found widely distributed in the world at the same time and their significance is not yet clear.

RS virus is also a significant pathogen in cattle and infects chimpanzees readily – early isolates were termed *chimpanzee coryza agent*. Both goats and sheep may be infected naturally, and there is evidence that several other domestic and rodent species are susceptible, either naturally, or after some adaptation.

Clinical features and pathogenesis

The most serious illness caused by RS virus is *bronchiolitis* in young babies, in whom the bronchiolar inflammation acts as a one-way valve leading to hyperinflation of the lungs (very characteristic on X-ray), but it is also associated with minor upper tract infections and non-specific 'failure to thrive'. The peak incidence is in those under 1 year of age, and there are (possibly as a consequence) annual winter epidemics. This infection is potentially life-threatening, particularly in those with bronchopulmonary dysplasia or congenital heart defects, or in those who are immunosuppressed or immunodeficient. In normal babies it is rarely fatal where medical staff have the experience and facilities for appropriate management. RS virus has been recovered from some victims of the *sudden infant death syndrome* (SIDS). Although it may have contributed to the death it is clear that other factor(s) are also significant.

The main clinical feature is bronchiolitis, but the upper respiratory tract remains infected, and this makes it possible to confirm the diagnosis. If RS virus is present in the nasopharynx and there is clinical evidence of lower respiratory tract involvement, RS virus is likely to be responsible.

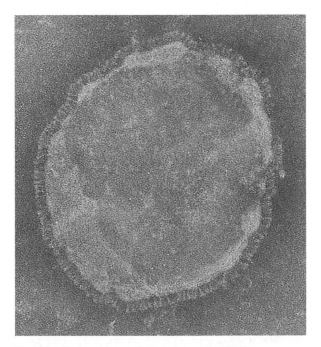

Fig. 50.2 Electron micrograph of respiratory syncytial virus. Phosphotungstic acid stain, ×200 000.

Recovery is apparently complete, although it has been suggested that the infection predisposes to chronic respiratory tract disease (asthma, bronchiectasis, etc.). This has yet to be confirmed although studies are in progress.

The sequelae to the use of an inactivated vaccine (see below) have led to the suggestion that some of the severity of bronchiolitis is due to hypersensitivity induced by an earlier infection. Studies in various centres have neither confirmed this theory nor fully excluded it. There is much still to learn about the pathogenesis of RS virus.

In older children and adults, the virus causes only minor infections, possibly because their air passages are larger. Re-infections are common and in adults may cause no more than a cold. However, the failure of acute infections to immunize, even in the immunocompetent, highlights the difficulty of producing a vaccine.

There have been reports of severe illness, with some fatalities, in old people's homes as well as in the elderly living in the community. The under-recognition of RS in these groups may be due to the difficulty in confirming a virological diagnosis in adults and the elderly (see below). An associated neurological syndrome has also been described, but whether RS virus is the cause is unproven.

Laboratory diagnosis

During the acute phase of illness virus may be readily demonstrated in nasopharyngeal secretions (which are usually copious) by immunofluorescence, enzyme immuno-assays or culture.

Rapid diagnosis in less than 1 h with commercially available conjugated monoclonal antibodies can be made reliably by immunofluorescence, provided an adequate number of desquamated respiratory cells are collected in the secretions. Generally, similar results can be obtained with enzyme immuno-assays. Such assays may be less sensitive when compared to culture, but the virus grows slowly and positive results will come too late to influence management. While antigen detection and culture methods are good for diagnosing RS virus infections in infants and young children, they are less reliable in adults and the elderly because the levels of virus or antigen are less in adult secretions compared with infants.

Serology using complement fixation is generally not helpful. Many of the patients are too young to respond reliably and even adults do not always produce a detectable rise in serum antibody levels. However, immuno-assays based on the G and F proteins seem to offer a more reliable serological test, especially in adults where other options are limited, but they are not yet widely or commercially available.

Treatment

Appropriate management includes use of oxygen, if indicated, and tube feeding to maintain energy intake if the baby has difficulty in suckling. Most babies can be managed symptomatically by these measures. The only specific antiviral drug available for chemotherapy is (t)ribavirin. In vivo there is some evidence of efficacy when given as a small-particle aerosol, although it is apparently not effective when given by intravenous infusion. The evidence of efficacy by any route is not overwhelming. This may be because the most affected parts of the lungs are also the least well aerated and therefore least accessible to the aerosolized drug. The drug is expensive and its recommended use is confined to those babies who are at high risk from rampant RS virus because they have congenital heart or lung abnormalities. Even in these babies the virus may have caused damage before the drug can be given.

Recently, hyperimmune RS virus immunoglobulin and humanized monoclonal antibodies have become available for prevention and/or treatment of RS infections. These preparations are very expensive and their use may be difficult to justify except in groups at very high risk, such as in very premature babies or those with pre-existing bronchopulmonary dysplasia.

Epidemiology

In temperate climates in both the northern and southern hemispheres, RS virus causes a substantial winter epidemic every year. In the Newcastle upon Tyne/Tyne and Wear conurbation (total population about 1 million), the annual number of virologically confirmed diagnoses regularly exceeds 500. Similar figures are obtained elsewhere where adequate facilities for diagnosis exist. Most infected babies reach hospital, and the failure to recover it from babies with 'colds' attending well-baby clinics in Newcastle upon Tyne has suggested that comparatively few cases go unrecognized.

Why it induces an epidemic every October/November is unknown. In other regions of the world the pattern can be markedly different. In Hong Kong, a semitemperate area, there is an equally clear epidemic, but in the hot and humid months of the summer. Therefore, RS virus epidemics do not always correspond to the same short-term climatic factors (temperature, humidity, etc.), and sporadic cases occur anyway throughout the year. The virus is distributed all over the world, but its activities in tropical, overcrowded and poor areas are under-recorded so far.

The significance, if any, of subtypes in explaining these RS virus phenomena is still under investigation.

Control

A formalin-inactivated crude whole-virus vaccine was tried in the 1960s. It induced good levels of circulating antibody but failed to protect the recipients, who actually became more ill than placebo controls when subsequently exposed to RS virus. As with measles, this may have been due to the vaccine failing to induce the right protective antibodies. Subsequently, several live vaccines based on cold adaptation, temperature-sensitive mutants or administration by a different route (intramuscularly) were tried but none has proved satisfactory (through either insufficient attenuation or inadequate immunogenicity).

A major obstacle in developing a good vaccine is the fact that the peak of disease occurs within the first year of life, and thus a safe vaccine immunogenic to such young and immunologically immature recipients is difficult to prepare. The increasing recognition that RS virus causes morbidity in the elderly may lead to consideration of the preparation of an adult vaccine, possibly an easier challenge to meet. In the future, genetic engineering offers new ways to prepare vaccines that contain only the relevant antigens in an appropriate viral or bacterial vector, but at present (2002) there is no satisfactory vaccine.

Newly discovered paramyxoviruses: Nipah and Hendra viruses

During 1998–99, an outbreak of respiratory disease in pigs associated with encephalitis in humans occurred in Malaysia. There were over 200 human cases, with 105 deaths. The causative agent was found to be a paramyxovirus given the name Nipah. It is distinct genetically from all the other paramyxoviruses and is most closely related to Hendra, another recently (1994) discovered paramyxovirus causing epidemic fatal respiratory disease in horses and which can be transmitted to man, resulting in at least one fatal infection.

The taxonomic position of these new viruses has yet to be established, but they will most probably be put in a separate genus within the *paramyxoviridae*. Fruit bats appear to be the natural reservoir of both viruses, with transmission to mammals (including man) an exceptional event. Nevertheless, these discoveries underline the fact that new pathogens capable of causing disease in man continue to emerge and we must be prepared for the unexpected.

RECOMMENDED READING

Mandell G L, Bennett J E, Dolin R (eds) 2000 *Principles and Practice of Infectious Disease*, 5th edn. Churchill Livingstone, Philadelphia

Zuckerman A J, Banatvala J E, Pattison J R (eds) 2000 *Principles and Practice of Clinical Virology*, 4th edn. Wiley, Chichester

51

Arboviruses: alphaviruses, flaviviruses and bunyaviruses

Encephalitis; yellow fever; dengue; haemorrhagic fever; miscellaneous tropical fevers; undifferentiated fever

A. D. T. Barrett and S. C. Weaver

The name 'arbo' (arthropod-borne) virus has been used for many years to denote viruses transmitted biologically by arthropod (mainly insect) vectors. However, it is now recognized that there are many different taxa of arboviruses. Indeed, there are more than 500 individual arbovirus species that are now officially classified in six virus families. Many arboviruses are highly pathogenic and are classified at biosafety level 3 (BSL-3) or BSL-4 (UK, Category 3 or 4 pathogens). As there are many similarities in their transmission cycles and in the diseases that they cause, they will be considered together in this chapter.

Arboviruses were defined by a World Health Organization Scientific Group as 'viruses that are maintained in nature principally, or to an important extent, through biological transmission between susceptible vertebrate hosts by haemotophagous arthropods or through transovarian and possible venereal transmission in arthropods; the viruses multiply and produce viraemia in the vertebrates, multiply in the tissues of arthropods, and are passed on to new vertebrates by the bites of arthropods after a period of extrinsic incubation.'

Certain viruses within the six families containing arboviruses are not transmitted by arthropods, but are maintained in nature within rodent reservoirs that may transmit infection directly to humans. These include the *Hantavirus* genus of the family *Bunyaviridae*.

DESCRIPTION

Classification

Arboviruses are classified within six families (Table 51.1). Most are members of the families Togaviridae, Flaviviridae and Bunyaviridae; some are assigned to the families Reoviridae (the genera *Coltivirus*, e.g. Colorado tick fever virus, and *Orbivirus*, e.g. Bluetongue viruses), Orthomyxoviridae (e.g. Thogotovirus) and the Rhabdoviridae (members of the genera *Vesiculovirus*, e.g. vesicular stomatitis

virus, and *Lyssavirus*). Within the Togaviridae, only one (*Alphavirus*) of the two genera contains arthropod-borne viruses; the other genus *Rubivirus*, contains rubella virus, which is not arthropod-borne, as its sole member (see Chapter 52). The Flaviviridae contains three genera (*Flavivirus*, *Pestivirus* and *Hepacivirus*) but only the *Flavivirus* genus contains arthropod-borne viruses. Pestiviruses only infect vertebrate animals (e.g. bovine viral diarrhoea virus) and hepatitis C virus is described in Chapter 52. The Bunyaviridae consists of five genera (*Bunyavirus*, *Hantavirus*, *Nairovirus*, *Phlebovirus* and *Tospovirus*), containing a total of over 300 species, and represents the largest virus family. The *Tospovirus* genus contains plant viruses that are transmitted by vectors (thrips) while the *Hantavirus* genus contains viruses that are transmitted by rodents rather than arthropods.

Many arboviruses show close relationships with other arboviruses. The classification of arboviruses into individual species has been made on the basis of neutralization or other serological tests where the virus shows a four-fold or greater difference in neutralization titre from all other viruses. Clusters of viruses that show antigenic overlap in haemagglutination inhibition (HI), enzyme immunosorbent assay (ELISA) or complement fixation (CF) tests are termed serogroups or antigenic complexes. In recent years the molecular properties and nucleotide sequences of genomes of viruses have increasingly contributed to classification. Table 51.2 lists some of the important members.

Properties

Arboviruses share common biological attributes (see Table 51.1).

1. Most induce fatal encephalitis 1–10 days after intracerebral inoculation of suckling mice aged less than 48 h; some also induce fatal encephalitis after intracerebral inoculation of weaned mice aged 3–4 weeks.

Table 51.1   Characteristic properties of arboviruses

Property	Arbovirus family (principal genus)					
	Togaviridae (*Alphavirus*)	Flaviviridae (*Flavivirus*)	Bunyaviridae (*Bunyavirus*)[a]	Rhabdoviridae (*Rhabdovirus*)[b]	Reoviridae (*Reovirus*)[c]	Orthomyxoviridae
Symmetry[d]	Cubic	Cubic	Helical	Bullet-shaped	Cubic	Cubic
Total diameter (nm)	60–65	40–60	80–100	180×85	60–80	15–120
Nucleic acid	(+)ssRNA	(+)ssRNA	(−)ssRNA and ambisense	(−)ssRNA	dsRNA	(−) ssRNA
Molecular weight ($\times 10^6$)	4.2–4.4	4.2–4.4	0.3–3.1	3.5–4.6	0.2–3.0	
No. of molecules	1	1	3	1	10–12	6–7
No. of viruses	28	68	318	63	77	2
Inactivation by diethyl ether or sodium deoxycholate	+	+	+	+	−	+

ssRNA, single-stranded RNA; dsRNA, double-stranded RNA.
[a] Other important genera: *Nairovirus*, *Phlebovirus* (arthropod-borne); *Hantavirus* (not arthropod-borne).
[b] See Chapter 58.
[c] See Chapter 54.
[d] All have enveloped virions (except Reoviridae).

Table 51.2   Some important arboviruses

Family and genus	Number of members	Some important members	Comments
Togaviridae			
Alphavirus	28	Western equine encephalitis	Mosquito-borne
		Eastern equine encephalitis	
		Venezuelan equine encephalitis	
		Chikungunya	
		Ross River	
Flaviviridae			
Flavivirus	68	St Louis encephalitis	Mosquito-borne
		Japanese encephalitis	
		Murray Valley encephalitis	
		Yellow fever	
		Dengue	
		Ilheus	
		West Nile	
		Louping ill	Tick-borne
		Powassan	
		Tick-borne encephalitis	
		Kyasanur Forest	
		Omsk haemorrhagic fever	
Bunyaviridae	318		
Bunyavirus	172	La Crosse	California (CAL) serogroup
		Snowshoe hare	
		Oropouche	
Phlebovirus	51	Rift Valley fever	
		Punta Toro	
		Sandfly fever	
		Toscana	
Nairovirus	34	Crimean-Congo haemorrhagic fever	
Hantavirus	15	Sin Nombre (not arthropod-borne)	

2. Haemagglutinin for erythrocytes of geese or newly hatched chicks. Most arboviruses are capable of agglutinating erythrocytes (haemagglutination) and this ability is inhibited by antiserum against viruses within the same serogroup. Seroreactivity against viruses from dissimilar serogroups is generally weak or of low titre. ELISA and CF tests can also detect arbovirus antigens.

3. Many arboviruses multiply in continuous polyploid tissue cultures of mammalian cells incubated at 37°C, such as grivet monkey kidney (Vero) and baby hamster kidney (BHK).

4. Many arboviruses, such as dengue and Ross River viruses, multiply in continuous tissue cultures of mosquito cells when incubated at 34°C or lower temperatures; *Aedes albopictus* C6–36 mosquito cells are often used. In general, mosquito-borne viruses do not replicate in tick cell cultures and vice versa. Multiplication is often detected by immunofluorescence tests.

5. Mosquito-borne arboviruses multiply after oral feeding or intrathoracic injection of several *Aedes* and *Culex* mosquito species, after incubation at 4–28°C (depending on the mosquito species), and mosquitoes transmit virus by biting susceptible vertebrates; virus multiplication in mosquito tissues is revealed by specific immunofluorescence, particularly in salivary glands and in central nervous tissue. Intrathoracic susceptibility of mosquitoes to dengue and California serogroup agents is 10–100 times higher than mammalian tissue cultures or suckling mice. Some arboviruses, including members of the *Bunyavirus* and *Phlebovirus* genera of the Bunyaviridae, *Flavivirus* genus of the Flaviviridae and some members of the *Vesiculovirus* genus of the family Rhabdoviridae, are also transmitted transovarially by vectors. Ticks do not normally transmit mosquito-borne arboviruses; mosquitoes do not normally transmit tick-borne arboviruses. Sandfly-borne viruses are transmitted only by sandflies (*Phlebotomus* spp. and *Lutzomyia* spp.).

6. Tick-borne arboviruses multiply after oral feeding to larval or nymphal ixodid ticks (hard ticks of the genera *Dermacentor* and *Ixodes*). The virus is transferred trans-stadially to the next developmental stage (nymph or adult, respectively), which then transmits virus by biting susceptible vertebrates.

REPLICATION

The replication of the various arboviruses differs significantly and is one of the major criteria used in their classification.

Alphaviruses

Alphaviruses enter cells by receptor-mediated endocytosis. Several different protein receptors have been identified, including the high-affinity laminin receptor. Following a drop in pH that occurs in endosomes, the virion fuses with an endosome membrane via the E1 envelope glycoprotein. The nucleocapsid is then released into the cytoplasm where it binds to ribosomes, and the non-structural proteins are translated directly from the genomic RNA. RNA replication occurs in complexes comprised of the non-structural proteins and cellular proteins, which are associated with cytoplasmic membranes. Genomic RNA of around 11.5 kb is messenger-sense (positive strand), and serves as a template for full length negative-sense RNA synthesis; these negative-sense RNAs are a template for the production of positive-sense genomic RNA, as well as a subgenomic mRNA designated 26S that encodes the structural proteins. Both of these RNAs are capped at the 5′ end and polyadenylated at the 3′ end. Regulation of positive- versus negative-strand synthesis occurs via changes in the non-structural protease activity mediated by different cleavage patterns of the non-structural polyprotein. The 26S message is translated to yield a polyprotein comprised of the capsid and envelope glycoproteins. The capsid is cleaved co-translationally in the cytoplasm via its own protease activity, and the remaining polyprotein enters the endoplasmic reticulum where it is processed through the secretory pathway to yield glycosylated E2 and E1 protein heterodimers in the plasma membrane. Genomic RNA combines in the cytoplasm with 240 copies of the capsid protein to form a nucleocapsid, and nucleocapsids interact with the cytoplasmic tail of the E2 envelope protein to mediate budding, whereby 240 E2/E1 protein heterodimers and a portion of the plasma membrane are incorporated into the mature virion of about 70 nm.

Flaviviruses

Morphologically, flaviviruses are similar to alphaviruses in several respects but are smaller, with a diameter of approximately 50 nm. The molecular biology of flaviviruses is different from the alphaviruses and has resulted in the viruses being classified into different virus families, the Flaviviridae and Togaviridae, respectively. Flavivirus virions have three structural proteins; the viral RNA genome is encapsidated by a small core protein and there are two proteins, termed the membrane (M) and envelope (E), on the outside of virus particles. The E protein is the major protein of the virus. It is normally glycosylated, has haemagglutination activity and is the target of neutralizing antibodies. Note that the

NS3 protein (see below) contains the majority of T cell epitopes. The virus genome is one single-stranded, positive-sense RNA molecule that is 11–12 000 nucleotides in length. Unlike alphaviruses, flaviviruses do not have a poly A tail at the 3′ terminus of the genome. The 5′ one-third of the genome encodes the three structural protein genes while the remaining two-thirds of the genome encodes seven non-structural protein genes (NS1, NS2A, NS2B, NS3, NS4A, NS4B and NS5). NS2B and the amino terminus of NS3 function together as a serine protease, while NS5 encodes the RNA-dependent RNA polymerase of the virus. Flaviviruses replicate in the cytoplasm of cells. Since the genome of flaviviruses is positive-sense RNA, the input virion RNA is translated as a single open reading frame to generate a polyprotein precursor that is rapidly post-translationally processed by viral and cellular proteases to yield the structural and non-structural proteins that enable the virus to replicate. Unlike alphaviruses, flavivirus particles assemble by budding through Golgi vesicles and contain prM, a precursor to M protein. However, mature virions are produced at the cell surface where the 'pr' portion of prM is cleaved by the cell enzyme furin to yield the mature M protein found in virions.

Bunyaviruses

Like the Flaviviridae and Togaviridae, members of the Bunyaviridae are icosahedral enveloped viruses. However, Bunyaviruses have a diameter of 100–120 nm and are therefore larger than the alphaviruses and flaviviruses. Although alphaviruses, flaviviruses and bunyaviruses all have RNA genomes totalling approximately 11–12 000 nucleotides, the Bunyaviruses have a tripartite genome where the genetic material of the viruses is divided between three pieces of single-stranded RNA termed large (L), medium (M) and small (S) segments. The L RNA encodes the RNA-dependent RNA polymerase that is also termed the L protein. The M RNA encodes two glycoproteins, termed G1 and G2, that are found on the surface of virions and the *Bunyavirus, Tospovirus* and *Phlebovirus* genera have a non-structural protein, NSm, whose function is unknown. The S RNA encodes a nucleocapsid (N) protein. The *Bunyavirus* genus also contains a non-structural protein, termed NSs, in an overlapping reading frame while the *Phlebovirus* and *Tospovirus* genera also contain the NSs gene. The tripartite genome enables bunyaviruses to undergo genetic reassortment whereby a cell infected by two or more bunyaviruses can result in progeny viruses containing the segments from different viruses. Reassortment has been shown to take place in nature between closely related bunyaviruses and is considered to be a process that contributes to genetic variation and evolution.

Unlike alphaviruses and flaviviruses, the bunyaviruses have a negative-sense RNA genome. Thus, virions have to contain the virus RNA-dependent RNA polymerase so that the virus genome can be transcribed in cells to generate mRNAs of different viral genes. In addition, the NSm gene of the *Tospovirus* genus and the NSs gene of the *Phlebovirus* and *Tospovirus* genera are encoded as genes in the positive-sense orientation. Thus, the S and M RNA segments of Tospoviruses and the S RNA of Phleboviruses are termed ambisense RNAs to denote that the open reading frames of the genes are in opposite orientations. Bunyaviruses replicate in the cytoplasm of cells and, like the flaviviruses, assemble by budding through Golgi vesicles.

PATHOGENESIS

Natural vertebrate infection by arboviruses is initiated when mosquitoes or other arthropods deposit saliva in extravascular tissues while blood-feeding. In the case of alphaviruses, murine model systems using needle inoculations indicate that the initial site of replication is the Langerhans cell. Alphavirus replication appears to stimulate:

- the migratory response of the Langerhans cell to the lymph nodes
- the accumulation of leucocytes in the draining lymph node, where local replication produces viraemia.

Arboviruses induce high titres of *viraemia* in susceptible vertebrates 1–4 days after parenteral inoculation or following bites by infected arthropods; viraemia persists for up to several days and serves as a source of infective blood meals for other biting arthropods. Invasion of the central nervous system (CNS) via the olfactory nervous tract may ensue in some infections while other viruses cross the blood–brain barrier. In alphaviral infections accompanied by rash and arthritis, virus replication and necrosis occurs in the epidermis and possibly the muscles, tendons and connective tissue. Infection of macrophages may mediate musculoskeletal pathology via suppression of cytokine induction. Wild bird and mammal reservoir hosts regularly exhibit viraemia without symptoms.

Antibodies are first detected when the fever subsides, usually within 5–10 days after infection, and may persist for many years. Antibodies are of the IgM class for 1–7 weeks after infection; subsequently they are of the IgG class.

Arboviruses capable of producing encephalitis typically cause a spectrum of disease:

- inapparent infection
- acute encephalitis.

Within the central nervous system, arboviruses multiply in and induce necrosis of neurones, which in turn become surrounded by microglia, forming glial knots. There is also evidence of apoptosis for some virus infections. An age-dependence of CNS disease has been observed for many arboviruses, and animal model systems indicate that age-dependent apoptosis of neurones may explain this phenomenon. Perivascular cuffing with mononuclear cells affects many cerebral blood vessels. Usually there is concomitant meningitis with accumulation of mononuclear cells in the subarachnoid space and hyperaemia of adjacent capillaries. It is important to note that although many subjects become infected with encephalitis viruses, relatively few develop illness manifested as meningitis or encephalitis. Invasion of the CNS appears to be a critical determinant in the pathogenesis and is in part due to the level of viraemia.

There is little information about the role of the immune system, although it may have a role in the pathogenesis of dengue haemorrhagic fever and dengue shock syndrome, which is seen in young children who are experiencing a second dengue virus infection. Antigen–antibody complex formation has been thought to underlie the syndrome, which is associated with:

- increased capillary permeability
- shock
- haemorrhage.

However, it is known that the uptake of virus into macrophages is enhanced in the presence of antibody, as the virus–antibody complexes bind to Fc receptors. In this way there is likely to be a great increase in the uptake of virus and hence the release of virus from macrophages.

CLINICAL FEATURES

The tissue tropism of arboviruses can be divided into three categories:

- infections of the CNS (e.g. encephalitis, aseptic meningitis)
- infections of the visceral organs (e.g. hepatitis and haemorrhagic fevers)
- febrile infections.

Arbovirus infections of humans become clinically manifest according to the target organ principally infected (Table 51.3). These include the following syndromes.

Encephalitis

For many arboviruses, encephalitis is most common in children and/or the elderly. Illness leading to encephalitis typically has an abrupt onset within 1 week of infection, with headache, fever, myalgia, dysthesias, and sometimes lethargy, chills, dizziness, nausea, vomiting and prostration. Inflammation of the throat, cervical lymphadenitis and abdominal tenderness are also common. Symptoms usually subside after several days, but may recrudesce later. Progression to encephalitis may occur rapidly, or a prodromal illness may last 1 week or more. Severe CNS disease is accompanied by neck stiffness, motor weakness and paralysis, meningismus, cranial nerve palsy, confusion, convulsions and somnolescence, leading to coma. Rigidity or weakness of the limbs may occur along with reduction in reflexes. White blood cells, predominantly lymphocytes, and elevated glucose may occur in the cerebrospinal fluid (CSF), which can exhibit elevated pressure. Peripheral blood cell counts may be elevated with a left shift. During most outbreaks of arboviral encephalitis, a proportion of cases develop aseptic meningitis only, without significant neuronal involvement, while up to 50% of cases recover from acute encephalitis to suffer from neuropsychiatric sequelae that may last from months to years. These sequelae vary from physiological impairment to mental disorders.

Yellow fever

Yellow fever is caused by a mosquito-borne flavivirus that is found in tropical South America and Africa. The disease is characterized by the sudden onset of headache and fever with temperatures exceeding 39°C, and is accompanied by generalized myalgia, nausea and vomiting, after an incubation period of 3–6 days. Jaundice may appear by the third day of illness, but frequently this is mild or absent. Haematemesis and melaena may occur from bleeding into the gastro-intestinal tract and epistaxis and bleeding gums may also be noted. Albuminuria and oliguria may also begin suddenly during the first week of illness. In severe cases, death may occur from 3 to 6 days after the onset of illness, and midzonal necrosis is observed in the liver. The case fatality rate is estimated at 20% but may be as high as 50%. Mild cases may develop fever, headache and myalgia only, without gastro-intestinal upsets, jaundice or albuminuria. In such cases, the diagnosis is frequently achieved only by demonstration of rising levels of antibody or occasionally by the isolation of virus from the blood.

Dengue

Dengue is caused by four serologically related flaviviruses called dengue-1, dengue-2, dengue-3 and dengue-4. These viruses are found in most tropical parts

Table 51.3 Clinical syndromes associated with selected arboviruses and their geographical distribution

Syndrome	Genus	Serogroup (vector)	Causative arbovirus serotype		Geographical distribution
Encephalitis or aseptic meningitis	*Alphavirus*	(mosquito)	EEE	Eastern equine encephalitis	Eastern Canada, USA, Caribbean
			VEE	Venezuelan equine encephalitis	Central and South America
			WEE	Western equine encephalitis	Western Canada and USA, Caribbean
	Flavivirus	(mosquito)	JE	Japanese encephalitis	Orient (Japan to Malaysia)
			MVE	Murray Valley encephalitis	Australia
			SLE	St Louis encephalitis	Canada, USA, Central America
		(tick)	LI	Louping ill	Scotland, Northern Ireland
			POW	Powassan	Canada, Northern USA
			TBE	Tick-borne encephalitis complex	Central and northern Europe, Siberia
	Bunyavirus	CAL (mosquito)	LAC	La Crosse	USA
			SSH	Snowshoe hare	Canada
Yellow fever	*Flavivirus*	(mosquito)	YF	Yellow fever	Tropical Africa, Caribbean, tropical South America
Dengue	*Flavivirus*	(mosquito)	DEN	Dengue (four types)	Entire tropical zone
Haemorrhagic fever	*Alphavirus*	(mosquito)	CHIK	Chikungunya	East Africa, India, South-east Asia
	Flavivirus	(mosquito)	DEN	Dengue (four types)	India, Philippines, South-east Asia, Oceania
		(tick)	KFD	Kyasanur Forest disease	India
			OMSK	Omsk haemorrhagic fever	Siberia
	Nairovirus	CCHF (tick)	CCHF	Crimean-Congo haemorrhagic fever	Central and Southern Africa, Asia, Europe
Miscellaneous tropical fevers	*Alphavirus*	(mosquito)	CHIK	Chikungunya	East Africa, India, South-east Asia
			RR	Ross River[a]	Australia, Oceania
	Flavivirus	(mosquito)	ILH	Ilheus	Caribbean, South America
			WN	West Nile	Central and Northern Africa
	Bunyavirus	SIM (mosquito)	ORO	Oropouche	Caribbean, South America
	Phlebovirus	PHL (mosquito)	RVF	Rift Valley fever	Northern, Eastern and Southern Africa
		PHL (sandfly)	PT	Punta Toro	Central America
		PHL (sandfly)	SFN	Sandfly fever - Naples	Mediterranean
	Vesiculovirus	VS (sandfly)	VSI	Vesicular stomatitis - Indiana	USA, Central America[b]
Undifferentiated fever	*Coltivirus*	CTF (tick)	CTF	Colorado tick fever	Western USA[c]

[a] Ross River virus infections frequently exhibit polyarthralgia.
[b] See Chapter 58.
[c] See Chapter 54.

of the world, including Africa, Asia and Central/South America. The disease dengue presents as an acute febrile illness with chills, headache, retro-ocular pain, body aches and arthralgia in more than 90% of apparent cases, accompanied by nausea or vomiting and a maculopapular rash resembling measles lasting 2–7 days in about 60% of cases. Illness usually persists for 7 days followed with fever remitting after 3–5 days followed by relapse ('*saddleback fever*'), and pains in the bones,

muscles and joints sufficiently severe to earn the epithet '*breakbone fever*'. Rash occurs more commonly in patients less than 14 years of age. Complete recovery is the rule. The incubation period is 5–11 days.

Dengue haemorrhagic fever

This is a less common manifestation of dengue, with about 5000 cases per year, mainly affecting children. It is occasionally accompanied by a shock syndrome, known as dengue shock syndrome, with a case fatality rate of 50%. These two severe forms of dengue are observed in patients who undergo successive infection with two different dengue viruses (e.g. a primary dengue-1 infection followed by a secondary infection with dengue-2 virus). After an acute onset, fever of 40°C, accompanied by vomiting and anorexia, enlarged liver and petechiae persists for 5–10 days. This is followed by a complete recovery unless shock supervenes; this occurs in 7–10% of cases from 2 to 7 days after onset, usually accompanied by haematemesis and melaena. Although dengue haemorrhagic fever with shock syndrome was initially recognized in South-east Asia in 1951, it has since occurred in the south-west Pacific, Caribbean and South American countries.

Miscellaneous tropical fevers

These comprise elevation of temperature beyond 39°C, together with any combination of headache, myalgia, malaise, nausea or vomiting, and sometimes accompanied by maculopapular rash or polyarthralgia, i.e. a dengue-like syndrome, but without haemorrhagic manifestations or the shock syndrome. Tropical fevers arise from infection with a wide variety of arboviruses (Table 51.3).

Undifferentiated fever

An example from the USA is Colorado tick fever (genus *Coltivirus*) in which symptoms of chilliness, headaches, retro-orbital pain and generalized aches, especially in the back and limbs, appear 3–6 days after bites by infected *Dermacentor andersoni* ticks in wooded areas of the Rocky Mountain region. Fever of 39–40°C often shows a biphasic course, with eventual defervescence within 1 week, followed by complete recovery.

Hantavirus pulmonary syndrome

This syndrome, due to the hantavirus Sin Nombre, was first recognized in south-western USA during 1993. The sudden onset of fever, myalgia, headache, cough and nausea or vomiting is accompanied by rapid respirations exceeding 20 per min, temperature above 38°C and hypotension. Extensive interstitial and alveolar infiltrates are observed on radiographic examination of the lungs, accompanied by reduced oxygen saturation below 90 mmHg. Fatal cases develop progressive pulmonary oedema with hypoxia and severe hypotension (systolic blood pressure below 86 mmHg) and die 2–16 (mean 8) days after onset of symptoms; the case fatality rate may exceed 50%. Non-fatal cases usually recover within 1–3 weeks.

General principles

Certain epidemiological principles apply to human illnesses induced by arboviruses:

- For each syndrome, several different virus families may be involved, as in encephalitis due to western equine encephalitis (WEE), Japanese encephalitis (JE) or La Crosse (LAC) virus infections.
- There is a high proportion of subclinical infections to clinical illnesses, e.g. 64:1 to 209:1 for St Louis encephalitis (SLE) virus, but this proportion is considerably lower for dengue and miscellaneous tropical fevers.
- There may be localization of a particular virus within a particular geographic zone such as: (a) Powassan (POW) virus in forested areas of eastern North America; (b) WEE virus in irrigated farmlands of western North America and Argentina, where SLE virus is also prevalent; and (c) Murray Valley encephalitis (MVE) virus in Australia. However, dengue is distributed widely throughout tropical regions of each continent and in Oceania.
- Virus transmission by the bite of culicine mosquitoes or ixodid ticks occurs after ingestion of relatively small titres (0.1–10 plaque-forming units) of virus in blood meals from naturally infected viraemic vertebrates after extrinsic incubation periods from less than 1 to 3 weeks at usual summertime temperatures.
- Viraemia develops asymptomatically in birds (some alphaviruses and mosquito-borne flaviviruses) and in mammals (some alphaviruses, bunyaviruses, tick-borne flaviviruses and orbiviruses) at titres sufficient to infect engorging mosquitoes or ticks. However, some vertebrates are dead-end hosts due to low viraemias that prevent infection of engorging vectors (e.g. humans infected with JE virus).

LABORATORY DIAGNOSIS

Diagnosis of arbovirus infections depends on:

- the isolation of virus from blood, CSF or tissues
- detection of arbovirus-specific RNA in, blood, CSF or tissue
- serology.

Although virus isolation is an important aspect of diagnosis, it should be noted that this is normally a very slow process and is unlikely to generate results until after an acute virus infection. Detection of virus-specific RNA by reverse transcriptase polymerase chain reaction (RTPCR) is a rapid approach to diagnosis but is dependent on the availability of oligonucleotide primers that will specifically amplify a region of the genome of a given virus. Given the large number of arboviruses, there has to be significant differential diagnosis prior to selection of appropriate primers. Similarly, enzyme-linked immunosorbent assays (ELISAs) can be used to detect serum antibodies from patients. However, these assays are dependent on availability of virus and/or antigens for use in ELISAs. One procedure that is commonly used to identify arbovirus infections is indirect immunofluorescence as this can give a result in a few hours.

Virus isolation

The causative virus can be isolated from blood collected during the initial 3-day febrile illness induced by viruses such as dengue, Ross River and yellow fever, when viraemia titres are at a maximum. Some arboviruses can also be isolated from CSF or brain biopsy, or from brain at autopsy of fatal encephalitis cases. Liver may yield virus isolation from fatal cases of yellow fever. The isolation procedures are as follows:

1. Inoculate mammalian tissue cultures, e.g. Vero or BHK, and incubate at 37°C for 14 days or until cytopathic effect is evident. Identify the virus in the cell culture supernate by neutralization or ELISA tests using appropriate polyclonal or monoclonal antibodies, or by indirect immunofluorescence of virus-infected cells from the cell culture.

2. For mosquito-borne viruses, inoculate continuous cultures of mosquito cells (e.g., *Aedes albopictus* C6/36) and incubate at 28°C for up to 14 days; examine cells for arbovirus antigen by immunofluorescence.

3. Inoculate acute-phase blood from dengue patients intrathoracically into mosquitoes and incubate at 30°C for 14 days. Detect viral antigen in head squashes by direct immunofluorescence.

4. Inoculate acute-phase blood, CSF, or brain or liver suspensions intracerebrally into suckling mice aged less than 48 h and examine daily up to 14 days for development of encephalitis (hunching, ruffled fur, convulsions, spasticity and, eventually, death). Extracts of brains from moribund mice are tested by haemagglutination inhibition tests and virus identification completed by neutralization tests in suckling mice or by plaque reduction in mammalian (e.g. Vero or BHK) tissue cultures.

Arbovirus–specific RNA detection

Viral RNA is extracted from serum or suspensions of tissues from patients, or from tissue culture cells or mosquito homogenates. This is amplified by RTPCR and the products analysed by restriction digestion and/or determination of the nucleotide sequence of the PCR product and comparison with nucleotide sequences found in Genbank or other nucleotide sequence databases.

Serology

Serological tests frequently offer the only available means of laboratory diagnosis of encephalitis. The detection of a four-fold or greater rise of antibody titre by HI or ELISA tests on paired sera collected during the initial week and several days later after defervescence provides good, but not definitive, evidence of concurrent infection. Antibodies detected by CF first appear 2 or more weeks after onset and become undetectable by 3 years. Note that HI and CF results are usually not as specific as those obtained by neutralization. Virus-specific IgM antibody may be detected within 1 day of onset of clinical symptoms using an IgM capture ELISA test. IgM antibody wanes 6 weeks after onset and is replaced by IgG antibodies. IgM antibodies are indicative of a recent infection.

TREATMENT

Currently, no specific anti-arboviral therapeutic agent is available. Patients with encephalitis are managed supportively, using anticonvulsants as required, and ice packs are applied when indicated to reduce hyperthermia. Elevated intracranial pressure can also be treated, and airway protection may be needed in patients exhibiting loss of consciousness, along with hyperventilation accompanied by anaesthesia and sedation. Regulating serum sodium and osmolarity can minimize brain swelling. Nosocomial infections, especially pneumonia, should be prevented and treated aggressively when they occur. Similarly, in dengue and haemorrhagic fevers, supportive nursing measures are employed, including intravenous infusions when indicated to replace fluids and electrolytes. Ribavirin is the only agent that is effective against non-HIV RNA viruses. It shows activity against some bunyaviruses and alphaviruses but is not therapeutic in humans against flavivirus infections.

EPIDEMIOLOGY

Natural cycles

Arboviruses are maintained in natural transmission cycles involving reservoir hosts and arthropod vectors, typically:

- ticks
- mosquitoes
- other biting flies.

With the exception of dengue viruses, arboviruses are zoonotic pathogens that utilize wild animals as reservoir hosts. Many arboviruses also use non-human animals as amplification hosts during epidemics and humans are often tangentially infected, *dead-end hosts* during these outbreaks. Mosquitoes or other arthropods become infected by engorging on a viraemic vertebrate host. In mosquitoes, infection begins in the midgut epithelium and spreads to the haemocoel or open body cavity where it may disseminate to other tissues and organs, including the salivary glands. Finally, this extrinsic incubation period is completed when replication in salivary gland acinar cells leads to virus release into the apical cavities and salivary ducts. Transmission may then occur upon a subsequent blood meal, when mosquitoes deposit saliva in extravascular tissues while probing to locate a venule. Infection of the vertebrate then leads to viraemia and the opportunity for infection of additional vectors.

Examples of natural cycles (illustrated in Figs 51.1–3) are:

- Human–mosquito cycle as in dengue and urban yellow fever (Fig. 51.1). Urban vectors of dengue viruses are typically the highly peridomestic and anthrophilic *Aedes aegypti*, but peridomestic *Ae. albopictus* has also been implicated; humans are the vertebrate reservoirs for rural and urban dengue.

- Mosquito–bird cycle as in SLE (Fig. 51.2). Vectors are typically *Culex* mosquitoes and birds serve as reservoirs; humans are infected tangentially and are dead-end hosts.
- Mosquito–mammal cycle, as in Venezuelan equine encephalitis (Fig. 51.3). Enzootic transmission cycles occur in tropical forests or swamps, where *Culex* (*Melanoconion*) spp. vectors transmit among rodent reservoir hosts. Equine epizootics emerge when critical mutations that permit equine amplification occur, followed by human cases in agroecosystems. Human infections also occur with sylvatic forms of the virus when people enter neotropical forests where continuous rodent–mosquito cycles occur.

Epidemiological aspects of arbovirus infections with major impact on human health are described according to syndrome and infecting serotype (see also Table 51.2).

Alphaviruses

Western equine encephalitis virus (WEEV)

WEEV was first isolated from the brain of a horse with fatal encephalitis. It has caused periodic outbreaks of

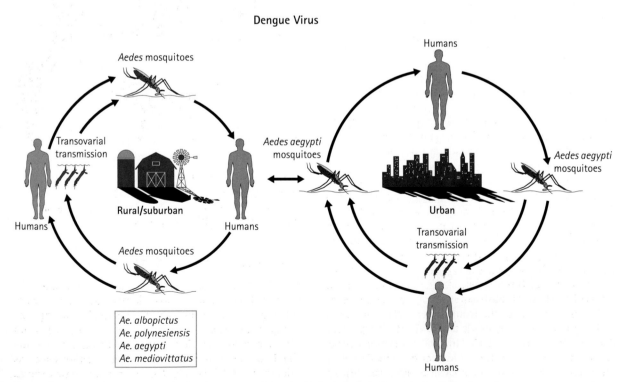

Fig. 51.1 Natural cycle of arbovirus infection: human–mosquito cycle of infection, e.g. dengue and urban yellow fever viruses.

St Louis encephalitis

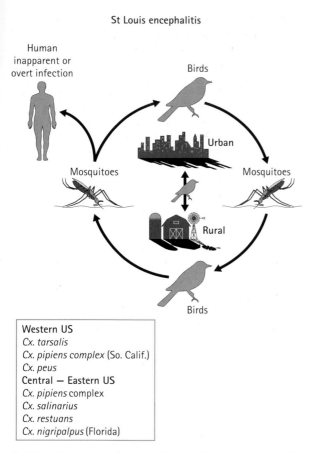

Western US
Cx. tarsalis
Cx. pipiens complex (So. Calif.)
Cx. peus
Central — Eastern US
Cx. pipiens complex
Cx. salinarius
Cx. restuans
Cx. nigripalpus (Florida)

Fig 51.2 Natural cycle of arbovirus infection: bird–mosquito cycle of infection, e.g. St. Louis encephalitis.

Venezuelan equine encephalitis

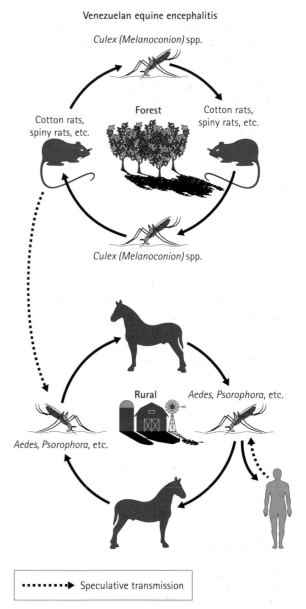

⋯⋯▶ Speculative transmission

Fig 51.3 Natural cycle of arbovirus infection: mammal–mosquito cycle, e.g. Venezuelan equine encephalitis.

equine and human encephalitis in the western half of North America, as well as in Brazil and Argentina. WEEV is found from the Mississippi Valley to California and northwards to western Canada. The mean incidence of WEE cases throughout the USA between 1966 and 1985 was 17 per year, constituting 7% of the total reported cases of arbovirus encephalitis. In North America, cases occur only during June to September, when mosquitoes are abundant. Outbreaks of infection occur at intervals of a few years and are preceded by epizootic peaks of encephalitis among horses. The principal mosquito vector species in Canada and the western USA is *Culex tarsalis*. Ducks and other water birds constitute the principal natural reservoirs. Humans and equines are considered dead-end hosts because they produce little viraemia. Although all age groups may be involved, encephalitis due to WEE virus and California serogroup agents commonly affects children, in whom the disease is often severe; SLE virus is most often seen in persons aged 55 years or more.

Eastern equine encephalitis virus (EEEV)

EEEV was also first isolated in 1933 from the brain of a horse with fatal encephalitis. Human and horse cases of encephalitis have occurred repeatedly during the summer in Atlantic coastal areas extending from Massachusetts and New Jersey southwards to Florida and Texas, as well as in a few inland locations such as Michigan and Wisconsin. Occasionally, disease extends northwards into the Province of Quebec, Canada.

During the 20-year period from 1966 to 1985 in the USA, EEE caused a mean of four cases of encephalitis per year, constituting 2% of the total cases of arbovirus encephalitis. Illness affected mainly humans aged less than 14 years and over 55 years, with overall case fatality rates as high as 69%. Surviving cases usually have severe neurological sequelae. Most human cases occur during late August and September, about 3 weeks after the peak of horse cases. Antigenically distinct forms of EEEV also occur throughout South and Central America, but are not associated with human disease. In North America, EEEV is maintained enzootically in hardwood swamp habitats, where the mosquito *Culiseta melanura* transmits among passerine birds. During years of hyperenzootic transmission, horses and humans residing near the swamp habitats become infected via different vectors such as *Aedes* spp. (*Cs. melanura* feeds almost exclusively on birds). Equines and humans are considered dead-end hosts because they develop little viraemia, and outbreaks are therefore confined to regions of enzootic activity.

Venezuelan equine encephalitis virus (VEEV)

VEEV was first isolated in 1938 from a horse in Venezuela. Periodic, sometimes widespread outbreaks involving up to hundreds-of-thousands of humans and equines have occurred since, primarily in northern South America, with one outbreak extending as far north as Texas in the USA in 1971. During outbreaks, VEEV is transmitted among equines by a variety of mosquitoes such as *Aedes* spp. and *Psorophora* spp. Equines are extremely effective amplifying hosts because they develop high-titred viraemia and are attractive to large numbers of mosquitoes. Antigenically related viruses occur in sylvatic and swamp habitats through much of the neotropics and subtropics, as far north as Florida, USA and as far south as northern Argentina. These viruses can cause febrile illness and encephalitis in humans that enter these foci, and one antigenic subtype (designated ID) can mutate to become capable of initiating widespread outbreaks. Rates of encephalitis (generally 5–15% of symptomatic cases) and mortality (around 0.5%) are generally lower than for EEEV, with most fatal cases occurring in young children. However, neurological sequelae are common.

Ross River virus (RRV)

RRV infection was first described in 1928 in Australia, where the disease is known as epidemic polyarthritis. Since that time numerous outbreaks have occurred in Australia and the South Pacific. In Australia, epidemic polyarthritis occurs primarily during the summer and autumn as sporadic cases and small outbreaks. Several thousand cases are typically reported each year in Australia, mostly involving vacationers and others travelling in rural areas. RRV is maintained in a zoonotic vertebrate–mosquito cycle, with *Culex annulirostris* and *Aedes vigilax* serving as the principal vectors in Australia, with flying foxes and marsupials implicated as reservoir hosts. Human infections have also been documented in New Guinea, the Solomon Islands, New Caledonia, Fiji, American Samoa and the Cook Islands. During 1979–1980, a large, explosive epidemic of Ross River polyarthritis swept across the South Pacific, with 40–60% of the population affected on some islands. *Aedes polynesiensis* was implicated as the vector, and epidemiological studies suggested a human–mosquito–human transmission cycle.

Chikungunya virus (CHIKV)

CHIKV was first isolated during a 1952 epidemic in Tanzania. In Swahili, 'chikungunya' means 'that which bends up', and refers to the posture assumed by patients suffering from severe joint pains. CHIK has probably occurred sporadically in India and South-east Asia for at least 200 years, and also occurs in most of sub-Saharan Africa, India, Indonesia and the Philippines. Its origin has been traced to East Africa. In Africa, a sylvatic transmission cycle occurs between wild primates and arboreal *Aedes* mosquitoes, while urban CHIK epidemics in India and South-east Asia causing hundreds-of-thousands of cases involve *Ae. aegypti* transmission in a human–mosquito–human cycle. Unlike dengue, which is endemic in many of these Asian cities, CHIKV disappears and reappears at irregular intervals. The mechanism of virus maintenance during inter-epidemic periods or re-introduction is unknown.

O'nyong-nyong virus (ONNV)

ONNV, derived from the description by the Acholi tribe, meaning 'joint breaker', was first isolated during a 1959–1962 epidemic affecting 2 million people in Uganda, Kenya, Tanzania, Mozambique, Malawi and Senegal. Another major outbreak involving an estimated one million cases occurred in 1996 in the Rakai, Mbarara and Masaka districts of Uganda, and the bordering Bukoba district of northern Tanzania. Attack rates are generally high and all age groups are affected during ONN epidemics. An antigenically closely related virus, Igbo-Ora, isolated from febrile patients in Nigeria, has been shown to be a strain of ONN virus. The transmission cycle of ONNV involves *Anopheles funestus* and *Anopheles gambiae* mosquitoes; ONNV is the only known alphavirus with *Anopheles* vectors.

Flaviviruses: mosquito-borne

St Louis encephalitis virus (SLEV)

SLEV was first isolated from the brain of a person dying with acute encephalitis in St Louis, Missouri. SLE activity is widely distributed throughout the USA, from the Ohio and Mississippi Valleys extending westwards through Colorado to California and Washington, northwards into the contiguous Canadian Provinces of Ontario, Manitoba and Saskatchewan, eastwards to Ohio and southwards to Florida and Texas. In common with WEE, SLE soon became prevalent in arid areas of the north-western and south-western USA, which have been developed for irrigation farming, due to the breeding of massive populations of the principal mosquito vector *Cx. tarsalis* in semipermanent collections of water in grassy locations. During the largest outbreak of the past quarter-century, in 1975, when 1815 of 2113 (86%) of confirmed cases of arbovirus encephalitis were due to SLEV, the Chicago metropolitan area was heavily affected for the first time. Substantial SLE outbreaks affected the Houston, Texas, metropolitan area in 1964 and 1986, where attack rates and case fatality rates were highest among persons over 55 years of age. Metropolitan Los Angeles in coastal southern California was first affected by SLEV, with 26 human cases of encephalitis in 1984. Mosquito vectors in California, the Rocky Mountains and plains states comprise mainly *Cx. tarsalis*, but *Cx. pipiens* and *Cx. quinquefasciatus* are important along the Mississippi Valley and eastwards. The salt marsh mosquitoes *Cx. restuans* and *Ae. sollicitans* may be important vectors in some localities.

Japanese encephalitis virus (JEV)

JEV was first isolated from the brain of a fatal case of encephalitis in Tokyo, Japan in 1935. JEV continues to cause epidemics of encephalitis, affecting children, particularly in India, Korea, China, South-east Asia and Indonesia, with case fatality rates often exceeding 20%. Approximately 50 000 cases occur each year, of which 15 000 are fatal. The ratio of apparent to inapparent infection is between 1:50–1:400 depending on geographical area. *Cx. tritaeniorhynchus* mosquitoes are the principal vectors, and maximum virus isolation rates from mosquitoes occur during late July simultaneously with human and equine epidemics. Important vertebrate reservoirs are black-crowned night herons and other water birds, while pigs are considered to be an amplifying host. In Malaysia, *Cx. gelidus* is an important vector as well as *Cx. tritaeniorhynchus*. In northern Thailand cases of encephalitis due to JEV have been diagnosed each year since the late 1960s, with most cases occurring during the rainy season in June, July and August. The case fatality rate of virologically confirmed cases is 33%, and about one of every 300 humans infected with JEV develops encephalitis.

West Nile virus (WNV)

WNV was first isolated from a febrile human in the West Nile district of Uganda in 1937. The virus has a wide geographic distribution, including Southern Europe, Africa, central and south Asia and Oceania. Genetic studies have shown that the related Kunjin virus, which is found in Australasia, is a subtype of WNV. Although WNV infects a wide variety of animals, including horses, cattle and humans, the major vertebrate hosts are wild birds and it is thought that migratory birds are important in the spread of the disease as they maintain high-titre viraemia over long periods. Both mosquitoes and ticks have been reported as vectors; the principal vectors are considered to be mosquitoes of the *Culex* genus. Both sylvatic and urban transmission cycles have been reported, with *Cx. pipiens* implicated as the major urban vector. WNV is usually recognized as causing a febrile illness; however, encephalitis is seen in patients over 50 years of age. Epidemics vary in size, with the largest reported in Israel and South Africa, including an epidemic of 3000 clinical cases in South Africa in 1974 and an equine epidemic in North Africa in 1998. In the late summer of 1999, the first outbreak of WN was reported in the Western hemisphere, in New York. A total of 62 clinical cases was reported, mostly in the elderly, including seven fatalities. During 2000 the virus spread to 11 states along the east coast of the USA and infects at least 60 bird species. It is anticipated to spread widely in the USA in the coming years.

Murray Valley encephalitis virus (MVEV)

MVEV was first isolated from the brain of a fatal case of encephalitis at Mooroopna, Victoria, Australia. MVEV caused epidemics of encephalitis in irrigated farming regions of the Murray-Darling River basin of south-eastern Australia during the summer months (January to March) of 1951 and 1974, with case fatality rates approaching 40%. MVEV was isolated from *Cx. annulirostris* mosquitoes only during 1974 but not during intervening years, which suggests epidemic introduction of virus into this dry temperate region. In the irrigated Ord River region of Western Australia, encephalitis due to MVEV has been recognized in 1974, 1978, 1981 and 1986, although the virus is endemic in this tropical region. Another endemic focus exists in the Gulf of Carpentaria region of Queensland. Natural cycles of transmission of MVEV involve *Cx. annulirostris* as the principal mosquito vector and water birds as reservoirs.

Yellow fever virus (YFV)

YFV was first isolated in Ghana, West Africa, from the blood of a male patient with fever, headache, backache and prostration. YFV is found mostly in tropical Africa and tropical South America. There are two epidemiological patterns: in the sylvatic cycle, virus is transmitted among monkeys by mosquitoes (*Haemagogus* and *Sabethes* species in South America and *Aedes* species in Africa). Man is infected incidentally when entering the area, e.g. to work as foresters. In the urban cycle, human-to-human transmission is via *Ae. aegypti*, which breeds close to human habitation in water, in pits and in scrap containers such as oil drums. No urban YF has been reported in South America since 1954.

In the Americas, the majority of YF cases are reported in Peru and Bolivia and involve males aged 15–45 years who are agricultural and forest workers. During 1995 there were at least 490 cases in Peru, representing the largest epidemic in South America in 40 years. YF usually occurs from December to May and peaks during March and April, when populations of *Haemagogus* mosquitoes are highest during the rainy season.

YF is endemic in many parts of West, Central and East Africa, principally between latitudes 15°N and 15°S, extending northwards into Ethiopia and Sudan. Continuing activity has been encountered in Nigeria, with occasional outbreaks in other parts of West Africa. There are relatively few outbreaks in East Africa. The last major outbreak was in Kenya in 1993 with 54 cases and a case fatality rate of 50%. *Ae. africanus* is the principal vector in Africa.

Dengue (DEN) viruses

DEN infection is endemic in all tropical regions between latitudes 23.5°N and 23.5°S. Four serologically related viruses termed dengue-1, dengue-2, dengue-3 and dengue-4 cause the disease *dengue*. However, the febrile clinical symptoms associated with dengue are similar to those of other arboviruses from other families, including the alphaviruses Chikungunya (CHIK) and Ross River (RR), and the bunyaviruses Oropouche (ORO), Rift Valley fever (RVF) and Toscana (TOS). This has resulted in confusion in the diagnosis of dengue versus other viruses that induce a dengue-like disease. In particular, the high incidence of dengue has resulted in some arbovirus outbreaks being misdiagnosed as dengue. These latter agents are differentiated from dengue viruses by serological procedures.

Dengue viruses are thought to have originated in a sylvatic cycle involving mosquitoes and monkeys. However, endemic viruses have evolved and are now maintained in nature by a cycle involving humans as both reservoirs and definitive hosts, and domestic mosquitoes, principally *Ae. aegypti*, as vectors. However, other mosquito species can also transmit the viruses.

Dengue has caused numerous outbreaks throughout the south-west Pacific region since it was first encountered among servicemen during the Second World War, when the average monthly attack rate of 54 per 1000 peaked to 197 per 1000 during the wet season. Subsequently, in the south-west Pacific, multiple dengue viruses have affected Tahiti, with haemorrhagic dengue first encountered in 1971. In addition to *Ae. aegypti* other species have been implicated as vectors, including *Ae. scutellaris hebrideus* in New Guinea, *Ae. polynesiensis* in Tahiti and *Ae. cooki* in Niue. Cases of imported dengue occurred in Hawaii during 1943 and 1944, probably through the inadvertent transport of dengue-infected mosquitoes on ships returning from dengue-endemic Pacific islands. Currently, Hawaii is dengue-free, with the absence of *Ae. aegypti*.

Dengue activity continues in many tropical countries of the Pacific rim, including northern Australia. Most South-east Asian countries, including Indonesia, Malaysia, Thailand, Vietnam, China, the Philippines and India, experience repeated epidemics of dengue due to all four viruses, with most cases occurring between June and November. Mostly children are affected; in some outbreaks up to 25% may develop haemorrhagic fever. Most epidemics occur in urban areas and villages where *Ae. aegypti* is abundant, but not in rural environments. Up to 100 million infections are thought to occur each year, with the majority in children. As such, dengue is considered to be a major public health problem.

Dengue is endemic throughout tropical Africa, including Nigeria in the west and Mozambique in the east, and also in Middle Eastern countries such as Saudi Arabia. Dengue disease does not tend to be severe in Africa and dengue haemorrhagic fever is rare.

Caribbean countries have been involved in epidemic waves of dengue since 1827, with little evidence of clinical dengue during interepidemic periods. All four dengue viruses have been implicated in outbreaks affecting residents of Caribbean islands and adjacent portions of Central and South America. Each year cases of dengue are imported into continental USA following visits to dengue-endemic Caribbean countries. Although most infections occur among travellers returning from the Caribbean, small numbers of cases (less than 30 per year) of indigenous dengue are reported among residents of south Texas who live near the border with Mexico. The semi-tropical climate in this area allows

Ae. aegypti to be prevalent during the nine warmer months each year. In 1985, *Ae. albopictus* was introduced from Asia into the Americas via used motor tyre casings that had been imported for retreading into Houston, Texas, from Japan, South Korea and several South-east Asian countries. The mosquito rapidly established itself in Texas and spread into mid-west, northeast and north-west states in the USA and also spread south into Mexico and other countries. A peridomestic mosquito, *Ae. albopictus,* was first identified as a dengue vector in Malaysia during the 1960s, and it transmits dengue both in the human–mosquito cycle and by transovarial transfer. However, to date, there have been few reports of dengue virus transmission in the Americas by *Ae. albopictus.*

Flaviviruses: tick-borne

Powassan virus (POWV)

POWV, the sole North American tick-borne flavivirus, was first isolated from the brain of a fatal human case of encephalitis in Powassan, Ontario, Canada. To date, POWV has been recognized as the cause of approximately 30 cases of encephalitis and four deaths among residents of forested areas of Ontario, Quebec and Nova Scotia in Canada, plus Massachusetts, New York State and Pennsylvania in the USA. All cases occurred between May and October. Principal tick vector species in Ontario are *Ixodes cookei*, which feeds on groundhogs, and *I. marxi*, which feeds on tree squirrels; both these mammals serve as reservoirs.

Tick-borne encephalitis viruses (TBEV)

Tick-borne encephalitis is used to describe a serocomplex of related viruses that are transmitted by ticks and cause similar diseases. These include central European (also known as Western subtype) TBE that causes central European encephalitis and Russian spring–summer encephalitis (also known as Far Eastern subtype of TBEV). In addition, a third subtype termed Siberian TBE has been described mainly on the basis of genetic studies. Russian spring–summer encephalitis is found in eastern Europe and parts of Asia and causes a more severe disease than the central European encephalitis that is found in western Europe and Scandinavia. The case fatality rate of central European encephalitis is usually below 10% while it can reach 30% for Russian spring–summer encephalitis. In Britain and Ireland (plus some parts of France and Scandinavia) a mild form of TBE is caused by a related virus called louping ill. The latter virus also infects sheep and grouse and gets its name because it induces a leaping gait in infected sheep. Louping ill

virus rarely infects humans. Human infections by TBEV may range in severity from mild biphasic meningoencephalitis, which is characteristic of the central European TBEV and louping ill virus, to a severe form of polio-encephalomyelitis that is characteristic of Russian spring–summer encephalitis virus. In Britain and other European countries, natural cycles involve *I. ricinus* ticks as vectors, and mice, shrews and other small rodents as reservoirs, with infection transferred tangentially to sheep or other farm animals, and also to humans. In Siberia, *I. persulcatus* ticks serve as vectors. Recently, additional viruses have been described from Spain, Turkey and Bulgaria that are related to louping ill virus and are members of the TBE complex and cause TBE-like disease symptoms in sheep and other animals.

In addition to the encephalitic viruses described above, the TBE complex also contains two viruses associated with haemorrhagic fever: Omsk haemorrhagic fever and Kyasanur Forest disease viruses. The former was first identified during the Second World War in Omsk and causes occasional outbreaks in Russia while the latter is only found in India and causes regular outbreaks of haemorrhagic fever.

Bunyaviruses: Bunyavirus genus

California (CAL) serogroup

There are at least 14 viruses that are related antigenically to the prototype California encephalitis virus. In the USA, encephalitis and aseptic meningitis arise commonly from infections with La Crosse virus (LAC), which was first isolated from the brain of a fatal case of encephalitis at La Crosse, Wisconsin. Other viruses occasionally associated with aseptic meningitis are snowshoe hare (SSH) virus, which was first isolated from the blood of a snowshoe hare in Montana, and Jamestown Canyon (JC) virus, which was first isolated from *Culiseta inornata* mosquitoes collected at Jamestown Canyon, Colorado. In central Europe, febrile illness sometimes associated with aseptic meningitis arises from infection with Tahyna (TAH) virus, which was first isolated from *Ae. caspius* mosquitoes collected near Tahyna, in the former Czechoslovakia.

Currently, CAL serogroup viruses are the commonest arboviruses associated with encephalitis in the USA. The highest attack rates occur in states adjoining the Great Lakes from Minnesota and Wisconsin through Illinois and Indiana to Ohio, affecting mainly children aged less than 15 years. Abundant tree holes in wooded areas provide optimum breeding sites for the principal mosquito vector *Ae. triseriatus*, but rainwater collected in disused motor tyres has proved a suitable breeding ground for *Ae. triseriatus* in suburban locations. Since adult mosquitoes die in winter, CAL serogroup viruses survive through transovarial transmission. Principal vertebrate reservoirs are tree squirrels and chipmunks.

Oropouche (ORO)

This virus is the only human pathogen in the Simbu serogroup and was first isolated in Trinidad in 1955. Outbreaks of ORO fever, a febrile illness, have been reported in Brazil since 1961, involving urban transmission by the midge *Culicoides paraensis*. Subsequently, a single outbreak was reported in Panama in 1989 while cases of ORO fever have been reported in Peru since 1992.

Bunyaviruses: Phlebovirus genus

Rift Valley fever virus (RVFV)

RVFV was first isolated in 1930 from sheep during an epizootic causing abortion and death in the Rift Valley near Lake Niavasha, Kenya, but is present from South Africa to Egypt. The virus infects many large domestic animals and a wide variety of mosquito species, with sheep, cattle, buffaloes and rodents as reservoirs. The virus is epizootic with long inter-epizootic periods. Outbreaks of RVF occurred in Egypt during 1977 involving an estimated 200 000 human cases and 600 deaths. Subsequently, RVF has been reported in tropical West Africa from 1987 onwards.

Sandfly fever (phlebovirus) group

These viruses are distributed throughout the European and North African countries surrounding the Mediterranean Sea, extending eastward through Israel and Iran to West Pakistan and central India. Sandfly fever – Naples (SFN) and Sicilian (SFS) – viruses were first isolated from the sera of US servicemen in those localities during an outbreak during the Second World War.

Epidemics of dengue-like fever occur during the sandfly season (June to September) and affect mainly visitors rather than residents. Natural vectors are *Phlebotomus papatasi* and other phlebotomine sandflies. Isolation of virus from male sandflies collected during July suggests transovarial transfer of virus. The natural cycle of sandfly fever appears to involve solely man as definitive host and reservoir, with sandflies as vectors.

Toscana virus (TOSV)

TOSV was first isolated from sandflies collected in Tuscany, Italy, and is transmitted by *Phlebotomus perniciosus* sandflies, and can be transferred transovarially.

Natural reservoirs of TOSV appear to be small rodents (*Apodemus sylvaticus*).

Bunyaviruses: Nairovirus genus

Crimean–Congo haemorrhagic fever virus (CCHFV)

CCHFV was originally described as two separate viruses: Crimean haemorrhagic fever virus was isolated from the serum of a man with fatal haemorrhagic fever near Samarkand, Uzbekistan, and Congo virus was detected in the serum of a child with fever and arthralgia in Zaire. Subsequently, antigenic and genetic studies found that the two viruses were identical. CCHFV is distributed widely throughout tropical Africa, from Mauritania to Uganda and Kenya, the Middle East and West Pakistan, and southwards to South Africa. It is also found in parts of Asia, including parts of China. The geographic distribution of CCHFV corresponds to that of *Hyalomma* spp. ticks, which have yielded numerous virus isolations from field-collected specimens. Human infection is relatively rare but mortality rates up to 50% have been reported.

Bunyaviruses: Hantavirus genus

Unlike the other genera in the *Bunyaviridae*, the members of the *Hantavirus* genus are rodent-associated viruses. They are zoonotic viruses of rodents (mainly mice or voles) that excrete virus in urine for prolonged periods. Virus is transmitted to humans by contact with aerosols of rodent urine.

Hantaan (HTN) and Puumala (PUU) viruses

These viruses induce:

- Severe illness, termed *haemorrhagic fever with renal syndrome* (HFRS), due to HTN virus in Japan, Korea, China and Siberia and PUU virus in Scandinavia.
- Mild illness, termed *nephropathia epidemica* due to PUU virus in Scotland, France, Belgium and Germany, the Balkans and Greece.

Hantaan virus was first identified in soldiers serving in Korea in 1951 and was later termed Hantaan virus after the Hantaan river area where the virus was first described. Principal vertebrate reservoirs comprise *Apodemus agrarius* rodents in Asia and *Clethrionomys glareolus* (bank vole) in Europe.

Sin Nombre virus (SNV)

SNV induces hantavirus pulmonary syndrome (HPS), a severe acute respiratory illness with a case fatality rate exceeding 50%. Initially encountered in May 1993 in the Four Corners region of the USA (Arizona, Colorado, New Mexico and Utah), additional cases have since occurred elsewhere in the USA and Canada. The principal rodent reservoir is *Peromyscus maniculatus* (deer mouse) but other rodents are hosts of other HPS-causing viruses. For example, Black Creek Canal virus is found in cotton rats (*Sigmadon hispidus*) in Florida. Subsequently, related viruses have been described in South America, each with a distinct rodent host.

This was the first occasion on which molecular methods were employed successfully to identify an unknown arbovirus before the virus was isolated. Initially, Hantavirus group antibodies were detected in sera from human cases and rodents. Total RNA was extracted from lung and liver of fatal human cases and seropositive rodents. Positive bands were detected by RTPCR using primers designed to detect Prospect Hill (North American) and PUU-like hantaviruses, but not Hantaan and Seoul-like (Asian) hantaviruses, within 3 weeks after death of the initial human cases. Several months later, SNV, genomically distinct from Prospect Hill and other hantaviruses, was isolated from tissue suspensions, initially from *P. maniculatus* and subsequently from humans.

CONTROL

Strategies for prevention of arbovirus infections depend on either vector control or active immunization with vaccine.

Vector control

This is possible for mosquito-borne viruses in urban and suburban localities; suppression of populations of vector mosquito species can halt virus transmission during epidemics. This can be achieved by:

- The use of insecticides to kill adult mosquitoes ('adulticiding'), e.g. aerial sprays of malathion, although this may kill many other insect species.
- The elimination of breeding sites of domestic *Ae. aegypti* by removal of objects such as tin cans and motor tyres that could contain rainwater, both near human habitations and in public parks and drainage systems, has prevented occurrence of dengue in Singapore and urban yellow fever in metropolitan areas in Caribbean countries.
- The chemical control of larvae, termed 'larviciding', by use of temephos granules or malathion in oil for even coverage of small breeding sites, has reduced mosquito vector populations substantially in irrigated localities in California and elsewhere.

- The biological control of larvae is attempted by microbiological agents such as *Bacillus thuringiensis israeliensis*, larvivorous fish, flatworms or mermethid nematodes, or insect growth regulators such as the juvenile hormone mimic methoprene.
- Personal protection against bites by mosquitoes involves a combination of wearing protective clothing, preferably impregnated with permethrin, screening of dwellings to prevent entry of mosquitoes and frequent application of mosquito repellants such as diethyl toluamide to exposed skin areas. For tick-borne viruses, protective clothing should be worn outdoors, followed by rigorous inspection to remove attached ticks from skin.

Vaccines

To date relatively few vaccines have been developed to control arbovirus diseases.

Alphaviruses

There are no commercially licensed vaccines for use in humans. However, formalin-inactivated vaccines have been developed for eastern and western equine encephalitis viruses. These vaccines are used to immunize horses, and researchers who work with the viruses. A live Venezuelan equine encephalitis vaccine, known as TC-83, is also administered to horses and researchers who work with the virus. TC-83 is associated with significant adverse reactions in human vaccinees and is not suitable for use in the general population. There is also an experimental killed Ross River virus vaccine.

Flaviviruses

Vaccines have been licensed against yellow fever, Japanese encephalitis and tick-borne encephalitis.

A live *yellow fever* vaccine, termed 17D, was developed in the 1930s by 176 passages of wild-type strain Asibi through chicken tissue. One dose of vaccine administered subcutaneously and containing 5000 to 200 000 pfu of virus gives protective immunity 10 days after immunization and immunity lasts for at least 10 years. The World Health Organization recommends immunization every 10 years to maintain immunity and the vaccine can be given to children over 9 months of age. Immunization is contra-indicated in immunocompromised individuals and pregnant women. Over 300 million doses of vaccine have been administered, with only 21 cases of post-vaccinal encephalitis reported. It is one of the finest vaccines ever developed.

Both live and killed vaccines have been developed to control *Japanese encephalitis*. Formalin-inactivated vaccines were developed in the 1940s based on virus grown in mouse brain. Although these vaccines continue to be used there is a risk of allergic reaction following immunization. Thus, there is a move to develop killed vaccines based on virus grown in Vero monkey kidney cell culture. Two doses of killed vaccine given 7–28 days apart are required for protective immunity. A booster is given at 1 year and subsequently every 3–4 years to maintain immunity. A live vaccine has also been developed: SA14-14-2 was generated in the People's Republic of China by 126 passages of wild-type strain SA14 in primary hamster kidney cell culture. The vaccine is given as two doses and has been administered to over 100 million people in China without any reports of adverse reactions. To date the vaccine has not been used outside China. In addition, a live vaccine is used to immunize pigs.

A formalin-activated tick-borne encephalitis vaccine based on virus grown in embryonated chicken eggs was developed in the 1970s to control *central European TBE*. The vaccine was subsequently improved by transferring manufacture to primary chick embryo fibroblast cell culture. Two doses are given, 2 weeks to 3 months apart followed by a booster given 9 months to 1 year after the second dose. Boosters are recommended every 3 years. The vaccine has proved to be very efficacious, with few adverse reactions, and has resulted in the near elimination of TBE in Austria. It is unclear if the vaccine is efficacious against Russian spring–summer encephalitis.

There are no vaccines available to prevent dengue. However, a number of candidate live vaccines are currently undergoing human trials.

Bunyaviruses

Although there are no commercially available vaccines against diseases caused by bunyaviruses, a number of experimental live and killed vaccines have been developed against Rift Valley fever.

RECOMMENDED READING

Barrett A D T 2001 Japanese encephalitis. In: Service M W (ed.) *The Encyclopedia of Arthropod-transmitted Infections*. CAB International, Wallingford, UK

Elliott R M (ed.) 1996 *The Bunyaviridae*. Plenum Press, New York

Karabatsos N 1985 *International Catalogue of Arboviruses including certain other viruses of vertebrates*, 3rd edn. American Society for Tropical Medicine and Hygiene, San Antonio

Ksiazek T G, Peters C J, Rollin P E et al. 1995 Identification of a new North American hantavirus that causes acute pulmonary insufficiency. *American Journal of Tropical Medicine and Hygiene* 52: 117–123

Monath T P (ed.) 1988 *The Arboviruses: Ecology and Epidemiology*, Vols 1–5, CRC Press, Boca Raton

U.S. Department of Health and Human Services 1999 *Biosafety in Microbiological and Biomedical Laboratories*, 4th edn. U.S. Government Printing Office, Washington DC

Weaver S C 1997 Vector biology in virus pathogenesis. In Nathanson et al. (ed.) *Viral Pathogenesis*, Lippincott-Raven, Philadelphia, pp. 329–352

Weaver S C 2001 Eastern equine encephalitis. In: Service M W (ed.) *The Encyclopedia of Arthropod-transmitted Infections*. CAB International, Wallingford, UK

Weaver S C 2001 Venezuelan equine encephalitis. In: Service M W (ed.) *The Encyclopedia of Arthropod-transmitted Infections*. CAB International, Wallingford, UK

52

Togavirus and hepacivirus

Rubella and hepatitis C viruses

P. Morgan-Capner and P. N. Simmonds

RUBELLA

Rubella (German measles) was first described in the 18th century and was considered a mild illness with only occasional complications. However, in 1941, an Australian ophthalmologist, Sir Norman Gregg, described the association between maternal rubella in pregnancy and congenital abnormalities in the infant. He noted an increased incidence of congenital cataracts in children. When questioned the mothers gave a history of having had rubella in early pregnancy when there had been an epidemic in Australia. Since then the importance of maternal rubella for the fetus has been confirmed by many studies.

Description

Rubella virus was first isolated in cell culture in 1962. It is a single-stranded RNA virus with an envelope, and is classified as a togavirus, being the only member of the genus *Rubivirus*. Virions are pleomorphic in appearance and 50–70 nm in diameter with a nucleocapsid of icosahedral symmetry. Rubella is inactivated by many chemical agents. The single-stranded RNA is infective, and replication occurs in the cytoplasm of infected cells. Virions acquire the envelope by budding from cell membranes either into intracellular vesicles or to the exterior. There are three major virion polypeptides: C and the envelope glycoproteins E1 and E2. No major antigenic difference between virus strains has been demonstrated. The virus envelope carries a haemagglutinin (E1), present as 5–6-nm projections, which will agglutinate the erythrocytes of 1-day-old chicks, pigeons, sheep and humans, a characteristic which is utilized in the haemagglutination inhibition test for specific antibodies. Experimentally, infection can be transmitted to rhesus monkeys, rabbits and some other animals, but humans are the only naturally infected species. Virus can be isolated in a range of primary and continuous cell lines, e.g. Vero, RK13 and BHK-21 cells, but in only some cell lines, such as RK13, does a cytopathic effect occur.

In other cell lines the presence of virus must be demonstrated by immunofluorescence with specific antibody or by resistance to superinfection with another unrelated virus such as echovirus 11. Only one antigenic type of rubella virus is recognized, although minor differences can be found between strains.

Clinical features

Postnatal rubella

The incubation period for postnatal primary rubella is 12–21 days, with an average of 16–17 days. Virus may be excreted in the throat for up to a week before and after the rash, and this covers the period of infectivity. The characteristic clinical features are:

- A macular rash, which usually appears first on the face and then spreads to the trunk and limbs. Particularly in childhood the rash may be fleeting and perhaps 50% of infections in children are asymptomatic. In adults, asymptomatic rubella is less common.
- General features such as minor pyrexia, malaise and lymphadenopathy also occur, with the suboccipital nodes being those most commonly enlarged and tender.
- Arthralgia is uncommon in children but may occur in up to 60% of adult females. The joints commonly involved are the fingers, wrists, ankles and knees and, although arthralgia usually only lasts a few days, it may occasionally persist for some months.
- Encephalitis and thrombocytopenia are rare complications of rubella and usually recovery is complete.

Unlike a number of other virus infections, rubella appears to present little danger to the immunocompromised patient, in whom the clinical features are similar to those seen in normal individuals.

Rubella re-infection is diagnosed when an antibody response is demonstrated in someone who has either had natural rubella or has been successfully immunized. Such re-infections are seldom clinically apparent and are usually found when someone is investigated after contact with rubella. It is very uncommon for fetal infection and damage to occur in subclinical re-infection. It can be difficult, however, to distinguish serologically between subclinical primary rubella, which is of major risk to the fetus, and re-infection. The rare re-infection that is clinically apparent must be assumed to present a risk to the fetus similar to that of primary rubella.

Rubella is notoriously difficult to diagnose clinically, as other virus infections, such as some enteroviruses and human parvovirus B19, can present with identical clinical features. For correct diagnosis laboratory investigation is essential and a history of rubella is an unreliable indicator of immunity unless it has been serologically confirmed.

Congenital rubella

If the fetus is infected during a primary maternal infection a wide spectrum of abnormalities may occur. The classical congenital rubella syndrome (CRS) triad consists of abnormalities of the eyes, ears and heart.

Abnormalities of the eyes, which may be bilateral or unilateral, include cataracts, micro-ophthalmia, glaucoma and pigmentary retinopathy, which may result in blindness.

Bilateral or unilateral sensorineural deafness may be present at birth, although it may not be detected until later in life; it may increase in severity as the child gets older.

There are many possible heart defects, with patent ductus arteriosus, pulmonary artery and valvular stenosis, and ventricular septal defect being most common.

The baby will often have a low birth weight due to intra-uterine growth retardation. A purpuric rash due to thrombocytopenia may be present at birth but this usually resolves, as does hepatosplenomegaly. Microcephaly, psychomotor retardation and behavioural disorders are manifestations of central nervous system involvement. Rarely, a persistent infection of the central nervous system occurs called *progressive rubella subacute panencephalitis*, which is similar clinically to the *subacute sclerosing panencephalitis* due to measles virus. Other problems which may not be present at birth but which may present later in life include pneumonitis, diabetes mellitus, growth hormone deficiency and abnormalities of thyroid function.

The fetus may be so severely affected that intra-uterine death with abortion or stillbirth occurs. Many infected babies, however, are born with no abnormalities, and the risk to the fetus depends on the gestational period in which primary rubella occurs. If maternal rubella occurs:

- In the first trimester the risk is considerable, as more than 70% of babies will be affected and have some or many of the abnormalities described above.
- In the fourth month of pregnancy the risk reduces to approximately 20%, and the only abnormality likely to be seen is sensorineural deafness.
- After the 16th week of pregnancy, although fetal infection still occurs, congenital abnormalities are very infrequent and no more likely to occur than in an apparently uncomplicated pregnancy.
- Before conception is unlikely to harm the fetus.

Pathogenesis

Rubella virus is transmitted by the air-borne route. Infection is established in the upper respiratory tract, and, towards the end of the incubation period, a viraemia occurs and seeds the target organs such as the skin and joints. Most of the clinical features are probably a consequence of the host's immune response to the virus, e.g. virus can be demonstrated not only in individual lesions of the macular rash but also in unaffected skin. During the viraemia the virus is able to infect the placenta and cross this barrier to infect the differentiating cells of the fetus. If such fetal infection occurs in early pregnancy a persistent infection is likely. The congenital abnormalities arise from a number of effects of the virus infection. Cell division is slowed, cell differentiation is disordered and damage to small blood vessels may occur. Such effects may lead to the abnormalities seen at birth, but the persistence of infection may result in the clinical problems presenting later in life, either due to direct damage, such as late-onset deafness, or because of immunopathological mechanisms, such as pneumonitis. Virus can persist for many years in babies infected during early gestation, but persistent infection is rare in later pregnancy when the babies are not damaged.

Diagnosis

Postnatal rubella

Clinical diagnosis is notoriously unreliable, and laboratory investigation is required if a diagnosis of rubella has important implications, such as in the pregnant patient. As subclinical rubella may occur, pregnant women should also be investigated if they are exposed to someone with possible rubella. Investigation by virus isolation is not indicated as it is unreliable and time-consuming. Serological diagnosis is the method of choice, using techniques to detect total rubella antibody or rubella-specific IgG, and rubella-specific IgM. In primary rubella, specific antibody becomes detectable about the time of the rash, although there may be a delay of 7–10 days, and rapidly increases in concentration (Fig. 52.1). Specific IgM usually, but not always, precedes specific IgG by 1–2 days but, unlike specific IgG, which persists for life, specific IgM is usually only detectable for 1–3 months. Thus, seroconversion may be demonstrated if a serum is obtained soon after contact, prior to the illness, and is examined in parallel with a sample collected at or soon after the rash; primary infection is confirmed by the development of specific IgM. If serum is collected after the rash or more than 12–14 days after contact, any total rubella antibody or specific IgG may have resulted from recent infection or infection many years previously. Tests for specific IgM must be used to determine if the infection was recent.

Tests for total rubella antibody or rubella-specific IgG are also used for serological screening to ascertain susceptibility and whether rubella immunization is indicated. Many assays of appropriate sensitivity and specificity are available. False-positive results must be avoided as a susceptible woman would not be immunized and may not be investigated if contact or illness occurs.

Congenital rubella

The majority of babies with congenital rubella syndrome excrete large amounts of virus for the first few months of life and, indeed, are highly infectious for their attendants. Thus, virus isolation in cell culture from throat swab or urine is indicated, although many laboratories may not have appropriate cell lines readily available. A more sensitive and widely available technique in the first 3–6 months of life is serological testing for specific IgM. Maternal IgM does not cross the placenta so the detection of specific IgM is diagnostic of intra-uterine infection. Specific IgG crosses the placenta from the mother so its detection in the early months of life is no help in diagnosis. Maternal IgG has a half-life in the infant of 3–4 weeks, however, so persistence to the age of 9–12 months is diagnostic of congenital rubella. It is uncommon for the specific IgM to persist to 1 year of age. Occasionally, if an older child presents with deafness, a diagnosis of possible congenital rubella may be suspected. It is impossible, however, to discriminate specific IgG resulting from intra-uterine infection from that persisting after postnatal infection or immunization, so the reliable diagnosis of congenital infection in older children is impossible.

Epidemiology

Rubella has a worldwide distribution, with infection being endemic in all countries which have not had a highly successful infant immunization policy. Outbreaks usually occur in spring and early summer, with major epidemics occurring every 4–8 years. Infection is common in childhood. Before immunization in the UK, 80–85% of young adults would have had rubella. Currently, only 2–3% of young adult females are susceptible.

Control

Passive prophylaxis

There is little evidence that administering normal human immunoglobulin after contact reduces the risk of maternal rubella and fetal infection, although it may attenuate the illness.

Active prophylaxis

Attenuated live rubella virus vaccines have been widely available since the early 1970s. They are safe, although occasional fleeting rashes and arthralgia occur. Seroconversion occurs in over 95% of susceptible vaccinees and protection persists for more than 20 years. Although vaccine virus may be isolated from the throat of vaccinees, there is no evidence of transmission to susceptible contacts. As it is a live virus vaccine, administration in pregnancy is contra-indicated, and pregnancy should be avoided for the month following immunization. Although the vaccine virus has been shown to infect the fetus, there is no evidence of teratogenicity, so if a susceptible pregnant woman is inadvertently immunized she should be reassured that the risk to her baby is very remote. It is advisable, however, that all women of childbearing age are screened for rubella antibody before immunization so that only susceptible women are offered vaccine.

The objective of rubella immunization is to eradicate congenital rubella. Two possible approaches are possible. In the UK it was decided in the early 1970s to target the vaccine at girls aged 11–14 years and susceptible adult women, identified by screening all pregnant

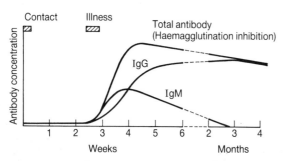

Fig. 52.1 Serological response in primary rubella.

women and women attending such facilities as family planning clinics, occupational health services and on the initiative of general practitioners. Such a policy was adopted because of uncertainties about the duration of protection and the belief that women would have better protection from having had natural rubella; 50% of adolescent girls would have had natural rubella. It was also thought that vaccine-induced protection would be boosted by occasional exposure to natural rubella. It became apparent in the late 1980s that such a policy would never achieve eradication as 10–20 cases of congenital rubella and 100–200 terminations of pregnancy still occurred each year in the UK. In the second approach, which was adopted in 1988, all children are immunized in an attempt to eradicate rubella from the community and so avoid exposure of any pregnant woman who is susceptible. Thus, the immunization schedule was augmented by offering rubella vaccine together with mumps and measles vaccine (MMR vaccine) to all children at 15 months of age. For the first few years, MMR vaccine was also offered to children at school entry as a 'catch-up' programme. In the late 1990s, a second dose of MMR vaccine was introduced at 3–5 years of age to 'boost' immunity in those who had received one dose, and to reach some of the children who had missed a first dose. This strategy has now almost eliminated congenital rubella in the UK, as it has done in the USA. To achieve such success, however, means that there must be at least a 90% uptake of vaccine in infancy.

HEPATITIS C VIRUS

Hepatitis C virus (HCV), discovered in 1989, was the elusive agent sought by scientists worldwide throughout the previous two decades that caused post-transfusion non-A non-B hepatitis. The rapid development of serological screening assays for HCV infection made possible by this discovery, and its adoption for blood donor screening, has virtually eliminated the transmission of HCV by blood transfusion, and indeed of transfusion-associated hepatitis.

Infection with HCV is widespread throughout the world, and is particularly associated with risk groups for parenteral (blood-borne) exposure. Amongst these, drug users sharing needles are numerically the most significant in western countries. HCV infection is frequently persistent, and leads to the development of significant liver disease, such as cirrhosis and hepatocellular carcinoma only after a long asymptomatic carrier phase. HCV is currently the subject of intensive efforts to develop effective antiviral treatment for chronic infection, and protective vaccines.

Properties

Structure

HCV is a small, enveloped virus with a single-stranded RNA genome of positive (coding) polarity (Fig. 52.2). HCV has been visualized in the plasma of HCV-infected individuals as small (50 nm) round particles. The surface of the virus particle contains a number of small surface projections thought to be formed from complexes of the virally encoded envelope glycoproteins E1 and E2. The RNA genome is approximately 9400 bases in length, of which over 98% contains protein-coding sequence. In common with many other small RNA viruses, the gene sequences of HCV are translated in a single block to produce a large (>3000 amino acid) polyprotein. During and after translation, proteases cleave this precursor into a total of nine mature proteins, which are involved in virus replication (NS2–NS5B), or form structural components of virus particle (core, E1 and E2).

Replication

Information on the replication of HCV and its assembly into infectious virus particles remains limited because it has proven (nearly) impossible to culture the virus in vitro. However, investigation of individual HCV-encoded proteins and comparison with related viruses has allowed the functions of most to be ascertained (Fig. 52.2). For example, NS5B is the RNA polymerase required by HCV for replication of its genetic material through a negative-stranded intermediate. NS3 contains protease and helicase activities; the former is required for the majority of cleavage reactions in the processing of the polyprotein after translation. The three proteins at the left hand end of the genome are structural proteins. Multiple copies of the core protein presumably assemble to form a nucleocapsid that packages the viral RNA, while E1 and E2 are synthesized on internal membranes within the infected cell, become heavily glycosylated and form the HCV envelope as the nucleocapsid buds out of the cell.

The extreme ends of the HCV genome are non-coding, and play a number of roles in the transcription and translation of the virus genome. Details of the factors that initiate and regulate HCV transcription remain unclear at present, although the non-coding ends are likely to be involved in protein complexes with NS5B, NS3 and other HCV and cellular proteins to mediate binding and initiation of RNA copying. The 5' untranslated region plays an important role in directing the translation of the HCV polyprotein from an internal (methionine) codon. RNA secondary structure formation apparently allows the direct binding of the host cell

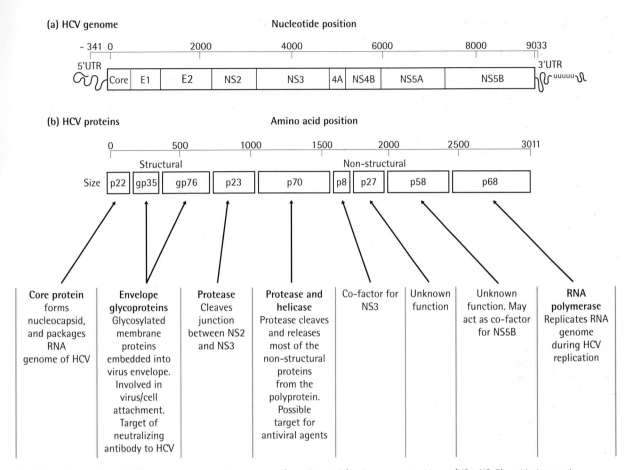

Fig. 52.2 Organization of HCV genome, showing **a** the structural (core, E1 and E2) and non-structural genes (NS2–NS5B), and **b** the proteins produced from them by proteolytic cleavage of the translated polyprotein. The properties and functions of the HCV proteins, where known, are summarized below.

ribosome to internal sequences in the 5′ untranslated region, bypassing the conventional attachment to the (modified) end of the RNA molecule, as is found in the translation of cellular mRNAs.

The principal targets of HCV replication in vivo are:

- hepatocytes
- perhaps haemopoietic cells such as B lymphocytes
- perhaps stem cells in bone marrow.

Details of the mechanism of HCV entry into the cells are currently unclear, as is the nature of the cellular proteins to which HCV binds. After entry, it is likely that the RNA genome is translated, a process which generates the RNA replicating and unwinding enzymes such as NS5B, NS5A and NS3 required for genome replication. The genomic RNA is likely to be transcribed into a full-length negative-polarity copy, which in turn acts as

the template for the production of multiple positive-stranded RNA copies. These can be used for further rounds of transcription, or for the production of further viral proteins. Factors that regulate negative- and positive-strand synthesis and the use of the latter transcripts for translation remain undetermined, and are likely to be complex.

Translation of the HCV polyprotein takes place in association with the endoplasmic reticulum. Although the core protein remains within the cytoplasm after cleavage from E1, E1 and E2 are embedded in the endoplasmic reticulum membrane, and their extracellular domains are glycosylated. Details of the subsequent stages of capsid assembly and maturation, the insertion of HCV RNA, and the budding of HCV through the endoplasmic reticulum into extracytoplasmic space and release from the cell await further studies.

Classification

HCV shows the greatest similarity in structure, size and genome organization with flaviviruses. Together, these viruses are classified as members of the *Flaviviridae* (Table 52.1), a family that also includes pestiviruses, viruses structurally closely related to HCV that infect a number of domestic and wild species of ruminants such as pigs, sheep and cows. The Flaviviridae are currently divided into three genera: the hepacivirus genus includes HCV as well as a number of recently discovered viruses that infect humans and non-human primate species. The most similar virus to HCV is GB virus-B, originally isolated from a captive tamarind, in which it causes acute hepatitis and liver disease similar to that of HCV in humans. It is currently under evaluation as a possible experimental model for HCV vaccines and antiviral treatment.

Particular attention is also drawn to hepatitis G virus or GB virus-C. This virus is widely distributed in humans and was originally thought to be a further agent involved in post-transfusion and chronic hepatitis of unexplained aetiology. This association has subsequently been disproved, and infection appears to be entirely asymptomatic, despite being persistent in a significant proportion of those it infects. Its genome shows a number of similarities to that of HCV, including a 5′ untranslated region that has similar ribosomal binding and internal initiation to that of HCV, while the coding region contains homologues to its structural and non-structural proteins. However, it lacks a protein corresponding to the core protein of HCV that forms the nucleocapsid. This has led to considerable speculation on how HGV/GBV-C might assemble to form complete virus particles. Viruses similar to HGV/GBV-C are widely distributed in a range of non-human primate species.

Virus stability

HCV is inactivated by exposure to chloroform, ether and other organic solvents, and by detergents. The effectiveness of a number of virus-inactivating procedures has been demonstrated by studies of the infectivity of products manufactured from plasma, e.g. the factor VIII and IX concentrates used to treat haemophiliacs. For example, HCV infectivity can be removed efficiently by:

- dry heat treatment at 80°C
- wet heat treatment at 60°C
- organic solvents (n-heptane)
- detergents.

Serological diagnosis

Chronic infection with HCV is associated with the presence of both plasma viraemia and antibody to HCV. Methods to detect both antibody and HCV directly have been used for diagnosis of HCV infection.

The technical simplicity of antibody testing has favoured its use for general screening and diagnostic testing. Antibody tests for HCV are based upon cloned HCV RNA sequences of HCV genotype 1a, originally derived from an experimentally infected chimpanzee. Recombinant proteins expressed from these clones have formed and remain the basis for almost all assays for antibody to HCV since then. While the original, first generation, assay was restricted to antigens expressed from the NS3 and NS4A regions of the genome, subsequent assays have incorporated additional antigens from the core, NS3 and NS5 regions to produce assays of greater sensitivity and specificity for antibody to HCV. The incorporation of antigen from the core and NS3 regions in these second and third generation assays also gives a greater sensitivity for antibody elicited by infection with non-genotype 1 infections.

Testing for antibody to HCV is normally carried out as a two-stage procedure. An enzyme-linked immunosorbent assay (ELISA) format is used for initial testing of serum or plasma from patients or blood donors. Repeatedly reactive samples are then re-tested by a second ELISA in a different format or by a supplementary assay such as the Ortho recombinant immunoblot assay that contains a number of separate HCV antigens. Currently used serological tests for anti-HCV are now highly sensitive and specific in most patient groups, although individuals who are immunosuppressed, such as those co-infected with HIV, those on

Table 52.1	Members of the flavivirus family
Genus	Examples
Hepacivirus (four members)	Hepatitis C virus GB Virus B GB Virus C (or HGV), GBV-A and other homologues in non-human primates
Pestivirus (four members)	Bovine viral diarrhoea virus, types I and II Swine vesicular disease virus (fomerly hog cholera virus) Border disease virus and less well characterized variants in other ruminant species
Flavivirus (68 members) (*some examples*)	Tick-borne encephalitis virus, louping ill virus Japanese encephalitis virus Dengue virus, serotypes 1-4 Yellow fever virus

renal dialysis and transplant patients, and those with congenital immunodeficiencies can produce false-negative serological test results. In these cases, direct detection methods for HCV, such as the polymerase chain reaction (PCR) to detect viral RNA should be considered.

Direct detection methods

While current screening and supplementary serological tests will detect the vast majority of chronic, established infections, there remains a considerable window period in HCV infection between exposure and development of antibody detectable by the best current ELISA methods (Fig. 52.3). For this reason, further direct detection methods for the detection of HCV antigens or RNA sequences are required for the effective diagnosis of HCV infection in acute hepatitis, or for diagnosis of HCV in immunosuppressed individuals who do not mount a detectable antibody response. More recently, genome detection methods have also been adopted in addition to serological tests for the routine screening of blood donors for HCV in most western countries.

Direct detection methods are based upon the detection of:

- HCV RNA sequences by PCR or other nucleic acid amplification methods.
- Viral antigens by ELISA.

The most commonly used method for direct detection of HCV is the PCR. Diagnostic PCR methods are commercially available and are capable of high sensitivity and specificity for the detection of HCV RNA sequences in plasma (or liver biopsy) specimens. Alternative, non-PCR-based methods, such as transcript-mediated amplification, have recently been developed and provide comparable sensitivity to PCR. An alternative to nucleic acid detection is the use of ELISA-based methods for the detection of viral protein in plasma, such as the Ortho assay for HCV core protein. Although this method achieves comparable sensitivity to PCR in the diagnosis of acute, preseroconversion HCV infections, it is unreliable for samples containing anti-HCV.

Direct virus detection is the only reliable method of following the effect of treatment with antiviral drugs on

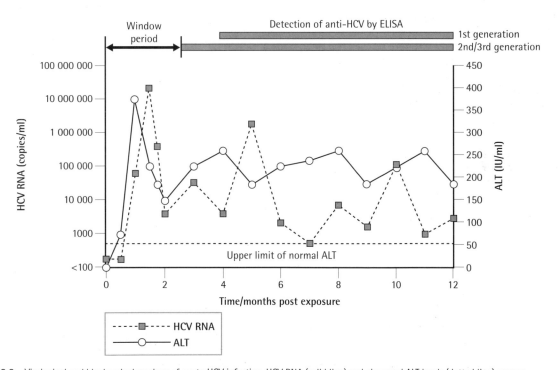

Fig. 52.3 Virological and biochemical markers of acute HCV infection. HCV RNA (solid line) and abnormal ALT levels (dotted line) appear approximately 50 days after exposure to HCV in a typical individual. The subsequent development of chronic hepatitis is indicated by persistent viraemia and by fluctuating abnormal ALT levels. Antibody to HCV first appears after the onset of acute hepatitis, in this example leading to 'window periods' of around 100–150 days for the first generation serological assay (containing only NS3 and NS4 proteins) and approximately 60–80 days for second and third generation assays (containing additional NS3 (NS5) and core proteins).

patients with chronic infection since normalization of biochemical liver function tests is not always associated with virus clearance. Similarly, chronic HCV infection with associated disease is known in patients with normal liver function tests. Quantification of the virus genome titre is now increasingly possible with commercial tests based on PCR, other amplification methods or hybridization, and has been used as a predictor for response to antiviral therapy (see Treatment).

Genetic variation

Nucleotide sequences of HCV frequently show substantial differences from each other. This has led to the current genotypic classification of HCV, in which variants from a variety of geographical locations can be classified into six main genotypes and a number of subtypes (Fig. 52.4). Genotypes show approximately 30% sequence divergence from each other, differences that greatly modify their antigenic properties and their biology.

Some genotypes of HCV (types 1a, 2a, 2b) show a broad worldwide distribution, while others such as type 5a and 6a are only found in specific geographical regions (South Africa and South-east Asia, respectively). HCV infection in blood donors and patients with chronic hepatitis from countries in western Europe and the USA frequently involves genotypes 1a, 1b, 2a, 2b and 3a. The relative frequencies of each may vary geographically, such as the trend for more frequent infection with type 1b in southern and eastern Europe, and the association of genotype 1a and 3a with infection through drug use. HCV genotypes can be identified by analysis of sequences from the 5′ untranslated region or from coding regions. Methods for rapid genotyping of HCV have been developed and play a role in the pretreatment assessment of patients receiving antiviral treatment (see Treatment).

Epidemiology

In western Europe, Australia and North America, most HCV-infected patients have a history of parenteral exposure to the virus, and the majority are (or have been) injecting drug users. The seroconversion rate in this group has been estimated at 20% per year and so long-term drug users are almost invariably infected with HCV. Drug use was uncommon before the 1960s and so drug users tend to be younger than patients infected through other routes such as transfusion. Most drug users have asymptomatic infection with no history of jaundice, but have chronic hepatitis; few have overt clinical signs or symptoms of liver disease or liver failure.

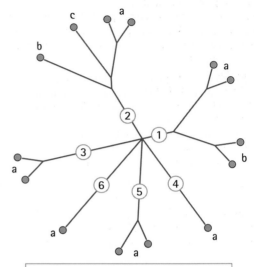

(1) a
Widely distributed in northern Europe and USA. Associated with IDUs

(1) b
Commonest genotype worldwide. Older age groups, risk factors generally ill-defined

(2) abc
Found predominantly in older HCV-infected individuals from Mediterranean countries and Far East

(3) a
Widely distributed in IDUs, particularly from Europe

(4) a
Widely distributed in Middle East. Associated with past medical treatment (e.g. bilharzia injections)

(5) a
Found commonly only in South Africa

(6) a
Found in IDUs in Hong Kong, Vietnam and, more recently, in Australia

Fig. 52.4 Comparison of complete genome sequences of the common genotypes of HCV plotted as a phylogenetic tree, showing the six main genetic groups (genotypes 1–6) and a number of the commoner subtypes (a, b, c). The distribution of the different genotypes in the principal risk groups for HCV infection is indicated. IDU, intravenous drug users.

Other blood-borne routes of HCV transmission include:

- blood transfusion before 1991 (when universal donor screening was initiated)
- recipients of pooled plasma products such as factor VIII, anti-D and immunoglobulin manufactured before the adoption of virus inactivation procedures (1986 onwards)
- transplant recipients
- haemodialysis patients
- health care workers from needle-stick injuries
- tattooing and acupuncture
- in countries of high prevalence, the use of unsterilized needles for cultural rituals, medical treatment or vaccination programmes.

The lowest frequencies of HCV infection are found in Scandinavian and other northern European countries, such as the UK (0.3–0.4%), with slightly higher prevalences in North America (1%) and Australia. Prevalence is intermediate in eastern and southern European countries, even higher in Japan, and most prevalent in the Middle East; frequencies of HCV infection of up to 30% have been recorded in areas of Egypt. In this latter case, bilharzia treatment using re-usable and unsterile needles in the 1960s has been identified as the main source of infection.

There is little evidence for non-parenteral transmission of HCV. For example, there is little convincing evidence for transmission by sexual contact where compounding factors have been removed. Mother-to-child transmission of HCV occurs at frequencies between 3 and 10% in the majority of studies. Transmission occurs generally at birth, presumably through contact with blood (recent evidence suggests that elective Caesarian section may prevent transmission).

Clinical features

Hepatitis C infection causes an indolent and slowly progressive liver disease that is asymptomatic until the development of decompensated liver disease, and often, liver cancer.

Acute hepatitis

Exposure to HCV usually results in an asymptomatic infection without jaundice, and the majority of individuals become chronic carriers of the virus. Most studies have reported an interval of around 8 weeks to the development of abnormal liver function tests (such as elevated alanine aminotransferase [ALT] levels), although viraemia can be detected earlier (Fig. 52.3). Clinically, hepatitis caused by HCV is indistinguishable from that caused by other hepatitis viruses; jaundice

may develop, but more usually symptoms are non-specific, e.g. fatigue, anorexia and nausea. Viraemia can be detected in the early stages of acute hepatitis, appearing at the same time or slightly earlier than abnormal ALT levels, while seroconversion for antibody may be delayed for several weeks or months after the onset of hepatitis. Histological features of acute HCV are similar to those associated with acute HAV and HBV infection; liver biopsy is rarely indicated to make a diagnosis of acute HCV infection.

Chronic hepatitis

The frequency of chronic infection following exposure to HCV ranges from 50 to 80%. Persistent infection with HCV is generally associated with persistent and progressive hepatitis, with fluctuating or continuously abnormal ALT levels. Although viraemia is invariably detected in patients with chronic hepatitis, there is no correlation between the level of viraemia and the severity of liver disease, ALT levels or other biochemical abnormalities associated with hepatitis.

HCV infection causes a range of characteristic histological changes in the liver, although few allow a specific diagnosis of HCV infection to be made. These include:

- lymphoid follicles within the portal tracts
- a dense periportal inflammatory process
- bile duct damage, lobular hepatitis, with lymphocyte infiltration within sinusoids surrounding the hepatocytes.

Liver histology in HCV infection is commonly classified as chronic persistent and chronic active hepatitis with or without cirrhosis, although more informative scoring systems such as the Knodell score have also been devised.

The percentage of chronically infected individuals who progress to cirrhosis and liver failure is not known. When chronic hepatitis does progress to clinically significant liver damage, then progression is almost invariably very slow, although faster progression may be observed in the context of immunosuppression. Particularly aggressive HCV-associated liver disease has been observed in immunosuppressed organ transplant recipients, and in patients with inherited immunodeficiency states. Cirrhosis is rarely observed within 10 years of infection, and as few as 20% of infected patients have cirrhosis after 20 years follow-up. Cirrhosis may be complicated by liver failure (decompensated cirrhosis), manifested as jaundice, portal hypertension and variceal bleeding; these manifestations of liver failure are shared with other forms of cirrhosis. Hepatocellular carcinoma frequently complicates chronic hepatitis C, although it is rare within 15 years of initial infection. In many western countries, such as Spain and Italy, and in Japan, HCV infection is found in 60–90% of cases of hepatocellular carcinoma.

Extrahepatic manifestations

In a minority of infected patients, HCV may be responsible for extrahepatic clinical manifestations and disease. These include certain types of vasculitis and glomerulonephritis caused by immune complex deposition. Associations between HCV infection and Sjögren's syndrome, essential mixed cryoglobulinaemia and membranoproliferative glomerulonephritis type 1 have been suggested.

Treatment

α-Interferon (IFN) or, more recently, α-IFN combined with ribavirin, is widely prescribed for the treatment of chronic hepatitis associated with HCV infection. Although most physicians have used 3–6 megaunits thrice weekly for 6–12 months, it seems likely that treatment response may be enhanced by the use of higher doses for longer durations. For example, higher frequencies of response, particularly amongst those infected with genotype 1, have been achieved by high-dose interferon administration (e.g. 6 MU three times a week for 12 months), alone or in combination with ribavirin.

Prior to the availability of PCR tests for HCV RNA, serum transaminases served as surrogate markers of response to treatment. Most physicians still rely on serum alanine transaminase (ALT) to monitor interferon treatment, and the principal aim of treatment is the normalization of ALT levels. The application of qualitative and quantitative PCR assays now permits virological assessment of response. These have shown that:

- persistently elevated ALT is associated with persistent HCV RNA positivity
- normalization of ALT is frequently associated with RNA clearance
- biochemical relapse is associated with reappearance of RNA
- viral RNA may be detected in the follow-up serum of patients with apparent biochemical remission.

Three patterns of response are observed (Fig. 52.5). In a typical study, approximately 50% of treated patients have persistently elevated ALT and remain RNA-positive despite treatment, while the remaining 50% respond with normalization of ALT, and RNA becoming undetectable. At least half of this latter group relapse during therapy or when therapy is withdrawn. The treatment objective is a sustained response and this implies persist-

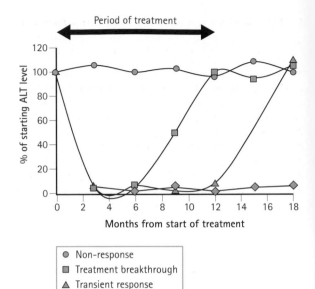

Fig. 52.5 Outcomes of α-IFN therapy in chronic hepatitis C. Non-responders are those where biochemical improvement is not observed during or after cessation of treatment. Among those initially responding to α-IFN and showing normalization of serum transaminases, a proportion will relapse during therapy (treatment breakthrough) and some will relapse at conclusion of therapy (transient response). The desired outcome is a complete response, where ALT levels remain in the normal range 12 months or longer after the cessation of treatment. In general, HCV RNA levels parallel ALT normalization, with individuals showing treatment response becoming PCR-negative; those showing a complete response may become permanently non-viraemic and virologically cured.

ently normal ALT with RNA clearance after treatment is concluded, but fewer than 20% achieve this objective. In an attempt to improve response rates, and to avoid the unnecessary treatment of potential non-responders, clinical and virological features associated with sustained response have been defined.

Several clinical studies have catalogued a variety of factors (including virus genotype) that correlate with severity of liver disease, and which show predictive value for the response to antiviral treatment. Historically, most information is related to IFN monotherapy, although it is likely that most factors will show similar influences on the outcome of IFN/ribavirin-combined therapy. Factors that have been frequently shown to influence response to IFN treatment include:

- patient age
- duration of infection
- the presence of cirrhosis before treatment. Sustained response is seldom observed for patients with cirrhosis and portal hypertension

- HCV genotype and pre-treatment level of circulating viral RNA in plasma also have a major influence on frequency of response to both monotherapy and combined treatments.

A consistent finding is the greatly increased rate of long-term response found upon treating patients infected with genotypes 2a, 2b and 3a compared with type 1. With standard monotherapy, normalization of ALT levels (>12 months) is typically observed in 15–20% of patients infected with type 1, compared with 40–50% of those with type 2 and 3 infections. Using multivariate analysis, the following have been shown to be each independently associated with a reduced chance of response:

- infection with type 1b
- the presence of cirrhosis
- high pre-treatment virus load.

Differences in responsiveness between type 1 and non-type 1 genotypes are also observed in patients treated with IFN/ribavirin combination treatment. Two recent studies reported frequencies of sustained virological and biochemical responses in type 2- and 3-infected individuals of 73% and 69%, respectively, after 6 months of treatment, compared with 30% and 16% in those infected with type 1. Interestingly, prolonging combination treatment to 12 months significantly improved the frequency of response in those infected with type 1 (16–>28%), but not non-type 1 genotypes (69–>66%). The mechanism by which different genotypes might differ in responsiveness to treatment remains obscure, particularly as it remains unclear whether IFN has a directly antiviral action, or whether it acts as an immunomodulatory agent and enhances immune responses to HCV infecting cells in the liver. It is unlikely that the greater response rates achieved with types 2 and 3 are simply secondary to differences in disease severity.

Pre-treatment assessment of genotype will undoubtedly allow for more appropriate patient selection for treatment, or be used to calculate the necessary dose and duration to obtain a sustained clearance of viraemia. The observation that 12 months of treatment with IFN and ribavirin is only of benefit for patients infected with type 1 provides an example of the value of genotype determination in avoiding unnecessarily prolonged treatment in many patients, and therefore greatly reducing treatment side-effects and costs. This, and other instances where knowledge of the infecting genotype influences the dose and duration of treatment, has led to the current recommendation that genotype determination should be carried out as a routine component of any assessment of patients for treatment.

Recently, pre-treatment variables such as virus genotype have been incorporated into cost-benefit analyses of HCV treatment to develop policies for more effective management of HCV infection. However, predictions of cost-effectiveness will also be improved when we know more about the natural history of infection, such as the proportion of individuals who will progress to end-stage liver disease and the influence of HCV genotype on this progression.

Liver transplantation

Liver transplantation is indicated for patients with decompensated HCV cirrhosis, and for some patients with HCC complicating HCV infection. Liver transplantation does not cure HCV infection, and re-infection of the graft is probably inevitable.

Prevention

Screening of blood donors has proved to be effective at preventing transmission of HCV infection through blood transfusion. A combination of blood donor screening and virus inactivation has virtually eliminated HCV transmission by blood products such as clotting factor concentrates and immunoglobulins.

The main continuing risks for HCV transmission are injecting drug abuse and the use of unsterile needles for medical and dental procedures, tattooing and other percutaneous exposures. Much of this could be prevented by education, greater availability of disposable needles, and, for drug abusers, by needle exchange programmes. Many of the public health measures adopted to prevent transmission of HIV by parenteral routes will assist efforts at controlling HCV.

Immunization

The development of a vaccine for HCV faces a series of formidable obstacles, amongst which viral heterogeneity and the difficulty in evaluating candidate vaccines in suitable animal models are the most acute. Despite these difficulties, encouraging results have been obtained using recombinant envelope proteins (E1 and E2), which induce a short-lived specific anti-E1 and E2 response in immunized chimpanzees, and transient protection from challenge with the same virus strain. There is, however, little prospect of an effective vaccine for human use in the coming decade.

Infection with HCV is a growing medical problem worldwide. A combination of public health preventative measures, improved diagnosis, screening, antiviral treatment and immunization will undoubtedly all be required to combat its spread in the future.

RECOMMENDED READING

Best J M, Banatvala J E 2000 Rubella. In: Zuckerman A J, Banatvala J E, Pattison J R (eds) *Principles and Practice of Clinical Virology*, 4th edn. Wiley, Chichester

Blight K J, Kolykhalov A A, Reed K E, Agapov E V, Rice C M 1998 Molecular virology of hepatitis C virus: an update with respect to potential antiviral targets. *Antiviral Therapy* 3: 71–81

Hepatitis C virus 1999 *Journal of Hepatology* 31: Suppl. 1 (whole issue)

Houghton M 2000 Strategies and prospects for vaccination against the hepatitis C viruses. *Current Topics in Microbiological Immunology* 242: 327–339

Liang T J, Hoofnagle J H (eds) *Hepatitis C*. Academic Press, San Diego

Miller E, Cradock-Watson J E, Pollock T M 1982 Consequences of confirmed maternal rubella at successive stages of pregnancy. *Lancet* ii: 781–784

Reesink H W (ed.) *Hepatitis C Virus*, 2nd revised and enlarged edition. CH-4009 Karger, Basel

Simmonds P 1997 Clinical relevance of hepatitis C virus genotypes. *Gut* 40: 291–293

53

Arenaviruses and filoviruses

Lassa, Junin, Machupo, Sabia and Flexal virus haemorrhagic fevers; Marburg and Ebola fevers

C. A. Hart

ARENAVIRUSES

Properties

Members of the family *Arenaviridae* have a single-stranded ambisense RNA genome. The genome has two segments: L (large) and S (small), of 7200 and 3400 nucleotides, respectively. The virions are spherical enveloped particles with diameters ranging from 90 to 100 nm on cryoelectron microscopy (Fig. 53.1a). The genome is encapsidated in a helical nucleocapsid. The lipid envelope is derived from the host plasma membrane and T-shaped glycoprotein spikes extend 7–10 nm from its surface. Virions are relatively unstable and infectivity is abolished by ultraviolet or gamma irradiation, heating to 56°C, exposure to detergents or other lipid solvents and pH outside the range 5.5–8.5.

The virions (Fig. 53.1) contain not only virus genome but also host ribosomes (both 28S and 18S rRNA),

which give the virus its characteristic grainy morphology (Fig. 53.1b) and the family name (arena is Latin for sand). The S segment is always more abundant and encodes the nucleoprotein (NP) and the two glycoproteins (GP-1 and GP-2). The L segment encodes the viral RNA polymerase, L (at the 3′ end) and a zinc-binding protein, Z (at the 5′ end). For both the L and S segments the intergenic spaces are predicted to form hairpins that are important in transcription termination.

The arenaviruses that affect humans are grouped as New World and Old World viruses (Table 53.1). Lymphocytic choriomeningitis virus (LCM) is a rare cause of disease in humans. Mice excrete the virus persistently and, although classed as an Old World arenavirus, it has a worldwide distribution as mouse has moved with man. The phylogeny of the arenaviruses is usually determined by comparison of NP gene sequence (a portion of the 3′ terminus). This confirms the distinction between Old and New World viruses and shows, for

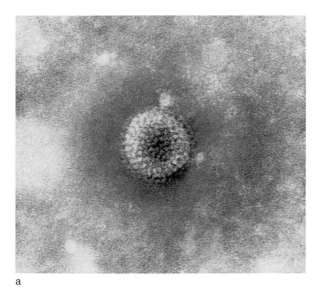

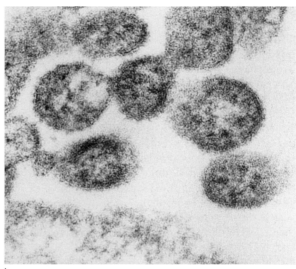

a   b

Fig. 53.1 **a** Lassa fever virus. **b** Lassa fever virus cross-section showing granular appearance of cell ribosomes.

Table 53.1 Old and New World arenaviruses

	First isolated	Human disease	Rodent host	Distribution
Old World				
Lymphocytic Choriomeningitis	1934	Mild to severe meningitis	*Mus musculus*	Worldwide
Lassa	1975	Asymptomatic to severe VHF	*Mastomys natalensis*	West Africa
Ippy	1970	Not known	*Mas. natalensis*	Central African Republic
Mopeia	1977	Not known	*Mas. natalensis*	South Central Africa
Mobala	1983	Not known	*Praomys jacksoni*	Central African Republic
New World				
Junin	1958	Argentinian VHF	*Calomys musculinus*	Argentina
			C. laucha	
			Akodon azari	
Machupo	1965	Bolivian VHF	*C. callosus*	Bolivia
'Tacaribe' complex	1963	Not known[a]	*Artibeus bato*	West Indies
Ampari	1966	Not known	*Oryzomys goeldii*	
			Neacomys guianae	Brazil
Parana	1970	Not known	*O. buccinatus*	Paraguay, USA
Tamiami	1970	Asymptomatic	*Sigmodon hispidus*	USA
Pichinde	1971	Not known	*O. albigularis*	Columbia
			Thomasomys fuscatus	
Latino	1973	Not known	*C. callosus*	Bolivia
Flexal	1977	VHF[a]	*Neacomys* spp.	Brazil
Guanarito	1991	Venezuelan VHF	*Oryzomys* spp.	Venezuela
Sabia	1994	Brazilian VHF	Not known	Brazil
Whitewater Arroyo	2000	VHF, severe	*Neotoma albigula*	USA (California)

VHF, Viral haemorrhagic fever.
[a] Moderate laboratory associated infection described.

example, that Junin and Machupo are closely related and that Sabia is distinct from all other New World arenaviruses but shares a common ancestor.

Replication

Arenaviruses can replicate in a number of mammalian hosts and in most tissues. Growth is restricted in terminally differentiated cells such as lymphocytes or macrophages. Arenaviruses are usually maintained in artificial culture in BHK-21 (baby hamster kidney), Vero E7 (African green monkey kidney) or mouse L cells. LCM has been shown to bind by GP-1 and GP-2 to a surface glycoprotein (160-kDa) on rodent fibroblasts, but its structure and normal functions are unknown. Entry appears to be by viropexis through smooth-walled vesicles. The endocytotic vesicles then become acidified, causing conformational changes in GP-1 and GP-2, leading to fusion of the viral envelope with the vesicle membrane and escape of the nucleocapsid into the cell cytoplasm. Viral transcription and replication take place in the cytoplasm, but there is a suggestion that the nucleus may also be involved, perhaps in providing capped cellular mRNA for priming arenavirus transcripts. NP and L mRNAs can be transcribed from

genomic RNA, whereas GP and Z mRNAs are transcribed only from antisense transcripts of the genome. The stem-loop hairpins act to separate genes on both the L and S segments, but transcription termination is apparently not a function of the secondary structure of the loop, as there are transcription terminations on the distal part of each loop.

The L (RNA polymerase: 250 kDa) protein catalyses production of both transcripts and new genomes and is non-structural (not in the mature extracellular virion). The Z protein (zinc binding: 11–14 kDa) is involved in viral transcription and also acts as a structural protein, perhaps in linking the internal hydrophilic tail of the glycoproteins to the nucleocapsid. The nucleoprotein NP (63 kDa) is the most abundant protein, with 1500–2000 copies per virion. The surface glycoproteins GP-1 and GP-2 are produced as a precursor protein (GP-C) on the rough endoplasmic reticulum. The protein is glycosylated and cleaved to GP-1 (43 kDa) and GP-2 (35 kDa) in the golgi and delivered to the cell surface. Together they form the T-shaped spikes and there are about 650 copies of each per virion.

There is only limited information on arenavirus assembly and release. Unlike many RNA viruses, arenaviruses have no matrix protein. Cross-linking studies indicate that the hydrophilic tail of GP-2 associates with NP and that Z interacts with NP. The assembled virus, together with host ribosomes, is released by budding. Arenaviruses are able to establish persistent infection in cell lines.

Clinical features and pathogenesis

Lymphocytic choriomeningitis virus

LCM virus has a worldwide distribution, reflecting the propensity for international travel of the domestic mouse (*Mus musculus*). Most human infections are acquired by contact with laboratory mice or hamsters. LCM is a rare illness but may present as:

- an undifferentiated febrile illness
- aseptic meningitis
- encephalitis.

The incubation period is 1–2 weeks and the illness is of short duration. It can vary from mild disease with headache and fever to neck stiffness, myalgia and photophobia. Long-term effects, including persistent headache, paralysis and psychological changes have been described. Although persistent infection and T cell reactivity to epitopes on GP-2 associated with disease manifestation have been described in mice, there is no evidence of either in human infections.

Lassa fever

This has an incubation period of 1–3 weeks with a gradual onset of fever, headache and muscle and joint pain. Pharyngitis with a non-productive cough is a common feature. In severe cases there is vomiting, diarrhoea and a raised haematocrit. Within a few days the patient will become increasingly febrile and complain of abdominal and retrosternal pain. The patient is lethargic, with oedema of the face and neck and enlarged lymph nodes. Oedema and bleeding may occur together or independently. Recovery takes 1–3 weeks.

Fatal cases show:

- maintained fever
- rapid deterioration over the first 2 weeks, associated with hypovolaemia, hypotension, pleural effusion, ascites and anuria
- bleeding from the gums, nose, intestine or vagina is linked to platelet dysfunction
- acute neurological changes, varying from unilateral or bilateral deafness (which occurs in a third of patients) to signs of encephalopathy, including generalized seizures, dystonia and neuropsychiatric changes.

Infection in pregnancy (third trimester) is particularly severe, with a 20% mortality rate and 87% fetal/neonatal loss. In children infection is associated with a 'swollen baby' syndrome of widespread oedema, abdominal distension and bleeding.

Blood platelet and lymphocyte counts fall early in the illness. Endothelial cells are damaged, which leads to extravascular fluid loss and thus oedema. Endothelial cell damage, together with platelet loss and dysfunction, lead to the haemorrhagic manifestations. Lassa virus antibodies are produced but this is not necessarily associated with viral clearance. Viraemia can persist for weeks and reaches high levels in severe and fatal cases.

South American haemorrhagic fever

Argentinian, Bolivian, Venezuelan and Brazilian haemorrhagic fevers are caused by Junin, Machupo, Guanarito and Sabia viruses, respectively. Flexal and Tacaribe viruses have caused laboratory-acquired haemorrhagic fever and very recently a variant (c.89% similar) of Whitewater Arroyo virus has caused three fatal cases of Venezuelan haemorrhagic fever in California, USA. The incubation is 1–2 weeks and illness begins with a 'flu-like' prodrome. In severe disease petechiae develop and there can be bleeding from the gastro-intestinal tract. There is fluid leak through damaged vascular endothelium, leading to hypotension, oliguria and hypovolaemic shock. Encephalopathy occurs in a large proportion of patients. The mortality varies between outbreaks but is in the range 5–30%. Virus becomes disseminated throughout the body and there is leucopenia and thrombocytopenia. There is neurological involvement in about half the cases. Haemorrhage results from both capillary damage and platelet dysfunction. Raised levels of tumour necrosis factor-α (TNF-α) and thrombopoietin are proportional to disease severity. There is often bone marrow hypoplasia, perhaps related to low levels of erythropoietin.

Diagnosis

Diagnosis depends upon an initial clinical suspicion of infection, which will also involve obtaining a history of potential contact from travel or contact with infective material. Specific diagnosis depends upon detection of the virus, its antigens or genome. A specific immune response may provide retrospective diagnosis or information on population prevalence of infection.

Arenaviruses can be isolated from:

- blood or serum in acutely infected patients or for up to 2 (Junin, Machupo) to 4 (Lassa) weeks subsequently in severe cases

- throat swabs, breast milk, cerebrospinal fluid (CSF), urine or a variety of tissues taken by biopsy or at autopsy.

Cell culture (BHK, Vero) is the most convenient and efficient mode of *isolation*, although animals (suckling mice, guinea-pigs, hamsters) have been used. The arenaviruses that cause haemorrhagic fever are all in hazard group 4 and culture should not be attempted, except in designated high security laboratories.

Antigen detection from blood by immunofluorescence assays (IFA) or enzyme-linked immunosorbent assay (ELISA) is useful for early diagnosis and prognosis. Early IFA positivity is correlated with risk of death.

Genome detection is by reverse transcriptase polymerase chain reaction (RTPCR) amplification, with or without confirmation by DNA hybridization. A strategy involving overlapping primers to amplify the whole of the S segment followed by restriction endonuclease digestion of amplicons has been shown to detect Old and New World arenaviruses, providing both diagnosis and identification. RTPCR is highly sensitive and specific, and is particularly valuable for early diagnosis. As little as >0.01 pfu of Junin virus, for example, can be detected in blood using such a strategy.

For *antibody detection*, ELISA is the most useful test and can be adapted to detect a specific IgM response. In human cases of LCM virus infection the CSF shows changes typical of viral meningitis. LCM virus can be grown from CSF, blood or brain.

Treatment

Immunotherapy by infusion of convalescent plasma is beneficial, especially if given early in the infection. For example, it has been associated with a decrease in mortality from 16% to 1% in Junin haemorrhagic fever. However, the efficacy is related to the concentration of neutralizing antibodies, and approximately 10% of those receiving immunotherapy develop a neurological syndrome 4–6 weeks later.

Ribavirin given early in the infection (within 6 days) is effective in both animal models and human infection with Lassa fever virus. There is anecdotal evidence of benefit in treating Junin and Sabia virus infections. Intravenous rather than oral ribavirin should be given.

In addition, *fluid, electrolyte and osmotic balances* must be maintained and evidence of development of shock sought, so as to allow rapid resuscitation.

Epidemiology and transmission

Each of the arenavirus infections is zoonotic and, in common with many zoonoses, the animal reservoir host is largely unaffected. In general, arenaviruses persistently infect only two of the rodent families:

- the *Muridae* (house mice, *Mastomys* and *Praomys*) inhabit the same ecosystem as man
- the *Cricetidae* (voles, deer-mice, gerbils) inhabit open grasslands and it is only when they invade man's territory or vice versa that human infections occur.

It is noteworthy, for example, that the peak period for Junin infections is harvest time in Argentina. It is thought that infection in the reservoir host occurs in utero or shortly after birth and that a persistent infection becomes established, with continued virus excretion in saliva and urine. Human infection usually occurs via inoculation into cuts and grazes or inhalation of dust contaminated with urine or saliva from infected rodents. Tacaribe virus is the only virus isolated from outside these two rodent families, being excreted by the fruit bat *Artibeus*. The reservoir hosts for the different arenaviruses are shown in Table 53.1.

Lassa fever virus is excreted persistently by the multimammate rat, *Mastomys natalensis*. The first case to be described was a nurse who may have become infected from her patients in 1969, in Nigeria. Infection also occurred in a laboratory worker who made the first isolation of the virus. Thus it is clear that both person-to-person transmission and laboratory-acquired infection can and do occur. Subsequently a number of outbreaks have occurred with case-to-case transmission and mortality rates in excess of 40%. It is estimated that Lassa fever causes 5000 deaths each year in West Africa. However, in these endemic areas it is clear from serosurveys that infection is widespread and can be very mild. Person-to-person transmission is associated with:

- blood and body fluid contact
- inoculation injuries rather than by the respiratory route.

Argentinian haemorrhagic fever (Junin) is found in the provinces of Buenos Aires, Cordoba, Santa Fe and La Pampa. It is seasonal (April to June), but cases or epidemics occur every year, with 100–4000 cases being reported annually. In untreated individuals mortality ranges from 15 to 30%. Nosocomial infections and laboratory-acquired infections have been described for many of the New World arenaviruses.

Control

A Junin virus vaccine has been produced and is proving effective in Argentina. A vaccinia-recombinant Lassa fever vaccine, expressing each of the structural proteins, has been shown to be highly effective in macaques. Prophylaxis in contacts by using ribavirin has also shown some benefit. It is not possible at present to control the natural reservoirs, although the increases in human cases noted when the rodent population increases suggest that it might be a useful approach. The only protection available is against contamination with rodent excreta. It ought to be possible in colonies of laboratory animals to protect handlers against LCM virus infection but this is a very difficult task in the endemic areas of Africa and South America for the haemorrhagic fever viruses. Suspected and confirmed cases must be cared for in strict isolation in designated hospitals to prevent exposure of the attendant staff to the high levels of virus present in acutely ill patients, especially those with Lassa fever.

FILOVIRUSES

Properties

The family *Filoviridae* is grouped with Rhabdoviridae and Paramyxoviridae within the order Mononegavirales. This is because each of these families of negative-strand RNA viruses has a similar genomic organization. *Marburg* and *Ebola*, the two members of the Filoviridae, are enveloped viruses with a single-stranded, unsegmented, helical negative sense RNA genome. Virions are approximately 80 nm in diameter but vary in length up to 14 000 nm. Marburg is more uniform, with a mean length of 865 nm, but Ebola is more variable (mean 1250 nm). Virions usually appear as long threads (filo is Latin for a thread) but they can be U-shaped, branched or 6-shaped (Fig. 53.2). The genome is approximately 19 kb long, the largest among the Mononegavirales. The non-coding leader (3′) and trailer (5′) ends of the genome are highly conserved among the different filoviruses. There are seven structural genes encoding (from 3′ to 5′) the nucleoprotein (NP), a phosphoprotein (VP35), a matrix-like protein (VP40), a surface glycoprotein (GP), a minor nucleocapsid protein (VP30), a membrane-associated hydrophobic protein (VP24) and the viral RNA polymerase (L). Some genes are separated by intergenic regions but others have short overlaps between them and the next. There is one overlap (VP30–VP24) in the Marburg genome but three in Ebola Zaire.

Embedded in the viral envelopes are glycoprotein spikes (homotrimers of the 120–160-kDa GP in the case of Marburg), that protrude 7 nm above the virion surface. Ebola also secretes a non-structural glycoprotein (sGP) that has c. 300 N-terminal amino acids in common with GP but a different C-terminus. The

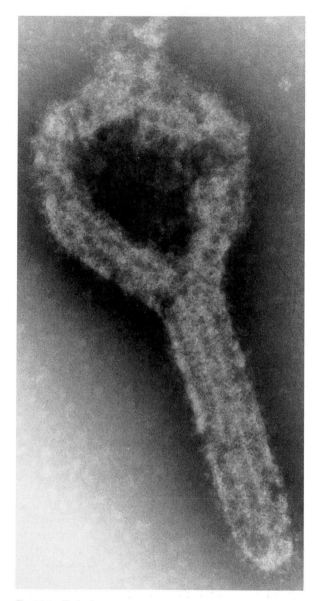

Fig. 53.2 Ebola virus.

differences between the two viruses are summarized in Table 53.2.

Human filovirus disease was first described in 1967 in Marburg (Germany) and shortly afterwards, it is presumed, as part of the same outbreak, in Frankfurt and Belgrade. In each case infection was related directly or indirectly to blood or tissues of vervet monkeys (*Cercopithecus aethiops*) imported to laboratories from Uganda via London. There have been five subsequent episodes, involving one or more case of Marburg infection (Table 53.3). Outbreaks of severe haemorrhagic fever occurred almost simultaneously in Nzara, Sudan

Table 53.2 Differences between Marburg and Ebola viruses

	Ebola	Marburg
Antigenic cross-reactivity	No	No
Subtypes	4	1
Glycoprotein (GP) (kDa)	140	170
Terminal sialylation of carbohydrates	Yes	No
Secreted GP (sGP)	Yes	No
Nucleoprotein (kDa)	105	95
Transcriptional editing	Yes	No
Gene overlaps	2–3	1
Mean virion size (nm)	80 × 1250	80 × 865
Peak infectivity virion length (nm)	805	665
Secondary spread common	Yes	No

(June 1976) and Yambuku, Zaire (August 1976). The filovirus responsible was named Ebola after a small nearby river in Zaire. The two outbreaks were not linked epidemiologically and it was subsequently demonstrated that two different subtypes, Ebola (Sudan) and Ebola (Zaire), were responsible. In 1989, macaques imported from the Philippines and held in a quarantine facility in Reston, Virginia died from similar haemorrhagic fever. Ebola (Reston) was isolated from the macaques. Four employees of the facility became infected asymptomatically. In 1994 a Swiss zoologist who investigated a troup of chimpanzees that had died of haemorrhagic fever developed VHF. This was due to a new subtype of Ebola (Côte d'Ivoire). In 1994 two outbreaks of VHF

Table 53.3 Filovirus infections

Place	Year	Virus/subtype	Cases (mortality)	Epidemiology
Germany/Yugoslavia	1967	Marburg	32 (23%)	Imported Vervet monkeys
Zimbabwe/South Africa	1975	Marburg	3 (33%)	Index infected in Zimbabwe, two secondary cases in companion and nurse
Southern Sudan	1976	Ebola/Sudan	284 (53%)	Origin in cotton factory (bat-infested), nosocomial spread
Northern Zaire	1976	Ebola/Zaire	318 (88%)	Unknown origin, nosocomial spread by needlestick etc.
England	1976	Ebola/Sudan	1 (0%)	Laboratory infection by needlestick
Tandala, Zaire	1977	Ebola/Zaire	1 (100%)	Sporadic case
Southern Sudan	1979	Ebola/Zaire	34 (65%)	Nzara, same site as 1976
Kenya	1980	Marburg	2 (50%)	Index travelled in area that was source of Vervet monkeys in 1967, secondary infection in doctor who survived
Kenya	1987	Marburg	1 (100%)	Traveller to Mount Elgon Cave (bat-infested)
USA	1989	Ebola/Reston	4 (0%)	Monkeys imported from Philippines fatally infected, four humans asymptomatically infected
Russia	1990	Marburg	1 (0%)	Laboratory-acquired
USA	1990	Ebola/Reston	0 (0%)	Imported monkeys from Philippines to same quarantine facilities in Virginia and Texas. No humans infected
Italy	1992	Ebola/Reston	0 (0%)	Imported monkeys from Philippines. No human infections
Gabon	1994	Ebola/?Zaire	44 (63%)	Unknown origin, identified retrospectively
Côte D'Ivoire	1994	Ebola/Côte d'Ivoire	1 (0%)	Conducted autopsy on dead chimpanzee
Liberia	1994	Ebola/Côte d'Ivoire	1 (0%)	Serological diagnosis only
Kikwit, Zaire	1995	Ebola/Zaire	317 (78%)	Source unknown, secondary family and nosocomial cases
Gabon	1996	Ebola/Zaire?	37 (57%)	Butchering dead chimpanzee plus family spread
Gabon	1996	Ebola/Zaire?	60 (75%)	Index case a hunter, secondary spread to close contacts
South Africa	1996	Ebola/Zaire	2 (50%)	Doctor treating patients in Gabon flew to South Africa, infected nurse who died
USA	1996	Ebola/Reston	0 (0%)	Imported monkeys from same facility in Philippines
Philippines	1996	Ebola/Reston	0 (0%)	Home to roost
Democratic Republic of Congo	1999	Marburg	86 (57%)	Community outbreak
Gulu, Uganda	2000	Ebola/?Zaire	400 (40%)	Community and nosocomially-acquired

occurred in Gabon, one in hunters who had butchered a chimpanzee. The Ebola virus that was isolated was related to, but distinct from, Ebola (Zaire). Phylogenetic analysis using the entire GP gene shows that Ebola and Marburg are 72% different and that the four Ebola sub-types, Sudan, Zaire, Reston and Côte d'Ivoire, have 47% nucleotide sequence differences from each other.

Replication

Filoviruses can be grown in a variety of cell lines, including Vero (especially E-6 clone), MA104 and SW13 cells, but culture requires category 4 containment. Although it is known that the asialoglycoprotein on hepatocytes is a receptor for Marburg virus, this molecule is not expressed on many of the other cells infectable by filoviruses. The mode of entry is not known but is presumed to involve membrane fusion. Filovirus replication takes place in the cytoplasm and large inclusions are formed. Mature virus is released as nucleocapsids bud through areas of plasma membrane rich in GP. It is thought that the process is orchestrated by VP40, the matrix-like protein, and/or VP24. In general the replication rates of Ebola (Sudan and Reston) are slower than the others, with a less dramatic cytopathic affect.

Clinical features and pathogenesis

After an incubation period of 4–10 days there is a rapid onset of:

- fever
- malaise
- myalgia
- severe frontal headaches.

Bradycardia and conjunctivitis occur early in the disease. It progresses rapidly with:

- nausea, vomiting, abdominal pain and diarrhoea to haematemasis and melaena
- frank haemorrhagic manifestations, including petechiae, ecchymoses and uncontrollable bleeding from venepuncture sites, within 5–7 days of onset.

Often a maculopapular rash appears around day 5, which is followed by desquamation. Death due to shock usually occurs 6–9 days after onset, with rates of 50–80% for Ebola, a little less for Marburg (Table 53.3). Infection of pregnant women usually results in abortion with fatal infection of the neonate. Recovery in survivors is slow, with weight loss, prostration and amnesia for the period of acute infection.

The filoviruses replicate in the liver and most other tissues in the body. The cause of death is related to both the haemorrhagic diathesis and the increased vascular permeability that causes fluid and blood loss into the extravascular spaces, resulting in shock. The haemorrhagic diathesis is related to both endothelial cell damage and probably platelet dysfunction. The endothelial damage seems to be mediated by the membrane glycoprotein (GP) since transfection of GP from Ebola (Zaire), but not Ebola (Reston), into human endothelial cells causes their complete disruption. During filovirus haemorrhagic fever there is a marked lymphopenia but a neutrophilia with a predominance of band forms. The secretory glycoprotein (sGP) appears to bind to Fc gamma receptor (CD16b) on neutrophils, and inhibit some neutrophil activities. Interestingly, asymptomatic Ebola infection in humans is linked to a strong inflammatory response characterized by high levels of circulating chemokines and cytokines. Although GP is a major target for an immune response, it has an external peptide domain (highly conserved) close to the transmembrane domain that has homology to an immunosuppressive domain in retroviruses. Humoral antibodies are produced within 10–14 days but they are usually nonneutralizing. Persistent infection has been demonstrated in convalescent patients.

Diagnosis

Virus can be isolated from blood by cell culture (Vero E-6 usually). Inclusions develop which can be demonstrated by immunofluorescence. Virus can be visualized by electron microscopy, either after culture or directly in blood in the early stages of infection. ELISA techniques are available for detection of either viral antigen or specific IgM. A recently described RTPCR test amplifying a conserved region of the L gene has proved to be the most sensitive and specific method for rapid diagnosis.

Treatment

Supportive treatment is all that can be offered to patients. Ribavirin has no effect on filovirus replication in vitro. Neither passive immunization nor interferon therapy appears effective. In a mouse model, inhibitors of S-adenosyl-L-homocysteine hydrolase were very effective even in immunosuppressed animals.

Epidemiology and transmission

Both Ebola and Marburg are undoubtedly zoonotic and disease appears to be more severe in primary than secondary cases. The nature of the reservoir host is unclear. Although a number of cases have been acquired from chimpanzees and monkeys it is unlikely that they are the definitive host, since they also develop severe or fatal infection. Persistent infection in bats has been achieved experimentally, and contact with bats was a risk factor for infection in Sudan and Mount Elgon. A recent study has demonstrated the presence of the Ebola virus genome and, in one case, nucleocapsid in the organs of small rodents in the Central African Republic, although virus was not grown. Species included *Mus setulosus, Praomys* spp., and a shrew, *Sylvisorex ollula*. Transmission appears to be associated with contamination from blood-stained body fluids or tissues. Although air-borne spread has been demonstrated, for example with Ebola (Reston) in monkeys, this does not seem to play a major role in human spread. Nosocomial spread is common, particularly affecting nurses and doctors. Transmission by sexual intercourse has been described from one case, to his wife, 83 days after initial infection.

Control

In hospital settings spread is controlled by patient isolation, use of protective clothing and strict attention to safe disposal of needles, syringes and blood and other body fluids. Filovirus infectivity is destroyed by:

- heating at 60°C for 30 min
- UV and gamma irradiation
- formalin (1%)
- lipid solvents
- β-propiolactone
- hypochlorite or phenolic disinfectants.

There is no safe and effective vaccine; however, a DNA vaccination strategy (GP genes) has proved highly effective in preventing Ebola infection in monkey models.

RECOMMENDED READING

Fields B N, Knipe D M, Howley P M (eds) 1996 *Virology*, 3rd edn. Plenum Press, New York

Richman D D, Whitley R J, Hayden F G (eds) 1997 *Clinical Virology*, Churchill Livingstone, New York

54

Reoviruses

Gastroenteritis

U. Desselberger

The *Reoviridae* constitute a diverse family of viruses that infect humans, many mammals, other vertebrates (including birds), plants and insects. The genus *Rotavirus* is recognized as the most important cause of infantile gastro-enteritis throughout the world. Viruses in the genera *Orbivirus* and *Coltivirus* infect various species of insects and can thus be described as arboviruses; they are discussed in Chapter 51.

CLASSIFICATION

Four out of the nine genera of the *Reoviridae* family infect humans:

- *Orthoreovirus* – reovirus types 1, 2, and 3
- *Orbivirus* and *Coltivirus* – various serogroups
- *Rotavirus* – several groups, multiple serotypes.

All reoviruses have a double-shelled capsid, no envelope and measure 75–80 nm in diameter. The main features are listed in Table 54.1. The RNA genome consists of 10–12 segments of double-stranded RNA. Functionally, reoviruses can be regarded as negative-stranded RNA viruses, as the virion-associated RNA polymerase early in replication only transcribes from the negative strand and as isolated viral RNA is not infectious. All reoviruses replicate in the cytoplasm of infected cells and form intracytoplasmic inclusion bodies. Whereas orthoreoviruses and rotaviruses are relatively stable over a wide pH range, orbiviruses and coltiviruses lose infectivity at low pH.

REPLICATION

Attachment is via a specific protein component of the outer capsid, e.g. $\sigma 1$ of orthoreoviruses or VP4 of rotaviruses, to a cellular receptor (the β-adrenergic receptor and sialoglycoproteins for orthoreoviruses, and sialoglycoproteins and integrins for rotaviruses). The viral protein–receptor interaction leads to a conformational change in the viral capsid, which enters the cell by receptor-mediated endocytosis or direct penetration. In the cytoplasm the outer capsid is removed (uncoating), but the viral RNA remains in the inner capsid (subviral particle). RNA is transcribed by the virion-associated, RNA-dependent RNA polymerase complex to produce messenger RNA (mRNA, plus sense) molecules from each RNA segment. The mRNA molecules, which are capped but not polyadenylated, leave the subviral particle and are translated to generate the various viral proteins. They also act as templates for RNA replication, which is completed by the RNA polymerase complex using single-stranded plus sense RNA

Table 54.1 Classification and features of genera of the Reoviridae infecting man

	Reovirus genus			
	Orthoreovirus	*Rotavirus*	*Orbivirus*	*Coltivirus*
Size (nm)	80	75	80	80
No. of RNA segments	10	11	10	12
Molecular weight of genomes (Da)	15.5×10^6	12.2×10^6	12.7×10^6	$\sim 18 \times 10^6$
Host range	Humans, other vertebrates	Humans, other vertebrates	Humans, other vertebrates, arthropods	Humans, other vertebrates, arthropods

segments as templates which are packaged within new core structures. Particle assembly takes place in the cytoplasm, and aggregates of core particles and subviral particles may be detected histologically as inclusion bodies. Mature virions (double-shelled particles) are formed in the endoplasmic reticulum and are released after cellular lysis. Double infection of cells with closely related reoviruses leads to a viral progeny carrying various combinations of different segments from both parents; those viruses are defined as reassortants.

ASSOCIATION WITH CLINICAL ILLNESS

The first human isolates of the *Reoviridae* were made from both respiratory secretions and faeces but could not be associated with disease – hence the name *reo*viruses (*r*espiratory *e*nteric *or*phan) was proposed. However, orthoreoviruses cause systemic disease (meningitis and encephalitis) in mice, and this virus–host system has been used extensively to dissect different steps and mechanisms of viral pathogenesis at a molecular level. Viral pathogenicity turns out to be a multifactorial phenotype. Although most of the human population is exposed to and develops antibodies against orthoreoviruses from an early age, there is still no clear link between these viruses and illness in man.

The orbiviruses include several serogroups which infect humans and which are transmitted by a variety of insects (ticks, midges and mosquitoes). In the blood the virus is associated with erythrocytes, and in this way is hidden from immune responses. Clinically, patients experience a febrile illness, with rashes in 10% and leucopenia in two-thirds of the cases. Infections of the central nervous system leading to meningitis or encephalitis are seen in 3–7% of laboratory-certified cases (see Chapter 51).

The coltiviruses are also transmitted by insects (ticks, mosquitoes), and rodents are considered to be the main animal reservoir. Man is usually infected by insect bite and develops a febrile illness with gastro-intestinal symptoms (20%), rash (10%) and meningitis/encephalitis (3–7%) (see Chapter 51).

Rotaviruses are the main viral cause of acute gastroenteritis in infants and young children, and will therefore be reviewed in more detail below.

ROTAVIRUSES

Rotavirus infections are usually mild to moderately severe in developed countries but can become very severe and cause high mortality in developing countries. Rotaviruses also cause diarrhoea in the young of a wide variety of mammals and birds. In the early 1980s, a rotavirus (*a*dult *d*iarrhoea *rota*virus, ADRV) was identified as the cause of outbreaks of diarrhoea in children and adults in different parts of China.

Description and classification

Morphologically, rotaviruses are polyhedrons of 75 nm diameter displaying characteristic sharp-edged double-shelled capsids, which in electron micrographs (Fig. 54.1) look like spokes grouped around the hub of a wheel (Latin, *rota*) The name 'rotavirus' was derived from this appearance which is pathognomonic. More detailed structural studies have shown (Figs 54.2 and 54.3) that the double-shelled capsid is penetrated by a large number of channels and that it carries on the surface 60 protrusions that consist of dimers of VP4 (viral protein 4) molecules (see below).

The genome of rotaviruses is located inside the inner core and consists of 11 segments of double-stranded RNA (Table 54.1) that can be easily extracted from viruses and separated by polyacrylamide gel electrophoresis (PAGE, Fig. 54.4). All segments, except one, code for only one virus-specific protein (VP), and gene–protein assignments have been completed for several rotavirus strains.

RNA segments 1, 2 and 3 code for the inner core proteins VP1, VP2 and VP3, respectively; VP2 is the main scaffolding protein (core layer). RNA segment 6 codes for the inner capsid protein, VP6, which forms a middle layer interacting with the core protein VP2 and the outer capsid proteins (see below); VP6 carries epitopes specifying groups and subgroups. So far, seven different groups (A–G) have been identified; for groups A–E complete lack of serological cross-reactivity has been proven. Within a group, all viruses share common VP6 antigens but may be further differentiated into subgroups. Thus, within group A there are at least four subgroups (I; II; I+II; non-I, non-II), which are identified by specific antisera and monoclonal antibodies. Most of the human rotaviruses are of group A; the Chinese ADRV is of group B; group C rotaviruses cause occasional outbreaks in humans. The outer capsid (third layer) is formed by two proteins, VP7, a glycoprotein (encoded by RNA 7, 8 or 9, depending on strain), and VP4 (encoded by RNA 4). Both surface proteins carry neutralization-specific epitopes that define serotypes. VP4 is post-translationally cleaved into the VP5* and VP8* subunits; proteolytic cleavage is essential for infectivity. Six non-structural proteins (NSP1–NSP6) are coded for by RNAs 5, 7, 8 or 9 (depending on strain), 10 and 11 (encoding NSP5 + NSP6), and have various functions during replication, mainly in morphogenesis.

So far, 14 different VP7-specific serotypes (G types, derived from *g*lycoprotein) and over 20 different VP4-

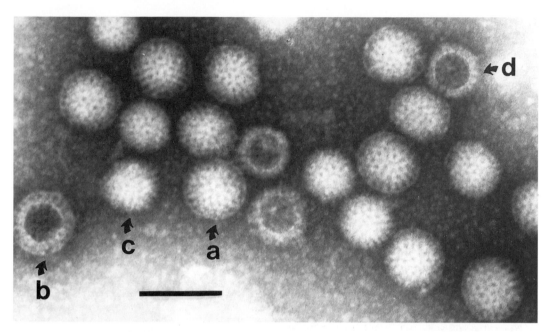

Fig. 54.1 Rotavirus particles in the faeces of a child admitted to hospital with acute gastro-enteritis. Negative staining with 2% potassium phosphotungstate, pH 7.0. The scale bar represents 100 nm. Examples of four different morphological forms are arrowed: **a** double-shelled (ds) particle containing RNA; **b** ds particle without RNA ('empty'; core penetrated with stain); **c** single-shelled (ss) particle containing RNA; **d**, ss empty particle. (By courtesy of M. Jenkins, Regional Virus Laboratory, East Birmingham Hospital.)

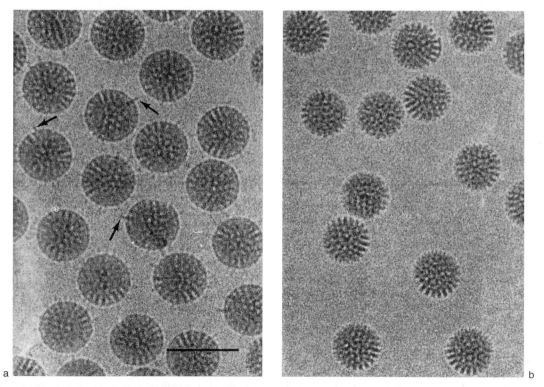

Fig. 54.2 **a** Double-shelled and **b** single-shelled rotavirus particles visualized by cryo-electron microscopy. The arrows indicate spikes (VP4) protruding from the surface of double-shelled particles. The scale bar represents 100 nm. (From Prasad et al. 1988 *Journal of Molecular Biology* 199: 269–275, with permission from the authors and publishers.)

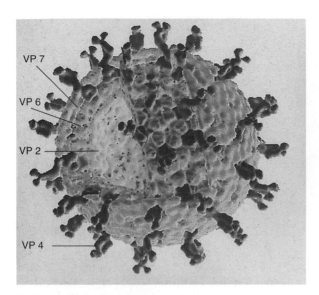

Fig. 54.3 Diagram of the three-dimensional structure of rotavirus particles derived from cryo-electron microscopy images. Core layer (VP2); inner capsid (VP6); outer capsid (VP7; with inserted dimeric VP4 spikes) shown as a whole particle with partial removal of capsid layers to illustrate the interaction of VP2 with VP6, VP6 with VP7, VP4 with VP7 and VP6. The outer and inner capsids are perforated by 132 holes of three types of symmetry. (From Yeager M et al. 1994 *EMBO Journal* 13: 1011–1018 by permission of Oxford University Press.)

specific types (P types, derived from *p*rotease-sensitive protein) have been distinguished. Whilst the correlation between G serotypes and genotypes is complete, not all P types have been confirmed as serotypes yet, and therefore the P serotype designation differs from the P genotype designation, e.g. strain Wa being designated as A/human/Wa(G1P1A[8]) etc. As VP7 and VP4 are coded for by different RNA segments, they can segregate independently, and a large variety of different G–P-type combinations of rotaviruses have been observed after reassortment in vitro and in nature in vivo. For example, G3 types carry P determinants of at least five different P types (P[2], P[3], P[8], P[12] and P[16]), and P[8] types at least four different G types (G1, G3, G4 and G9). Certain G and P types are only found in humans (e.g. G9, G12; P[4], P[8]) or only in animals (e.g. G11, G13; P[7], P[15], P[16]); other G and P types are found in *both* humans and animals (e.g. G3, G6, G10; P[3], P[6], P[11]). Certain G/P combinations (e.g. G3P[3], G4P[6] or G10P[11]) have been observed in *both* humans and animals, raising the possibility of zoonotic transmission (see below). Animals from which rotavirus can be readily isolated are cattle, sheep, horses, pigs, dogs, cats and mice, but also elks, rabbits, monkeys and many others.

Electrophoresis of genomic RNA segments (PAGE) has been used to establish so-called 'electropherotypes'

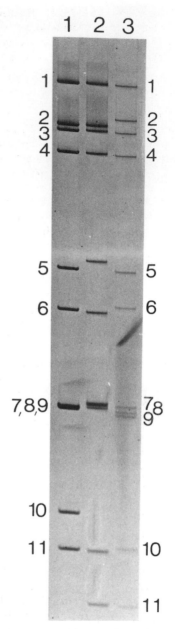

Fig. 54.4 Profiles of genomic RNA of rotaviruses. RNA extracted from purified rotavirus particles was separated by electrophoresis on a polyacrylamide gel. RNA segments (1–11) are labelled at both sides. A 'short' electropherotype RNA is shown in track 1; two 'long' electropherotype RNAs differing in the migration rate of corresponding segments are shown in tracks 2 and 3. (By courtesy of F. Hundley, Institute of Virology, Glasgow.)

of rotavirus isolates (Fig. 54.4). Besides 'long' and 'short' electropherotypes (differing in the rates of relative migration of RNA segments 10 and 11), various minor differences in the migration of corresponding segments have been recognized. These differences have been utilized extensively in epidemiological studies, but for many surveillance purposes and for vaccine development serological classification remains essential.

Pathogenesis and immunity

Rotaviruses replicate exclusively in the differentiated epithelial cells at the tips of the villi of the small intestine. New virus is produced after 10–12 h. Progeny virus is released in large numbers into the intestinal lumen ready to infect other cells. Biopsies show atrophy of the villi with reactive crypt hyperplasia and lymphocytic infiltrates in the lamina propria. The cellular damage leads to malabsorption of nutrients, electrolytes and water, and the crypt hyperplasia to hypersecretion. An osmotic and secretory diarrhoea with vomiting and dehydration results. It has been established that the product of RNA 4, VP4, holds a central position for replication, spread and pathogenicity of rotaviruses, but that products of other RNA segments also contribute to the development of disease. In particular, NSP4 (encoded by RNA segment 10) has been recognized as a viral enterotoxin.

The infection is followed by a local, humoral and cell-mediated immune response and is normally overcome within a week. Rotavirus-specific IgA enteric antibodies, which are secreted into the gut, are the best known correlate of protection. Infection with one serotype provides homotypic, and re-infection leads to partial heterotypic, protection. In the immunodeficient host, however, a persistent infection can occur with severe chronic diarrhoea.

Clinical features

The onset of symptoms is abrupt after a short incubation period of 1–2 days. Diarrhoea and vomiting are seen in the majority of infected children and last for 2–6 days. Although symptoms of respiratory tract infection are frequently observed at the time of rotavirus infections, there is no evidence that rotaviruses replicate in the respiratory tract. Clinical symptoms can range from mild to very severe, in part depending on the rotavirus strain. Asymptomatic infections of neonates with 'nursery strains' are not uncommon. It has been estimated that about half of all gastro-enteritis cases in children requiring admission to hospital are caused by rotaviruses. Infection has been detected in older children and adults, but is usually asymptomatic. Only in the elderly have outbreaks of diarrhoea due to rotavirus infection been observed. Rotavirus infections can be life-threatening if children are already malnourished. Five million children under the age of 2 years die from diarrhoeal disease in developing countries each year; rotavirus infections account for about 20% of these deaths.

Laboratory diagnosis

At the peak of the disease as many as 10^{11} virus particles per millilitre of faeces are present. Therefore, the diagnosis is not difficult. Agglutination tests using latex particles coated with rotavirus-specific antibody and different forms of enzyme-linked immunosorbent assay (ELISA) are most commonly used. Electron microscopy, when routinely applied to the diagnosis of viral diarrhoea in infants and young children, will easily detect the characteristic virus particles (see Fig. 54.1) and also particles of other gastro-enteritis viruses (caliciviruses, astroviruses and enteric adenoviruses (see Chapters 56 and 42). Group, subgroup, and G and P serotypes of rotaviruses are determined by ELISA with monoclonal antibodies. Recently, reverse transcription polymerase chain reaction (RTPCR) with gene- and type-specific primers has been widely applied as a very reliable typing procedure. Most human group A rotaviruses are of subgroup II and types G1P[8], G3P[8] or G4P[8], or of subgroup I and type G2P[4]. In the majority of cases there are sufficient numbers of virions in faeces to allow identification of RNA profiles by PAGE (Fig. 54.4). Although they are fastidious, rotaviruses can be propagated in secondary or continuous cultures of monkey kidney cells. To ensure success it is necessary to incorporate trypsin in the culture medium. Cell culture, however, is not used for routine diagnosis.

Epidemiology

Rotavirus infections occur worldwide. Most symptomatic infections are seen in children under 2 years of age; by the age of 3 years, more than 90% of children have been infected by most of the major serotypes. In family outbreaks there may be evidence of subclinical infection in older children and adults who may be the source of infection for young children in family or nursery outbreaks. The release of enormous numbers of virions during the acute stage contributes to the easy transmission of the virus. Only a few virus particles are sufficient to cause disease in the susceptible host. Longer-lasting outbreaks may be maintained by the ability of the virus to survive outside the body for some time. In temperate climates there is a pronounced seasonal incidence, with peaks in the winter months occurring with 'clockwise precision'. In tropical areas infections occur evenly throughout the year.

Various surveys in different parts of the world have shown that at any time there is co-circulation of genomically and serologically different rotaviruses. In tropical and subtropical regions, high prevalence of G/P constellations are seen which are rare in temperate climates (e.g. G8P[6], G9P[11]). G9P[6] viruses have recently emerged in a number of countries of several continents.

At the molecular level, several factors have been identified that can explain the genomic and antigenic variability of co-circulating rotavirus strains:

- Like the genomes of other viruses that depend on virion-associated, RNA-dependent RNA polymerases for their replication, rotavirus genomes undergo frequent point mutations that accumulate in time and give rise to lineages and sublineages.
- Rotaviruses, like other segmented RNA viruses, undergo extensive reassortment in doubly infected cells. This has been shown to occur both in vitro and in vivo. If RNA segments coding for subgroup- and serotype-specific proteins are involved, antigenic shift can occur in reassortants (mechanisms 1 and 2 are also seen in influenza A viruses; see Chapter 49).
- Rotaviruses may be transferred into humans from animal species, and this may contribute to the genomic variability. Human group A rotavirus isolates have been described, the genome of which is very closely related to that of cat and cattle rotaviruses. ADRVs of group B may have been derived recently from animals, perhaps rats. On the other hand, human group C rotaviruses are significantly different from animal group C rotaviruses.
- Rotaviruses establishing chronic infections in immunodeficient hosts undergo various forms of genome rearrangements, resulting in highly atypical RNA profiles. Evidence is now emerging that such rearrangements may occur more frequently than originally thought.
- Various combinations of these factors may occur, e.g. reassortment of viruses with rearranged genomes, or point mutations combined with reassortment.

Treatment and control

Therapy consists mainly of oral, sometimes intravenous, rehydration with fluids of specified electrolyte and glucose composition (see Table 30.2, p. 299). Antimotility drugs (codein phosphate, loperamide) are generally not advised for use in children, but recently developed enkephalinase inhibitors (e.g. racecadotril) which decrease gut secretion but not motility have been given successfully to children.

As with any infectious agent transmitted by the faecal–oral route, attention to hygienic measures such as handwashing and disinfection of contaminated surfaces and safe disposal of faeces are very important.

For a variety of reasons, rotavirus infections have so far resisted prevention by widespread vaccination. Co-circulation of several serotypes at a time occurs in populations at risk (see above), which is also reflected in polytypic serum antibody responses. Furthermore, it is not fully clear to what extent vaccination with one rotavirus serotype cross-protects against other serotypes. However, polyvalent 'cocktail' vaccines containing two or more different serotypes have been shown to have a significant effect on preventing severe disease. One of them, a rhesus rotavirus-based tetravalent human reassortant vaccine (RRV-TV, RotaShield™), had been licensed in the USA in 1998 for universal use, and over 1.5 million doses (three doses per child at the ages of 2, 4 and 6 months) were administered over the following year. However, the vaccine had to be revoked and taken off the market when a strong epidemiological link between application of the first (and second) dose of the vaccine and the development of gut intussusception became apparent.

A number of different candidate vaccines of live-attenuated rotavirus of bovine or human origin, including bovine rotavirus monoreassortants carrying human VP7 genes of different serotypes, are currently being evaluated. Baculovirus-expressed virus-like particles, DNA-based vaccines and micro-encapsidated viral proteins or cDNAs are also being explored. It is hoped that (an) efficient rotavirus vaccine(s) will become available in the not too distant future.

RECOMMENDED READING

Burke B, Desselberger U 1996 Rotavirus pathogenicity. *Virology* 218: 299–305

Desselberger U 1998 Reoviruses. In: Mahy B and Collier L (eds) *Topley and Wilson's Microbiology and Microbial Infections*. 9th edn. Vol. 1: Virology. Edward Arnold, London

Desselberger U 1999 Rotavirus infections. Guidelines for treatment and prevention. *Drugs* 58: 447–452

Desselberger U 2000 Viruses associated with acute diarrhoeal disease. In: Zuckerman A J, Banatvala J E, Pattison J R (eds) *Principles and Practice of Clinical Virology*, 4th edn. Wiley, Chichester

Estes M K 1996 Rotaviruses. In: Fields B N, Knipe D M, Howley P M (eds) *Virology*, 3rd edn Lippincott Raven, Philadelphia

Murphy T V, Garguillo P M, Massoudi M S et al. 2001 Intussusception among infants given an oral rotavirus vaccine. *New England Journal of Medicine* 344: 564–572

Salazar-Lindo E, Santisteban J, Chea-Woo E, Gutierrez M 2000 Racecadotril in the treatment of acute watery diarrhoea in children. *New England Journal of Medicine* 343: 463–467

Velazquez F R, Matson D O, Calva J J et al. 1996 Rotavirus infections in infants as protection against subsequent infections. *New England Journal of Medicine* 335: 1022–1028

55

Retroviruses

Acquired immune deficiency syndrome; lymphoma

P. Simmonds and J. F. Peutherer

The family Retroviridae contains many viruses from widely different host species. They have been studied in the laboratory for many years, initially because some are associated with tumour production in their natural hosts. Indeed, a wide variety of tumours are caused by the oncovirus genus, including leukaemias and lymphomas, sarcomas, breast and brain tumours, auto-immune disease and blood disorders. The host species include birds, mice, cattle, pigs and several primates. Despite intense effort, it was not until 1980 that the first human retrovirus was isolated from the T cells of patients with T cell leukaemia – the *human T lymphotropic virus type-1* or HTLV-I. Since then, the cause of the acquired immune deficiency syndrome (AIDS) has been shown to be a retrovirus, also with a predilection for T cells but differing significantly from HTLV-I. It is known as the *human immunodeficiency virus type 1* or HIV-1. Infection with this virus has become pandemic and is a major cause of mortality in sub-Saharan Africa and other developing countries. Infection with the related HIV-2 is restricted largely to West Africa and shows a lesser pathogenicity.

DESCRIPTION

All retroviruses have an outer envelope consisting of lipid and viral proteins; the envelope encloses the core, made of other viral proteins, within which lie two molecules of viral RNA and the enzyme reverse transcriptase, an RNA-dependent DNA polymerase. The virions have a diameter of about 100 nm and, in thin section, differences can be seen in the appearance of the core; those with a central condensed structure are known as type C particles while those with an eccentric bar structure are type D particles (Fig. 55.1).

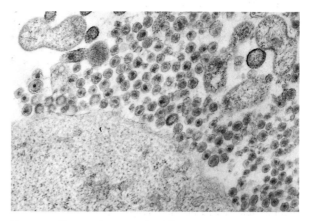

Fig. 55.1 Electron micrograph of HIV. Thin section of infected T lymphocyte. There are numerous virions lying outside the cell membrane.

Virus stability

HIV is inactivated by:

- heat, in the autoclave or hot air oven
- glutaraldehyde 2%
- hypochlorite (10 000 ppm.); 1 in 10 dilution of domestic bleach
- other disinfectants, including alcohols.

The chemicals will inactivate at least 10^5 units of virus within a few minutes, but it is important to remember that disinfectants are inactivated in the presence of organic material.

The survival of HIV has been investigated. It has been shown that:

- virus may survive for up to 15 days at room temperature
- at 37°C virus can survive for 10–15 days
- over 60°C virus is inactivated 100-fold each hour.

These are the limits of survival. However, the results underline the need for cleanliness and disinfection when dealing with blood and infected secretions.

CLASSIFICATION

The family Retroviridae was originally divided into the subfamilies *Oncovirinae*, *Spumavirinae* and *Lentivirinae*, based on their biological properties and appearances in cell cultures. However, the availability of nucleotide sequences from a large number of human and animal retroviruses has indicated that viruses referred to as oncoviruses belong to several distinct groups. In the new classification of retroviruses there are five groups, including two corresponding to the original lentiviruses and spumaviruses, a group containing HTLV-I and -II and the B/D group that contains a number of oncogenic viruses from other animals (Fig. 55.2).

The human viruses HTLV-I and HTLV-II are related to the simian viruses STLV-I and -II that are widely distributed in Old and New World monkeys. In common with HTLV-I, they can cause lymphomas in some pri-

mates. STLV-I shows approximately 90% similarity to HTLV-I at the sequence level. A more distantly related virus is found in cows (bovine leukaemia virus). Three major lineages of HTLV-I have been identified within human populations.

The spumaviruses have been detected in various species, including cats, cattle and primates, but are not associated with disease. The name is derived from the foamy or vacuolated appearance of infected cells in culture. There is no evidence for widespread infection of humans with spumaviruses.

The lentiviruses are so named due to their association with slowly progressive diseases. Visna and maedi of sheep were the first to be recognized; they are different clinical presentations of the same virus. The genus includes a virus causing arthritis and encephalitis in goats, equine infectious anaemia virus, and feline, bovine and simian viruses. HIV-1 and -2 are more closely related to lentiviruses infecting Old World primates. HIV-2 is almost identical to simian immunodeficiency virus (SIV) found in sooty mangabeys, and it is likely that human infection originated through cross-species transmission. Similarly, HIV-1 corresponds closely to SIV variants infecting chimps in Central Africa that are the probable source of the human virus.

The genome organization is similar for all retroviruses in that their genomes contain in the same order the genes *gag*, *pol* and *env*, which code for the three groups of structural proteins (Figs 55.3 and 55.4). The long terminal repeat sequences (LTR) at both ends of the genome contain promoter and enhancer sequences. There are important differences between the types in the nature and arrangement of the genes involved in the regulation of the replication cycle. There are at least six regulatory genes in HIV and at least two in HTLV-I. In HIV, *tat* codes for a protein that has a general stimulating effect on the synthesis of all viral proteins through its binding to a region in the LTR that promotes transcription of viral mRNAs. The *rev* gene product has a regulatory effect, switching on viral protein synthesis by favouring the production of full-length RNA molecules rather than the spliced RNA from the regulatory genes. There is evidence that the product of other transactivating genes, such as that of cytomegalovirus, can also act on the same sequence within the LTR of HIV. The four proteins coded for by the *gag* gene of HIV are all found in the virion (Fig. 55.4), including p24. The *pol* gene products are a protease, endonuclease, integrase and reverse transcriptase. The *env* gene codes for a large protein that is glycosylated and cleaved to gp41, the transmembrane protein and gp120, the external envelope glycoprotein present on the envelope as a trimer with many glycosylation sites. Both HIV-1 and -2 show considerable sequence variability, which has allowed their

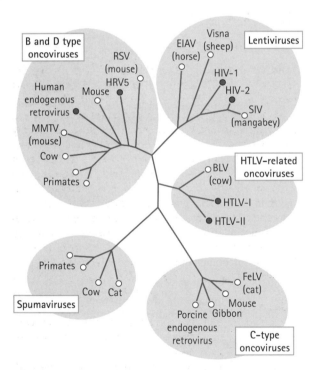

Fig. 55.2 Tree of sequences from the retroviral *pol* gene showing relatedness of retroviruses infecting humans and a range of animal species. Sequences form five main groups, in which human retroviruses are found in three. Viruses previously classified as oncoviruses comprise three genetically distinct groups (C-type, B/D-type and HTLV-related). For animal retroviruses the host species and names of familiar viruses are indicated (MMTV, Moloney murine tumour virus; RSV, Rous sarcoma virus; BLV, bovine leukaemia virus; FeLV, feline leukaemia virus; EIAV, equine infectious anaemia virus). The tree includes sequences of endogenous retroviruses found in the germline of the host (human and pig).

classification into a number of subtypes that show marked differences in geographical distribution and association with different risk groups (see below). HIV variants are currently classified into at least eight subtypes (A–H) that differ from each other by 20–30% in nucleotide sequence. In addition, in areas with more than one subtype in circulation, viruses with recombinant genomes have been described.

REPLICATION

Retroviruses differ from other RNA viruses in that they replicate and produce viral RNA from a DNA copy of the virion RNA. The best studied method of attachment of HIV to cells is by the interaction of the external envelope glycoprotein gp120 with part of the CD4 molecule of T helper lymphocytes and other cells. Attachment is followed by interaction of the HIV envelope with a second (co-) receptor. Membrane proteins used by HIV-1 and -2 in this second step include the chemokine receptors, CCR5 and CXCR4. These are expressed on a wide range of lymphoid and non-lymphoid cells, whose ligands are chemotactic cytokines such as macrophage inflammatory protein-1α involved in inflammatory responses. After this second binding step, entry of the virus occurs by fusion of the viral envelope with the cellular membrane, a step that requires exposure of a hydrophobic domain in gp41. Once the RNA is released into the cytoplasm, the reverse transcriptase acts to form the double-stranded DNA copy, which is circularized, enters the nucleus and is spliced into the host cell DNA (see Chapter 9). Once inserted into the host DNA, infection with HIV is permanent. The virus may stay latent or enter a productive cycle. Transcription of mRNA from the provirus is by the host RNA polymerase to produce viral mRNA and RNA. Proteins are synthesized and processed to form the virion components (Figs 55.3 and 55.4). Virions are assembled

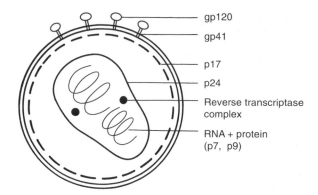

Fig. 55.4 Diagram of HIV to show location of structural proteins.

at the cell membrane where envelope and core proteins have located. The internal structure of the virion matures as the virion buds from the cell. In the productive growth cycle the host cell is destroyed.

CLINICAL FEATURES

HTLV–1 infection

Adult T cell leukaemia/lymphoma (ATL) was first recognized in Japan, and the isolation of the virus HTLV-I reported in 1980. The disease is an acute T cell proliferative malignancy; clinically, the features are leukaemia, generalized lymphadenopathy and hepatosplenomegaly with bone marrow and skin involvement. It is now clear that other less dramatic forms exist, including a variant that runs a slow course, associated with adenopathy and splenomegaly. Another disease, a non-Hodgkin T cell lymphoma, is also recognized. The T cells involved carry the CD4 antigen. HTLV-I is the cause of a neurological disease, *tropical spastic paraparesis*, a slowly progressive myelopathy with spastic or ataxic features. Pathologically, areas of demyelination with lymphocytic inflammation and perivascular cuffing are seen. Males are at greater risk of developing ATL. A form of uveitis is also recognized.

No acute disease is apparent at the time of seroconversion. The period of latency until ATL arises lasts for many years, often decades.

During the latent period viral proteins are expressed, as there are steady high titres to various proteins, particularly the *gag* proteins. The virus is genetically stable and little cell-free virus is produced. However, during the latent period, virus is present as integrated provirus and is replicated with the cell DNA as the cell divides. The viral DNA provirus is present within the tumour cells, which contain monoclonally integrated HTLV-I provirus at random sites. There are no transforming

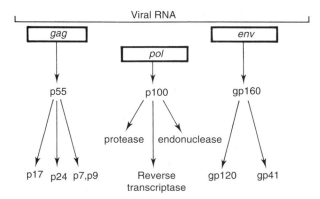

Fig. 55.3 The genomic organization of HIV structural genes and their protein products.

genes; the T cell proliferation is the result of the action of the viral *tax* gene. This can activate transcription of cellular genes including those for interleukin-2 and its receptor, and cause cell proliferation. It is not known what triggers this effect after the long latency in the 1–4% of those infected who develop disease. Antibody to the *tax* protein can block the stimulation of cell division; loss or decay of immune control may be important.

HTLV-II is not linked to a particular disease, although the first isolation was from a patient with a rare T hairy-cell leukaemia.

HIV and AIDS

In contrast to HTLV-I, a great deal is known about the association of HIV with disease; Fig. 55.5 summarizes the clinical stages.

The acute seroconversion illness resembles glandular fever, with adenopathy and flu-like symptoms. Although most patients will experience some symptoms, only 5–10% show the full picture. Even fewer have the rare encephalitic presentation.

Persistent generalized lymphadenopathy (PGL) is present in 25–30% of patients who are otherwise asymptomatic (Table 55.1). The enlarged lymph nodes are painless and symmetrical in distribution. The rate of progression of patients with PGL to AIDS is no greater than in those without adenopathy.

The *acquired immune deficiency syndrome (AIDS)* presents in many ways, all due to the underlying severe loss of the ability to respond to infectious agents and to control tumours. The features classified as group IV include what was known as the *AIDS-related complex* or ARC. This label was applied to patients with constitutional symptoms of fever, weight loss and diarrhoea and minor opportunistic infections. Without treatment, such patients will progress rapidly to AIDS. The clinical fea-

Table 55.1 Classification of HIV infection and AIDS (Communicable Disease Center, USA)

Group I	Seroconversion illness
Group II	Asymptomatic
Group III	Persistent generalized lymphadenopathy
Group IV	
	A – Constitutional disease
	B – Neurological disease
	C – Secondary infectious disease
	D – Secondary cancers
	E – Other conditions

tures of AIDS are varied and reflect the specific agents involved: a diagnosis is made if the conditions listed in Table 55.2 are present.

Oral hairy leucoplakia appears to be unique to HIV-infected patients. The margins of the tongue show white ridges of fronds on the epithelium. An association with Epstein–Barr virus and papilloma viruses has been proposed.

Table 55.2 Group IV disease (Communicable Disease Surveillance Centre, London)

Not Aids indicator disease
Zoster
Oral candidiasis
Oral hairy leucoplakia
Seborrhoeic dermatitis
Other infections – strongyloidiasis, nocardiasis, pulmonary tuberculosis
Constitutional symptoms
Peripheral neuropathy and myelopathy
Thrombocytopenia

Aids indicator disease
Bacterial infection, multiple or recurrent in child aged less than 12 years
Candidiasis of oesophagus, trachea, bronchi, lungs
Coccidioidomycosis
Cryptococcosis
Cryptosporidiosis
Histoplasmosis
Isosporiasis
Mycobacteriosis – disseminated or extrapulmonary
Pneumocystis carinii pneumonia
Toxoplasmosis of brain
Salmonellosis-recurrent septicaemia
Cytomegalovirus, e.g. retinitis
Herpes simplex virus for more than 1 month; or bronchi, lung or oesophagus involved
Progressive multifocal leuco-encephalopathy
HIV dementia
Kaposi's sarcoma
Lymphoma – Burkitt's or immunoblastic or primary in brain
Lymphoid interstitial pneumonia/pulmonary lymphoid hyperplasia in child aged less than 12 years
Wasting syndrome

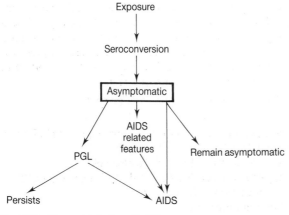

Fig. 55.5 Stages of infection with HIV.

Kaposi's sarcoma was one of the earliest diseases used to define AIDS. This rare tumour had been known for many years; it usually occurred at a single site and was not aggressive. In AIDS patients the tumour arises in many sites, including the skin, mouth, gut and eye. The tumours arise from endothelial cells of blood vessels, causing bluish–purple, raised irregular lesions. The aetiological agent is thought to be human herpesvirus 8 (see p. 419). The tumours were seen only in homosexual men; the incidence has now declined.

Pneumocystis carinii pneumonia was another presentation found in many of the first patients recognized. This opportunist pathogen was known to cause infections in the immunocompromised, but the diagnosis in young men with no explanation for their immunosuppression was the first clue to the recognition of AIDS.

Toxoplasma gondii infections can manifest at various sites, but are always associated with compromised patients. The brain is an important site.

HIV dementia develops in 25% of patients with AIDS and is marked by a gradual loss of cognition, progressing to overt dementia. Brain scans show a loss of tissue, with widening of sulci and ventricles.

In developing countries many of the same infections are seen but there is an emphasis on local problems. *Mycobacterium tuberculosis* infections are an enormous problem in many regions, with the development of strains of the organism resistant to many antibiotics. Many patients show profound weight loss, perhaps accompanied by chronic diarrhoea; the term *slim disease* has been given to this presentation.

Paediatric AIDS cases suffer from many of the problems of adults. However, children infected early in life or at birth are at risk of recurring bacterial infections as they have never acquired immunity to the organisms. Lymphoid interstitial pneumonia and pulmonary lymphoid hyperplasia are presentations seen only in young children.

PATHOGENESIS OF HIV INFECTION AND AIDS

The major virological and immunological features of the acute and persistent stages are represented in Fig. 55.6. The incubation period in the acute stage is from 1 to 2 months. This is preceded by a period of intense, unrestrained viral replication, reflected in the presence of high numbers of viral RNA genomes and p24 antigen in the circulation. After entering the body, virus is taken up by cells such as dendritic cells that carry the viral receptors. Within 24–48 h infected cells are present in the regional lymph nodes; virus can be detected in the blood and circulating lymphocytes by 5 days. As the immune system responds, both p24 antigen and RNA copy

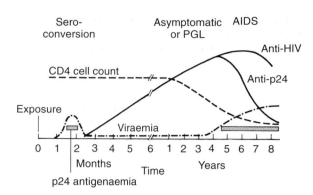

Fig. 55.6 Events in HIV infection. ☐ p24 antigenaemia.

number decrease, so that by 6–12 months p24 antigen is usually undetectable and the RNA load has stabilized at a lower level; in some it may be undetectable. The decline in RNA copy number is usually by at least $3–4 \log_{10}$, and the effectiveness of the immune system in controlling virus replication at this time forecasts when the virus will escape control and symptoms appear. Temporary increases in the RNA level can be seen during intercurrent infections, immunizations and pregnancy.

Patients with AIDS are profoundly immunosuppressed. It was recognized early that the ratio of T helper to cytotoxic T cells (CD4:CD8) was markedly reduced. In fact, the ratio is upset in the acute stages, but is restored as the patient's response controls the virus.

In peripheral blood, lymphoid tissue and other tissues such as brain where HIV replication occurs, HIV targets CD4 positive (CD4+) cells and cells of the monocyte––macrophage lineage; the latter may act as an important reservoir of virus. Macrophages are also important in carrying the virus into the central nervous system across the blood–brain barrier.

The proportion of infected CD4+ cells and the level of circulating virus rise as the infection progresses, reflecting increasing virus replication until the patient becomes symptomatic. Activation of latently infected lymphocytes can be achieved by contact with foreign antigen and lectins such as phytohaemagglutinin. Activation of uninfected CD4+ cells is also important in increasing their sensitivity to infection.

Destruction of CD4+ cells is caused by:

- Viral replication
- Syncytium formation via membrane gp120 binding to cell CD4 antigen
- Cytotoxic T cell lysis of infected cells
- Cytotoxic T cell lysis of CD4+ cells carrying gp120 released from infected cells
- Natural killer cells
- Antibody-dependent cell cytotoxicity.

A few cases have been described in whom T cell responses to viral components appear to be present in the absence of anti-HIV or virus. Such patients may have been exposed to the virus on many occasions but seem to be immune to it.

Analysis of the viral genomes from a patient shows that there are several different viral genomes present at any time and that these change with time. Virus isolated in culture may be different from the predominant variants in the blood. Viruses isolated in the later stages of infection have been shown to grow more rapidly, to higher titres and to form syncytia (giant cells) more readily than virus isolated in the early stages. Regions of the envelope glycoproteins show most variation and this could affect the ability of antibody to react with the viruses. While this could be relevant to the progression of the infection, it has implications for the development of vaccines.

Disease progression. There are host genetic differences influencing the risk of disease progression, e.g. HLA haplotype A1B8DR3 has been linked to rapid development and severe disease. There is also an age effect, with evidence of fast progression in some infants and in the elderly. Table 55.3 lists a number of laboratory markers that are associated with progression. The most useful in assessing the state of a patient's immune system is the absolute CD4+ cell count. Although this can vary, a downward trend is indicative of progression: when the count reaches 200 the patient is severely compromised and the diagnosis of AIDS is made even in the absence of an AIDS indicator disease. The most accurate prognostic marker of disease progression is the plasma viral load. High viral loads and the presence of p24 antigen all correlate with progression, as does a change to a more cytopathic phenotype of HIV isolates grown in lymphocyte culture. The switch to so-called syncytium-inducing variants is accompanied by a change in co-receptor use of virus isolates from CCR5 to CXCR4.

The numbers progressing to AIDS have been studied over many years, although the use of specific therapy has changed the outcome. Untreated, from initial infection the results were:

- 5% within 3 years
- 20–25% by 6–7 years
- 5–10% each year
- <5% asymptomatic for more than 10 years
- 2% asymptomatic for more than 12 years.

When it became possible to measure viral load, it was established that:

- 13% of patients with a viral RNA copy number of <1500/ml will develop AIDS within 9 years
- 93% progression in 9 years with RNA copy number >55 000/ml.

Table 55.3 Laboratory markers associated with progression of HIV infection

Number of CD4 lymphocytes
Increasing proportion of infected CD4 cells
Increasing titre of virus in plasma (HIV RNA copy number)
p24 antigen in plasma
Isolation of virus in culture - rapid growth, syncytium formation
Loss of antibody to p24
Elevated β_2-microglobulin level
Elevated serum neopterin level
Elevated serum soluble interleukin-2 level
Loss of cutaneous hypersensitivity

Paediatric infection

In most cases, infection is transmitted to the baby in the perinatal period when the child's immune system is immature. This results in a major difference from the picture seen in older children and adults in that the initial replicative phase is not limited by the immune response and high levels of viral RNA persist. The RNA counts are often more than 100 000/ml at 2 months. About three-quarters will show a steady decline thereafter of 0.6 $\log_{10}$ each year; however, by age 9–16 years, a third are still asymptomatic and show little impairment of immune function. The other quarter of the children have high levels of viral RNA and develop early onset disease and death by 20–24 months. The mother often has advanced disease during the pregnancy and some of these children may have been infected before birth. It has been suggested that this group of rapid progressers can be identified by detection of virus by RNA polymerase chain reaction (PCR) and culture within 48 h of birth. Analysis of the child's RNA can show that it differs from that of the mother, suggesting that replication has occurred by the time of sample collection or that a minor maternal variant has been transmitted to the baby.

LABORATORY DIAGNOSIS

HIV infection

Both direct and indirect diagnostic methods are available to make a laboratory diagnosis of HIV infection. The infection is invariably persistent, and it is possible to diagnose infection through detection of antibodies to the virus (anti-HIV), or to detect the virus itself. Of these, the most sensitive assay is reverse transcriptase PCR for viral nucleic acid, which can detect a single copy of RNA or proviral DNA from infected cells.

Various tests are used in different circumstances. Thus, to date the main approach to the diagnosis of infection in patients and for screening populations, e.g. blood donors, has been by testing for anti-HIV. However, when serological tests are inappropriate, such as during the early acute stage and in infants who still carry maternal anti-HIV, direct detection methods are required.

Tests for anti-HIV

This was the first practical approach and many different assays are now available, most using enzyme tracing of the reaction (enzyme-linked immunosorbent assay; ELISA). All current tests use HIV antigens derived from cloned recombinant HIV *gag, pol* and *env* genes expressed in *Escherichia coli*, or synthetic peptides. *Western* or *immunoblotting* has been used extensively as a confirmatory assay. Most current assays can detect antibody to both HIV-1 and HIV-2 antigens. A first positive result must be confirmed by at least two other different assays with different viral antigens, and a second serum sample checked to confirm that the original sample was correctly identified.

As all who are infected with HIV remain so, a positive test for anti-HIV indicates that the patient is infected. Most patients will seroconvert within 2–3 months (Fig. 55.6) but some may take longer. Thus there is a window before antibody tests can detect infection.

PCR

Both HIV RNA and DNA sequences can be detected by PCR. RNA sequences are found in extracellular virus particles in plasma. Levels of RNA can be assayed as copy numbers and indicate the extent of virus replication in the patient. Measurement of plasma virus load is now essential for monitoring disease progression and response to antiviral therapy (see below). A number of commercial assays have been developed, e.g. the Roche Monitor™ and Bayer Nuclisens™ assays, to provide accurate and standardized viral load measurements in clinical laboratories.

HIV proviral DNA is synthesized in infected cells, and can be detected readily in peripheral blood mononuclear cells of infected individuals. This method is principally used to diagnose infection in infants born to HIV-infected mothers. As infection is often acquired perinatally, a negative test result at 3 months or later is required to exclude infection. In horizontally transmitted infections, detection of proviral DNA can be used to diagnose an acute infection before seroconversion, although detection of plasma viral RNA is more often used.

Tests for p24 antigen

p24 antigen is part of the virion core and it can be found in the blood when there is active viral replication. Antigenaemia is usually of short duration at the time of initial infection, and may not be detected in all cases (Fig. 55.6). As the antibody response builds up antigen tests become negative. However, late in infection, p24 antigen may reappear until most patients give a positive result. Tests for p24 antigen are now used less often since the introduction of PCR assays for viral RNA load estimation for monitoring disease progression. Similarly, p24 antigen detection is rarely used for the diagnosis of acute infection before seroconversion for antibody, or detecting infection in neonates.

Virus isolation

Isolation of HIV is slow, taking from 3 to 6 weeks. The usual sample is blood, from which the lymphocytes are separated and co-cultured with phytohaemagglutinin-stimulated donor lymphocytes. Virus presence is detected by assays for reverse transcriptase and p24 antigen in the culture fluids. With the advent of PCR, there are now few, if any, diagnostic uses of virus isolation.

HTLV-I

Assays for the detection of antibody to HTLV-I are available: as with HIV, confirmation by other assays or immunoblot must be attempted, although interpretation can be difficult. Confirmatory tests are able to distinguish between HTLV-I and HTLV-II. Detection of HTLV proviral sequences by PCR can also be used as a confirmatory test, and to distinguish HTLV-I and HTLV-II.

TREATMENT

HTLV-I infection

Interferon and inhibitors of reverse transcriptase may have a role, but further evaluation is neded.

HIV infection and AIDS

Specific therapy for HIV infection has been available for some years since the inhibitory effect of zidovudine on the viral reverse transcriptase (reverse transcriptase inhibitor; RTI) was discovered. It was established that zidovudine therapy could lead to an improvement in the patient's health, with weight gain, a reduction in viral load and partial recovery of CD4+ cell numbers. However, the improvement seldom lasted longer than

6 months, as drug-resistant mutants were selected. A similar response is seen with other RTIs used alone. More recently, a second point of attack against HIV has been exploited with the development of drugs active against the viral protease (protease inhibitor).

The major advance has come with the application of combination therapy, where RTIs are given with a protease inhibitor. At present, the compounds available are:

- nucleoside analogue RTIs: zidovudine; didanosine (ddI); abacavir; zalcitabine (ddC); stavudine; lamivudine
- non-nucleoside RTIs: nevirapine; delavirdine; efavirenz
- protease inhibitors: indinavir; ritonavir; nelfinavir; saquinavir; amprenavir.

Initial therapy is now a combination of two RTIs and a protease inhibitor. A typical combination is:

- zidovudine 200 mg three times a day
- lamivudine 150 mg twice a day
- indinavir 800 mg three times a day or nelfinavir 750 mg three times a day.

It is essential that the drugs are started together and that the regime is adhered to strictly. It is important to know if the drugs have been used before by that patient and if the patient is infected with drug-resistant virus. Each drug should be given at its optimum dosage and schedule. If a drug is to be replaced because of prior use, known resistance or development of resistance, an alternative should be chosen that does not show cross-resistance with the drug being replaced.

Selection of a patient for therapy can be made on the basis of the following:

- clinical state deteriorating
- plasma viral load high or rising
- CD4+ count falling or less than 200
- acute stage of initial infection to reduce early viral replication, achieve a lower stable RNA load, preserve immune function and reduce risk of viral mutation.

The aims of therapy are to:

- produce the maximum lasting reduction in viral load
- preserve or improve immune function
- reduce clinical problems
- prolong life
- reduce infectivity, if possible.

Measurement of the plasma viral load is the best means of assessing the effectiveness of the chosen therapy. It is combined with CD4+ counts to estimate the state of the immune system. These should be assayed when therapy is started, at 1 month and 3–4-month intervals thereafter. If there is a response, the RNA load will decrease within a few days, will drop by 1 $\log_{10}$ at 2–8 weeks and be <50 by 4–6 months. If these objectives are not achieved, or the viral load increases after a time on therapy, or the clinical state deteriorates, a new combination regime should be started. It may be necessary to assess the resistance pattern of the patient's virus before selecting the new drugs.

It is important to continue with the prophylaxis and prompt treatment of opportunistic infections such as *Pneumocystis carinii* and *Toxoplasma gondi*. Some patients have problems with compliance to the drug regime and some suffer significant side-effects. About 50% of those on long-term therapy will suffer a redistribution of body fat – the lipodystrophy syndrome. Many patients have been treated for years with a good quality of life as a result of these advances. The major problem is the emergence of resistance.

The prophylaxis of perinatal infection and accidental exposure is described below.

The cost of the drugs is high – many thousands of pounds each year. This cost may be affordable for the relatively low number of cases in the developed world but is an impossible burden for the rest of the world where the great majority of patients are located.

TRANSMISSION AND EPIDEMIOLOGY

HTLV–I and HTLV–II

The three lineages of HTLV-I strains are linked to Melanesia, to Central Africa and to various countries, the Cosmopolitan group. The latter includes viruses from Japan, North and West Africa and the Caribbean, which can be distinguished. HTLV-I and the simian virus, STLV-I, are closely related and it is proposed that human infection occurred many thousands of years ago in Africa and that the presence of the virus in many different parts of the world is related to the migration of ancient peoples. The slave trade may account for foci found in the West Indies and the southern USA.

Where it is found the virus is endemic in certain communities. In parts of Japan, the prevalence of antibody can be 27%, with a rising trend from 7 to 8% in the 20–39-year age group to 52% in females and 32% in males by 80 years. In the Caribbean, the rates are in the range of 5–10%, with clusters in communities and families. In other regions, infection has been found in parenteral drug misusers and prostitutes.

The virus is cell-associated in the host, so transmission will occur when infected cells are transferred. This can occur during intercourse. Breast milk is also a source. Transfer of infected lymphocytes during blood transfusion and sharing injecting equipment by drug misusers are other recognized routes.

HTLV-II is transmitted by the same routes. The strains found in drug misusers in different countries are related.

Transmission of HIV-1 and HIV-2

The World Health Organization estimates that worldwide more than 40 million people have been infected with HIV and that 16 million have died. How has this virus spread so widely?

Virus is present in the blood, semen, and cervical and vaginal secretions, and these sources are important in transmission. Virus may also be present in cerebrospinal fluid (CSF), saliva, tears and urine, but at lower titres than in blood. There is no epidemiological evidence that these are significant sources for transmission. Free virus is present at high titre during the early stage of infection and increases in titre in the blood in the later stages of the disease; there is evidence of a greater risk of transmission from such patients.

To transmit, virus has to reach susceptible cells at the point of entry, e.g. Langerhan's cells in mucous membranes, or after entering the circulation.

The three important routes of transmission of HIV are:

- by unprotected, penetrative sexual intercourse
- from mother to child
- by blood and blood products.

Sexual intercourse

Heterosexual transfer of virus is the route by which the great majority of infections are spread, accounting for 90% of the global total: most live in the developing world. Both sexes are affected equally. Overall the estimated risk of transmission from one unprotected exposure is 0.1–0.2% for vaginal intercourse. The probability of transfer is increased if either partner has ulcerative genital or other sexually transmitted disease. Any trauma during intercourse will also facilitate transfer, by allowing direct access of the virus to susceptible cells and the circulation. Sex workers are at high risk due to their large number of partners; they are often an important reservoir. Transmission may be more likely from male to female.

AIDS was first recognized in homosexual men in the USA. Most early studies established that unprotected anal intercourse was a particular risk, especially to the passive, receptive partner. The estimated risk from a single exposure is 0.1–0.3%.

Transmission during oral sexual contact has been documented, but is not a major route.

Mother to child

Most perinatal transmission occurs late in pregnancy or during birth. The most likely source is cells and virus in the cervix and vagina, as the baby passes through the birth canal. The risk of transmission varies from 13 to 32% in the developed world to 25–48% in the developing world. Prolonged and difficult labour is a factor. Breast milk is another possible source. It is difficult to be precise about the contribution of this route, but estimates ranging from 14–30% have been made.

Blood and blood products

All blood for transfusion and the preparation of products such as Factor VIII for haemophiliacs is screened for anti-HIV by sensitive assays. This eliminates almost all the risk, but as there is a delay of some weeks before the tests become positive, it is important to screen donors for possible exposure to risk. Preparation of blood products from large pools of donations was a major factor in contaminating the product as even one infected donation could introduce virus to all the material. Transplanted organs have been implicated in a few cases.

Intravenous drug misuse is a risk factor in about one-quarter of AIDS cases in the USA and to a varying extent elsewhere in the world. The risk rises with the volume of blood injected and the frequency of sharing contaminated equipment. The withdrawal of blood before injection increases contamination. The virus can spread very rapidly so that most misusers in an area become infected in a few months. Those infected in this way can spread the virus to their sexual partners. Drug and sexual routes merge when misusers support their habit by prostitution.

Occupational exposure of health care workers to infected patients has resulted in transmission in a relatively small number of cases. The route is via accidental penetrating injuries with needles and sharps contaminated with blood. The risk from a needle stick is 1 in 200–300; up to 1998, less than 200 instances had been established or suspected in North America and Europe. Contamination of eyes and mucous membranes is another possible route, but this is seldom confirmed. Transmission from health care workers to patient has been suspected in only a few cases.

HIV-2 is transmitted by the same routes as HIV-1.

General. The majority of infected individuals have a recognized exposure to a known source of infection. In some this may be difficult to establish. However, there is no evidence that HIV can spread by casual contact and by inhalation.

Studies of people exposed to the virus on many occasions have shown that a few show no evidence of infection, and remain negative for anti-HIV. The resistance of these individuals is of great interest to understanding protective immunity.

Epidemiology of HIV

The extent of spread of infection can be measured by the numbers of cases identified clinically and by serological testing. Much more evidence can be obtained from seroprevalence surveys of particular groups or the general population. The availability and collection of samples impose limits. Surveys have been performed on patients attending hospitals, antenatal clinics, sexually transmitted disease clinics and blood donors. Specific groups such as drug misusers and prostitutes can be targeted; non-invasive sampling, e.g. collecting saliva, may make these studies more feasible. Repeat testing over time will give an indication of the trend of infection in that population. Such studies are important in monitoring the effect of intervention strategies and forecasting the demand for health services.

HIV was isolated in the early 1980s, but the first identified cases date to the 1960s. During the 1970s, the virus began to spread widely in some populations and groups by the routes described above.

In *North and South America, Europe and Australia*, at least 30–40% of cases are in gay men. Parenteral drug misusers are the other major risk group in these areas. Virus of subtype B is closely associated with these groups and accounts for at least 50% of all infections. The other cases are in the heterosexual partners of bisexual men, drug misusers and men and women from other areas of the world. Infected blood caused some cases before screening was introduced. The estimated prevalence in the populations is from 0.05 to 0.35%, with less than 0.01% in antenatal patients. The numbers of infections in risk groups can change as health education programmes are introduced; however, their success can vary and advice may be ignored if the perception of risk changes. There have been 1.4 million deaths so far in these areas.

Regions of *Africa* have suffered the greatest epidemic spread of the virus, particularly in most of the countries of the sub-Saharan region. It is estimated that 70% of the world total of infections are in this area. Population prevalences range from 1.5 to 18%, with 2–40% of antenatal patients infected. The viruses circulating here are of subtypes C, A, D and E. Of these, C has spread rapidly and now accounts for 50% of all infections. There is some evidence that subtype C may be able to transmit more easily by heterosexual contact than subtype B, due to its greater affinity for the receptors of Langerhan's cells.

Almost 90% of AIDS deaths have occurred in Africa (13.7 million). The virus continues to spread, and there were an estimated 3.8 million new infections in 1999. The social and economic consequences of this epidemic are devastating, with the loss of parents and wage earners. The high infant mortality will have profound effects in the future.

HIV was introduced into *South and South-east Asia* later than in the rest of the world, and so far there have been 1.2 million deaths from AIDS. Infection is spreading rapidly, with an estimated 1.3 million new infections in 1999. The earliest infections were in drug misusers, but this did not lead to wide spread outside the risk group. The situation changed with the introduction of subtype C virus, and there is now rapid heterosexual transmission of this strain. Prevalences from 0.45 to 3.5% have been estimated, with 1–10% in antenatal patients. Without effective intervention large numbers of cases and deaths will occur, with all the expected human and socio-economic consequences. Throughout the region, subtypes A, B, C, D and E have been found.

As a result of the wide circulation of different subtypes in some populations, recombinant viruses have been identified. AC and AD recombinants have been found. Studies in Tanzania suggest that 15% of the virus population in the country is recombinant and that these viruses can be transmitted. A few recombinants have been isolated from areas in the East.

The existence of different subtypes of HIV, and recombinants, is important for two reasons. Firstly, assays for anti-HIV and viral nucleic acid must be able to recognize all types. Secondly, vaccine developers must take account of the various types and establish the spectrum of protection of candidate vaccines.

CONTROL

Sexual transmission

Until a vaccine is available, the emphasis in controlling the spread of infection must be on risk reduction by avoiding unprotected penetrative intercourse with partners of unknown status. Despite knowledge of the major routes of infection, there has only been limited success in reducing sexual transmission. Globally the problem is enormous and efforts are hampered by the poverty and lack of resources of the countries worst affected. The use of condoms and vaginal antiseptics could have an impact, but they need to be available and acceptable to the local population.

In the areas of the world with low levels of infection, early efforts to encourage safe practices had an effect on the spread of the virus among gay men in the Americas and Europe, but this was not always maintained as the perception of the risks changed as a result of declining rates of infection and, more recently, as the latest therapies appeared to be succeeding and prolonging survival. Also, it is difficult to persuade the heterosexual majority that safe practices are relevant to them.

Mother to child transmission

This can be reduced by identifying infected mothers and giving specific therapy in the later stages of pregnancy and to the baby after birth. It has been shown that zidovudine alone can reduce the transmission rate by a factor of three if given:

- Orally to the mother from weeks 14 to 34 of the pregnancy
- Intravenously to the mother during labour
- Orally to the child for 6 weeks after delivery.

If the mother is already being treated, zidovudine should be part of her treatment, even if she has had it before. Transplacental transfer of the drug is important, perhaps aided by phosphorylation of the drug in the placenta. Most transmissions are believed to occur close to, or during, delivery. Thus simpler treatment regimes may be effective. Oral therapy for the mother for 1 month, during delivery and for a short period post-partum may halve the rate. Further studies are needed to establish the most appropriate regimes for the developing world.

As exposure to infected genital secretions is the source of the virus, avoiding prolonged rupture of the membranes before delivery can reduce risk. Caesarean section may have a similar effect, but is of limited applicability.

Breast-feeding is another possible route. However, studies of children protected by specific therapy at and after birth do not show that there is a significant extra risk of infection by this route. Even without therapy, the advantages of breast-feeding if no other adequate nutrition is available far outweigh any risk of infection Where alternative nutrition is available, the baby may not be breast-fed.

Exposure to blood

Drug injectors can avoid risk by not injecting, or can reduce risk by using only clean equipment. Screening of all blood donors should eliminate almost all possibility of transmission. Factor VIII and other blood products are heat-treated, if possible, to inactivate HIV. All organ donors must be screened.

Occupational risk in the health care setting can be controlled by the implementation of safe working practices to prevent accidental injury and contamination with blood and body fluids. The use of gloves, masks and eye protection is important in situations such as surgical procedures where bleeding and spattering are pos-

sible. The risk must be assessed in other situations. Safe disposal of used needles, scalpel blades and other sharps is an essential requirement. The sensitivity of HIV to heat and various disinfectants has been described above.

If an accidental exposure occurs, any wound should be washed with soap and water, or mucous membranes flushed with water. The accident must be reported so that, if necessary, prophylaxis can be started as soon as possible. The risk must be assessed through knowledge of:

- The HIV status of the source patient; if unknown, can the source be tested?
- Is the source on therapy for HIV? Any evidence of drug resistance?
- The nature of the exposure, e.g. injury or contamination of skin or mucous membranes.

Knowledge of the status of the source patient is essential. The patient may be known to be antibody-positive or to have AIDS. If on therapy, it is important to know the regimen, and if there is any evidence of drug resistance. The risk of infection from splashing on to mucous membranes or skin is harder to quantify, but is certainly less than with penetrating injuries. An intact skin is an effective barrier, but abrasions and diseases such as eczema may impair this protection.

If a sharp injury is reported the nature of the injury has to be assessed:

- needlestick or cut with sharp instrument
- depth of penetration
- volume of blood involved
- if blood vessel entered.

If there is an indication of risk, therapy must be started within 1–2 h, and not later than 48–72 h. If no professional advice is available, e.g. at night, prophylaxis should be started and advice obtained and a decision made about continuing with the drugs within 12–24 h. The victim should be involved in the decision, with discussion of the risks and the possible side-effects of the drugs.

Zidovudine alone can reduce the transmission rate, but should now be combined with another RTI (e.g. lamivudine) and a protease inhibitor. The combination of drugs can be varied with knowledge of any drug resistance in the source. Therapy should be continued for 4 weeks and the victim followed with testing for virus for the next 6 months. A few cases of transmission have been seen in cases given prophylaxis.

Vaccines

Much effort has been devoted to the development of a vaccine to provide protection against infection. By analogy with hepatitis B and other viruses, and understanding of the attachment mechanisms of HIV to cells, most emphasis has been placed on vaccines containing the viral *env* protein gp160, gp120 or gp41 prepared by recombinant DNA cloning and expression, or as synthetic peptides known to be important epitopes for neutralizing antibodies. Several prototypes are undergoing evaluation.

RECOMMENDED READING

De Thé G and Gersain A (eds) 1996 HTLV 1995. *Journal of the Acquired Immune Deficiency Syndrome and Human Retrovirology* 13: (Suppl 1)

Fields B N, Knipe D M, Howley P M (eds) 1996 *Virology* 3rd edn. Lippincott-Raven, Philadelphia

Grubman S, Gross E, Lerner-Weiss N et al. 1995 Older children and adolescents living with perinatally acquired human immunodeficiency virus infection. *Pediatrics* 95: 657–663

Martin J C, Bandres J C 1999 Cells of the monocyte-macrophage lineage and pathogenesis of HIV-1 infection. *Journal of Acquired Immune Deficiency Syndromes* 22: 413–429

UK Health Departments 1998 *Guidance for Clinical Health Care Workers; Protection against Infection with Blood-Borne Viruses.* Recommendations of the Expert Advisory Group, Her Majesty's Stationery Office, London

Various authors 2000 – A Year in Review 2000 *AIDS* 14 (Suppl 3)

Internet site

Information on therapy: www.hivatis.org

56

Caliciviruses and astroviruses

Diarrhoeal disease

D. Cubitt

The introduction of electron microscopy for the examination of faecal samples led, in the 1970s, to the discovery of a number of viruses that cause diarrhoeal disease in humans and animals. The viruses discussed here are *Norwalk-like viruses* and the *Sapporo-like* human *caliciviruses* that form two distinct genera of the Caliciviridae, and viruses belonging to the family Astroviridae. Evidence that they cause diarrhoeal disease has been provided by epidemiological surveys, human volunteer experiments and laboratory investigations.

Diagnosis of caliciviruses is still dependent on the use of electron microscopy, except in a few research laboratories that have developed in-house enzyme immuno-assays (EIA) or reverse transcription polymerase chain reactions (RTPCRs). Recently an EIA (Dako Ltd) that detects all eight serotypes of human astrovirus has become available. The application of these techniques has demonstrated that caliciviruses and astroviruses have a worldwide distribution and that outbreaks of infection involving infants and the elderly are common. Caliciviruses are a major cause of food- and water-associated outbreaks of diarrhoea and vomiting, affecting individuals of all age groups.

Recently, astroviruses have been implicated as a cause of extensive outbreaks of food-borne infection in Japan.

DESCRIPTION

The properties of the viruses are summarized in Table 56.1.

Morphology

Human caliciviruses (HuCVs) have a characteristic surface morphology (Fig. 56.1), formed by the 32 cups or 'calices' formed by 90 dimers arranged in a $T=3$ symmetry. Three distinct appearances can be observed depending upon the orientation of the particles (Fig. 56.2). Factors such as freezing and thawing, the presence of proteolytic enzymes or incorrect staining can affect the appearance of the particles, which may then be indistinguishable from small round structured viruses (SRSVs). The morphology may be masked also by the presence of antibodies.

Table 56.1 Properties of human caliciviruses (HuCVs) and astrovirus

	HuCV (Sapporo-like)	HuCV (Norwalk-like)	Astrovirus
Nucleic acid	ssRNA	ssRNA	ssRNA
Protein	VP1	VP1	VP1, VP2, VP3?
Molecular weight	65 000	60 000–70 000	29 000–39 000
Lipid	None	None	None
Buoyant density (g/cm³)	1.38–1.4	1.38–1.41	1.36–1.38
Morphology	See Figs 56.1 and 56.2	See Fig. 56.3	See Fig. 56.4
Diameter (nm)	30–35	30–38	28–35
Antigenic strains	> 4	> 12	8
Replication	Cytoplasm	?	Cytoplasm
Host range	Man	Man	Man
Transmission	Faecal-oral, air-borne, contaminated food, and water		

ssRNA, single-stranded RNA.

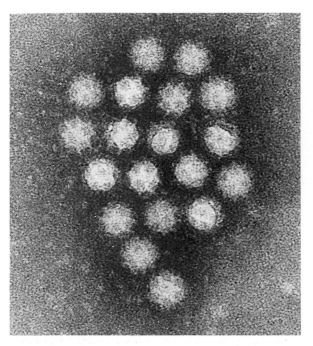

Fig. 56.1 HuCVs, displaying characteristic cupped surface morphology. ×300 000. (From Cubitt W D et al. 1987 *Journal of Infectious Diseases* 156: 806–813.)

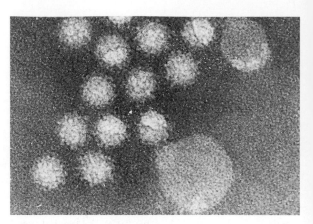

Fig. 56.3 SRSVs resembling Norwalk agent. ×300 000. (From Cubitt W D et al. 1987 *Journal of Infectious Diseases* 156: 806–813.)

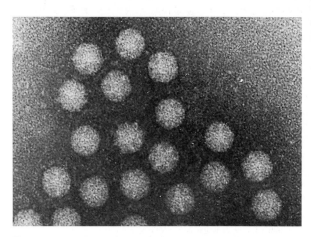

Fig. 56.4 Astroviruses, showing surface star. ×280 000.

Norwalk-like viruses have a similar structure when studied by cryo-electron microscopy but the tips of the capsomeres are bent and partially obscure the hollows, resulting in an amorphous surface structure with a ragged outline (Fig. 56.3). Complete virions measure 35–40 nm in diameter with a solid inner shell at a radius of 11.5–15.5 nm surrounding the RNA.

Astroviruses can be recognized by a five- or six-pointed star on their surface (Fig. 56.4), but this is generally evident on only a minority of particles in a preparation. The particles have a radius of 35 nm and are surrounded by a hair-like fringe.

Physicochemical and physical properties

The properties of the Norwalk-like and Sapporo-like caliciviruses are identical (Table 56.1). Astroviruses

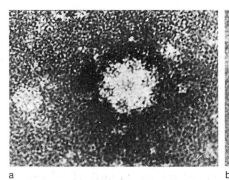

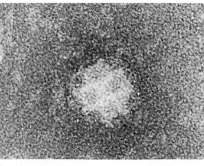

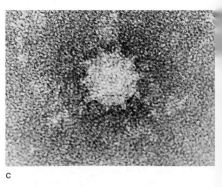

a   b   c

Fig. 56.2 Electron micrograph showing calicivirus morphology when viewed (**a–c**) along the two-, five- and three-fold axes of symmetry. ×450 000. (From Cubitt W D et al. 1979 *Journal of Clinical Pathology* 32: 786–793.)

have similar properties but appear to be more resistant to inactivation, withstanding acid (pH 3.0), 50ºC for 1 h and 60ºC for 5 min.

Genome organization

It is now known that morphologically typical HuCVs and many SRSVs are members of the family Caliciviridae. Based on differences in their genomic organization (Fig. 56.5a), human caliciviruses have been characterized within two genera of the Caliciviridae:

- Sapporo-like viruses, e.g HuCV Manchester
- Norwalk-like viruses, e.g. Norwalk virus.

Non-structural proteins are encoded by ORF (open reading frame) 1 and structural proteins by ORF2. ORF3 encodes a minor structural protein. Caliciviruses possess highly conserved regions within ORF1 encoding a helicase (2C), a protease (3C) and the RNA-dependent RNA polymerase 3D. These serve as suitable sites to direct primers for RTPCR. More recently, primers have been designed to amplify regions within ORF2 that encode the antigenic domains. Phylogenetic analyses of the human caliciviruses show that there are at least four

distinct clades within the Sapporo-like viruses and two major clades within the Norwalk-like viruses.

Astroviruses have a unique genomic arrangement (Fig. 56.5b) and constitute a new family, the Astroviridae.

Antigenic properties

At least four antigenically and genetically distinct strains of Sapporo-like viruses have been identified: Sapporo, Houston, London and Stockholm. The use of immune electron microscopy and EIA has demonstrated that there are numerous strains of Norwalk-like viruses.

There are eight strains of astrovirus that have been identified with specific antisera. The use of a monoclonal antibody has shown that all serotypes share a group antigen. Types 6–8 were first reported in 1994–95.

Host range

In-vivo studies with strains of HuCV and Norwalk virus suggest that they are not readily transmitted to other species, although other caliciviruses have been identified in primates, domestic and farm animals, birds, fish, reptiles, amphibians and insects, and some are known to cross species barriers. There are two reports suggesting that primates can undergo subclinical infection when fed with HuCV or Norwalk agent. In both these cases, animals showed a significant antibody response and were found to be excreting small numbers of virus particles in faeces. Similar experiments have not been conducted with human astroviruses.

Human volunteer studies with caliciviruses (Norwalk, Hawaii and Snow Mountain agents) and astroviruses have shown that some adults became infected after they had been challenged with faecal filtrates containing virus. Pre-existing antibody to Norwalk virus did not confer immunity to subsequent challenge with the virus.

Replication

Attempts to propagate enteric caliciviruses in vitro have generally been unsuccessful.

Astroviruses can be readily propagated in a human intestinal cell line CaCo2, and in HT-29 cells provided trypsin is incorporated in the medium. Immunofluorescence shows that replication occurs within the cytoplasm and that a protein is present in the nucleolus at an early stage in the replication cycle. Electron microscopical examination of thin sections of infected cells shows the presence of crystalline arrays of particles adjacent to cytoplasmic vacuoles.

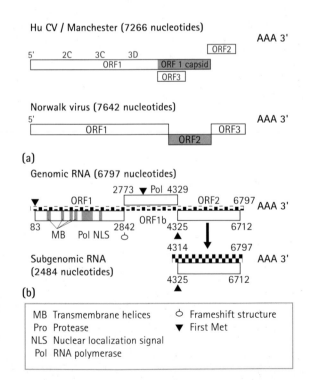

Fig. 56.5 a Genomic organization of the two genera of human caliciviruses: Sapporo-like (Manchester strain) and Norwalk-like (Norwalk Virus). b Genomic arrangement of astrovirus. (From Murphy et al. 1995 by kind permission of Springer-Verlag publishers.)

PATHOGENESIS AND CLINICAL FEATURES

Human volunteer studies with Hawaii and Norwalk viruses have shown that replication occurs in the jejunum. Light microscopy showed that the villi in the proximal part of the small intestine were broadened and blunted, and the enterocytes covering the damaged villi were cuboidal and vacuolated. At the same time the numbers of intra-epithelial lymphocytes and neutrophils were increased. Electron microscopical studies showed that epithelial cells remained intact but the microvilli were disarranged and reduced in length. A similar histopathological picture has been found in calves experimentally infected with a bovine calicivirus ('Newbury agent 2').

The only data on astrovirus infection in humans come from the examination of duodenal biopsies obtained from infants with symptoms of gastro-enteritis. Electron microscopical examination of thin sections showed the presence of arrays of virus particles in epithelial cells of the lower third of the villi.

Clinical features

The clinical features of infection with calicivirus and astrovirus are shown in Table 56.2. The symptoms are similar, but vomiting, sometimes projectile, is more frequently reported in calicivirus infections. In some outbreaks of calicivirus infection involving adults the illness resembles 'gastric flu', i.e. diarrhoea, headache, fever, aching limbs and malaise.

The incubation period for HuCVs is between 12 and 72 h, and slightly longer, 3–4 days, for astrovirus. Illness lasts typically for between 1 and 4 days with excretion of detectable numbers of particles for the same period. Application of RTPCR has shown that virus may continue to be shed for up to 2 weeks. Occasionally, symptoms may persist for periods of up to 2 weeks.

In patients with severe combined immune deficiency disease, persistent excretion of caliciviruses, astroviruses and rotaviruses can occur, either individually or simultaneously; in one report a patient was found to be excreting five different enteric viruses over a period of several weeks before he died.

Symptoms of illness are generally mild and seldom require admission to hospital. However, when outbreaks occur among debilitated elderly patients or infants with other underlying problems, intravenous rehydration may be necessary; fatalities are extremely rare.

LABORATORY DIAGNOSIS

Specimens required

Faecal samples should be collected as soon as possible after the onset of symptoms and stored at 4°C. Paired serum samples should be obtained, the first taken as soon as possible after onset of symptoms and a further sample 10–14 days later. Blood samples from infants can be obtained by finger or heel pricks and dried on filter papers.

Laboratory tests

Until recently the only widely available test for the diagnosis of caliciviruses and astroviruses was electron microscopy, which requires skilled operators and expensive capital equipment. All the viruses are small and are often difficult to recognize. The sensitivity of electron microscopy and virus particle recognition are increased by solid phase immune electron microscopy (SPIEM), which relies on particles being captured by antibodies bound to the grid. Conventional IEM, in which virus reacts with antibodies in a fluid phase, resulting in aggregates of particles, is also of value, provided particles are not totally masked by excess antibody. IEM can also be used to measure antibody responses.

Table 56.2 Clinical features recorded in outbreaks

Virus	No. of cases	Cases presenting with symptom (%)						
		Vomiting	Diarrhoea	Fever	Abdominal pain	Nausea	Aching limbs	Headache
HuCV/Norwalk[a]	30	66	83	47	70	100	73	83
HuCV/Snow Mountain[a]	59	71	70	32	67	72	NS	68
HuCV/UK	181	52	66	65	60	NS	56	NS
HuCV/UK	9	100	22	NS	33	NS	NS	NS
HuCV/Sapporo	250	42	96	18	77	NS	NS	NS
Astrovirus	14	74	30	30	49	NS	NS	NS

NS, not stated.
[a] Morphological appearance = SRSV.

Enzyme immuno-assays

Several research laboratories, particularly in the UK, USA and Japan, have developed assays for the detection of calicivirus antigens and to measure antibody responses to them. However, these tests rely on scarce reagents obtained from well documented outbreaks or from human volunteer studies. Monoclonal and polyclonal antibodies to HuCVs and some SRSVs are being raised and assays should soon become available to diagnostic laboratories. Several strains of calicivirus, e.g. Norwalk, Hawaii, Toronto and Mexico, have been expressed in baculovirus and found to assemble as virus-like particles, which has enabled sensitive EIAs to be developed by research centres.

A specific and sensitive EIA that detects all eight serotypes of human astrovirus is commercially available (IDEIA-Astrovirus, Dako Ltd).

RTPCR

The success in obtaining the complete sequence of three caliciviruses (Norwalk and Southampton in 1991 and Manchester in 1995) has enabled primers to be designed, directed to the highly conserved 3D region of ORF1. Application of the technique is becoming more widespread for the diagnosis of outbreaks of gastroenteritis, but it is apparent that a single set of primers will not detect all strains of HuCV. Sufficient genomic variability exists between strains to use sequence data for detailed epidemiological investigation of outbreaks, e.g. associating a particular source of oysters with an outbreak of gastro-enteritis.

RTPCR has been applied for the diagnosis of astrovirus using primers directed to conserved regions within ORF2. Primers have been designed that are group-specific and others that can differentiate between the serotypes.

EPIDEMIOLOGY

Age distribution

Tests for antigen and sero-epidemiological surveys indicate that HuCVs and astroviruses have a worldwide distribution. All age groups can be affected, but outbreaks of morphologically typical HuCV and astrovirus infection most commonly involve:

- infants
- school children
- the elderly.

In contrast, SRSV outbreaks are more prevalent among adults and the elderly, although there are several reports of episodes in paediatric wards.

Modes of transmission

The various routes of transmission are shown in Fig. 56.6. Epidemiological studies can identify two characteristic epidemic curves for an outbreak. In one (Fig. 56.7), when most cases appear at about the same time, this usually results from a *point source*, e.g. contaminated food or water. In the other (Fig. 56.8), cases occur in smaller numbers over a longer period, often with short intervals between the occurrence of cases. This is characteristic of person-to-person spread.

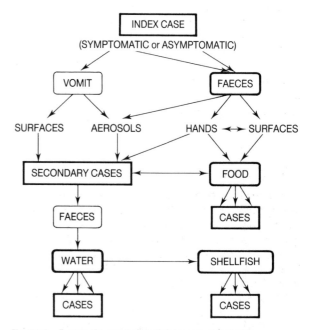

Fig. 56.6 Routes of transmission of viruses associated with gastro-enteritis.

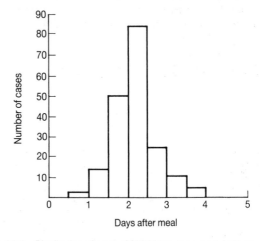

Fig. 56.7 Distribution of cases of SRSV following a meal, indicative of a point source of infection.

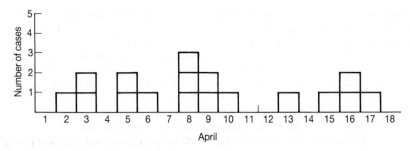

Fig. 56.8 Distribution of cases of astrovirus infection in a geriatric ward, indicative of person-to-person spread.

Faecal–oral route

Affected individuals may excrete large numbers of particles in their faeces and/or vomit ($>10^9$ particles per gram). Human volunteer studies indicate that stored viruses can remain viable for several years and that the infectious dose is 10–100 particles. It is therefore important to recognize that even apparently minor contamination of hands, work surfaces, taps, carpets, etc., can be a major source of infection. This is illustrated by the number of people who can become ill when food is contaminated by a single handler (Table 56.3).

Respiratory route

There is strong epidemiological evidence that inhalation of aerosols of vomit or faecal material, from bed linen or nappies, can result in infection. At present, however, there is no evidence that virus replicates in the respiratory tract.

Cold foods

Cold foods which undergo extensive handling during their preparation are a major source of outbreaks of SRSV infection. It is important to note that the foods involved, e.g. sandwiches, iced cakes, melons and salads, are not generally considered as potential causes of food poisoning. It is therefore likely that the true extent of the problem has escaped attention.

Shellfish

Numerous outbreaks of gastro-enteritis due to caliciviruses and, occasionally, astroviruses have been caused by the consumption of *bivalve shellfish*, i.e. oysters, clams, mussels, cockles and scallops. The reason for the problem is that they are harvested from estuarine or coastal waters polluted with faecal material, which is greatly concentrated by the filter-feeding bivalves. Methods to cleanse them prior to consumption, i.e. holding them in tanks of ultraviolet-irradiated, circulating filtered water, although successful in removing bacteria, are ineffective in freeing them of viruses. A further problem is that shellfish are frequently eaten raw or after minimal cooking.

Water

Outbreaks of calicivirus and astrovirus infection associated with the consumption of untreated water, contaminated municipal drinking water or ice have been reported in the USA, UK and Australia. In the developing world, where water is often untreated, the problem is likely to be far greater.

Asymptomatic excretors

Epidemiological investigation and volunteer trials have shown that asymptomatic excretion of caliciviruses and

Table 56.3	Food- and water-borne infections		
Virus	Source	Origin	Attack rate (%)
SRSV	Asymptomatic food handler; salads	USA	220/383 (57)
SRSV	Asymptomatic food handler; melon	UK	239/280 (85)
SRSV	Caterers; cold foods	Japan	835/3000 (46)
HuCV	Oysters	UK	500/1700 (29)
SRSV	Oysters	Japan	63/121 (52)
SRSV	Cockles and mussels	UK	>130/>300
SRSV	Drinking water	USA	495/647 (76)
	Secondary home contacts		719/1740 (41)

astroviruses is not uncommon. Such individuals may serve as an important reservoir of infection, particularly in situations such as hospitals or the catering industry.

TREATMENT

At present there is no specific treatment for infections with these agents. Severe dehydration in infants or elderly debilitated patients should be managed in hospital with parenteral fluid replacement.

CONTROL

Control of food–borne outbreaks

The following guidelines for the management of an outbreak associated with food have been proposed in the UK by the Public Health Laboratory Service Working Party on Viral Gastro-enteritis:

- Staff who develop or have had symptoms such as diarrhoea and/or vomiting should be excluded from work until 48 h after recovery.
- If kitchen or adjacent areas have been fouled (e.g. by vomitus) then (a) the area should be thoroughly cleaned and disinfected with a 10 000 ppm hypochlorite solution, and (b) all food to be eaten uncooked should be destroyed.
- The importance of hygienic practices, particularly hand-washing, should be re-inforced.
- High-risk foods such as bivalve shellfish should be excluded from the kitchen, and other foods that require much handling (e.g. salads and sandwiches) should be bought in or obtained from other branches if at all possible.
- Unnecessary kitchen traffic should be stopped: the kitchen should not be used as a short cut for other staff, particularly during the period of an outbreak.

Management and prevention of hospital outbreaks

- Ensure that both bacteriological and virological investigations are instigated at the same time.
- Whenever possible, affected patients should be isolated and infected nursing, medical and support staff excluded from work.
- All staff and patients on an affected ward should be screened as asymptomatic infections are common.
- Particular attention should be paid to hand-washing; 70–90% methanol or ethanol has been shown to be effective against astroviruses and rotaviruses even in the presence of faeces.
- Bed-pan washers need to be examined to ensure they are working efficiently.
- In some outbreaks it may be necessary to close wards to new admissions until all patients have stopped excreting virus and no new cases have occurred for a period of 72 h.
- Staff movement from affected to unaffected wards should be restricted, group activities stopped and visits by children discouraged.

RECOMMENDED READING

Carter M J, Cubitt W D 1995 Norwalk and related viruses. *Current Opinion in Infectious Disease* 8: 403–409

Caul E O 1996 Viral gastroenteritis: small round structured viruses, caliciviruses and astroviruses. Part II. The epidemiological perspective. *Journal of Clinical Pathology* 12: 959–964

Cowden J M, Wall P G, Adak C, Evans H, le Baigue S, Ross D 1995 Outbreaks of foodborne infectious intestinal disease in England and Wales; 1992 and 1993. *Public Health Laboratory Service Communicable Disease Report* 5, review 8

Kapikian A Z (ed.) 1994 *Viral Infections of the Gastrointestinal tract*, 2nd edn. Marcel Dekker, New York, pp 471–518, 549–569

Monroe S S, Ando T, Glass R I 1999 International Workshop on Human Caliciviruses. *The Journal of Infectious Diseases.*181 (Suppl. 2) S249–391

Willcocks M M, Carter M J, Madeley C R 1992 Astroviruses. *Reviews in Medical Virology* 2: 97–106

Internet site

www.iah.bbsrc.ac.uk/caliciviridae/index.html

57

Coronaviruses

Upper respiratory tract disease

J. M. Darville and E. O. Caul

The relatively short history of the coronaviruses began in the early 1930s when an acute respiratory infection of domesticated chickens was shown to be caused by a virus now known as avian infectious bronchitis virus (IBV). Similarly, in the early 1950s, it was shown that colonies of mice maintained for laboratory research were endemically infected with a virus that in some circumstances caused outbreaks of fatal hepatitis. This virus was termed mouse hepatitis virus (MHV). A longer history, however, may be claimed for feline infectious peritonitis virus (FIPV), which has been associated by retrospective diagnosis with a case reported in the literature in 1912.

In the 1960s, research with human volunteers at the Common Cold Unit near Salisbury showed that colds could be induced by nasal washings that did not contain rhinoviruses. Subsequent in-vitro work using organ cultures revealed the presence of enveloped viruses in these washings. Electron microscopical studies demonstrated a unique morphology for these viruses, and comparative studies demonstrated a similarity to the previously described IBV and MHV. The term *coronavirus* was adopted for these agents in 1968, reflecting their morphology in the electron microscope after negative staining, and in 1975 the name Coronaviridae was accepted for the family. It is now evident that coronaviruses are widespread in nature, infect a range of hosts with variable tissue tropisms and are highly species-specific. Although in humans they appear to be limited to infections of the respiratory and probably the enteric tracts, their involvement in systemic disease in other animals has, over the years, given rise to the suspicion that they may also cause more severe human disease. Evidence for central nervous system (CNS) involvement in man is now emerging and research in this area is expanding.

PROPERTIES

Morphology and structure

The most studied coronaviruses are IBV and MHV. The particles are pleomorphic and enveloped, varying between 60 and 220 nm in diameter, although this measurement has been found to be affected by the choice of negative stain used for electron microscopy. Widely spaced club-shaped surface projections or peplomers (composed of surface or S protein) of approximately 20 nm in length are seen in all species. These give the particles their characteristic fringed appearance, reminiscent of the solar corona, when negatively stained (Fig. 57.1). It is from this unique appearance that the name of the virus (Latin, *corona* = crown) is derived. There is some variation in the morphology and spacing of the peplomers. Bovine coronavirus (BCV) has a distinct inner fringe of short peplomers of haemagglutinin esterase, as well as the outer fringe. This double fringe is also seen

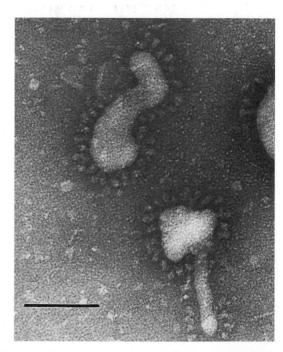

Fig. 57.1 Particles of HCoV serogroup 229E grown in human fibroblast cells and stained with 1.5% phosphotungstic acid. The bar represents 100 nm.

in other coronaviruses of the same antigenic group, including human coronavirus (HCoV) OC43.

The genome is encoded in non-segmented single-stranded positive-sense RNA of approximately 30 kb, making these the largest known RNA virus genomes. In the virion this is complexed with nucleoprotein (N) in an extended helical nucleocapsid of 9–11 nm diameter. This is enclosed within a lipoprotein envelope in association with a transmembrane protein (M). Coronaviruses also have a small membrane minor protein required for virus replication. S protein is the major inducer of neutralizing antibody, although haemagglutinin esterase also induces it while monoclonal antibodies raised against M protein can neutralize infectivity in the presence of complement. Antigenic variation is a feature of the S protein while the N protein is relatively conserved. In addition to the four or five proteins described, reports of other minor proteins have been made but these are not consistent.

Many coronaviruses have the ability to haemagglutinate, a property that has been used in their diagnosis.

Taxonomy

Viruses of the order Nidovirales have similarities in the organization and expression of their genomes. In particular, all produce nested mRNAs (Latin *nidus* = nest). The order comprises the two families Coronaviridae and Arteriviridae. The former contains two genera, *Coronavirus* and *Torovirus*. Toroviruses are well recognized animal pathogens, while agents shown by sequencing to be toroviruses have been detected in human infantile gastro-enteritis. The Arteriviridae contains one genus, *Arterivirus*, which has no known human species.

It is now accepted that there two species of human coronavirus (HCoV) causing respiratory disease, rather than two strains of one species. Human enteric coronavirus (HECV) is a likely third species. Also firmly recognized are coronaviruses of chickens (causing bronchitis), mice (hepatitis, gastro-enteritis and encephalitis), pigs (gastro-enteritis and encephalomyelitis), dogs, turkeys, cattle, horses (all gastro-enteritis), rats (pneumonia and swelling of salivary glands) and cats (peritonitis). In addition, coronavirus-like particles have been demonstrated in the faeces of cats, monkeys and rabbits both with enteritis and in health. In all probability they infect all or most higher animal species.

The confirmed species of coronavirus may readily be distinguished from each other by their limited host range. Serological studies of the N, M and S proteins (see below) have revealed antigenic relationships, allowing classification into two mammalian (Table 57.1) and two avian groups.

Table 57.1 Antigenic relationships of mammalian coronaviruses

Group 1
Human coronavirus (HCoV) 229E
Porcine transmissible gastro-enteritis (TGEV)
Canine coronavirus (CCV)
Feline infectious peritonitis virus (FIPV)
Porcine epidemic diarrhoea virus (PEDV)

Group 2
Human coronavirus (HCoV) OC43
Rat coronavirus (RCV)
Rat sialodacro-adenitis virus (SDAV)
Porcine haemagglutinating encephalomyelitis virus (HEV)
Bovine coronavirus (BCV)
Mouse hepatitis virus (MHV)

Unclassified
Human enteric coronavirus (HECV)
Rabbit coronavirus (RbCV)
Mink coronavirus (MkCV)
Cheetah coronavirus (ChCV)

Cultivation

Some avian and mammalian coronaviruses can be cultivated in fertile eggs or in cell culture with relative ease. The study of many coronaviruses, including HCoV, has, however, been hampered by a relative difficulty in cultivation. The traditional method of cultivating HCV has been in fetal tracheal organ culture. However, HCoV strains related to 229E may be isolated more readily in human diploid cells and strains related to OC43 may be adapted to grow in them after initial isolation in organ culture. Recently, a wider range of cell lines capable of supporting coronavirus replication has been developed.

REPLICATION

Coronaviruses attach to either protein or carbohydrate moieties of glycoprotein receptors on host cells via their S (and haemagglutinin esterase) proteins. After fusion of the viral envelope with the host cell membrane the core penetrates the cell. An RNA-dependent RNA polymerase translated from the genomic RNA makes the negative strand template from which it then synthesizes a series of 3′ co-terminal nested genomic mRNAs. The viruses replicate in the cytoplasm with a growth cycle of 10–12 h. They bud not from the plasma membrane but from the rough endoplasmic reticulum (where the M protein localizes) into intracytoplasmic vesicles. These are transported via the Golgi apparatus to the plasma membrane through which they are released by exocytosis. Viral infection may result in cell lysis, but fusion of adjacent cells leading to the formation of *syncytia* can also occur and the virus may have a potential for persistence. The optimum temperature for the replication of HCV is 33°C, reflecting its usual habitat in the upper respiratory tract.

CLINICAL FEATURES AND PATHOGENESIS

Coronaviruses show:

- marked species specificity
- strong tissue tropism.

They usually infect via the gut and/or respiratory tract. In animals, infections of the liver and CNS are well recognized. While some remain in these sites others can spread to specific organs. Different isolates of the same coronavirus type show different tropisms for the gut and respiratory tract. This tropism is determined by the S protein and by the type and distribution of receptors. All species may replicate in the respiratory tract to some extent. Coronaviruses can also infect neural cells, in which they may persist, and macrophages.

Human coronavirus

The only significant condition known to follow HCoV infection is upper respiratory tract disease, and it is estimated that coronaviruses cause up to 30% of 'common colds'. This figure is based on serological responses to OC43 and 229E antigens and could well be higher depending on the prevalence of unclassified human coronaviruses. Statistically, when compared with rhinoviruses, coronaviruses cause:

- more coryza
- more discharge
- less pharyngitis
- less coughing.

However, individual cases cannot be attributed to either virus group on clinical grounds.

In some cases infection is mild or even subclinical. In contrast, there is some suspicion that coronaviruses may cause severe lower respiratory tract infection in the very old and the very young, including premature infants. However, although coronaviruses have been detected in such cases they have also been detected in control groups and so at present the association remains tentative. There is some evidence that they may cause pneumonia in imunocompromised patients. Coronavirus infections of the upper respiratory tract have been linked in several studies with wheezing attacks, especially in asthmatic children in whom the virus may persist.

Although the morbidity caused by HCoV infection is trivial to the individual, it is economically important as illness is so widespread in the community that the virus is a major contributor to time lost from work and from academic studies.

The incubation period is from 2 to 4 days, and virus is detectable at the onset of symptoms and for 1–4 days thereafter. Symptoms outlast virus shedding and typically persist for a week, probably as a result of secondary bacterial infection.

After infection, humoral and local serological responses are detectable and cellular immune responses probably develop. These are presumed to be responsible for clearing the virus. Despite this, however, re-infection commonly occurs, and this can happen as little as 4 months after infection with the same serotype. Detectable antibody usually disappears after about 1 year.

CNS involvement

HCoVs can replicate in, persist in and activate neural cell lines of human origin and models of putative human CNS diseases have been developed. Molecular evidence also suggests that HCoVs often reach the CNS. These viruses are undoubtedly neuro-invasive and they may have a role in the aetiology of multiple sclerosis, but whether their presence is causative or incidental is presently unclear.

Non-human coronaviruses

In other animals coronaviruses regularly infect and cause disease beyond the mucosal surfaces. In infected adult mice, for example, hepatitis is sometimes a consequence of reactivation.

In rats and mice, MHV strain JHM has been shown to cause demyelinating disease via an auto-immune mechanism. This is dependent on factors such as the maturity of the central nervous and immune systems. Inevitably perhaps, the coronaviruses too have been added to the list of agents, viral and otherwise, that have been implicated in the aetiology of human multiple sclerosis, none with any substantial supporting evidence.

The cause of an encephalomyelitis in pigs has been shown to be a coronavirus, haemagglutinating encephalomyelitis virus. Feline infectious peritonitis virus frequently infects populations of most species and all ages, and there is evidence for a carrier state. Although usually asymptomatic, the infection may cause severe peritonitis through antibody-dependent enhancement of infectivity and is usually fatal.

Pathogenesis

It is presumed that the major pathogenic process, at least in HCoV infection, is the direct cytolysis of infected cells as a result of viral replication. However, the ciliostasis observed in organ culture may also be a contributory factor in vivo. Since HCoV can cause disease on re-infection soon after primary infection, it cannot be excluded that humoral antibody or some other component of the immune response has some role in causing or aggravating acute disease, but no evidence for this exists. That coronaviruses have the potential to cause disease by immunopathological mechanisms is shown in the examples already given of CNS disease in mice and rats and of peritoneal disease in cats.

LABORATORY DIAGNOSIS

There is no clinical requirement for laboratory diagnosis since human respiratory tract infections with coronaviruses appear to be mild. At present, therefore, laboratory diagnosis has essentially research and epidemiological applications.

Virus isolation

Members of the OC43 group of HCoV will only grow on primary inoculation in *organ culture* (hence the designation). Virus growth may be detected by indirect means, such as passage to suckling mouse brain (resulting in fatal encephalitis and yielding a complement-fixing antigen from brain tissue) or by the demonstration of a haemagglutinin. Passage to diploid cell cultures may result in a cytopathic effect while infection of human volunteers may result in clinically apparent respiratory disease. Premature inhibition of ciliary motion in organ cultures, i.e. ciliostasis, can be seen. Furthermore, increasing numbers of characteristic particles due to replication can be demonstrated by electron microscopy.

In contrast to the OC43 group, the 229E group can be cultivated directly in human diploid cells such as W138 or human embryo kidney. The cytopathic effect, often described as 'tatty', resembles the non-specific degeneration of aged cultures with individual cells rounding and detaching from the cell monolayer. However, overlays such as agarose or methylcellulose may reveal the development of plaques by some strains while others produce syncytia.

Serology

Antibodies to HCoV have been detected by complement fixation, by haemagglutination inhibition (some strains) and by neutralization. The last is always a complex procedure and is especially so with these viruses. More recently, reliable enzyme-linked immunosorbent assay (ELISA) tests for detecting anti-HCoV antibody have been developed. ELISA is now the preferred technique

although its use is still limited to research and epidemiology. Antibody is a marker of past infection but, as re-infections are well documented, such antibody cannot be regarded as reflecting immunity.

Rapid techniques

Although not yet of any practical value in monitoring HCoV disease the methods developed for the rapid diagnosis of other agents have been applied to HCoV. For example, ELISAs have been used to detect antigens in respiratory secretions. Since coronavirus antigens are associated with cell membranes the virus can be detected using techniques based on monoclonal antibody immunofluorescence, as are other respiratory viruses. Finally, reliable reverse transcriptase polymerase chain reaction techniques for detecting coronavirus RNA are now widely available.

TREATMENT AND PREVENTION

The treatment of coronavirus infections, in common with most viral infections, remains *symptomatic* only. Indeed, since disease in humans is almost invariably mild, coronavirus infection ranks low on the list of candidates for specific antiviral chemotherapy. Although ribavirin has an in-vitro effect against coronaviruses there is no record of this drug being used in vivo. Recombinant α-interferon has been used to prevent infection in volunteers in experimental studies. Effective vaccines have been produced to control some of the economically important coronavirus infections of animals.

EPIDEMIOLOGY

Studies using both virus isolation and serology have shown that HCoV infections occur wherever in the world they have been sought. Similarly, HCoV activity can be widespread in the community and in widely separated areas. Rates of infection are similar in all age groups and there are no other factors, e.g. sex or socioeconomic status, known to influence the frequency of infection. Given the above, coronaviruses behave in the same way as other human respiratory viruses.

Infection with HCoV is markedly seasonal, with peaks of disease usually occurring late in winter or early spring. However, the exact timing of the peak can vary within the season, as it does with respiratory syncytial virus, and occasionally peaks of infection have been observed outside the usual season.

The two serogroups 229E and OC43 display an unusual periodicity. Each group becomes prevalent every 2–3 years with only sporadic isolates being made of the non-dominant type within the same community. However, the cycles do overlap, so that in a single season 229E might predominate in one region and OC43 in another. This short-term cycling indicates that, despite the diversity that exists within the OC43 serogroups at least, there are functionally few serotypes of HCoV. Were it not for the ease with which re-infection occurs, this might be thought to indicate the feasibility of control by vaccination.

Transmission

HCoV infects the respiratory tract by the air-borne route, i.e. by the inhalation of droplets or aerosols generated by the coughs and sneezes of infected individuals. There is some evidence that fomites are a secondary factor in transmission.

HUMAN ENTERIC CORONAVIRUS

In 1975 simultaneous reports of the discovery of corona-virus-like particles in human faeces were made in Bristol, UK, and in southern India. It was at first suggested that these particles were derived from host cells or mycoplasmas. However, it was soon shown that they could be propagated in human fetal intestinal organ cultures with a replication cycle indistinguishable from that of HCoV. The agent has now been adapted to grow in a range of cell lines and subjected to detailed analysis. Although a causative association of *human enteric coronavirus* (HECV) with human enteric disease has yet to be proven, coronaviruses are significant agents of enteritis in other animals. Two serotypes of HECV may exist, one of which is reported to cross-react serologically with HCoV strain OC43.

Other than the labour-intensive organ culture method described above, the only means of detecting HECV is by electron microscopy. The introduction of other techniques awaits the confirmation and upgrading of the virus as a pathogen.

HECV appears to be endemic throughout the world, with a high prevalence in the developing countries, where there may be some seasonal variation. In western countries the prevalence is high in travellers from third world countries and in low socio-economic groups, and is markedly higher in male homosexuals than in the normal population. Although it has not been proved that HECV is spread by the enteric or faecal–oral route, there is strong circumstantial evidence that this is so; transmission by contaminated water may also be possible. The observed high prevalence among western male homosexuals may be explained by oral–anal–genital contact.

CONTROL

Given the economic impact of the common cold, HCoV infections, like those with rhinoviruses, are obvious targets for control. However, the ease of re-infection suggests that the development of conventional vaccines would be an unrewarding approach, which might indeed create further problems through postulated immune-mediated pathogenic mechanisms. Nevertheless, in the veterinary field, effective vaccines have been developed to protect animals of economic importance from outbreaks of infection in which flocks or herds can be devastated. For example, both attenuated and inactivated vaccines are available to protect chickens from IBV, and live vaccines are used in sows to give their piglets lactogenic immunity to porcine transmissible gastro-enteritis virus. There is, however, a need for improved vaccines.

RECOMMENDED READING

Ashley C, Caul E O 1989 Human enteric coronaviruses. In: Farthing M J G (ed.) *Viruses and the Gut (Proceedings of the Ninth BSG: SK & F International Workshop 1988)*. Smith, Kline and French Laboratories, Welwyn Garden City, pp 91–95

Cavanagh D 2000 Coronaviruses and toroviruses. In: Zuckerman A J, Banatvala J E, Pattison J R (eds) *Principles and Practice of Clinical Virology*, 4th edn. John Wiley and Sons Ltd, London, pp 345–356

Lavi E, Schwartz T, Jin Y-P, Fu L 1999 Nidovirus infections: experimental model systems of human neurologic diseases. *Journal of Neuropathology and Experimental Neurology* 58: 1197–1206

Luby J P, Clinton R, Kurtz S 1999 Adaptation of human enteric coronavirus to growth in cell lines. *Journal of Clinical Virology* 12: 43–51

McIntosh K 1997 Coronaviruses. In: Richman D D, Whitley R J, Hayden F G (eds) *Clinical Virology*. Churchill Livingstone, New York, pp 1123–1132

Murphy F A, Gibbs E P J, Horzinek M C, Studdert M J 1999 1. Coronaviridae and 2. Arteriviridae. In: *Veterinary Virology* 3rd edn. Academic Press, San Diego, pp 495–508, 509–515

Resta S, Luby J P, Rosenfield C R, Seigel J D 1985 Isolation and propagation of a human enteric coronavirus. *Science* 229: 978–981

Siddell S G (ed.) 1995 *The Coronaviridae*. Plenum Press, New York

Siddell S, Wege H, ter Muelen V 1983 The biology of coronaviruses. *Journal of General Virology* 64: 761–776

Sturman L S, Holmes K V 1983 The molecular biology of coronaviruses. *Advances in Virus Research* 28: 35–112

Tyrrell D A J, Alexander D J, Almeida J D et al. 1978 Coronaviridae: second report. *Intervirology* 10: 321–328

Internet sites

www.stanford.edu/group/virus/corona/virushome.html
www.ncbi.nlm.nih.gov/ICTVclb/Ictv/fs_coron.htm

58

Rhabdoviruses

Rabies

S. Sutherland

The hosts of viruses constituting the family Rhabdoviridae include mammals, reptiles, birds, fish, insects and plants. By definition, members of the family must be enveloped, single-stranded RNA viruses, with bullet-shaped or rod-shaped morphology. As with other virus families its members are unrelated serologically unless they form part of a distinct genus. About 80 viruses have vertebrate hosts with many found in invertebrates also. Most of these rhabdoviruses have not as yet been fully categorized, but two genera are known whose members have important roles in animal or human disease. The smaller genus, with which this chapter is concerned, has been designated *Lyssavirus*, the name being derived from the Greek word for madness or frenzy. This genus has rabies virus as its prototype. The larger genus, named *Vesiculovirus*, whose members are associated with the disease vesicular stomatitis, is particularly prevalent among horses, cattle and pigs in the Americas.

Rabies has been recognized in humans and animals for many centuries, even before biblical times, as a distressing disease that develops rapidly into an acute encephalomyelitis, often frenzied initially, then subsiding into delirium, coma and death. A prominent feature in humans is *hydrophobia* – fear of water and inability to swallow it. Figure 58.1 shows part of a case report from Edinburgh dated 1747.

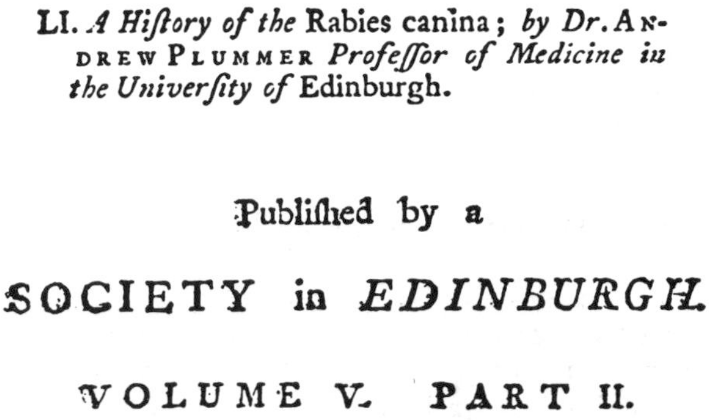

THE VIRUS

The genus *Lyssavirus* includes rabies virus and six other rabies-related viruses. They have been isolated in Africa, mainly from various animal and insect species (Table 58.1).

Rabies virus typically is bullet-shaped (Fig. 58.2) and measures 75×180 nm. Established as a transmissible agent by Pasteur, it was shown in 1931 by the collodion filtration method to be an ultramicroscopical particle, and was first visualized by electron microscopy in 1962. Its inner nucleoprotein core of single-stranded RNA enclosed in nucleoprotein (N) with helical symmetry pro-

LI. *A History of the* Rabies canina; *by Dr.* ANDREW PLUMMER *Profeſſor of Medicine in the Univerſity of* Edinburgh.

Publiſhed by a

SOCIETY in EDINBURGH.

VOLUME V. PART II.

Printed by W. and T. RUDDIMANS, for Meſſrs. HAMILTON and BALFOUR, Bookſellers.

M. DCC. XLVII.

A Young Gentleman, about ſeventeen Years of Age, who had been Apprentice to a Surgeon in the Country, and had come to *Edinburgh* for his Improvement, about the Beginning of *December* 1728, was bit by a Dog in the middle Finger of the right Hand, about the Middle of the Nail. At firſt he ſaid the Dog belonged to a Perſon of his Acquaintance; which Dog had no Symptoms of Madneſs at the Time : But afterwards he affirmed, that he was bit by a ſmall Dog, which he obſerved ſtraggling on the Streets, when he was endeavouring to catch him; and that he never knew what became of the Dog.

Fig. 58.1 Rabies case report, Edinburgh 1747. (By courtesy of Dr A. G. Dempster, University of Otago, New Zealand.)

vides the group antigen for the genus. This antigen may have a role in cell-mediated immunity. The RNA has a molecular weight of 4.5×10^6 and is of negative sense. The enzyme RNA-dependent RNA polymerase is essential for the initiation of replication, and is enclosed within the virion in association with the ribonucleoprotein core.

Table 58.1 Lyssaviruses

Species	Serotype/genotype	Source	Occurrence
Rabies (prototype)	1	Carnivores, cattle, man, bats (warm-blooded animals)	Worldwide
Lagos bat (rabies-like)	2	Fruit-eating bats, cats	West Africa
Mokola (rabies-like)	3	Shrews, man, cats, dogs, rodents	Africa
Duvenhage (rabies-like)	4	Man, bats (insectivorous)	South Africa, Europe
European bat lyssavirus 1	5	Bats, man	Europe
European bat lyssavirus 2	6	Bats, man	Europe
Australian bat lyssavirus	7	Bats, man	Australia

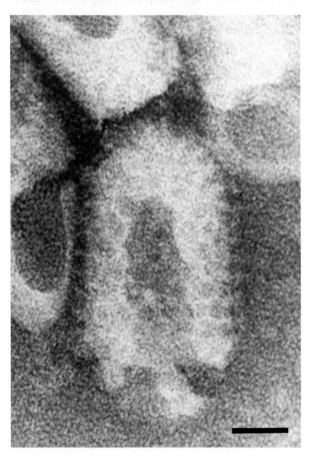

Fig. 58.2 Rabies virus particle. Bar, 30 nm. (By courtesy of Dr Joan Crick, Animal Virus Research Institute, Pirbright, UK.)

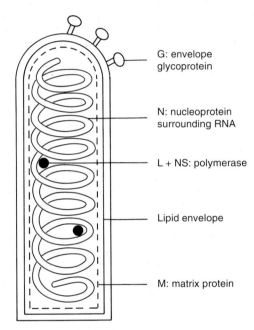

Fig. 58.3 Diagram of rabies virus.

- G: envelope glycoprotein
- N: nucleoprotein surrounding RNA
- L + NS: polymerase
- Lipid envelope
- M: matrix protein

The viral membrane or matrix (M) protein lies between the core and the outer lipoprotein envelope, which is fringed with projections (Fig. 58.3). Extraction of the outer envelope releases a glycoprotein (G) that can induce the formation of neutralizing antibody. Such antibody is more serotype- than group-specific and can have a protective effect if circulating in the blood in sufficient amount at, or even shortly after, the time of a biting incident by a rabid animal. Molecular analysis of the G protein in virulent and avirulent variants has detected an amino acid substitution at site 333, where arginine has replaced glutamine or isoleucine, in the more pathogenic variant.

Rabies virus is rapidly inactivated at 60°C. It can remain viable for some days at 4°C, for longer periods when stored as infected brain tissue suspended in 50% glycerol at 4°C and indefinitely when stored at or below −70°C or in a freeze-dried state. It is sensitive to lipid solvents, β-propiolactone, detergents and proteolytic enzymes.

REPLICATION

Virus replication will occur in all warm-blooded animals, of which rabbits, guinea-pigs, rats and mice are useful for primary isolation. Growth also occurs in the chick or duck embryo and in a range of cell cultures, including baby hamster kidney and mouse neuroblastoma cells, human diploid lung fibroblasts, chick embryo fibroblasts and Vero monkey kidney cells, though with minimal cytopathic effects. The last three are among cell lines used in vaccine production.

Virus attaches via the glycoprotein of the envelope. In neural tissue virus attachment occurs at neuromuscular junctions via the acetylcholine receptors. However, while this may account for the localization and spread of the virus within the nervous tissue, there must be other receptors since the host cell range is broad and not confined to the central nervous system. Entry is by endocytosis; transcription of five messenger RNA species is catalysed by the virion RNA polymerase. The corresponding viral proteins are: N, the nucleoprotein; L and NS, together forming the polymerase; M, the internal membrane protein; and G, the protein which is glycosylated and inserted into the viral envelope (Fig. 58.3). Viral RNA is replicated on a positive-strand template by a viral polymerase. Only negative strands are enclosed in new virions. The M protein appears to be important in packaging the RNA and protein N and linking it to the envelope. Virions are formed by budding at the endoplasmic reticulum of the cell. The virus affects cell protein synthesis and the cell will die but, before this stage, it is possible to detect viral antigens by immunofluorescence or immunoprecipitation tests. Accumulation of cytoplasmic viral protein inclusions (*Negri bodies*) may be visible by light microscopy after appropriate staining. This has long been a useful diagnostic feature.

Newly isolated strains from animals are capable of killing laboratory animals such as mice within 10–20 days after intracerebral inoculation. The appearance of eosinophilic Negri bodies, particularly in nerve cells of the hippocampus, brain stem or cerebellum, and specific rabies immunofluorescence confirm the diagnosis. Such strains, stemming from Pasteur, are called 'wild' or 'street' viruses. Serial animal passage may select out attenuated strains of lesser virulence called 'fixed' viruses. They are usually no longer able to multiply when injected extraneurally, but reversion to greater virulence is possible by the use of an alternative host.

CLINICAL FEATURES AND PATHOGENESIS

Rabies may present as a:

- predominantly encephalitic disease – *furious rabies*
- paralytic illness – *dumb rabies*.

In humans, about two-thirds suffer the encephalitic form and die within 7 days, the rest initially present as para-

lytic then develop encephalitis, and death may not occur for 2–3 weeks. Survival is exceedingly rare.

The incubation period in humans, mostly pinpointed from the time of a bite, can be very variable. It may be less than a week after head and neck wounds, when the virus site of entry is close to the brain, or range up to several years. Molecular studies have identified cases with incubation periods of 4 and 6 years. The average is between 1 and 3 months, with a shorter duration in children than adults. Initial virus replication is considered to occur in the tissues at the point of entry, persisting there for 48–72 h. The virus then spreads to gain access to the nerves via the motor end plates. Once within the nerve fibres it is out of reach of any circulating antibody as it travels along the axons towards the central nervous system. The manifestations of illness are:

- initially, fever, malaise and headache
- then, symptoms related to the wound site, e.g. tingling, pain, lumbar weakness and ascending paralysis after leg bites, and numbness, hyperaesthesia and pain with increasing shoulder weakness after hand or arm bites.

The prodromal symptoms include malaise, headache, fever, and a profound sense of apprehension and feelings of irritation with paraesthesia at the wound sites. There are complaints of dry throat, cough and thirst, but patients will not drink. High fever, rigors, difficulty in swallowing and revulsion to water predominate, followed by bizarre behaviour, excitement, agitation, hallucinatory seizures, laryngeal spasms, choking and gagging, intermingled with lucid intervals. This state, the furious form of rabies, gradually subsides into delirium, convulsions, coma and death. Sometimes only the dumb form is seen, with symmetrical ascending paralysis followed by coma and death.

Clinically, the disease may resemble other types of acute encephalomyelitis although there is often a history of exposure to, or an unprovoked attack by, a deranged animal. Tetanus with its severe spasms may confuse but it does not induce CSF changes.

The predominantly neurological mode of spread has some experimental support, since section of the main nerve trunk proximal to the inoculation site can prolong the incubation period, as can the use of drugs such as colchicine, which inhibit axonal flow. Experimentally, pathogenicity has been related to the capacity of a strain to induce cell fusion in neuroblastoma cells.

Despite an inflammatory reaction from the developing encephalomyelitis accompanied by considerable virus multiplication, observable damage to the nerve cells in the brain appears minimal, though if survival is sufficiently prolonged, specific Negri bodies will appear. Non-specific changes include a parenchymal microglial response and perivascular cuffing, with lymphocyte and plasma cell infiltration in the grey matter of the brain stem and spinal cord. From the brain the virus spreads via efferent nerves to most body tissues, including:

- salivary glands, with multiplication in the acinar cells and extrusion into the saliva
- conjunctival cells, with release into tears and exudates
- the kidneys, with excretion in the urine
- lactating glands and milk after pregnancy.

Virus has also been found in the suprarenal glands, pancreas, myocardium and at the base of hair follicles, as in the neck. Study of saliva, corneal impression smears, conjunctival exudate or hair follicle biopsy from the nape of the neck, all by immunofluorescence, may provide an initial diagnosis.

LABORATORY DIAGNOSIS

The history may be so characteristic that early laboratory confirmation of rabies, often a problem in itself, is not requested. Difficulties can arise when information about exposure to a rabid animal is not elicited, as shown in the USA where more than a fifth of deaths due to rabies are in this category. It is worth remembering that when any visits, particularly to known rabies-endemic areas, have been made up to a year or more before a death which is ascribed to encephalitis, post-mortem examination of brain and cord tissue should include a search for rabies virus.

Because of risks from contact and handling, the British Advisory Committee on Dangerous Pathogens, in line with World Health Organization (WHO) safety recommendations, has classed rabies virus as a hazard group 4 pathogen on the basis that it can cause severe human disease and is dangerous for any person in contact, but effective prophylaxis is available. Regulations provide that high-risk diseases such as rabies and viral haemorrhagic fevers should be treated in secure isolation units, and the virological investigation of specimens from such patients is permitted only in specially designated laboratories. Similarly, for suspect rabid animals there is a designated veterinary laboratory. Stringent government regulations allow propagation of rabies virus only in designated category 4 laboratories.

Where rabies is endemic, wild animals or bats captured after biting incidents should be sent immediately for laboratory confirmation of rabies, but post-exposure treatment of persons bitten should not be delayed pending a laboratory diagnosis. Domesticated dogs and cats, particularly if previously vaccinated against rabies, may be observed in isolation for up to 10–14 days. If they survive

for that time it is unlikely they were incubating rabies at the time of the incident but, if they succumb quickly, antirabies treatment of persons bitten should be started without waiting for laboratory confirmation. Britain, being free from indigenous rabies, usually offers vaccine only to persons bitten while abroad, but may make an exception for anyone bitten by a bat.

Diagnostic methods

1. Identification of rabies antigen by specific immunofluorescence:
   - Ante mortem – in salivary, corneal or conjunctival smears or skin biopsy from the nape of the neck. Negative results, which are frequent, do not exclude rabies.
   - Post mortem – in impression smears of the cut surface of the salivary gland, hippocampus, brain stem or cerebellum.

2. Virus isolation:
   - Ante mortem – from saliva or CSF.
   - Post mortem – from salivary gland or brain tissue extract by mouse intracerebral inoculation. Cell culture inoculation may be used, but cytopathic changes are minimal and viral antigen must be looked for by specific immunofluorescence.

3. Histological examination of fixed brain tissues by staining or immunofluorescence, including a search for Negri inclusions.
4. Fluorescent tests or enzyme-linked immuno-sorbent assay (ELISA) on serum or CSF for evidence of specific antibody. This would not, however, be present until 7–10 days or more had elapsed since the onset of illness.
5. Amplification of DNA following reverse transcription of viral RNA is the most sensitive technique now in use and can be used on saliva to give the best ante mortem results. When combined with the use of restriction enzymes, species-specific variants can be identified, allowing useful molecular epidemiology to trace the source of the virus in those cases without a history of exposure.
6. A latex agglutination test has been used on saliva from rabid dogs and gives 99% specificity and 95% sensitivity when compared with the immunofluorescent antibody test on brain smears.

EPIDEMIOLOGY

During the period 1946–2000 there were 20 human cases of rabies in the UK. All were infected in other countries, 19 the result of dog bites and one from cat scratches and bites. Of the 12 cases since 1975 none had received any post-exposure treatment. In Europe, between 1977 and 1994, 198 human cases were reported, of which 21 had been infected elsewhere. Russia and Romania have reported the majority (70) of the 104 European cases since 1989. World surveys of rabies report about 35 000–50 000 cases annually, with the highest numbers in Asia, particularly in India. In Asia, 90% of cases result from dog bites.

Among animals the disease may spread via two intercommunicating pathways, urban and sylvatic.

- The *urban* mode, more immediately dangerous for humans, diffuses among domestic or scavenger dogs and cats, a situation prevailing in Third World countries.
- The *sylvatic* mode, as it affects small carnivores and mustelids, provides less opportunity for contact with humans. Its main focus in different regions may be confined to separate species, e.g. foxes in continental Europe, Canada and northern parts of the USA, racoons along the eastern seaboard, skunks in the mid-western states and coyotes in the southern states of the USA, and the mongoose in the West Indies. Spread to other species or to humans, though a potential threat, appears unusual. Perpetuation of the disease comes particularly from salivary excretion of the virus during the early stages of illness, combined with the biting tendencies of carnivores.

Dogs, and to a lesser extent cats, are the main sources of human infection so that control of such animals by surveillance, with elimination of strays and the initiation of vaccination programmes, as has occurred in the USA and many European countries, has considerably reduced the incidence of human rabies in these countries. In areas without the benefit of these programmes the incidence of both human and animal disease is much greater.

As well as the involvement of terrestrial animals there is widespread rabies infection in numerous species of bats. This was first noted in Brazil in about 1916 when it was realized that both cattle and humans could develop rabies after being bitten by blood-sucking vampire bats. A similar situation was then found to exist in many Central and South American countries and also in the West Indies, with considerable mortality in cattle. Some human and animal infections may have followed the eating of infected carcasses.

Reports, initially from the USA in 1953, have shown that many species of insectivorous and fruit-eating bats may also harbour rabies viruses, with excretion and transfer of infection when they are sick. It is now believed that affected vampire bats, although thought to be mostly carriers, do ultimately succumb to the disease. Spread can readily occur in some bat colonies from the close contact among large numbers congregating together.

Most viruses isolated from bats in the western hemisphere resemble the classic serotype 1 rabies virus, though in cross-protection and neutralization tests, as would be expected, minor antigenic differences are found. As dog rabies is brought under control in the USA and Europe, a proportionate increase in bat rabies infections has been identified. Of 21 human rabies cases indigenous to the USA from 1990 to 1997, 19 (90%) were bat variants even though a history of bat bites was obtained in only one. Bites by bats are assumed to be the usual mode of transmission to humans, though in two reported fatal cases in the USA, in 1956 and 1958, direct inhalation of virus while working in bat-infested caves in Texas led to the disease.

In continental Europe the fox provides the main animal reservoir, but rabies-like viruses have also been recovered occasionally from bat species in Germany since 1954. Infected bats have also been identified in the former Yugoslavia, Turkey, the former USSR, Poland, Finland, the Czech Republic, Denmark, Holland, France, Switzerland and Spain. No interchange of viruses between bats and animals such as foxes has so far been observed. The European bat viruses EBR1 and EBR2 more closely resemble the serotype 4 Duvenhage virus from South Africa than the American bat viruses, which are serotype 1 rabies viruses. A bat virus closely related to rabies has been responsible for at least two human deaths in Australia, which is officially rabies-free.

In the UK the system of 6 months' quarantine for imported canines and felines was introduced in 1886, together with measures for the muzzling of dogs. By 1902 these steps had succeeded in freeing the country from rabies. The disease was re-introduced in 1918 via a dog brought back illegally from Europe. The disease was again eliminated from animals by 1922. Since that time the UK has been free from indigenous rabies despite two incidents in 1969 and 1970 when dogs released from quarantine developed rabies but, fortunately, there was no further spread. The quarantine barrier was extended to include most other imported animals with an additional proviso that quarantined dogs and cats must be injected, under veterinary supervision, with an acceptable animal rabies vaccine on entry to quarantine and again after 1 month.

In September 1998 the Report of the Advisory Group on Quarantine recommended that quarantine should be replaced by a system ensuring that an imported animal was electronically identifiable by microchip, vaccinated against rabies, blood-tested to confirm immunity, free of tapeworms and ticks and certified as such. As a result of these recommendations, the Pet Travel Scheme (PETS) was piloted from 28 February 2000. This allows pet dogs and cats from western Europe and assistance dogs from Australia to enter without quarantine provided they have complied with the above scheme. At present pets from other locations are still subject to quarantine and vaccination regulations, but in future the PETS is likely to be extended. In Britain, foxes do not appear to have been involved, and laboratory studies of bat species have not shown the presence of rabies or rabies-like viruses so far.

Transmission

Rabies virus does not penetrate intact skin and, if deposited on it from saliva, would become inactivated through such factors as temperature, time and the process of drying. The portal of entry from the infected saliva of a rabid animal are:

- abrasions or scratches on the skin
- mucous membranes exposed to saliva from licks
- most frequently via deep penetrating bite wounds.

The amount of virus excreted in saliva is variable. Bites through clothing may reduce the amount of virus reaching the wound so that not every person bitten by a rabid animal necessarily develops the disease. Uncommon routes include:

- inhalation while in bat-infested caves
- aerosols released during centrifugation of infected materials in the laboratory
- ingestion of the flesh of rabid animals. High doses of virus would be necessary in such instances
- corneal transplants.

Despite the excretion of virus in saliva and conjunctival exudates and occasional misguided attempts at mouth-to-mouth resuscitation, humans do not figure as spreaders of rabies. Transfer via infected corneal transplants has, however, been reported on at least eight occasions in five countries.

IMMUNOPROPHYLAXIS

The risk of infection must first be assessed to take account of the type of exposure, the animal involved and whether rabies is known to be present in that species in the geographical area where the injury occurred. Since there is no effective antiviral drug, post-exposure immunoprophylaxis must be started as soon as possible after the bite or other type of exposure. The following procedures are recommended in the UK and USA for those who have not previously had a full intramuscular vaccine course:

1. Thorough wound cleaning with soap solution or a detergent and running water for 5 min followed by application of 40–70% alcohol or tincture or aqueous solutions of iodine or quaternary ammonium compounds. Scrubbing should be avoided and suturing delayed if possible.

2. Passive treatment with antirabies immunoglobulin, preferably human, 20 IU/kg body weight given half in and around the wound and half in the gluteal muscle.

3. Active immunization with inactivated whole virus vaccine (cell culture-grown), containing at least 2.5 IU/dose, given into the deltoid muscle. The complete course of post-exposure vaccination recommended in the UK comprises five intramuscular 1-ml doses on days 0, 3, 7, 14 and 30. The WHO also approves two alternative schedules: (a) the 2–1–1 regimen in which a 1-ml intramuscular dose given into each deltoid muscle on day 0 is followed by one dose on days 7 and 21; and (b) an intradermal 2–2–2–0–1–1 regimen in which two doses of 0.1 ml are given on days 0, 3 and 7 and one dose of 0.1 ml on days 30 and 90.

In individuals previously immunized against rabies, passive prophylaxis is not given but two booster doses are given on days 0 and 3.

Vaccination

Pasteur introduced vaccination after exposure to rabies in 1885 on the basis that a long incubation period should allow time for immunity to develop before the onset of symptoms. His vaccine was a crude extract of rabbit spinal cord containing virus 'fixed' as a result of serial passage. A well publicized early success established the procedure, still in use despite various vicissitudes. A phenolized brain suspension formed the basis of the *Semple vaccine*, used in the UK from 1919 until 1966. Its drawbacks included a variable but generally low potency, which necessitated a considerable number of daily, often painful, injections, with an antibody response mainly of the IgM class. There was also the disadvantage that the amount of myelin in its nervous tissue content sensitized a proportion of those being immunized, estimated to range from 1 in 500 upwards, so that many went on to develop an allergic type of encephalomyelitis. When the risk of a possible exposure to a rabid animal was assessed as only marginal, it was a matter of debate whether the risk of rabies was greater than the risk of allergic encephalomyelitis.

A *suckling mouse brain vaccine* was developed and contains much less myelin. It is claimed to have a five-fold reduction or more in the incidence of allergic encephalomyelitis, and is widely used in Latin American countries. A non-neurogenic *duck embryo vaccine* was used in the UK from 1966 to 1976. A purified version has shown increased potency, but this vaccine has been superseded by cell culture vaccines, of which there are several types. Those available worldwide, though not necessarily used because of their high cost, include:

- diploid cell vaccine
- rabies vaccine adsorbed
- purified chick embryo cell vaccine
- Vero cell vaccine.

These all have good immunogenicity and safety.

The diploid cell vaccine is the only one licensed in the UK for both pre- and post-exposure prophylaxis and is the only vaccine recommended for intradermal administration. Severe reactions are rare after use, though up to 20% may report minor local effects, and a smaller proportion report systemic, influenza-like or sensitization effects. Intradermal vaccine is not recommended while antimalarials are in use because these may interfere with the immune response. Immuno-suppressed persons may show a poor response and should have antibody levels checked.

In the UK, stocks of vaccine and of human rabies immune globulin are held and distributed mainly through the Public Health Laboratory Service in England and Wales and from designated centres in Scotland and Northern Ireland.

Several vaccine types and modes of delivery have been used in animals. Those used in dogs and cats are given intramuscularly, and require boosting every 1–3 years depending on the vaccine type. Attempts have been made to control the infection in wild animals by the use of live-attenuated vaccines delivered orally. By carefully selecting desirable baits, such as chicken heads for foxes, successful vaccination programmes have been carried out in several European countries.

Work continues on a number of recombinant and subunit vaccines, and on alternative antibody preparations for use in humans.

CONTROL

Because rabies has a worldwide distribution its complete elimination would need the eradication of infection from all susceptible animal species. First steps in this direction have been the use of vaccine-impregnated baits to reduce rabies in foxes in Europe and Canada and racoons in the USA. Since most human exposure has resulted from contact with infected dogs and cats, vaccination of domestic dogs and cats combined with post-exposure prophylaxis for those exposed in specific incidents to suspect rabid animals and pre-exposure for those who may come in contact with such animals in the course of their work has reduced the number of human cases in many countries. Pre-exposure vaccination is recommended for the following groups:

- laboratory workers handling the virus
- those handling imported animals at animal quarantine centres, zoos, research centres and ports
- veterinarians and their technical staff
- animal health inspectors
- licensed bat handlers
- travellers to enzootic areas if work involves handling animals or patients with rabies
- those travelling more than a day's journey from modern medical treatment.

Pre-exposure immunization requires two injections of 1 ml of vaccine, given into the deltoid muscle 4 weeks apart. A test for neutralizing antibody is advised 4 weeks later. A re-inforcing dose is given at 12 months. A booster should be given after any potential exposure. Those at high risk of exposure should have periodic antibody testing and boosting as required every 6 months to 2 years.

Clear signs of case reduction have come from the developed countries that have applied this scheme, and now the need is to extend the procedure to other, particularly enzootic, regions where dogs are the major reservoir of the virus. Past attempts to control wildlife rabies by such draconian measures as shooting and gassing have had short-lived effects. Species vary in their susceptibility to rabies and live vaccine strains that may be used for one species may be unsuitable for another. Extension to canine and other species may become feasible when suitable oral vaccine strains are identified. A number of vectors, such as vaccinia, racoon poxvirus, fowlpox, canarypox and adenovirus, have been used to express a recombinant rabies glycoprotein gene with successful induction of neutralizing antibody in a variety of animal species.

RECOMMENDED READING

Baer G M 1994 Rabies – an historical perspective. *Infectious Agents and Disease* 3: 168–180
Department of Health 2000 Memorandum on Rabies Prevention and Control.
Porterfield J S 1989 *Viruses of Vertebrates*, 5th edn. Baillière Tindall, London, pp 214–229
Rupprecht C E, Dietzschold B, Koprowski H (eds) 1994 Lyssaviruses. *Current Topics in Microbiology and Immunology* 187

Smith J S 1989 Rabies virus epitopic variation: use in ecologic studies. *Advances in Virus Research* 36: 215–253
Smith J S, Fishbein D B, Rupprecht C E, Clark K 1991 Unexplained rabies in three immigrants in the United States. *New England Journal of Medicine* 324: 205–211
Winkler W G, Bogel K 1992 Control of rabies in wildlife. *Scientific American* June: 56–62

59

Transmissible spongiform encephalopathies (prion diseases)

Scrapie; bovine spongiform encephalopathy; Creutzfeldt–Jakob disease; variant Creutzfeldt–Jakob disease

J. W. Ironside

INTRODUCTION

The transmissible spongiform encephalopathies, or prion diseases, are a unique group of fatal neurodegenerative disorders occurring in humans and animals that take their name from two major characteristics:

1. All are experimentally transmissible to a variety of mammals. The precise nature of the transmissible agents involved is unknown (see below), but they possess physical and chemical properties that are quite distinct from those of conventional viruses and bacteria. One hypothesis concerning these agents suggests that they are composed entirely of protein, without any nucleic acid, for which the term *prion* (proteinaceous infectious particle) is used. No evidence of a conventional host immune reaction has been found in these diseases.

2. The diseases caused by these agents are characterized in all species by spongiform change in the central nervous system (CNS). This consists of numerous small vacuoles (10–200 μm) that are formed within neuronal cell bodies and their processes. Neuronal death and a reactive proliferation of astrocytes and microglia also occur, and an abnormal form of prion protein (PrP^{Sc}) accumulates within the CNS both as diffuse deposits and in the form of amyloid plaques.

SCRAPIE

The first animal spongiform encephalopathy to be described was *scrapie*, an endemic disorder of sheep and goats. It has been present in Europe for at least two centuries. Affected animals become ataxic and wasted, and often rub or scrape the fleece off the sides of their bodies, hence the name. The first experimental transmission of scrapie from affected to healthy sheep by intraocular injection of spinal cord homogenate was reported in 1936. Scrapie can be transmitted from ewe to lamb, but there is no evidence to suggest that this occurs in utero. Natural transmission is thought to occur at parturition, or by scarification or via the oral (alimentary) route. The placenta from an infected ewe is one known source of infection that can contaminate the farm environment. There is no epidemiological evidence to indicate that scrapie is pathogenic to man.

The transmissible agent: virus or prion?

The scrapie agent has been the subject of intense research and is by far the best characterized of the transmissible spongiform encephalopathy agents. Although its precise nature is uncertain, it is subviral in size and notoriously resistant to inactivation by many physical and chemical agents, including:

- heat
- exposure to ionizing or ultraviolet radiation
- DNAase, RNAase
- formaldehyde and glutaraldehyde.

The agent has been studied by experimental transmission following inoculation into mice and hamsters, in which around 20 strains of the scrapie agent have now been identified. These strains are defined on the basis of their incubation period and on the nature and distribution of the pathology in the brain when transmitted under identical conditions to genetically similar animals. Incubation periods range from 60 days to more than 2 years, which is close to the natural life span of mice and hamsters. The incubation period is influenced by:

- the route of inoculation (intracerebral inoculation is the most efficient mode of infection; oral or parenteral routes are less efficient)
- the dose of the injected inoculum and its infective titre.

Host genetic factors also influence the incubation period (susceptibility) of these diseases and it has recently been recognized that the major host gene involved is the prion protein gene.

Electron microscopical studies of extracts from scrapie-infected brain have revealed abnormal fibrillary structures named scrapie-associated fibrils, which comprise a modified form of the normal host prion protein (PrP^C). PrP^C is expressed in a variety of cells, including neurones in the CNS, where it may act as a copper-binding protein, and is thought to play a role in synaptic function. This protein has a molecular weight of 33–35 kDa and is highly conserved through a wide range of species, but its amino acid sequence varies from one species to another. This variation is thought to influence the species barrier, a factor that regulates the success of disease transmission from one species to another under experimental conditions.

During the course of scrapie infection PrP^C appears to undergo a conformational change to convert to PrP^{Sc}. This abnormal isoform has a relatively high beta-pleated sheet conformation, which renders it partially resistant to digestion with proteinase K and allows it to aggregate in the form of scrapie-associated fibrils in the brain. In the prion hypothesis, conversion of the PrP^C to PrP^{Sc} is thought to occur by a direct interaction, which sparks off a catalytic conversion. This conversion has been replicated experimentally in a cell-free system, but it remains to be demonstrated that this biochemical change accounts for all the biological properties of the scrapie agent. Many of the physical and chemical features of the scrapie agent can be explained by the prion hypothesis. However, the mechanisms by which the various strains of scrapie agent have different effects in genetically identical mice are unclear; some research groups continue to believe that a second molecule, not prion protein, determines the strain of the infectious agent.

Pathogenesis

Transmission of scrapie to experimental hamsters and mice can be achieved by inoculation of infected brain tissue into a number of sites in the body; the most rapid onset of disease in experimental animals occurs following intracerebral inoculation. With peripheral inoculation spread of infection appears to occur along sympathetic nerve fibres, which connect via the splanchnic nerve complex to the spinal cord. Infection then spreads to the brain at a rate of around 1 mm/day, and there is evidence to support transport of the scrapie agent within neurones. Peripheral inoculation of the agent may also be followed by a phase of accumulation and replication in the lymphoreticular system, mainly in follicular dendritic cells. In the spleen, there is a postulated 'neuro-immune' connection that allows access to the splanchnic plexus and then to the CNS. In the brain, the mechanisms through which spongiform change occurs are unknown, although dilatation of neuronal lysosomal, Golgi and endoplasmic reticulum structures has been suggested.

Bovine spongiform encephalopathy and other animal prion diseases

Scrapie-like diseases have been recorded in an increasing number of captive or domesticated animals (Table 59.1), the most significant of which is bovine spongiform encephalopathy (BSE). BSE was first identified in 1985 in the UK and spread rapidly throughout the cattle population to affect around 1% of all adult cattle by 1992. It appears that this epidemic resulted from:

- Oral ingestion of the scrapie agent via contaminated meat and bone meal in cattle feed.
- Changes in the rendering processes by which these feeds were produced in the 1980s allowed the scrapie agent to persist as a contaminant.
- Recycling of contaminated cattle carcasses in the meat and bone meal subsequently fed to cattle appears to have fuelled the epidemic.

Table 59.1 Animal diseases caused by scrapie and related agents

Disease	Occurrence	Hosts
Scrapie	Common in many countries worldwide	Sheep and goats
Transmissible mink encephalopathy	Very rare, mostly in farms in the USA	Mink
Chronic wasting disease	Isolated foci in Colorado and Wyoming	Mule deer and elk
Bovine spongiform encephalopathy	Widespread epidemic in dairy cattle in the UK, smaller outbreaks in other countries	Domestic cattle
Unnamed spongiform encephalopathy	Small number of exotic ungulates in zoos	Nyala, gemsbok, greater kudu, Arabian oryx, Eland
Feline spongiform encephalopathy	Small numbers of domestic cats in the UK and a few large cats in zoos	Domestic cats, cheetah, lion, puma, ocelot, tiger

The incidence of the disease is now declining as a result of a ban on the use of bovine organs as foodstuffs for other animals. Experimental studies on BSE indicate that it represents a single agent strain. In addition to transmission to cattle, this strain of agent has also transmitted by foodstuff to domestic cats, large cats and exotic ungulates in zoos (Table 59.1). There is now good evidence to indicate that the BSE agent has also spread to humans, causing a new disease known as variant Creutzfeldt–Jakob disease (CJD; see below).

HUMAN PRION DISEASES

Creutzfeldt and *Jakob* first described a human transmissible spongiform encephalopathy in the 1920s; the commonest form of this disease now bears their name. Since then, an ever-widening spectrum of human prion diseases has been identified, with three main subgroups, comprising:

- idiopathic
- familial
- acquired.

The identification of prion protein and sequencing of the human prion protein gene on chromosome 20 have allowed considerable advances in our understanding of human transmissible spongiform encephalopathies (Table 59.2).

Diagnosis of human prion diseases

The diagnosis of human prion diseases requires a range of clinical, biochemical, genetic and pathological studies. Analysis of the prion protein gene is essential to identify cases of familial CJD with a pathogenic muta-

Table 59.2 Human spongiform encephalopathies classified by aetiology	
Sporadic disorders	CJD (around 90% of all cases)
Inherited disorders	CJD (around 10% of all cases) Gerstmann-Sträussler-Scheinker syndrome Fatal familial insomnia
Transmitted from human to human	Kuru Iatrogenic CJD (less than 1% of all cases)
Transmitted from bovines to human	Variant CJD
CJD, Creutzfeldt–Jakob disease.	

tion. Genetic studies have also demonstrated a naturally occurring polymorphism at codon 129 in the prion protein gene, which is important in determining disease susceptibility. At present, there is no form of screening test for human prion diseases and no specific treatment is available. A definitive diagnosis depends on the examination of the brain, which is usually performed at autopsy. Brain biopsy is not performed as a routine investigation, since the procedure can compromise an already ill patient and the neurosurgical instruments used have to be destroyed if the diagnosis is confirmed in order to prevent iatrogenic infection via subsequent neurosurgical procedures.

Neuropathology

It is recommended that all suspected CJD cases should be investigated by autopsy, with appropriate permission for retention and examination of the brain to allow confirmation of the clinical diagnosis and accurate subclassification of the individual case. The principal neuropathological features of human transmissible spongiform encephalopathies are:

- spongiform change
- neuronal loss
- astrocytosis
- amyloid plaque formation (Fig. 59.1).

In recent years, the enormous increase in our knowledge of the biochemistry and molecular biology of the transmissible agents responsible for this group of diseases has allowed the development of a range of techniques to detect PrP^{Sc} accumulation within the CNS. PrP^{Sc} deposition can be detected by immunocytochemistry in the CNS, and can occur in a variety of patterns, including amyloid plaques, perivacuolar deposition around areas of spongiform change, perineuronal and axonal deposition. PrP^{Sc} can also be detected by Western blot techniques, which allow further study of the PrP^{Sc} isotype in terms of its glycosylation and molecular weight following digestion with proteinase K (Fig. 59.2).

Sporadic CJD

CJD occurs most commonly as a sporadic disorder, affecting around 1/million population/year in most recent epidemiological studies. CJD usually presents as a rapidly progressive dementia of less than 1 year's duration, which is often accompanied by other neurological abnormalities, including cerebellar dysfunction, pyramidal and extrapyramidal signs, cortical blindness and akinetic mutism. Many of these features evolve as the disease progresses, and electro-encephalography often shows characteristic diffuse periodic synchronous

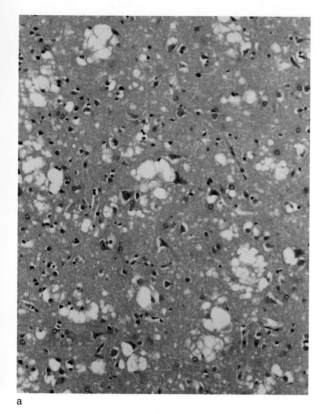

a

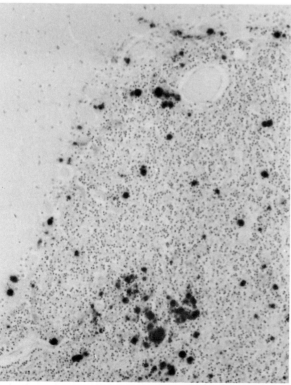

b

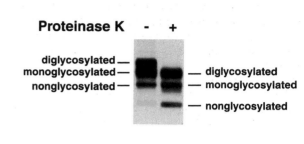

a

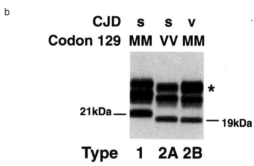

b

Fig. 59.2 Western blot analysis of prion protein (PrP) in post-mortem CJD brain. PrP from CJD brain occurs in three glycoforms resulting in diglycosylated, monoglycosylated or non-glycosylated PrP, which can be separated by Western blotting. Proteinase K treatment (+) destroys the normal form of the prion protein, but in CJD it only partly denatures the disease-associated protein, which has an increased mobility (shown in **a**). Two main subtypes of the abnormal protein can be identified (**b**): Types 1 and 2 are found in sporadic CJD (s) irrespective of their genotype at the codon 129 genotype. Examples of two types (MM1 and VV2 are shown here). All cases of variant CJD (v) thus far tested are methionine homozygotes (MM), and have had a type 2 PrP characterized by the predominance of the diglycosylated glycoform (*), termed type 2B. The type 2 cases found in sporadic CJD, where the monoglycosylated glycoform predominates, are termed type 2A.

Fig. 59.1 **a** Spongiform change in the cerebral cortex in a case of sporadic CJD consists of numerous small cyst-like spaces which tend to coalesce in the neuropil and around neurones (centre). Haematoxylin and eosin stain, ×200. **b** In this case of sporadic CJD, PrP accumulation in the cerebellum has occurred in the form of numerous plaques which stain intensely on immunocytochemistry for PrP. ×250.

discharges. The peak incidence is in the seventh decade of life, but the disease has also been described in teenagers and may occasionally present in the ninth decade. The disease is untreatable and invariably fatal; most patients survive for only 4 months after the onset of major symptoms.

A naturally occurring methionine/valine polymorphism at codon 129 in the prion protein gene is of major influence in determining susceptibility to sporadic CJD (Table 59.3). The mechanism for this influence on disease susceptibility is unclear. The cause of this disorder remains unknown; it might possibly reflect selective exposure to an unidentified ubiquitous agent, perhaps causing disease only in genetically susceptible individu-

als, or a somatic mutation involving the prion protein in the CNS (Fig. 59.3). No specific occupational or dietary risk factors exist for sporadic CJD. The distribution of

Table 59.3   Prion protein gene codon 129 polymorphism in CJD

Codon 129 genotype	Methionine/ Methionine	Methionine/ Valine	Valine/ Valine
Normal population	37%	51%	12%
Sporadic CJD	75%	11%	14%
Variant CJD	100%	0%	0%

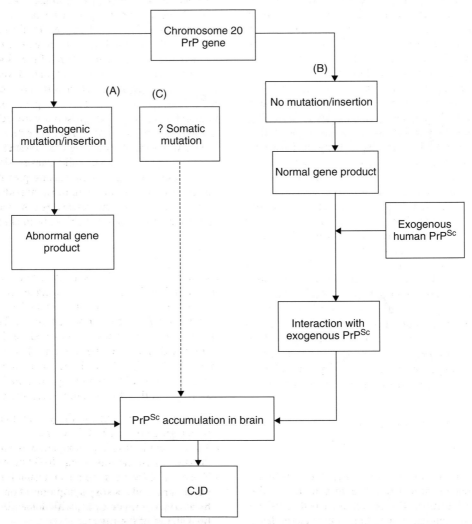

Fig. 59.3   Postulated mechanisms of PrP^Sc accumulation in CJD. In A, an inherited PrP gene mutation results in familial CJD. In B, exogenous human PrP^Sc interacts with the normal host precursor protein, resulting in PrP^Sc accumulation. This mechanism is thought to operate in iatrogenic CJD. The cause of sporadic CJD is unknown, but proponents of the prion hypothesis have suggested that a somatic mutation in a neurone (C) might initiate the process of PrP^Sc accumulation in the brain. This 'rare event' might also explain the low incidence of sporadic CJD.

sporadic CJD on a worldwide basis is markedly different from that of scrapie, particularly in Australia, where scrapie has been eradicated for many decades, but sporadic CJD occurs at a similar frequency to the UK, where scrapie is endemic.

FAMILIAL PRION DISEASES

Around 10% of cases of CJD occur as inherited disorders; these are associated with mutations or insertions in the open reading frame of the human prion protein gene on chromosome 20 (Fig. 59.3). In recent years, many new mutations and insertions have been identified in this gene in familial prion diseases. Gerstmann–Straussler–Scheinker syndrome (GSS) is the best known example of an inherited human transmissible spongiform encephalopathy. In this very rare disorder, which occurs as an autosomal dominant disease affecting middle-aged adults, cerebellar ataxia, nystagmus and gait abnormalities are prominent clinical features, with dementia occurring only towards the end of the illness. The neuropathology is characteristic, with enormous multicentric PrP amyloid plaques present throughout the CNS and a widespread loss of neurones, which is particularly severe in the cerebellum and basal ganglia. However, these changes are not entirely specific; similar features may occur in both sporadic and other familial cases of CJD. GSS was the first human disease found to be associated with a mutation in the PrP gene; a codon 109 proline-to-leucine mutation was first identified in 1989 and has subsequently been found in several GSS families, including the original kindred described in 1936. Fatal familial insomnia is an extremely rare inherited disorder, characterized clinically by disturbances of sleep and autonomic function with relative intellectual preservation in middle age. This disorder is associated with a unique PrP genotype (codon 178 asparagine, 129 methionine/methionine), and neuropathological changes which predominantly involve the thalamus. The relationship between the genotype, neuropathology and clinical features of this enigmatic disorder await further study.

ACQUIRED PRION DISEASES

Iatrogenic CJD

CJD can occur as an iatrogenic disorder following accidental transmission from one human to another (Fig. 59.3). Iatrogenic CJD was first described in 1974 in a corneal graft recipient. Since then, other examples of iatrogenic CJD have involved central inoculation of contaminated material from a human CJD victim to another patient, for example following the implantation of inade-

quately decontaminated intracerebral electrodes, or via human dura mater grafts. In the UK, the commonest form of iatrogenic CJD occurs in recipients of human growth hormone derived from cadaveric pituitary glands, at an approximate incidence of 1 in 10 000 at-risk individuals, with an average age at death of 25 years and incubation periods of up to 20 years. This variant of CJD is unusual in its clinical features, in which a cerebellar syndrome predominates with prominent ataxia, gait and visual disturbances; gross cerebellar atrophy and a predominant accumulation of PrP within the cerebellum are characteristic neuropathological features.

Kuru

Kuru was a disease occurring in the Fore tribe of Papua New Guinea, apparently in association with practices related to ritualistic cannibalism. It still remains uncertain as to whether the brain was actually eaten, but it was handled after death by members of the tribe, particularly females and children, who went on to develop this disorder. The name *kuru* means shivering or trembling in the local dialect, which reflects the predominant clinical manifestations of a progressive cerebellar syndrome accompanied by dementia. The incubation period of the disease was variable, ranging from around 5 to 40 years. No evidence of mother-to-child transmission occurred in this disease, although its increasing prevalence made it the primary cause of death in most individuals within the tribes in the 1960s. The disease is now virtually extinct since cannibalistic practices have been abandoned.

Variant CJD

The emergence of BSE as a new epidemic in cattle had potential implications for human disease, under the assumption that this disorder may be transmitted to humans through the food chain. A National CJD Surveillance Project was established for the UK in May 1990, based at the Western General Hospital, Edinburgh. In 1996, the CJD Surveillance Unit identified a new variant form of CJD, which by 2002 had affected over 100 people in the UK, five in France and one in Ireland.

- The age of onset is unusually young (mean 27 years), with a range from 12 to 74 years.
- The clinical illness is prolonged, with an average duration of 14 months (range 6–39 months).
- The clinical features are also unusual for CJD, with psychiatric and sensory symptoms at onset, followed by ataxia and myoclonus, with dementia only in the final stages of the illness.
- All variant CJD patients so far are methionine homozygotes at codon 129 in the prion protein gene (Table 59.3).

The neuropathological features are relatively uniform and consist of massive accumulations of PrP^{Sc} throughout the brain, with the formation of multiple amyloid plaques surrounded by spongiform change, known as florid plaques. Variant CJD also differs from other forms of human prion disease in that PrP^{Sc} can be detected in lymphoid tissues (in follicular dendritic cells) both during the clinical illness (Fig. 59.4) and in the late preclinical illness. This observation is consistent with variant CJD being acquired by the oral route (see below), and has implications for the possible transmission of the variant CJD agent by surgical instruments used on lymphoid tissues, e.g. in tonsillectomies. This finding has also given rise to concerns that the agent may be present in the blood of individuals who are in the preclinical incubation phase of the illness. To reduce this potential risk, leucodepletion of blood for transfusion has been instigated in the UK, and plasma products are sourced from other countries.

Experimental strain typing studies in mice have shown that the transmissible agent in variant CJD is identical to the BSE agent. Furthermore, biochemical analysis of the PrP^{Sc} from the brain in cases of variant CJD has shown a similar banding pattern in Western blot preparations to PrP^{Sc} from BSE in cattle, which is distinct from sporadic CJD (Fig. 59.2). These findings provide strong support for the hypothesis that variant CJD is causally linked to BSE, but the precise route of exposure is not yet confirmed. Since it is highly likely that the BSE agent entered the human food chain in the UK in the 1980s, a dietary exposure seems most likely. Recently, a statistically significant increase in the incidence and death rate for variant CJD has been reported in the UK. However, because the incubation period for this new disease is unknown and the number of individuals exposed to the BSE agent is uncertain, it is difficult to predict future numbers of variant CJD cases. Continuing disease surveillance will be required to help refine these estimates.

CONCLUSION

A group of human and animal fatal neurodegenerative disorders is caused by unconventional transmissible agents. They result in spongiform change, neuronal loss, reactive gliosis and amyloid plaque formation in the affected brain. Extensive investigations on the nature of the infectious agent in these disorders have so far failed to reach any conclusion. The prion hypothesis, which states that the transmissible agent is composed entirely of PrP^{Sc}, has gained much favour at present since it appears to explain many of the transmissible and genetic aspects of these remarkable diseases. PrP^{Sc} is derived from a larger precursor host glycoprotein (PrP^{C}) which is normally expressed in neurones and is encoded by a gene on chromosome 20 in humans. Human prion diseases occur as sporadic, familial and acquired diseases. The commonest of these is sporadic CJD, the underlying cause for which is unknown. Familial prion diseases occur as inherited disorders which are invariably associated with mutations or insertions in the human prion protein gene. A large body of evidence exists to support the claim that susceptibility to both iatrogenic and sporadic human diseases is controlled by a naturally occurring polymorphism at codon 129 in the PrP gene; individuals who are homozygous at this locus account for the large majority of CJD patients. A new variant form of CJD has been identified in the UK, which is causally linked to exposure to the BSE agent. The incidence of this disease is now increasing in the UK, but the likely number of future cases in the UK population is uncertain.

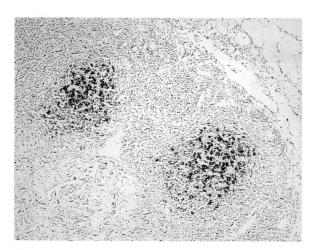

Fig. 59.4 Section of a tonsil from a patient with variant CJD stained to show the prion protein. The dark stain demonstrates accumulation of the prion protein in the follicular dendritic cells within germinal centres in the tonsil. Accumulation of prion protein in lymphoid tissues does not occur in sporadic CJD.

RECOMMENDED READING

Bruce M E, Will R G, Ironside J W et al. 1997 Transmissions to mice indicate the 'new variant' CJD is caused by the BSE agent. *Nature* 389: 498–501

Collinge J, Sidle K C L, Meads J et al. 1996 Molecular analysis of prion protein strain variation and the aetiology of "new variant" CJD. *Nature* 383: 685–690

Collinge J, Palmer M S (eds) 1998 *Prion Diseases.* Oxford, Oxford University Press

Ironside J W 1998 Prion diseases in man. *Journal of Pathology* 186: 227–234

Ironside J W, Head M W, Bell J E et al. 2000 Laboratory diagnosis of variant Creutzfeldt-Jakob disease. *Histopathology* 37: 1–9

Van Duijn C M, Delasnerie-Laupretre N, Masullo C et al. 1998 Case-control study of risk factors of Creutzfeldt-Jakob disease in Europe during 1993–1995. *Lancet* 351: 1081–1085

Will R G, Ironside J W, Zeidler M et al. 1996 A new variant of Creutzfeldt-Jakob disease in the UK. *Lancet* 347: 921–925

Internet sites

National Creutzfeldt-Jakob disease Surveillance Unit: www.cjd.ed.ac.uk
Department of Health: www.doh.gov.uk/cjd
BSE Inquiry: www.bse.org.uk

PART 5
FUNGAL PATHOGENS, PARASITIC INFECTIONS AND MEDICAL ENTOMOLOGY

60

Fungi

Thrush; ringworm; subcutaneous and systemic mycoses

E. G. V. Evans

Fungi constitute a large, diverse group of heterotrophic organisms, most of which are found as saprophytes in the soil and on decaying plant material. They are eukaryotic, with a range of internal membrane systems, membrane-bound organelles, and a well defined cell wall which is composed largely of polysaccharides (glucan, mannan) and chitin. They show considerable variation in size and form, but can be divided into three main groups:

- *Moulds (filamentous fungi)*, which are composed of branching filaments, *hyphae*, that grow by apical extension, forming an interwoven mass, the

mycelium; in most fungi the hyphae have regular cross-walls (septa) but in lower fungi these are usually absent (Fig. 60.1). In some higher fungi the hyphae may be compacted together to form a fungal tissue from which macroscopic structures such as mushrooms and toadstools are formed. Moulds reproduce by means of spores produced, often in large numbers, by asexual cell division (Fig. 60.2) or as a result of sexual reproduction. Many fungi can produce more than one type of spore, depending on the growth conditions. The precise method of spore production and the type(s) of spore produced are

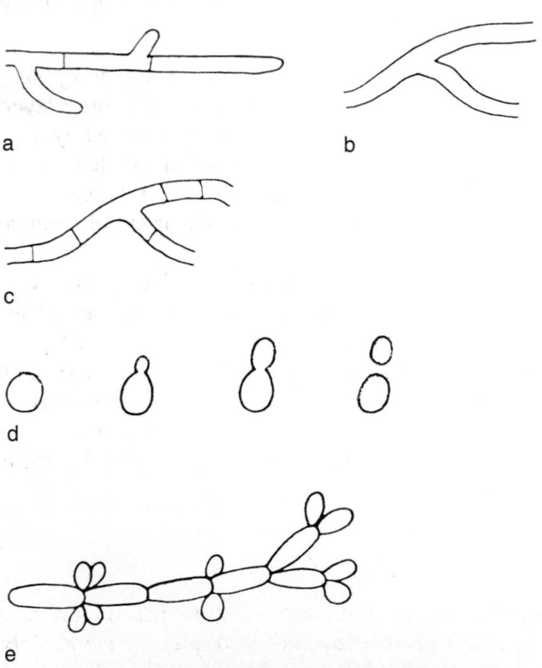

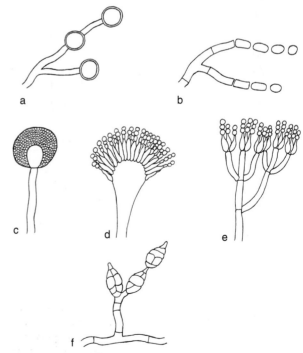

Fig. 60.1 Diagrammatic representation of vegetative forms of fungi: **a** hyphal tip with lateral branching; **b** aseptate (coenocytic) hypha; **c** septate hypha; **d** yeast cells showing stages in budding; **e** yeast pseudomycelium (pseudohypha). (From Evans E G V, Gentles J C 1985 *Essentials of Medical Mycology*. Churchill Livingstone, Edinburgh.)

Fig. 60.2 Types of asexual spores produced by moulds: **a** chlamydoconidia; **b** arthroconidia; **c** sporangium of *Mucor* species, containing sporangiospores; **d, e** sporing heads of *Aspergillus* and *Penicillium* species, respectively, with unicellular conidiospores; **f** multicelled conidia of *Alternaria* species.

unique to each individual fungal species. In laboratory cultures, moulds mainly produce asexual spores.

- *Yeasts*, which are predominantly unicellular and oval or round in shape. Most reproduce by an asexual process called *budding* in which the cell develops a protuberance, which enlarges and eventually separates from the parent cell. Some yeasts produce chains of elongated cells (*pseudomycelium*) that resemble the mycelium of moulds; some species also produce true mycelium (Fig. 60.1). A small number of yeasts reproduce by fission.
- *Dimorphic fungi*, which are capable of changing their growth to either a mycelial or yeast phase, depending on the growth conditions.

The classification of fungi is based primarily on the method of sexual reproduction, although morphology and the method of asexual reproduction are also important. The fungal kingdom, containing moulds and yeasts, is organized into four divisions or phyla, one of which is an artificial group that contains fungi with no known sexual phase. All the divisions contain human pathogens.

Identification of moulds is based on a detailed study of their macroscopic and microscopic morphology and, in particular, the type of spores they produce. Yeasts are primarily identified according to their ability to ferment sugars and to assimilate carbon and nitrogen compounds.

FUNGAL DISEASES OF MAN

Fungal pathogens

About 180 of the 250 000 known fungal species are recognized to cause disease (*mycosis*) in man and animals. Most are moulds, but there are a number of pathogenic yeasts and many are dimorphic. Dimorphic fungi usually assume the mould form when growing as saprophytes in nature and the yeast form when causing infection. In the laboratory, the tissue form can be induced by culture at 37°C on rich media such as blood agar, whereas the mould form develops when incubated at a lower temperature (22–27°C) on a less rich medium such as Sabouraud (glucose–peptone) agar.

Some fungi can establish an infection in all exposed individuals, e.g. the systemic pathogens *Histoplasma capsulatum* and *Coccidioides immitis*. Others, such as *Candida* and *Aspergillus* species, are opportunist pathogens which ordinarily cause disease only in a compromised host. In some mycoses the form and the severity of the infection depend on the degree of exposure to the fungus, the site and method of entry into the body, and the level of immunocompetence of the host.

Some fungi may cause serious, occasionally fatal, toxic effects in man, either following ingestion of poisonous toadstools or consumption of mouldy food that contains toxic secondary metabolites (*mycotoxins*). Allergic disease of the airways may result from inhalation of fungal spores.

Epidemiology

Most fungal infections are caused by fungi which grow as saprophytes in the environment. Some yeasts are commensals of man and cause endogenous infections when there is some imbalance in the host. Only ringworm (dermatophyte) infections are truly contagious.

Many fungal diseases have a worldwide distribution, but some are endemic to specific geographical regions, usually because the causal agents are saprophytes restricted in their distribution by soil and climatic conditions.

Types of infection

Superficial mycoses

Diseases of the skin, hair, nail and mucous membranes are the most common of all fungal infections and have a worldwide distribution.

- *Ringworm* is a complex of diseases affecting the keratinous tissues of hair, nail and the horny layer (stratum corneum) of the skin; it is caused by a group of closely related mould fungi called *dermatophytes* which can colonize and digest keratin. Ringworm infections occur in both man and animals.
- Yeast infections affect the skin, nail and mucous membranes of the mouth and vagina, and are usually caused by commensal *Candida* species, notably *Candida albicans*. Infection is generally endogenous in origin but genital infection can be transmitted sexually. The yeast *Malassezia furfur*, a skin commensal, can cause an infection of the skin called *pityriasis versicolor*.

Subcutaneous mycoses

Mycoses of the skin, subcutaneous tissues, fascia and bone, which show slow localized spread, occur mainly in the tropics and subtropics; they result from the traumatic inoculation of saprophytic fungi from soil or decaying vegetation into the subcutaneous tissue. The principal subcutaneous mycoses are mycetoma, chromomycosis and sporotrichosis.

Systemic mycoses

Deep-seated fungal infections generally result from the inhalation of air-borne spores produced by the causal moulds, present as saprophytes in soil and on plant material. They are mostly caused by dimorphic fungi and occur mainly in the Americas. The principal diseases are:

- coccidioidomycosis (caused by *C. immitis*)
- blastomycosis (*Blastomyces dermatitidis*)
- histoplasmosis (*H. capsulatum*)
- paracoccidioidomycosis (*Paracoccidioides brasiliensis*).

Systemic mycoses caused by pathogens such as *Aspergillus, Candida* and *Cryptococcus* species have a more widespread distribution. These infections are being seen with increasing frequency in patients compromised by disease or drug treatment. In transplant patients, for example, these fungi are among the most frequent causes of mortality due to infection.

Incidence

The incidence of all the mycoses is related directly to factors that affect the degree of exposure to the causal fungi, e.g. living conditions, occupation and leisure activities.

- Ringworm of the foot (*athlete's foot*), with associated infections of nails and groin, occurs most commonly in swimmers, sportsmen and industrial workers who use communal bathing facilities.
- Animal ringworm is an occupational hazard for farmers, veterinarians and others closely associated with animals.
- Agricultural workers in warm climates who wear little protective clothing frequently contract subcutaneous infections following minor injuries from thorny vegetation.
- Systemic mycoses occur most frequently in workers in agriculture or the construction industry and following disturbance of soils containing the causal agents. The incidence of infections due to opportunistic pathogens has increased with developments in medical and surgical practice and with the increased number of immunocompromised individuals.

Pathogenesis and immunity

Knowledge of the pathogenesis of fungal infections and the mechanisms of immunity to fungal disease is still relatively limited, but it is clear that infection most often arises due to deficiencies in the host rather than because of any inherent pathogenic properties of the fungus.

Antigenic variation on the surface of *Candida* cells may help the organism to avoid host defences. Cellular immunity is suppressed by cell wall mannan of *Candida* species, the capsular mucopolysaccharide of *Cryptococcus neoformans* and melanin, which is produced by a number of pathogenic fungi. However, the importance of various fungal antigens and fungal enzymes such as proteinases in the disease process has yet to be elucidated fully.

Diagnosis

Diagnosis is based on a combination of clinical observation and laboratory investigation.

Clinical investigation

Superficial and subcutaneous mycoses often produce characteristic lesions that strongly suggest a fungal aetiology, but they may also closely resemble and be confused with other diseases. Also, the appearance of lesions may be modified beyond recognition by previous therapy, e.g. with topical steroids.

The first indication that a patient may have a systemic mycosis is often their failure to respond to antibacterial antibiotics. Since early diagnosis considerably increases the chances of successful treatment, it is important that the possibility of fungal involvement should be considered from the outset, particularly in those known to be at risk of developing a fungal infection. Computed tomography scanning is widely used to help diagnose *Aspergillus* infections and other invasive mycoses.

Laboratory diagnosis

Laboratory diagnosis depends on:

- recognition of the pathogen in tissue by microscopy
- isolation of the causal fungus in culture
- the use of serological tests
- detection of fungal DNA by the polymerase chain reaction (PCR).

It is important that the correct type of specimen, together with adequate clinical data, is sent to the laboratory so that the appropriate investigations can be carried out. Information on factors such as travel or residence abroad, animal contacts and the occupation of the patient will enable the laboratory staff to direct their investigations towards a particular fungus or group of fungi when appropriate.

Types of specimen. Skin scales, nail clippings and scrapings of the scalp that include hair stubs and skin scales are the most suitable specimens for the diagnosis of ringworm; these are collected into folded paper squares for transport to the laboratory. Swabs should be taken from suspected *Candida* infections from the mucous membranes and preferably sent to the laboratory in 'clear' transport medium. For subcutaneous infections the most suitable specimens are scrapings and crusts, aspirated pus and biopsies. In suspected systemic infection, specimens should be taken from appropriate sites.

Direct microscopy. Most specimens can be examined satisfactorily in wet mounts after partial digestion of the tissue with 10–20% potassium hydroxide. Addition of Calcofluor white and subsequent examination by fluorescence microscopy enhances the detection of most fungi since the fluorescent hydroxide-Calcofluor binds to the fungal cell walls. Gram films may also be used for the diagnosis of yeast infections of mucous membranes. Giemsa staining of smears is advised for detection of the yeast cells of *H. capsulatum* because of their small size.

Histology. Invasive procedures are required to obtain specimens for histological examination. While sometimes necessary to provide firm evidence of invasive disease, such procedures are often impracticable on patients who are already seriously ill. Haematoxylin and eosin staining is seldom of value for demonstrating fungi in tissue and specific fungal stains such as periodic acid–Schiff (PAS) and Grocott–Gomori methenamine–silver (GMS) are widely used.

Culture. Most pathogenic fungi are easy to grow in culture. Sabouraud glucose agar and 4% malt extract agar are most commonly used. These may be supplemented with chloramphenicol (50 mg/l) to minimize bacterial contamination and cycloheximide (500 mg/l) to reduce contamination with saprophytic fungi. Many fungal pathogens have an optimum growth temperature below 37°C. Consequently, cultures are incubated at 25–30°C and 37°C. With some dimorphic pathogens, enriched media such as brain–heart infusion or blood agar are used to promote growth of the yeast phase.

Many fungi develop relatively slowly and cultures should be retained for at least 2–3 weeks (in some cases up to 6 weeks) before being discarded; yeasts usually grow within 1–5 days. Moulds are identified by their macroscopic and microscopic morphology. Yeasts are identified by sugar fermentation and their ability to assimilate carbon and nitrogen sources. Commercial kits are available for the identification of medically important yeasts.

Culture may provide unequivocal evidence of fungal infection when established pathogens are isolated or when fungi are recovered from normally sterile sites. However, when commensals such as *Candida* species are isolated, results must be interpreted according to the quantity of the fungus isolated, the source and clinical evidence.

Serology. The most common tests for fungal antibodies are:

- immunodiffusion
- countercurrent immuno-electrophoresis (CIE)
- whole cell agglutination
- complement fixation
- enzyme-linked immunosorbent assay (ELISA).

For antigen detection:

- latex particle agglutination
- ELISA.

PCR. Detection of fungal DNA in clinical material, principally blood, serum, broncho-alveolar lavage fluid and sputum, is increasingly used for diagnosis.

Treatment

There are relatively few therapeutically useful antifungal agents compared to the large number of antibacterial agents that are available (see Chapters 5 and 66). Since fungi and man are both eukaryotes most substances that kill or inhibit fungal pathogens are also toxic to the host. Antifungal agents vary considerably in their spectrum of activity (see Table 5.4, p. 55). Most exploit differences in the sterol composition of the fungal cell membrane, although caspofungin, a polypeptide of the echinocandin type, interferes with β-glucan synthesis in the fungal cell wall.

Most antifungal agents are available only for topical use. Relatively few can be administered systemically:

- Amphotericin B and caspofungin are given parenterally because of poor absorption from the gastro-intestinal tract.
- Fluconazole, itraconazole, voriconazole and flucytosine are available for oral or parenteral administration.
- Terbinafine and griseofulvin are usually administered orally.
- Amphotericin B is the treatment of choice in life-threatening disease, despite its toxicity; liposomal and lipid-complex formulations are less toxic but expensive.
- A combination of amphotericin B and flucytosine reduces the likelihood of the emergence of resistance to flucytosine. Combinations of azole drugs and amphotericin B are seldom used therapeutically.
- New antifungals, voriconazole and caspofungin are being evaluated for use in systemic mycoses.

Antifungal prophylaxis may be used to help prevent opportunistic infections in patients undergoing transplants or cardiac surgery and those with haematological malignancies. Oral or topical antifungals are also used to prevent recurrent vaginal candidosis.

Primary or acquired resistance is not a major problem. About 12% of clinical isolates of yeasts are resistant to flucytosine and resistance may also develop during therapy. More importantly, resistance to azole antifungals is increasingly encountered, especially after prolonged fluconazole therapy of oropharyngeal *Candida* infections in patients with acquired immune deficiency syndrome (AIDS). Some yeast species (e.g. *Candida krusei*, *Candida glabrata*) are inherently resistant to triazoles such as fluconazole. Consequently, sensitivity testing is carried out for flucytosine and fluconazole and for any drugs failing to produce the expected therapeutic response.

SUPERFICIAL INFECTIONS

Ringworm

Ringworm infections are common diseases of the stratum corneum of the skin, hair and nail; they are also referred to as *dermatophytosis* or *tinea*, a name that is qualified by the site affected, e.g. *tinea pedis* or *tinea capitis* for infections of the feet or scalp, respectively.

Ringworm infections are caused by about 20 species of dermatophyte fungi which are grouped into three genera: *Trichophyton*, *Microsporum* and *Epidermophyton* (Tables 60.1 and 60.2); some species are restricted to, or are more common in, certain parts of the world. Most ringworm infections in Europe are caused by *Trichophyton rubrum*, *T. mentagrophytes*, *T. tonsurans*, *T. verrucosum*, *Epidermophyton floccosum* and *Microsporum canis*.

Some dermatophytes are primarily animal pathogens which may also infect man (Table 60.2); a few species are saprophytes of keratinous material in soil, but these only occasionally infect man and animals. Infections are spread by direct or indirect contact with an infected individual or animal. The infective particle is usually a fragment of keratin containing viable fungus. Indirect transfer may occur via the floors of swimming pools and showers or on brushes, combs, towels and animal grooming implements. Dermatophytes can remain viable for long periods of time and the interval between deposition and transfer may be considerable.

Table 60.1 Common dermatophyte pathogens of man

Species	Common site(s) of infections	Main area of distribution
Epidermophyton floccosum	Groin, feet (nail)	Worldwide
Microsporum audouinii	Scalp (body)	Africa, America and Europe
M. ferrugineum	Scalp (body)	Africa, Balkans and Asia
Trichophyton mentagrophytes var. *interdigitale*	Feet, (nail, groin)	Worldwide
T. concentricum	Body	South Pacific
T. rubrum	Feet, nail, groin, body	Worldwide
T. schoenleinii	Scalp (body, nail)	Eurasia and North Africa
T. soudanense	Scalp (body)	Africa
T. tonsurans	Scalp, body (nail)	Europe and America
T. violaceum	Scalp, body (nail)	Africa and Eurasia

Parentheses indicate secondary sites of infection.

Table 60.2 Common dermatophyte species of animals

Species	Animals commonly affected	Main area of distribution
Microsporum canis	Cat, dog	Worldwide
M. distortum	Cat, dog	Australasia, USA
M. nanum	Pig	Worldwide
M. persicolor	Bank field voles	Europe
Trichophyton mentagrophytes var. *mentagrophytes*	Rodents (horse, cat, dog)	Worldwide
T. equinum	Horse	Worldwide
T. erinacei	Hedgehog	UK, New Zealand
T. quinckeanum	Mice	Europe, North America
T. simii	Monkey, chicken	India
T. verrucosum	Cattle	Worldwide

In addition to exposure to the fungus, some abnormality of the epidermis, such as slight peeling or minor trauma, is probably necessary for the establishment of infection.

In industrialized countries, scalp ringworm is relatively uncommon, and is caused by dermatophytes of both human and animal origin, although *T. tonsurans* scalp infections are on the increase in Europe. However, the use of communal bathing facilities has resulted in a considerable increase in the incidence of foot ringworm and associated nail and groin infections. These now comprise about 75% of all ringworm infections diagnosed in temperate zones.

In developing countries, particularly in warm climates, scalp, body and groin infections predominate, with *T. rubrum* and *T. violaceum* among the most common causes.

There is no evidence of natural immunity, although some may be genetically predisposed to it. Scalp ringworm is predominantly a disease of children and foot ringworm a disease of adults, particularly adult men. Resistance to infection is partly determined by the production of inhibitory fatty acids and the rate of epithelial cell turnover, but the development of active T cell-mediated immunity and, in follicular infections, phagocytosis by neutrophils, also play a part.

Dermatophytes invade keratin by enzymic digestion and mechanical pressure; the hyphae grow into newly differentiated keratin as it is formed, keeping pace with the keratin growth. In tissue the dermatophytes take the form of branching hyphae, which may eventually break up into arthroconidia, particularly in infected hair.

Many dermatophyte species produce two types of asexual spore: *macroconidia* and *microconidia* (Fig. 60.3). Classification into the three genera *Trichophyton*, *Microsporum* and *Epidermophyton* is based on the morphology of the macroconidia, although the identification of species is also based on the shape and disposition of the microconidia and the macroscopic appearance of the colony. Biochemical tests can also be used to differentiate some species.

Pathogenesis

Lesions vary considerably according to the site of the infection and the species of fungus involved. Sometimes there is only dry scaling or hyperkeratosis, but more commonly there is irritation, erythema, oedema and some vesiculation. More inflammatory lesions with weeping vesicles, pustules and ulceration are usually caused by zoophilic species.

In skin infections of the body, face and scalp, spreading annular lesions with a raised, inflammatory border are usually produced. Lesions in body folds, such as the groin, tend to spread outwards from the flexures. In foot ringworm, infection is often confined to the toe clefts,

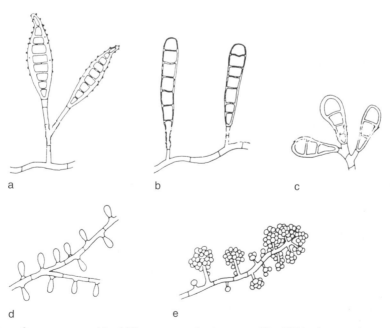

Fig. 60.3 Dermatophyte spore forms: **a** macroconidia of *Microsporum* species; **b** macroconidia of *Trichophyton* species; **c** macroconidia of *Epidermophyton* species; **d** microconidia along sides of vegetative hyphae (*en thyrses*); **e** microconidia in grape-like bunches (*en grappe*). (From Evans E G V, Gentles J C 1985 *Essentials of Medical Mycology*. Churchill Livingstone, Edinburgh.)

but it can spread to the sole; sometimes, painful secondary bacterial infection occurs in the toe clefts.

In nail infection, the nail becomes discoloured, thickened, raised and friable; most nail infections are due to *T. rubrum* and involve toenails.

In scalp infections there is scaling and hair loss, the extent of which depends on the causal fungus. Some zoophilic species give rise to a highly inflammatory, raised suppurating lesion called a *kerion*; kerions may also occur in the beard area of adults. It is important that scalp ringworm is recognized and treated promptly since it can lead to scarring and permanent hair loss.

In scalp infection the fungus invades the hair shaft and then the hyphae break up into chains of arthroconidia. In some species (e.g. *T. tonsurans*, *T. violaceum*) the arthroconidia are retained within the hair shaft (*endothrix* invasion), whereas in others (e.g. *Microsporum* species, *T. verrucosum*) they are produced in a sheath surrounding the hair shaft (*ectothrix* invasion; Fig. 60.4). The pattern of hair invasion affects the clinical appearance of the lesion:

- In endothrix infection the hair breaks off at, or just below, the mouth of the follicle to give what is described as *black dot* ringworm.

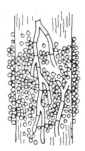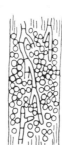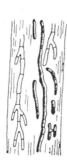

a   b   c

Fig. 60.4 Diagrammatic representation of various forms of hair invasion by dermatophytes as seen in longitudinal and transverse sections of hair shaft: **a** ectothrix (e.g. *M. audouinii, M. canis* and *T. mentagrophytes*) with hyphae sparsely distributed within hair shaft and a sheath of arthroconidia on the outside; **b** endothrix (e.g. *T. tonsurans* and *T. violaceum*) with heavy arthroconidia formation completely filling hair shaft; **c** favus (*T. schoenleinii*) showing sparse hyphal growth and formation of air spaces. (From Evans E G V, Gentles J C 1985 *Essentials of Medical Mycology.* Churchill Livingstone, Edinburgh.)

- In ectothrix infection the hair usually breaks off 2–3 mm above the mouth of the follicle, leaving short stumps of hair.
- In *favus*, caused by *T. schoenleinii*, fungal growth within the hair is minimal. The hair remains intact, but intense fungal growth within and around the hair follicle produces a waxy, honeycomb-like crust on the scalp.

Infections of the groin, hands and nails are nearly always secondary to infection of the feet and are usually (except in developing countries) caused by *T. rubrum*, *T. mentagrophytes* or *E. floccosum*. Mixed infections also occur.

Occasionally, patients with inflammatory infections develop a secondary rash known as an *id* reaction, which is thought to be an immunological reaction to fungal antigens. In patients with foot ringworm this takes the form of a vesicular eczema of the hands, whereas patients with scalp ringworm (especially kerion) develop a follicular rash, usually on the trunk or limbs. These secondary lesions do not contain viable fungus and they disappear spontaneously when the infection subsides.

Laboratory diagnosis

Ringworm infections may be reliably diagnosed in the laboratory by direct microscopical examination and culture of skin, crusts, hair and nail.

Collection of samples. Skin, hair and nail samples are best collected into folded squares of black paper or card, which can be fastened with a paper clip. The use of paper allows the specimen to dry out, which helps reduce bacterial contamination and provides conditions under which specimens can be stored for 12 months or more without appreciable loss in viability of the fungus.

Nail samples should be collected by taking clippings from any discoloured, dystrophic or brittle parts of the nail and, importantly, by scraping material from underneath the nail. The sample should be taken from as far back as possible from the free edge of the nail.

Scales from skin lesions should be collected by scraping outwards with a blunt scalpel from the edges of the lesions, where most viable fungus is likely to be. Specimens from the scalp should include hair stubs, the contents of plugged follicles and skin scales. Infected hairs are usually easy to pluck from the scalp with forceps. Cut hairs are unsatisfactory since the focus of infection is usually below or near the surface of the scalp.

Wood's lamp. This is a source of long-wave ultraviolet light that can be used to detect fluorescence in infected hair. It is especially useful for the detection of inconspicuous scalp lesions, and to select infected hairs for laboratory investigation.

Hairbrush sampling. Adequate material from minimal lesions may be obtained by brushing the scalp with a sterilized plastic hairbrush or scalp massage pad; this is then used to inoculate an appropriate culture medium by pressing the brush or pad spines into the agar.

Processing of specimens. If there is insufficient material for both microscopy and culture, the sample should be used for culture, since this is generally the more sensitive procedure (except for nails).

The specimen should first be examined macroscopically; hair samples are examined under a Wood's lamp. Material from representative parts, and any fluorescent hairs, are divided up into 1–2-mm fragments with a sterile scalpel blade before microscopical examination and culture.

Direct microscopy. Microscopy of wet-mounts of keratinous material in potassium hydroxide is simple and reliable. The preparation is allowed to stand for 15–20 min to digest and 'clear' the keratin. Dermatophytes are seen in skin and nail as branching hyphae, which often appear slightly greenish in colour and run across the outlines of the colourless host cells. With Calcofluor (see above) the cell outlines fluoresce white.

Culture. Small fragments of keratinous material are planted or scattered on Sabouraud glucose or 4% malt extract agar and incubated at 27–30°C for up to 3 weeks; room temperature is adequate but the dermatophytes grow more slowly. Only *T. verrucosum* grows well at 37°C.

Identification is based on colonial appearance and colour, pigment production, and the micromorphology of any spores produced. Special tests exist for differentiating certain morphologically similar species. Thus, the ability of *T. mentagrophytes* to produce urease within 2–4 days distinguishes it from *T. rubrum*, and the ability to grow on rice grains distinguishes *M. canis* from *M. audouinii*.

Treatment and prevention

Topical therapy is satisfactory for most skin infections, but oral antifungals are required to treat infections of the nail and scalp, and severe or extensive skin infections.

Topical agents include azole compounds, terbinafine, amorolfine and ciclopirox olamine. Oral griseofulvin is useful for scalp, skin and fingernail infections, but gives poor results in toenail infections, even after 18 months' therapy. Terbinafine and itraconazole have largely replaced griseofulvin for the treatment of nail infections because of their much better cure rates and shorter periods of treatment (around 85% cure for toenails after 3 months' therapy).

Relatively little has been done to control the spread of ringworm. The prophylactic use of antifungal foot powder after bathing helps to reduce the spread of infection among swimmers. Foot-baths containing antiseptic solutions, which are commonplace in swimming pools, are of no value.

Superficial candidosis

Superficial *Candida* infections involving the skin, nails and the mucous membranes of the mouth and vagina are very common throughout the world. *Candida albicans* accounts for 80–90% of cases, but other species, notably *C. tropicalis*, *C. krusei*, *C. glabrata*, *C. parapsilosis*, *C. guilliermondii* and *C. lusitaniae* may occur.

Candida species, usually *C. albicans*, are found in small numbers in the commensal flora (mouth, gastrointestinal tract, vagina, skin) of about 20% of the normal population. The carriage rate tends to increase with age and is higher in the vagina during pregnancy. Commensal yeasts are more prevalent among hospital patients. Yeast overgrowth and infection occur when the normal microbial flora of the body is altered or when host resistance to infection is lowered by disease. Infection is most likely when several factors operate together to compound their effects, and in some cases deep-seated candidosis may result (p. 585).

Immunity depends on non-specific and immunological defences. In superficial infections the non-specific inhibitory factors include inhibitors in serum such as unsaturated transferrin, and epithelial proliferation. Specific immunity largely depends on the appearance of sensitized T lymphocytes and phagocytes, particularly neutrophils.

On Sabouraud glucose agar *Candida* species grow predominantly in the yeast phase as round or oval cells, 3–8 mm in diameter. A mixture of yeast cells, pseudomycelium and true mycelium is found in vivo and under micro-aerophilic growth conditions on nutritionally poor media. *C. glabrata* does not form either mycelium or pseudomycelium.

Pathogenesis

Mucosal infection. This is the commonest form of superficial candidosis. Discrete white patches develop on the mucosal surface, and may eventually become confluent and form a curd-like pseudomembrane.

In oral candidosis white flecks appear on the buccal mucosa and the hard palate and, although these are adherent, they can be removed; the surrounding mucosa is red and sore. Infection may spread to the tongue. This form of oral candidosis occurs most frequently in infancy and old age, or in severely immunocompromised patients, including those with AIDS. Other forms of oral candidosis occur:

- Lesions in the occluded area under the denture in those who wear dentures.
- Painful infection of the tongue in some individuals receiving antibiotic therapy.
- Chronic infection with extensive leucoplakia and infection of the angles of the mouth (*angular cheilitis*).

In vaginal candidosis, itching, soreness and a non-homogenous white discharge accompany typical white lesions on the epithelial surfaces of the vulva, vagina and cervix. Sometimes the mucosa simply appears inflamed and friable. The perivulval skin may become sore and small satellite pustules may appear around the perineum and natal cleft. Vaginal candidosis is common, especially during pregnancy; most women will have at least one episode during their lifetime, and some suffer recurrent attacks.

Chronic, intractable oropharyngeal candidosis, which may extend to give oesophageal infection, is very common in AIDS patients, although the use of combinations of antiretroviral drugs has reduced its incidence. The appearance of this infection can be the indicator of the transition from human immunodeficiency virus (HIV)-positive status to full-blown AIDS.

Skin and nail infection. *Candida* infections of the skin almost invariably occur at moist sites such as the axillae, groin, perineum, submammary folds and occasionally the toe clefts. In infants, *Candida* species are often secondary invaders in napkin dermatitis. Infection of the finger webs, nail folds and nails is associated with frequent immersion of the hands in water and is an occupational disease, e.g. among housewives, nurses and barmaids. Superficial infections occasionally occur on the penis after intercourse with females with vaginal thrush. *Candida* may also infect the outer ear.

Chronic mucocutaneous candidosis. This is a rare form of candidosis, which usually becomes apparent in childhood and takes the form of a persistent, sometimes granulomatous, infection of the mouth, skin and nails. Some of those who develop this condition have subtle defects in lymphocyte or neutrophil function.

Laboratory diagnosis

Specimens of skin and nail are collected in the same way as for suspected ringworm. For infections of the mouth or vagina, scrapings taken with a blunt scalpel or a spatula from areas with white plaques or erythema are better than swabs if the material is to be processed immediately. However, swabs are more convenient for transport to the laboratory, and they are better for collecting vaginal discharge. Swabs should first be moistened with sterile water or saline before taking the sample and should be sent to the laboratory in 'clear' transport medium.

In Gram-stained smears of mucous membrane samples the fungus is seen as budding Gram-positive yeast cells; mycelium is usually present except in the case of *C. glabrata*. Contrary to popular belief, the presence of *Candida* mycelium in clinical material does not confirm infection with the organism, particularly as it may have developed in the period between collection and processing of the sample.

Candida species grow well on Sabouraud medium or on blood agar at 25–37°C; typical yeast colonies appear within 1–2 days. *C. albicans* isolates can be identified by the germ tube test: after incubation in serum at 37°C for 1.5–2 h *C. albicans* produces short hyphae known as *germ tubes*. Other yeasts may be identified with one of the commercial kits, or by fermentation and assimilation tests.

Quantification of growth, especially in the case of vulvovaginal samples, may help the clinician to distinguish between commensal carriage and infection.

Treatment and prevention

Most superficial infections respond well to topical therapy with an imidazole. In oral candidosis, nystatin, amphotericin B or miconazole may be effective in lozenge or gel form. Most cases of vaginal candidosis can be treated successfully with a single application of a topical imidazole or with oral fluconazole or itraconazole. Intermittent prophylaxis with an oral azole or vaginal pessaries is of benefit in controlling recurrent vaginal candidosis.

Treatment of chronic paronychia involves a combination of antifungal therapy, nail care and avoidance of prolonged exposure to water by use of protective gloves; patients should dry their hands carefully after washing. Regular application of an azole lotion or an azole given orally, sometimes in conjunction with a topical steroid and an antibacterial agent, is the most appropriate therapy but it may take several months to cure the condition; antifungal creams or ointments are less effective.

Oral therapy is essential for the treatment of intractable chronic *Candida* infections; treatment is given until remission is achieved but in some patients (e.g. those with AIDS) relapse is common and intermittent or prolonged therapy may be required. This may, however, lead to the development of resistance, as occasionally happens with fluconazole.

Pityriasis versicolor

This is a mild, chronic infection of the stratum corneum which produces a patchy discoloration of the skin caused by lipophilic yeasts of the genus *Malassezia*. The yeasts are common members of the normal skin flora and most infections are thought to be endogenous. Disease is probably related to host or environmental factors. It is very common in the tropics and, although it occurs in all age groups, it is most prevalent in young adults.

The organism requires lipids for growth and media containing Tween and lipid supplements have been specifically developed. On normal skin and in conditions such as dandruff and seborrhoeic dermatitis (in which its precise role is uncertain), it occurs as an oval or bottle-shaped yeast, which characteristically produces buds on a broad base. In pityriasis versicolor the organism produces predominantly round yeast cells and short hyphae. The optimum growth temperature is about 30°C but in culture the colonial morphology and growth rate vary with the strain species and the medium. All forms of *Malassezia* are Gram-positive.

Pathogenesis

Small, well demarcated, non-inflammatory, scaling macules are usually present on the upper trunk or neck; these may appear hypopigmented or hyperpigmented, depending on the degree of pigmentation of the surrounding skin. The lesions tend to spread and coalesce, and occasionally they spread to other sites.

Laboratory diagnosis

The diagnosis can be confirmed reliably by direct microscopy of skin scales and culture is unnecessary. Demonstration of clusters of the characteristic round yeast cells (5–8 μm in diameter) with short, stout hyphae, which may be curved and occasionally branched, is diagnostic.

Treatment

Pityriasis versicolor responds well to topical therapy with 1% selenium sulphide or azoles such as ketoconazole in cream, lotion or a shampoo. Oral azole therapy is sometimes used for recalcitrant or widespread infections. Relapse is common, particularly in hot climates.

Other superficial infections

Skin and nail

Certain non-dermatophyte moulds may cause infection of skin and nail. It is important that these are recognized since they are often resistant to the agents used to treat ringworm and superficial candidosis.

In the UK, about 5% of fungal nail infections are caused by non-dermatophyte moulds. *Scopulariopsis brevicaulis*, a ubiquitous saprophyte of soil, is the most common, although other saprophytic moulds such as *Fusarium*, *Aspergillus* and *Penicillium* species are also occasionally implicated. There is some debate as to whether these moulds are primary pathogens of nails – infection usually follows trauma and in many cases they are found in nails along with a dermatophyte.

Two other moulds, *Scytalidium dimidiatum*, a pathogen of fruit trees, and *Scy. hyalinum*, a soil fungus, occasionally cause infection of nails and sometimes skin in the tropics. Infections are diagnosed by microscopy and culture, as for ringworm infections. However, both species are sensitive to cycloheximide and will not grow if this antibiotic is included in the medium.

Non-dermatophyte mould infections do not respond to existing antifungal agents. Attempts may be made to remove the nail with topical 40% urea paste.

Tinea nigra. This is a superficial, asymptomatic skin disease characterized by pigmented macules of variable size, usually on the palms and soles. It is caused by a black mould, *Exophiala werneckii*, and occurs mainly in the tropics. Tinea nigra is not contagious but is contracted by contact with the fungus in soil.

Diagnosis is made easily by recognition of the dark-coloured hyphal elements on microscopical examination of skin scrapings in potassium hydroxide. On Sabouraud agar the fungus develops as grey, yeast-like colonies, which gradually become more mycelial and darker coloured with age.

Tinea nigra responds well to treatment with keratolytic agents such as Whitfield's ointment.

Hair

White piedra. This disease, caused by the yeast *Trichosporon beigelii*, results in soft, white, greyish or light-brown nodules on the hair shafts, mainly in the axillae. The hair often breaks at the point of infection, leaving hairs with a clubbed or swollen end. Shaving of the affected area is usually sufficient to effect a cure.

Black piedra. This condition, caused by *Piedraia hortae*, is characterized by the presence of black, hard nodules up to 1 mm in diameter, mainly on the hairs of the scalp. It occurs in humid, tropical climates. Crushing the nodules reveals the sexual reproductive phase, club-shaped asci, each with eight ascospores. Culture is not necessary. Shaving to remove infected hairs is a satisfactory treatment.

Otomycosis

About 10–20% of chronic ear infections are due to fungi. The commonest causes are species of *Aspergillus*, in particular *A. niger*. The fungi are easy to see in material from swabs or scrapings and grow readily in culture.

Treatment with topical antifungals is usually successful, although relapse is common. Any concurrent bacterial infection or other underlying abnormality should also be treated.

Mycotic keratitis

Fungal infections of the cornea are secondary to injury, bacterial infection and treatment with antibacterial agents and steroids. They occur most often in hot climates and are caused by common saprophytic moulds, in particular *Aspergillus* and *Fusarium* species. Culture results should be interpreted with care since these opportunist pathogens are also encountered as contaminants. Superficial swabs are of no value for laboratory investigation and scrapings should be taken from the base or edge of the ulcer. The branched, septate hyphae may be rather sparse in potassium hydroxide mounts and some of the material should also be stained with PAS or methenamine–silver techniques.

Treatment is with topical antifungal agents, in particular natamycin.

SUBCUTANEOUS INFECTIONS

Mycetoma

Mycetoma is a chronic, granulomatous infection of the skin, subcutaneous tissues, fascia and bone, which most often affects the foot or the hand. It may be caused by one of a number of different actinomycetes (*actinomycetoma*) (see Chapter 20) or moulds (*eumycetoma*). The disease is most prevalent in tropical and subtropical regions of Africa, Asia and Central America. Infection follows traumatic inoculation of the organism into the subcutaneous tissue from soil or vegetable sources, usually on thorns or splinters. Consequently, the disease occurs most frequently in male agricultural workers, in whom minor skin injuries are common.

A large number of organisms have been implicated in this disease, including species of *Madurella, Exophiala, Acremonium, Pseudallescheria, Actinomadura, Nocardia* and *Streptomyces*. Within host tissues the organisms develop to form compacted colonies (grains) 0.5–2 mm in diameter, the colour of which depends on the organism responsible; for example, *Madurella* grains are black and *Actinomadura pelletieri* grains are red.

Pathogenesis

Localized swollen lesions, which develop multiple draining sinuses, are usually found on the limbs, although infections occur on other parts of the body. There is often a long period between the initial infection and formation of the characteristic lesions; spread from the site of origin is unusual but may occur, particularly from the foot up the long bones of the leg.

Laboratory diagnosis

The presence of grains in pus collected from draining sinuses or in biopsy material is diagnostic. The grains are visible to the naked eye and their colour may help to identify the causal agent. Grains should be crushed in potassium hydroxide and examined microscopically to differentiate between actinomycetoma and eumycetoma; material from actinomycetoma grains may be Gram-stained to demonstrate the Gram-positive filaments. Samples should also be cultured, at both 25–30°C and 37°C, on brain–heart infusion agar or blood agar for actinomycetes and on Sabouraud agar (without cycloheximide) for fungi. The fungi that cause eumycetoma are all septate moulds that appear in culture within 1–4 weeks, but their identification requires expert knowledge. Serological precipitin tests have been used to differentiate between eumycetoma and actinomycetoma and to identify specific causal agents, but they are of little value for diagnosis and are not in routine use.

Treatment

The prognosis varies according to the causal agent, so it is important that the identity is established. Actinomycetoma responds well to rifampicin in combination with sulphonamides or co-trimoxazole, but an average of 9 months' therapy is required. In eumycetoma, chemotherapy is ineffective and radical surgery is usually necessary. However, some antifungals have yet to be properly evaluated in this condition.

Chromoblastomycosis

This disease, also known as *chromomycosis*, is a chronic, localized disease of the skin and subcutaneous tissues, characterized by crusted, warty lesions usually involving the limbs. The disease is mainly encountered in the tropics. The principal causes are *Fonsecaea pedrosoi, F. compacta, Phialophora verrucosa* and *Cladosporium carrionii*. Like mycetoma, the disease is seen most often among men in rural areas.

Laboratory diagnosis

The dark-coloured fungal elements are relatively easy to see on microscopical examination of skin scrapings, crusts and pus. Culture on Sabouraud agar at 25–30°C yields slow-growing, greenish grey to black, compact, folded colonies. Cultures should be incubated for 4–6 weeks. Specific identification of these closely related fungi is usually left to a reference laboratory. Serological tests are not used routinely.

Treatment

Treatment is usually unsatisfactory but in preliminary trials promising results have been obtained with terbinafine and with itraconazole either alone or in combination with flucytosine. Early, solitary lesions may be excised.

Phaeohyphomycosis

This is a general term given to non-specific solitary subcutaneous lesions caused by any black fungus. Diagnosis is often made at surgery, and treatment is by excision. These fungi may also cause opportunistic, deep-seated infections, such as brain abscesses, which require therapy with amphotericin B and flucytosine.

Sporotrichosis

Sporotrichosis is a chronic, pyogenic granulomatous infection of the skin and subcutaneous tissues which may remain localized or show lymphatic spread. It is caused by *Sporothrix schenckii*, a saprophyte in nature. The disease occurs mainly in Central and South America, parts of the USA and Africa, and Australia; it is rare in Europe.

S. schenckii is a dimorphic fungus. In nature and in culture at 25–30°C, it develops as a mould with thin (1–2 μm) septate hyphae; spore-bearing hyphae carry clusters of oval spores. The yeast phase is formed in tissue and in culture at 37°C, and is composed of spherical or cigar-shaped cells (1–3 × 3–10 μm).

Pathogenesis

Sporotrichosis most frequently presents as a nodular, ulcerating disease of the skin and subcutaneous tissues, with spread along local lymphatic channels. Typically, the primary lesion is on the hand with secondary lesions extending up the arm. The primary lesion may remain localized or disseminate to involve the bones, joints, lungs and, in rare cases, the CNS. Disseminated disease usually occurs in debilitated or immunosuppressed individuals.

Laboratory diagnosis

Diagnosis is confirmed by isolation of the causative organism by culture of swabs from moist, ulcerated lesions or pus aspirated from subcutaneous nodules; biopsy specimens may be necessary in some cases. Direct microscopy is of little value since so few of the small *S. schenckii* yeast cells are present in diseased tissue. The mycelial phase develops within 7–10 days on Sabouraud agar or blood agar at 25–30°C; the yeast phase develops in 2 days at 37°C. Identification depends on the micromorphology of the mould phase and its conversion to the yeast phase at 37°C.

A latex agglutination test is of value for the diagnosis of the extracutaneous forms of sporotrichosis. The test has poor prognostic value since titres change little after successful therapy. A skin test with sporotrichin antigen is positive in almost all patients with cutaneous sporotrichosis.

Treatment

Prolonged therapy is usually required. For the cutaneous form, treatment with potassium iodide or itraconazole is satisfactory. In disseminated disease, intravenous amphotericin B is required.

Other subcutaneous mycoses

Rhinosporidiosis is a chronic, granulomatous disease of the mucocutaneous tissues, with the appearance of large polyps or wart-like lesions in the nose or conjunctiva. Most reported cases have been from India and Sri Lanka, although the disease is also seen in South America. It was thought to be caused by a fungus, *Rhinosporidium seeberi*, but all attempts at isolation from clinical material failed. Molecular studies have shown that the organism responsible is not in fact a fungus, but a primitive aquatic bacterium.

Several other fungi, including *Loboa loboi*, *Basidiobolus haptosporus* and *Conidiobolus coronatus*, occasionally cause subcutaneous infections, usually in the tropics. Surgical excision is often curative in rhinosporidiosis and *L. loboi* infections; antifungal therapy may be of use for the other infections, but the newer drugs have not been properly evaluated.

SYSTEMIC MYCOSES

Coccidioidomycosis

This is primarily an infection of the lungs caused by *Coccidioides immitis*, a dimorphic fungus found in the soil of semi-arid areas, mainly in the south-west USA and northern Mexico. Agricultural workers with a higher exposure risk and dark-skinned people are especially prone to the disease. In endemic regions over 90% of inhabitants may exhibit positive skin tests and infection rates of 20% or higher have been recorded among newcomers to the areas in their first year of residence. Recovery usually confers lifetime immunity.

In culture and in soil *C. immitis* grows as a mould, producing large numbers of barrel-shaped arthroconidia (4 × 6 μm diameter), which are easily dispersed in wind currents. In the lungs the arthroconidia form spherules (30–60 μm diameter) which contain numerous endospores (2–5 μm diameter). Endospores are released by rupture of the spherule wall and develop to form new spherules in adjacent tissue or elsewhere in the body. In culture the mycelial colony is initially moist and white but changes within 5–12 days to become pale grey or brown.

Pathogenesis

C. immitis usually causes an asymptomatic or self-limiting pulmonary illness, but a progressive and sometimes fatal secondary disease occasionally develops. Primary pulmonary coccidioidomycosis develops 7–28 days after infection. Skin rashes develop in up to 20% of those with the primary disease and indicate a good prognosis. In some cases primary infection may result in a chronic, cavitating, pulmonary infection which may resolve after several years, or may progress to the disseminated form. Localized subcutaneous infection may result from direct inoculation of the fungus through the skin or may be secondary to pulmonary disease.

Disseminated infection occurs in about 1% of those who contract the primary pulmonary disease; it is more common in immunocompromised individuals (e.g. organ transplantation, lymphoma, AIDS), and in Filipinos, Negroes and American Indians. When dissemination occurs, it involves virtually every tissue of the body, including the CNS, skin and joints. The prognosis for disseminated coccidioidomycosis is generally poor, particularly in immunosuppressed individuals and those with meningeal involvement.

Laboratory diagnosis

Microscopical examination of sputum, pus and biopsy material is helpful since the relatively large size and numbers of mature spherules present makes their detection and identification comparatively straightforward. Material for culture should be inoculated onto test-tube slopes of Sabouraud agar and incubated at 25–30°C for at least 3 weeks. The fungus can be identified by its colonial morphology and the presence of numerous thick-walled arthroconidia formed in chains from alternate cells of the fine, septate hyphae.

The arthroconidia are highly infectious and are a serious danger to laboratory staff. Consequently, Petri dishes should *never* be used for isolation of the organism and all procedures should be carried out in Category 3 containment facilities. Preparations for microscopy should be made only after wetting the colony to reduce spore dispersal.

Skin tests with coccidioidin, a culture filtrate antigen from the mycelial phase of *C. immitis*, or spherulin, an extract of the spherules, are useful although cross-reactions may occur in patients with histoplasmosis and blastomycosis. The skin test does not distinguish present from past infection and a negative skin test does not preclude infection with *C. immitis*.

Serological tests play an important part in diagnosis. The precipitin test is most useful for detection of early, primary infection or exacerbation of existing disease; precipitins appear 1–3 weeks after infection but are seldom detectable after 2–6 months, or in patients with disseminated coccidioidomycosis. The latex agglutination test gives similar results to the precipitin test, but is less specific. The complement fixation test is most useful for detecting disseminated disease: complement fixing antibodies appear 2–3 months after infection and persist until death or recovery.

Treatment

Intravenous amphotericin B is the standard therapy, but oral fluconazole, itraconazole or ketoconazole are also used. Therapy is for at least a year. Intrathecal therapy with amphotericin B is used in the meningeal form, but oral fluconazole is now often used as an alternative. Ketoconazole and itraconazole are also useful.

Histoplasmosis

H. capsulatum is found in soil enriched with the droppings of birds and bats, and infection results from the inhalation of spores. The major endemic areas for histoplasmosis are the Mississippi and Ohio river valleys of the eastern USA, where the prevalence of infection may be as high as 95%. It also occurs in other parts of the USA and many other temperate and tropical areas. A similar organism, *H. duboisii*, which may be a variant of *H. capsulatum*, is mainly restricted to the continent of Africa.

The fungus grows in soil and in culture at 25–30°C as a mould and as an intracellular yeast in animal tissues. The yeast phase cells (2–3 × 3–4 μm) can also be produced in vitro by culture at 37°C on blood agar or other enriched media containing cysteine. In culture the mould colonies are fluffy, white or buff-brown; the mycelium is septate and two types of unicellular asexual spores are usually produced: large round, tuberculate macroconidia

(8–14 μm in diameter) are most prominent and are diagnostic, but smaller broadly elliptical, smooth-walled microconidia (2–4 μm in diameter) are also present in primary isolates. *H. duboisii* is morphologically identical to *H. capsulatum* in its mycelial phase but the yeast phase has larger cells (12–15 μm diameter).

Pathogenesis

Most infections are asymptomatic and are detected only when individuals develop a positive skin test reaction. Sometimes an acute influenza-like illness develops with fever and a non-productive cough. These infections are usually self-limiting, but patients are frequently left with discrete, calcified lesions in the lung.

A chronic form of histoplasmosis occurs mainly in adults; large cavities develop directly from primary lesions in the lung or by reactivation of old lesions. The clinical picture closely resembles tuberculosis; in some cases the infection may disseminate to give acute generalized disease.

Occasionally, patients develop an acute progressive form of the disease, with widespread infection of the reticulo-endothelial system and dissemination to other organs of the body. The rate of progression of the disease varies considerably, but generally the prognosis is poor.

Disseminated infection occurs most often in old age and infancy, or in individuals with impaired immune responses, e.g. due to neutropenia, haematological malignancy, AIDS or high-dose steroids.

Laboratory diagnosis

Microscopy of smears of sputum or pus should be stained by the Wright or Giemsa procedure. Blood smears may be positive for *H. capsulatum*, especially in patients with AIDS. Liver or lung biopsies stained with PAS or methenamine–silver may provide a rapid diagnosis of disseminated histoplasmosis in some patients. *H. capsulatum* is seen as small, oval yeast cells, typically packed within macrophages or monocytes.

Specimens should be cultured on Sabouraud agar at 25–30°C to obtain the mycelial phase. Mycelial colonies develop within 1–4 weeks but cultures should be retained for 6 weeks before discarding. The fungus is identified by its colonial morphology and the presence of the characteristic macroconidia and microconidia. Culture at 37°C for the yeast phase is not used for primary isolation but conversion from the mould to yeast phase is useful to confirm the identity of isolates. Mould cultures of *H. capsulatum* are a hazard to laboratory staff and consequently test-tube slopes rather than Petri dishes should be used for isolation.

A histoplasmin skin test has been used, but a positive result does not differentiate between active and past infection, and false-positive reactions can occur in patients with other fungal infections; furthermore, skin testing induces humoral antibodies that complicate the interpretation of subsequent serodiagnostic tests.

Serological tests are useful, but cross-reactions can occur, mainly with *C. immitis*. The complement fixation test, with histoplasmin or killed whole yeast cells as antigen, is positive in up to 96% of culturally proven cases. Generally, titres of 8 are regarded as presumptive evidence of infection, and titres of 32 or above indicate active disease. Low titres or negative results do not exclude infection. The precipitin test gives positive results in up to 85% of infected patients; there are few problems with cross-reactions, but positive results should be confirmed by a complement fixation test. The latex agglutination test is useful for detection of acute histoplasmosis but is of less value than the other tests.

Antibody tests fail to detect antibodies in up to 50% of immunosuppressed individuals. Tests for antigen detection by radio-immunoassay or ELISA are useful, but are not widely available.

Treatment

Intravenous amphotericin B for up to 3 months is the treatment of choice for most forms of disseminated histoplasmosis; this is followed by oral itraconazole for 6–24 months in immunocompromised patients. Ketoconazole and itraconazole give good results in less ill cases.

Blastomycosis

Blastomycosis occurs mainly in the central and mid-western states of the USA and eastern Canada. It is caused by *Blastomyces dermatitidis*, which has been isolated from the environment on only a few occasions; its exact ecological niche has yet to be established. Infection results from inhalation of spores and most infections appear to be contracted sporadically in cool, wet climatic conditions. The disease is seen most often among men aged 30–50 years.

B. dermatitidis is a dimorphic fungus. In culture at 25–30°C it grows as a mould with a septate mycelium. The colony varies in texture from floccose to smooth and from white to brown in colour. Asexual conidia are produced on lateral hyphal branches of variable length; the conidia are 2–10 μm in diameter and some may be dumb-bell shaped. In tissue and in culture at 37°C the fungus grows as a yeast (8–15 μm diameter) which characteristically produces broad-based buds from a single pole on the mother cell.

Pathogenesis

The disease is slowly progressive and if left untreated has a poor prognosis, although a subclinical pulmonary form of the disease, similar to that seen in coccidioidomycosis and histoplasmosis, probably exists.

Primary pulmonary disease is usually relatively mild, but within a few weeks the disease may disseminate to other tissues. The chest radiograph can resemble that of tuberculosis or carcinoma. In disseminated infection the chronic pulmonary disease persists, and abscesses and granulomatous lesions are found in most organs and body tissues, including bone. Disseminated blastomycosis has been described in immunosuppressed patients. Chronic cutaneous lesions occur in about 80% of patients with pulmonary infection; the characteristic secondary skin lesions are typically raised, with a well demarcated edge. It is from these skin lesions that the diagnosis is most often made. Primary cutaneous infection resulting from the introduction of the fungus to the skin is rare and produces a localized, self-limiting lesion.

Laboratory diagnosis

Direct microscopy of pus, scrapings from skin lesions, or sputum usually shows thick-walled yeast cells 8–15 μm in diameter, which characteristically produce buds on a broad base; the buds remain attached until they are almost the size of the parent cell, often forming chains of three or four cells. In biopsy material the yeasts are best seen in sections stained with PAS or methenamine–silver.

B. dermatitidis will grow in culture on Sabouraud agar (or blood agar) without cycloheximide, to which the fungus is sensitive. The mycelial phase develops slowly at 25–30°C and cultures must be retained for 6 weeks before discarding. Test-tube slopes rather than Petri dishes are used for culture. Identification is usually confirmed by subculture at 37°C to convert it to the yeast phase.

Most skin and serological tests are unreliable because of poor sensitivity and cross-reaction with histoplasmosis and coccidioidomycosis. An ELISA test that appears to be more than 90% specific has been developed.

Treatment

Intravenous amphotericin B is used to treat all forms of blastomycosis and is the drug of choice in serious infection. Itraconazole follow-on therapy is given once the patient improves. Hydroxystilbamidine was formerly used in localized disease or when amphotericin B failed or proved too toxic. Ketoconazole or itraconazole are also effective and are now the drugs of choice in less serious, extra-CNS blastomycosis.

Paracoccidioidomycosis

This is a chronic, granulomatous infection, caused by *Paracoccidioides brasiliensis*, which may involve the lungs, mucosa, skin and lymphatic system. The disease is fatal if untreated.

P. brasiliensis enters the body via the lungs; it grows as a saprophyte in nature but the precise reservoir is unknown. The disease occurs most frequently in humid mountain forests of South and Central America. Most infections are seen in rural workers 20–40 years of age.

P. brasiliensis grows in the mycelial phase in culture at 25–30°C, and in the yeast phase in tissue or at 37°C on brain–heart infusion or blood agar. The mould colonies are slow-growing with a variable colonial morphology, although most are white and velvety to floccose in texture with a pale brown reverse. Spore production is usually sparse and best seen in 8–10-week cultures. Asexual conidia may be produced but are not characteristic, and identification depends on conversion from the mycelial to the yeast phase. The yeast phase consists of oval or globose cells 2–30 μm in diameter, with small buds attached by a narrow neck encircling the parent cell.

Pathogenesis

Paracoccidioidomycosis usually presents as an ulcerative, granulomatous infection of the oral and nasal mucosa and the adjacent skin. The lymphatic system, spleen, intestines, adrenals and liver are also often involved. Primary skin lesions are rare. There is evidence of prolonged latent infection before overt disease develops, and a mild, self-limiting pulmonary form of paracoccidioidomycosis probably exists.

Laboratory diagnosis

Microscopy of sputum or pus, crusts and biopsies from granulomatous lesions usually reveals numerous yeast cells showing the characteristic multipolar budding, which is diagnostic. Tissue sections should be stained with PAS or methenamine–silver. In culture the mycelial and yeast phases both develop slowly and cultures must be retained for 6 weeks before discarding. The mould phase can be isolated on Sabouraud agar supplemented with yeast extract at 25–30°C, but colonies may take 15–25 days to appear. Blood agar (without cycloheximide) and incubation at 37°C is recommended for isolation of the yeast phase.

Skin tests are of limited diagnostic value because of poor sensitivity and cross-reactivity with other systemic mycoses. Serological tests are useful for diagnosis and for monitoring the response to therapy. Precipitin tests and complement fixation tests, when used together, detect about 98% of infections. Cross-reactions are rare, particularly with the precipitin test.

Treatment

The choice of therapy depends on the site of infection and its severity. Amphotericin B is the drug of choice for serious infections although it is not effective on its own and needs to be given with sulpha drugs or azoles, preferably itraconazole. Oral ketoconazole and itraconazole have also given good results.

Cryptococcosis

Cryptococcosis, caused by the capsulate yeast *Cryptococcus neoformans*, is most frequently recognized as a disease of the CNS, although the primary site of infection is the lungs. The disease occurs sporadically throughout the world but it is now seen most often in patients with AIDS.

There are four serotypes of *C. neoformans* (A, B, C, D) which represent two varieties of the organism, namely, *C. neoformans* var. *neoformans* (A, D) and *C. neoformans* var. *gattii* (B, C). Most infections are caused by *C. neoformans* var. *neoformans*, which is commonly found in the excreta of wild and domesticated birds throughout the world. Pigeons carry *C. neoformans* in their crops and counts of over 10^7 cells per gram of pigeon faeces have been found. The birds themselves do not appear to become infected, probably because of their high body temperature. *C. neoformans* var. *gattii* is associated with the flowers of *Eucalyptus camaldulensis* (red river gum tree) and infections coincide with the distribution of the tree.

Pathogenesis

Infection follows inhalation of the cells or basidiospores of *C. neoformans* which, in nature, are thought to be small, allowing the organism to enter deep into the lung. The disease is more common in men than women.

A mild, self-limiting pulmonary infection is believed to be the commonest form of cryptococcosis. In symptomatic pulmonary infection there are no clear diagnostic features. Lesions may take the form of small discrete nodules, which may heal with a residual scar or may become enlarged, encapsulated and chronic (*cryptococcoma* form). An acute pneumonic type of disease has also been described.

The meningeal form of cryptococcosis can occur in apparently healthy individuals, but occurs most frequently in patients with abnormalities of T lymphocyte function, including those with Hodgkin's disease, sarcoidosis, collagen disease and neoplasms. Around 3–20% of individuals with AIDS develop cryptococcosis. Chronic meningitis or meningo-encephalitis develops insidiously with headaches and low-grade pyrexia, followed by changes in mental state, anorexia, visual disturbances and eventually coma. The disease may last from a few months to several years, but the outcome is always fatal unless it is treated. AIDS patients with cryptococcosis generally develop a chronic meningeal form with milder symptoms.

Although predominantly a disease of the CNS, lesions of the skin, mucosa, viscera and bones may also occur; in its disseminated form, the disease may resemble tuberculosis. Rarely, lesions of skin and bones may occur without any evidence of infection elsewhere.

Laboratory diagnosis

C. neoformans is readily demonstrated in cerebrospinal fluid (CSF) or other material by direct microscopy, culture or serological tests for capsular antigen. The yeast load is generally higher in patients with AIDS. The cellular reaction and chemical changes in CSF usually resemble those seen in tuberculous meningitis. The yeast cells of *C. neoformans* are round, 4–10 μm in diameter, and are surrounded by a mucopolysaccharide capsule. The width of the capsule varies and is greatest in vivo and on rich media in vitro.

In unstained, wet preparations of CSF mixed with a drop of India ink or nigrosine, the capsule can be seen as a clear halo around the yeast cells. Capsulate yeasts are seen in the CSF of about 60% of patients with cryptococcosis (higher in AIDS), but the capsule may be difficult to visualize in some cases. Sputum, pus or brain tissue should be examined after digestion in potassium hydroxide and here the capsulate yeasts are often delineated by the cellular debris. For examination of tissue sections it is best to use a specific fungal stain such as PAS; alcian blue and mucicarmine stain the capsular material, enabling the organisms to be differentiated from *H. capsulatum* and *B. dermatitidis*.

The yeast is easily cultured from CSF although large volumes or multiple samples may be required in some cases; in AIDS patients it is also useful to culture blood. On Sabouraud agar (without cycloheximide) cultured at 25–30°C and 37°C, colonies normally appear within 2–3 days, but cultures should not be discarded for 3 weeks. In culture, *C. neoformans* appears as creamy–white to yellow–brown colonies, which are mucoid in strains with well developed capsules and dry in strains that lack prominent capsules. Buds appear at any point on the cell surface but mycelium or pseudomycelium are not normally produced. Preliminary identification depends on demonstration of the capsule but this may be absent or difficult to see. *C. neoformans* can be identified with commercial kits or can be distinguished from other yeasts by its lack of fermentative ability, its ability to produce urease, to grow at 37°C and to assimilate inositol.

The latex agglutination test for the detection of cryptococcal polysaccharide antigen in CSF or blood is highly sensitive and specific for the diagnosis of cryptococcal meningitis and disseminated forms of the disease, and gives better results than microscopy and culture. In AIDS, the test is positive in well over 90% of infected patients and titres of over 10^6 may be detected. Antigen may also be detected by ELISA.

A whole-cell agglutination test for serum antibody is positive in less than 50% of proven cases of cryptococcal meningitis, since antibodies are rapidly neutralized by the large amounts of capsular antigen released during evolution of the infection. Antibodies may subsequently reappear in patients after successful treatment, but not usually in AIDS patients. Consequently, the progress of the disease and the response to therapy can be monitored by using antigen and antibody tests in combination.

Treatment

In immunocompetent individuals, cryptococcosis may be treated with oral fluconazole or itraconazole. Intravenous amphotericin B in combination with flucytosine is usually the treatment of choice for immunocompromised individuals. Intrathecal amphotericin B may also be used in severe meningeal disease. Patients with AIDS commonly relapse after the initial course of therapy and many react badly to the drugs.

Amphotericin B therapy is usually followed by oral fluconazole, sometimes for prolonged periods. Fluconazole can be administered orally and is useful if amphotericin B proves too toxic; it is also used as a maintenance therapy to control cryptococcosis in AIDS patients. Itraconazole may be used as an alternative follow-on therapy. Resistant strains *of C. neoformans* have emerged in AIDS patients after prolonged therapy with fluconazole.

Individuals at risk of developing cryptococcosis should avoid contact with bird droppings.

Aspergillosis

There are more than 100 species of *Aspergillus* but only a few have been implicated in human disease: the most important are *A. fumigatus, A. niger, A. flavus, A. terreus*

and *A. nidulans*. All grow in nature and in culture as mycelial fungi with septate hyphae and distinctive sporing structures; the spore-bearing hypha (conidiophore) terminates in a swollen cell (vesicle) surrounded by one or two rows of cells (sterigmata) from which chains of asexual conidia are produced (Fig. 60.2).

Aspergillus spores are ubiquitous and in winter months counts may reach 600 spores/m³ of air in the UK. The fungus is particularly prevalent in decaying vegetation, such as mouldy hay, and counts of more than 10^7 spores/m³ of air have been recorded inside farm buildings.

Pathogenesis

Allergic aspergillosis. Allergy to *Aspergillus* species is usually seen in atopic individuals with elevated IgE levels; about 10–20% of asthmatics react to *A. fumigatus*. Asthma with eosinophilia is a more chronic form, which manifests as episodes of lung consolidation and fleeting shadows on chest radiography; the fungus grows in the airways to produce plugs of fungal mycelium which may block off segments of lung tissue and which, when coughed up, are a diagnostic feature. Allergic alveolitis follows particularly heavy and repeated exposure to large numbers of spores. Breathlessness, fever and malaise appear some hours after exposure, and repeated attacks result in progressive lung damage. A well known example of this form of the disease is *Maltster's lung*, which occurs in workers who handle barley on which *A. clavatus* has sporulated during the malting process.

Aspergilloma. In this form of aspergillosis, also referred to as *fungus ball*, the fungus colonizes preexisting (often tuberculous) cavities in the lung and forms a compact ball of mycelium, eventually surrounded by a dense fibrous wall.

Aspergillomas are usually solitary. Patients are either asymptomatic or have only a moderate cough and sputum production. Occasional haemoptysis may occur, especially when the fungus is actively growing, and haemorrhage following invasion of a blood vessel is one of the fatal complications of this condition. Surgical resection is most often used to treat this condition.

Invasive aspergillosis. This form occurs in severely immunocompromised individuals who have a serious underlying illness. Neutropenia is the most common predisposing factor and *A. fumigatus* is the species most frequently involved. This infection is responsible for significant mortality in bone marrow transplant patients.

The lung is the sole site of infection in 70% of patients, but dissemination of infection to other organs occurs in many cases. There is widespread destructive growth of *Aspergillus* species in lung tissue and the fungus invades blood vessels, causing thrombosis; septic emboli may spread the infection to other organs, especially the kidneys, heart and brain. Invasive aspergillosis has a poor prognosis and is often diagnosed post mortem.

Endocarditis. *Aspergillus* species may rarely cause endocarditis in immunosuppressed patients and those who have undergone open heart surgery. The condition has a poor prognosis and successful therapy depends on a combination of antifungal treatment and surgical removal of infected tissue.

Paranasal granuloma. *A. flavus* and *A. fumigatus* may colonize and invade the paranasal sinuses and the infection may spread through the bone to the orbit of the eye and brain. This condition is seen most often in warm dry climates and is common in parts of the Sudan and northern India.

Laboratory diagnosis

The value of the laboratory in diagnosis varies according to the clinical form of aspergillosis; the diagnosis of invasive disease is particularly difficult.

Direct microscopy. In potassium hydroxide preparations (preferably with Calcofluor to enhance detection) of sputum the fungus appears as non-pigmented septate mycelium, 3–5 μm in diameter, with characteristic dichotomous branching and an irregular outline; rarely the characteristic sporing heads of *Aspergillus* species are present.

- In allergic aspergillosis there is usually abundant fungus in the sputum and mycelial plugs may also be present.
- In aspergilloma, fungus may be difficult to find on microscopy.
- In invasive aspergillosis, microscopy is often negative.

Biopsy may provide a definitive diagnosis, although many clinicians are reluctant to undertake this procedure because of the associated risk. In tissue sections *Aspergillus* species are best seen after staining with PAS or methenamine–silver.

Culture. *Aspergillus* species grow readily at 25–37°C on Sabouraud agar without cycloheximide; colonies appear after 1–2 days. Isolates can be identified by their colonial appearance and micromorphology. The ability of *A. fumigatus* to grow well at 45°C can be used to help identify this species or to isolate it selectively.

Since aspergilli are among the commonest laboratory contaminants, quantification of the amount of fungus in sputum helps to confirm the relevance of a positive culture. However, all isolates from neutropenic patients *must* be taken seriously and acted upon.

Large quantities of fungus are usually recovered from the sputum of patients with allergic aspergillosis but cultures from those with aspergilloma or invasive disease are commonly negative or yield only a few colonies. Blood cultures are negative in invasive disease.

Skin tests. Skin tests with *A. fumigatus* antigen are useful for the diagnosis of allergic aspergillosis. All patients give an immediate type I reaction and 70% of those with pulmonary eosinophilia also give a delayed type III arthus reaction.

Serological tests. Immunodiffusion, CIE and ELISA are widely used for the detection of antibodies in the diagnosis of all forms of aspergillosis, particularly aspergilloma and allergic bronchopulmonary aspergillosis.

Antigen detection has also been used successfully for diagnosis of invasive aspergillosis by techniques such as ELISA and latex agglutination. However, with ELISA sensitivity is currently <80%.

PCR. This is now increasingly used for diagnosis of invasive aspergillosis but its precise value is still being assessed.

All available serological and PCR tests lack sensitivity and are best used along with other laboratory tests and computed tomography, which is very useful in invasive aspergillosis.

Treatment

Allergic forms of aspergillosis are treated with corticosteroids. Aspergilloma is treated by surgical excision because antifungal therapy is of little value, but because of the significant morbidity and mortality with this procedure, it is reserved for those with episodes of life-threatening haemoptysis and immunocompromised patients. In invasive aspergillosis, the treatment of choice is intravenous amphotericin B (conventional or liposomal). Oral or intravenous itraconazole is an alternative but has yet to be fully evaluated. It has given good results in some cases for continuing therapy in those who have responded to initial amphotericin B therapy. Caspofungin is reserved for those unresponsive to, or intolerant of, other therapies.

Systemic candidosis

Systemic candidosis is an iatrogenic infection encountered among certain groups of hospital patients, who carry more yeasts in the mouth and gastro-intestinal tract than the normal population. The highest numbers of yeasts occur:

- in patients treated with antibiotics or steroids
- in immunosuppressed patients
- after surgical procedures such as organ transplants or heart surgery.

Several factors predispose to yeast overgrowth:

- natural receptive states (infancy, old age, pregnancy)
- changes in local bacterial flora (e.g. secondary to antibiotics)
- changes to epithelial surfaces (e.g. due to moisture, local occlusion, trauma)
- T lymphocyte defects (primary or secondary to disease, e.g. AIDS or immunosuppression)
- neutropenia (primary or secondary to disease or immunosuppression)
- endocrine disease (e.g. diabetes mellitus)
- miscellaneous conditions (e.g. zinc or iron deficiency).

Infection may be localized, e.g. in the urinary tract, liver, heart valves (endocarditis), meninges or peritoneal cavity, or may be widely disseminated and associated with a septicaemia (*candidaemia*). Deep-seated candidosis is difficult to diagnose and treat, and for some forms the prognosis is poor.

Candidaemia is seen mainly in postoperative or immunosuppressed patients; in some patients it clears spontaneously, or disappears when contaminated intravenous catheters are removed. However, some patients with candidaemia, notably those treated with cytotoxic drugs or corticosteroids, develop generalized or localized deep-seated infection.

Common sites of involvement in disseminated infection include the kidney, liver, spleen, brain and gastrointestinal tract; pulmonary infections are rare. One common sign of deep-seated candidosis is the presence of white lesions within the eye (*Candida* endophthalmitis). *Candida* endocarditis usually follows surgery for valve replacement, but also occurs in drug addicts and occasionally in patients on immunosuppressive therapy.

Infection of the kidney is usually blood-borne and ascending infection is thought to be rare. Bladder infections are usually associated with the presence of an indwelling urinary catheter; the infection often clears when the underlying cause is corrected.

C. albicans accounts for most cases of systemic candidosis, but infections due to *C. tropicalis*, *C. lusitaniae*, *C. glabrata*, *C. krusei* and *C. parapsilosis* are seen increasingly; *C. glabrata* and *C. krusei* are important pathogens because they are unresponsive to fluconazole. *C. parapsilosis* is responsible for about 25% of cases of yeast endocarditis and *C. glabrata* is often involved in infections of the urinary tract. The mycological features of these organisms have been outlined in the section on superficial candidosis (p. 575).

Laboratory diagnosis

Diagnosis of deep-seated candidosis is difficult and many cases are revealed post mortem. There are no distinctive clinical signs to indicate *Candida* infection, unless endophthalmitis is present, although some patients develop a macular skin rash. Hepatosplenic candidosis (a common deep-seated form) has a characteristic computed tomography scan appearance.

Candida species may be present as commensals in the absence of infection, so that isolation from clinical material, except from sites that are normally sterile, is of little significance. Similarly, antibodies to *Candida* species can be detected in uninfected individuals because of their exposure to commensal yeasts, although a rise in antibody titre or high titres may be of diagnostic significance. In suspected systemic candidosis, samples from as many sources as possible should be examined by direct microscopy and culture. Results should always be interpreted in the light of clinical findings.

Direct microscopy. Appropriate samples are examined microscopically in potassium hydroxide or after Gram staining. In tissue sections, the fungus is seen best if stained with PAS or methenamine–silver. Mycelium is often abundant but the presence of mycelium in sputum or urine does not confirm that the yeast is present as a pathogen.

Culture. *Candida* species grow readily in culture at 37°C on common isolation media, such as Sabouraud agar (p. 576). Blood cultures provide the most reliable evidence of systemic infection, although repeated attempts to isolate the organism may be necessary. Transient candidaemia is not uncommon, especially in patients with indwelling intravenous catheters, but isolation of *Candida* from blood should certainly not be disregarded in immunocompromised patients.

Isolation of the yeast from otherwise sterile sites provides reliable evidence for the diagnosis, but cultures obtained from urine, faeces and sputum are of less value unless done quantitatively over a period of time. Cell counts of the yeast in urine in excess of 10^4 per ml are usually taken to indicate urinary tract infection, except in those with an indwelling urinary catheter.

Since *Candida* species multiply rapidly in clinical material it is important that specimens are processed as soon as possible after collection.

Serological tests. Currently available tests lack specificity and sensitivity, and the results must be interpreted with care. The most widely used tests are immunodiffusion, CIE and ELISA for detection of antibodies to somatic extracts of *C. albicans* and *C. parapsilosis*. A positive test does not necessarily indicate infection since the antigens used do not differentiate between antibodies formed during mucosal colonization and those produced during deep infection. Similarly, a negative antibody test does not necessarily rule out the possibility of deep-seated candidosis in immunocompromised patients who are incapable of mounting an adequate antibody response; in such cases ELISA gives better results.

Antigen tests, based mainly on ELISA, passive haemagglutination or latex agglutination, that detect cell wall mannan or cytoplasmic components, have been developed and are used for diagnosis. Although there is a need to improve sensitivity, antigen detection is useful for serodiagnosis of some forms of systemic candidosis.

PCR. This is now used to diagnose invasive candidosis, although its precise value is still being evaluated.

Treatment

The treatments of choice for most forms of systemic candidosis are:

- intravenous amphotericin B (conventional or liposomal)
- intravenous or oral fluconazole.

Both drugs can be used in combination with flucytosine, but flucytosine is not used alone since resistance may develop during treatment. Ketoconazole and intravenous itraconazole have also been used successfully. Removal of existing intravenous catheters is desirable if feasible, especially in non-neutropenic patients.

Zygomycosis

Zygomycosis, also referred to as *mucormycosis* or *phycomycosis*, is a relatively rare, opportunistic infection caused by saprophytic mould fungi, notably species of *Rhizopus*, *Mucor* and *Absidia*. The fungi responsible are characterized by having broad, aseptate mycelium, with large numbers of asexual spores inside a sporangium which develops at the end of an aerial hypha.

The best known form of the disease is rhinocerebral zygomycosis, a rapidly fulminating infection which is almost invariably associated with acute diabetes mellitus, or with debilitating diseases such as leukaemia or lymphoma. There is extensive cellulitis with rapid tissue destruction, most commonly spreading from the nasal mucosa to the turbinate bone, paranasal sinuses, orbit and brain. The condition is rapidly fatal if untreated and, although the prognosis has improved over recent years, most diagnoses are still made at necropsy.

Pulmonary and disseminated infections can occur in severely immunocompromised individuals. Primary cutaneous infections have also been reported, but these are extremely rare and usually occur in patients with severe burns. Subcutaneous forms of zygomycosis are less serious.

Laboratory diagnosis

Recognition of the fungus in tissue by microscopy is considerably more reliable than culture, but material such as nasal discharge or sputum seldom contains much fungal material and examination of a biopsy is usually necessary for a firm diagnosis. Direct examination of curetted or biopsy material in potassium hydroxide may reveal the characteristic broad, aseptate, branched mycelium and sometimes distorted hyphae. However, they are seen much more clearly when stained with methenamine–silver; the hyphae of these fungi do not stain with PAS.

The fungi are readily isolated on Sabouraud agar at 37°C, but isolation is of little diagnostic significance in the absence of strong supporting clinical evidence of infection.

There are no established serological tests.

Treatment

Successful treatment depends on early diagnosis of the infection to allow prompt therapy with high doses of intravenous amphotericin B (conventional or liposomal), control of any diabetes and aggressive surgical intervention.

Pneumocystosis

Molecular studies indicate that *Pneumocystis carinii* is a fungus, but its morphology, behaviour and response to antimicrobial agents are more typical of a protozoon. It has yet to be fully embraced by mycologists. The organism was originally described as a cause of atypical pneumonia in malnourished infants, but came to prominence in the 1980s as a common cause of pneumonia, which was commonly fatal, in patients with AIDS. The advent of reliable antiretroviral therapy has considerably reduced the incidence of the disease in HIV-positive individuals. Around 10–40% of HIV-negative patients undergoing immunosuppressant treatments for malignancy, connective tissue disease or organ transplantation also develop *P. carinii* pneumonia, with mortality rates of 40–50%.

Serological and PCR studies indicate that exposure to *P. carinii* is very common: over 90% of immunocompetent children appear to have had a primary, presumably subclinical, infection and asymptomatic hospital patients have shown evidence of latent infection. In addition to pneumonia, other as yet unrecognized forms of *Pneumocystis* infection may exist.

Diagnosis usually depends on the identification of typical octonucleate 'cysts' in material obtained from the lung, since serology is unreliable. Simple expectorated sputum commonly fails to reveal evidence of the organism, and broncho-alveolar lavage or biopsy may be needed to establish the diagnosis.

In the immunocompromised, *P. carinii* is demonstrated by fluorescent antibody staining of bronchial lavage fluid smears. Molecular diagnosis by PCR methods is being introduced in some centres.

P. carinii is sensitive to co-trimoxazole, which is the treatment of choice. It is also used prophylactically, but patients with AIDS or those undergoing solid organ or bone marrow transplant may suffer unacceptable side-effects to the high doses used. Several alternative drugs are used in patients who do not respond to standard therapy; these include pentamidine, atovaquone, trimetrexate and the combination of clindamycin and primaquine. Pentamidine is most effective when given intravenously, but to minimize the risks of toxic side-effects it is sometimes instilled into the lungs by nebulizer, especially when used for prophylaxis.

Other opportunist fungi

Penicillium marneffei causes serious disseminated disease with characteristic papular skin lesions in AIDS patients in South-east Asia. The fungus is dimorphic, forming yeast-like cells that are often intracellular, resembling histoplasmosis, in infected tissues. It is associated with the bamboo rat (*Rhizomys sinensis*) and has been isolated from their burrows and internal organs. Treatment is with amphotericin B, followed by itraconazole to prevent relapse.

Almost any fungus may invade a severely immunocompromised host and infections with many common fungi, including *Fusarium* species, *Trichosporon beigelii* and *Pseudallescheria boydii*, have been reported. Diagnosis is made by culture of the causative organism from clinical specimens and serological tests play little part. Tissue sections are often not very helpful since the causal fungi either have no special features to enable identification, or they resemble other fungal pathogens.

Infections are usually treated speculatively, and sometimes successfully, with amphotericin B.

RECOMMENDED READING

Ajello L, Hay R J 1998 *Microbiology and Microbial Infections* 9th edn, Vol. 4 *Medical Mycology*. Arnold, London

Clayton Y, Midgley G 1985 *Medical Mycology*. Pocket Picture Guide Series. Gower, London

Evans E G V, Gentles J C 1985 *Essentials of Medical Mycology*. Churchill Livingstone, Edinburgh

Evans E G V, Richardson M D (eds) 1989 *Medical Mycology. A Practical Approach*. Oxford University Press, Oxford

Kibbler C C, Mackenzie D W R, Odds F C (eds) 1996 *Principles and Practice of Clinical Mycology*. Wiley, Chichester

Kwon-Chung K J, Bennett J E 1992 *Medical Mycology*. Lea & Febiger, Philadelphia

Odds F C 1988 *Candida and Candidosis*, 2nd edn. Baillière Tindall, London

Richardson M D, Warnock D W 1993 *Fungal Infection: Diagnosis and Management*. Blackwell Scientific, Oxford

Warnock D W, Richardson M D (eds) 1991 *Fungal Infection in the Compromised Patient*, 2nd edn. Wiley, Chichester

Internet sites

Wide range of information on all aspects of fungal infections: www.mycology.adelaide.edu.au/

Information on a range of fungal infections and treatment: www.clinical-mycology.com/

Information on antifungal drugs and modes of action: www.vet.purdue.edu/bms/courses/mcmp611/chmrx/antifuhd.htm

WWW Virtual Library of mycology images: hivinsite.ucsf.edu/akb/1997/section6.html

Wide range of information on all aspects of fungal infections: fungusweb.utmb.edu/mycology

Links to many sites about *Candida* and other yeasts: www.panix.com/~candida/#ed

Information on *Aspergillus* and the diseases it causes: www.aspergillus.man.ac.uk/

61

Protozoa

Malaria; toxoplasmosis; cryptosporidiosis; amoebic dysentery; sleeping sickness; Chagas' disease; leishmaniasis; giardiasis; trichomoniasis

D. Greenwood

Infection with pathogenic protozoa exacts an enormous toll of human suffering, notably, but not exclusively, in the tropics. Numerically the most important of the life-threatening protozoan diseases is malaria, which is responsible for at least 1 million deaths a year, mostly in young children in tropical countries.

Pathogenic protozoan parasites are conveniently dealt with by placing them in four groups: *sporozoa, amoebae, flagellates* and a miscellaneous group of other protozoa that may cause human disease (Table 61.1).

Table 61.1 Principal protozoan pathogens of man

Group	Species	Disease
Sporozoa	*Plasmodium falciparum*	Malignant tertian malaria
	P. vivax	Benign tertian malaria
	P. ovale	Benign tertian malaria
	P. malariae	Quartan malaria
	Toxoplasma gondii	Toxoplasmosis
	Isospora belli	Diarrhoea
	Cryptosporidium parvum	Diarrhoea
	Cyclospora cayetanensis	Diarrhoea
Amoebae	*Entamoeba histolytica*	Amoebic dysentery
	Naegleria fowleri[a]	Meningo-encephalitis
	Acanthamoeba spp.[a]	Keratitis
	Balamuthia mandrillaris[a]	Encephalitis
	Blastocystis hominis[b]	Pathogenicity doubtful
Flagellates	*Giardia lamblia*	Diarrhoea, malabsorption
	Trichomonas vaginalis	Vaginitis, urethritis
	Trypanosoma brucei gambiense	Sleeping sickness
	T. brucei rhodesiense	Sleeping sickness
	T. cruzi	Chagas' disease
	Leishmania spp.	See Table 61.4
Others	*Babesia microti*[a]	Babesiosis
	B. divergens[a]	Babesiosis
	Balantidium coli[a]	Balantidial dysentery
	Encephalitozoon cuniculi[a]	Microsporidiosis
	Enterocytozoon bieneusi[a]	Microsporidiosis
	Nosema connori[a]	Microsporidiosis

[a] Organisms rarely encountered in human disease.
[b] Taxonomic status uncertain.

SPOROZOA

This group includes the malaria parasites and related coccidia, which exhibit a complex life cycle involving alternating cycles of asexual division (*schizogony*) and sexual development (*sporogony*). In malaria parasites, the sexual cycle takes place in the female anopheline mosquito (Fig. 61.1).

Malaria parasites

Description

Four species are encountered in human disease: *Plasmodium falciparum*, which is responsible for most fatalities; *P. vivax* and *P. ovale*, both of which cause *benign tertian malaria* (febrile episodes typically occurring at 48-h intervals); and *P. malariae*, which causes *quartan malaria* (febrile episodes typically occurring at 72-h intervals). The appearances of trophozoites of the four species as seen in Romanowsky-stained films of peripheral blood are illustrated in colour plates 1–6 (p. 591).

Life cycle. When an infected mosquito bites, *sporozoites* present in the salivary glands enter the bloodstream and are carried to the liver, where they invade

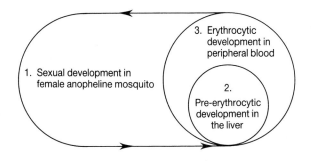

Fig. 61.1 Schematic representation of the life cycle of malaria parasites.

589

liver parenchyma cells. They undergo a process of multiple nuclear division, followed by cytoplasmic division (*schizogony*) and, when this is complete, the liver cell ruptures, releasing several thousand individual parasites (*merozoites*) into the bloodstream. The merozoites penetrate red blood cells and adopt a typical 'signet-ring' morphology (colour plate 2).

In the case of *P. vivax* and *P. ovale*, some parasites in the liver remain dormant (*hypnozoites*), and the cycle of pre-erythrocytic schizogony is completed only after a long delay. Such parasites are responsible for the relapses of tertian malaria that may occur up to 2 years after the initial infection.

In the bloodstream, the young ring forms (*trophozoites*) develop and start to undergo nuclear division (*erythrocytic schizogony*). Depending on the species, about 8–24 nuclei are produced before cytoplasmic division occurs, and the red cell ruptures to release the individual merozoites, which then infect fresh red blood cells (colour plate 1).

Instead of entering the cycle of erythrocytic schizogony, some merozoites develop within red cells into male or female *gametocytes*. These do not develop further in the human host, but when the insect vector ingests the blood, the nuclear material and cytoplasm of the male gametocytes differentiate to produce several individual *gametes*, which give it the appearance of a flagellate body (*exflagellating male gametocyte*). The gametes become detached and penetrate the female gametocyte, which elongates into a zygotic form, the *ookinete*. This penetrates the mid-gut wall of the mosquito and settles on the body cavity side as an *oocyst*, which is yet another multiplicatory phase within which numerous *sporozoites* are formed. When mature, the oocyst ruptures, releasing the sporozoites into the body cavity, from where some find their way to the salivary glands.

P. falciparum differs from the other forms of malaria parasite in that developing erythrocytic schizonts form aggregates in the capillaries of the brain and other internal organs, so that only relatively young ring forms are found in peripheral blood.

The cycle of erythrocytic schizogony takes 48 h, except in the case of *P. malariae*, in which the cycle occupies 72 h. Since febrile episodes occur shortly after red cell rupture, this explains the characteristic periodic fevers. However, with *P. falciparum*, the cycles of different broods of parasite do not become synchronized as they do in other forms of malaria, and typical tertian fevers are not usual in falciparum malaria.

Laboratory diagnosis

Acute falciparum malaria is a medical emergency that demands immediate diagnosis and treatment. To establish the diagnosis, a drop of peripheral blood is spread on a glass slide. The smear should not be too thick; a useful criterion is that print should be just visible through it. The smear is allowed to dry thoroughly and stained by Field's method. This is an aqueous Romanowsky stain, which stains the parasites very rapidly, and haemolyses the red cells, so that the parasites are easy to detect despite the thickness of the film.

With experience, the species of malaria can usually be determined from a thick blood film, but some of the characteristic features used to establish the identity of the parasites (Table 61.2), such as the typical stippling of the red cell that accompanies infection with *P. vivax* or *P. ovale*, are better observed in a conventional thin

Table 61.2 Differential characteristics of human malaria parasites as seen in Romanowsky-stained thin films of peripheral blood (see also colour plates 1–6)

Species	Morphology of trophozoite	Morphology of red cell	Stippling of red cell	Morphology of gametocyte	No. of merozoites in mature schizont
P. falciparum	Ring forms only	Normal	Maurer's spots[a]	Crescentic	(16–24)[b]
P. vivax	Rings, becoming amoeboid during development	Enlarged	Schüffner's dots	Large, round	16–24
P. ovale	Rings, becoming compact during development	Slightly enlarged; sometimes oval with fimbriate edge	James's stippling[c]	Round	8–12
P. malariae	Rings, becoming compact, stretched across red cell	Normal or slightly shrunken	(Ziemann's dots)[d]	Small, round	8–12

[a] Maurer's spots (or clefts) are relatively scanty and accompany more mature ring forms.
[b] Mature schizonts of *P. falciparum* are rarely seen in peripheral blood.
[c] James's stippling is similar to the intense stippling of Schüffner's dots.
[d] Ziemann's dots are rarely seen, except in intensely stained preparations.

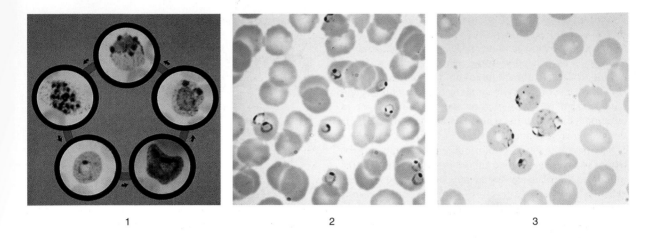

1   2   3

Plate 1   Stages in the erythrocytic cycle of *Plasmodium vivax*.

Plate 2   Ring form trophozoites of *P. falciparum*.

Plate 3   Trophozoites of *P. falciparum*. Note peripheral location of the parasites (*appliqué* or *accolé* forms) and light stippling of the red cells (*Maurer's spots*).

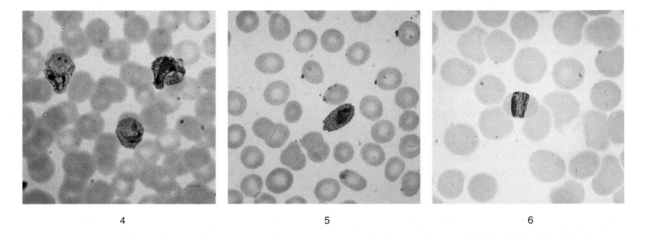

4   5   6

Plate 4   Amoeboid trophozoites of *P. vivax*. Note the marked enlargement of the parasitized red cells and the intense stippling (*Schüffner's dots*).

Plate 5   Trophozoite of *P. ovale*. Note the fimbriate, oval-shaped red cell and marked stippling (*James' stippling*).

Plate 6   Band-form trophozoite of *P. malariae*.

blood film stained by one of the many modifications of Giemsa's or Leishman's stain. The water used to dilute the stain should be at pH 7.2 (not 6.8 as used for haematological purposes).

Various other diagnostic tests have been devised for the rapid diagnosis of falciparum malaria. Some are available as simple 'dipstick' tests, which are sufficiently reliable to be used by inexperienced staff (perhaps even by patients themselves) or in field conditions where microscopy is not available. They are not foolproof, and may remain positive for some time after successful treatment. Moreover, they detect only *P. falciparum* infections. Visualization of the parasites in Romanowsky-stained peripheral blood films remains the most reliable method.

Pathogenesis

Malaria is characterized by severe chills, high fever and sweating, often accompanied by headache, muscle pains and vomiting. Falciparum malaria, unlike the other forms, may progress (especially in primary infections) to coma, convulsions and death. This condition, *cerebral malaria*, is associated with the adherence of parasitized red blood cells to the endothelium of brain capillaries. However, the precise mechanism for the pathological sequelae that follow, including the marked increase in the production of tumour necrosis factor that occurs, is not known with certainty.

Falciparum malaria is notoriously varied in its presentation, so that a definitive laboratory diagnosis is most important. Various systems may be affected. Severe anaemia and renal failure are common complications and hypoglycaemia, pulmonary oedema and gastroenteritis may be present.

Individuals that are homozygous or heterozygous for the sickle cell gene have a much reduced susceptibility to infection with *P. falciparum*, and this has provided a selective advantage for the maintenance of sickle cell disease in holo-endemic areas. Similarly, individuals whose red cells lack the antigen known as the *Duffy factor* are protected from infection with *P. vivax*. In parts of tropical Africa, where most of the population are Duffy factor-negative, *P. vivax* is rare, although the related *P. ovale* is found, especially in West Africa.

Treatment

For many years the standard treatment for acute malaria was chloroquine. However, resistance to that drug in *P. falciparum* (and, less commonly, in *P. vivax*) is now widespread and alternative agents often have to be used. The most reliable alternative to chloroquine is quinine (or quinidine), the traditional remedy that has been available for centuries in the form of cinchona bark. Some antibiotics, including tetracyclines and clindamycin, exhibit anti-malarial activity and are used as an adjunct to quinine therapy.

Alternative agents include mefloquine and halofantrine. These drugs are active against chloroquine-resistant strains, but resistance to them is increasing in prevalence, and both are associated with occasional problems of toxicity. Derivatives of artemisinin (a natural product from the plant *Artemisia annua*), including artemether and sodium artesunate, are being successfully used in some countries.

Treatment of acute malaria with chloroquine, quinine or other antimalarials will not eliminate parasites in the liver. For this purpose the 8-aminoquinoline drug primaquine must be used. This agent carries the risk of precipitating haemolysis in individuals who are deficient in the enzyme glucose-6-phosphate dehydrogenase.

Prophylaxis

Chloroquine and the antifolate drugs pyrimethamine (often combined with sulfadoxine or dapsone) and proguanil have been widely used for antimalarial prophylaxis, but the widespread occurrence of resistance to these agents has made it difficult to offer definitive advice to travellers, particularly those going to regions in which *P. falciparum* is prevalent. One solution has been to suggest a combination of antifolate drugs, together with either chloroquine or mefloquine. Such cumbersome regimens invite lapses in compliance and increase the risk of side-effects, particularly if a sulphonamide is used; moreover, they are not completely protective. For these reasons some authorities recommend a simple prophylactic regimen such as daily proguanil, or weekly mefloquine, together with advice to bring any fever to medical attention. The combination of daily proguanil and weekly chloroquine is also widely recommended. Whatever prophylactic advice is given, it should be combined with recommendations to avoid exposure to mosquito bites: wearing long clothing in the evening when the insects are most active; use of insect repellents; and sleeping under mosquito netting impregnated with insecticide.

Because parasites in the pre-erythrocytic stage of development escape the action of prophylactic drugs, prophylaxis should continue for at least 4 weeks after leaving a malarious area. This will effectively prevent the development of falciparum malaria, although long-term relapses of other types may occur up to 2 years after exposure.

Coccidia

The coccidia are related to malaria parasites and share alternating sexual and asexual phases of development. They are not, however, transmitted by insects and infection is usually acquired by ingesting mature oocysts.

Toxoplasma gondii

This is a coccidian parasite of the intestinal tract of the cat that is transmissible to many other mammals. Serological evidence suggests that human infection is common, presumably as a transient febrile illness or a subclinical attack, and is of worldwide occurrence. Occasionally, more severe infection occurs: intra-uterine toxoplasmosis is an important cause of stillbirth and congenital abnormality; ocular disease is a rare but serious condition; and cerebral toxoplasmosis sometimes occurs in immunocompromised patients, probably as a result of reactivation of latent infection.

Mature oocysts excreted by infected cats contain two sporocysts, within which *tachyzoites* develop. On ingestion the tachyzoites pass to the bloodstream and lymphatics to invade macrophages, in which they multiply (see colour plate 7). As the immune response develops, other cells are infected and tissue cysts containing slowly metabolizing *bradyzoites* are formed. Infection is acquired by ingestion of oocysts, or of tissue cysts in undercooked meat. Intra-uterine infection is acquired transplacentally.

It is not usually possible to demonstrate toxoplasmas in clinical material. Diagnosis of acute infection is made by demonstration of a rising titre of serum antibodies to *T. gondii*. The *Sabin–Feldman dye exclusion test* recognizes the ability of serum antibody to kill viable toxoplasmas. Other serological tests, including an enzyme-linked immunosorbent assay (ELISA), are available and have the advantage that they avoid the use of live toxoplasmas. The polymerase chain reaction has proved useful, particularly in the diagnosis of intra-uterine and cerebral infections.

The combination of pyrimethamine and a sulphonamide is effective against active tachyzoites. Spiramycin is also effective and may be preferred during pregnancy. Clindamycin, azithromycin and atovaquone, usually in combination with pyrimethamine, offer alternatives in patients with cerebral toxoplasmosis.

Isospora belli

This coccidian parasite usually causes mild, self-limiting diarrhoea, but it is occasionally associated with more severe infection, particularly in patients with AIDS. It is more common in areas of poor sanitation. The characteristic oocysts can be seen in faecal 'wet' mounts, but are poorly refractile and easily missed. Co-trimoxazole is usually effective if antimicrobial treatment is necessary.

Cryptosporidium parvum

Cryptosporidia are common animal parasites. One species, *Cryptosporidium parvum*, causes diarrhoea in man. Infection is usually water-borne or acquired from animals. Large numbers of oocysts are often present in faeces; they are partially acid-fast and can be demonstrated by modifications of the Ziehl–Neelsen method with carbol–fuchsin or auramine as the primary stain.

The infection usually responds to symptomatic treatment, with fluid replacement if necessary. In severely immunocompromised patients, cryptosporidia may cause severe life-threatening diarrhoea for which the combination of paromomycin (an aminoglycoside) and azithromycin appears to offer some benefit.

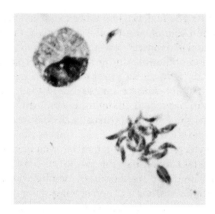

Plate 7 Tachyzoites of *Toxoplasma gondii* in a macrophage (top left) and lying free (bottom right.)

Cyclospora cayetanensis

Unlike cryptosporidia, cyclospora develop intracellularly in the gut mucosa. The immature oocysts are excreted in the faeces as round bodies about 10 μm in diameter, with a characteristic 'mulberry' appearance. They are more variably acid-fast than are cryptosporidia.

Cyclospora cayetanensis causes diarrhoea and is associated with poor sanitation. As with other coccidian parasites, infection is more severe in the immunocompromised. Mild infection is treated symptomatically, with rehydration if necessary. Co-trimoxazole appears to be effective in serious infection.

Sarcocystis species

The animal parasites *Sarcocystis bovihominis* and *S. suihominis* occasionally invade the intestinal tract or muscle of humans. Infection is usually subclinical and discovered accidentally.

AMOEBAE

Entamoeba histolytica

This is the most important amoebic parasite of humans. The amoebae invade the colonic mucosa, producing characteristic ulcerative lesions and a profuse bloody diarrhoea (*amoebic dysentery*). Systemic infection may arise, leading to abscess formation in internal organs, notably the liver. Such disease may arise in the absence of frank dysentery.

Laboratory diagnosis

In acute amoebiasis, blood-stained mucus, or colonic scrapings from ulcerated areas, are examined by direct microscopy. The material should be examined within 2 h of collection. *Entamoeba histolytica* may be recognized by its active movement, pushing out finger-like pseudopodia and sometimes progressing across the microscope field. If mucosal invasion has occurred, the amoebae usually contain ingested red blood cells, but these may be absent if infection is confined to the gut lumen. The nucleus is not usually visible in unstained 'wet' preparations, but in fixed smears stained with haematoxylin, it is seen as a delicate ring of chromatin with a central karyosome (Fig. 61.2).

Typical amoebic trophozoites may also be seen in aspirates of liver abscess. The pus often has a distinctive red–brown 'anchovy sauce' appearance. Since the amoebae actively multiply in the walls of the abscess, they are most likely to be found in the last few drops of pus drained from the lesion.

In the intestinal carrier state active amoebae are usually absent, but the encysted form, by which infection is spread, may be found. They are spherical, about 10–15 μm in diameter, and contain one to four of the nuclei typical of *Entamoeba* species: a circular ring with a central dot. Young, uninucleate cysts may also contain a large glycogen vacuole and, in fresh specimens, cysts of all stages of development may exhibit one or more thick, blunt-ended *chromatoidal bars* (Fig. 61.2).

Although demonstration of active amoebae or cysts is the best way to make a definitive diagnosis, serology is also sometimes helpful, particularly in systemic disease. Various immunodiagnostic tests have been described, but they are usually performed only in reference centres. Culture of *E. histolytica* is unhelpful as a diagnostic procedure.

Treatment

Not all strains of *E. histolytica* are invasive and some (now classified as *E. dispar*) never cause disease. Nevertheless, it is not possible readily to distinguish pathogenic from non-pathogenic strains in asymptomatic cyst excreters and, at least in areas of the world in which amoebiasis is uncommon, it is prudent to treat all excreters, particularly if they are food handlers. For this purpose, diloxanide furoate is often used.

Acute amoebiasis is usually effectively treated with metronidazole or tinidazole. Chloroquine is also useful in amoebic liver abscess. Older drugs, including emetine and dehydroemetine, are effective, but more toxic.

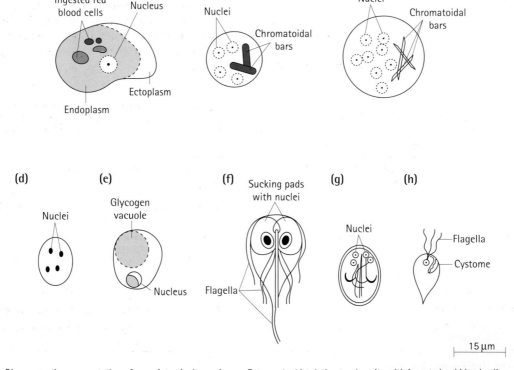

Fig. 61.2 Diagrammatic representation of some intestinal parasites: **a** *Entamoeba histolytica*, trophozoite with ingested red blood cells; **b** *E. histolytica*, mature cyst; **c** *E. coli*, mature cyst; **d** *Endolimax nana*, mature cyst; **e** *Iodamoeba bütschlii*, mature cyst; **f** *Giardia lamblia*, trophozoite; **g** *G. lamblia*, mature cyst; **h** *Chilomastix mesnili*, trophozoite.

Non-pathogenic intestinal amoebae

Although there are occasional reports of diarrhoea associated with other intestinal amoebae, notably *Dientamoeba fragilis* (an amoeba flagellate), most occur as commensals and are important only because of potential confusion with *E. histolytica*. The differential characteristics of non-pathogenic intestinal amoebae are compared with those of *E. histolytica* in Table 61.3. The greatest opportunity for confusion arises with the other intestinal *Entamoeba* species, *E. hartmanni* and *E. coli* (Fig. 61.2). *E. hartmanni* is morphologically identical to *E. histolytica*, but is smaller and the trophozoite never contains ingested red blood cells. *E. coli* is somewhat larger than *E. histolytica*, particularly in the cyst form. The trophozoites are more sluggish than those of *E. histolytica*, and mature cysts contain up to eight nuclei; chromatoidal bars, if present, are fine and pointed, rather like slivers of broken glass.

Blastocystis hominis, an organism commonly found in faeces and formerly thought to be a yeast, is probably a form of amoeba. Any pathogenic role is the subject of dispute, but it has been associated with diarrhoea in the absence of other known pathogens. Metronidazole is said to be useful if true infection is suspected.

Free-living amoebae

Environmental amoebae belonging to the genus *Naegleria* (usually *N. fowleri*) have occasionally been implicated in meningo-encephalitis. Rare cases of granulomatous encephalitis caused by *Balamuthia mandrillaris* and *Acanthamoeba* species have also been described, often, but not exclusively, in immunocompromised patients. The outcome in all kinds of amoebic encephalitis is ordinarily fatal, although amphotericin B has been successfully used in infections with *N. fowleri*. *Acanthamoeba* spp. more commonly cause keratitis, sometimes following use of contaminated cleaning fluids for soft contact lenses. Optimal antimicrobial chemotherapy remains to be defined, but topical propamidine in combination with neomycin or other agents has been used.

FLAGELLATES

Giardia lamblia (syn. G. intestinalis; G. duodenalis)

This intestinal parasite lives attached to the mucosal surface of the upper small intestine. Vast numbers may be present, and their presence may lead to malabsorption of fat and chronic diarrhoea. Young infants may be particularly severely affected. Infection is usually water-borne.

The trophozoite is kite-shaped, with two nucleated sucking pads, and four pairs of flagella (Fig. 61.2). Trophozoites may be found in duodenal aspirate, but examination of faeces usually reveals the cyst form by which the disease is transmitted. This is oval, about $10 \times 8 \mu m$, and contains up to four nuclei as well as the remains of the skeletal structure of the trophozoite (Fig. 61.2).

Table 61.3 Differential characteristics of intestinal amoebae

Species	Trophozoites Size (μm)	Ingested red blood cells	Cysts Size (μm)	No. of nuclei[a]	Chromatoidal bars	Nuclear morphology
Entamoeba histolytica[b]	10–40	+	10–15	4	Solid, blunt-ended	Fine ring of chromatin with central karyosome
E. hartmanni	4–10	–	6–10	4	As above	As above
E. coli	10–40	–	15–25	8	Slender, pointed	As above, but karyosome may be eccentric
E. gingivalis[c]	10–25	–	No cyst stage			
Iodamoeba bütschlii	10–20	–	10–15	1	None	Chromatin massed at one end of ring
Endolimax nana	5–12	–	5–8	4	None	Small shadowy masses of chromatin
Dientamoeba fragilis	5–10	–	No cyst stage			Ring containing several chromatin granules

[a] Refers to mature cyst.
[b] Including *E. dispar*.
[c] *E. gingivalis* is a commensal of the mouth.

Cysts of other, non-pathogenic, intestinal protozoa, including *Chilomastix mesnili*, *Enteromonas hominis* and *Retortamonas intestinalis*, may be mistaken for *G. lamblia*, but they are usually smaller and lack the regular oval shape and characteristic internal morphology. These non-pathogenic protozoa may also be found as trophozoites during microscopy of diarrhoeic faeces, but the most common intestinal flagellate is *Trichomonas hominis*, which is recognizable by its undulating membrane. There is no cyst form.

Giardiasis can be treated with 5-nitroimidazoles such as metronidazole, or, on the rare occasions when this fails (and re-infection is excluded), with mepacrine (quinacrine). Surprisingly, the anthelminthic, albendazole, also appears to be effective.

Trichomonas vaginalis

T. vaginalis is a flagellate protozoon with four anterior flagella and one lateral flagellum which is attached to the surface of the parasite to form an undulating membrane. There is no cyst form; the parasite is transmitted by sexual intercourse.

As the name suggests, *T. vaginalis* is predominantly a vaginal parasite, although urethritis may occur in the male consorts of infected women. The organism is responsible for a mild vaginitis, with discharge, which ordinarily responds to treatment with metronidazole or tinidazole.

T. vaginalis is readily identified by its characteristic motility in untreated 'wet' films of vaginal discharge and can be cultivated in appropriate culture media.

Trypanosomes

In contrast to the flagellates already described, trypanosomes have a complex life cycle involving an insect vector. The diseases that are caused in humans, African trypanosomiasis (*sleeping sickness*) and South American trypanosomiasis (*Chagas' disease*), are restricted in distribution according to the habitat of the insect host.

African trypanosomiasis

African sleeping sickness is caused by trypanosomes that are subspecies of *Trypanosoma brucei*, an important aetiological agent of *nagana* in cattle in tropical Africa. Tsetse flies (p. 618) act as the insect vector. The human parasites are *T. brucei gambiense*, which occurs in riverine areas of west and central Africa, and *T. brucei rhodesiense*, a parasite of the savannah plains of east Africa, where cattle and wild antelope act as reservoirs of infection.

Pathogenesis. Following the bite of an infected tsetse fly, a localized *trypanosomal chancre* may appear transiently, but invasion of the bloodstream rapidly occurs. The parasites multiply in blood, and at this stage there may be non-specific symptoms with occasional febrile episodes and some lymphadenitis. Swollen lymph glands in the posterior triangle of the neck (*Winterbottom's sign*) are often present in *T. brucei gambiense* infection. If untreated, the disease inexorably progresses to involve the central nervous system (CNS) with the classic signs of sleeping sickness and, ultimately, death.

Infection with *T. brucei rhodesiense* tends to follow a more acute, fulminating course over a period of a few months, whereas *T. brucei gambiense* infection usually progresses slowly, sometimes over several years.

Laboratory diagnosis. During the parasitaemic stage scanty trypanosomes may be found in peripheral blood in unstained 'wet' mounts or in smears stained by the Giemsa or Leishman methods. Examination of lymph node exudate may be helpful. Once the disease has progressed to involve the CNS, examination of cerebrospinal fluid reveals a lymphocytic exudate, often with *morula cells* (plasma cells) and scanty motile trypanosomes.

The parasites have a characteristic morphology: they are elongated, about 20–30 μm in length, with a single anterior flagellum arising via an undulating membrane from a basal body situated near a posteriorly placed kinetoplast (Fig. 61.3 and colour plate 8).

In-vitro cultivation is unreliable, but animal inoculation is sometimes useful, particularly with *T. brucei rhodesiense*, which infects laboratory mice more readily than *T. brucei gambiense*.

Various immunodiagnostic tests have been described, but they are not as reliable as direct microscopy in establishing a definitive diagnosis.

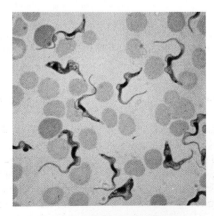

Plate 8 Trypomastigotes of *Trypanosoma brucei rhodesiense* in mouse blood.

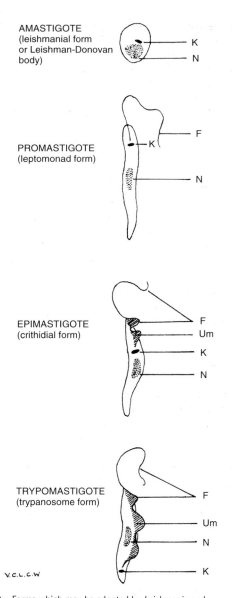

AMASTIGOTE
(leishmanial form
or Leishman-Donovan
body)

K
N

PROMASTIGOTE
(leptomonad form)

F
K
N

EPIMASTIGOTE
(crithidial form)

F
Um
K
N

TRYPOMASTIGOTE
(trypanosome form)

F
Um
N
K

V.C.L.C.W

Fig. 61.3 Forms which may be adopted by *Leishmania* and *Trypanosoma* spp. In parentheses are given the terms for the forms under the old nomenclature now superseded. F, flagellum; K, kinetoplast; N, nucleus; Um, undulating membrane.

Treatment. In the early, parasitaemic stage the infection is amenable to treatment with suramin or pentamidine, but if the disease has progressed to sleeping sickness, the trivalent arsenicals, melarsoprol or tryparsamide, are used. Less toxic alternatives are clearly required; encouraging results have been obtained with eflornithine in *T. brucei gambiense* infections, but use of this compound is threatened by difficulties of availability. Surprisingly, the drug is not effective in disease caused by *T. brucei rhodesiense*.

South American trypanosomiasis

Chagas' disease, caused by *T. cruzi*, is quite different from African trypanosomiasis. The insect vectors are various species of reduviid bugs (p. 617). The trypanosomes are not transmitted by the bite, but are present in the bug's faeces, which the unwitting sleeper rubs into the bite wound. The trypanosomes enter the bloodstream, but do not multiply there; instead, they invade cells of the reticulo-endothelial system and muscle, where they lose their flagellum and associated undulating membrane and adopt a more rounded shape (Fig. 61.3). This morphological form is called an *amastigote*, and suggests a phylogenetic relationship with *Leishmania* species (see below). The amastigotes multiply in muscle and are liberated from ruptured cells as trypanosomal forms (*trypomastigotes*), which disseminate the infection and provide the parasitaemia needed to infect fresh reduviid bugs when they next feed.

Pathogenesis. Chagas' disease is a chronic condition, characterized by extensive cardiomyopathy, sometimes with gross distension of other organs (e.g. mega-oesophagus and megacolon). Death is usually from heart failure.

Laboratory diagnosis. Trypomastigotes may be seen in peripheral blood, but are often extremely scanty. They are shorter than those of the *T. brucei* group and have a characteristically large kinetoplast (colour plate 9). Unlike the African trypanosomes, *T. cruzi* can be grown in vitro in the rich blood agar medium also used to isolate leishmania (see below). Biopsy of skeletal muscle may be performed but is usually of little value. The appearance of amastigotes in heart muscle is shown in colour plate 10.

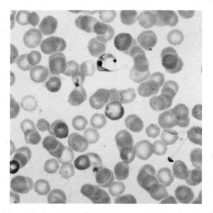

Plate 9 Trypomastigote of *T. cruzi* in blood. Note the prominent kinetoplast and the 'C' shape adopted by the parasite.

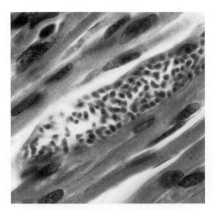

Plate 10 Amastigotes of *T. cruzi* in heart muscle

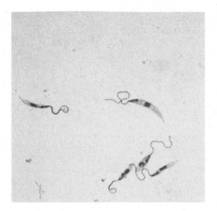

Plate 12 Promastigotes of *L. tropica* from laboratory culture in Novy, MacNeal and Nicolle's (NNN) medium.

T. cruzi is infective to laboratory mice. Alternatively, a procedure known as *xenodiagnosis* may be used: uninfected reduviid bugs are allowed to feed on the patient, and after about 3–4 weeks the gut contents of the bug are examined for trypanosomes.

Immunofluorescence, ELISA and other tests may be used for presumptive serological diagnosis, but false-positive results are common. Assays based on the polymerase chain reaction have been developed and appear to be more specific.

Treatment. There is no reliable antimicrobial chemotherapy for Chagas' disease, but the nitrofuran derivative nifurtimox and the imidazole compound benznidazole have been used with modest success.

Leishmania species

Leishmania species are intracellular parasites of the reticulo-endothelial system. They are related to try-

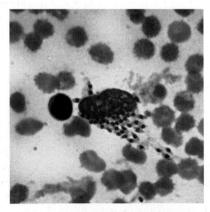

Plate 11 Amastigotes of *Leishmania tropica* in a ruptured macrophage from a cutaneous lesion (*Oriental sore*).

panosomes, but exist in only two morphological forms: *amastigotes* (non-flagellate forms), which occur in the infected lesion, and *promastigotes* (flagellate forms that lack an undulating membrane), which occur in the insect vector or in laboratory culture (Fig. 61.3 and colour plates 11 and 12).

The parasites are transmitted by sandflies (p. 618) in various parts of the world, including the Middle East, India, South America, the Mediterranean littoral and parts of Africa.

Pathogenesis

Several distinct types of disease are recognized (Table 61.4), although they are caused by morphologically identical parasites. The taxonomic relationships between the various forms have still not been entirely clarified. *Cutaneous leishmaniasis (oriental sore)* is the least troublesome, causing a boil-like swelling on the face or other exposed part of the body. The central part of the lesion may become secondarily infected with bacteria, but the leishmania organisms reside in the raised, indurated edge of the lesion. The sore usually heals spontaneously, leaving a scar, but with some species a more severe *disseminated cutaneous leishmaniasis* may occur. Parasites of the *Leishmania mexicana* complex may cause a destructive lesion of the outer ear (*Chiclero's ulcer*).

In *mucocutaneous leishmaniasis (espundia)*, which is associated with the *L. braziliensis* complex, disfiguring lesions of the mouth and nose may be caused. However, the most serious form of leishmaniasis is *visceral leishmaniasis (kala azar)*, which is a life-threatening disease involving the whole of the reticulo-endothelial system. A late complication of kala azar, *post-kala azar dermal leishmaniasis*, may be confused with leprosy or other skin conditions.

Table 61.4 *Leishmania* species involved in human disease

Species	Form of disease	Common names	Main geographical distribution
Leishmania tropica	Cutaneous	} Oriental sore, Baghdad boil, Delhi boil, etc.	Middle East, central Asia
L. major	Cutaneous		Africa, Indian subcontinent, central Asia, Ethiopia, Kenya
L. aethiopica	Cutaneous, DCL		
L. donovani	Visceral		Middle East, Africa, Indian subcontinent
L. infantum[a]	Visceral	} Kala azar, Dum-dum fever	Mediterranean coast, Middle East, China
L. chagasi	Visceral		Tropical South America
L. mexicana complex	Cutaneous, DCL	Chiclero's ulcer	Central America, Amazon basin
L. braziliensis complex	Mucocutaneous	Espundia	Tropical South America
L. peruviana	Cutaneous	Uta	Western Peru

DCL, disseminated cutaneous leishmaniasis.
[a] *L. infantum* may be a subspecies of *L. donovani*.

Laboratory diagnosis

In the cutaneous or mucocutaneous form of the disease, typical intracellular amastigotes may be recognized in Giemsa-stained smears of material obtained from tissues at the margin of the lesion (colour plate 11). Free amastigotes are commonly seen because of rupture of the macrophage host cell. Material should also be cultured in Novy, MacNeal and Nicolle's (NNN) medium or a modification thereof. This is a rabbit blood agar containing antibiotic to prevent bacterial contamination and a buffered salt overlay solution in which the parasites grow as promastigotes (colour plate 12). Incubation is maintained for up to 3 weeks at room temperature (*not* 37°C).

In kala azar, spleen puncture is the most reliable method of diagnosis, but sternal marrow aspirate is safer and is usually preferred. Smears and cultures are made and examined as for cutaneous leishmaniasis.

Various serological tests have been designed, but demonstration of the parasite by microscopy or culture is preferable whenever possible.

Treatment

The pentavalent antimony compounds sodium stibogluconate and meglumine antimoniate have been used traditionally in all forms of leishmaniasis, but they are toxic and therapy often fails. Amphotericin B is effective, but poorly tolerated, and the less toxic liposomal formulation is preferred. Antifungal azoles and paromomycin (aminosidine) have been used with some success in cutaneous forms of disease. There are hopes that a new phosphocholine derivative, miltefosine, will prove useful in kala azar.

OTHER PATHOGENIC PROTOZOA

Babesia species

Babesiae are predominantly animal parasites related to the piroplasmas that cause theileriasis in wild and domestic animals in many parts of the world. They are intracellular parasites living within red blood cells and are transmitted by ixodid ticks (p. 620). In stained blood films they superficially resemble young ring forms of plasmodia.

Human infection is uncommon. European cases have mostly been in patients whose resistance was impaired by lack of a functioning spleen; the causative parasite was usually *Babesia divergens*. In contrast, babesiosis caused by *B. microti* has been reported in otherwise healthy persons in parts of the USA.

The disease in immunocompetent individuals is usually self-limiting, so that specific treatment is not required. Optimal treatment for more serious cases has not been properly defined, but the combination of quinine with clindamycin has been successfully used.

Balantidium coli

Balantidium coli is the only ciliate protozoon that is pathogenic to man. It is a common parasite of the pig, and human infections have usually been traced to contact with these animals. The infective form is a large (about 50 μm in diameter), thick-walled cyst. The trophozoite inhabits the lumen of the gut and may attack the colonic mucosa in much the same way as *E. histolytica*, to cause balantidial dysentery. Many highly motile ciliate trophozoites are readily seen in untreated 'wet' films of diarrhoeic faeces.

Treatment has not been fully defined, but tetracyclines and metronidazole are said to be effective.

Microsporidia

These animal and insect parasites are represented by several genera, including *Encephalitozoon,* *Enterocytozoon* and *Nosema.* They are, on rare occasions, implicated in opportunistic infections of immunocompromised patients, especially those with acquired immune deficiency syndrome (AIDS). Infections of the eye, meninges and other organs have been reported. Albendazole may be useful in treatment, but is not always curative.

RECOMMENDED READING

Chiodini P L, Moody A, Manser D W 2000 *Atlas of Medical Helminthology and Protozoology*, 4th edn. Churchill Livingstone, Edinburgh
Cook G C (ed.) 1996 *Manson's Tropical Diseases*, 20th edn. W B Saunders, London
Gilles H M 2000 *Essential Malariology* 4th edn. Arnold, London
Goodgame R W 1996 Understanding intestinal spore-forming protozoa: cryptosporidia, microsporidia, isospora, and cyclospora. *Annals of Internal Medicine* 124: 429–441
Herwaldt B L 1999 Leishmaniasis. *Lancet* 354: 1191–1199
Leber A L 1999 Intestinal amoebae. *Clinical Laboratory Medicine* 19: 601–619
Peters W, Pasvol G 2001 *Tropical Medicine and Parasitology*, 5th edn. Wolfe, London
World Health Organization 1991 *Basic Laboratory Methods in Medical Parasitology*. WHO, Geneva
World Health Organization 1990 *Practical Chemotherapy of Malaria. Technical Reports Series*, No. 805. WHO, Geneva

CD-ROMs

Wellcome Trust 1998 *Malaria* 2nd edn (Topics in International Health series). CAB International, Wallingford
Wellcome Trust 2000 *Leishmaniasis* (Topics in International Health series). CAB International, Wallingford

Internet sites

London School of Hygiene and Tropical Medicine Malaria Centre. www.lshtm.ac.uk/centres/malaria/resources.html
Ohio State University. *Parasites and Parasitological Resources.* www.biosci.ohio-state.edu/~parasite/home.html
University of Western Australia: *Malaria. An on-line resource.* www.rph.wa.gov.au/labs/haem/index.html
US Centers for Disease Control and Prevention, Division of Parasitic Diseases. www.cdc.gov/ncidod/dpd/professional/default.htm
World Health Organization. *Protective Measures against Malaria:* www.who.int/ith/english/protect.htm

62

Helminths

Intestinal worm infections; filariasis; schistosomiasis; hydatid disease

D. Greenwood

Medical helminthology is concerned with the study of parasitic worms. These creatures are responsible for an enormous burden of infection throughout the world and, although few helminthic infections are life-threatening, their impact on human health is incalculable. Most helminths have no independent existence outside the host and are therefore truly parasitic. Since they rely on the host for sustenance, it is not in their interest to cause the host harm; consequently they do not usually exhibit great virulence and are characterized more by the novel methods that they have evolved to prevent rejection by the host defences. The pathogenic manifestations of helminthic disease, which can none the less be considerable, are ordinarily due to physical factors related to the location of the worms, their life-style or their size (see Chapter 13).

There are two major groups of helminths: *nematodes*, or roundworms, and *platyhelminths*, or flatworms. Flatworms are, in their turn, represented by two classes: *trematodes* (flukes) and *cestodes* (tapeworms).

NEMATODES

The principal nematode parasites of man are conveniently considered under two headings: intestinal nematodes and tissue nematodes.

Intestinal nematodes

Infection with intestinal roundworms (Table 62.1) is generally associated with conditions of poor hygiene. Such infections are extremely common, particularly throughout the tropics and subtropics, although several are also found in temperate regions. Low worm burdens are generally asymptomatic, but heavy infections may cause problems, especially in young children where they have been associated with impaired development.

Ascaris lumbricoides

This is the common roundworm, which infects over a billion people in the world. The adults are large and fleshy, rather like a garden worm and, as with many nematodes (other than the hookworm group), the smaller male can be recognized by his characteristically crooked tail. The eggs (ova) are produced in huge numbers; they are thick-walled, bile-stained and typically exhibit a corrugated albuminous coat (Fig. 62.1a). In the absence of a male worm, the female will produce infertile eggs, which tend to be more elongated and irregular than the fertile variety (Fig. 62.1b).

In warm, moist conditions, infective larvae develop within fertile eggs, but do not hatch. Such eggs can survive for long periods in soil. If ingested, the eggs

Table 62.1 Principal intestinal nematodes of man

Species	Common name	Relevant examination
Ancylostoma duodenale	Hookworm	Stool concentration (ova)
Ascaris lumbricoides	Common roundworm	Stool concentration (ova)
Enterobius vermicularis	Threadworm	Peri-anal swab (ova), adult worms on stool
Necator americanus	Hookworm	Stool concentration (ova)
Strongyloides stercoralis	–	Stool concentration (larvae) or culture
Toxocara canis[a]	Dog roundworm	Serology
Trichostrongylus spp.	Hookworm	Stool concentration (ova)
Trichuris trichiura	Whipworm	Stool concentration (ova)

[a] Not an intestinal parasite of man; causes visceral larva migrans (see text).

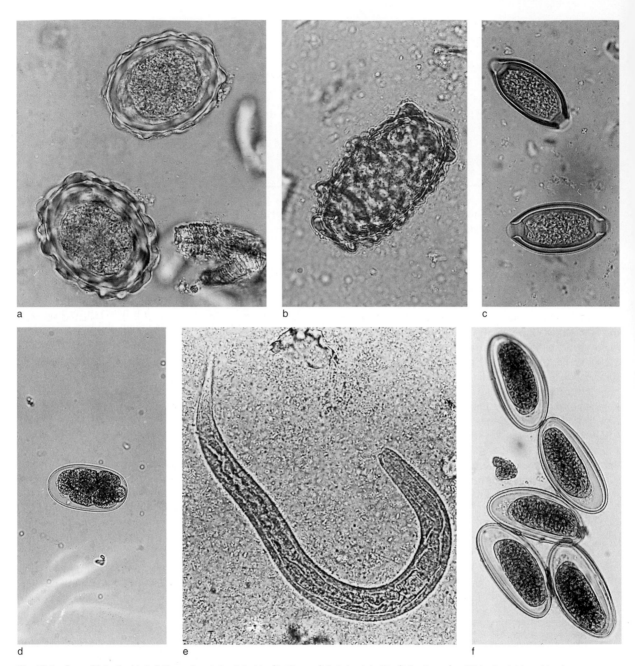

Fig. 62.1 Eggs of intestinal helminths: **a** *Ascaris lumbricoides* (fertile eggs); **b** *A. lumbricoides* (infertile egg); **c** *Trichuris trichiura;* **d** hookworm; **e** *Strongyloides stercoralis* (larva); **f** *Enterobius vermicularis.*

hatch in the duodenum and the larvae penetrate the gut mucosa to reach the bloodstream. They are carried to the pulmonary circulation, where they gain access to the lung and undergo two moults before migrating via the trachea to the intestinal tract. Having completed their round-trip, they mature in the gut lumen and live for several years.

Ascaris lumbricoides is a well adapted parasite that is not usually pathogenic in the ordinary sense. However, pneumonic symptoms may accompany the migratory phase and the adult worms may invade the biliary and pancreatic ducts. Moreover, heavy infection with these large worms can cause intestinal obstruction. Allergy is also sometimes a problem.

The dog ascarid, *Toxocara canis*, may accidentally infect man. Larvae hatch in the small intestine and penetrate the gut wall, but they are unable to complete their migratory phase. Instead, they find their way to remote parts of the body, a condition known as *visceral larva migrans*. Occasionally the larvae reach the eye and cause serious retinal lesions. Larvae of several other roundworms, including *Angiostrongylus, Gnathostoma* and *Anisakis* species, are occasionally implicated in visceral larva migrans in some parts of the world.

Trichuris trichiura

This is the common whipworm, often found together with ascaris. The adults live with the head (the 'whip' end of the worm) embedded in the colonic mucosa. Each female lays thousands of characteristic 'tea-tray' eggs (Fig. 62.1c) every day. Like those of ascaris, they develop infective larvae in warm, moist conditions, but the ova do not hatch outside the body. However, after ingestion and hatching, there is no migratory phase and adult worms develop directly in the large intestine.

Infection is usually trivial, though massive infections can cause rectal prolapse in young children, and a form of dysentery is described.

Hookworm

The two human hookworms, *Ancylostoma duodenale* and *Necator americanus*, are widely distributed throughout the tropics and subtropics. The two species produce indistinguishable thin-walled eggs (Fig. 62.1d) which hatch in soil. The larvae undergo several moults before infective larvae are produced. These are capable of penetrating unbroken skin, and in this way they gain access to the bloodstream to begin a migratory phase similar to that of ascaris. When they reach the gut they attach by their mouthparts to the mucosa of the small intestine.

Hookworms ingest blood and, moreover, move from site to site in the gut mucosa, leaving behind small bleeding lesions. These two facts are responsible for the chief pathological manifestation of heavy infection with hookworms: iron deficiency anaemia.

Larvae of animal hookworms, notably the dog hookworm, *A. caninum*, may penetrate human skin, but do not migrate further. They do, however, cause irritation by wandering locally through subcutaneous tissue to cause *cutaneous larva migrans*.

Trichostrongylus species

Various species of *Trichostrongylus* have been associated with human disease, particularly in the Middle East. The eggs are similar to those of hookworm, but are more elongated.

Strongyloides stercoralis

This parasite is also related to the hookworms, but differs in several important respects. There is a distinct free-living phase in the life cycle, during which males and females reproduce. Human infections arise after penetration of infective larvae through skin and there is a migratory phase involving the lungs. However, human infection appears to be restricted to female worms, which attach to the gut mucosa and produce eggs that contain fully developed larvae; these hatch within the intestinal lumen so that larvae, not eggs, are found in faecal samples (Fig. 62.1e). Infection can persist for many years, probably because some larvae can develop sufficiently within the body to initiate a fresh cycle of development and cause auto-infection.

Symptoms are usually benign, but in debilitated individuals larvae may be activated to penetrate the gut wall and invade other organs, a serious condition known as *hyperinfection*.

Enterobius vermicularis

This is the common threadworm, which infects children throughout the world. It has the simplest life cycle of all intestinal worms. Adults live in the large intestine and are occasionally found in the appendix. Mature, gravid females crawl through the anus at night and lay their eggs in the peri-anal area. The eggs are characteristically flattened on one side (Fig. 62.1f) and usually contain fully developed larvae. Ingestion of these eggs initiates a fresh infection. Symptoms are restricted to itching (*pruritus ani*) associated with the deposition of eggs.

Since eggs are not discharged by the worm into faeces, faecal examination is not appropriate in the laboratory diagnosis of threadworm infection. The diagnosis is established by finding the characteristic threadworms on the surface of formed stools, or by examination of swabs (or Sellotape impressions) of unwashed peri-anal skin for the characteristic ova.

Treatment of intestinal nematode infections

In endemic areas, the need to treat intestinal worm infections has to be balanced against the severity of symptoms (if any), the inevitability of re-infection, and the use of scarce medical resources. In the industrially developed world, where the infections are less common and mostly imported, a more liberal approach to treatment can be adopted.

Table 62.2 Spectrum of activity of drugs used in the treatment of intestinal nematode infections

Drug	Ancylostoma duodenale	Necator americanus	Ascaris lumbricoides	Strongyloides stercoralis	Trichuris trichiura	Enterobius vermicularis
Piperazine	–	–	+++	–	–	+++
Levamisole	++	++	+++	–	–	–
Pyrantel pamoate	++	++	+++	+	++	+++
Thiabendazole	++	++	+++	++	–	++
Mebendazole	++	++	+++	+	++	+++
Albendazole	+++	++	+++	++	++	+++

From Greenwood D (ed.) 2000 *Antimicrobial Chemotherapy*, 4th edn. Oxford University Press, Oxford.
+++, highly effective; +, poorly effective; –, no useful activity.

The range of options is listed in Table 62.2. Most effective (and expensive) are the benzimidazole derivatives, especially albendazole and mebendazole.

Tissue nematodes

This group includes the filarial worms, the Guinea worm (*Dracunculus medinensis*) and *Trichinella spiralis* (Table 62.3).

Filarial worms have a complex life cycle involving developmental stages in an insect vector. They vary considerably in their pathogenic effects, but some are responsible for disabling diseases that have a major impact on communities living in endemic areas.

Wuchereria bancrofti

This filarial worm is transmitted by the bite of various species of mosquito throughout the tropical belt of the world. It is believed that over 100 million people are infected. The larvae invade the lymphatics, usually of the lower limbs, where they develop into adult worms. Presence of the adult worms causes lymphatic blockage and gross lymphoedema, which sometimes leads to the bizarre deformities associated with bancroftian filariasis, *elephantiasis*.

Embryonic forms (*microfilariae*) are liberated into the bloodstream. They retain the elastic egg membrane as a sheath, which covers the whole larva (Fig. 62.2a). Microfilariae remain in the pulmonary circulation during the day, emerging into the peripheral circulation only at night, to coincide with the biting habits of the insect vector. The physiological basis of this nocturnal periodicity is not understood, but it can be reversed by altered sleep patterns in, for example, night-shift workers. Moreover, strains of *Wuchereria bancrofti* encountered in some Pacific islands do not exhibit a nocturnal periodicity. Aside from these exceptions, blood for examination for *W. bancrofti* must be taken during the night, optimally between midnight and 2 am.

Loa loa

This worm is restricted in distribution to central and western parts of tropical Africa, where it is transmitted by biting flies (*Chrysops* species; pp. 618–619). The adult worms live in subcutaneous tissue and wander round the body, provoking localized reactions known as *Calabar*

Table 62.3 Principal tissue nematodes of man

Species	Intermediate host	Geographical distribution	Relevant examination
Wuchereria bancrofti	Mosquitoes	Tropical belt	Night blood
Loa loa	*Chrysops* spp.	West and Central Africa	Day blood
Brugia malayi	Mosquitoes	South-east Asia	Night blood
Mansonella perstans	*Culicoides* spp.	Tropical Africa, South America	Blood
M. ozzardi	*Culicoides* spp.	West Indies, South America	Blood
Onchocerca volvulus	*Simulium* spp.	Tropical Africa, Central America	Skin shavings
M. streptocerca	*Culicoides* spp.	West and Central Africa	Skin shavings
Dracunculus medinensis	Water fleas	Africa, Indian subcontinent	Adult worm when mature
Trichinella spiralis	None[a]	Worldwide	Muscle biopsy, serology

[a] Pork forms the chief reservoir.

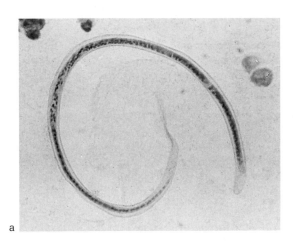

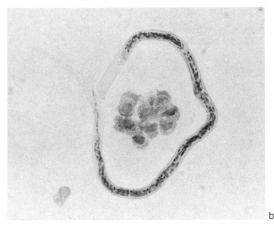

a

b

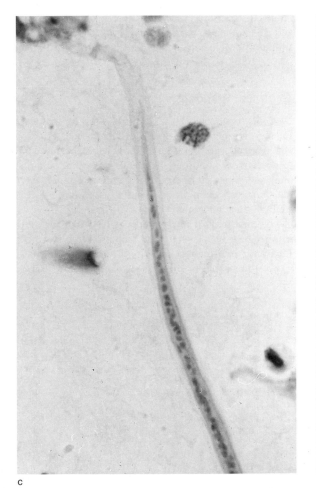

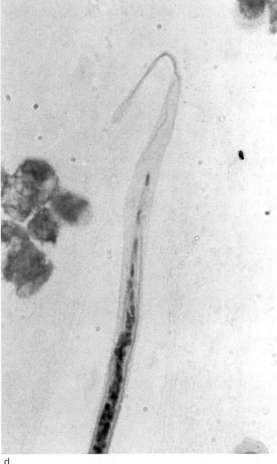

c

d

Fig. 62.2 Sheathed microfilariae of **a** *Wuchereria bancrofti* and **b** *Loa loa*; **c** tail of microfilaria of *W. bancrofti* showing tip devoid of somatic nuclei; **d** tail of microfilaria of *L. loa* showing nuclei extending to tip of tail.

swellings and sometimes migrating across the front of the eye.

The sheathed microfilariae of *Loa loa* (Fig. 62.2b) exhibit diurnal periodicity, so that, unlike those of *W. bancrofti*, they appear in peripheral blood only during the day.

Brugia malayi

This parasite is probably related to *W. bancrofti*. It is transmitted by mosquitoes in parts of India, the Far East and South-east Asia. Adult worms inhabit the lymphatics and, like *W. bancrofti*, can cause elephantiasis. Microfilaraemia usually shows a nocturnal periodicity.

Onchocerca volvulus

This filarial worm is common in parts of tropical Africa and Central America. It is transmitted by *Simulium damnosum* and related species of black-fly (p. 619). Adult worms develop in subcutaneous and connective tissue, and often become encapsulated in nodules, which form on bony parts of the body, such as the hip, elbow and (particularly in central America) the head. The microfilariae are not found in blood, but live in the superficial layers of the skin causing itching and, in heavy chronic infections, gross thickening of the skin. The eye is commonly invaded by microfilariae, which may cause corneal and retinal lesions that lead to blindness. Because the vector breeds by rivers, the condition is known as *river blindness*.

If nodules are present, diagnosis can be made by finding macroscopic worms within an excised nodule. Otherwise, superficial slivers of skin, taken from calves, buttocks and shoulders, are suspended in a drop of saline and examined microscopically for motile microfilariae.

Mansonella species

Mansonella perstans is widespread throughout tropical Africa and parts of South America; the related *M. ozzardi* is restricted to parts of the West Indies and South America. They are transmitted by biting midges (*Culicoides* species; p. 618). The unsheathed microfilariae appear in the bloodstream and exhibit no periodicity. They are generally regarded as non-pathogenic.

M. streptocerca causes skin infections similar to those of *O. volvulus*, although the symptoms are usually milder. It is restricted to parts of western and central Africa.

Differential characteristics of microfilariae

The microfilariae of filarial worms can be differentiated in stained preparations of clinical material by various criteria, the most useful of which are the presence or absence of a sheath and the disposition of the somatic nuclei in the tip of the tail (Table 62.4 and Fig. 62.2c and d). Giemsa stain is suitable for the demonstration of somatic nuclei, but hot (60°C) haematoxylin is necessary to stain the sheath.

Treatment of filariasis

Diethylcarbamazine (DEC) has been used for many years for the treatment of all forms of filariasis. It effectively kills microfilariae, but is not reliably lethal to adult worms. It is relatively non-toxic, but death of the microfilariae is often accompanied by a severe allergic reaction (*Mazzotti reaction*), especially in onchocerciasis. Suramin kills the adult worms, but is much more toxic than DEC.

The treatment of onchocerciasis has been revolutionized by use of the veterinary anthelminthic ivermectin. This drug is effective in a single oral dose and is less likely than DEC to elicit a severe reaction. Periodic

Table 62.4 Differential features of human microfilariae

Species	Site in human host	Periodicity	Sheath	Nuclei in tip of tail	Length (μm)
Wuchereria bancrofti	Blood	Nocturnal[a]	Present	Absent	250–300
Loa loa	Blood	Diurnal	Present	Present	250–300
Brugia malayi	Blood	(Nocturnal)[b]	Present	Present[c]	200–250
Mansonella perstans	Blood	Non-periodic	Absent	Present	150–200
M. ozzardi	Blood	Non-periodic	Absent	Absent	180–220
Onchocerca volvulus	Skin	Non-periodic	Absent	Absent	250–300
M. streptocerca	Skin	Non-periodic	Absent	Present	180–240

[a] Subperiodic forms occur in the Pacific Islands.
[b] Partial nocturnal periodicity.
[c] Two small, well separated nuclei in the tip of the tail.

administration of ivermectin, together with vector control measures, has had an important impact on onchocerciasis in endemic areas.

Ivermectin and albendazole are effective in other forms of filariasis, though neither drug kills adult worms. Since they exhibit activity against intestinal nematodes, including *A. lumbricoides*, these may be incidentally expelled during treatment. Albendazole is being used, alone or in combination with ivermectin, in campaigns aimed at eradicating lymphatic filariasis.

Dracunculus medinensis

This is the *Guinea worm*. The infective larvae develop within water fleas of the genus *Cyclops*, and human infection is normally acquired through infected drinking water. The larvae penetrate the gut mucosa and grow to maturity in connective tissue, usually of the lower limbs. The male is small and insignificant, but the female may reach a length of 1 m. After fertilization, the female worm incubates the larvae to maturity and, when ready to give birth, emerges to the skin surface to provoke an intensely irritating blister. When the sufferer immerses the blister in water, the uterus of the female worm bursts, liberating up to 1 million larvae, which are ingested by water fleas to continue the cycle.

Attempts can be made to wind out the dead worm over several days, but breakage of the worm often occurs, and pyogenic cocci may be carried into the tissues to cause a cellulitis. Chemotherapy is not usually helpful, other than to treat secondary bacterial infection. Prevention is the best approach; health education campaigns and the provision of safe water have much reduced the prevalence of this disease, and complete eradication is now possible.

Trichinella spiralis

Unlike most parasitic worms, *Trichinella spiralis* has an extremely wide host range. Human infections are usually acquired by eating undercooked pork products, although other meat, including bear and walrus meat, has been incriminated. The infected larvae lie dormant in skeletal muscle (Fig. 62.3) and are released when the meat is digested. Male and female worms develop to maturity attached to the mucosa of the small intestine. The female is viviparous, producing numerous larvae during a life-span of only a few weeks. The larvae penetrate the gut wall and migrate to skeletal muscle, where they enter the quiescent phase. Most of the symptoms of trichinosis, which can be severe, even life-threatening, are associated with the migration of larvae.

Mebendazole is said to be effective against the adult worms and the larvae, but treatment is unsatisfactory.

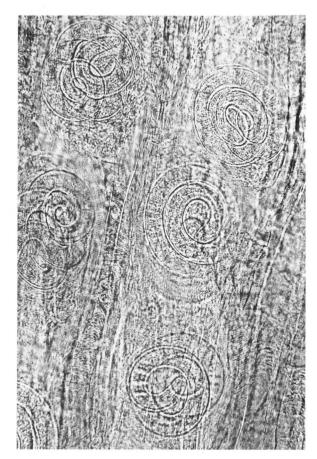

Fig. 62.3   Larvae of *Trichinella spiralis* in muscle.

Symptoms usually develop only during the invasive stage, and measures to control the sequelae of invasion are more important than anthelminthic therapy.

TREMATODES

The flukes (Table 62.5) are a diverse group of worms that share a similar life cycle involving a snail host and, often, a second intermediate host that provides the vehicle for the transmission of infection. Most flukes have a restricted geographical distribution that reflects the habitat of the appropriate type of snail.

Most trematodes are hermaphrodite, but the most important human flukes, the schistosomes, are differentiated into separate sexes.

Life cycle

When excreted, trematode eggs often contain a fully developed ciliated organism called a *miracidium*,

Table 62.5 Principal trematode parasites of man

Species	Common name	Intermediate host		Geographical distribution	Relevant examination
		First[a]	Second		
Clonorchis sinensis	Chinese liver fluke	*Bithynia* sp.	Freshwater fish	Far East	Stool concentration
Fasciola hepatica	Sheep liver fluke	*Lymnaea* sp.	Vegetation	Worldwide	Stool concentration, serology
Fasciolopsis buski	Giant intestinal fluke	*Segmentina* sp. etc.	Water chestnut	Far East	Stool concentration
Paragonimus westermani	Lung fluke	*Semisulcospira* sp.	Crabs and crayfish	Chiefly Far East	Sputum
Schistosoma mansoni	Bilharzia sp.	*Biomphalaria*	None (water)	Africa, West Indies, South America	Stool concentration, rectal biopsy
S. haematobium	Bilharzia	*Bulinus* sp.	None (water)	Africa	Terminal urine (midday)
S. japonicum	Bilharzia	*Oncomelania* sp.	None (water)	Far East	Stool concentration, rectal biopsy

[a] The first intermediate host is a snail in each case.

although in some species immature eggs are produced which require a period of development before the miracidium is formed. In water, the miracidium escapes, either through a lid-like *operculum* in the egg shell, or (in the case of the schistosomes) by osmotic rupture of the egg. The miracidium penetrates the appropriate species of snail and undergoes several stages of asexual reproduction before emerging as a free-swimming body called a *cercaria*. The cercariae encyst in the muscle of fish (*Clonorchis sinensis*), crabs and crayfish (*Paragonimus westermani*), water chestnuts (*Fasciolopsis buski*), or vegetation (*Fasciola hepatica*), and man becomes infected by ingesting the encysted metacercariae. In the case of *Schistosoma* species, the cercariae remain in water and penetrate unbroken skin to gain access to the body.

Clonorchis sinensis (syn. Opisthorchis sinensis)

This is the Chinese liver fluke. Infection is acquired from uncooked freshwater fish, notably carp. The metacercariae excyst in the small intestine and pass into the bile ducts, where they mature. Typical small, flask-shaped eggs with a prominent operculum (Fig. 62.4a) are excreted in large numbers into the faeces.

Infection is commonly asymptomatic, but fibrosis of the bile ducts with impairment of liver function may occur in heavy, chronic infections. As with most fluke infections, praziquantel is emerging as the drug of choice for treatment.

A closely related fluke, *Opisthorchis felineus*, which is a parasite of the cat, has been associated with human disease in parts of eastern Europe.

Fasciola hepatica

This is the cosmopolitan liver fluke of sheep. Human infections have usually been associated with eating wild watercress from infected sheep pastures. The adult worm is larger than *C. sinensis*, and lighter infections can cause biliary fibrosis and obstructive jaundice. The large, immature eggs with an indistinct operculum (Fig. 62.4b) may be found in faeces, but are usually scanty.

Unlike other trematode infections, fascioliasis does not reliably respond to praziquantel, and treatment with the veterinary anthelminthic triclabendazole or the more toxic chlorophenol derivative bithionol may be required.

Paragonimus westermani

This is the lung fluke, which is found in parts of the Far East. Closely related species have occasionally been implicated in human disease in parts of Africa and South America. Human infection follows ingestion of raw, infected muscle of freshwater crabs and crayfish. The metacercariae penetrate through the gut wall and diaphragm to reach the lung, where they develop to maturity. Occasionally the larvae find their way to the brain. Pulmonary infection usually provokes the production of sputum, in which the characteristic large eggs (Fig. 62.4c) can be found, often associated with flecks of altered blood. Praziquantel is used for treatment.

Intestinal flukes

Several genera of intestinal flukes cause human infection, particularly in the Far East. *Fasciolopsis buski* is

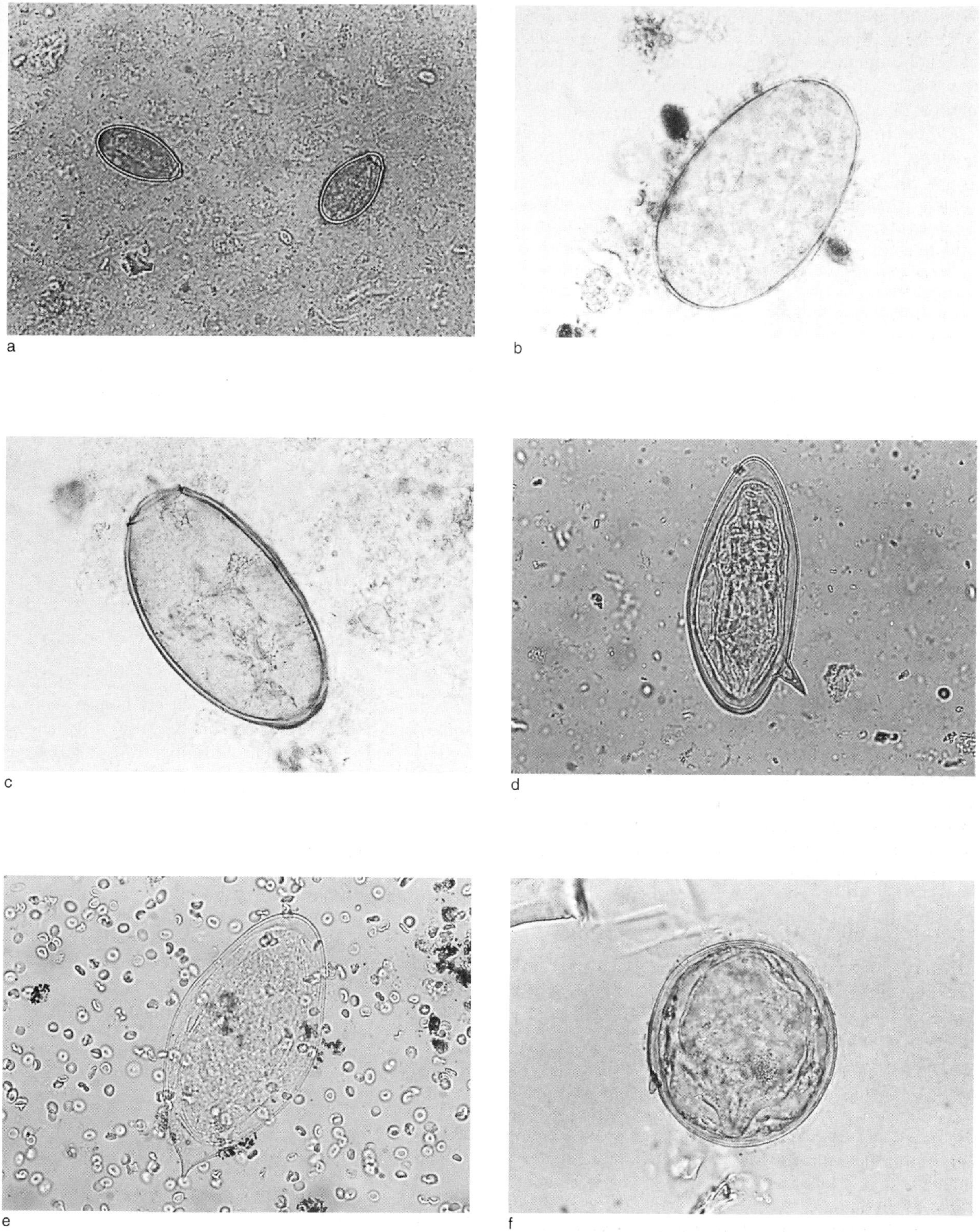

Fig. 62.4 Eggs of trematodes: **a** *Clonorchis sinensis*; **b** *Fasciola hepatica*; **c** *Paragonimus westermani*; **d** *Schistosoma mansoni*; **e** *S. haematobium*; **f** *S. japonicum*.

found in restricted foci in China and South-east Asia. Infection is often acquired by the habit of opening water chestnuts with the teeth. The adult flukes live attached to the wall of the small intestine, and produce a large number of eggs that resemble those of *F. hepatica*.

Other intestinal flukes include *Gastrodiscoides hominis*, *Heterophyes heterophyes*, *Metagonimus yokogawai* and various species of *Echinostoma*. Infection is usually asymptomatic unless the worm burden is large. Such evidence as exists suggests that praziquantel is effective in these cases.

Schistosoma species

The schistosomes, or *blood flukes*, also known as *bilharzia* after the discoverer, Theodor Bilharz, are the most important of the pathogenic trematodes. At least 200 million people are infected, principally in Africa, where *Schistosoma mansoni* and *S. haematobium* are widespread, and *S. intercalatum* is encountered in some areas. *S. mansoni* is also found in parts of the West Indies and South America; *S. japonicum* and the related *S. mekongi* are restricted to the Far East.

Human infection follows exposure to cercaria in water harbouring infected snails. The cercariae penetrate the skin, often causing a transient dermatitis, called *swimmer's itch*. Once in the bloodstream, the schistosomula migrate to the liver, where they develop into mature male and female worms. The integument of the mature male worm is adapted in the form of two long flaps, the *gynaecophoral canal*, in which the female is held. The mature worms migrate to the small veins of the rectum (*S. mansoni, S. intercalatum, S. japonicum* and *S. mekongi*) or the bladder (*S. haematobium*). Eggs, which contain a fully developed miracidium, are passed through the rectal mucosa onto the surface of colonic faeces or through the bladder wall into the urine.

The ova of *S. mansoni* (Fig. 62.4d) are large (c. 140 μm long) and possess a characteristic lateral spine, while *S. haematobium* (Fig. 64e) and *S. intercalatum* have a terminal spine. The smaller, more rounded eggs of *S. japonicum* and *S. mekongi* do not have a prominent spine, but may exhibit a rudimentary nipple-like appendage (Fig. 62.4f).

Pathogenesis

The adult worms adopt the subterfuge of coating themselves with host antigens to evade attack by host defences and, in themselves, the adults are innocuous. Most of the serious manifestations of schistosomiasis are associated with the deposition of eggs, with the formation of granulomata and fibrotic lesions of the liver, bladder or other organs. Such effects may herald malig-

nant changes. Heavy infection with *S. mansoni* may give rise to *schistosomal dysentery*, while *S. haematobium* infections are commonly accompanied by a marked haematuria.

Laboratory diagnosis

Ova of rectal schistosomes can be sought on the surface of formed faeces. Blood-stained mucus should be examined, if present. Alternatively, microscopical examination of snips of rectal mucosa teased out in a drop of saline on a microscope slide may reveal viable or calcified eggs.

For the diagnosis of infection with *S. haematobium*, the last few drops of urine at the end of micturition (*terminal urine*) are most likely to be rich in ova. Excretion is said to be maximal around midday.

To test for viability of the eggs after treatment, ova can either be hatched in water (the motile miracidia can be seen with the help of a hand-lens) or the eggs can be examined microscopically for the characteristic flickering movement of excretory 'flame-cells'.

Various serodiagnostic tests, including enzyme-linked immunosorbent assay (ELISA), are available, but are no substitute for demonstration of the ova. Antigen detection methods have also been developed.

Treatment

Praziquantel is effective against all the human schistosomes and is the drug of choice. Because of its lack of toxicity and simplicity in administration it has been used, together with molluscicides and water purification, in control programmes.

Other compounds are more selective in their action: metriphonate (an organophosphate compound) is active against *S. haematobium*; oxamniquine is effective in *S. mansoni* infection.

CESTODES

The species of tapeworm most commonly involved in human infection are listed in Table 62.6.

Taenia species

Taenia saginata, the *beef tapeworm*, is much more prevalent than the related *T. solium*, the *pork tapeworm*. Both have a relatively simple life cycle, alternating between man and the intermediate host. Human infection is acquired by eating raw or undercooked beef or pork containing the encysted larval stage, the *cysticercus*. The larvae hatch in the small intestine, and attach to the

Table 62.6 Principal cestode parasites of man

Species	Common name	Intermediate host	Relevant examination
Taenia saginata	Beef tapeworm	Cattle	Mature segments on stool
T. solium	Pork tapeworm	Pig	Mature segments on stool
Diphyllobothrium latum	Fish tapeworm	Cyclops spp./fish	Ova in stool
Hymenolepis nana	Dwarf tapeworm	None	Ova in stool
Echinococcus granulosus[a]	Hydatid worm	Sheep, man	Radiology; serology

[a] Dog tapeworm; man is one of the intermediate hosts.

mucosal surface by four suckers on the head (*scolex*) of the worm. The scolex of *T. solium* additionally carries a crown of hooklets. The worm grows backwards from the head, first producing immature segments (*proglottids*), which continue to develop as they become more distant from the head. When sexually mature, the proglottids, which exhibit both male and female characteristics, cross-fertilize one another, and eggs start to be produced in the uterine canal. This becomes grossly distended as more eggs are produced, so that the fully gravid segments at the end of the worm become nothing more than bags full of eggs. The complete chain of segments is known as a *strobila*, and may measure 10 m or more.

Eggs are not laid. They are retained within the proglottids, which become detached from the end of the worm and are passed with the faeces. Animals become infected by ingesting the eggs from pastures which are contaminated with inadequately treated sewage or, possibly, by birds that scavenge in untreated sewage.

Considering the size of the worm, infection is usually remarkably asymptomatic. However, in the case of *T. solium*, eggs may hatch in the human host and form cysticerci. When these lodge in the brain, they may cause a serious epileptiform disease, *cerebral cysticercosis*.

Laboratory diagnosis

Taenia infection is usually diagnosed by finding the typical segments in faeces. Since eggs are not laid, faecal examination for ova is inappropriate. *T. saginata* can usually be differentiated from *T. solium* if the segment is pressed between two microscope slides and examined macroscopically. In the case of *T. saginata*, numerous branchings of the central uterine canal are evident, whereas there are usually far fewer branchings with *T. solium* (Figs 62.5a and b). The eggs (Fig. 62.6a) are thick-walled and contain an *oncosphere* with six hooklets. The eggs of *T. saginata* and *T. solium* are indistinguishable.

Treatment

A single dose of praziquantel is usually successful. Niclosamide is also used, but this drug causes the worm to disintegrate, with the consequent theoretical (but unproven) risk of auto-infection in the case of *T. solium* through the intraluminal release of eggs. Treatment of cerebral cysticercosis is problematical, but albendazole and praziquantel have been successfully used.

Diphyllobothrium latum

This is the *fish tapeworm*, which is prevalent in lakeland areas where freshwater fish is eaten raw. The life cycle is reminiscent of that of the trematodes. The mature adult worm, which may attain a length of 10 m, lays numerous operculate eggs within which a ciliated body called a *coracidium* develops. This hatches in water and is ingested by the water flea (*Cyclops* species). After a period of development, the larva awaits ingestion by a freshwater fish in which it invades the muscle as an infective *plerocercoid larva* or *sparganum*.

Human infection is usually asymptomatic, although a form of pernicious anaemia caused by competition for dietary vitamin B_{12} has been described.

The characteristic immature eggs have an indistinct operculum (Fig. 62.6b) and are usually present in large numbers in faeces. Occasionally, a length of the worm may break off and be passed in the stool.

Niclosamide or praziquantel is used for treatment.

Hymenolepis nana

In contrast to the enormous length of *Taenia* species and *D. latum*, *Hymenolepis nana* is only 2–4 cm long, and is consequently known as the *dwarf tapeworm*. It has a very simple life cycle with no known intermediate host. The characteristic 'poached egg' ova (Fig. 62.6c) are directly infective, and it is surprising that infection is not more common.

Infection is usually asymptomatic; heavy infections can be treated with praziquantel or niclosamide.

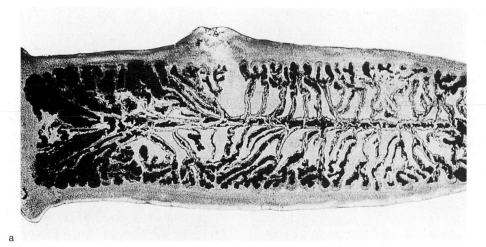

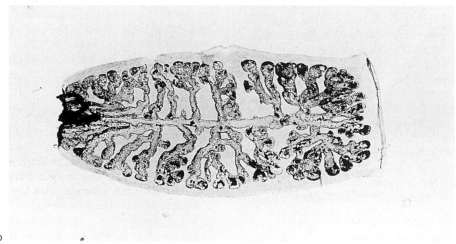

Fig. 62.5   Segments of **a** *Taenia saginata* and **b** *T. solium*. The uterine canal has been injected with Indian ink to show the branchings.

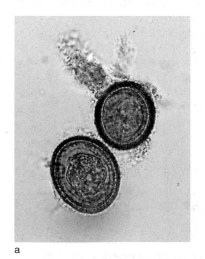

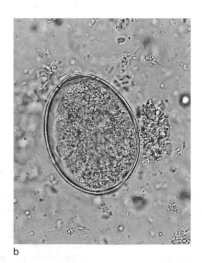

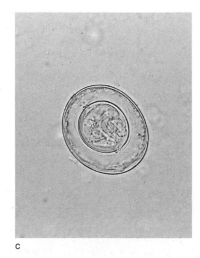

Fig. 62.6   Eggs of cestodes: **a** *Taenia* species; **b** *Diphyllobothrium latum*; **c** *Hymenolepis nana*

A slightly larger species, *H. diminuta*, is occasionally found in man. This is a parasite of small rodents and is transmitted by their fleas.

Echinococcus granulosus

This is the tapeworm of the dog and other canine species and, unusually, humans are an intermediate host. It is a small worm, consisting usually of just four segments and measuring only a few millimetres in length. Sheep are the usual intermediate hosts. Other animals, including man, may become infected, especially in sheep-farming areas, where the cycle of transmission is maintained between sheep and dogs.

After ingestion of the eggs, which resemble those of *Taenia* species, larvae hatch in the small intestine, penetrate the gut mucosa and are carried by the bloodstream to various organs (commonly the liver), where they are filtered out by the capillaries. The larva starts to grow, eventually forming a cystic cavity, the *hydatid cyst*. The inner wall of the cyst contains the *germinal layer*, from which develop *brood capsules* that bud off and fall into the cyst cavity. Within these brood capsules new scolices develop, and some of these may initiate the formation of daughter cysts within the main cavity. The young cyst may die and calcify, but it often continues to grow inexorably, eventually seriously compromising the function of the organ in which it is situated.

In certain parts of the world, notably the arctic regions of North America and Siberia, infection with a related canine tapeworm, *E. multilocularis*, is encountered. The hydatid cyst infiltrates the surrounding tissue, making it difficult to remove surgically.

Laboratory diagnosis

The diagnosis is usually made on clinical and radiological evidence. Examination of the cyst fluid (*hydatid sand*) reveals the typical invaginated scolices (Fig. 62.7), but diagnostic puncture of cysts is not recommended because of the risk of spillage (see below).

Imaging techniques supported by serological tests offer the best means of diagnosis. ELISA is the preferred

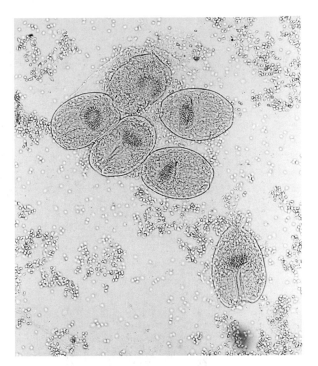

Fig. 62.7 Scolices of *Echinococcus granulosus* from hydatid cyst.

laboratory method, but other serodiagnostic tests are also available. A skin test with antigen derived from hydatid fluid (*Casoni test*) was formerly used, but is unreliable.

Treatment

Cysts of *E. granulosus* can often be removed surgically, but accidental spillage of viable scolices into body cavities may cause an anaphylactic reaction and, moreover, is likely to lead to the development of fresh cysts. For this reason the hydatid cyst is first injected with a scolicidal agent, such as hypertonic saline or ethanol.

The relative impermeability of the cyst militates against successful chemotherapy, but some success has been obtained with benzimidazole derivatives, notably albendazole, and with praziquantel.

RECOMMENDED READING

Cook G C (ed.) 1996 *Manson's Tropical Diseases*, 20th edn. W B Saunders, London
Crompton D W T 1999 How much helminthiasis is there in the world? *Journal of Parasitology* 85: 397–403
Fleck S L, Moody A H 1988 *Diagnostic Techniques in Medical Parasitology*. Wright, London

Muller R 1975 *Worms and Disease: A Manual of Medical Helminthology.* Heinemann, London
Peters W, Pasvol 2001 *Tropical Medicine and Parasitology*, 5th edn. Wolfe, London
Stoll N R 1947 This wormy world. *Journal of Parasitology* 33: 1–18 (reprinted *Journal of Parasitology* 1999; 85: 392–396)

World Health Organization 1991 *Basic Laboratory Methods in Medical Parasitology.* WHO, Geneva

CD-ROM

Wellcome Trust 1999 *Schistosomiasis* (Topics in International Health series). CAB International, Wallingford

Internet sites

University of Cambridge Department of Pathology. *Helminth infections of man*
www.path.cam.ac.uk/~tjs16/General_Parasitology/Hm.helminths.html
Ohio State University. *Parasites and Parasitological Resources*:
www.biosci.ohio-state.edu/~parasite/home.html
US Centers for Disease Control and Prevention, Division of Parasitic Diseases: www.cdc.gov/ncidod/dpd/professional/default.htm

63

Arthropods

Arthropod–borne diseases; ectoparasitic infections; allergy

D. Greenwood

Arthropods are animals with jointed legs, segmented bodies and chitinous exoskeletons. They are hugely diverse and incredibly numerous – over 850 000 species have been described (probably only a tenth of the true number) and a swarm of locusts alone may contain 10^9 individuals. Strictly speaking, the term 'arthropod' includes lobsters, crabs, millipedes and centipedes, but these seldom cause much serious mischief and most medical interest centres on insects and arachnids. A simplified classification scheme is shown in Table 63.1.

MEDICAL IMPORTANCE OF ARTHROPODS

Insects and other arthropods are mainly of importance in human disease in three ways:

• as vectors of the agents of bacterial, viral or parasitic infection

• as parasites in their own right, spending part or all of their life-span on man

• as instigators of allergic responses that vary in severity.

In addition, many arthropods have a considerable nuisance effect because of their biting or stinging habits, and these occasionally give rise to serious, even life-threatening, reactions.

The larvae (maggots) of some common flies that feed on decomposing matter have been used for centuries to treat infected lesions. There has been renewed interest in this phenomenon, since the maggots not only scavenge dead tissue, but also appear to secrete factors conducive to wound healing.

Abnormal fear of insects or other arthropods (e.g. arachnophobia; excessive fear of spiders) is well recognized, as are delusions of infestation with these creatures. The mere mention of head lice can make people

Table 63.1 Simplified classification of arthropods of medical importance

Class	Members of class	Medical importance
Insects	Ants, bees, wasps (Hymenoptera)	Venomous bites and stings
	Beetles (Coleoptera)	Some secrete fluids causing blisters
	Bugs (Hemiptera)	Bites; vectors of Chagas' disease
	Butterflies and moths (Lepidoptera)	Urticaria (caterpillars)
	Cockroaches (Dictyoptera)	Mechanical vectors of disease
	Fleas (Siphonaptera)	Ectoparasites; vector of plague
	Flies and gnats (Diptera)	Vectors of many viral and parasitic diseases; myiasis
	Lice (Phthiraptera)	Ectoparasites; vectors of typhus, trench fever, relapsing fever
Arachnids	Spiders and scorpions	Venomous bites and stings
	Ticks	Vectors of rickettsiae, borreliae
	Mites	Scabies; allergy; vectors of scrub typhus, rickettsialpox
Pentastomes	Tongue worms	Animal parasites; human infestations rare
Myriapods	Centipedes and millipedes	Some cause painful bites or secrete fluids causing blisters
Crustacea	Crabs, crayfish	Intermediate host of lung fluke
	Copepods	Intermediate host of fish tapeworm and Guinea worm

scratch their scalps. Distinguishing between the real and the imaginary can test the diagnostic acumen of the attending physician. Persistent cases may need psychiatric referral.

Arthropods as disease vectors

Mechanical transmission

Insects such as flies, ants and cockroaches that are attracted by food can transmit pathogenic micro-organisms passively. The common house fly, *Musca domestica*, is a particular nuisance because of its predilection for decaying matter, its mobility and its habit, shared by a number of other flies, of regurgitating food material and defecating on food. Flies undoubtedly play a role in the transmission of diseases such as shigellosis and trachoma.

Intermediate hosts

A wide variety of arthropods act as obligatory hosts in the transmission of viral, bacterial, protozoal and helminthic disease. Their role in individual diseases is dealt with in appropriate chapters elsewhere in the book.

Arthropods as ectoparasites

Many insects, ticks and mites pester man to obtain a blood meal or spend part or all of their life in association with human beings. Several fleas, lice and mites are among those that are adapted in various ways for life on man. Occasionally, man acts as the host of the larval stages of certain insects, causing a condition known as *myiasis*.

Arthropods as allergens

Biting or stinging insects and other arthropods can give rise to severe reactions in hypersensitive individuals. Anaphylactic reactions and multiple stings need immediate treatment with adrenaline. The hairs of several caterpillar species found in various parts of the world are irritant and may give rise to urticaria if brushed against. Contrary to popular belief, the bites of mosquitoes (gnats), fleas and some other insects are painless. The intense irritation that may develop is an immunological reaction elicited in most, but not all, subjects. Persons travelling to malarious areas should beware of claiming that they never get bitten and hence do not need protection.

House dust mites (usually *Dermatophagoides pteronyssinus* in Europe; more commonly *D. farinae* in Japan and America) flourish in centrally heated homes with wall-to-wall carpeting. They feed on flakes of skin and have been incriminated as a cause of asthma in atopic subjects. The allergens, which include a cysteine protease, are secreted in the mites' faeces.

INSECTS

Insects are the most numerous and familiar form of arthropod life. They are characterized by having six legs and segmented bodies. The legs (and wings, if present) are carried on the thoracic segment between the head, which bears sucking or biting mouthparts, and the abdomen. Most insects, apart from lice and bugs, undergo complete metamorphosis, developing from eggs to adults through morphologically distinct larval and pupal (chrysalis) stages.

Ants, bees and wasps (Hymenoptera)

These insects have little medical relevance apart from their propensity to retaliate to disturbance with defensive bites or stings. These can be serious if the subject is hypersensitive, but are usually trivial. Particularly notorious are the African honey bees, *Apis mellifera scutellata*, and the South American fire ants, *Solenopsis* spp., both of which have been introduced into the USA. Ants also forage wherever food is to be found and frequently infest kitchens and food stores.

Beetles (Coleoptera)

Some beetles act as intermediate host of the dwarf tapeworm *Hymenolepis diminuta*, an uncommon human parasite of minor importance. Otherwise, their only real medical significance lies in the fact that the body fluids of certain beetles can cause blistering of the skin. One such beetle, 'Spanish fly', is the source of cantharidin, a vesiculating agent.

Bugs (Hemiptera)

The bugs of importance in human medicine are blood-sucking species. Most familiar throughout the world is the bed bug, *Cimex lectularius*, together with its tropical cousin, *C. hemipterus*. They have a body that is flattened dorsoventrally and from a distance they resemble brown lentils. Bed bugs live in cracks and crevices of walls, floorboards and furniture, from where they emerge to take a periodic blood meal whenever it is on offer. The adults are long-lived and can survive up to a year without a blood meal. They are usually spread between premises in infested furniture. There is no evidence that they transmit disease.

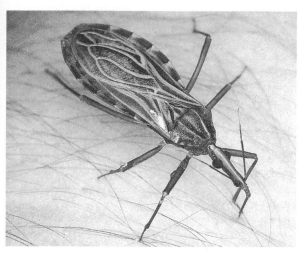

Fig. 63.1 A reduviid bug feeding on human skin. These insects transmit Chagas' disease in South America. (Photograph courtesy of Dr H.-J. Grundmann, University of Nottingham Medical School.)

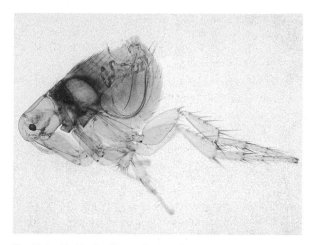

Fig. 63.2 The Rat flea *Xenopsylla cheopsis*, vector of plague.

Reduviid bugs (colloquially known as *kissing bugs* or *assassin bugs*) transmit Chagas' disease in South America (see p. 597). Various species of *Triatoma*, *Rhodnius* and *Panstrongylus* are implicated. They are about 2.5 cm in length – much larger than bed bugs – and, unlike them, they have wings (Fig. 63.1). They are usually active at night, settling on the face of an unsuspecting sleeper to take a blood meal and to defecate. The infective trypanosomes are in the hindgut and the bitten person becomes infected by rubbing the bug's faeces into the irritating bite wound.

Butterflies and moths (Lepidoptera)

Adult butterflies and moths are of no medical significance, although some tropical moths may feed on the discharge from the eyes of mammals, including man. The hairs of certain caterpillars can cause skin rashes, as noted above.

Cockroaches (Dictyoptera)

Cockroaches are of little medical significance, although they can harbour pathogens and infest food stores. Laboratory workers in the tropics are familiar with their habit of removing the blood from blood slides left exposed on the bench.

Fleas (Siphonaptera)

Fleas are small blood-sucking parasites. Their laterally flattened bodies and lack of wings enable them to negotiate the hairs and feathers of their animal hosts. Well developed hind legs enable them to jump from host to host (Fig. 63.2). Many fleas will feed on man if given the opportunity, as those who have been attacked by the common cat flea *Ctenocephalides felis* bear witness. However, the species that is adapted for life on man is the human flea, *Pulex irritans*, which is still common throughout the world. Female fleas of another species, *Tunga penetrans*, attack man once they have been fertilized. The fleas burrow into the skin, or under the toenails, of the human host and are known as *jiggers*. The abdomen of the gravid female becomes grossly distended with eggs, causing pain, irritation and, sometimes, secondary infection. Jigger fleas are common in dry, sandy soil, mainly in Africa and parts of central and South America.

Human fleas are seldom implicated in the transmission of disease, but some other species are important disease vectors. Most notorious is the rat flea, *Xenopsylla cheopsis*, which is the most important, but not the sole, vector of plague (p. 329). Some forms of typhus are also transmitted by *X. cheopsis* and other fleas (pp. 369–370).

Flies and gnats (Diptera)

Dipterous insects are strong and active flyers, with a pair of wings used for flying and an additional vestigial pair, known as *halteres*, which are used as organs of balance. The developmental cycle from egg to adult fly involves complete metamorphosis. As well as being among the most annoying of insect pests, many biting flies have an obligate role in the transmission of a wide variety of important infections (Table 63.2). The larvae of certain flies may also infest wounds; others are able to penetrate skin to cause myiasis (see below).

Table 63.2 Principal infections associated with biting flies, mosquitoes and midges

Type of insect	Diseases transmitted
Biting midges (*Culicoides* spp.)	Filariasis (*Mansonella* spp.)
Blackflies (*Simulium* spp.)	Onchocerciasis
Deerflies (*Chrysops* spp.)	Loiasis
Mosquitoes:	
Anopheline (*Anopheles* spp.)	Malaria; bancroftian filariasis
Culicine (*Culex, Aedes, Mansonia* spp.)	Bancroftian and brugian filariasis; yellow fever, dengue and other arboviruses
Sandflies (*Phlebotomus, Lutzomyia* spp.)	Leishmaniasis; Oroya fever; sandfly fever
Tsetse flies (*Glossina* spp.)	African trypanosomiasis

Mosquitoes

Mosquitoes are readily recognized by a long needle-like proboscis (Fig. 63.3). Adult males and females both feed on plant juices, but the female needs blood for the development of her eggs, and is also a voracious predator on a wide variety of vertebrate animals throughout the world. Mosquitoes of importance in human medicine are divided into two broad types: *anopheline* mosquitoes, numerous species of which transmit malaria (p. 589), and *culicine* mosquitoes, which are the vectors of many so-called *arbovirus* infections (p. 484). Both anopheline and culicine mosquitoes also act as the intermediate hosts of certain filarial worms (p. 604).

Female mosquitoes lay their eggs on water; larvae and pupae are both aquatic. Most anopheline mosquitoes prefer relatively large expanses of water that do not dry up, but many culicine mosquitoes, particularly *Aedes* spp., will breed in small pockets of water, such as tree-holes, water butts, etc. The adults have a wide flight range and may be found several kilometres from their breeding ground. Mosquitoes capable of transmitting malaria are found throughout the world, even within the Arctic Circle, but indigenous disease is nowadays restricted to the tropical and subtropical belt.

Midges

Biting midges are tiny flies that are able to cause a nuisance out of all proportion to their size. The females attack in swarms, usually in the evening, and may give rise to painful reactions. Like mosquitoes, they are mostly aquatic. One genus, *Culicoides* spp., transmits filarial worms of *Mansonella* spp. (p. 606).

Sandflies

Sandflies are tiny flies that are well able to penetrate most mosquito netting. They are more demanding in their habitat than mosquitoes and have a restricted flight range, so that the diseases they transmit – notably kala azar and other forms of leishmaniasis (p. 598), bartonellosis (p. 325), and sandfly fever (p. 498) – tend to be localized in distribution. Female flies suck blood, usually at night, and breed in dark, moist areas, often in or around human dwellings. Species associated with disease transmission in Africa, the Middle East, Asia and the Mediterranean littoral belong to the genus *Phlebotomus*. In Central and South America, *Lutzomyia* spp. act as vectors of leishmaniasis and Oroya fever, a form of bartonellosis.

Other biting flies

Although flies that are capable of inflicting a painful bite, such as *Stomoxys calcitrans*, the stable fly, are found throughout the world, species that are important vectors of human disease are restricted in distribution to areas of the tropics. The tsetse flies, *Glossina* spp., are found in the so-called 'fly-belts' of sub-Saharan Africa, where they are responsible for trypanosomiasis in man as well as in cattle and other animals (p. 596). Unusually, both males and females feed on blood. The vectors of human trypanosomiasis ('sleeping sickness') in areas of West Africa are riverine species such as *Glossina palpalis*, whereas *G. morsitans*, which prefers the savannah plains and woodlands, is the principal vector in the eastern part of the continent.

Other biting flies responsible for transmission of disease in Africa include species of *Chrysops* (*deer flies* or *mango flies*) and *Simulium* (*black-flies*).

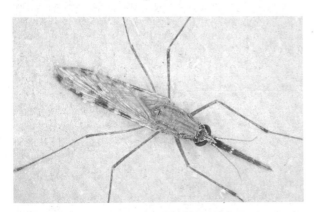

Fig. 63.3 A female anopheline mosquito, the vector of human malaria. (Photograph courtesy of Dr H.-J. Grundmann, University of Nottingham Medical School.)

Chrysops spp. belong to the tabanid group and are related to horse flies, which themselves can evoke a severe reaction in man although they are not known to transmit disease. The species that act as vectors of the filarial worm *Loa loa* (p. 604), *Chrysops dimidiata* and *C. silacea*, breed in marshy areas of the rain forests of tropical West and Central Africa. The females are said to be attracted by the smoke of fires and inflict a painful bite.

The breeding grounds of black-flies are the banks of rivers, where females attach their eggs to vegetation. They are small, hump-backed flies that often attack in swarms. Only the female feeds on blood. *Simulium damnosum* and *S. naevi* are important vectors of onchocerciasis (*river blindness*; p. 606) in parts of tropical Africa. Related species transmit the disease in Central and South America.

Myiasis

Given the chance, many common flies will lay their eggs on the exposed tissues of ulcers and sores, which consequently become the breeding ground for maggots. The condition is known as *semi-specific myiasis* to distinguish it from *specific myiasis*, in which man (and other animals) act as obligate hosts for the larval stage of development. *Accidental myiasis* is said to occur when larvae are ingested with food, or invade orifices such as the urogenital tract.

Myiasis is of great economic importance in animal husbandry throughout the world, but human infestation is largely a problem of the tropics. Specific myiasis in Africa is most commonly caused by *Cordylobia anthropophaga* (the *tumbu fly*). In Central and South America *Dermatobia hominis* (the *human bot fly*) is the usual culprit. *C. anthropophaga* lays its eggs in soil or dust, but *D. hominis* attaches its eggs to other insects, including mosquitoes, that visit man. When the larvae hatch they burrow into the skin of individuals with whom they are in contact. The larvae remain there breathing through spiracles at the posterior end until they are ready to pupate and emerge. Larvae of another African fly, *Auchmeromyia luteola* (the *Congo floor maggot*), also parasitize man, but do not penetrate the skin, preferring instead to suck the blood of unsuspecting sleepers.

Cutaneous myiasis is a transient condition causing boil-like lesions in the skin. The body of the larvae is furnished with spines (Fig. 63.4), which make them difficult to remove, but covering the posterior spiracles with paraffin oil prevents them from breathing and encourages them to emerge with the help of digital pressure. Care should be taken not to allow the lesion to become secondarily infected with bacteria.

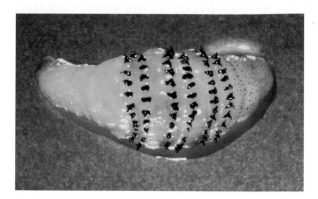

Fig. 63.4 Larva of *Dermatobia hominis*, from a case of human myiasis.

Lice (Phthiraptera)

Lice are wingless insects that undergo incomplete metamorphosis during their development. The ones that parasitize man are blood-sucking species with flattened bodies and short legs that are adapted to cling to hairs. Body lice and head lice are considered to be variants of the same species, *Pediculus humanus*, though the body louse, *P. humanus corporis*, is somewhat larger than the head louse, *P. humanus capitis*, and there are other minor differences. A third species, *Phthirus pubis*, is quite distinct morphologically, living up to its common description as the 'crab' louse (Fig. 63.5). Head lice are usually confined to the hairs of the scalp, but body lice live in clothing covering the body, rather than on the skin itself. *Ph. pubis*, as the name suggests, is usually found on pubic hairs, but may also infest other hairy parts, including eyelashes. All types attach their characteristic eggs (*nits*) to body hairs, and effective treatment involves removal of the nits as well as dealing with the adults.

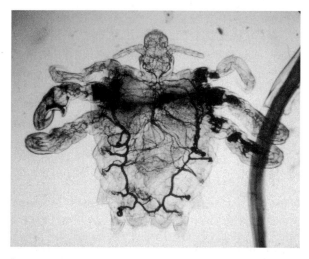

Fig. 63.5 *Phthirus pubis*, the human 'crab' louse.

Crab lice are not known to be involved in disease transmission, but body and head lice are the classic vectors of epidemic typhus (p. 372) and relapsing fever (p. 349). Lice also cause irritation, and continuous scratching may lead to various forms of infective dermatitis.

Lice are very common throughout the world and head lice, in particular, often spread quickly between school children, even in affluent areas. Treatment with insecticides such as permethrin, malathion and carbaryl may be effective, but resistance occurs. There are also fears about the possible neurotoxicity of malathion and the mutagenic potential of carbaryl. Repeated 'wet-combing' with a fine-tooth comb after shampooing the hair may eventually succeed in eliminating the infestation, although re-infection from untreated family members or school contacts is common. Aqueous solutions of malathion or carbaryl may also be used to treat crab lice, but the whole body should be treated. Since the infestation is transmitted by intimate contact, sexual partners should also be investigated.

ARACHNIDS

This group includes spiders, scorpions, ticks and mites. Unlike insects, the adult forms have eight legs and they are invariably wingless. They have two main body regions – cephalothorax and abdomen – which in mites and ticks are fused to give the appearance of a single segment. They develop by incomplete metamorphosis, and immature forms resemble small versions of the adults. However, ticks and mites only acquire the full complement of eight legs as they mature from first-stage larvae to nymphs during their progression to adulthood.

Mites

Despite their name, mites are variable in size, though many, including those commonly implicated in human disease, are so small as to be almost invisible to the naked eye. Parasitic varieties include *Sarcoptes scabiei* (the *itch mite*), and *Demodex folliculorum* (the *blackhead mite*). Other species occupy a wide variety of natural habitats. Certain species may cause an intense pruritus or dermatitis when man comes into contact with them; some transmit scrub typhus and rickettsialpox (p. 372). House dust mites have attracted considerable attention as a precipitating cause of atopic disease (see above).

The human itch mite, *S. scabiei*, is related to mites causing mange in various animals. It is the cause of scabies, an infestation of the skin that is still very prevalent in many countries. After fertilization on the surface of the skin, the gravid female mite burrows into the epidermis, eventually leaving behind a trail of about 40 eggs. The larvae usually hatch in 3–4 days, leave the burrow and pass through nymphal stages to reach adulthood in hair follicles. Burrowing females cause intense itching, often in folds of skin, especially between the fingers, and there may be secondary bacterial infection. Elderly and immunocompromised patients may develop a severe crusting infestation known as *Norwegian scabies*, which may be confused with psoriasis.

Application of an aqueous solution of malathion or permethrin is often successful therapy, but household contacts should also be treated. Norwegian scabies can be additionally treated systemically with the anthelminthic agent ivermectin, which is widely used in animal husbandry for the control of ectoparasites.

Demodex folliculorum, the blackhead mite, has an elongated body adapted for its life in sebaceous follicles, commonly around the nose or eyelids. They seldom cause much pathology, but can be treated with permethrin application or sulphur preparations.

Ticks

Ticks are essentially large mites, but they are much more important as vectors of human disease. They are conveniently classified into two main families: *hard (ixodid) ticks*, which have a chitinous shield (*scutum*) on the back (Fig. 63.6), and *soft (argasid) ticks*, which lack this feature. In addition, the head parts of soft ticks are hidden on the ventral surface and are not visible from above. Ticks are obligate blood-feeders. They parasitize a very wide variety of animals in nature and many will attack man, given the opportunity. The initial bite is usually painless, but it can give rise to a serious reaction. In some countries, notably Canada, the USA and Australia, *tick paralysis*, a poorly understood condition

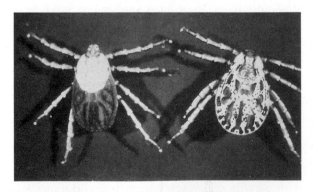

Fig. 63.6 *Dermacentor andersoni*, the vector of Rocky Mountain spotted fever and a cause of tick paralysis. These are known as 'hard ticks' because of the presence of the dorsal scutum, prominent in the male (right), but much reduced in the female (left).

associated with the bite of ixodid ticks, is occasionally reported. It is likely that a neurotoxin is responsible.

Ixodid ticks, which transmit many rickettsiae of the spotted fever group (pp. 369–370), as well as the agents of Q fever (p. 376), Lyme disease (p. 350), tularaemia (p. 335), babesiosis (p. 599) and some arboviruses (Table 51.3, p. 489), are very tenacious. Adults, especially the females, gorge on blood for long periods, and efforts to remove them manually often leave the head embedded in the skin. However, the various developmental stages – larvae, nymphs and adults – may not remain on the same host and some of the most important species involved in human disease transmission, such as *Dermacentor andersoni* and *Ixodes ricinus*, are known as *three host ticks*. Larvae that acquire micro-organisms remain infected through the nymphal and adult stages (*trans-stadial transmission*); the adult can, in turn, pass on infection through the egg (*transovarial transmission*). Thus, transmission of infection to new hosts may be very efficient.

Argasid ticks prefer to attack the host at night and do not remain attached to the host after feeding. They are relatively long-lived and inhabit dry, dusty environments, mainly in hot countries. The most important species from a medical point of view is *Ornithodoros moubata*, the main vector of tick-borne borreliosis (relapsing fever) in tropical Africa (p. 349). Other species of *Ornithodoros* transmit American forms of relapsing fever and some are notorious for their voracious feeding habits and extremely painful bites.

Spiders and scorpions

Although all spiders kill their prey by injecting venom, the toxin is usually innocuous to man and the mouthparts (*chelicerae*) are seldom robust enough to allow penetration of human skin. The sting of scorpions, which is carried at the end of an elongated extension of the abdomen, can penetrate skin, but the venom is usually of low potency (though sufficient to make children ill) and the sting itself relatively painless.

Some spiders and scorpions do have painful bites or stings and a few can cause serious, occasionally fatal, illness by virtue of powerful neurotoxins. The most dangerous spider is the Australian funnel web spider, *Atrax robustus*, but species of *Latrodectus* (*black widow spider*) found in many areas of the world, including southern Europe, can also inflict a serious bite. The venom of some *Lycosa* and *Loxosceles* spiders encountered in the USA and South America may cause tissue necrosis.

The most dangerous scorpions belong to the large Buthidae family. Buthid scorpions with dangerous stings are most commonly found in parts of North Africa, the Middle East, the southern states of the USA and Central America. They are nocturnal creatures and sting as a defensive reaction. Most human cases of scorpion bite occur when the arthropod seeks shelter in shoes or other clothing.

Spider and scorpion wounds seldom need more than supportive treatment. Antivenoms are sometimes available in areas where dangerous species are prevalent. Intravenous calcium gluconate has been successfully used to relieve the painful muscle spasm associated with bites of the black widow spider.

Other arthropods

Pentastomes (*tongueworms*) are important parasites of animals, but human infestation is very rare. A few species of centipede can inflict a painful bite and some millipedes can secrete a fluid capable of raising blisters. Crustaceans (crabs and crayfish) are of interest in human medicine mainly as intermediate hosts of *Paragonimus westermani*, the lung fluke (p. 608). Copepods (*water fleas*) are similarly important only as hosts of the guinea worm, *Dracunculus medinensis* (p. 607), and the fish tapeworm, *Diphyllobothrium latum* (p. 611).

RECOMMENDED READING

Burgess N R H, Cowan G O 1993 *A Colour Atlas of Medical Entomology*. Chapman & Hall, London

Goddard J 2000 *Infectious Diseases and Arthropods*. Humana Press, Totowa, New Jersey

Kettle D S 1984 *Medical and Veterinary Entomology*. Croom Helm, London

Service M W 2000 *Medical Entomology for Students*. Cambridge University Press, Cambridge

Smith K G V (ed.) 1973 *Insects and Other Arthropods of Medical Importance*. British Museum (Natural History), London

Zinsser H 1934 *Rats, Lice and History*. Routledge, London

Internet site

Iowa State University *Entomology Index of Internet Resources*: www.ent/iastate.edu/list/
(Includes an extensive listing of medical entomology sites.)

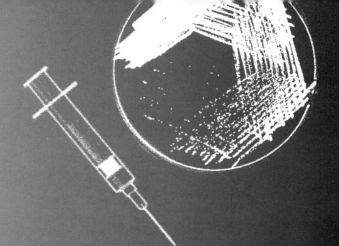

PART 6

DIAGNOSIS, TREATMENT AND CONTROL OF INFECTION

64
Infective syndromes

R. C. B. Slack

Throughout this book, infections have been dealt with as appropriate according to the micro-organisms involved. In this chapter, the study of infection is considered by syndromes associated with the major organs in order to emphasize the variety of microbes that may attack different body systems. The subject is presented in broad outline, and the reader should refer back to earlier chapters for a more extensive account of specific themes.

In infectious diseases, as in other branches of clinical practice, a diagnosis may be obvious and require little investigation, e.g. a case of chickenpox during an epidemic, or may only be established after laboratory and radiological examination, as with a patient with pyrexia of unknown origin (PUO). Figure 64.1 shows a flow chart of a rational approach to diagnosis and management of a patient with infection. In practice, treatment is

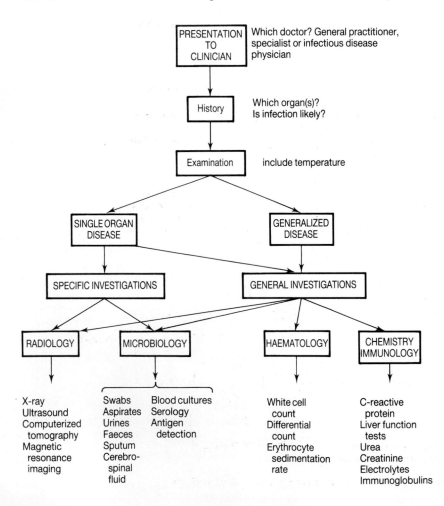

Fig. 64.1   Flow diagram for the diagnosis of infection.

often started before isolating and identifying the pathogen and in many viral conditions the exact cause can only be determined during convalescence, either by serological tests or after prolonged growth in tissue culture. The availability of rapid methods of diagnosis and new chemotherapeutic agents has made the study of infectious disease even more important.

SPECIFIC SYNDROMES

Upper respiratory tract

The upper respiratory tract is frequently the site of general and localized infections. Indeed, this group of ailments is amongst the most common presenting to domiciliary practice. It is the primary site of infection for most viral diseases, which are spread by sneezing, coughing or direct contact with materials contaminated by respiratory secretions. Although the majority of such symptoms are viral in origin, secondary bacterial infection may often follow, particularly in the very young and malnourished. Resident bacteria in the upper respiratory tract such as *Haemophilus influenzae*, *Streptococcus pyogenes* and *Str. pneumoniae* are the most common causes. Figure 64.2 shows the anatomical sites of respiratory infection and the appropriate specimens which may be taken for microbiology.

Sore throat

Bacterial acute tonsillitis or pharyngitis is commonly due to *Str. pyogenes* (group A), and a few are caused by groups C and G. Viruses are even more common causes of sore throats, especially the milder, non-exudative forms. However, it is important to make a definitive diagnosis of streptococcal pharyngitis for two reasons:

1. *Str. pyogenes* remains sensitive to penicillin, which should be used for treatment.

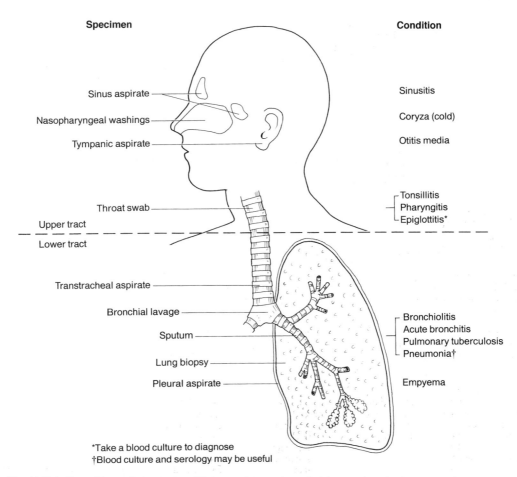

Fig. 64.2 Microbial infections of the respiratory tract and the appropriate specimens for laboratory investigation.

2. Group A β-haemolytic streptococci, if untreated, may give rise to septic complications such as a peritonsillar abscess, or to immune complex disease (glomerulonephritis, rheumatic fever).

On the other hand, since *Str. pyogenes* may account for only 20% of patients presenting with typical symptoms, many courses of antibiotics would be prescribed unnecessarily if all suspected cases were treated. Even in experienced hands it is difficult to predict on clinical grounds alone which cases are streptococcal. This has led to three approaches:

1. Treat all children with a penicillin, or erythromycin if allergic. Adults are treated if the throat looks very inflamed or if there is pus on the tonsils.
2. Swabs are taken for culture of streptococci and antibiotics are started as above but stopped if *Str. pyogenes* is not found.
3. Swabs are taken for rapid diagnosis (by antigen detection) and penicillin commenced only if the throat swab is positive.

There are pros and cons to each method. One drawback to early use of antibiotics is that the patient may react to the drug. If ampicillin is used, there is a strong chance of a skin reaction if the sore throat is the harbinger of glandular fever. In defence of the antibiotic lobby, there is no doubt that complications of streptococcal disease are seen far less commonly where there is access to medical service and pharmacies. However, these improvements have occurred in concert with better housing and social conditions.

There is little need to make a virological diagnosis as specific therapy is not available. However, epidemiological studies of patients with throat symptoms have revealed how common and varied are the viruses in the respiratory tract.

In the severely ill child with toxaemia and a membrane, diphtheria must be considered and treatment should not await laboratory confirmation. Moreover, the laboratory needs to do special tests to isolate and identify *Corynebacterium diphtheriae*, and communication (by telephone, if possible) between the clinician and laboratory is essential. Other corynebacteria such as *C. ulcerans* and *Arcanobacterium haemolyticum* may rarely cause ulcerated sore throats. In the sexually active, gonococcal pharyngitis should not be missed and again the laboratory needs to be told as they will use special selective media for *Neisseria gonorrhoeae*.

Common cold (coryza)

This common complaint, characterized by a nasal discharge (acute rhinitis) which is usually watery with scanty cells, afflicts humans of all ages who congregate together. Since there are many types of rhinoviruses, coronaviruses, adenoviruses, etc., and since immunity may be short-lived, individuals in a crowded environment, such as at school and university or travelling on public transport, may suffer three or four clinical infections a year. Most of these do not seek medical help knowing that there is little to offer. This is a condition for which many 'alternative' remedies are tried, from garlic to peppermint and vitamin supplements.

Bacterial superinfection with pneumococci and *H. influenzae* can occur in the nasopharynx but is only symptomatic when the sinuses or middle ear are involved. Pharyngitis and, occasionally, tracheobronchitis may occur with a cold or develop in more susceptible individuals. Respiratory syncytial virus (RSV) may cause upper respiratory symptoms in children and adults, but in those contracting the virus for the first time (usually infants under 1 year of age) acute bronchiolitis is common.

Sinusitis and otitis media

Direct extension of a viral or bacterial infection from the nasopharynx into frontal and maxillary sinuses in adults and into the middle ear in children is not uncommon. Obtaining adequate material for microbiology is difficult and requires the expertise of ear, nose and throat specialists. In most cases of acute sinusitis or otitis media the microbial cause is not found. It is assumed that severe pain and discharge of pus from the nose or ear is suggestive of bacterial infection and antibiotics are usually given to cover streptococci (mainly *Str. pneumoniae*) and *H. influenzae*. In adults with recurrent or chronic sinusitis, anaerobes (peptostreptococci or bacteroides) are often found in sinus washings.

Lower respiratory tract

Epiglottitis

Although situated in the upper part of the respiratory tract, *epiglottitis* behaves like a serious systemic infection which requires urgent admission to hospital and treatment. The diagnosis should be made clinically in a toxic child (usually under 5 years old) with respiratory obstruction and stridor. The most useful investigation is blood culture, which invariably grows *H. influenzae* type b unless antibiotics have been given or the child immunized. The epiglottis, which is swollen and cherry-red in appearance, should only be examined by skilled paediatricians prepared for a respiratory arrest. A lateral radiograph shows a soft tissue swelling in the throat.

Laryngotracheobronchitis

In adults, some viral infections cause acute laryngitis with voice loss or tracheitis with a dry cough. Respiratory tract infection in children is usually generalized and presents as *croup*. This may lead to respiratory obstruction and, as with haemophilus epiglottitis, urgent admission to hospital is necessary. The condition may be caused by a variety of respiratory viruses, with para-influenza viruses, adenoviruses and enteroviruses the most common. RSV can also cause croup, but more commonly this virus attacks infants in the first few months of life. In the UK there are winter epidemics of *acute bronchiolitis* due to RSV. This clinical syndrome starts as a cold which is followed by wheezing. In older children, asthmatic attacks are often precipitated by viral respiratory infections.

Whooping cough

Pertussis may be confused with croup, and, as special specimens need to be taken, the laboratory must be informed. A pernasal swab in special transport medium is required, and *Bordetella pertussis* will only grow on enriched culture media in conditions of high humidity.

Acute bronchitis

Acute exacerbation of chronic obstructive airways disease (COAD) is the commonest adult lower respiratory infection. It is invariably due to pneumococci, non-encapsulated haemophili, or both. Sometimes, acute bronchitis follows a viral infection. Although often examined, expectorated sputum from ambulatory patients with COAD is almost always a waste of effort.

Cystic fibrosis patients have frequent exacerbations and, in those situations, sputum examination is valuable because the causative bacteria (*Staphylococcus aureus, H. influenzae, Pseudomonas aeruginosa* or *Burkholderia cepacia*) may show variable antimicrobial resistance and appropriate therapy is essential.

Acute pneumonias

It is sometimes possible on clinical and radiological grounds to distinguish between *lobar pneumonia* (pneumococcal), *bronchopneumonia* (staphylococcal and klebsiellal) and *'atypical' pneumonias* (mycoplasmal and chlamydial). This division is of importance in guiding primary treatment, but should not give the clinician a blinkered view in investigation as some cases will invariably not follow a textbook! Expectorated sputum is often poorly collected and may not yield the pathogen. Blood cultures should always be taken from pneumonia patients but may not yield an organism,

especially if antibiotics have been started. *Antigen detection* in urine or sputum by fluorescent antibodies, immuno-electrophoresis, latex agglutination or enzyme-linked immunosorbent assay (ELISA) is a useful method for rapid diagnosis but may lack sensitivity. New amplified DNA detection methods are likely to improve diagnostic accuracy in respiratory infections. At present most cases of 'atypical' pneumonia are diagnosed by obtaining acute and convalescent sera and finding a significant titre or a rising titre of antibodies. *Legionnaires' disease* may be diagnosed by culture of *Legionella pneumophila* from sputum or a biopsy, but this has too low a sensitivity. Urine antigen detection by ELISA or DNA amplification of respiratory secretions have become more widely available methods of diagnosis. However, as with most pneumonias treatment must often be given on clinical suspicion.

Chronic chest disease

Tuberculosis must always be considered in any patient with fever, prolonged cough and weight loss. Again, a request for examination for mycobacteria must be included on the request card.

In the immunocompromised, various opportunist pathogens may give rise to respiratory infection. *Pneumocystis carinii* is demonstrated by fluorescent antibody staining of bronchial lavage. Fungal infections are diagnosed by growth of the pathogen or by serology. Special investigations are required for all these situations and unless the diagnosis is considered the laboratory cannot assist the clinician.

Gastro-intestinal infection

Acute diarrhoea with or without vomiting is a common complaint. Microbial causes, either by multiplication in the intestine or from the effects of preformed toxin, are the most important reasons for acute gastro-intestinal upset in an otherwise healthy individual. The aetiology of inflammatory bowel disease such as ulcerative colitis has not been established, although a patient may present with symptoms similar to an infectious diarrhoea but usually the natural history and chronicity of the condition make the distinction obvious.

Although many new causes of bowel infection have been discovered in the past 25 years the majority of food-related and short-lived episodes do not yield a microbial cause. In part this is due to the wide range of viruses, bacteria and protozoa which may be sought (Table 64.1). A search for all causes involves extensive and expensive laboratory effort, and this is often considered unnecessary for a condition which is usually self-limiting and relatively harmless.

Table 64.1 Common microbial causes of infectious intestinal disease

Viruses	Rotavirus
	Astrovirus
	Calicivirus (SRSV)
Bacteria	*Salmonella* spp.
	Campylobacter spp.
	Shigella spp.
	Escherichia coli (ETEC, VTEC)
	Vibrio cholerae
	V. parahaemolyticus
	Yersinia enterocolitica
Protozoa	*Cryptosporidium parvum*
	Entamoeba histolytica
	Giardia lamblia

SRSV, small round-structured viruses.
ETEC, enterotoxigenic *Esch. coli*; VTEC, Verotoxigenic *Esch. coli*.

Toxin-mediated disease of microbial origin ranges in severity from relatively trivial episodes of food poisoning caused by:

- enterotoxin-producing strains of *Staph. aureus,*
- *Clostridium perfringens*
- *Bacillus cereus,*

to the life-threatening systemic diseases:

- botulism caused by *Cl. botulinum,*
- severe *pseudomembranous colitis* caused by *Cl. difficile* (often antibiotic-associated).

There are, in addition, many non-microbial causes of food poisoning, such as that due to the ingestion of certain toadstools, undercooked red kidney beans or various types of fish (*ciguatera toxin, scombrotoxin*); most notorious is the puffer fish which, during part of its reproductive cycle, produces a neurotoxin that is responsible for more than 100 deaths a year in Japan, where the delicacy *fugu* is enjoyed.

It may be possible on clinical grounds to distinguish between patients with dysentery, in which bloody diarrhoea and mucus are found, and those with watery diarrhoea, due to the toxic effects of the pathogen on the small intestinal mucosa, leading to accumulation of fluid in the bowel. Some conditions, such as staphylococcal food poisoning and some viral illnesses, present largely with vomiting. A specific cause is also suspected if there is a history of foreign travel, if the case forms part of an outbreak which is food- or water-associated, or if the individual has a relevant food history.

Travellers' diarrhoea encompasses many clinical and microbial causes, but the commonest organisms implicated are enterotoxigenic strains of *Escherichia coli*

(ETEC). However, a host of microbes must be considered. Some, such as salmonellae, are found worldwide; others, such as vibrios, have a more limited distribution.

More chronic intestinal infections contracted in warmer climates usually do not present with diarrhoea but with vague abdominal symptoms. Many helminths and protozoa are found on screening faeces for other pathogens.

Urinary tract infections

The diagnosis of urinary tract infection cannot be made without bacteriological examination of the urine because many patients with the frequency–dysuria syndrome have sterile urine and, conversely, asymptomatic bacteriuria is a common condition. Infection is most commonly caused by members of the Enterobacteriaceae (Table 64.2), but there are great variations in antimicrobial susceptibility, and control of chemotherapy requires laboratory examination. Occasionally, *Mycobacterium tuberculosis* invades the kidney and appropriate tests must be carried out if this is suspected.

Infection in the urinary tract may be confined to particular anatomical sites, e.g. urethritis or renal abscess. Alternatively, the urine may become infected and, in cases of obstruction or reflux, bacteria may ascend from the bladder to give rise to kidney infections. *Urethritis* is really a genital infection and is most commonly due to sexually transmitted organisms such as chlamydiae or *N. gonorrhoeae*. Confirmation depends on obtaining, by swabbing or scraping, a sample of urethral discharge for microscopy and culture. *Metastatic abscesses* in the kidney and *perinephric abscesses* cannot usually be diagnosed by urine examination, although pyuria may be present. Specific radiological or surgical exploration is necessary, as with any localized infection.

Throughout most of their life-span women suffer far more attacks of urinary tract infection than men. In young adult women who become sexually active, frequency and dysuria are common reasons for seeking

Table 64.2 Common causes of urinary tract infection (approximate percentages)

Organism	Domiciliary	Hospital
Escherichia coli	70–80	50
Proteus mirabilis	10	1–5
Klebsiella spp.	1–5	5–10
Staphylococcus saprophyticus	10–15	0
Staph. epidermidis	1–5	10–20
Enterococci	1–5	10–20
Other coliforms	<1	5–10
Pseudomonas aeruginosa	1–2	5–10

medical attention. Only about one-half of these yield an organism in 'significant' numbers, usually defined as above 10^7 organisms per litre. The commonest cause by far is *Esch. coli* (Table 64.2), some strains of which possess specific uropathogenic determinants. It has been suggested that many of the culture-negative infections are due to coliforms which are present in small numbers in urine. Infection of the urine is common and may be asymptomatic in many elderly patients.

Infections of the central nervous system

Meningitis

Meningeal irritation may occur in association with other acute infections (*meningism*) or with non-infective conditions such as subarachnoid haemorrhage. In the early stages of meningococcal disease, signs of meningitis may be absent, yet examination of the cerebrospinal fluid (CSF) yields *N. meningitidis*. Thus, CSF and blood cultures should be examined from all suspected cases. There are contra-indications to performing a lumbar puncture in any patient with raised intracranial pressure because of the danger of herniation through the foramen magnum (*coning*). Thus, lumbar puncture should only be carried out in hospital. In fulminating disease, especially if it is meningococcal, it is prudent to give penicillin as soon as the diagnosis is suspected and before admission. This has led to a greatly reduced yield by culture of suspected cases. Antigen and DNA detection have become increasingly important in confirming the diagnosis.

It is often possible to consider the likely pathogen on clinical and epidemiological grounds. *H. influenzae* type b occurs almost always in infants from 6 to 24 months of age, although use of the Hib vaccine in many countries has almost made this a disease of the past. *Str. pneumoniae* is seen generally in the very young and the elderly. *Meningococcal meningitis* is characteristically a disease of children and young adults. In the neonate, coliforms (mainly *Esch. coli* K1), *Listeria monocytogenes*, group B streptococci and pneumococci may be found. In infants a few months old, salmonella meningitis is an important condition in some countries with a warm climate.

If no readily cultivated organism is found, but the CSF shows an increase in cells, the syndrome of *aseptic meningitis* is present. Table 64.3 shows some of the causes of this condition. If the symptoms are short in duration, viruses are most likely. If the child has been unwell for more than 1 week, *tuberculous meningitis* must be considered. This is one of the most difficult and important microbiological diagnoses to make.

Table 64.3	Causes of aseptic meningitis
Viruses	Enteroviruses (echoviruses, polioviruses, coxsackieviruses) Mumps (including post-immunization) Herpes (herpes simplex and varicella-zoster) Arboviruses
Spiral bacteria	Syphilis (*Treponema pallidum*) Leptospira (*Leptospira canicola*)
Other bacteria	Partially treated with antibiotics Tuberculous (*Mycobacterium tuberculosis*) Brain abscess
Fungi	*Cryptococcus neoformans*
Protozoa	*Acanthamoeba, Naegleria,* *Toxoplasma gondii*
Non-infective	Lymphomata, leukaemias Metastatic and primary neoplasms Collagen-vascular diseases

In the immunocompromised, listeria meningitis may be seen in the adult and *Cryptococcus neoformans* in all age groups, but particularly those with human immunodeficiency virus (HIV) infection. Central nervous system disease in patients with acquired immune deficiency syndrome (AIDS) is a very complicated differential diagnosis (Table 64.4).

Cerebral infections

Encephalitis may extend into the meninges with signs and CSF findings of an aseptic meningitis. Many viral infections may, however, only infect the brain cortex and

Table 64.4	Causes of neurological damage in HIV-infected patients	
Direct HIV infection		Subacute encephalomyelitis (AIDS-dementia complex)
Opportunist infections		
	Viruses	Cytomegalovirus Herpes simplex Varicella-zoster Papovavirus
	Bacteria	*Treponema pallidum* (syphilis)
	Fungi	*Cryptococcus neoformans*
	Protozoa	*Toxoplasma gondii*
Malignancy		
	Primary	Brain lymphoma
	Secondary	Kaposi's sarcoma Systemic lymphoma

clinical symptoms may be vague: loss of consciousness, fits, localized paralysis. This can also occur in toxaemia, cerebral malaria, electrolyte disturbances or vascular accidents.

In western Europe, herpes simplex or varicella–zoster viruses are the most common causes of encephalitis, but in many parts of the world arboviruses such as Japanese B encephalitis virus are important.

Abscesses in the brain or subdural space may arise from haematogenous spread during bacteraemia or by direct extension, either through the cribriform plate from the nasopharynx or from sinuses or the middle ear. They may be clinically silent or present as a space-occupying lesion accompanied by fever and systemic upset. Skilled radiological scanning by computerized axial tomography (CAT) or magnetic resonance imaging (MRI), if available, and early neurosurgical intervention will reduce complications and, if appropriate systemic antibiotics are given for a prolonged period, the success rate is nowadays good.

Skin and soft tissue infections

Human skin acts as an excellent barrier to infection. Some parasites, such as hookworm larvae and schistosome cercariae, can penetrate skin to initiate infection. This may also be true of some bacteria, notably *Treponema pallidum*, although in primary syphilis the spirochaete probably enters through minute abrasions which are present even in healthy skin. Primary skin infection such as *impetigo* is due to *Staph. aureus* or *Str. pyogenes*, or both, gaining access to abrasions, usually in children. This may occur in association with ectoparasite infestation, in particular, scabies. *Dermatophyte* fungi are specialized to grow well in keratinized tissue.

Skin lesions are a feature of some virus infections, such as warts, herpes simplex and molluscum contagiosum. In other virus diseases, including rubella, measles, chickenpox (and, before its eradication, smallpox), a characteristic rash follows the viraemic phase of the illness. *Wound infections* may be accidental or postoperative and many organisms can cause sepsis. Even after surgery many wounds are infected with the endogenous flora of the patient. Swabs, or preferably pus, obtained directly from the wound or abscess, are adequate to find the causative organisms. *Anaerobic* sepsis most commonly occurs following amputations or in contaminated traumatic wounds, particularly if the blood supply has been compromised or the bowel perforated. In classic *gas gangrene*, bubbles of gas may be felt in the wound and surrounding tissues, and the muscle and fascia have a black necrotic appearance. Less florid examples of anaerobes causing extensive cellulitis are more commonly seen and the laboratory should be requested to look carefully for anaerobes in all situations where deep wounds may be contaminated with endogenous flora.

Genital tract infections

In the male, acute urethritis is a common condition which is usually due to a sexually transmitted microbe such as *N. gonorrhoeae, Chlamydia trachomatis* or *Ureaplasma urealyticum*. If untreated these organisms can cause prostatitis or epididymitis, and gonorrhoea may produce unpleasant consequences such as urethral stricture or sterility. Genital ulcers in both sexes may be due to herpes simplex virus, syphilis or chancroid (*H. ducreyi*).

The more complicated female reproductive organs are subjected to many more infections with a greater scope for sequelae. Vaginitis may present as vaginal discharge or irritation and often these symptoms are due to infections that are not always exogenously acquired. *Trichomonas vaginalis* is the most common sexually acquired microbe, although both *N. gonorrhoeae* and chlamydia may also present as discharge. Thrush due to *Candida* species is especially common in pregnancy and in diabetics. It is usually an endogenous condition due to disturbances in the normal commensal flora. Another cause of vaginal discharge, but usually without inflammatory cells and irritation, is associated with an alteration of local pH with proliferation of *Gardnerella vaginalis* and anaerobic spiral bacteria, now termed *Mobiluncus* species. The alkaline conditions and characteristic amines found in *bacterial vaginosis* allow a diagnosis to be easily made on examination of the patient. This condition, which used to be called nonspecific vaginitis, is a common condition in sexually active women, although probably not a venereal disease in the usual sense.

The endocervical canal is the site of infection with *N. gonorrhoeae* and *C. trachomatis* in the sexually mature woman. During parturition both organisms may be passed to the baby's eyes to give rise to *ophthalmia neonatorum*. The cervix may also be infected with human papillomavirus (HPV), and this is associated with a high risk of cervical cancer. HPV commonly causes warts on the external genitalia, peri-anally as well as in the vagina and cervix. Herpes, chancroid and syphilis may cause ulcers in parts of the genital tract which are not visible without a speculum.

Ascending genital infection due to gonococci or chlamydia is a common sequela. In cases of *acute gonococcal salpingitis* there is usually fever and pelvic pain. On vaginal examination, there is referred lower abdominal pain on moving the cervix (*cervical excitation*) and tenderness in the iliac fossa on abdominal palpation. Signs and symptoms in cases due to *C. trachomatis* are much less pronounced, and some women develop chronic *pelvic inflammatory disease* (PID) without having suffered a recognizable acute episode. PID, although most often initiated by these two common sexually transmitted pathogens, is usually a polymicrobial infection, in which endogenous commensals, particularly anaerobes, play an important role.

Infection may progress outside the fallopian tubes to give rise to *pelvic abscesses*, especially in the pouch of Douglas, and peritonitis. Spread across the peritoneal cavity may give rise to *perihepatitis*, which was first described in gonorrhoea as the Fitz-Hugh–Curtis syndrome, but also occurs in chlamydial disease.

Eye infections

Various microbes may cause acute conjunctivitis. Ophthalmia neonatorum may be due to gonococci or chlamydia. In the newborn, *Staph. aureus* is commonly found in 'sticky eyes', either as a primary cause of conjunctivitis or after infection with another pathogen. In older infants and children, *H. influenzae* and *Str. pneumoniae* are common. Chlamydiae give rise to *trachoma*, the commonest cause of blindness in the world, and to a milder form of inclusion blennorrhoea in sexually active individuals.

Primary viral conjunctivitis often occurs in epidemics when certain types of adenovirus are implicated. This is usually a mild condition with few sequelae compared with the keratitis due to herpes simplex virus or in shingles when the ophthalmic division of the trigeminal nerve is infected with varicella–zoster virus.

Corneal damage due to fungi as well as herpesviruses is seen in immunosuppressed patients, and keratitis caused by free-living amoebae (*Acanthamoeba* species), though rare, is becoming more common, particularly in wearers of contact lenses.

Penetrating injuries of the eye and ophthalmic surgery may introduce a wide range of bacteria and fungi into the chambers of the eye which may give rise to *hypopyon* (pus in the eye). This condition requires prompt surgical drainage and instillation of appropriate antibiotics such as gentamicin. *Ps. aeruginosa* and *Proteus* species are among the more common organisms isolated.

Infections of the back of the eye (choroidoretinitis) are seen in many diverse infectious diseases (Table 64.5).

Table 64.5	Causes of choroidoretinitis
Viruses	Cytomegalovirus, rubella
Bacteria	*Treponema pallidum*
Protozoa	*Toxoplasma gondii*
Helminths	*Toxocara canis, Onchocerca volvulus*

SYSTEMIC AND GENERAL SYNDROMES

Pyrexia of unknown origin

PUO may be defined as a significant fever (greater than 38°C) for a few days without an obvious cause, i.e. no apparent infection of an organ or system. In the classic studies of PUO only patients with persistent fever for at least 3 weeks were included. These chronic cases are often due to non-infective causes such as malignancy (especially lymphomata) or auto-immune and connective tissue diseases (such as systemic lupus erythematosus).

In determining an infective aetiology some of the most important questions to be asked of the patient are:

1. Have you been abroad recently?
2. What is your occupation (especially, is animal contact involved)?
3. What immunizations have you had – in particular, have you had BCG?
4. Have you or your family ever had tuberculosis?
5. Are you taking or have you recently had any drugs (especially antibiotics)?

Character of fever

The individual with suspected PUO should be admitted to hospital so that measurements can be made regularly by skilled staff. Rarely, malingerers may be found out and drug reactions discovered by controlling intake. Rhythmical fevers such as the quartan fever (every 72 h) of *Plasmodium malariae* or undulant fever of *Brucella melitensis* may be rarely found and point to the aetiology. More commonly, fevers are intermittent with rises at the end of the day and falls after rigors or extensive sweating.

The degree of temperature depends also on the host response as well as the pyrogens produced by microbes. Generally, the older the patient the less able they are to mount a pyrexia. Many elderly patients with septicaemia may have normal or subnormal temperatures whereas infants can have fevers of 40°C and febrile convulsions with otherwise mild respiratory viral infections.

Endocarditis

Infections of the tissue of the heart usually involve damaged valves, either after rheumatic fever or with atheroma. Another important group of patients are those who have had heart surgery, in particular prosthetic valve replacements. In addition, intravenous drug addicts or patients who have had indwelling vascular devices are liable to bacteraemia and, occasionally, endocarditis may follow. The most common causative organisms are listed in Table 64.6.

Table 64.6 Common causes of infective endocarditis (approximate percentages)

Organism	Non-operative	IVDA/surgery
Viridans group of streptococci	70	35
Enterococci	5	3
Other streptococci (group G, F)	10	<1
Staphylococcus epidermidis	10	25
Staph. aureus	5	25
Gram-positive rods (diphtheroids)	<1	5
Haemophilus spp. and other fastidious Gram-negative organisms[a]	<1[b]	<1
Gram-negative bacilli (coliforms, Pseudomonas spp.)	0	5
Coxiella burnetii (Q fever)	<1[b]	0
Chlamydia psittaci	<1	0
Fungi (Candida spp.)	<1	2

IVDA, intravenous drug abusers.

[a] Neisseria, Brucella, Cardiobacterium, Streptobacillus spp.
[b] These are rough UK figures; in some parts of the Middle East, brucellae and Q fever cause significant numbers of infective endocarditides.

Septicaemia

It is not clinically useful to distinguish between *bacteraemia*, organisms isolated from the bloodstream, *septicaemia*, which is a clinical syndrome, and *endotoxaemia*, which is circulating bacterial endotoxin. The spectrum of clinical disease ranges from hypotensive shock and disseminated intravascular coagulation (DIC) with a high mortality, to transient bacteraemia, which may occur in healthy individuals during dental manipulations.

The vascular compartment is sterile and usually intact. Microbes gain entry from breakages of blood vessels adjacent to skin or mucosal surfaces or by phagocytic cells carrying organisms into capillaries or the lymphatic system. Active multiplication within the bloodstream probably only occurs terminally, but in many cases of septicaemia there are high numbers of bacteria recovered from blood cultures, which often only sample 10 ml at a time. This occurs from a heavily contaminated site such as an indwelling urinary catheter which releases bacteria into veins on movement. Septic shock may be due to Gram-negative lipids (endotoxins) or Gram-positive toxins (e.g. staphylococcal enterotoxin), which are usually proteins. The end result of both is to initiate a cascade of events involving cytokines, especially tumour necrosis factor and interleukin-2, vascular mediators and platelets, which combined lead to DIC and hypotension. This process becomes irreversible and produces failure of all major organs. Patients die from a variety of terminal events which make up the syndrome of *septic shock*. The main microbial causes are listed with approximate frequency in Table 64.7.

Clinical features may occasionally suggest the aetiological agent, e.g. the characteristic purpuric rash of meningococcal disease and the black lesions (*ecthyma gangrenosum*) seen on the skin of compromised patients with pseudomonas septicaemia, but in the majority of bacteraemias the agent can only be determined after blood culture. Sometimes, prior antibiotic therapy may render cultures negative and new methods of antigen detection or gene probes may be useful. Non-specific investigations such as those shown in Fig. 64.1 may

Table 64.7 Major causes of septicaemia (approximate percentages)

Organism	Community-acquired	Hospital-acquired	Sources and comments
Escherichia coli	35	30	UTI (catheters), biliary tract
Other enterobacteria	5	10	UTI, chest
Pseudomonas spp.	5	5	UTI, immunocompromised
Other Gram-negative rods	2	5	Ventilator pneumonia
Neisseria meningitidis	3	0	Characteristic skin rash
Staphylococcus aureus	30	25	Vascular, postoperative
Staph. epidermidis	<1	20	Vascular devices
Streptococcus pneumoniae	10	0	Pneumonia
Str. pyogenes	5	2	Skin, soft tissue
Other Gram-positive cocci	2	0	Skin
Listeria monocytogenes	<1	0	Bowel, foods
Clostridium spp.	<1	0	Bowel, gangrenous wounds
Bacteroides spp.	3	1	Bowel, pelvis, wounds
Mixed infection	10	7	Bowel, intensive care

Data from Dr P. Ispahani, Nottingham Public Health Laboratory, UK.
UTI, urinary tract infection.

offer some help that the cause of the illness is infective. C-reactive protein (CRP), an acute-phase protein which is often greatly elevated in the serum during bacterial infections, may be the most useful of these but, as with peripheral leucocyte counts, there are a significant number of errant results.

Imported fevers

An important group of patients with fever are those who have recently returned from abroad. In whichever country a doctor may practise, travellers with unfamiliar disease will be encountered. A knowledge of medical geography is useful but conditions vary greatly within one country and with time. Up-to-date information is held, often on computer, by communicable disease centres and tropical disease hospitals and schools. The World Health Organization and the Centers for Disease Control, Atlanta, USA, publish international notification data and maps. Undoubtedly the most important condition to diagnose is malaria due to *Plasmodium falciparum*, which may be rapidly fatal without appropriate treatment in the non-immune subject. The wide distribution of drug resistance in *P. falciparum* has led to difficulties in giving adequate prophylaxis and in treating an acute attack. Other common febrile illnesses

which are imported into northern countries are typhoid and paratyphoid. These do not usually present with diarrhoea so the possibility of an enteric fever may not be considered. It is also obvious, but sometimes overlooked, that the fever may not be related to the travel history and that the cause is a microbe which could have been caught at home.

Imported infections

Table 64.8 lists some of the more common causes of infectious diseases imported from tropical countries into temperate regions where the diseases are not normally transmitted. There are three groups of patients which are considered separately, but the separation of diseases and microbes is not exclusive:

1. Short-term travellers or *tourists* who usually visit major cities or special holiday areas and stay in good accommodation and have minimal contact with the indigenous population.
2. Long-term visitors who may be engaged in lengthy overland trips or be working abroad as *expatriates*.
3. *Immigrants* who were brought up abroad and visit or have residence in the host country: also settled immigrants who pay short-term visits to their country of origin.

Table 64.8 Some important infective conditions imported to temperate regions from the tropics

Causative organism	Tourists[a]	Expatriates[a]	Immigrants[a]
Viruses	Hepatitis A Influenza	HIV Yellow fever (Other arboviruses)	Hepatitis B Haemorrhagic fever
Rickettsiae and chlamydiae	Tick typhus	Q fever	Trachoma
Bacteria	Legionnaires' Disease Toxigenic *Escherichia coli*	Brucellosis Shigellosis	Tuberculosis, enteric fever Cholera
Protozoa	Cryptosporidiosis Falciparum malaria Cutaneous leishmaniasis	Giardiasis Malaria (all) Schistosomiasis	Amoebiasis Vivax malaria Kala azar (visceral leishmaniasis)
Helminths	–	Tapeworm Stronglyloidiasis Filariasis	Roundworm Hookworm
Ectoparasites (ticks, mites and insects)	Ticks	Myiasis Jigger flea	Scabies
Fungi	–	Dermatophytosis Histoplasmosis	Mycetoma

[a] These categories are not mutually exclusive.

Individuals who travel abroad vary in their risk behaviour and their exposure to potential pathogens. Generally, advice given by travel operators, tourist offices, embassies and medical sources has greatly improved in the past few years. Companies sending out expatriate workers tend to look after their staff well. Nevertheless, many tourists (up to 50% in some studies) have episodes of travellers' diarrhoea, which in some cases results in admission to hospital. The major groups who are missed in preventative programmes are overland travellers and immigrants returning to their homeland, often with young families who have never been exposed to the infectious risks of their parents' home. Immigrants returning for visits to malarious areas seldom take prophylactic advice, believing themselves to be immune, but protective immunity wanes with prolonged absence.

Cryptogenic infections

Some of the commonly encountered sites of infection which may give rise to fever, and must be considered in the differential diagnosis of PUO, are listed in Table 64.9.

Table 64.9 Some common sites of infection in pyrexia of unknown origin

Abdomen	Subphrenic abscess
	Appendix abscess
	Ileal tuberculosis
	Pelvic abscess
Liver and biliary tract	Intrahepatic abscess
	Empyema of gallbladder
	Ascending cholangitis
	Cholecystitis
	Viral hepatitis
Kidney and urinary tract	Perinephric abscess
	Renal tuberculosis
	Pyelonephritis (especially children)
Bones	Vertebral osteomyelitis
	Tuberculosis
	Prosthetic infections
Cardiovascular	Endocarditis
	Graft infections
Respiratory	Tuberculosis
	Empyema and lung abscess
Nervous system	Cryptococcal or tuberculous meningitis
	Brain or spinal abscess

RECOMMENDED READING

Armstrong D, Cohen J (eds) 1999 *Infectious Diseases.* Mosby, St Louis

Christie A B 1987 *Infectious Diseases: Epidemiology and Clinical Practice,* 4th edn. Churchill Livingstone, Edinburgh, Vols 1 and 2

Conlon C, Snydman D 2000 *Colour Atlas and Text of Infectious Diseases,* Mosby, St Louis

Long S S, Pickering L K, Prober C G (eds) 1997 *Principles and Practice of Paediatric Infectious Diseases,* Churchill Livingstone, New York

Mandell G L, Bennett J E, Dolin R 2000 *Principles and Practice of Infectious Diseases,* 5th edn. Churchill Livingstone, New York

Shanson D C 1998 *Microbiology in Clinical Practice,* 4th edn. Arnold, London

Weatherall D J, Ledingham J G G, Warrell D A 1996 *Oxford Textbook of Medicine,* 3rd edn. Oxford University Press, Oxford

65

Diagnostic procedures

R. C. B. Slack

The role of the laboratory in assisting clinicians in the diagnosis of infection is illustrated in the specimen flow diagram shown in Fig. 65.1. The choice of specimen depends on following the principles outlined in Chapter 64. The microbiology laboratory requires enough information on the request card accompanying the specimen to use the optimal methods necessary for identification of potential pathogens in particular infective syndromes. At the most basic level, it is obvious that, when a swab is received in the laboratory, it is necessary to know if it comes from the throat or the vagina! But additional information is also essential: is the patient being investigated for pharyngitis or diphtheria; for vaginal discharge or septic abortion? Furthermore, the specimen must be obtained with care and transported to the laboratory without delay in an appropriate manner. The value of the result is in direct proportion to the attention given to these details, as well as to the skill and efficiency of the laboratory. For further details of laboratory methods, including specimen containers and culture media used, the reader is encouraged to consult the companion volume *Practical Medical Microbiology* listed in the recommended reading section.

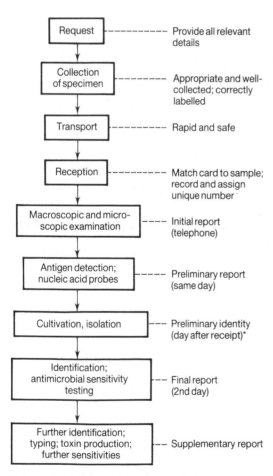

* viruses, fungi and some bacteria may take longer

Fig. 65.1 Steps in the isolation and identification of pathogens from an infected patient.

COLLECTION OF SPECIMENS

Samples for microbiological examination need to be carefully collected, if possible without contamination with commensals or from external sources. Some points to remember with specimens from individual sources are shown in Table 65.1. It is essential to use sterile containers which are leak-proof and able to withstand transportation through the post if necessary. It is more convenient for both the clinician and microbiologist if the laboratory provides request cards, containers and an efficient transport system. There is a need for staff to be aware of safety regulations and for all parties to understand who has responsibility for each step of the process and how to minimize handling by untrained people. Special precautions required for 'high-risk' specimens need to be defined by the laboratory and hospital management. Storage of clinical material must be separate from food and drugs, and this may necessitate provision of additional refrigerator space and transport facilities.

Table 65.1 Some important points to remember in the collection of specimens for microbiological examination

Respiratory secretions

Nasal swab (anterior)	Only for carriage of staphylococci and streptococci
Nasopharyngeal swab	For pertussis and meningococci
External ear swab	Wide range of microbes, including fungi
Myringotomy and sinus samples	As for abscesses – including anaerobes
Throat (pharyngeal) swab	Specify if only for streptococci; mention if diphtheria possible; use special transport media for virology
Saliva	Used for antibody detection (gingival swab); otherwise discard
Laryngeal swab	Specify if for mycobacteria
Expectorated sputum	Often poorly collected; specify mycobacteria, legionellae, pneumocystis
Transtracheal aspirate, bronchoscopy specimens, lung biopsy	Specify likely diagnosis; ask for specific tests
Pleural fluid	Treat as pus; always look for mycobacteria

Gastro-intestinal specimens

Vomitus	Only for virology
Gastric washings	For mycobacteria (particularly in children)
Gastric biopsy	For *Helicobacter pylori*
Duodenal/jejunal aspirates	Protozoa (*Giardia lamblia*, microsporidia, etc.)
Liver aspirates	As for pus (anaerobes); consider amoebae
Spleen puncture	For *Leishmania* spp.
Rectal biopsy	Schistosomiasis
Rectal swab	Only for gonococci and chlamydia
Colonic biopsy	Histopathological diagnosis of amoebiasis, pseudomembranous colitis (*Clostridium difficile*)
Colonic scrapings	Protozoa; amoebic trophozoites (deliver to laboratory immediately)
Faeces	Specify possible diagnosis; ask for clostridial toxins, parasite examination if suspected
Peri-anal swab	For eggs of threadworm

Urine

Mid-stream (MSU)	Suitable for most patients
Clean catch	Infants and elderly – increased contamination
Suprapubic aspirate	Infants and neonates
Ureteric/bladder washout	To localize infection
Prostatic massage	Collect samples before, during and at end of micturition
Terminal urine	Schistosome ova, chlamydia DNA amplification
Complete early morning or 24-h urine	Mycobacteria (tubercle)

Central nervous system

Cerebrospinal fluid by spinal tap	For meningitis collect sample for protein and glucose – test blood sugar simultaneously, specify virology, fungi or syphilis serology
Ventricular tap	Specify if through an indwelling shunt or catheter
Brain abscess	As for pus (include anaerobes)

Skin and soft tissue

Skin scraping/nail clipping	Dermatophyte fungi
Skin swab	Rarely valuable without pus
Skin snips	Onchocerciasis – seek advice
Vesicle fluid	Suitable for electron microscopy for viruses
Wound swab	Obtain pus if possible; record site
Pus, tissues, aspirates	Describe site and any relevant operative details

Genital

Urethral swab	Pus for gonococci, scrape for chlamydia
Vaginal swab (adult)	Candida, trichomonas, bacterial vaginosis or chlamydia DNA
Vaginal swab (prepubertal)	State age; caution required if abuse possible
Cervical swab	Separate media for chlamydia
Ulcer scrape	Immediate dark-ground microscopy; separate media for virology or chancroid
Uterine secretions	Specify puerperium or post-abortion
Pelvic aspirates	As for pus
Laparoscopy specimens	Include chlamydia specimen

Table 65.1 (*Continued*)

Eye	
Conjunctival swab	Separate virology; scrape for chlamydia
Aspirates	As for pus
Blood	
Culture	Strict aseptic technique; take large sample in special media before antibiotics
Bone marrow	Valuable for leishmania, mycobacteria, brucella
Film	Malaria (thick and thin), filaria, borrelia, trypanosomes
Whole blood	Filaria (day or night samples as appropriate)
Serum antigen	Rapid diagnosis of many microbial diseases (e.g. hepatitis B)
Serum antibody	Retrospective diagnosis of common viral diseases, syphilis and other selected infections; need rising titre or specific IgM

Food and water

The examination of non-clinical specimens is beyond the scope of this book and readers are referred to appropriate reading. However, an outbreak of gastro-intestinal disease inevitably leads to the question of identifying the source. When disease is due to preformed toxins, as with staphylococcal food poisoning, faecal examination is unhelpful, and the diagnosis can only be made by testing the food. Frequently, the offending item has been discarded and the examination of food and water related to specific patients is often unrewarding. Routine sampling of water sources and potentially contaminated food such as poultry at various critical points of production is essential in maintaining good public health.

TRANSPORT

Many microbes may perish on transit from the host's body to a laboratory incubator. Some contaminants, especially coliforms, may overgrow the pathogen and so mask its presence. These two constraints make it essential that any material for cultivation of microbes is transported as quickly as possible to the laboratory in a manner expected to protect the viability of any pathogens. Such problems may be minimized by the use of antigen or gene probe detection because of the relative stability of the chemical structures identified.

The ideal situation is to bring the patient to the laboratory for specimen collection or take the laboratory to the clinic. Both approaches are used for special purposes but are obviously inconvenient for many patients and inappropriate and costly for complicated techniques such as virus isolation which need specialized (and safe) facilities.

To overcome any drawbacks due to delay in reaching the microbiology department the following methods may be used:

1. *Transport media* (Table 65.2).
2. *Boric acid*. The addition of boric acid to urine at a concentration of 1.8% (v/w) will stop bacterial multiplication but lower concentrations are ineffective and higher ones may kill the pathogen.
3. *Dip slides*. These provide a convenient way of inoculating urines at the clinic. They comprise small plastic spoons or strips holding a thin layer of agar which is dipped into the urine and then put in a screw-topped bottle for transport. The agar adsorbs a fixed

Table 65.2 Types of transport medium

Type of organism	Medium	Comments
Bacteria	Stuart's semi-solid agar	Contains charcoal to inactivate toxic material
Anaerobic bacteria	Various systems, including gassed-out tubes and anaerobic bags	Not widely used, but essential for some strict anaerobes
Viruses	Buffered salts solution containing serum	Contains antibotics to control bacteria and fungi
Chlamydiae	Similar to viral transport medium, but without agents that inhibit chlamydiae	Chlamydial antigen media contain detergent to lyse infected cells
Protozoa, helminths	Merthiolate-iodine-formalin	Kills active protozoa, but preserves cysts and ova in a form suitable for concentration and microscopy

volume of urine and, after incubation, colony counts of bacteria give a semi-quantitative estimation of numbers.

4. *Refrigeration.* Storage at 4°C before processing will prevent multiplication of most bacteria. However, delicate microbes such as neisseriae may not survive whereas certain organisms, notably listeriae, flourish at low temperatures.

5. *Freezing.* Temperatures of −70°C or below, which can be achieved in liquid nitrogen or special deep freezes, will preserve many microbes, providing they are protected by a stabilizing fluid such as serum or glycerol.

RECEPTION

The importance of good documentation cannot be overstressed. No matter how well the specimen was taken, transported and processed in the laboratory, the end result depends on communication between people. The clinician making the request must give complete details on the request card and specimen to reduce errors. Staff receiving specimens in the laboratory must match them with the cards and record them into a book or computer. This is usually done by assigning a unique number to each specimen and labelling both the specimen and the request. When parts of the specimen are separated from the original bottle, e.g. after centrifugation of serum, the laboratory number becomes the only recognizable identification. Transcription errors are especially important for requests for human immunodeficiency virus (HIV) or syphilis serology, which may have disastrous consequences and medicolegal implications if wrong results are given. Transcription mistakes in laboratories are far more common than is supposed: studies in chemical pathology departments have shown a significant number of 'errors', amounting to 5% of the total samples.

EXAMINATION

Looking at clinical material with the naked eye or hand-lens should be part of the examination of a patient at the bedside. Sadly, many doctors delegate this to nurses or to the laboratory staff. Many unnecessary laboratory tests could be avoided if unsuitable specimens were rejected on the ward or in the general practitioner's surgery. These would include: crystal-clear urine from patients with 'cystitis'; well formed stools from patients with 'diarrhoea'; and mouth washings or saliva from patients with respiratory symptoms.

It was once common practice to carry out certain basic investigations in ward side-rooms, and kits offering 'near-patient testing' are becoming available. However, there are cogent arguments against bedside pathology, including issues of safety, time, competence and quality control.

Microscopy

Microscopy is an important part of the examination of many specimens. For bacteriology, the Gram and Ziehl–Neelsen stains are usually sufficient, but for the demonstration of fungi or parasites special stains or concentration techniques may be required. 'Wet' mounts, i.e. unstained preparations of fluid material, are widely used in looking at cells in urine, cerebrospinal fluid (CSF), faeces and vaginal secretions. None of these procedures takes more than 5 or 10 min and all are inexpensive in reagent costs and capital equipment. They are therefore ideal rapid methods and new diagnostic techniques have to be judged against microscopy. An initial report, such as 'Gram-negative diplococci and pus cells seen' from meningitic CSF, can be issued within minutes of receiving the specimen and will aid the clinician in confirming the diagnosis and starting appropriate antibiotics.

Similarly, a rapid diagnosis of falciparum malaria can be life-saving. Indeed, suspected pyogenic meningitis and falciparum malaria are among the few conditions for which it is clearly justifiable to call upon emergency laboratory services outside normal working hours.

Electron microscopy requires more elaborate preparation than does light microscopy and it is therefore much slower. It is, however, valuable in the relatively rapid diagnosis of certain viral infections, including viral diarrhoea. The non-specific nature of electron microscopy gives it an advantage over virus-specific techniques in that any type of viral agent, if present in sufficient numbers, may be recognized.

Non-culture methods

There are many situations where isolation of microbes in vitro or in tissue culture is impossible or is insufficiently sensitive to make a microbiological diagnosis. Some microbes are so fastidious or slow-growing that useful information cannot be given to clinicians. The isolation of many viruses requires laborious tissue culture methods that are too slow to influence patient management. Microscopy is usually of low sensitivity, e.g. the threshold of detection of acid-fast bacilli in sputum is about 10^5 microbes per millilitre. Microscopy also has low specificity; for example, Gram staining of faeces would yield millions of Gram-negative rods, but it is not possible to recognize those that are pathogenic by this means.

To overcome these deficiencies probes have been developed which combine a part that reacts with a specific microbial structure and a part that will produce a signal (colour, fluorescence or radio-activity) after the reaction. Many microbes are detectable in this way. Antibodies labelled with fluorescent molecules are widely used in diagnostic virology, e.g. for respiratory secretions to find respiratory syncytial virus. Enzyme-linked antibodies are available as enzyme-linked immunosorbent assay (ELISA) kits for chlamydia detection, and many other *immunoprobes* are commercially produced or under investigation. The explosion in molecular biology has led to the widespread availability of DNA and RNA probes, which have changed from complicated research techniques requiring radio-isotopes to relatively simple methods that can be carried out with minimal expertise. Use of the *polymerase chain reaction* (see p. 71) has greatly increased the sensitivity of nucleic acid probes. Provided a unique sequence of nucleotides is used, the method is highly specific. None the less, as the new technology becomes more commonplace traditional methods will not be discarded. It is more likely that it will complement them.

One of the chief advantages of probes – their specificity – is also one of their major disadvantages. For example, in the investigation of diarrhoea, it would be impossibly laborious to have to use a separate probe for each of the possible microbial causes. The advent of 'chip' technology may overcome this deficiency. Furthermore, use of probes leaves little scope for detection of the unexpected and hampers the discovery of previously unsuspected aetiological agents of disease.

Serology

In situations in which microbial isolation is impossible and probes are unavailable, evidence of infection may be obtained by finding a rise in antibody titre or the presence of specific IgM. Serology is still the most common method of diagnosing the causes of 'atypical' pneumonia (mycoplasmal pneumonia, psittacosis, Legionnaires' disease), syphilis, brucellosis and many viral infections, including HIV. It is preferable to take a blood sample early in the illness (the *acute serum*) and another 10–14 days after the onset (the *convalescent serum*); a four-fold or greater rise in antibody titre in the second specimen is diagnostic of acute infection. With some infections, such as HIV and hepatitis B and C, much longer times must elapse.

Isolation of micro-organisms

The basis of the study of medical microbiology was laid over a century ago by the isolation of microbes in pure culture outside the host animal. The methods used by the fathers of bacteriology have been adapted, simplified and, in some cases, automated for the modern diagnostic laboratory. The principles remain the same: use sterile equipment and media (with cell lines if necessary) and add clinical material. After incubation at 37°C, for a variable time, from a few hours for enterobacteria to weeks for mycobacteria and some viruses and fungi, a visible effect will be produced. This might be colonies growing on agar or a cytopathic effect (CPE) in tissue culture. The skill of microbiology is in identifying the microbes responsible for the effect.

There are limits to the methods that can be used in a routine hospital laboratory to isolate microbes. The choice of media used is dictated by the specimen and by the clinical condition of the patient. For example, in some areas of the world there is little point in looking for *Corynebacterium diphtheriae* in every throat swab, so that the specific media needed are not routinely used. It is therefore incumbent on the doctor to make sure that the laboratory is alerted to look for diphtheria bacilli in any suspicious case. Similarly, clinicians need to know which microbes are routinely sought from particular specimens so that they can make a special request if they suspect the unusual.

'New' causes of illness are often found and new methods of investigating old diseases regularly appear on the market. It is a difficult decision for the laboratory manager to assess at what point a 'new' pathogen becomes sufficiently important to be routinely sought, or to balance the advantages of new (and expensive) technology against cheap and well tried techniques.

Identification

The full identification of each microbe isolated in a clinical laboratory is both uneconomic and unnecessary. Short-cuts must be made to satisfy the clinical demand of a final report which the doctor can understand and which is available in time to influence management of the patient. In practice, most laboratories use simple and incomplete methods of identification, depending on the level of useful information required. Typing of isolates is for epidemiological or other special reasons, and this is usually done in national reference centres using standardized methods.

Examples of the extent of identification are shown in Table 65.3. This shows that the same organism may not be identified even to the genus level, or it may have extensive genetic investigation depending on the reason for the request. In a cost-conscious climate you get what you pay for and what the service thinks you need!

Table 65.3 Examples of bacterial identification in medical laboratories

Reason for request	Extent of identification	
	Example 1	Example 2
Test of sterility	Bacteria present	
Initial blood culture report	Gram-negative rod	Gram-positive cocci
Urine examination	'Coliforms'	Staphylococci
Wound swab	Escherichia coli	Staphylococcus aureus
Outbreak epidemiology	Esch. coli O157	Staph. aureus phage type 80/81
Pathogenicity tests	Esch. coli O157 Vero toxin-producing	Staph. aureus enterotoxin A-positive

Antimicrobial sensitivity testing

One advantage of good bacterial identification is that it helps greatly in choosing antibiotics and in some situations in-vitro tests of susceptibility are unnecessary. However, the widespread occurrence of bacterial resistance, even in genera such as *Neisseria* and *Haemophilus* in which sensitivity to β-lactam antibiotics was previously assumed, has meant that tests are often performed on all significant clinical isolates of bacteria. The relevance of information generated in the extremely artificial conditions of the laboratory is discussed in Chapter 66.

As there are technical problems in carrying out sensitivity tests at the same time as the primary culture, the report will be delayed for at least 24 h after isolation of the pathogen. Tests of slow-growing bacteria such as mycobacteria take much longer and tests involving fungi, viruses and protozoa are not ordinarily available. In general, all patients with acute symptoms will receive treatment before the report returns to the doctor so that the result will merely confirm that correct treatment had been chosen. Sometimes, the laboratory report will allow speculative antimicrobial therapy to be modified, e.g. by allowing one or more drugs in a precautionary mixture to be discontinued.

A frequent difficulty facing microbiologists is which, out of a rapidly increasing number of agents, should be tested and, of those tested, which should be reported. Most laboratories test a few representative compounds from among the many penicillins, cephalosporins, aminoglycosides, tetracyclines, quinolones, etc., and restrict those reported to the clinician to two or three agents selected for their appropriateness in the particular infection. In this way, institutional antibiotic policies are re-inforced and the impact of the promotional activities of pharmaceutical companies is lessened. If the primary agents are unsatisfactory for any reason, a telephone call to the laboratory will establish what other agents have been tested, or what further tests may be useful.

REPORTS OF RESULTS

Just as it is important to obtain as accurate a result as possible, so it is vital to transfer the information rapidly to the user of the laboratory in a form that is easily intelligible. Laboratory workers need to tailor their reports to suit their customers and to recognize their needs. Trained microbiologists are used to the vagaries of microbial taxonomy and the profusion of antibiotics with similar names, but physicians and surgeons are easily confused by laboratory jargon and changes in nomenclature. On the other hand, clinicians rightly expect laboratory reports to be explicit and helpful. As in so many spheres of health care, a spirit of mutual respect and co-operation is in the best interests of the patients, and this is most likely to happen if microbiologists regularly visit the wards and if clinicians are encouraged to discuss problems with laboratory staff.

In these days of computers and facsimile machines it is attractive to use the latest technology to transfer results, but the personal touch is essential, particularly for important results such as positive blood or CSF cultures. Clinicians dealing with difficult problems enjoy the reassurance that the laboratory has found the cause of a patient's illness and advice on management is generally well received. Seeing the problem for oneself and discussing it with the responsible doctors is the ideal. The telephone is a satisfactory substitute in many cases and is far preferable to a report form printed by a computer and arriving after the crisis is over. It behoves us all to communicate better and faster.

NOTIFICATION OF INFECTIOUS DISEASES

In addition to making a clinical diagnosis and treating the individual there is a need with some infectious diseases to determine the source and prevent further spread. In some countries there are public health laws specifying the method of reporting these. The list of *notifiable diseases* in England and Wales is shown in Table 65.4. This reporting system requires a clinical diagnosis, although laboratory confirmation may be sought separately. In England and Wales each health district has a consultant responsible for communicable disease control, who is usually the 'proper officer' for the local government authority. Notifications are sent by this officer to the Office of National Statistics (ONS) and the Communicable Disease Surveillance Centre (CDSC).

There is also an obligation, which in some circumstances may be statutory, for laboratories to report isolates of certain pathogens to central authorities for surveillance purposes. For HIV/AIDS infection the system is voluntary and confidential, yet over 90% of cases are reported to CDSC. In an outbreak, or where the pathogen is highly infectious, it is essential for the head of the laboratory to inform both the clinician looking after the patient and local communicable disease control staff. In this way a co-ordinated approach can be made to prevent further spread of infection.

Table 65.4 List of notifiable diseases in England and Wales

Acute encephalitis	Ophthalmia neonatorum
Acute poliomyelitis	Paratyphoid fever
Anthrax	Plague
Cholera	Rabies
Diphtheria	Relapsing fever
Dysentery (amoebic or bacillary)	Rubella
Food poisoning	Scarlet fever
Leprosy	Smallpox
Leptospirosis	Tetanus
Malaria	Tuberculosis
Measles	Typhoid fever
Meningitis	Typhus
Meningococcal septicaemia	Viral haemorrhagic fever
(without meningitis)	Viral hepatitis
Mumps	Whooping cough
	Yellow fever

RECOMMENDED READING

Baron E J, Finegold S M 1990 *Bailey and Scott's Diagnostic Microbiology.* C V Mosby, St Louis

Collee J G, Fraser A G, Marmion B P, Simmons A 1996 *Practical Medical Microbiology*, 14th edn. Churchill Livingstone, Edinburgh

Johnson F B 1990 Transport of viral specimens. *Clinical Microbiology Reviews* 3: 120–131

Murray P R, Baron E J, Pfaller M A 1999 *Manual of Clinical Microbiology*, 7th edn. American Society for Microbiology, Washington, DC

66

Strategy of antimicrobial chemotherapy

R. C. B. Slack

In the previous chapter the work of the laboratory in assisting doctors in making a definitive microbiological diagnosis was described and summarized in Figure 65.1. Ideally, management of an infection should involve these stages plus choice of an appropriate antimicrobial agent (if necessary) and follow-up tests of cure. Chapter 5 listed the different classes of antimicrobial agents from which the doctor may prescribe. The objectives of an antibiotic strategy are to implement clinical guidelines which cover the treatment of an individual patient and policies based on these which will have a maximum public health effect. These

include cost-effectiveness and limiting the spread of antibiotic resistance.

CHOICE OF TREATMENT

Infections are so common in general practice that it is not practical for each patient to be fully investigated and a rational choice of antimicrobial agent made on the results. Because many have a viral aetiology and most respond rapidly to simple symptomatic relief, the choice is not which agent to use but whether to prescribe at all. Many

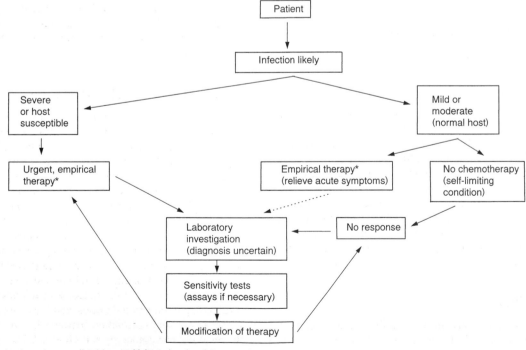

*Choice based on predictable sensitivity or local resistance patterns.
Broken line indicates a course of action that will depend on circumstances

Fig. 66.1   General strategy of antimicrobial chemotherapy.

patients who make the effort to see a doctor expect drug treatment. Although the time taken to educate the public and convince the individual is often longer than that needed to write a prescription, it is important that prescribers do not yield to pressure if antibiotics are not indicated. Figure 66.1 shows a flow diagram of choice of antibiotics which is applicable to many common conditions. There are three main points in the diagram:

1. Patients may be categorized on clinical grounds into those with mild, moderate or severe infection and also into those who were previously healthy or have underlying disease which may affect their response to therapy; for example, impaired immunity or the presence of a foreign body. In the latter situation it is more important to send specimens to the laboratory and start empirical therapy to cover likely pathogens.

2. The organisms causing many common clinical syndromes have predictable antibiotic sensitivities, allowing a rational choice to be made.

3. The results of laboratory tests may lead to modification or withdrawal of chemotherapy.

Although 'best guess' or empirical therapy is commenced before the results of laboratory tests are available, it is wrong to argue that this approach is incorrect since early administration of an antimicrobial is sometimes life-saving.

LABORATORY MONITORING

Susceptibility tests

As well as providing routine tests of sensitivity on individual isolates, the laboratory should provide a general picture of the prevalence of different pathogens occurring in the local population and their pattern of resistance. Different lists should be prepared and regularly circulated to general practitioners, hospital consultants and specialized units. The methods used and limitations of susceptibility testing are outlined in Chapter 5. Sometimes individual patients will need to be monitored for the efficacy of treatment and to determine if failure has occurred due to acquired resistance or replacement with a more resistant organism. This is especially important in the assessment of new agents in clinical trials.

Antibiotic assay

Rapid methods are now available to determine the amount of antibiotic in serum and other body fluids during treatment. These assays can be used to monitor the adequacy of dosage or to avoid possible toxic effects of overdosage.

In practice, it is necessary to carry out such assays only in a small minority of patients in hospital: those who are seriously ill with infections such as endocarditis; those receiving potentially toxic agents such as aminoglycosides and vancomycin; and those who may be compromised with regard to absorption or excretion of the drug.

The interpretation of the results of antibiotic assays may be difficult if the patient is receiving multiple antibiotics. In such cases, the power of the body fluid to inhibit or kill the infecting organism in vitro may be a more useful measurement of adequate dosage; for example, in bacterial endocarditis, the patient's serum should kill the causative organism at a dilution of 1 in 4 or more.

It is important to know the relationship of the sample being assayed to the time of dosage: maximum or *peak* levels are usually measured in serum 0.5–1 h following a dose; minimum or *trough* levels are from a sample taken shortly before the next dose.

Assays should always be carried out in close collaboration with the microbiologist to ensure the correct timing of samples and to avoid errors of interpretation.

Assay of urine

Urine samples may be screened for antibacterial activity. This can be of value in determining patient compliance with treatment and also in interpreting the culture result in relation to possible inhibition by residual antibiotic.

Clinical correlation of laboratory tests

The epithet *sensitive* or *resistant* is a clinical description; in laboratory tests it is usual to select a concentration of the agent which is known to be easily attained in serum, other body fluids or tissue after normal recommended dosage. Organisms susceptible to this, or lower concentrations, are regarded as sensitive; those able to grow are resistant. These terms relate to the *minimum inhibitory concentration* (MIC) of the microbe (see p. 59). The correlation between this interpretation and clinical results is generally good, but not perfect. Discrepancies may be due to a failure to attain adequate concentrations at the site of infection, resulting in clinical failure. However, there are many factors on which the outcome of the host–parasite relationship in infection depends, and it would be surprising if a complete correlation between in-vitro tests and the results of chemotherapy was observed. The best correlation occurs with penicillin treatment of acute gonorrhoea in males, where outcome is easy to assess and single-dose therapy is standard.

PREDICTABLE SENSITIVITY

Once the identity of an infecting organism is known, the sensitivity pattern is often predictable with a fair degree of accuracy. Not surprisingly, however, the susceptibility of common pathogens may change with time. Thus, predictable sensitivity of micro-organisms, while useful, is a changing concept and will have local variations, so that the advice of local microbiologists should be sought.

Organisms with predictable sensitivity patterns

Streptococcus pyogenes is a good example of an organism that has retained a sensitivity pattern that has changed little in 50 years. Thus, penicillin is always the drug of choice for the treatment of haemolytic streptococcal infections. Other β-lactam antibiotics are also uniformly active against *Str. pyogenes*. Erythromycin is an alternative if the patient cannot be given penicillin because of allergy, but an increasing number of strains in some areas show some resistance to this antibiotic in vitro.

Until recently, most strains of *Str. pneumoniae* were highly sensitive to penicillin. An increasing number of penicillin-resistant pneumococci are now found in cases of invasive disease in some institutions, and are posing a major problem worldwide.

Table 66.1 Examples of organisms and antimicrobial agents for which susceptibility is *usually* predictable

Organism	Antimicrobial agents normally active
Streptococci	Penicillin, erythromycin, vancomycin
Enterococci	Ampicillin, vancomycin
Anaerobic cocci	Penicillin, erythromycin, metronidazole
Staphylococci	Flucloxacillin, clindamycin, fusidic acid, gentamicin, vancomycin
Haemophilus influenzae	Co-amoxiclav, tetracycline, cefotaxime, erythromycin
Escherichia coli / *Proteus mirabilis*	Gentamicin, cefotaxime, co-amoxiclav, ciprofloxacin
Pseudomonas aeruginosa	Gentamicin, ceftazidime, azlocillin, ciprofloxacin, imipenem
Bacteroides fragilis	Metronidazole, cefoxitin, co-amoxiclav
Rickettsiae / Chlamydiae	Tetracyclines, macrolides, rifampicin
Mycoplasmas	Tetracyclines, erythromycin
Candida albicans	Nystatin, amphotericin B, azoles
Herpes simplex virus	Aciclovir

Table 66.2 Examples of organisms and antimicrobial agents for which resistance is usually predictable

Organism	Antimicrobial agents *NOT* normally active
Streptococci / Enterococci	Aminoglycosides, nalidixic acid, aztreonam
Staphylococci	Most penicillins[a], nalidixic acid, aztreonam
Escherichia coli	Penicillin, vancomycin, erythromycin, metronidazole
Klebsiella spp.	Most penicillins, erythromycin, metronidazole
Pseudomonas aeruginosa	Most penicillins and cephalosporins, erythromycin, metronidazole
Anaerobes	Aminoglycosides, aztreonam, nalidixic acid, fluoroquinolones

[a] Except methicillin and isoxazolylpenicillins.

Reproducible patterns of sensitivity to antimicrobial drugs can be shown for many other groups of bacteria and offer a useful guide to the choice of chemotherapy (Table 66.1). However, exceptions to these patterns occur and resistant variants may become prevalent in some localities, particularly under the pressure of intensive antibiotic usage.

In the same way that organisms may exhibit predictable sensitivity to some agents, they may be predictably resistant. Some examples are shown in Table 66.2.

ORGANISMS OF VARIABLE SENSITIVITY

Many groups of pathogenic bacteria, notably staphylococci and enterobacteria, vary unpredictably in their sensitivity to antimicrobial drugs. With these organisms there is a greater need to carry out sensitivity tests on individual isolates.

Staphylococci

Staphylococci, including coagulase-negative strains, show great variability in susceptibility, and this can severely limit choice of antibiotics. Four main kinds of staphylococci may be encountered:

1. *Penicillin-sensitive strains.* Before the widespread use of penicillin in the 1940s, most *Staphylococcus aureus* isolates were sensitive. Usually these strains are

susceptible to other antistaphylococcal agents (macrolides, aminoglycosides and fusidic acid). Penicillin-sensitive strains now account for about 10% of isolates.

2. *β-lactamase-producing strains*. Staphylococcal penicillinase confers resistance to all penicillins except methicillin, the isoxazolyl group (cloxacillin etc.) and nafcillin. These strains usually retain susceptibility to cephalosporins. Most *Staph. aureus* and *Staph. epidermidis* strains found in clinical practice belong to this group.

3. *Methicillin-resistant strains (MRSA)*. Methicillin, the first penicillinase-stable penicillin, is used as the test compound to identify these strains in the laboratory. Strains of *Staph. aureus* resistant to methicillin are also resistant to virtually all β-lactam agents. MRSA have epidemiological significance as a group and have been isolated from hospital outbreaks in different countries. Many of these epidemic strains are multi-resistant, exhibiting resistance to aminoglycosides, macrolides and other antistaphylococcal agents, including the topical compound, mupirocin, which has been used to eradicate the organism from carriers of MRSA. Vancomycin, teicoplanin or linezolid may be the only agents available for treatment.

4. *Other antibiotic-resistant strains*. Multiple resistance to antistaphylococcal antibiotics may be seen in strains which are methicillin-sensitive. They are found in similar situations to MRSA, namely hospital units with severely debilitated patients and problems with cross-infection. Such resistance patterns are more common in coagulase-negative staphylococci.

Enterobacteria

Escherichia coli includes many strains of variable sensitivity, but among the general population in the UK most strains (about 60%) are sensitive to ampicillin and amoxicillin, and an even higher proportion are sensitive to cephalosporins, co-amoxiclav (the combination of amoxicillin and clavulanic acid) and trimethoprim.

Variable sensitivity is also a feature of other enterobacteria. Multi-resistant typhoid is a particular problem in many countries where the disease is endemic. If there is doubt about the clinical response, or the sensitivity of the strain, laboratory tests should be carried out.

Other organisms

Several pathogens which were formerly reliably sensitive to standard agents, including neisseriae, *Haemophilus influenzae*, pneumococci, enterococci, mycobacteria and *Plasmodium falciparum*, are now commonly resistant to first-line therapy. In some cases, options for treatment of infection with these organisms have become severely constrained.

ANTIBIOTIC POLICIES AND THE CONTROL OF RESISTANCE

The benefits of the use of antibiotics, not only in medicine but also in animal husbandry, must be taken into account in considering the merits of restrictive policies undertaken to control antibiotic resistance.

There is, without doubt, a problem of resistance among many commonly occurring micro-organisms. Indeed, difficulties are already being experienced with infections highly refractory to therapy with available agents. However, most of the problems of resistance occur among patients susceptible to colonization by resistant strains within closed communities such as hospitals. This is most marked in areas of intensive care, where large amounts of antibiotics are used in highly susceptible patients with low immunity to infection. In the general community, multiple resistance to antibiotics is presently not a major problem, but the spread of MRSA out of hospitals into nursing and residential homes may herald a change in this situation.

Accordingly, attention should be directed to those hospital units in which the problem of resistance is significant and which may be the most important source of spread to the general community. As resistance in bacteria has many of the features of an epidemic disease, the application of classic rules for the prevention of infection may prevent the spread of antibiotic-resistant organisms from such units.

Restrictive policies

The use of antibiotics by general practitioners and clinicians is influenced by the prescribing habits of other medical colleagues and by the promotional efforts of the pharmaceutical companies. Thus, an ordered and systematic use of antimicrobial drugs might be of benefit in the general strategy of chemotherapy. Since the use of antibiotics acts as a powerful selective factor in the emergence and spread of resistant micro-organisms, restriction of use should have the opposite effect and reduce the proportion of resistant organisms in a community. The acceptance of this thesis has encouraged restrictive policies involving temporary bans on the use of certain antibiotics. Such policies may also lead to a reduced chance of prescription error and some cost benefits.

Rotational policies

Periodic changes of antibiotics used in treatment might also help to avoid the emergence of resistant strains by altering the selective pressures and discouraging opportunistic pathogens such as *Pseudomonas* and *Acinetobacter* species. Such a rotational policy might help to retain the therapeutic value of antibiotics over a longer period. The availability of a large range of clinically useful antibacterial substances (Table 66.3) makes this kind of policy more practicable.

PROPHYLACTIC USE OF ANTIBIOTICS

The unnecessary prophylactic use of antibiotics should be discouraged since this may result in increased selection of resistant variants or superinfection with resistant flora. However, there are several circumstances in which chemoprophylaxis is clearly beneficial.

A widely accepted use of antimicrobial agents for the prevention of infection is in patients who have suffered from rheumatic fever, or are thought otherwise to be at risk of rheumatic carditis to prevent further streptococcal infection. Among other indications for chemoprophylaxis are the use of peri-operative antibiotics in patients undergoing joint replacement to reduce the chance of potentially disastrous infection. Similarly, patients undergoing lower bowel resection receive peri-operative treatment with combinations of agents intended to suppress the lower bowel flora. The clinical and laboratory evidence for the benefit of these kinds of prophylaxis is now well established.

Table 66.3 Main groups of antibiotics available for clinical use

Antibacterial agent	Route of administration	Antibacterial spectrum[a]	Some indications for therapy
Phenoxymethylpenicillin	O	+	Streptococcal infections
Benzylpenicillin	P	+	Community-acquired pneumonias/meningitis
Ampicillin Amoxicillin }	O, P	+ and −	Respiratory, hepatic, biliary infections
Flucloxacillin	O, P	+	Staphylococcal infections
Co-amoxiclav	O, P	+ and −	Infections due to β-lactamase-producing organisms
Imipenem	P	+ and −	Serious infections with mixed organisms
Cephalosporins	O, P	+ and −	Respiratory and urinary infections; staphylococcal infections
Aminoglycosides	P	−	Gram-negative coliform infections; endocarditis (with penicillin) pseudomonas infections
Macrolides	O, P	+	Streptococcal and staphylococcal infections and those due to legionellae, campylobacters, chlamydiae and coxiellae
Tetracyclines	O, P	+ and −	Respiratory infections and those due to chlamydiae, mycoplasmas and rickettsiae
Chloramphenicol	O, P	+ and −	Serious infections due to *Haemophilus influenzae*, salmonellae and rickettsiae
Fusidic acid	O, T	+	Staphylococcal infections
Glycopeptides	O, P	+	Resistant staphylococcal infections; *Clostridium difficile* enteritis
Trimethoprim Co-trimoxazole }	O, P	+ and −	Urinary and respiratory infections; salmonellosis
Imidazoles	O, P	+ and −	Anaerobic infections
Sulphonamides	O, T	+ and −	Intestinal and eye infections
Fluoroquinolones	O, P	+ and −	Urinary infections; pseudomonal infections; salmonellosis

O, oral; P, parenteral; T, topical; +, mainly active against Gram-positive bacteria; −, mainly active against Gram-negative bacteria.
[a] See also Table 5.1, p. 46.

Chemoprophylaxis is also justified in preventing pneumococcal infection in splenectomized patients and pneumocystis pneumonia in people with human immuno-deficiency virus (HIV). In healthy individuals who are close contacts of infectious diseases such as meningococcal meningitis, short courses of antibiotics are justified to prevent acquisition of the organism or to eradicate carrier status. Travellers to regions in which malaria is endemic should take antimalarial prophylaxis.

HOST FACTORS INFLUENCING RESPONSE

In most individuals with normal immune systems an antimicrobial drug assists in a more rapid recovery from infection, but the choice of agent is often not critical providing it has some effect on the causative organisms. In very serious infections or when the patient is at a disadvantage because of impaired or absent immunity, the role of the antibiotic becomes more important and more care should be taken in its selection, dosage and administration.

Problems of toxicity

The final choice of the most appropriate antimicrobial drug may be influenced by the history and responses of the patient. Known hypersensitivity to a drug such as penicillin means that neither this antibiotic nor other penicillins can be safely given and alternatives must be used. Side-effects such as nausea, vomiting, diarrhoea or pruritis may be severe enough to warrant a change in treatment. Some antibiotics have potentially serious side-effects, such as the ototoxicity of the aminoglycosides, and care must be taken to avoid these by laboratory monitoring of drug levels, since such toxicity is usually dose-related. Intercurrent disease may require modification of the dosage of certain antibiotics because of specific organ deficiency, e.g. liver failure or impaired renal function. Ototoxicity of the aminoglycosides must always be borne in mind in patients who have poor renal function.

Failure to reach the site of infection

The absorption of oral antibiotics varies widely from patient to patient and, if poor, may be a cause of treatment failure. Alternatively, infection may be localized within a large collection of pus or at an anatomical site that is penetrated by antibiotics with difficulty. Obstruction to the flow of body fluids may likewise militate against success; this is important in infections of the urinary tract, biliary system and the central nervous system. In some of these cases more radical interference may be indicated to relieve the obstruction.

Alteration of normal flora

Antibiotic therapy may upset the patient's microflora and result not only in the selection of resistant strains of commensals, such as staphylococci on the skin, or *Esch. coli* in the intestinal tract, but also colonization with species not normally present. This can lead to antibiotic-induced infection, such as candidosis. Diarrhoea is frequently associated with antibiotic therapy, and reflects disturbance of the normal bowel flora. In a few patients the clinical condition can be severe and proceed to pseudomembranous colitis associated with the toxins of *Clostridium difficile* (see p. 240).

Intravenous administration

When antibiotics are given intravenously, they should normally be administered directly into the vein and not added to other infusion fluids; otherwise adequate blood levels of the drug may not be attained owing to excretion outpacing administration. There is also the possibility of incompatibility between the antibiotic and the contents of the fluid. In all cases, the manufacturer's instructions and recommendations about the administration of the drug should be closely followed.

COMBINATIONS OF ANTIBIOTICS

The clinical benefits of the use of combinations of antibacterial agents tend to be exaggerated. The combination of two or more agents has been long accepted in the treatment of tuberculosis, so limiting the selection of mutants resistant to the individual components. The use of β-lactam antibiotics with an aminoglycoside in the treatment of streptococcal endocarditis is also accepted, since the mixture is more bactericidal than the individual components.

A combination of a β-lactam antibiotic with a β-lactamase inhibitor may prevent destruction of the antibiotic. Thus, the enzyme inhibitor clavulanic acid in combination with amoxicillin (co-amoxiclav) restores the activity of the antibiotic against many β-lactamase-producing bacteria.

Potentiation of the antibacterial effect by combinations is referred to as *synergy*; some combinations exhibit a lesser effect than the individual components, and this is called *antagonism*. These interactions are generally displayed in vitro, and it is difficult to establish evidence of advantages or disadvantages in the patient. Thus, the combination of trimethoprim and sulphamethoxazole (co-trimoxazole) can be shown to be synergistic in the test tube, but it has been difficult to demonstrate any clinical benefit, and trimethoprim is now often used on its own to avoid the chance of toxic reactions to sulphonamides.

ANTIVIRAL THERAPY

An increasing number of agents are being used in the prophylaxis or treatment of viral infections (see Chapter 5).

Aciclovir is the most widely used agent at present, and is prescribed for the treatment of herpes simplex and herpes zoster. This drug can be given orally, but in severely ill patients it is administered intravenously; for example, in treating herpes encephalitis. Aciclovir is also used in the prophylaxis and treatment of varicella, particularly in immunocompromised patients. The related compound ganciclovir is available for the treatment of cytomegalovirus infection, but is associated with considerable toxicity.

Amantadine is active against influenza A virus, but not against influenza B virus. This drug, and the related rimantadine, have been chiefly used for the prophylaxis of influenza. The new agents, zanamivir and oseltamivir, are active against both A and B viruses and have been used to modify infection and prevent spread of influenza.

Ribavirin (tribavirin) is useful in the treatment of respiratory syncytial virus infections in children, hepatitis B and C and some haemorrhagic fever viruses, such as Lassa fever.

Zidovudine (azidothymidine) is an inhibitor of HIV and is used in the management of patients with acquired immune deficiency syndrome (AIDS). There are a number of new anti-retroviral agents often used in combination (see p. 57).

ANTIFUNGAL THERAPY

Superficial fungal infections are very common. Systematic fungal disease is relatively rare in the UK, except in patients who are immunosuppressed or otherwise compromised. There are few effective antifungal agents that can be used systemically (see Table 5.4, p. 55) and some have considerable toxicity.

For many years the chemotherapy of superficial fungal infections depended on preparations of benzoic, salicylic or undecanoic acid. More effective is griseofulvin, given orally, sometimes over long periods, for the treatment of dermatophytoses; the new allylamine, terbinafine, seems to be at least as effective in these conditions. Nystatin and other polyenes are used for the topical treatment of superficial candidosis (thrush). Imidazoles such as clotrimazole are also used in the treatment of vaginal yeast infections.

Amphotericin B is used parenterally for the treatment of systemic candidosis, cryptococcccal infections and aspergillosis. Flucytosine is also active against yeasts and has been used in combination with amphotericin B.

Amphotericin B is toxic and treatment has to be carefully monitored to obtain the most satisfactory clinical results. New liposomal formulations of the drug appear to be safer and more effective.

Ketoconazole, and triazoles such as itraconazole and fluconazole, also have a fairly wide range of antifungal activity, and are being used more widely in the treatment of systemic fungal disease because of their relative lack of toxicity, although the development of resistance may be a problem.

CHEMOTHERAPY OF SYSTEMIC INFECTIONS

Serious generalized infection

Patients with serious and often overwhelming generalized infection include those with *bacterial shock syndrome* and others with the symptomatology of acute infection without localizing signs. These syndromes may be related to postoperative infection, to instrumentation, or to the aggravation of a previously mild infection (e.g. extension of a middle ear infection to the brain). Generalized infection may also follow a reduction in the natural resistance of the patient. Such a situation may arise in renal failure, immune deficiency states, in blood dyscrasias and in neoplastic disease. Specific measures used in the treatment of these diseases may further reduce resistance to infection and the clinical features characteristic of infection may be muted or absent.

Appropriate specimens should be submitted to the laboratory before treatment is begun, in an effort to isolate the causative organisms. However, these patients may require immediate treatment and often there will be little indication of the nature of the infecting organism; more than one species may be involved, especially when the source of the infection is within the abdomen. Empirical chemotherapy must therefore cover Gram-positive cocci, Gram-negative bacilli and anaerobes such as bacteroides. A combination of amoxicillin, an aminoglycoside and metronidazole is suitable. Co-amoxiclav improves the spectrum of amoxicillin and allows omission of the metronidazole. Alternatively, an expanded-spectrum cephalosporin such as cefotaxime can be used. Therapy may be subsequently changed according to the results of laboratory tests. If the patient fails to respond after treatment for 3 days, the use of alternative agents should be considered.

In some patients in intensive care and in the immunocompromised, the possibility of systematic fungal infection or activation of dormant viruses, such as cytomegalovirus, must be considered.

It must always be remembered that bacterial toxins are unaffected by antibacterial therapy. Supportive treatment will include correction of fluid and electrolyte imbalance and appropriate treatment of any co-existing organ failure. In future, immunotherapy such as the use of anti-endotoxin preparations may find a place in treatment.

Infective endocarditis

Whenever possible, treatment of endocarditis should be related to the results of sensitivity tests made on the organism isolated from the blood. Formerly, viridans streptococci were the most common isolates and penicillin was the drug of choice. Viridans streptococci are now isolated from only about one-third of patients and the organisms from the remainder are usually relatively resistant to penicillin. In a proportion of cases believed to be infective on clinical evidence, no organism can be isolated and treatment must be empirical.

It seems to be important to kill all the organisms growing in heart valve tissue since the normal body defences find it difficult to penetrate this site to assist the antibiotic. Bactericidal therapy with a penicillin in combination with an aminoglycoside is usually indicated. It is sometimes helpful to carry out bactericidal tests against the causative organism and it may also be useful to monitor the progress of the patient by assays of the bactericidal activity of the serum against the causative organism.

After operations for the replacement of heart valves it may be difficult to isolate an organism and there may be doubt as to whether or not infection has become superimposed. The risk of withholding treatment, however, is so great that empirical treatment may be indicated, and as staphylococcal infection may occur in such circumstances, it is best to include an antistaphylococcal antibiotic.

For the prevention of bacterial endocarditis in patients at risk following dental extraction, 3 g of amoxicillin, given orally 1 h before surgery, is recommended.

Rare causes of infective endocarditis in which blood cultures are negative include infections with *Coxiella burnetti* or certain chlamydiae. The diagnosis of these conditions depends largely upon serological evidence as it is difficult to isolate the organisms. An aetiological diagnosis is important, as treatment with an appropriate antibiotic, usually tetracycline, may be life-saving.

Urinary tract infections

Uncomplicated cystitis

Uncomplicated urinary infections and asymptomatic bacteriuria are common in adolescent and adult women seen in general practice and maternity clinics. Most infections are due to *Esch. coli*, and most are sensitive to a wide range of drugs. In most cases eradication of the organism is achieved after a short course of therapy with an oral agent such as trimethoprim. The remainder will often respond to a second course of treatment, but if the bacteriuria still persists, fuller urological investigation is required since failure of treatment is more usually related to an abnormality of the urinary system than to resistance of the organism.

Recurrence of bacteria within weeks of a short course of treatment is quite common, and patients should have their urine bacteriologically examined 3–7 days after the cessation of any antibacterial treatment and again after 1 month.

Infections following catheterization

Infection of the urinary tract sometimes occurs after instrumentation such as catheterization or cystoscopy; it is almost unavoidable if indwelling catheters are used. Often the strains causing these infections are derived from the hospital environment, and include resistant strains of Gram-negative bacilli, sometimes in mixed culture. Frequently, the patient is not greatly inconvenienced by such infection, and chemotherapy is not indicated in most areas. If therapy is required, elimination of the organisms can be difficult, particularly if there is residual pathology or a degree of urinary obstruction. Sensitivity tests must be carried out to assist in the choice of therapy. The most useful agents are cephalosporins, trimethoprim and ciprofloxacin; for more serious or refractory cases, in which there is the hazard of systemic spread of the infection, parenteral treatment with an aminoglycoside or an expanded-spectrum cephalosporin must be considered.

Recurrent infection

In chronic pyelonephritis and recurrent bacteriuria it may be important to control infection by continuous treatment with antibiotics such as trimethoprim. Unfortunately, some patients may become re-infected with resistant species so that alternative drugs must be used. Thus, long-term therapy may require periodic bacteriological reassessment and sensitivity tests on the flora isolated to indicate when changes in therapy are required.

Prostatitis

Prostatitis is common in men over a wide age range and it is often difficult to obtain categorical evidence of bacterial infection; examination of seminal fluid, prostatic secretions and urine specimens may help. Treatment with trimethoprim, ciprofloxacin or erythromycin is sometimes beneficial as these drugs penetrate well into the prostate, but short-term use is rarely curative.

Prophylaxis during prostatectomy is now well established; cephalosporins such as cephradine or cefotaxime have been used for this purpose.

Respiratory infections

Respiratory tract infections are extremely common, and, although many are primary virus infections, those that are more severe and prolonged usually indicate secondary bacterial invasion. Laboratory diagnosis of these conditions is important since effective treatment depends on use of an antibiotic specifically active against the causative organisms.

Upper respiratory tract infections

A number of bacteria may be associated with sore throat, pharyngitis and sinusitis, including *Str. pyogenes, Str. pneumoniae, H. influenzae* and Vincent's organisms. The most important infections from the point of view of the development of sequelae are those due to *Str. pyogenes*, for which the treatment of choice is penicillin given for at least 7 days to ensure eradication of the organism. All the other important bacterial pathogens will also respond to this treatment, with the exception of *H. influenzae*, for which treatment with amoxicillin, tetracycline, co-trimoxazole or erythromycin is appropriate.

If for some reason a penicillin cannot be prescribed, the antibiotic of choice is erythromycin or co-trimoxazole. Ampicillin and amoxicillin should be avoided if there is any likelihood of glandular fever because these antibiotics tend to cause a rash and prolong the disease. Tetracyclines should be avoided in young children because of the risk of discoloration of developing teeth.

Lower respiratory tract infections

Lobar pneumonia is most frequently caused by pneumococci and penicillin is the drug of choice; erthyromycin or cefotaxime are good alternatives as are some of the newer fluoroquinolones such as levofloxacin or moxifloxacin. Infections due to klebsiellae or other organisms will require treatment with antibiotics according to the results of sensitivity tests; cefotaxime or cefuroxime are usually effective if laboratory confirmation is not available. Other coliform bacilli are rarely involved in pulmonary infections although they often colonize the upper respiratory tract; they seldom require specific treatment.

Among atypical pneumonias, mycoplasma infections respond best to a tetracycline or erythromycin; legionella infections respond to erythromycin, alone or combined with rifampicin.

Bronchopneumonia is most frequently associated with pneumococi or haemophilus, so that amoxicillin, tetracycline or trimethoprim should be effective. More rarely, bronchopneumonia is caused by *Staph. aureus* and flucloxacillin, fusidic acid or clindamycin is urgently required for treatment.

Acute exacerbations of chronic bronchitis are almost invariably associated with either *Str. pneumoniae* or *H. influenzae*. Amoxicillin, tetracycline or trimethoprim is usually effective.

In bronchiectasis, lung abscess or cystic fibrosis, antimicrobial treatment should be prescribed according to laboratory culture and sensitivity test results. Combinations of antibiotics may be effective in some of these patients. In pulmonary tuberculosis, combination treatment, usually with rifampicin, isoniazid and pyrazinamide, is mandatory.

Meningitis

A Gram film and cell count of cerebrospinal fluid (CSF) will usually differentiate viral from bacterial meningitis. If bacteria cannot be seen, initial treatment is with cefotaxime or ceftriaxone. This choice ensures adequate treatment of infections with Gram-negative bacilli (most common in neonates) and of infections with *Neisseria meningitidis, H. influenzae* and *Str. pneumoniae*, which are the most common causes of meningitis in young children. Care must be taken to differentiate *Listeria monocytogenes* infection, as this organism is less sensitive to penicillin and cefotaxime; a combination of amoxicillin and gentamicin is usually used.

When the causative organism is isolated, therapy may be altered to penicillin for meningococcal or pneumococcal infections. *Pseudomonas aeruginosa* meningitis may occasionally occur as a nosocomial infection and should be treated with full doses of gentamicin plus a β-lactam agent such as azlocillin. It is rarely necessary to give intrathecal antibiotics.

Where there is increased CSF pressure, as in spina bifida, shunts are inserted to facilitate the circulation of fluid. These often become contaminated, usually with staphylococci, probably derived from the skin. Antistaphylococcal antibiotics are used to control the growth of the infecting organism in anticipation of replacement of the prosthesis.

Intestinal infections

Mild bacillary dysentery, salmonella food poisoning and other forms of bacterial diarrhoea do not ordinarily require chemotherapy. Indeed, such therapy may make intestinal carriage more likely and increase the risk of the selection of antibiotic-resistant strains. The most important treatment is correction of fluid balance.

Patients with invasive infection (e.g. typhoid and paratyphoid fever) and those with severe bacillary dysentery or cholera may warrant treatment (see appropriate chapters). Even potentially fatal intestinal infections with *Esch. coli* O157 fare worse with antimicrobials than fluids alone. This may be due to excess toxin release.

Many intestinal infections are due to viruses, for which there is presently no specific chemotherapy. Cryptosporidiosis is now being diagnosed more frequently, but is usually self-limiting except in the immunocompromised. Infection with other protozoa, such as *Giardia lamblia* or *Entamoeba histolytica*, requires treatment with metronidazole.

Spread of infection from the bowel may give rise to serious infections and associated toxaemia. If subphrenic, retrocolic or pelvic abscesses form, drainage is the most important aspect of treatment, but antibiotics can assist recovery of the patient. Cephalosporins or an aminoglyoside plus ampicillin are useful in empirical treatment, and metronidazole should be added if bacteroides is likely to be present. Acute peritonitis after non-specific inflammation of the bowel, such as appendicitis, is usually effectively treated with amoxicillin (with or without clavulanate) or cefotaxime combined with metronidazole.

Liver infections

Bacterial infections of the liver and portal pyaemia are best treated with large doses of cefuroxime, cefotaxime, or an antibiotic chosen on the basis of laboratory findings (e.g. ampicillin against enterococci). Liver abscesses occur most frequently by spread via the portal tract of intestinal Gram-negative bacilli, or by retrograde spread in the biliary passages of streptococci (especially *Str. milleri*) and anaerobes from the gallbladder. Ampicillin is selectively concentrated in the bile, and is often useful in treatment of cholecystitis. Amoebic abscess requires prompt and specific treatment with metronidazole, and its possibility should always be kept in mind, particularly in a patient who has been abroad.

Infection caused by the hepatitis viruses B and C has been treated by α-interferon with ribavirin and lamivudine with variable success.

Bone and joint infections

Most infections of bones and joints are due to *Staph. aureus*. Large doses of flucloxacillin should be given in combination with either fusidic acid or clindamycin unless antibiotic resistant strains are involved which may limit the choice to a glycopeptide or linezolid.

Penicillin in prolonged high dosage is the drug of choice for streptococcal arthritis. Where other organisms, such as *H. influenzae*, neisseriae or Gram-negative rods are involved, specifically directed therapy is required.

Genital tract infections

Venereal infections such as syphilis and gonorrhoea are traditionally treated with penicillin, but a proportion of isolates of gonococci are now resistant to this agent, in which case ceftriaxone, co-amoxiclav or ciprofloxacin should be used.

Non-specific infections of the genital tract are common in women; aerobic and anaerobic bacteria, *Candida* species or *Trichomonas vaginalis*, may be involved. Frequently, an abnormal flora is isolated in the absence of an inflammatory exudate, and it may be difficult to decide on the necessity for chemotherapy. Bacterial vaginosis is such a clinical syndrome associated with *Mobiluncus* spp. which responds to metronidazole or amoxicillin. Vaginal candidiasis is usually treated topically with nystatin or an anti-fungal imidazole. In trichomoniasis, metronidazole is indicated.

More serious pelvic infection in women is often associated with chlamydiae, and tetracycline or erythromycin is the drug of choice. Azithromycin is a useful single dose agent for uncomplicated genital infection due to chlamydiae. Infection of the Fallopian tubes usually involves anaerobic bacteria and metronidazole or co-amoxiclav may be prescribed.

Surgical wound infections

Most surgical infections are caused by the patient's own organisms, but some arise exogenously, often by cross-infection. In orthopaedic units, most exogenous infections are due to staphylococci, but in gastro-intestinal units, Gram-negative bacilli and anaerobes are more common. The situation may change from time to time as a result of ecological movements in the microbial flora within the unit, associated with selective pressures of antibiotic use.

Specimens from infected lesions should always be sent to the laboratory, since the identity of the isolate may have epidemiological significance as well as being of importance in the management of the patient. The microbiologist should always be informed of any therapy as this may affect the interpretation of bacteriological tests.

Superficial infections

Skin and soft tissue infections are common in general practice. Most are of bacterial origin, although some have a fungal or viral aetiology.

Common lesions such as boils, carbuncles, impetigo and infected wounds are associated with *Staph. aureus* and *Str. pyogenes*. Systemic treatment with appropriate antibiotics may be indicated in some patients, but topical treatment is often effective. The use of antibiotics commonly prescribed for systemic infections should be avoided in favour of topical antiseptics or topical antibiotics such as mupirocin.

RECOMMENDED READING

Finch RG, Greenwood D, Norrby SR, Whitley RJ 2002 *Antibiotic and Chemotherapy*, 8th edn. Churchill Livingstone, Edinburgh

Greenwood D (ed.) 2000 *Antimicrobial Chemotherapy*, 4th edn. Oxford University Press, Oxford

Kucers A, Crowe S M, Grayson M L, Hoy J F 1997 *The Use of Antibiotics*, 5th edn. Butterworth-Heinemann, Oxford

Mandell G L, Douglas R G, Dolin R (eds) 2000 *Principles and Practice of Infectious Disease*, 5th edn. Churchill Livingstone, New York

Internet sites

WHO Essential Drug Monitor: www.who.int/dap/edmonitor.html
British Society for Antimicrobial Chemotherapy: www.bsac.org.uk/

67

Epidemiology and control of community infections

D. Reid

When you can measure what you are speaking about and express it in numbers, you know something about it; when you cannot express it in numbers, your knowledge is of a meagre and unsatisfactory kind.

William Thomson, Lord Kelvin
(Popular Lectures and Addresses, 1891)

Good surveillance does not necessarily mean the making of right decisions but it reduces the chances of wrong ones.

Alexander Langmuir, 1963

Once is happenstance, twice is coincidence, the third time it's enemy action.

Ian Fleming
(Goldfinger, Jonathan Cape, 1959)

Attempts to observe and record diseases in order to devise means of determining their cause and control have a long history. Hippocrates (460–361 BC) 'the father of medical science' and Herodotus (484–425 BC) 'the father of history' both related environmental factors to health. Hippocrates, when writing of the occurrence of diseases, distinguished between the 'steady state', the 'endemic state' and the abrupt change in incidence, the 'epidemic'.

Probably the first public health measures based on case reports of infectious diseases taken by a European government occurred in 1348 when the Republic of Venice excluded ships with affected people on board in order to control outbreaks of pneumonic plague (the *black death*). Fifty years later, again in Venice, the concept of *quarantine* was introduced when ships from plague-stricken areas had to stay outside the harbours for 40 days (*quaranta giorni*).

Also because of the fear of a plague epidemic, the first of the *Bills of Mortality*, in which causes of death were recorded, was published in London in 1532. In 1662 John Graunt (1620–74), in his book *Natural and Political Observations Made Upon the Bills of Mortality*, was the first to count the number of persons dying in London from specific illnesses and to advocate the value of obtaining numerical data on a population in order to study the causes of disease (Table 67.1). In 1837 the office of the Registrar General was established to develop the work started by John Graunt; the English physician William Farr (1807–83) added reports to those

Table 67.1 Selection of causes of death in London taken from the Bills of Mortality, 1632	
Causes of death	Numbers
Chrisomes[a] and infancy	2268
Consumption[b]	1797
Fever	1108
Aged	628
Smallpox	531
Teeth	470
Abortive and stillborn	445
Bloody flux[c], scouring[d] and flux	348
Dropsy[e] and swelling	267
Convulsions	241
Childbed	171
Measles	80
Ague[f]	43
King's evil[g]	38

[a] A child who died during the first month of life or a child who died unbaptized.
[b] Usually pulmonary tuberculosis.
[c] Dysentery.
[d] Diarrhoea.
[e] Oedema.
[f] Malaria.
[g] Tuberculosis of the skin.

of the Registrar General which dealt with infectious diseases, occupational diseases, accidents or hazardous work conditions.

The importance of keen observation of disease in order to deduce the likely cause has been demonstrated on many occasions. In 1849, 34 years before the identification of *Vibrio cholerae* by Robert Koch (1843–1910), John Snow (1813–58), a London physician, proved by epidemiological observation that cholera is mainly spread by drinking infected water and not through the air in the form of miasmas as was commonly thought at the time. Similarly, William Budd (1811–80), a general practitioner from Devon, showed in 1873 how typhoid was caused, even though it was not until 1885 that the typhoid bacillus was first isolated in the

653

laboratory. More recently, William Pickles (1885–1969), a general practitioner in Wensleydale, Yorkshire, was able to elucidate many of the epidemiological characteristics of hepatitis and other infections well before microbiological advances were to confirm his observations.

From these beginnings the surveillance of infection has assumed national and international proportions. In the UK, information on microbial disease is collated in England and Wales by the Communicable Disease Surveillance Centre (CDSC) at the Central Public Health Laboratory, London, and in Scotland by the Scottish Centre for Infection and Environmental Health (SCIEH) at Ruchill Hospital, Glasgow. The Royal College of General Practitioners also undertakes regular recording of disease voluntarily reported by various practices. Elsewhere, national surveillance is carried out in different countries (e.g. at the Centers for Disease Control and Prevention (CDCP) in Atlanta, USA). On a worldwide basis the World Health Organization (WHO) provides important liaison and support. This international co-operation is vital as 'germs do not recognize boundaries'.

The most outstanding achievement of international surveillance was the development of a programme for smallpox eradication. The multidisciplinary approach adopted by the WHO, in which programmes were community-based with measurable goals and constant monitoring, resulted in the last endemic case being recorded in October 1977; smallpox was officially declared eradicated in December 1979.

EPIDEMIOLOGY: DEFINITIONS AND PRINCIPLES

Epidemiology is usually defined as *the study of the nature, distribution, causation, mode of transfer, prevention and control of disease*. It has also been regarded as 'the natural history of disease' or as 'the human face of ecology'. Closely linked with the study of epidemiology is the concept of surveillance, which is the most effective infection control technique available. Surveillance is defined as: *the epidemiological study of a disease as a dynamic process involving the ecology of the infectious agent, the host, the reservoirs, the vectors as well as the complex mechanisms concerned in the spread of infection and the extent to which this spread will occur*. The three main elements of surveillance of infection are:

1. The systematic collection of pertinent data
2. The orderly consolidation and evaluation of the data
3. The prompt dissemination of the findings, especially to those who can take appropriate action.

Surveillance provides for the recognition of acute problems requiring immediate local, national or international action, and for the assessment of specific problems by revealing trends or facilitating forecasts. It also provides a rational basis for planning and implementing efficient control measures and for their evaluation and continuing assessment. Although particularly appropriate to the study of infectious diseases, epidemiological principles are also used to elucidate the causes of non-communicable diseases.

The infectious process is a dynamic state involving three main factors: the micro-organism, the host and the environment (Fig. 67.1).

The micro-organism

Since few micro-organisms are harmful to humans the concept of *virulence* (i.e. the degree of pathogenicity of an infectious agent indicated by fatality rates and/or its ability to invade and damage the tissues of the host) must be recognized. The degree of virulence depends on *invasiveness* (i.e. the capacity of the organism to spread widely through the body) and *toxigenicity* (i.e. the toxin-producing property of the organism) (see Chapter 8). A second variable is the *dosage* of the organism, and this is closely related to the virulence. A small number of organisms of high virulence is usually sufficient to cause disease in a susceptible person, whereas if the organism is of low virulence it often fails to cause disease. A third variable is the *portal of entry*. Many organisms have a predilection for a particular tissue or organ. For example, the causal organism of typhoid fever, *Salmonella* Typhi, usually causes typhoid only when it enters the human body through the mouth in food or water.

The host

The reaction of the host to a micro-organism will depend on the ability to resist infection. The individual may not possess sufficient resistance against a particular

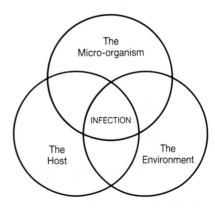

Fig. 67.1 The three main factors involved in the infectious process.

pathogenic agent to prevent contraction of infection when exposed to the organism. Alternatively, the individual may possess specific protective antibodies or cellular immunity as a result of previous infection or immunization. However, immunity is relative and may be overwhelmed by an excessive dose of the infectious agent or if the person is infected via an unusual portal of entry; it may also be impaired by immunosuppressive drug therapy, concurrent disease, or the ageing process.

Herd immunity

Herd immunity is an important element in the balance between the host population and the micro-organism and represents the degree to which the community is susceptible or not to an infectious disease as a result of members of the population having acquired active immunity from either previous infection or prophylactic immunization (see Chapter 69). Herd immunity can be measured:

1. *Indirectly* from the age distribution and incidence pattern of the disease if the disease is clinically distinct and reasonably common. This is an insensitive and inadequate method for those infections which manifest themselves subclinically.

2. *Directly* from assessments of immunity in defined population groups by antibody surveys (sero-epidemiology) or skin tests; these may show 'immunity gaps' and provide an early warning of susceptibility in the population. Although it may be difficult to interpret the data in absolute terms of immunity and susceptibility, the observations can be standardized and reveal trends and differences between various defined population groups in place and time.

The decision whether to introduce herd immunity artificially by immunization against a particular disease will depend on several epidemiological principles:

- the disease must carry a substantial risk
- the risk of contracting the disease must be considerable
- the vaccine must be effective
- the vaccine must be safe.

The effectiveness and safety of immunization programmes are monitored by observing the expected and actual effects of such programmes on disease transmission patterns in the community by appropriate epidemiological techniques.

The environment

The environment plays a major role in the causation, spread and control of infection. In the UK, the virtual disappearance of relapsing fever, plague and cholera, the rarity of indigenous typhoid fever and the relative infrequency of tuberculosis and bacillary dysentery are all indications of the improvements which have taken place in environmental conditions. The decrease in overcrowding and infestation, together with the demand for cleaner water supplies and better sanitation, have been of paramount importance in producing these dramatic advances. This is well illustrated in the case of tuberculosis, which was declining before the availability of chemotherapy and mass BCG vaccination in countries where socio-economic conditions were improving (Fig. 67.2). Paradoxically, better living conditions may unexpectedly create new problems; for example, poliovirus infection, previously experienced

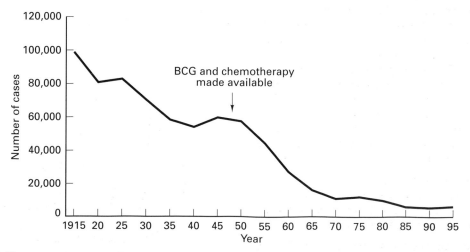

Fig. 67.2 Notifications of tuberculosis in England, Wales and Scotland, 1915–95.

mainly in early childhood, is usually postponed in more favoured communities to older ages when paralysis is a more likely complication unless there is an adequate immunization programme.

THE SPREAD OF INFECTION

Infection spreads in well defined epidemiological patterns. A knowledge of these will lead to an understanding of the best methods of control, or even eradication, and enables an estimate to be made of the likelihood of this happening.

Infection spread directly from one person to another

Among this group can be included such highly infectious diseases as measles. Infection is passed directly from a person with the disease to a susceptible contact. Diseases in this category are usually clinically apparent and healthy carriers are not a feature. When it is possible to diminish the number of susceptibles in the target population then eradication becomes feasible, as has happened with smallpox.

Infection in which healthy carriers are involved

Because apparently healthy individuals may harbour the bacilli responsible for such diseases as typhoid, paratyphoid and diphtheria, often for long periods after having acquired the infection, it is possible for such infections to be transmitted to others and the source remains undetected.

Infection in which persons harbour the organism before the onset of clinical illness

Organisms such as *Streptococcus pneumoniae* may not cause the person any harm until an event such as a skull fracture allows for the transfer of the bacterium from the middle ear to the cerebrospinal space where it can cause a potentially lethal meningitis.

Infection derived from animal sources

Diseases derived from animals, such as leptospirosis, Q fever, anthrax, rabies and brucellosis are known as *zoonoses*. These diseases are spread by direct contact with the animal concerned or indirectly by such means as the ingestion of infected milk, contact with infected bone products, etc.

Infections derived from environmental sources

The spread of legionellae from cooling towers and air conditioning units to cause Legionnaires' disease is an example of illness derived from an infected environment. By dealing appropriately with the infected source by use of biocides in the water the population is protected.

OUTBREAKS OF INFECTION

The crowding together of humans (or for that matter animals, fish or birds) provides the necessary conditions to allow micro-organisms to multiply and spread. When humans led nomadic lives there was less opportunity for outbreaks to occur; the main opportunities came when large numbers gathered for a pilgrimage or had other reasons for a meeting. These clusterings facilitated the spread of infection, resulting in outbreaks; the subsequent dispersal of the group enabled the causative organism to be carried elsewhere.

The threat of outbreaks in overcrowded and difficult conditions is particularly well illustrated in military history; on many occasions the germ has been as important in determining the outcome of a campaign as the sword or gun. The typhoid bacillus caused severe effects during both the American Civil War (1861–65) and the Boer War (1899–1902). The use of typhoid vaccine in the latter years of the First World War meant that the main impact of typhoid in this war subsided after 1916. Similarly, typhus was rife in the Civil War in Britain (1642–49), when both the Parliamentary and the Royalist armies were affected. The pandemic of influenza in 1918–19, in which about 700 million people were affected with approximately 22 million deaths, was a scourge of military camps and affected many servicemen returning home from the First World War.

Nomenclature of outbreaks

The term *outbreak* is often confused with other epidemiological terms used to enumerate infection:

1. *Sporadic case*: a person whose illness is not apparently connected with similar illnesses in another person.
2. *Outbreak*: the occurrence of cases of a disease associated in time or location among a group of persons. A *household outbreak* involves two or more persons resident in the same private household and not apparently connected with any other case or outbreak. A *general outbreak* involves two or more persons who are not confined to one private household.
3. *Epidemic*: the large-scale temporary increase in the occurrence of a disease in a community or region which is clearly in excess of normal expectancy.

4. *Pandemic*: the occurrence of a disease which is clearly in excess of normal expectancy and is spread over a whole geographical area, usually crossing national boundaries.

Types of outbreak

There are three main patterns of outbreak which may be revealed by the construction of graphs of occurrence of cases over time:

1. *The explosive outbreak*. This is characterized by the occurrence of a large proportion of cases in a relatively short period of time (Fig. 67.3); there is a sharp rise and fall in the number of infected persons, since the usual cause of such an event is a common source which infects the people concerned. This type of outbreak is also frequently termed *a common source outbreak* or a *point source outbreak*. This pattern of infection is often discovered when water or food becomes contaminated, although other vehicles of infection can also be responsible for this type of outbreak.

2. *Person-to-person spread*. Outbreaks caused by infections which are spread from person to person have a more protracted course, taking longer than explosive outbreaks to build up and to subside. An infective agent may be passed from person to person by a variety of routes. Diseases such as dysentery, hepatitis type A and gastro-enteritis, which are usually spread by the faecal–oral route, often follow this pattern of spread (Fig. 67.4).

3. *Explosive outbreaks with subsequent person-to-person spread*. This pattern is often apparent when there is contamination of a common water or food source and the initial cases subsequently infect their contacts. Thus, the pattern of the outbreak is a combination of that seen with an explosive outbreak, but followed by a slower decline (Fig. 67.5).

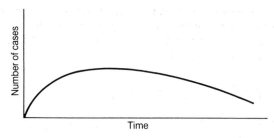

Fig. 67.4 Epidemic curve apparent when there is person-to-person spread of infection.

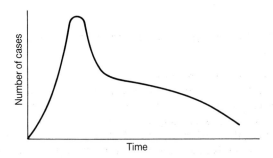

Fig. 67.5 Epidemic curve apparent when there is person-to-person spread subsequent to a common source outbreak.

Analysis of outbreaks

The investigation of an outbreak should be approached in a logical and methodical way. The cause may be elucidated by determining details of the *persons* involved, the *place* where they had been and the *time* when they became ill.

The fundamental pieces of information which should be sought whenever an outbreak occurs are as follows:

1. *WHO gets infected?* What is their age? For example, if a possible food-borne outbreak mainly affects children, could the source be milk or ice-cream?

2. *WHERE were those who became infected?* Where have they recently been? For example, in a hospital outbreak were they all in the same surgical ward? Could a member of the operating staff be a carrier of a pathogen? In a community outbreak of Legionnaires' disease were those affected living downwind from a contaminated source of infection? (Fig. 67.6.)

3. *WHEN did the infection occur?* By knowing the incubation period of the infection it may be possible to trace back to an event which was attended by all those affected.

4. *WHAT was the common factor?* For example, in a food poisoning episode, the ingestion of an article of food by most of those affected but not by those unaffected may be a vital piece of evidence.

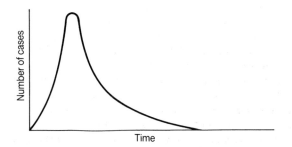

Fig. 67.3 Epidemic curve apparent when there is an explosive (common or point source) outbreak.

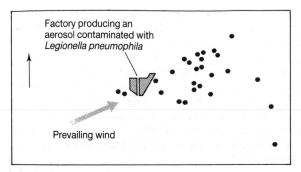

Factory producing an
aerosol contaminated with
Legionella pneumophila

Prevailing wind

Fig. 67.6 Occurrence of Legionnaires' disease in persons living downwind from a factory with an evaporative condenser contaminated with *Legionella pneumophila.*

5. *HOW did those involved become infected?* For example, abscess formation among recently immunized persons might be due to contaminated vaccine.

6. *WHY did the infection occur?* For example, the reheating of meat is often the cause of a *Clostridium perfringens* food poisoning outbreak.

Investigation of outbreaks

In the investigation of outbreaks it is important to have a standardized approach to the various steps involved. Such an approach might have the following as a basis:

1. *Verify the diagnosis.* It is always prudent to confirm that the clinical history is compatible with the diagnosis. Occasional 'pseudo-epidemics' can occur, sometimes resulting from contamination of specimens.

2. *Establish the existence of an outbreak.* The increased interest of an investigator or a change in the mechanism of reporting can sometimes result in an increase in the number of reports of illness. It is important to check the previous level of investigation of a clinical entity or alteration in laboratory methods.

3. *Establish the extent of an outbreak.* Often the number of cases notified is only a proportion of the total number of those affected. It is necessary to seek out the additional cases or vital information may be lost.

4. *Identify common characteristics or experiences of the affected persons.* An individual history from each confirmed or suspected case is required to detect any common factor among those affected (e.g. eating the same item of food).

5. *Investigate the source and vehicle of infection.* In addition to ascertaining the general characteristics of the material suspected as being the source or vehicle of infection, appropriate laboratory investigation will often have to be done. Good co-operation with the laboratory staff is vitally important.

6. *Analyse the findings.* The data should be analysed by the various epidemiological criteria, especially persons, time and place. Denominators should be obtained to calculate attack rates.

7. *Construct a hypothesis.* On the basis of the evidence a hypothesis should be constructed concerning the origin of the outbreak. This may be confirmed by laboratory findings but action to control the outbreak may be needed in advance of such findings.

Control of outbreaks

The investigation of an outbreak should be carried out as swiftly as possible so that adequate control measures can be started without delay. Knowledge of the *source of infection*, the *route of transmission* and the *person at risk* should allow appropriate action to be taken to achieve success.

Sources of infection

These may be:

- human cases or carriers
- animal cases or carriers
- the environment.

If the initial cases have readily identifiable clinical features (e.g. measles) then control is often easier as it is much more likely that the index case will be located. On the other hand, it is more difficult to control diseases in which apparently healthy carriers are responsible, as it is necessary to search for an infected person who may be asymptomatic.

It may be important to isolate the case or carrier, and possibly to institute appropriate treatment, until the patient is no longer infectious. The degree of isolation will depend on the type of disease as not all infections require strict isolation. For example, a patient with a highly infectious disease may require very strict isolation whereas the salmonella excreter will usually need only to cease food handling activities and observe a high standard of personal hygiene until free from infection. In contrast to 'isolation' the term 'quarantine' applies to restrictions on the healthy contacts of an infectious disease.

If an animal reservoir is responsible, action has to be directed at ensuring that the source of infection is eradicated, withdrawn from consumption, or rendered harmless (e.g. by the pasteurization of milk or the adequate cooking of meat).

When the environment is the source of an outbreak the control measures required will depend on the nature of infection and the mode of spread. In recent years, water-borne spread of Legionnaires' disease (e.g. from

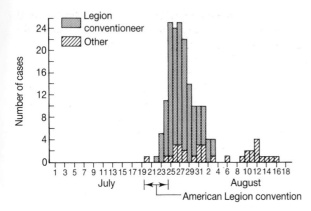

Fig. 67.7 Legionnaires' disease among those associated with a convention in a hotel in Philadelphia (July to August 1976): an example of an explosive outbreak.

shower heads, air-conditioning systems, or droplet spread from cooling towers) has become increasingly recognized (Fig. 67.7). Environmental measures, such as the use of biocides, can destroy the causative legionellae at their source and so prevent further cases.

The hospital setting is particularly dangerous since the presence of compromised patients can result in tragic consequences. Moreover, the increasing use of invasive techniques and the appearance of antibiotic-resistant strains of micro-organisms further compound the problem. In a survey of hospital patients in England and Wales 9% of all patients acquired infection while in hospital. The early detection of infection by effective surveillance, the emphasis on the cleanest possible environment and awareness among the staff of potential problems are among the measures that need to be stressed to control infection among hospital patients (see Chapter 68).

Route of transmission

Infection may be spread by:

- direct or indirect contact
- air-borne transmission
- percutaneous transmission
- food- and water-borne transmission
- insect-borne transmission
- transplacental transmission.

There are various ways in which the routes of transmission occurring during an outbreak may be blocked by measures appropriate to the route involved: effective handwashing; disinfection or disposal, if necessary, of the patient's belongings; and strict adherence to high standards of personal hygiene by the *contacts* of a case are important measures. When the disease is air-borne,

overcrowding should be avoided and, where appropriate, dormitory or ward beds should be well spaced out. The acquired immune deficiency syndrome (AIDS) is a good example of a disease which can be spread *percutaneously* via contaminated needles as well as by other routes. *Food* and *water* should be as free as possible from infection as these are major causes of outbreaks. To deal with *insect-borne transmission*, eradication policies and repellents should be considered. The *transplacental* route is important in the spread of diseases such as hepatitis B.

Persons at risk

Where indicated and feasible, susceptible persons at risk should be protected as soon as possible. Among the measures available, the following may need to be considered:

- immunization
- chemoprophylaxis for close contacts.

Immunity against several infectious diseases can be obtained either by active or passive immunization (see Chapter 69). Examples of rapid effective protection of communities by active immunization are the 'ring vaccination' policy used to protect close contacts of poliomyelitis and so stop more widespread dissemination of poliovirus, and the early (within 72 h of exposure) administration of measles vaccine to close contacts in an institution. Passive immunization, usually by means of human normal immunoglobulin or human specific immunoglobulin, gives rapid protection to contacts of hepatitis A and some other infections, although protection is short lived. Chemoprophylaxis is effective in the protection of close contacts of meningococcal infections and diphtheria.

MATHEMATICAL MODELS

Mathematical modelling techniques attempt to define by use of relatively simple estimates and assumptions, the dynamic conditions governing transmission of communicable agents. With the advent of powerful computers it is possible to calculate many values of likely variables and present them graphically. Details of the multiplication and growth rates of micro-organisms and the spread of infection under natural or experimental conditions need to be known. Measurable factors include:

- the number of infective persons or sources of introduction of infection
- the proportion of susceptible persons in a community at risk
- the duration of immunity

- the introduction of new susceptibles
- the removal rate of infective persons (by isolation, immunity or death)
- the response to vaccines and chemotherapeutic agents.

Mathematical models can be used to predict institutional outbreaks and epidemics. This approach has been used to forecast the number of cases of AIDS, vCJD and BSE that are likely to occur, the effect of control measures such as immunization or the number of cases over time.

ASSOCIATION AND CAUSATION OF INFECTION

A problem commonly encountered by microbiologists and epidemiologists is the attribution of an infectious disease to a particular micro-organism. How do we determine if the relationship is one of causation or merely a chance association? Koch addressed this when he formulated his 'postulates' in 1891. These state that:

1. The organism must always be found in the given disease
2. The organism must be isolated in pure culture
3. The organism must reproduce the given disease after inoculation of a pure culture into a susceptible animal
4. The organism must be recoverable from the animal so inoculated.

For many organisms pathogenic to man it is not possible to fulfil all of Koch's postulates; moreover, they are not applicable to the study of the transmission of infection within a population. For this purpose it is more appropriate to consider the following factors, suggested by the medical statistician Bradford Hill, to establish whether a disease is caused by a particular infectious agent:

1. *Strength*. What is the strength of the association? During the cholera epidemic in London in 1854 John Snow compared the death rates among persons drinking the sewage-polluted drinking water of the Southwark and Vauxhall Company and those receiving the purer water of the Lambeth Company; he discovered that the rate in the former was 14 times higher (Table 67.2). This strength of association allowed Snow to consider that polluted water was a cause of cholera, although at that time the causative organism itself had not been identified.

2. *Consistency*. Similar observations, made by different people at different times in different places, add confidence to a conclusion that causation is likely.

3. *Specificity*. If the association is limited to a specific group of persons, with a specific type of illness, who

Table 67.2 Deaths in London during the cholera epidemic of 1854 according to source of water supply

Water source	Number of houses supplied	Deaths
Southwark and Vauxhall Company (polluted)	10 000	71
Lambeth Company (non-polluted)	10 000	5

have all been subjected to the same specific infection, then a cause and effect relationship can be more strongly suspected.

4. *Temporality*. This can be of especial importance when persons in particular occupations become infected (e.g. leptospirosis in fishworkers). The history of working in a particular environment *before* infection rather than vice versa is particularly relevant.

5. *Biological gradient*. If a dose-response curve is apparent then the evidence for causation is much stronger.

6. *Plausibility*. Is the possibility biologically plausible? The likelihood of veterinary surgeons becoming ill with a zoonotic infection from affected cattle which they have recently been treating seems biologically plausible.

7. *Coherence*. If all the evidence is coherent (e.g. if the same micro-organism is isolated from the index case, the vehicle of transmission and from the victims) this is strong support for causation.

8. *Experiment*. Is the frequency of infection reduced if certain preventative measures are taken? The beneficial effects of the pasteurization of milk to diminish the number of cases of milk-borne salmonellosis is presumptive evidence of a zoonotic relationship.

9. *Analogy*. Has there been similar evidence in the past? The known capacity of the rubella virus to cause congenital abnormalities in the infants of infected mothers makes it easier to accept the possibility of other viruses causing similar problems if maternal infection occurs.

CONCLUSION

Because of the multifactorial causation of infection it is usually necessary to study the epidemiology of infection in a *multidisciplinary* manner. The microbiologist, the clinician, the epidemiologist, the infection control nurse, the veterinarian, the environmental health officer, and other appropriate personnel, must all be involved; the extent of the involvement will depend on the nature of the infection. Success will depend on the expertise and co-operation of these members of the team.

RECOMMENDED READING

Anderson R M, May R M 1991 *Infectious Diseases of Humans: Dynamics and Control*. Oxford University Press, Oxford

Chin J E (ed.) 2000 *Control of Communicable Diseases Manual*, 17th edn. American Public Health Association, Washington, DC

Eylenbosch W J, Noah N D 1988 *Surveillance in Health and Disease*. Oxford University Press, Oxford

Giesecke J 1994 *Modern Infectious Disease Epidemiology*. Edward Arnold, London

Grist N R, Ho Yen D O, Walker E, Williams G R 1993 *Diseases of Infection*, 2nd edn. Oxford University Press, Oxford

Hawker J, Begg N, Blair I, Reintjes R, Weinberg J 2001 *Communicable Disease Control Handbook*, Blackwell Science Ltd, Oxford

Last J M, Abrahamson J H (eds) 2001 *A Dictionary of Epidemiology*. Oxford University Press, Oxford

Mims C A, Nash A, Stephen J 2000 *Mims' Pathogenesis of Infectious Disease*, 5th edn. Academic Press, London

Reid D, Grist N R, Pinkerton I W 1986 *Infections in Current Medical Practice*. Butterworth, London

Pickles W N 1939 *Epidemiology in Country Practice*. Wright, Bristol (re-issued 1972 by the Devonshire Press, Torquay)

Internet sites

Centers for Disease Control and Prevention: www.cdc.gov/
PHLS/CDSC: www.phls.org.uk/
SCIEH: www.show.scot.nhs.uk/scieh/
WHO: www.who.int/
All have links to many other websites worldwide.

68

Hospital infection

R. C. B. Slack

The battle between man and microbe is at its most obvious in institutions where vulnerable people are crowded together. Historically, hospitals have a notorious reputation for infection. The hazards of puerperal sepsis and the horrors of septic infection in the pre-Listerian era have been well documented; admission to hospital in the mid-19th century was associated with the fear of gangrene and death.

Since then, surgical and medical techniques have developed dramatically, basic standards of building and hygiene have greatly improved, and the identification and treatment of most infecting micro-organisms have become possible. Despite such changes, infection acquired in hospitals remains a major cause of morbidity and mortality, leading directly or indirectly to an enormous increase in the cost of hospital care and to the emergence of new health hazards for the community. In the past two decades enormous advances in biomedical technology and therapeutics have produced greater numbers of highly susceptible patients requiring treatment in hospitals, and this is aggravated by the occurrence of transferable resistance to antibiotics in pathogenic bacteria and the emergence of new pathogens transmitted by a variety of routes. In spite of these advances in medical care, in many countries pressures on health care facilities and shortages of trained staff make it difficult to practise adequate infection control. There has also been a mistaken view among many health professionals that the advent of the antibiotic era made such precautions unnecessary, and many studies have shown poor compliance with simple hygiene.

CLASSIFICATION

To measure the extent of hospital-acquired infection and conduct surveillance the following definitions should be considered:

1. Community-acquired infections: either those contracted and developing outside hospitals which require admission of the patient (e.g. pneumococcal pneumonia) or those contracted outside hospital which become clinically apparent when the patient has been admitted to hospital for other reasons (e.g. chickenpox or zoster).

2. Infections contracted and developing within hospital (e.g. device-associated bacteraemias).

3. Infections contracted in hospital but not becoming clinically apparent until after the patient has been discharged (e.g. many postoperative wound infections).

4. Infections contracted by hospital staff as a consequence of their work, whether or not this involves direct contact with patients (e.g. hepatitis B).

On average, around 10% of all hospital patients will develop an infection as a result of their stay in hospital. Urinary, respiratory and wound infections are the most common.

FACTORS THAT INFLUENCE INFECTION

Hospital infection, also known as *nosocomial infection*, may be exogenous or endogenous in origin. The exogenous source may be another person in the hospital (*cross-infection*) or a contaminated item of equipment or building service (*environmental infection*). A high proportion of clinically apparent hospital infections are endogenous (*self-infection*), the infecting organism being derived from the patient's own skin, gastro-intestinal or upper respiratory flora.

Most infections acquired in hospital are caused by micro-organisms that are commonly present as commensals in the general population. Thus, contact with micro-organisms is seldom the sole or main event predisposing to infection. Various risk factors, alone or in combination, influence the frequency and nature of hospital infection.

Susceptibility to infection

Natural resistance to infection is lower in infants and the elderly, who often constitute the majority of hospital patients. Pre-existing disease, such as diabetes, or other conditions for which the patient was admitted to hospital, and the medical or surgical treatment, including immunosuppressive drugs, radiotherapy or splenectomy, may also reduce the patient's natural resistance to disease. Moreover, the natural defence mechanisms of the body surfaces may be bypassed either by injury or by procedures such as surgery, insertion of an indwelling catheter, tracheostomy or ventilatory support.

CONTACT WITH OTHER PATIENTS AND STAFF

In common with any large institution or workplace, the patients and staff of a hospital share many facilities in close or crowded conditions. Outbreaks of diarrhoeal and food-borne disease may be traced to a common source via the hospital water or food supplies. The specific role of hospitals in admitting infected patients or carriers for treatment clearly serves as a potential source of infection for others. Patients with comparable susceptibility to infection tend to be concentrated in the same area, e.g. in neonatal units, burns units or urological wards, where infected and non-infected patients may be cared for by the same staff, thus creating numerous opportunities for the spread of micro-organisms by direct contact. The more susceptible patients usually require the most intensive care with far more daily contacts with staff who act as vectors in the transmission of microbes like insects spreading parasites.

Inanimate reservoirs of infection

Equipment and materials in use in hospitals often become contaminated with micro-organisms which may subsequently be transferred to susceptible body sites on patients. Gram-positive cocci, derived from the body flora of the hospital population, are found in the air, dust and on surfaces where they may survive along with fungal and bacterial spores of environmental origin. Gram-negative aerobic bacilli are common in moist situations and in fluids, where they often survive for long periods, and may even multiply in the presence of minimal nutrients. An important example of this is legionellae in hospital domestic water supplies. Awareness of the common reservoirs of environmental and contaminating hospital micro-organisms provides the basis for maintaining standards of hygiene (cleaning, disinfection, sterilization) throughout the hospital as well as good engineering and building.

Role of antibiotic treatment

At least 30% of hospital patients receive antibiotics, and this exerts strong selective pressures on the microbial flora, especially of the gastro-intestinal tract, leading to the development of antibiotic-associated diarrhoea due to *Clostridium difficile*, one of the commonest causes of outbreaks of hospital infection. Sensitive species or strains of micro-organisms which normally maintain a protective function on the skin and other mucosal surfaces tend to be eliminated, whereas those that are more resistant survive and become endemic in the hospital population. This may restrict the range of agents available for treatment and may lead to the transmission of plasmid-mediated antibiotic resistance into strains that show increased virulence, survival and spread within the hospital.

MICRO-ORGANISMS CAUSING HOSPITAL INFECTION

The most important micro-organisms responsible for hospital infection are listed in Table 68.1.

Outbreaks of *Staphylococcus aureus* infection were often seen in surgical wards and maternity units before the advent of penicillinase-stable penicillins such as methicillin in the early 1960s. Some strains, such as the notorious phage type 80/81, demonstrated particular virulence and colonizing capabilities. Subsequently, epidemic or pandemic strains characterized by resistance to methicillin (MRSA) have been found in many hospitals worldwide, presenting a daunting challenge. Some strains are better able to colonize patients or staff than to produce

Table 68.1 Commonly occurring micro-organisms in hospital infection

Urinary tract infections	*Escherichia coli* *Klebsiella, Serratia, Proteus* spp. *Pseudomonas aeruginosa* *Enterococcus* spp. *Candida albicans*
Respiratory infections	*Haemophilus influenzae* *Streptococcus pneumoniae* *Staphylococcus aureus* Enterobacteriaceae Respiratory viruses Fungi (*Candida* spp., *Aspergilli*)
Wounds and skin sepsis	*Staph. aureus* *Str. pyogenes* *Esch. coli* *Proteus* spp. Anaerobes *Enterococcus* spp. Coagulase-negative staphylococci
Gastro-intestinal infections	*Salmonella* serotypes *Clostridium difficile* Viruses (Norwalk-like)

systemic disease. This illustrates the adaptation and evolutionary changes possible within common hospital bacteria revealed by careful epidemiological typing and observation. The changing patterns may be related to particular events and infection control measures, so that lessons can be learnt for future control and prevention.

With the advent of more elaborate surgery and intensive care, combined with the use of broad-spectrum antibiotics and immunosuppressive drugs, Gram-negative bacteria increased in importance. Many, such as *Pseudomonas aeruginosa*, are *opportunists* capable of causing infection in compromised patients. Such organisms may be found in the patient's own flora, or in damp environmental sites, including patient equipment and medicaments. They may exhibit natural resistance to many antibiotics and antiseptics, and have the ability to colonize traumatized skin such as burns and bed sores.

In recent years, groups of micro-organisms which formerly played no recognized part in hospital infection have emerged. These include the coagulase-negative staphylococci and *Acinetobacter baumanii* present in normal skin flora. Viral or fungal infection, particularly of the immunocompromised patient, has become more important. *Legionella pneumophila*, disseminated from environmental sources such as cooling towers and hot water systems, causes sporadic cases or outbreaks of respiratory infection in hospitals. Awareness of the risks of blood-borne viruses, including hepatitis B and C, human immunodeficiency virus (HIV) and of many agents such as cytomegalovirus, which can be transmitted by organ or cellular transplants, has increased in patients and in staff. The possible risk of iatrogenic spread of the prion causing Creutzfeldt–Jakob disease has persuaded the UK government to take stringent measures on decontamination of surgical instruments and the US blood transfusion service to ban British donors.

ROUTES OF TRANSMISSION

The hospital offers many opportunities for the exchange of microbes, many of which are harmless and a normal part of the balance between man and his environment. For there to be a significant risk of infection, several factors, including the right susceptible host and the appropriate inoculum of infecting micro-organism, must be linked via an appropriate route of transmission. Understanding of the sources and transmission routes of hospital infection enables efforts to be concentrated in more effective preventive measures.

Common routes of transmission for different micro-organisms are shown in Table 68.2.

Air-borne transmission

Infections may be spread:

- By air-borne transmission from the respiratory tract (talking, coughing, sneezing).
- From the skin by natural shedding of skin scales during wound dressing or bed-making.
- By aerosols from equipment such as respiratory apparatus and air-conditioning plants.

Table 68.2 Hospital infection: sources and spread

Route	Source	Examples of disease
1. Aerial (from persons)		
Droplets	Mouth	Measles, tuberculosis, pneumonia
	Nose	Staphylococcal sepsis
Skin scales	Skin exudate, infected lesion	Staphylococcal and streptococcal sepsis
2. Aerial (from inanimate sources)		
Particles	Respiratory equipment	Gram-negative respiratory infection
	Air-conditioning plant	Legionnaires' disease, fungal infections
3. Contact (from persons)		
Direct spread	Respiratory secretions	Staphylococcal and streptococcal sepsis
Indirect via equipment	Faeces, urine, skin and wound exudate	Enterobacterial and viral diarrhoea, *Pseudomonas aeruginosa* sepsis
4. Contact (environmental source)	Equipment, food, medicaments, fluids	Enterobacterial sepsis (*Klebsiella/Serratia/Enterobacter* spp.) *Ps. aeruginosa* and other pseudomonads
5. Inoculation	Sharp injury, blood products	Hepatitis B, HIV, malaria

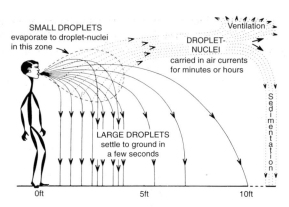

Fig. 68.1 Spread of respiratory infections by droplets and droplet nuclei.

Infectious agents may be dispersed as small particles or droplets over long distances (Fig. 68.1). Staphylococci survive well on mucosal secretions, skin scales and dried pus and may be redistributed in the air after initial settlement during periods of increased activity (Fig. 68.2). Gram-negative bacilli do not generally survive desiccation in air, and this route of transmission is therefore limited to conditions of high humidity such as ventilatory equipment, showers or other fine water aerosols.

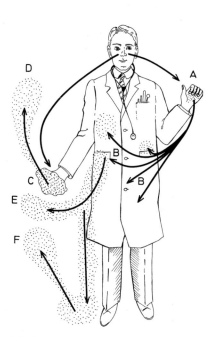

Fig. 68.2 Infection of the air with dust particles derived from nasal and oral secretions contaminating hands, handkerchief, clothing and surrounding surfaces: **A**, hand soiled with secretions from lips or nose-picking; **B**, clothing contaminated by hand; **C**, soiled handkerchief; **D**, infected dust from handkerchief; **E**, dust from clothing (e.g. from near handkerchief pocket); **F**, infected dust raised after settling on floor.

Contact spread

The most common routes of transmission for hospital infection are:

- By *direct* contact spread from person to person.
- By *indirect* contact spread via contaminated hands or equipment.

Human secretions as well as contaminated dust particles or fluids may be carried on thermometers, bed-pans, bed-linen, cutlery or other shared items. Hands and, to a lesser extent, clothing of hospital staff serve as vectors of Gram-negative and Gram-positive infection. Procedures involving contact with mucosal surfaces, e.g. insertion of a urinary catheter, may introduce micro-organisms from the contaminated hands of the operator or from the patient's own urethral flora into the normally sterile bladder.

Food-borne spread

Infection may originate in the hospital kitchen, or in special diets, infant feeds, kitchen or commercial supplies. Deteriorating hygiene standards may support the proliferation of flies, cockroaches and other insects or rodents which damage stored products and act as carriers of microbes.

Blood-borne spread

The accidental transmission of infections such as HIV, hepatitis B or C by needlestick or contaminated 'sharp' injuries has been well documented. In areas of high prevalence of malaria, syphilis and these viruses stringent precautions should be taken to minimize transmission between patients by strict use of single-use items and from health care workers to patients and vice versa by minimizing needlestick episodes.

Self-infection and cross-infection

The interaction between different sources of infection may be illustrated by the example of a patient undergoing lower bowel surgery. *Self-infection* may occur due to transfer into the wound of staphylococci (or occasionally streptococci) carried in the patient's nose and distributed over the skin, or of coliform bacilli and anaerobes released from the bowel during surgery. Alternatively, *cross-infection* may result from staphylococci or coliform bacilli derived from other patients or healthy staff carriers. The organisms may be transferred into the wound *during operation* through the surgeon's punctured gloves or moistened gown, on imperfectly sterilized surgical instruments and materials, or by airborne theatre dust. *Postoperatively*, organisms may be transferred in the ward from contaminated bed-linen, by air-borne ward dust or in consequence of a faulty wound dressing technique.

Of all the possible routes, by far the most likely in this example is self-infection from the patient's own bowel flora and it is therefore against this route that most specific preventive measures in colorectal surgery are directed. Understanding of possible sources of infection and the methods available to block transmission to susceptible sites forms the basis of hospital infection control.

Cross-infection is more often caused by 'hospital' strains selected for characteristics of antimicrobial resistance and virulence. An important example at present is MRSA, which can be easily identified by the microbiology laboratory, which should have a system for alerting the infection control team who need to collect the following basic epidemiological data:

- patient details
- the site and extent of infection
- the dates of admission, operative procedures, first recognition of infection
- specimens and laboratory isolates and typing results
- ward and staff details.

The clustering of cases according to a common surgical team or location in the ward may suggest a common source and may be the first firm indication of an outbreak of hospital infection.

Soon after admission to hospital, individuals commonly become contaminated with the 'hospital flora'. This has been shown with *Staph. aureus* in studies of patients before and during hospital treatment. Patients who need to stay longer in hospital, e.g. those requiring intensive care or the elderly, are less able to withstand infection and the risks of hospital infection are greater.

PREVENTION AND CONTROL

The infection control policy

The establishment of an effective infection control organization is the responsibility of good management of any hospital. There will normally be two parts:

1. An *infection control committee*, meeting regularly to formulate and update policies for the whole hospital on matters having implications for infection control, and to manage outbreaks of nosocomial infection.
2. An *infection control team* of workers, headed by the *infection control doctor* (usually the microbiologist), to take day-to-day responsibility for this policy.

The functions of this team include surveillance and control of infection and monitoring of hygiene practices, advising the infection control committee on matters of policy relating to the prevention of infection and the education of all staff in the microbiologically safe performance of procedures. The *infection control nurse* is a key member of this team. Close working links between the microbiology laboratory, infection control nurse and the different clinical specialties and support services (including sterile services, laundry, pharmacy and engineering) are important to establish and maintain the infection control policy, and to ensure that it is rationally based and that the recommended procedures are practicable. Some of the control measures in which the infection control team should be involved are shown in Fig. 68.3.

Sterilization

The provision of sterile instruments, dressings and fluids is of fundamental importance in hospital practice and is dealt with in detail in Chapter 7. Sterilization by heat in high-vacuum autoclaves has become accepted hospital practice. The development of these sterilizers for processing wrapped goods facilitated the provision of a centralized service of sterile supply to wards, complementing the existing theatre service. The availability of a wide range of prepacked single-use items (syringes, needles, catheters and drainage bags) sterilized commercially by γ-irradiation or ethylene oxide has further improved aseptic procedures and removed the need for reprocessing items that are difficult to clean and therefore impossible to sterilize.

Most fluids for topical use or intravenous administration are now prepared commercially or in regional units where standards of quality control and efficiency for bulk processes are more readily achieved than in individual hospital pharmacies.

Aseptic techniques

The provision of sterile equipment will not prevent the spread of infection if there is carelessness in its use. Wherever possible, *no-touch* techniques must be used, coupled with strict personal hygiene on the part of the operator. These routines are rigidly laid down in operating theatre practice and may be modified as required for other procedures such as wound dressing and insertion of intravenous catheters.

Cleaning and disinfection

The general hospital environment can be kept in good order by attention to basic cleaning, waste disposal and laundry. The use of chemical disinfectants for walls, floors and furniture is necessary only in special instances,

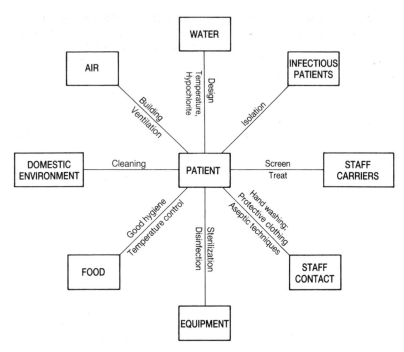

Fig. 68.3 Control measures to reduce exogenous hospital-acquired infection.

such as spillages of body fluids from patients with blood-borne virus infections. Ward equipment such as bed-pan washer/disinfectors and dishwashers should be monitored to ensure reliable performance, and cleaning materials such as mopheads and cloths should be heat-disinfected and stored dry after use. Precleaning of contaminated instruments and equipment, preferably by means of an automatic washing process with an ultrasonicator, is an essential step before disinfection or sterilization.

Skin disinfection and antiseptics

The ease of acquisition and transfer of transient hospital contaminants, particularly Gram-negative bacilli on the hands of staff, is an important factor in the spread of hospital infection. Thorough handwashing after any procedure involving nursing care or close contact with the patient is essential. Alcohol-based hand antiseptics or 'rubs' have been introduced in wards where routine handwashing with water and detergent is not practicable. Gloves may be worn for many dirty contact procedures, such as emptying a urinary drainage bag or bed-pan, although it should not be forgotten that the gloved hand may also become colonized by transient hospital flora.

Procedures for pre-operative disinfection of the patient's skin and for surgical scrubs are mandatory within the operating theatre. Dilute 'in-use' solutions of

antiseptics may readily become colonized with Gram-negative bacteria and should be replaced regularly. Ideally, *single-use* preparations should be used. Restriction should be placed on the indiscriminate use of antiseptics and disinfectants by means of a *disinfectant policy* agreed by pharmacists, microbiologists and key users, such as theatre staff.

Prophylactic antibiotics

Widespread and haphazard use of antibiotics hastens the emergence of antibiotic-resistant bacteria and increases both the incidence of toxic side-effects and the cost of treatment. However, rational antibiotic prophylaxis plays an important role in infection control. Specific indications include peri-operative prophylaxis in gastrointestinal and gynaecological surgery directed predominantly against anaerobic infection and for patients known to have bacteriuria at the time of urological surgery or instrumentation, directed against the urine isolate. An *antibiotic policy* which limits the choice of broad-spectrum agents is important both for prophylaxis and treatment (see Chapter 66).

Protective clothing

Different activities within the hospital require different degrees of protection to staff and patients. In operating theatres the wearing of sterile gowns, gloves, head gear and face masks minimizes the shedding of micro-organisms. The properties of fabrics available for theatre use have improved, and now include close-weave ventile fabrics that are comfortable to wear and allow evaporation of moisture. 'Total protection' of the operating site may be considered for certain high-risk clean surgery such as hip replacements, during which the surgical team may wear exhaust-ventilated suits and operate under conditions of ultraclean laminar air-flow.

For many ward procedures in which there may be soiling, or for simple *barrier nursing* of patients with communicable diseases, plastic aprons and gloves are used. Gloves, face masks and goggles are also indicated for specific procedures when blood contact is likely through splashes or aerosols, such as dental procedures. These are sometimes referred to as '*universal precautions*'.

Isolation

The isolation policy should list facilities and procedures needed to prevent the spread of specific infections to other patients (*source isolation*) and to protect susceptible or immunocompromised patients (*protective isolation*). Effective isolation demands a highly disciplined approach by all staff to ensure that none of the barriers to transmission (air-borne, direct and indirect contact) are breached. Multibedded rooms may be used, and even wards converted during hospital outbreaks, but the simplest solution wherever possible is to use single rooms.

'Cubicle' isolation, by which the patient is nursed alone in a room separated by a door and corridor from other patients, confers a substantial measure of protection. Preferably, each isolation room has its own toilet and washing facility. Clean, filtered air is supplied to the room, which should be at negative pressure (*exhaust-ventilated*) to the corridor for source isolation or at positive pressure (*pressure-ventilated*) to the corridor for protective isolation. If, however, there is a small airlock vestibule separating the room from the outer corridor, then exhaust ventilation of the airlock will give effective isolation for either situation. The vestibule or lobby should contain a wash basin and include space for gowning and equipment.

In some critical situations such as bone marrow transplant units, where air-borne contamination with environmental fungal spores is a problem, the efficiency of air filtration may be increased and laminar airflow maintained as a barrier around the patient. Stringent isolation, such as a plastic tent or 'Trexler' isolator, is required only for patients with highly contagious infections, such as those due to Lassa, Marburg and Ebola viruses, who are nursed in a *high-security isolation unit*.

Hospital building and design

The routine maintenance of the hospital building is important, ensuring that surfaces wherever possible are smooth, impervious and easy to clean. Major rebuilding works on or near the hospital site may generate dust containing fungal and bacterial spores, with implications for specialized units serving immunocompromised patients. Close communications with the works department and hospital administration are necessary to co-ordinate any protective action. When a new hospital or modification of existing building is planned, the infection control team should be closely involved in discussing the plans. In many countries, guidance on new building design exists to minimize potential hospital-acquired infection. Areas requiring special attention include operating theatres, kitchens, acute wards, laboratories and air-conditioning systems. The risk of Legionnaires' disease is reduced by installing water supplies that circulate below 20°C for the cold and above 60°C for the hot circuit.

Equipment

Any object or item of equipment for clinical use should be assessed to determine the appropriate method, frequency and site of decontamination. Wherever possible, heat processes are preferred, although this may be precluded for certain thermolabile items such as fibre-optic endoscopes (see Chapter 7).

Personnel

An occupational health service in hospitals should screen staff before employment and offer appropriate immunization. Hepatitis B vaccine should be given to all health care workers. Those at special risk performing exposure-prone procedures, such as invasive surgery, should be screened for blood-borne viruses. All staff (including medical students) should receive occupational health advice and protection. Staff who have contracted specific infections such as diarrhoea or following needlestick injury should report and be screened if necessary.

Monitoring

Routine microbiological monitoring of the environment is of little benefit, although monitoring of the physical performance of air-conditioning plants and machinery used for disinfection and sterilization is essential. In the event of an outbreak of hospital infection, more specific monitoring targeted at the known or likely causative micro-organism should be considered.

Microbiological screening of staff or patients is not undertaken routinely, but it may be needed for specific purposes: to detect carriers of MRSA and hepatitis viruses in those performing some types of surgery or where transmission to patients has occurred.

Surveillance and the role of the laboratory

The detection and characterization of hospital infection incidents or outbreaks rely on laboratory data that alert the infection control team to unusual clusters of infection, or to the sporadic appearance of organisms that may present a particular infection risk or management problem. This is sometimes referred to as the 'alert organism' system. Bacterial typing schemes and antibiograms (see Chapter 3) are very important in this regard. Regular visits to the wards are also important to record data on infected patients for whom specimens have not been received and to respond to problems as they occur. Such visits also serve to provide opportunities for practical teaching, which is another important element of the infection control team's responsibility.

EFFICACY OF INFECTION CONTROL

The evidence base in the literature for acceptable proof of efficacy for infection control measures is scant.

These include sterilization, hand-washing, closed-drainage systems for urinary catheters, intravenous catheter care, peri-operative antibiotic prophylaxis for contaminated wounds and techniques for the care of equipment used in respiratory therapy. Isolation techniques are assumed to be reasonable as suggested by experience or inference. Measures which are now considered to be ineffective include the chemical disinfection of floors, walls, sinks and routine environmental monitoring.

Effective surveillance and action by the infection control team have been shown to reduce infection rates. One important role of the team is to monitor compliance with practices known to be effective and to eliminate the many rituals or less effective practices which may even increase the incidence or cost of cross-infection. As further advances occur in medical care and limited health care resources are spread across hospital and community needs, innovations in infection control will need to be evaluated for efficacy and cost-effectiveness. With this understanding it is possible that hospital infection can be controlled and largely prevented. The dictum of Florence Nightingale, made over a century ago, that 'the very first requirement in a hospital is that it should do the sick no harm', remains the goal.

RECOMMENDED READING

Ayliffe G A J, Taylor L J, Babb J 1999 *Hospital Acquired Infection*, 3rd edn. Arnold, London
Ayliffe G A J, Fraise A, Mitchell K, Geddes A M 2000 *Control of Hospital Infection*, 4th edn. Arnold, London
Report 1995 *Hospital Infection Control. Guidance on the Control of Infection in Hospitals*. Department of Health and Public Health Laboratory Service, London
Wenzel R P (ed.) 1997 *Prevention and Control of Nosocomial Infection*, 3rd edn. Lippincott, Williams and Wilkins, Baltimore

Internet sites

Centers for Disease Control Hospital Infection Program: www.cdc.gov/ncidod/hip/
Department of Health England Healthcare Associated Infection: www.doh.gov.uk/hai/
Hospital Infection Society: www.his.org.uk/
Infection Control Nurses Association: www.icna.co.uk/
Medical Devices Agency: www.medical-devices.gov.uk
Thames Valley University Evidence Based Guidelines: www.epic.tvu.ac.uk/

69

Immunization

R. C. B. Slack

Immunization is only one of the measures that may be used for the control of infectious diseases (Table 69.1). It has dramatically and successfully rid the world of the scourge of smallpox. Its cost and efficacy must be assessed against other forms of defence, such as:

- environmental sanitation
- safe sewage disposal
- a secure water supply
- food hygiene
- clean air and adequate ventilation
- good animal husbandry with effective quarantine arrangements where necessary
- insect vector control
- improved nutrition.

Much of the morbidity and mortality of infection is still either not assuredly preventable by immunization or presents great difficulties. For example, many of the diarrhoeal diseases and respiratory infections that take a heavy toll of life and health among young children in poor and overcrowded communities are not amenable to control by specific vaccines. Nor are the common bacterial infections associated with haemolytic streptococci, staphylococci and coliform bacilli, or many virus infections. However, some spectacular successes can be claimed, and encouraging efforts are being made to extend the range of success.

Table 69.1 Approaches to the prevention of infectious disease: an indication of priorities

- Preventive engineering: water, sewage, ventilation, food production and food processing
- Surveillance and diagnostic awareness
- Prompt management: recognition, treatment, isolation and contact tracing where necessary
- Improvement and maintenance of good socio-economic conditions: housing, nutrition, education, medical and social care
- Increased resistance to infection by appropriate active immunization policies and in some special circumstances by passive immunization

---

RATIONALE OF IMMUNIZATION

The objective is to produce, without harm to the recipient, a degree of resistance sufficient to prevent a clinical attack of the natural infection and to prevent the spread of infection to susceptibles in the community. There is therefore both a personal gain from being immunized and a public health benefit to the population. The degree of resistance conferred may not protect against an overwhelming challenge, but exposure may help to boost immunity.

PASSIVE IMMUNIZATION

Artificial passive immunization is used in clinical practice when it is considered necessary to protect a patient at short notice and for a limited period. Antibodies, which may be antitoxic, antibacterial or antiviral, in preparations of human or animal serum are injected to give temporary protection. Human preparations are referred to as *homologous*, and are much less likely to give rise to the adverse reactions occasionally associated with the injection of animal (*heterologous*) sera. An additional advantage of homologous antisera is that, although they do not confer durable protection, their effect may persist for 3–6 months, whereas the protection afforded by a heterologous serum is likely to last for only a few weeks.

Antiserum raised in the horse against diphtheria toxin (*equine diphtheria antitoxin*) is available for the prophylaxis and treatment of diphtheria. A similar heterologous antiserum is available for emergency use in cases of suspected botulism and to protect those thought to be at risk. Equine tetanus antitoxin is still used in some countries, but it should be abandoned in favour of human tetanus immunoglobulin (see Chapter 22, p. 239). It is most important to give an intended recipient of equine serum a prior test dose to exclude hypersensitive subjects who may have been sensitized by a previous dose of equine serum and may suffer 'serum sickness'.

Pooled immunoglobulins

Protective levels of antibody to a range of diseases are present in pooled normal human serum. *Human normal immunoglobulin* (HNIG) is available for the short-term prophylaxis of hepatitis A in contacts or travellers who intend to visit countries where hepatitis A is common. However, active immunization is a much better alternative against hepatitis A for frequent travellers to areas where hepatitis A is common. HNIG also protects those with agammaglobulinaemia.

Specific immunoglobulins

Preparations of specific immunoglobulins are available for passive immunization against the following:

- tetanus (human tetanus immunoglobulin; HTIG)
- hepatitis B (HBIG)
- rabies (HRIG)
- varicella–zoster (ZIG)
- vaccinia (AVIG).

ACTIVE IMMUNIZATION

Types of vaccine

Toxoids

If the signs and symptoms of a disease can be attributed essentially to the effects of a single toxin, a modified form of the toxin that preserves its antigenicity but has lost its toxicity (a *toxoid*) provides the key to successful active immunization against the disease. This has been spectacularly successful with tetanus and diphtheria.

Inactivated vaccines

If the disease is not mediated by a single toxin, it may be possible to stimulate the production of protective antibodies by using the killed (inactivated) organisms. This is done as a routine with vaccines against pertussis (whooping cough), influenza and the inactivated polio (Salk) vaccine.

Attenuated live vaccines

In some cases, the inactivation procedure to make a killed vaccine destroys or modifies the protective antigenicity (*immunogenicity*) of the organisms. Hence, another approach is to use suspensions of living organisms that are reduced in their virulence (*attenuated*) but still immunogenic. This strategy has yielded mumps, measles and rubella vaccines (now combined), the live-virus polio (Sabin) vaccine, and yellow fever vaccine.

Sometimes it is possible to use a related organism with shared antigens. Thus, the vaccinia virus vaccine was used to eradicate smallpox, and a bovine tubercle bacillus was modified by Calmette and Guérin to make bacille Calmette–Guérin (BCG), which protects humans against tuberculosis and leprosy (see p. 209).

Special procedures

Some vaccines, such as influenza (virus) vaccine, can be refined by a process that removes unwanted protein and other reactive material but retains the important protective antigens. Some others must be conjugated to proteins to render them immunogenic. Some vaccines, such as hepatitis B vaccine, can be bio-engineered. There is much current interest in the possibility of developing *subunit vaccines* consisting of purified fragments of the major immunogenic components of micro-organisms, particularly viruses.

Immune response

Antibodies against the agents of some bacterial and viral infections may be present in the mother's blood and be passively acquired by the baby. This gives some protection to the infant at a time when it is poorly equipped to produce specific antibodies, but it may interfere to a varying extent with the infant's capacity to respond to the stimulus of injected or ingested vaccines in the very early months of life. Although the capacity of the infant to produce specific antibody to injected antigens is poorly developed in the first few months of life, this problem can often be resolved by the use of *adjuvants*. Thus, effective responses are produced to powerful antigens such as alum-adsorbed toxoids. Pertussis whole-cell vaccines have an adjuvant effect of their own, so the combination of adsorbed toxoids and whole-cell pertussis vaccine (the triple diphtheria, tetanus and pertussis vaccine; DTP) is an effective immunizing complex that can be given at 2, 3 and 4 months of age to cover the period when the lethal potential of pertussis is greatest (see Chapter 32). The tissues of the newborn respond effectively to BCG vaccine because the protection here is cell-mediated. The use of a high-potency measles vaccine at 6 months of age is likely to be exploited in countries where measles kills or severely injures the very young.

When a good specific antibody response is being sought to a toxoid or a killed antigen, the usual procedure is to give three doses of the antigen at spaced intervals. The first or 'priming' dose evokes a low level of antibody after a latent period of about 2 weeks, but the second dose elicits a much greater (secondary) antibody response, and this is further boosted by the third dose.

The efficacy of injected antigen preparations can be enhanced by slow-release agents such as mineral carriers which have adjuvant effects. With most antigens, the response is better if the first two doses are separated by an interval of a month or two. A third dose is generally recommended at some time thereafter, and further booster doses may be given to maintain immunity.

Duration of immunity

After an effective course of active immunization, a protective amount of antibody may persist in the blood for some years and a subsequent booster injection may maintain protection for a further decade. Much depends upon circumstances that will vary for different vaccines and different groups of people. The duration of active protection cannot be absolutely equated with the presence of demonstrable antibody because factors such as the sensitivity of the test and the actual protective role of the antibody detected have to be taken into consideration.

Age of commencement of active immunization

This must take account of the immaturity of the antibody-forming system in the very early months (see above) and the infectious challenges that a child may encounter early in life and in later years. The start of any immunization programme must be adjusted to the known epidemiology of the diseases that are prevalent in the country in which it is to be instituted, and it must also be related to any serious infective challenges that may be imported from time to time. Poliomyelitis is a good example of a disease that has been largely eradicated from many communities; however, the disease is quick to strike back if the immunization shield is lowered.

CONTROLLED STUDIES OF PROPHYLACTIC VACCINES

Combined field and laboratory studies aim to provide confidence in the efficacy of vaccines. A field trial can show only whether or not the actual preparation of vaccine used was successful under the circumstances prevailing at the time. Accordingly, trials require very sophisticated design and much care in their execution. They are very expensive. In order to satisfy the requirement for reproducibility, the method of preparation of the vaccine must be meticulously described and controlled. Much work continues to define and to refine laboratory tests for the protectiveness of a particular vaccine that might be correlated with its efficacy in field trials. The laboratory test that gives results most closely corresponding to the protective value in the field trials

may then be adopted as the test for standardizing future batches of vaccine.

Manufacturers of vaccines for commercial use are required in the UK and in many other countries to satisfy certain standards relating to the purity, safety, potency and stability of their products. In addition, the World Health Organization (WHO) has established internationally agreed requirements. At the national level, a system for continuing surveillance of the efficacy of prophylactic vaccines with continuing notification of any suspected adverse reactions is essential.

CONTRA-INDICATIONS TO THE USE OF VACCINES

In the delivery of an important immunization programme there is a balance between the rights of the individual (and often this is the carer not the person being immunized) and the benefit to the public. It is necessary not to take too legalistic view of theoretical hazards and thus err on the side of opting out. The risk of opting out of an immunization schedule should be clearly appreciated and shown to be greater than the adverse effects.

There are some useful general principles about contra-indications:

- do not give a vaccine to a patient with an acute illness
- do be sure that the postponed immunization is subsequently given
- do not give a live vaccine to a pregnant woman, unless there is a clear balance of risk in favour of vaccination
- avoid giving any vaccine in the first trimester of pregnancy
- do not give live vaccines to patients receiving immunosuppressive drugs or irradiation, or to patients suffering from malignant conditions of the reticulo-endothelial system – delay until after successful therapy when they are in remission.

Experience with human immunodeficiency virus (HIV) antibody-positive patients with or without the signs and symptoms of the acquired immune deficiency syndrome (AIDS) indicates so far that measles, mumps, rubella and polio (live virus) vaccines can be given, but that BCG vaccine should not be given. Inactivated vaccines, e.g. pneumococcal, are not contra-indicated and are of great benefit.

Hazards of immunization

Possible adverse reactions to immunization are:

- mild or moderate pain at the site of injection
- fever and malaise for a day or two after

- anaphylactic reactions are very rare but, as they may be fatal, doctors and nurses should be aware of the possibility and should be prepared for such an emergency by carrying drugs and equipment for resuscitation (a 'shock box') to all immunization sessions.

During the first few years of life when many vaccines are given, children tend to have various health problems that include occasional febrile convulsions and may, sadly, include an unexplained cot death or other tragedy. It is inevitable that some of these events will coincide with the period shortly after a vaccine was given to a child and the possibility of a causal relationship will be entertained. The probability of such a link certainly deserves to be considered, but it is most important to bear in mind that the issue is emotive and that ill-balanced or ill-informed adverse publicity can do irreparable harm to an immunization programme. For example, annual notifications of whooping cough in England and Wales dropped from more than 100 000 in the early 1950s to some tens of thousands in the late 1950s as the vaccine gained ground. By the early 1970s (and after modification of the vaccine to take account of a possible deficiency in its protective cover), whooping cough was largely controlled in the UK, with about 75% of children immunized. In the late 1970s, after some ill-informed adverse publicity, acceptance rates for the vaccine fell steeply to 30% or lower, and the uptake of other vaccines was also affected. Epidemics of whooping cough followed in the UK in 1978 and 1982, with tens of thousands of children affected and a number of deaths. As a result of efforts to restore confidence in pertussis vaccine, uptake figures increased in the 1980s and the disease again began to be brought under control. Preliminary results of tests with new (acellular) pertussis vaccines indicate that these are safe and probably more effective.

Over the past few years there has been considerable publicity about claims that autism and inflammatory bowel disease were associated with MMR vaccine. Although several well conducted studies have failed to confirm the original study that first drew attention to this hazard the media in the UK have supported the hypothesis and cover of the vaccine has fallen to the point that these three childhood infectious diseases may re-emerge. Mathematical models of measles show that if the number of susceptibles in the population exceeds 5% there is a possibility of transmission.

Children who are most vulnerable are likely to be least protected. Pertussis, polio and measles spread most effectively when living conditions are overcrowded and unhygienic. To some extent, these diseases depend upon population density for their spread. Some underprivi-

---

Table 69.2 Safety considerations

- Use a separate sterile syringe and needle
- Avoid errors: check the vial personally
- Check 'cold chain'
- Consider the patient's history: note pregnancy and various contra-indications
- Keep careful records, including batch number

---

leged groups in a community are in very real danger when the average rate of vaccine uptake falls, because they often represent the extreme end of the fall in vaccine cover.

In view of the stringency of the regulations that control the quality and efficacy of vaccines, the probability of error lies more with the vaccinator than with the producer. There is a special obligation to ensure that a vaccine is properly stored, properly reconstituted (if relevant) and properly administered (Table 69.2). Many preparations rapidly lose their potency if frozen and thawed or exposed to temperature variation. This means it is vital to maintain the 'cold chain' in which the vaccines are held between 2 and 8°C. The appropriate instructions and local protocols should be followed in detail. *An injectable vaccine must be given with a sterile syringe and needle, a separate sterile syringe and needle must be used for each injection, and the equipment must be properly disposed.* The dangers of contamination with blood-borne viruses such as HIV have led to the search for alternative methods of delivery by air jets or via mucosal surfaces.

Site of injection

This will vary with the vaccine to be given. Specific instructions should be followed. In general, and with the exception of BCG, injectable vaccines are given by intramuscular or deep subcutaneous injection. The anterolateral aspect of the thigh or upper arm is the preferred site for infants. Some doctors and nurses use the upper outer quadrant of the buttock, but fat in this area may interfere with the efficacy of the vaccine, especially hepatitis A and B. In future, the technological advances in delivery methods mentioned above will revolutionize the immunization clinics feared by countless school children.

HERD IMMUNITY

When most of the people in a community are immune to a particular infection that is spread from person to person, the natural transmission of the infection is effectively inhibited. Thus, if almost all children in a residential school have been immunized against measles, the school is most unlikely to have an outbreak of measles; even the few children who have not been immunized will enjoy a measure of protection afforded by the general herd immunity in that they will not be challenged within the school. This will only apply so long as the school population is largely composed of immune pupils and a non-immune pupil does not encounter a visitor who is infected with measles. If there is an influx of non-immunes, the level of herd immunity will fall and the general protection will be lost. When the pupils go into other communities at holiday times, the non-immune individuals are liable to get measles at their first contact with an infective case.

For herd immunity to operate well in a community or a country, vaccine uptake rates must exceed 90%. For some highly transmissible infections, such as measles, uptake rates above 95% are the target. Bear in mind that herd immunity operates only for infections transmitted from person to person. Tetanus is not transmitted in this way; a non-immune person is fully vulnerable to tetanus even if he or she is surrounded by fully immunized colleagues in a closed community (Fig. 69.1).

IMMUNIZATION PROGRAMMES

An immunization campaign carried out without provision for its continuation as a routine procedure will not give satisfactory results unless complete eradication of the disease is achieved. Thus, in planning immunization schedules, consideration must be given to ensuring that the general public is receptive and understands the policy. It is essential to secure the trust and co-operation of parents who have to bring their children to the doctor or clinic for a series of inoculations and who will undoubtedly seek reassurance that the benefits are considerable and the risks negligible. Parental consent must be obtained for each immunization.

In the planning and execution of a programme, immunological points that merit special attention are:

- the use of combined antigens and the simultaneous administration of killed and live vaccines
- the incorporation of adjuvants in killed vaccines and toxoids
- the age of commencement
- the dosage and spacing of antigens.

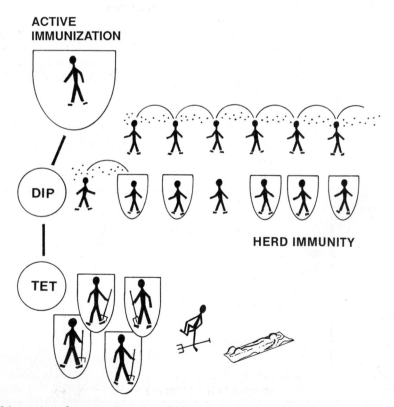

Fig. 69.1 If almost all of the members of a community receive active immunization against a disease that is normally transmitted from person to person, the resulting herd immunity confers some advantage even upon an occasional non-immune member because rapid transmission of the disease through the community is prevented. This is true for diphtheria, but not for tetanus, which is not dependent on person-to-person spread

IMMUNIZATION SCHEDULES

The provision of a programme of active immunization to a community should be governed by considerations of need, efficacy, safety and ease of administration. An overriding consideration is the cost and the availability of skilled manpower and the safe delivery and supply of vaccines. Circumstances vary widely in different countries, and priorities vary. The WHO Expanded Programme on Immunization (EPI) has been adopted by most countries of the world as a minimum schedule to protect children in parts of the world where transmission rates are particularly high. Single measles is given at about 9 months rather than the combined MMR given at 12–15 months in industrialized countries. This is a balance between mean age of infection and response to the vaccine. Also, the EPI recommends hepatitis B immunization from birth (see below).

In the UK, it is generally agreed that protection of the susceptible population against diphtheria, whooping cough and tetanus (with a triple vaccine), *Haemophilus influenzae* type b (with an inactivated conjugated Hib vaccine), *Neisseria meningitidis* group C (with protein conjugated to group polysaccharide as menC), poliomyelitis (with a live vaccine), and mumps, measles and rubella (with a combined live vaccine) merit priority in the very early years of life. BCG vaccine is offered to tuberculin-negative children at 10–14 years and in some high-risk populations

neonatally. In the UK it is now recommended that the DTP triple vaccine with the Hib vaccine and oral polio vaccine are started early, at 2 months, with further doses at 3 and 4 months (Table 69.3). This secures earlier protection against pertussis in the months when the disease is most dangerous to the young child.

NOTES ON SOME VACCINES IN COMMON USE

Adsorbed tetanus toxoid

The preparation in routine use in the UK is adsorbed onto an aluminium salt; it is more effective and less reactive than simple toxoid. It is a component of the triple DTP vaccine. A course of three injections given at intervals of about 4 weeks and boosters prior to, and on leaving, school, i.e. a total of five doses, should protect for life, although studies show that the elderly have low levels of protective antibody. Prevention of tetanus should be considered in relation to the management of wounds (see Chapter 22, p. 238).

Diphtheria toxoid

The adsorbed preparation used in the UK and incorporated into the triple DTP vaccine contains aluminium phosphate and affords good protection which is boosted at school entry age. This preparation is not used for

Table 69.3 Schedule of immunization for children in the UK

Age	Vaccine	Notes
During year 1	Diphtheria Tetanus Pertussis	DTP triple vaccine: start at 2 months; second dose at 3 months and third dose at 4 months intramuscularly
	Hib vaccine MenC Oral polio vaccine	Give at the same times as the DTP injections
During year 2	Measles Mumps Rubella	MMR vaccine: give one injection of the combined live vaccine at age 12–15 months
At 4–5 years	Diphtheria Tetanus Pertussis MMR Oral polio vaccine	Pre-school booster
At 10–14 years	BCG vaccine	After negative Heaf (tuberculin) test
At 13–18 years	Tetanus/low-dose diphtheria (Td) Oral polio	Booster Booster

adults; a dilute adsorbed diphtheria vaccine preparation is used for people who are more than 10 years old and is now incorporated with tetanus toxoid for school leavers as Td. Active immunization of adults against diphtheria is not practised in the UK as a routine, unless there is a potentially high occupational risk of encountering the organism in laboratory or clinical work, or unless a person has been in contact with a case of diphtheria or is travelling to an endemic area and protection is deemed necessary. A course of erythromycin gives further protection to a close contact, and this has replaced the use of diphtheria antitoxin in contacts. The falling level of immunity to diphtheria among adults in communities that regard themselves as having good preventive medical services gives some cause for concern and calls for continuing vigilance, particularly because of large outbreaks in eastern Europe.

Pertussis vaccine

The vaccines in general use are whole-cell preparations of killed *Bordetella pertussis*. Acellular vaccines containing antigenic components of the organism have been developed and are being assessed for their protective potency; results so far are very promising. The protection afforded by the whole-cell vaccines is generally acknowledged to be considerable, but the acellular vaccines seem to be more effective. Three injections are given at intervals of 1 month or more. Whole-cell pertussis vaccine is a component of the DTP triple vaccine, and has the added advantage of being an adjuvant in that combination.

Adverse reactions that may be associated with pertussis vaccine include soreness at the site of injection, irritability and pyrexia. Reactions such as persistent screaming, shock, vomiting and convulsions have been reported, but the association with pertussis vaccine is not invariably clear. Particular attention has been paid to a possible association of convulsions and encephalopathy and cerebral damage. It should be noted that unexplained convulsions occur in young children, especially during the period when the immunization programme is set, and that such an incident may occur by chance shortly after a vaccine has been given. Moreover, the age at which certain cases of cerebral damage begin to be apparent coincides with this age range. It is uncertain if there is a risk of permanent brain damage associated with whole-cell pertussis vaccine; if there is, it must be very small and it must be greatly outweighed by the known risk of neurological and other damage that may be life-threatening when the natural disease occurs. It is hoped that acellular pertussis vaccines, which are much less likely to cause reactions, will resolve the problem.

Haemophilus influenzae type b (Hib) vaccine

Invasive encapsulated strains of *H. influenzae*, almost always of serotype b, are associated with meningitis, bacteraemia, epiglottitis and other serious infections particularly affecting young children. The risks of severe morbidity and mortality are highest in children in the age range 3–18 months. Hib conjugate vaccines containing the capsular polysaccharide linked to a protein are immunogenic. The Hib vaccines used in the UK are given combined with DTP as part of the primary immunization. Children in the age range 1–4 years who have not received Hib vaccine can be protected by a single dose of Hib vaccine. Routine immunization of older children or adults with Hib vaccine is not generally recommended unless they are immunocompromised.

Meningococcal group C (MenC) vaccine

In 1999, following an increase in fatal cases of invasive meningococcal disease especially due to group C, the UK government was the first in the world to introduce MenC vaccine to the routine programme. Although it is now given as part of primary immunization at 2, 3 and 4 months, when the campaign started it was necessary to protect the whole population up to 18 years of age. The design of the antigen is similar to Hib in that the relatively poorly immunogenic polysaccharide is covalently linked to a protein carrier which produces a prolonged immune response in naïve infants. As with Hib there are few adverse reactions and the introduction universally to children has led to a great reduction in cases of meningitis.

Poliomyelitis vaccines

The control of poliomyelitis is one of the great success stories of active immunization, and the worldwide eradication of poliomyelitis is a goal of the WHO which has nearly been achieved. The Salk vaccine came first; this is a killed mixture of the three types of poliovirus (1, 2 and 3). A course of three injections is given at appropriate intervals.

The oral polio vaccine (OPV) favoured in the UK and many other countries is the live-attenuated form developed by Sabin. This is a mixture of the three types, and it is given orally on three occasions, usually at the same time as the triple DTP vaccine is given in the early months. As it is a live preparation, the vaccine must be stored and held according to the manufacturer's instructions. OPV colonizes the gut and gives rise to local and humoral antibodies. The faeces contain live virus for some time, and poliomyelitis caused by a vaccine strain is a rare, but recognized, hazard. Any non-immune contact in the household should be advised to be immunized at the same time, but difficulties in arranging this should not delay the primary job of getting the baby immunized. It is important to advise on the hygienic handling of the baby's nappies during the period of excretion of the virus (and at any other time, for that matter!).

Measles, mumps and rubella (MMR) vaccine

This is a mixture of live-attenuated strains of these three viruses in freeze-dried form; it has to be stored at 2–8°C (not frozen), reconstituted according to the manufacturer's instructions and used promptly. One injection of the mixture is given between 12 and 15 months in the UK schedule, and the second dose in the fifth year, before entry to school.

The measles component may give rise to fever or malaise and sometimes a rash about a week after inoculation. The mumps component may cause some parotid swelling, seen about 3 weeks after inoculation. Very occasional cases of mumps vaccine-associated meningoencephalitis occur; these generally occur at 3 weeks after use of the Urabe strain. It is usually benign, but there may be confusion with other more serious syndromes in this age group. The rubella component is not usually associated with reactions in this age group, though temporary malaise, mild fever and arthralgia occurring about the ninth day after vaccination have been noted in some older recipients of rubella vaccine.

It is hoped that high vaccine coverage with two doses of MMR vaccine in the UK schedule will eradicate measles, mumps and rubella in this country as it nearly has done in north America. Much depends upon public faith in the immunization programme, which has been undermined by media-led campaigns about the safety of MMR.

Rubella vaccine is offered to all seronegative women of child-bearing age and to seronegative professional attendants who might come into contact with pregnant women. Although rubella vaccine is not thought to be teratogenic, any woman of child-bearing age who is given the vaccine should avoid pregnancy for a month.

BCG

The attenuated strain of bovine tubercle bacillus known as bacille Calmette–Guérin (BCG) produces cross-immunity to human tuberculosis and has significantly contributed to the control of that disease and to the other important mycobacterial disease, leprosy, in many countries. An intradermal injection of the live-attenuated vaccine is given on the lateral aspect of the arm at the level of the deltoid insertion, but not higher, or on the upper lateral surface of the thigh. Instruction on the reconstitution of the freeze-dried vaccine, the dosage and the detailed technique of giving a truly intradermal injection, should be most carefully observed. With the exception of newborn children, any recipient of BCG vaccination should have been tested for hypersensitivity to tuberculin and found to be negative. Tuberculin tests include the *Mantoux test*, in which diluted tuberculin is injected intradermally, and the *Heaf test*, which is done with a multiple puncture apparatus (see Chapter 18). Be sure to appreciate the difference between the tuberculin test and a BCG vaccination; note that attention to detail in the sterilization of the Heaf apparatus is of crucial importance.

Hepatitis B vaccine

For the protection of groups of people considered to be at special risk of acquiring hepatitis B, a bio-engineered vaccine is now in common use. A course of three intramuscular injections is given (not into the buttock) at intervals of 1 and 5 months; thus, it takes 6 months to complete the course, and this is of practical importance. Following needlestick injuries or known contact with the virus it is possible to give an accelerated course although efficacy may not be as good. Protective antibody responses are generally achieved in about 90% of those given the vaccine, with a range of responses from weak to strong, but there is a worrying minority of non-responders (10–15% in those over 40 years of age). Antibody responses should be checked at least 6 weeks after completion of a course, and it may be prudent to give poor responders or non-responders a booster dose or a repeat course. Non-response rates are particularly worrying among patients on maintenance haemodialysis, for whom a higher dose preparation is available. In the general population, the protection afforded to responders is thought to last for about 5 years, when a booster dose of vaccine may be given. Established policy must await further experience with hepatitis vaccines, which in many countries are being given universally as part of the routine schedule. Great success has been claimed in China in reducing prevalence and preventing cancer.

Other vaccines

Various vaccines are available for the protection of special groups of people or for individuals in special circumstances (Table 69.4). The reader is referred to the appropriate chapters for more detailed consideration of such topics as:

- the prevention of tetanus in wounded patients
- the indications for pneumococcal vaccine

- the management of rabies
- the control of Q fever
- the protection of those at special risk from hepatitis B and varicella–zoster
- the protection of the immunocompromised such as HIV/AIDS patients.

PROTECTING THE TRAVELLER

An intending traveller to another country should seek advice in advance about the prevailing diseases and the precautions that should be taken. Advice on immunization is unlikely to be of much help if the traveller unwisely runs the risk of drinking raw water or eating uncooked salads and vegetables in a country where sanitation is inadequate and water supplies are insecure.

In advising travellers about exotic diseases, do not forget that diseases now uncommon in countries with developed medical services may still be common in countries that lack such services. If work in a hospital or health clinic is envisaged, include the risk of diphtheria and check immunity to tuberculosis, hepatitis B, measles and poliomyelitis. If the traveller is going to Central Africa or Central America, bear in mind the need for protection against yellow fever. Other vaccines that may be indicated include those that will afford some protection against typhoid. Some of the special vaccines listed in Table 69.4 may also merit inclusion, especially if the traveller's activities when abroad are likely to expose him or her to the relevant diseases. Japanese B encephalitis vaccine may provoke more adverse events than the risk entailed. Travellers to rural areas in the tropics must always put insecticides on the top of their list of necessities because although there is some progress in the development of an effective malaria vaccine none is available commercially. Practical, simple advice is often of more value than a typhoid or hepatitis immunization.

UNRESOLVED PROBLEMS

Nothing is perfect (Table 69.5). Some vaccines are more imperfect than others, and some circumstances pose special problems. The influenza virus has shifts and drifts in its antigenic pattern, so vaccines must be frequently updated. Then decisions have to be made on the patients who merit this special protection. As these include many old people and many patients with respiratory or cardiovascular impairment, the decisions are quite difficult. Most temperate climate countries immunize the elderly and vulnerable before winter and this has been shown in the US to reduce mortality and hospital admissions.

Cholera vaccines have had a chequered record, with very little evidence of real efficacy for the traveller, who is much better protected by a basic knowledge of hygiene. New developments with oral vaccines are more promising and may protect against ETEC (enterotoxigenic *Esch. coli*).

Acute purulent (bacterial) meningitis is a dramatic clinical problem. The MenC vaccine has afforded protection against group C meningitis, but a group B vaccine is not available at the time of writing (2001) and group B strains are more common in many areas.

We are still quite unclear about the place of pneumococcal vaccine (see Chapter 16). A polysaccharide vaccine produced against 23 types of pneumococci is recommended, particularly for the protection of patients who do not have a spleen or are about to be splenectomized in the course of therapy. It is also suggested that the vaccine may be of use, sometimes with additional penicillin prophylaxis, for the protection of various groups of patients against pneumococcal infections. Conjugate vaccines are available in some countries and have been considered in childhood programmes. At present they cover a limited range of serotypes (usually seven) and there is always the fear of strains not included in the vaccines becoming dominant.

Several vaccines have been developed against various herpesviruses, including herpes simplex, varicella–zoster and Epstein–Barr viruses. There have been many difficulties, but a live-attenuated varicella

Table 69.4 Vaccines for active immunization of people at special risk

Anthrax	Pneumococcal infection*
Cholera	Q fever
Hepatitis A*	Rabies
Hepatitis B*	Tick-borne encephalitis
Influenza*	Typhoid*
Japanese B encephalitis	Typhus
Meningococcal infection*	Varicella-zoster*
Plague	Yellow fever

The asterisk indicates that there are some problems (see text).

Table 69.5 Properties of an ideal vaccine

- Promotes effective immunity
- Confers lifelong protection
- Safe (no side-effects)
- Stable
- Cheap
- Seen to be good and effective by the public

vaccine has been developed which is useful for susceptible staff who work in paediatric or maternity wards.

A vaccine effective against HIV is being urgently sought in the fight against AIDS. There have been many disappointments, and there is now a glimmer of hope.

RECOMMENDED READING

Anonymous. Immunological products and vaccines. In: *British National Formulary*. British Medical Association and Royal Pharmaceutical Society of Great Britain, London (revised at intervals of about 6 months). Also www.bnf.org/

Department of Health, Welsh Office, Scottish Home and Health Department 2001 *Health Information for Overseas Travel*. HMSO, London

Department of Health, Welsh Office, Scottish Home and Health Department, DHSS (Northern Ireland) 1996 *Immunisation against Infectious Disease*. HMSO, London

Mackett M, Williamson J D 1995 *Human Vaccines and Vaccination*. Bios Scientific Publications, Oxford

Nicholl A, Rudd P (eds) 1989 *British Paediatric Association Manual on Infections and Immunizations in Children*. Oxford University Press, Oxford

Plotkin S, Orenstein W (eds) 1999 *Vaccines* 3rd edn. WB Saunders, Philadelphia

Root R K, Warren K S, Griffiss J M, Sande M A 1989 *Immunization*. Churchill Livingstone, New York

World Health Organization 2000 *International Travel and Health. Vaccination Requirements and Travel Advice*. WHO, Geneva

Internet sites

Centers for Disease Control and Prevention: www.cdc.gov/travel/ and www.cdc.gov.nip/

Department of Health (England): www.doh.gov.uk/hat/ and www.immunisation.org.uk/

Public Health Laboratory Service: www.phls.org.uk/

Scottish Centre for Infection and Environmental Health: www.show.scot.nhs.uk/scieh/ and www.fitfortravel.scot.nhs.uk/

World Health Organization: www.who.int/vaccines/ and www.who.int/ith/

INDEX

Note: page numbers in italic refer to figures and tables.

'A' antigen, hepatitis B virus, 439
Abiotrophia species, 174, 184
Abortion, 359, 364, 386, 453
Abortive viral infections, 93, 104–5
Abscesses
  antimicrobial therapy, 651
  intracranial, 630
  kidney, 628
  liver, 593, 651
  pelvic, 631
  post-injection, 217
  tonsillar, 178
Absidia, 587
Acanthamoeba, 595
Acellular pertussis vaccines, 316, 676
Acetamide, 284
Acetic acid, vaginal warts, 432
Acetylcholine receptors, rabies, 553
N-acetylmuramic acid units, 14
Acholeplasma laidlawii, *384*
Acholeplasma oculi, *384*
Achromobacter, 287
Aciclovir, 55–6, 648
  cercopithecine herpesvirus 1, 419, 420
  Epstein–Barr virus, 412, 414
  herpes simplex virus, 406, *644*
    plaque reduction assay, 59
  varicella-zoster virus, 410
Acid-fast staining, mycobacteria, 15, 22
Acidophilic (term), 21
Acinetobacter, 287
Acquired immunity, 110, 121, 130–45
  deficiency, 142–3
  diphtheria, 191
  parasitic infections, 156–8
  viral infections, 148
Acquired immune deficiency syndrome
  see AIDS; Human
    immunodeficiency virus
Acrosoxacin, 53
Actin, *Listeria monocytogenes* on, 195
Actinobacillus actinomycetemcomitans,
  221
Actinobacillus pneumotropica, 335
Actinomadura, 222, 223
Actinomyces, *11*, 28, 86, 221–2, 341–2
Actinomycetoma, 578
Actinomycosis, 221–2
Active immunity, 131
Acute bronchitis, 627
Acute haemorrhagic conjunctivitis, 459
Acute seroconversion illness, HIV, 530
Acute-phase proteins, 124–5
Acyclovir *see* Aciclovir
Adansonian classification, 26
Adaptive responses, bacteria, 43–4
Adefovir, 57
Adenocarcinomas, human papillomavirus,
  434
Adenovirus-associated viruses, 104, 398,
  450–1
Adenoviruses, 392–8
  morphology, *22*, 392–4
Adenylate cyclase, cholera toxin on, 297

Adhesion
  bacteria to cells, 17–18, 85–6, 87
  entero-aggregative *Escherichia coli*,
    HEp-2 cells, 272
  Mycoplasma, 379–80
  Salmonella, 253
  Str. pyogenes, 176
Adjuvants, 110, 671
  pertussis vaccine, 316
Adolescence, hepatitis B immunization,
  446
Adsorbed tetanus toxoid, 238, 675–6
Adsorption
  viruses to cells, 94–5
  see also Haemadsorption
Adult diarrhoea rotavirus, 522
Adult T cell leukaemia/lymphoma, 529–30
Aerobacter aerogenes, 275
Aerobactin
  dysentery, 260
  Escherichia coli, 266
  Klebsiella, 277
Aerobic bacteria, 41, *42*
Aeromonas, 301
Aerosols
  anthrax, 226–7
  antibiotics, 285
  hospital infections, 664–5
  Legionella, 319, 320
  ribavirin, 482
  Yersinia pestis, 330
Aerotolerant anaerobes, 41, *42*
Affinity maturation, 140
  B cells, 135
Afipia felis, 327
Africa, AIDS, 536
African tick bite fever, *370*
African trypanosomiasis, 596–7
Agar, 39
Agar immunoprecipitation test, 190, *191*
Age
  human immunodeficiency virus, 532
  immunization programmes, 672
  influenza, 471–2, 473
  Legionnaires' disease, 319
  Listeria monocytogenes, 197
  mycoplasmal pneumonia, 385
  Neisseria meningitidis, 246
  pyrexia, 631
  respiratory syncytial virus, 482
  susceptibility to infection, 123, 151–2
Agglutination, 115–16
  Brucella, 324
  infectious mononucleosis, 414
  leptospirosis, 355
  see also Latex agglutination
Agglutinogens, *Bordetella pertussis*, 311
  vaccines, 315
Aggressins, 83–4
Agricultural anthrax, 228–9
AIDS, 530, 531–4
  adenoviruses, 396, 397
  Africa, 536
  candidosis, 576

  central nervous system diseases, 629
  cryptococcosis, 583
  cytomegalovirus, 416
  Mycobacterium avium complex, 216,
    218
  pregnancy, prevention, 537
  South and South-east Asia, 536
  surveillance reporting, 641
  treatment, 533–4
  tuberculosis, 205
    epidemiology, 208
    treatment, 206-8
AIDS indicator diseases, *530*
AIDS-related complex, 530
Air filtration, 79
Air-borne transmission, prevention, 668
Air-conditioning systems, *Legionella*,
  320–1
Airway obstruction
  human papillomavirus infection, 433
  infectious mononucleosis, 413
  see also Croup
Alanine transaminase, hepatitis C virus,
  509, 510
Alastrim, 423–4
Albendazole, 58
  activity spectrum, *604*
  filariasis, 607
  giardiasis, 595
Alcaligenes, 287, 311–12
Alcohols, disinfection, 80
Aldehydes *see* Formaldehyde;
  Glutaraldehyde
'Alert organism' systems, 669
Aleutian disease virus, 450
Algae, 25
Alginate, *Pseudomonas aeruginosa*, 283,
  284
'Alkalescens-Dispar' bacteria, 265
Alkaline peptone water, 297
Allelic exclusion, 114
Allergens, arthropods as, 616
Allergic alveolitis, 221
Allergic aspergillosis, 584, 585
Allergic encephalomyelitis, rabies
  vaccine, 556
α-haemolysis, *Streptococcus*, 175
α-toxin, *Clostridium perfringens*, 233
Alphaviruses, *485*, 486, *489*, 492–4
Alternative pathway, complement, 125,
  126, 149
Alum-precipitated toxoid, anthrax
  vaccine, 229
Amantadine, 55, *56*, 57, 474, 648
Amastigotes
  Leishmania, 598
  Trypanosoma cruzi, 597
Ambisense RNAs, bunyaviruses, 487
Amikacin, 51, *52*, 224
Amines, bacterial vaginosis, 302
Aminoglycosides, *46*, 51, *52*, 186, 285,
  646, 647
Amoebae, 58, *589*, 593–5, 651
Amoxicillin, 47, 256, *646*

Amphoteric detergents, 81
Amphotericin B, 54, *55*, 571, 648
Ampicillin, 47, 222, 308, 626, *646*
Amplification
  gene probes, 32
  hepatitis C virus tests, 507
  see also Polymerase chain reaction
Amplified fragment length polymorphism, 35
Amyloid plaques, 563, 564
Anaemias
  B19 erythrovirus, 451, 452
  from parasitic infection, 154
  see also Haemolytic anaemia
Anaerobes, 41, *42*
  antibacterial agents, *46*, *644*
  non-sporing, 337–42
  specimen transport, *637*
  wounds, 630
Anaerobic culture, 339
  mycoplasmas, 383
Anaerobiospirillum, 342
Anal sexual intercourse, human
    immunodeficiency virus, 535
Anal warts, 432–3, 435
Anamnestic responses, pertussis false
    positives, 313–14
Anaphylatoxins, 127, 129, 162
Anaphylaxis, 143, 159, 673
Anaplasma, 375, 376
Ancylostoma duodenale (hookworm), *601*,
    602, 603, *604*
Anergic phase, Buruli ulcer, 218
Anginosus group, *Streptococcus*, 175, 184
Angiomatosis, bacillary, 327
Angular cheilitis, 576
Animals
  anthrax, 226–7
  arboviruses, 490, 491–2
  arenaviruses, 516
  bites, 334, 335, 553, 556
  Bordetella pertussis, experimental
      infection, 312–13
  Brucella, 322
  Campylobacter, 290, 291
  chlamydial infection, 366
  coronaviruses, 548
  Edwardsiella, 281
  Leptospira, 356, 357
  Listeria monocytogenes, 198
  Q fever, 377
  rabies, 553, 554, 556, 557
  retroviruses, 528
  Salmonella, 252, 257–8
Annealing, DNA, 27
Anogenital warts, 432–3, 435
Anopheline mosquitoes, 618
Ansamycin (rifabutin), 54
Antagonism, antibiotics, 647
Anthracoid colonies, *Bacillus cereus*, 229
Anthrax, 4, 225, 226–9
  vaccines, 5, 225, 229
Antibacterial agents, 46–54
Antibiotics, 46–60
  assay, 60
  historical aspects, 6

infections induced, 240–1, 647, 663
malaria, 592
pharyngitis, 626
pseudomembranous colitis, 240
resistance, 643, 644–5
  policies *vs*, 71, 645–6
  Salmonella typing, 252
  Staph. aureus, 48
  Staph. haemolyticus, 173
  tuberculosis, 208
  viridans streptococci, 186–7
  see also Methicillin-resistant
      Staphylococcus aureus
resistance genes, 32, 69–71
sensitivity tests, 58–60, 640
serum assay, 643
Staph. aureus, 171–2
therapy strategy, 642–52
urine assay, 643
Antibodies, 112–16, 135–6, 639
  anti-HIV antibody tests, 533
  arbovirus infections, 487
  bacterial infections, 162–3
  chlamydial infection, 365
  ELISA, 33
  Epstein–Barr virus, B cell activation,
      412–13, 414
  fluorescent labelling, 33
  hepatitis B, 443
  hepatitis C, 506–7
  historical aspects, 5–6
  homologous *vs* heterologous
      preparations, 670
  human herpesviruses 6 and 7, avidity
      tests, 418
  Legionella, 320
  micro-organism identification, 32
  Neisseria meningitidis, 244–5
  parasitic infections, 156–7, 159
  pertussis, 313–14
  Pseudomonas aeruginosa, 284
  rubella, 502–3
  specificity, 111–12
  Treponema, 347
  vs viruses, 148–9, 151
  Yersinia enterocolitica, 333
  see also Immunoglobulins; Monoclonal
      antibodies
Antifungal agents, 54–5, 571–2, 648
Antigenic determinants, 110, 111
Antigenic drift, 468, 473
Antigenic shift, 468, 473
Antigenic variation, 88
  Borrelia, 349
  mycoplasmas, 384
  parasites, 158–9
  rotaviruses, 526
  Str. pyogenes M proteins, 177
  viruses, 152
Antigen-presenting cells, 133–4, 139
  B cells as, 134, 148
Antigens, 110–12, 133–4
  adenoviruses, 393–4, 397
  defined, 6
  IgG response, 135
  IgM response, 135, 136

immunosuppression by, 159
lymphatic system on, 132
mycoplasmas, 384
processing pathways, 140
recognition, 116–17
tolerance to, 140, 141
viral, capping, 151
see also Capsular antigens;
    Superantigens
Antiglobulin conjugates,
    immunofluorescence, 33
Anti-HBs
  induction, hepatitis B vaccines, 445–6
  therapy, 441–2
    liver grafts, 442, 444, 445
    see also Hyperimmune
        immunoglobulins, hepatitis B
Antihelminthic agents, 58, *59*
Anti-HIV antibodies, tests, 533
Anti-I antibodies *see* Cold agglutinins
Antimalarials, 58, 557, 592
Antimony compounds, leishmaniasis, 599
Antiparasitic agents, 58
Antiprotozoal agents, 58
Antiretroviral drugs, 533–4
  antagonism by rifampicin, 208
  see also specific drugs
Antisepsis, 7, 73
Antiseptics, 79–81
Antisera, 6, 112, 136, 670
  gas gangrene, 234
Antistreptolysin O test, 186
Antitoxins
  botulism, 239, 240
  diphtheria
    serum levels, 190
    treatment with, 191
  equine, 239, 670
  tetanus, 239
Antituberculosis drugs, 206–8, 209, 219
Antiviral agents, 55–8, 648
  sensitivity tests, 59–60
Ants, 616
Aplastic crisis, B19 erythrovirus, 452,
    454
Apoptosis, viral replication and, 102–3
Arabinoglactan, mycobacteria, 15
Arachnids, *615*, 620–1
Arbitrarily primed PCR, 35
Arboviruses, 484–500
Arcanobacterium haemolyticum, *192*,
    194
Archaea, 9, 10
Archaebacteria, 25
Arcobacter butzleri, 288
Arenaviruses, 513–17
Argasid ticks, 620, 621
Argentinian haemorrhagic fever, 516
Armadillos, *Mycobacterium leprae*,
    210
Army camps *see* Military camps
Arsphenamine, 6
Artemisinin derivatives, 592
Arthritis
  B19 erythrovirus, 452
  mycoplasmas, 386–7

Arthritis
  rubella, 500
  Salmonella, 254
  see also Reactive arthritis
Arthrobacter, 195
Arthroconidia, *Coccidioides immitis*, 580
Arthropods, 7, 263, 490, 491–2, 615–21
Arthus reaction, 144
Ascaris lumbricoides, 601–3
  drugs *vs*, *604*
Aseptic techniques, 666
ASO test, 186
Aspergilloma, 584
Aspergillosis, 584–5
Aspergillus, 584–5
  otomycosis, 577–8
Aspergillus fumigatus, *55*, 585
Asplenia, *Streptococcus pneumoniae*
    prophylaxis, 188
Assassin bugs, 617
Assembly, viruses, 101–2
Association, *vs* causation, 660
Asthma
  allergic aspergillosis, 584
  human coronavirus, 548
Astroviruses, 539–45
Atheroma, *Chlamydophila pneumoniae*,
    365
Athlete's foot, 570, 572–4
Atmosphere, bacterial cultures, 41
  see also Anaerobic culture; Capnophilic
    organisms; Microaerophilic
    organisms
Attaching and effacing *Escherichia coli*,
    268, 272
Attenuated vaccines *see* Live-attenuated
    vaccines
Atypical pneumonias, 627
  antimicrobial therapy, 650
Auchmeromyia luteola, 619
Auramine stain, 33
Auto-antibodies, parasitic infections, 159
Autoclaves, 77
  anthrax spores, 226
Autocrine action, interleukin-2 on T cells,
    134
Autofluorescence, *Legionella*, *318*, 319
Auto-immunity, 145
Autolysin, *Str. pneumoniae*, 182
Autotransporters, 90
Autotrophs, 40
Auxotyping, *Neisseria gonorrhoeae*,
    243–4
Aviadenoviruses, 394
Avian infectious bronchitis virus, 546
Avian strains, influenza viruses, 469, 470
Azidothymidine *see* Zidovudine
Azithromycin, 52, 320, 367
Azlocillin, 47
Aztreonam, 49

B cell receptors, 115, 117, 132–3
B cells
  activation, 133, 134–5
  antibody response, 135

as antigen-presenting cells, 134, 148
  Epstein–Barr virus, 411, 412
  immunoglobulin production, 114–15
  interferons on, 147
  parasitic infections, 159
  tolerization, 141
  viral infections, 148
B virus (cercopithecine herpesvirus 1),
    419–20
B19 erythrovirus, 448, 449, 451–4
  receptors, *95*
Babesia, 599
Bacillary angiomatosis, 327
Bacillary dysentery, 260–4
Bacillary index, leprosy, 212
Bacillary peliosis, 327
Bacille Calmette–Guérin *see* BCG
    vaccine
Bacilli, 10, 18, 29
Bacillus, 29, 225–30
Bacillus anthracis, 225–9
Bacillus cereus, 225, 229–30
Bacillus globigi, sterilization testing, 230
Bacillus megaterium, *15*, 20
Bacillus pumilis, 230
Bacillus stearothermophilus, *42*, 77, *225*,
    230
Bacillus subtilis, *225*
Bacitracin, 51, 185, 307
Background staining, 21
Back-mutation, 65
Bacteraemia, 632–3
  Haemophilus influenzae, 305
  Listeria monocytogenes, 197
  Salmonella, 254, 256
  Str. pneumoniae, 183
  Str. pyogenes, 179
Bacteria
  cell anatomy, 10–18
  classification, 25–30
  genetics, 61–72
  growth, 18, 37–8
    vs resistance to sterilization, 76
  historical aspects, 4
  immunity, 161–5
  life cycle, 18–20
  pathogenicity, 83–92
  physiology, 37, 40–5
  viability, 44–5
Bacterial endocarditis *see* Endocarditis
Bacterial vaginosis, 302, 386, 630,
    651
Bacteriocins, 183
  Klebsiella, 276
  typing, 34
Bacteriophages, 61
  gene transfer by, 66–7
  see also Phage typing
Bacterium aerogenes, historical aspects,
    275
Bacteroides, 339, 340, *644*
Baits, rabies vaccines, 557
Balamuthia mandrillaris, 595
Balantidium coli, 599
Ballerup-Bethesda group (*Citrobacter*),
    281

Bangladesh, cholera types, 298
Bartonella, 325–7
Bartonella bacilliformis, 325–6
Bartonella clarridgeiae, 327
Bartonella henselae, 327
Bartonella quintana, 326–7, 369
Basic polypeptides, 124
Basidiobolus haptosporus, 579
Basidiomycetes, 28
Basophilic (term), 21
Basophils, 122
Bassi, Agostino, 4
Bats, 520, 555
Battey bacillus, 215–16
Bauer-Kirby test, 59
BCG vaccine, 677
  environmental mycobacteria and, 209,
    220
  leprosy, 213
  neonate, 671
  tuberculosis, *201*, 209
  UK vaccination scheduling, *675*
BCYE agar, *Legionella*, 318
Bed bugs, 616
Bees, 616
Beetles (Coleoptera), 616
Bejel (endemic syphilis), 346
Bengal subtype *V. cholerae*, 299
Benign tertian malaria, 589
Benzimidazoles, *59*
Benzylpenicillin, 47, *646*
β_2-microglobulin, 118
β-haemolysis, *Streptococcus*, 175
β-lactam antibiotics, 20, *46*, 47–51,
    284–5, 647
β-lactamases, 47, 647
  gene mutations, 70
  Klebsiella, 277
  Moraxella catarrhalis, 249
  Neisseria gonorrhoeae, 248
  Staphylococcus strains, 645
Bifidobacterium, 221, *341*
Biken test, 270
Bilharzia *see* Schistosomiasis
Biliary tract
  antimicrobial agents, 651
  Salmonella carriage, 256
  trematode infections, 608
Biochemical reactions, bacteria, 31,
    42
Biofilms, 16, 38, 86
  Staph. epidermidis, 172
Biopsy
  cervix, 434–5
  Helicobacter pylori, 294
  Rickettsia, 373
  zygomycosis, 587
Biotypes, *Corynebacterium diphtheriae*,
    189
Biotyping, bacteria, 33–4
Birds
  arboviruses, 490
  Campylobacter, 290
  chlamydial infection, 366
  influenza viruses, 473
    see also Avian strains

Bites
  animals, 334, 335, 553, 556
  black widow spider, 621
  insects, 616
BK virus, 429, 435–7
Black Creek Canal virus, 499
Black death, 330
Black dot ringworm, 574
Black piedra, 577
Black widow spider, 621
Black-flies (*Simulium*), 618, 619
Blackhead mite, 620
Blastocystis hominis, 595
Blastomycosis, 581–2
Blistering diseases, *Staphylococcus aureus*, 170
Blood, 6, 7
  hepatitis B, 441, 444-5
  hepatitis C virus, 508–9
  HIV, 535, 537
  Leptospira, 355
  malaria, 590
  specimen collection, *637*
Blood cultures, *637*
  brucellosis, 323–4
  Candida, 586
  enteric fever, 255
  Haemophilus influenzae, 307
  mycoplasmas, 387–8
  Str. pneumoniae, 185
Blood flukes *see Schistosoma*
Blood group O, echoviruses, 456
Blood smears, malaria, 590
  cockroaches, 617
Blood transfusion
  B19 erythrovirus infection, 454
  cytomegalovirus, 417, 418
  hepatitis B, 444
  hepatitis C, 509
    prevention, 511
  HIV, 535
  syphilis, 348
  variant CJD, precautions, 564
  Yersinia enterocolitica, 334
Blue-green algae, 25
Body cavity lymphomas, 419
Boiling, 79
Bone infection, antibiotics, 651
Bone marrow
  B19 erythrovirus, 451, 452, 453
  transplantation, polyomaviruses, 436
Bordetella, 311–17
Bordetella bronchiseptica, 311–12
Bordetella parapertussis, 311
Bordetella pertussis, 87, 91, 311
  see also Pertussis
Boric acid, urine specimens, 637
Bornholm disease, 459
Borrelia, 29, 343–5, 348–51
Borrelia afzeli, 350
Borrelia burgdorferi, *344*, 350–1
Borrelia garinii, 350
Borrelia recurrentis, *344*
Boston fever, 458
Bot fly (*Dermatobia hominis*), 619

Botulism, 239–40
  toxins, 92, 239, 240
Bound coagulase, *Staph. aureus*, 169
Boutonneuse fever, *369*
Bovine farcy, 223
Bovine papillomavirus, oncogenicity, 429
Bovine spongiform encephalopathy, 559–60
  variant CJD and, 564
Bovine tuberculosis
  epidemiology, 208
  see also Mycobacterium bovis
Bovis group, *Streptococcus*, 175, 184
Bowie–Dick test, 77
Brachyspira hyodysenteriae, 346
Bradyzoites, *Toxoplasma gondii*, 593
Branhamella catarrhalis, see Moraxella catarrhalis
Brazilian purpuric fever, 309
Breakbone fever, 489
Breast milk, HIV, 535
Brill–Zinsser disease, 372, 374
Britain
  leprosy, 210
  see also England and Wales; United Kingdom
Broiler chickens, 290, 291
Bronchial cilia, pertussis, 312
Bronchiolitis, 481–2
Bronchitis
  acute, 627
  see also Chronic obstructive airway disease
Bronchopneumonia, 627
  antimicrobial therapy, 650
Broth media
  atmospheric conditions, 41
  Corynebacterium diphtheriae biotypes, 189
  growth in, 38–9
  see also Dilution MIC titrations; Enrichment media
Brucella, 322–5
  intracellular parasitism, 163, 323
  Yersinia enterocolitica cross-reactions, 333
Brucellin test, 325
Brucellosis, 322, 323–5
  vaccines, 325
Brugia malayi, *604*, 606
Bruton's disease *see* X-linked infantile hypogammaglobulinaemia
Bubonic plague, 330, 331
Budd, William, on typhoid fever, 653
Budding
  virus release, 101–2
    immune response, 150
  yeasts, 569
Buffered charcoal yeast-extract agar, *Legionella*, 318
Bugs (Hemiptera), 616–17
Buildings, hospitals, 668
Bulbar paralysis, poliomyelitis, 458
Bullneck diphtheria, 190

Bunyaviruses, 484, *485*, 487
  epidemiology, 497–9
  syndromes, *489*
Burkholderia cepacia, 282, 286–7
Burkholderia mallei, 286
Burkholderia pseudomallei, 282, 286
Burkitt's lymphoma, *413*, 414
Burns, *Pseudomonas aeruginosa*, 285
Buruli ulcer, 216, 217–18
Buthid scorpions, 621

C4b-binding protein, *Streptococcus pyogenes*, 177
C5a peptidase, *Str. pyogenes*, 177
Caesarean section, neonatal herpes prevention, 405, 407
CagA (cytotoxin-associated gene protein), *Helicobacter pylori*, 293
Calabar swellings, 604–6
Calcium gluconate, for black widow spider bite, 621
Calcofluor, fungus microscopy, 571
Calculi, urinary tract infections
  mycoplasmas, 386
  Proteus, 280–1
Caliciviruses, 539–45
  carriage, 544–5
  epidemiology, 543–5
California serogroup bunyaviruses, 497–8
Calymmatobacterium granulomatis, 310
cAMP, cholera, 297
CAMP factor, 180–1
Campylobacter, 29, 288–91
  epidemiology, 290–1
  former *Bacteroides* spp., 340
Campylobacter coli, 288–91
Campylobacter fetus, 288
Campylobacter jejuni, 288–91
Candida
  culture appearances, 575
  resistance to antifungals, 572
  superficial infections, 569, 575–6
  systemic infections, 585–7
Candida albicans, 55, 570, *644*
Candida glabrata, 575, 586
Candida krusei, 586
Candida parapsilosis, 586
Candidaemia, 586
Canine parvoviruses, 448, 449, 450
Cannibalism, kuru, 563
Cantharidin, 616
Capnocytophaga, former *Bacteroides* spp., 340
Capnophilic organisms, *42*
Capping, viral antigens, 151
Capsids, 22–4, 30, 101
Capsomers, 22–4
  adenoviruses, 393
Capsular antigens, 34
  Pasteurella multocida, 334–5
Capsules
  Bacillus anthracis, 227
  bacteria, 11, 15, 16, 87–8
  Cryptococcus neoformans, 583

Str. pneumoniae, 182
    vaccines, 188
Str. pyogenes, 177
    swelling test *see* Quellung reaction
Carbapenems, 49
Carbaryl, 620
Carbohydrates, *Neisseria* identification, 243
Carbon isotopes, urea breath test, 294
Carbon source types, 40
Carcinoma
    hepatitis B, 441
    hepatitis C, 509-10
    human papillomaviruses, 434
        cervix, 107, 433, 434
    nasopharyngeal, *413*
Cardiolipin, reagin antibodies, 347
Carriage, 6
    infection from, 656
    see also named organisms
Carriers (of haptens), 110–11
Case finding, tuberculosis, 209
Caseation, 202
Casoni test, 613
Caspofungin, 54, 571
Castaneda culture system, *Brucella*, 323
Cat flea typhus, *370*
Cat scratch disease, 327
Catalase, 41, 88
Catering
    prevention of food poisoning, 258–9
    see also Kitchens
Catgut, *Clostridium tetani*, 236
Catheters (urinary), antimicrobials for infections, 649
Cats
    feline parvovirus disease, 450
    plague, 331
    rabies, 555–6
    Toxoplasma gondii, 593
Cattle
    bovine papillomavirus, 429
    bovine spongiform encephalopathy, 559–60
    Escherichia coli, 272
Causation, *vs* association, 660
Cavitation, tuberculosis, 203–4
CD system, T cells, 122
CD3, T cells, 117, *122*
CD4+ T cells, 117, 119, *122*
    activation, 134
    AIDS, 531–2
        treatment monitoring, 534
    immune function, 136, 139
    parasitic infections, 157
    subtypes, 137
    see also T_H cells
CD8+ T cells, 117, 119–20, *122*, 139–40
    activation, 134
    vs intracellular bacteria, 163–4
Cefaclor, 49
Cefalexin, 49
Cefotaxime, 49
Cefoxitin, 49
Cefpirome, 49
Ceftazidime, 49

Ceftriaxone, 49
    Neisseria gonorrhoeae, 248
Cefuroxime, 49
Cell culture vaccines, rabies, 556–7
Cell cultures (tissue cultures)
    arboviruses, 486, 491
    chlamydiae, 361, 366
    cytomegalovirus, 416, *417*
    herpes simplex virus, 405
    mycoplasmas, 382–3
        contamination with, 388
    Rickettsia, 373
Cell division, bacteria, *11*, 11, 12, 13
    planes, 29
Cell invasion, bacteria, 86–7
Cell walls, bacteria, 10–11, 13–15
    synthesis inhibitors, 47–51
    see also Spheroplasts
Cell-mediated hypersensitivity *see* Delayed-type hypersensitivity
Cell-mediated immune responses, 110, 131, 136–9
    antigen recognition, 117
    bacterial infections, 163
    chlamydial infection, 365–6
    Mycobacterium tuberculosis, 201
    viral infections, 149–50
Cellulitis, 179
    Vibrio vulnificus, 301
    see also Erysipeloid
Cellulose acetate, *Campylobacter* culture, 290
Centipedes, 621
'Central dogma' of molecular biology, 62
Central European encephalitis, 497
    vaccine, 500
Central nervous system, 629–30
    cercopithecine herpesvirus 1, 419–20
    Cryptococcus neoformans, 583
    herpes simplex virus, 403–4
    pertussis vaccine and, 676
    polioviruses, 457–8
    prion diseases, 560
    Whipple's disease, 224
Cepacia syndrome, 286
Cephalosporinase, *Enterobacter*, 278
Cephalosporins, 48–9, *50*, *646*
    activity spectrum, *46*
    Haemophilus influenzae, 308
    Neisseria gonorrhoeae, 248
Cercariae, 608, 610
Cercopithecine herpesvirus 1, 419–20
Cerebellar ataxia syndrome, 409
Cerebral cysticercosis, 611
Cerebral infections *see* Encephalitis
Cerebral malaria, 592
Cerebrospinal fluid, 629, *636*
    Cryptococcus neoformans, 583
    enteroviruses, 461
    herpes simplex virus
        detection, 405
        polymerase chain reaction, 404
    listerial meningitis, 197
    mumps virus, 477
    Neisseria meningitidis, 245
    Str. pneumoniae, 185

Cervix, 630
    carcinoma, human papillomaviruses, 107, 433, 434
    chlamydiae, 364
    intra-epithelial neoplasia, 433, 434
    warts, 432–3
Cestodes, 610–13
CF29K adhesin, *Klebsiella*, 277
CFA *see* Colonization factor antigens
Cfu, *see* Colony-forming units
Chagas' disease, 145, 597–8
    auto-antibodies, 159
    vector, 617
Chancre, 345
Chancroid, 309
Charcoal–blood agar, *Bordetella pertussis*, 311
Chemoprophylaxis, 646–7, 667
    diphtheria, 676
    endocarditis, 187, 649
    Escherichia coli enteritis, 273
    fungi, 571–2
    gas gangrene, 234
    Haemophilus influenzae, 309
    malaria, 592
    Neisseria meningitidis, 246
    in outbreaks of infection, 659
    prostatectomy, 650
    Streptococcus, 187
    tetanus, 239
    trachoma, 367
    tuberculosis, 209
Chemostat studies, 39
Chemotaxis
    Escherichia coli, 16
    inflammation, 130
    phagocytes, 128
Chemotrophs, 40
Chemotyping, bacteria, 35
Chickenpox *see* Varicella
Chickens
    Campylobacter enteritis, 290, 291
    Salmonella, 257–8
Chiclero's ulcer, *598*, 599
Chiggers, scrub typhus, 372, 374
Chikungunya virus (CHIKV), 494
Childbirth *see* Parturition
Children
    B19 erythrovirus, 454
    bacillary dysentery, 263
    botulism, 240
    cytomegalovirus, 415
    Haemophilus influenzae, 308
    listeriosis, 197
    para-influenza virus, 477
    polyomaviruses, 437
    rotaviruses, 525
    Salmonella, 253
    susceptibility to infection, 123
        viral, 151–2
    vaccines, 673
    see also Paediatric AIDS
Chilomastix mesnili, *594*, 595
Chimpanzees, RSV, 481
China, adult rotavirus, 522

Chinese liver fluke *see Clonorchis sinensis*
Chlamydia, 28, 30, 358–68
  antibiotics, *644*
  birds and mammals, 366
  diseases, 362–5
  epidemiology and management, 367
  eye infections, 362–3, 367, 631
  immune response, 365–6
  laboratory diagnosis, 366
  specimen transport, *637*
Chlamydia pecorum, 358
Chlamydia trachomatis, 358, 366, 630–1
Chlamydophila, 358–9
Chlamydophila abortus, 359
Chlamydophila caviae, 359
Chlamydophila pneumoniae, 358, 359, 364, 366, 367
Chlamydophila psittaci, 358, 364
Chloramphenicol, 51, *646*
  activity spectrum, *46*
  enteric fever, 256
  fungal culture, 571
  Haemophilus influenzae, 308
  Oroya fever, 326
  plague, 330–1
  Rickettsia, 373
Chlorhexidine, 80
Chlorine-releasing disinfectants (e.g. hypochlorites), 80
  enteroviruses, 456
  on hepatitis B virus, 440
  HIV, 527
Chloroplasts, 12
Chloroquine, *58*, 592
Chocolate agar, 305, 306–7
Cholecystectomy, *Salmonella* carriage, 256
Cholera, 297–300
  epidemiology, 298–9
  toxin, 90, 297
  treatment, 299
  vaccines, 299–300, 324, 678
  see also Snow, John
Cholesterol, mycoplasmas, 381
Chordopoxvirinae, 421
Choroidoretinitis, 631
Chromatoidal bars, amoebae, 594
Chromoblastomycosis, 578–9
Chromosomes, bacteria, 61
Chronic active hepatitis, 152
Chronic hepatitis
  hepatitis B, 438, 441
  hepatitis C virus, 509–10
  interferons for, 57, 443, 510
Chronic mucocutaneous candidosis, 576
Chronic obstructive airway disease
  acute exacerbation, 627
  antimicrobial therapy, 650
  Haemophilus influenzae, 306
Chronic syndrome, brucellosis, 323
Chronic wasting disease, prion-associated, 559
Chrysops, 618, 619
Cidofovir, *55*, 57, 417
Cilastatin, 49

Cilia, pertussis, 312
Cimex, 616
Cinchona bark, 6
Ciprofloxacin, 53
  anthrax, 228
  enteric fever, 256
  Neisseria meningitidis, 246
  Pseudomonas aeruginosa, 285
Cirrhosis, 441, 509
Citrobacter, 281
Citron bodies, 235
CJD *see* Creutzfeldt–Jakob disease
Class switching, antibody response, 135
Classical biotype, *Vibrio cholerae*, 297
Classical pathway, complement, 125, *126*, 149
Classifications
  arthropods, *615*
  hypersensitivity, 143
  micro-organisms, 25–30
    morphological *vs* molecular, 9
    rubella virus, 484
    Salmonella, 251
    vaccinia virus, 421
  plasmids, 68
  viruses, 26, *30*
Clavulanic acid, 49
Cleaning, 73, 79, 666–7
CLED agar, 300
Clerical procedures, 638
Clindamycin, 52, 186
Clofazimine, 212
Clonal selection, 132–3
Clones, bacteria, 33
Clonorchis sinensis, 608, *609*
Clostridium, 29, 231–41
Clostridium botulinum, 239–40
Clostridium difficile, 240–1
Clostridium novyi, 235
Clostridium perfringens, 231–5
Clostridium septicum, 235
Clostridium sporogenes, 235–6
Clostridium tetani, 236–9
  see also Tetanus
Clue cells, 302
Clumping factor, 169
CMV *see* Cytomegalovirus
CMV early antigen, 416, *417*
Co-aggregation, 86
Coagulase, *Staph. aureus*, 168, 169
Coagulase-negative staphylococci, 168, 172–3
Co-amoxiclav, 49, *646*, 647
  actinomycosis, 222
  Neisseria gonorrhoeae, 248
Cocci, 29
  Gram-negative anaerobic, 341
  Gram-positive, 340–1, 663
  morphology, 10, 11
Coccidia, 592–3
Coccidioidomycosis, 579–80
Cockroaches, 617
Coenocytism, 28
Cold agglutinins, 385
  mycoplasmas, 384, 387
Cold chains, vaccine storage, 673

Cold enrichment
  Yersinia, 332, 333
Cold sores, 402 *see also* Herpes simplex
Colds *see* Common cold
Coleoptera (beetles), 616
Coliforms, 265
Coliphages, T-even, morphology, *23*
Colistin, 54, 285
Colitis
  Clostridium perfringens, 235
  haemorrhagic, 267, 271
  pseudomembranous, 240–1
Colonies, 38
  anthracoid, 229
  defined, 10
  draughtsman, 185
  eugonic, 201
  growth phases in, 39
  identification of bacteria, 31
  medusa head, 225
  Pseudomonas aeruginosa, 283
  role of cell envelopes, 15
  spider, 222
Colonization, bacteria, 85–6
Colonization factor antigens, *Escherichia coli*, 85, 269
Colony-forming units, 38
Colorado tick fever, 490
Coltiviruses, *489*, 490, 521
Combination therapy, 647
  AIDS, 534
  hepatitis B, 444
  see also Antituberculosis drugs
Commensal micro-organisms, 3
  anaerobes, 337–8
  Clostridium, 231
  Neisseria, 242
  protective function, 124
  Staphylococcus, 168
Common cold, 464–5, 548, 626
Common source outbreaks, 657
Community-acquired infections, 662
Compartment for peptide loading (CPL), 134, 140
Complement, 125–7
  activation, 116
  deficiency, 142
  inflammation, *130*
  parasitic infections, 155, 158
  resistance, 89
  vs viruses, 149
Complement fixation (tests)
  Brucella, 324
  Coxiella burnetii, 377
  herpes simplex virus, 405
  histoplasmosis, 581
  immunoglobulins, *115*
  influenza virus detection, 472
  mumps, 478
  mycoplasmas, 387
Complement receptors, 116
Complementarity determining regions, 114
Condylomata acuminata, 432–3, 435
Conformational epitopes, 111

Congenital cytomegalovirus infection, 415–16
Congenital rubella, 502, 503
Congenital syphilis, 345
Congenital varicella, 409
Congo floor maggot, 619
Conidia, 19
Conidiobolus coronatus, 579
Conjugate vaccines
  Hib (*Haemophilus influenzae* type B), 308, 309
  Str. pneumoniae, 188
Conjugation, gene transfer, 66
Conjunctivitis, 631
  acute haemorrhagic, 459
  adenoviruses, 395–6, 398
  chlamydial, 362–3
  see also Ophthalmia neonatorum
Contact dermatitis, 145
Contact transmission, 665
Continuous cultures, 39
Controversies
  over spontaneous generation, 3
  vaccines, 673
Convulsions, pertussis vaccine and, 676
Cooling towers, *Legionella*, 320–1
Coombs and Gell classification, hypersensitivity, 143
Copepods, 621
Cordylobia anthropophaga, 619
Core protein assay, hepatitis C virus, 507
Cornea, 631
  herpes simplex virus, 403
  transplants
    iatrogenic CJD, 563
    rabies, 556
  see also Keratitis
Coronary artery disease, *Chlamydophila pneumoniae*, 365
Coronaviridae, 547
Coronaviruses, 546–50
  morphology, *23*
Corticosteroids, susceptibility to infection, 123
Corynebacterium, 29, 189–95
  pharyngitis, 626
Corynebacterium diphtheriae, 189–92
  lysogenic conversion, 67
  non-toxigenic, 190
  staining pattern, 21
  see also Diphtheria
Coryneform bacteria, 189
Co-stimulatory signal, T cell activation, 134, 135
Co-trimoxazole, *646*, 647
  enteric fever, 256
  Pneumocystis carinii, 588
'Cotton wool balls', 327, 328
Cough
  investigation, 627
  mycoplasmal pneumonia, 385
  see also Pertussis
Councilman bodies, 440
Counterimmuno-electrophoresis, B19 erythrovirus detection, 453
Coxiella burnetii, 369, 376–8

Coxsackieviruses, 456–7, 459, 461
Crab lice, 619–20
C-reactive protein, 124, 633
Crepitus, gas gangrene, 233
Creutzfeldt–Jakob disease, 560–4
Crimean–Congo haemorrhagic fever, 498
Crohn's disease, measles virus, 479
Cross-infection, 663, 665–6
  Escherichia coli enteritis, prevention, 273
  Listeria, neonates, 198
Cross-reactions
  antibodies with antigens, 111, 112
  auto-immunity, 145, 159
  Bord. pertussis serology, 313
  Brucella ELISA, 324
  Citrobacter, 281
  Guillain–Barré syndrome, 290
  herpes simplex and varicella-zoster viruses, 407
  mycoplasmas, 384
  Salmonella, 255
Croup, 477, 627
Crustacea, *615*, 621
Cryogenic freezing, 638
Cryoglobulinaemia, hepatitis C virus and, 510
Cryptic disseminated tuberculosis, 205
Cryptococcus neoformans, *55*, 583–4
Cryptogenic tetanus, 237
Cryptosporidium parvum, 58, 593
Culicine mosquitoes, 618
Culture, 30-31, 639
  anaerobic, 339
    mycoplasmas, 383
  continuous, 39
  identification, 31
  media, 39–40
    Leptospira, 353–4
  methods, *see* named micro-organisms
  Mycobacterium tuberculosis, 206
  Streptococcus, 185
  see also Non-culturability
Cutaneous larva migrans, 603
Cutaneous leishmaniasis, *598*, 599
Cyanobacteria, 41
Cyclic AMP, cholera, 297
Cycloguanil, 53
Cycloheximide, fungal culture, 571
Cycloserine, 51
Cyclospora cayetanensis, 593
Cystic fibrosis, 283, 627
Cysticerca, 610–11
Cysticercosis, 154
  cerebral, 611
Cystine-lactose-electrolyte-deficient agar, 300
Cystitis
  antimicrobial therapy, 649
  encrusted, *Corynebacterium urealyticum*, 193
  haemorrhagic, adenoviruses, 396
Cysts
  Entamoeba histolytica, 594
  Giardia lamblia, 595
  hydatid, 154, 613

Cytarabine, 437
Cytokines, 122, *130*, 137, *138*, 365
Cytolysis
  complement, 127
  mycobacterial infections, 164
  toxins, *91*
  viral, 93–103
Cytomegalic inclusion body disease, 416
Cytomegalovirus, 414–17
  ganciclovir *vs*, 57, 414, 417
Cytopathic effects, viruses, 103, 639
Cytoplasm, bacteria, 10
Cytoplasmic membranes
  bacteria, 12–13, 42
  mycoplasmas, 380–1
  viral fusion, 96
Cytotoxic hypersensitivity, 143–4
Cytotoxic T cells, 136, 137, 149–50
Cytotoxicity, immune, 136–7, 147, 155
Cytotoxin-associated gene protein, *H. pylori*, 293

D values, 75
Dalfopristin, 53
Dane particles, 438–9
Dangers *see* Hazardous substances/organisms
Dapsone, 212
Dark-ground microscopy, 20–1
  spirochaetes appearance, 29–30
Deafness
  Lassa fever, 515
  rubella, 502
Deamination, *Proteus*, 280
Death of micro-organisms, measurement, 74–5
DEC *see* Diethylcarbamazine
Decimal reduction values, 75
Decline phase of growth, 38
Decontamination, 73
Defective interfering particles, 105
Defence mechanisms
  avoidance, 87–9
  see also Innate immunity
Defined media, 40
Dehydration, treatment, 299
Delavirdine, 58
Delayed-type hypersensitivity, 137, 144–5
  leprosy, 212
Deletion mutations, *64*
Delta agent (hepatitis D virus), 24, 446–7
Dementia, AIDS, 531
Demodex folliculorum, 620
Denaturation temperature, 27
Dendritic cells, 134
Dendrograms, 26
Dengue, 488–90
  epidemiology, 496–7
  haemorrhagic fever, 488, 489–90
  natural cycle, 492
  shock syndrome, 488, 490
  virus isolation, 491
Densivirinae, 448

Dental plaque
  bacterial exopolysaccharides, 86
  Streptococcus, 184
Dental treatment
  actinomycosis, 222
  chemoprophylaxis, 187, 649
Deoxyribonucleases, *Streptococcus pyogenes*, 178
Dependoviruses, 398, 448, 450–1
Dermacentor andersoni, 620
Dermatobia hominis, 619
Dermatophytosis, 569, 572–8
  agents *vs*, 54, *55*
  tinea nigra, 577
  see also Ringworm
Detergents, 81
Developing countries, 2
  immunization programmes, 675
  rotaviruses, 525
  see also Tropics
Diagnosis
  flow chart, *624*
  procedures, 635–41
meso-Diaminopimelic acid, 14
Diaminopyrimidines, 53
  activity spectrum, *46*
Diarrhoea, 627–8
  adenoviruses, 396, 397
  antibiotics and, 241, 650–1
  Bacillus cereus, 229
  Campylobacter, 289
  cholera, 297
  coccidia, 593
  Escherichia coli, 267–73
  flagellates, 595
  rotaviruses, 525
  Vibrio vulnificus, 301
  see also Gastro-enteritis; Travellers' diarrhoea
Didanosine (dideoxycytidine), 58
Dienes phenomenon, 280
Dientamoeba fragilis, 594, *595*
Diethylcarbamazine, *59*, 606
Differential interference contrast microscopy, 21
Differential staining, 21
DiGeorge syndrome, 143
Digitonin inhibition, 383
Dihydrofolate metabolism, antibacterial agents, 53
Dilution MIC titrations, 59
Dimorphic fungi, 28, *55*, 569
Dip slides, 637–8
Diphtheria, 189–92, 626
  epidemiology, 191–2
  toxin, 91, 190
  treatment, 191
  triple vaccine, 671
  UK vaccination scheduling, *675*, 676
  see also Corynebacterium diphtheriae
Diphtheroids, 192–5
Diphyllobothrium latum, 611, *612*
Diploid cell cultures, coronaviruses, 549
Diploid cell vaccine, rabies, 557
Diptera, 617–19
Disc diffusion test, 59

Disinfectants, 79–81, 667
  hepatitis B, 440
  HIV, 527
  Mycobacterium tuberculosis, 201
Disinfection, 73, 74, 78–81, 666–7
  water systems, *Legionella*, 321
Disseminated intravascular coagulation, 164
Disseminated mycobacterial disease, 218–19
  see also Cryptic disseminated tuberculosis; Miliary tuberculosis
Distemper, measles and, 480
DNA, 61
  bacteria, 12
    synthesis inhibitors, 53–4
  microarrays, 72
  sequencing, 72
  viral, 24, *see also* named viruses
    retroviruses, synthesis, 100
    see also Genomes; Pathogenicity isles;
DNA composition, classification by, 27
DNA fingerprinting, 35, 69, 72
  Mycobacterium tuberculosis, 206
DNA homology, 27
DNA probes *see* Gene probes
DNA viruses
  partial double-stranded, 101
  single-stranded, 98
  see also Double-stranded DNA viruses
DNAases, *Str. pyogenes*, 178
Dogs
  canine parvovirus disease, 450
  rabies, 555–6
  tick-borne rickettsial fevers, 374
Donovan bodies, 310
Dormancy, bacteria, 18
Double-stranded DNA viruses, replication, 97
  partial double-stranded DNA viruses, 101
Double-stranded RNA, interferon inducer, 146
Double-stranded RNA viruses, 98
Doubling times, 38
Doxycycline, 375, 376
Dracunculus medinensis, *604*, 607
Draughtsman colonies, 185
Droplet infection, *665*
Drug users
  hepatitis B 444, 445
  hepatitis C, 508, 511
  HIV, 535
Drugs, type III reactions, 144
Dry heat, sterilization, 76, 77–8
DTP (diphtheria, pertussis, tetanus) vaccine, 671, 675–6
Duck eggs, 258
Duck embryo vaccine, rabies, 556
Duffy blood groups, malaria resistance, 155, 592
Dumb rabies, 553
Duplication mutations, *64*

Dysentery
  bacillary, 260–4
  balantidial, 599
  vs watery diarrhoea, 628
Dysgammaglobulinaemia, 143

EaggEC (entero-aggregative *Escherichia coli*), 267, 272–3
Ear *see* Deafness; Otitis media; Otomycosis
Early genes, poxviruses, 422
Early replicative phase, hepatitis B, 441
Eastern equine encephalitis
  epidemiology, 493–4
  vaccine, 499
Eaton agent, 384, 385, 387, 388
Ebola virus, 517–20
EBV *see* Epstein–Barr virus
EBV early RNA species, 412
EBV nuclear antigens, 412
  antibodies, 413
Echinococcus granulosus, 613
Echinococcus multilocularis, 613
Echoviruses, 456, 458, 461
  paralysis, 458
Eclipse phase, viral, 93–4
Ecthyma gangrenosum, 283
Ectoparasites, 3, 616
Ectothrix infections, 574
Eczema herpeticum, 403
Eczema vaccinatum, 427
Edwardsiella, 281
Efavirenz, 58
Effacing lesions, enteropathogenic *Escherichia coli*, 268
Effector molecules, injection by bacteria, 15
Eflornithine, 597
Eggs (cestodes), 611, *612*
Eggs (hen), vaccines, 474
Eggs (intestinal helminths), 601–2
Eggs (trematodes), *609*
Egypt, hepatitis C virus, 509
Ehrlichia, 375–6
EIEC (entero-invasive *Escherichia coli*), 267, 270
Eikenella corrodens, 287
El Tor *V. cholerae*, 297, 298
Elastase, 128
Electron microscopy, 638
  bacterial cell walls, 13
  fimbriae, 17
  flagella, 16
  rotaviruses, 525
Electronic information, viii
Electropherotypes, rotaviruses, 524–5
Electrophoresis
  counterimmuno-electrophoresis, 453
  pulsed-field gel, 34, *35*
  serum proteins, 112
  see also Gel electrophoresis
Elek test, 190, *191*
Elementary bodies, chlamydiae, 359, *360*, *361*, 362
Elephantiasis, 144

ELISA *see* Enzyme-linked
    immunosorbent assay
Ellinghausen–McCullough–Johnson–Harr
    is medium, 354
Elongation factor 2, diphtheria toxin on,
    190
Embryology, immune system, 131–2
Emergency diagnosis, 638
Empirical antimicrobial therapy, 643
    systemic sepsis, 648
Encephalitis, 629–30
    amoebae, 595
    arboviruses, 487–8, *489*
    herpes simplex virus, 403–4
    measles, 479
    mumps vaccine, 677
    pertussis vaccine and, 316, 676
    postvaccinial, 427
    serology, 491
    varicella, 409
    see also Transmissible spongiform
        encephalopathies
Encephalomyelitis
    rabies, 553
        vaccine, 556
Endemic infection
    cholera, 298–9
    coccidioidomycosis, 579–80
    HTLV-1, 534
    measles, 480–1
Endemic relapsing fever, 349–50
Endemic syphilis, 346
Endocarditis, 164, 184, 631, *632*
    antimicrobial therapy, 649
    Aspergillus, 585
    chemoprophylaxis, 187, 649
    Haemophilus, 310
    Listeria monocytogenes, 197
    Q fever, 377
Endocytosis, viruses, 95–6
Endoflagella, spirochaetes, 16
Endogenous infections, 7
    see also Opportunist pathogens;
        Self-infection
Endolimax nana, 594, *595*
Endometritis, chlamydial, 364
Endophthalmitis, *Candida*, 586
Endoscopy, *H. pylori*, 294
Endosomes, 128
Endospores, 18
    microscopy, 18
Endosymbiosis, 13
Endothelial cells
    Kaposi's sarcoma, 419
    Lassa fever, 515
Endothrix infections, 574
Endotoxin, 15, 89–90, 145, 164, 632
Energy metabolism, bacteria, 42
Energy source types, 40
England and Wales
    notifiable diseases, 641
    pertussis incidence, 314–15
Enkephalinase inhibitors, 526
Enrichment media, 40
Entamoeba coli, 594, *595*
Entamoeba dispar, 594

Entamoeba gingivalis, 595
Entamoeba hartmanni, 595
Entamoeba histolytica, 58, 593–4, *595*,
    651
Enteric fever, 252, 253–5, 256, 257, 633
    vaccines, 257
Enteritis
    Campylobacter, 289–91
    coronaviruses, 550
    Escherichia coli, 267–73, 273
    Yersinia enterocolitica, 333–4
Enteritis necroticans, 235
Entero-aggregative *Escherichia coli*, 267,
    272–3
Enterobacter, 277–8
Enterobacteriaceae, 250, 275
    antibacterial agents, *46*, 645
Enterobactin, *Esch. coli*, 266
Enterobius vermicularis, 601, *602*, 603
    drugs *vs*, *604*
Enterococcus, 174, 184
    antibiotics and, 187, *644*
    identification, 185
Entero-invasive *Esch. coli*, 267, 270
Enteromonas hominis, 595
Enteropathogenic *Esch. coli*, 267, 268
Enterotoxigenic *Esch. coli*, 267, 268–70
    heat-labile toxins, 90
Enterotoxins, 90, *91*
    antidotes, 273
    Staph. aureus, 169
Enteroviruses, 455–64
    epidemiology, 461–2
    new types, 457, 459–60
    paralysis, 458
        see also Poliomyelitis
    see also Hepatitis A
Env gene, retroviruses, 528
Envelope proteins, viral, 101–2
Environment
    Bacillus anthracis sampling, 228
    infection from, 655–6
    sources, 84–5
Environmental mycobacteria, 215–20
    BCG vaccine and, 209, 220
    contamination by, 220
    epidemiology, 220
Enzootic infection
    anthrax, 228
    rabies, 557
    typhus, 374
Enzyme immuno-assays
    caliciviruses, 543
    herpes simplex virus, 406
    respiratory syncytial virus, 482
Enzyme-linked immunosorbent assay
        (ELISA), 32–3, 639
    antibody detection, 33
    arboviruses, 491
    Brucella, 324
    coronaviruses, 549
    fungal infections, 571, 581, 582, 584,
        585
    hepatitis B, 442
    hepatitis C, 506
    Legionella, 320

parvoviruses, 453
rabies, 554
rotaviruses, 525
Treponema pallidum, 348
viral haemorrhagic fevers, 516
Enzymes
    bacteria
        antibodies *vs*, 162
        pathogenesis, 92
    viruses, 24
Eosinophils, 122, 129, 156, 157
EPEC (enteropathogenic *Escherichia
        coli*), 267, 268
Epidemic jaundice *see* Infectious hepatitis
Epidemic myalgia, 459
Epidemic polyarthritis, 494
Epidemic relapsing fever, 349–50
Epidemic strains, *Neisseria meningitidis*,
    243
Epidemic typhus, 372, 374
Epidemics, 656
    cholera, 298
    coxsackieviruses, 459
    echoviruses, 458
    enterovirus 71, 459–60
    influenza, 473
    measles, 480
    Neisseria meningitidis, 246, 247
    RSV, seasonal, 482
    Streptococcus group C and G, 182
Epidemiology, 653–61
    historical aspects, 7, 653–4
    plasmids, 68–9
    typing of bacteria, 33
Epidermal growth factor, *Trypanosoma*,
    159
Epidermodysplasia verruciformis, 432
Epidermolytic toxins, 170
Epidermophyton, 572
Epididymitis, chlamydial, 363
Epiglottitis, 305, 626
    danger of throat swabs, 307
Epimastigotes, *596*
Episomal DNA, bacteria, 11
Epithelioid cells, 144, 202
Epithelium
    cytomegalovirus, 414
    Epstein–Barr virus, 411–12
    influenza viruses, 471
    rhinoviruses, 466
Epitopes, 110, 111
Epizootic infection, anthrax, 228
Epstein–Barr virus, 411–14
    adults, 152
    latent infection, 105
    receptors, 95
    vaccines, 414
    X-linked recessive lymphoproliferative
        syndrome, 150
Equine antitoxins, 239, 670
Equine morbillivirus, 479
Eradication
    brucellosis, 325
    pertussis, 317
    poliomyelitis, 463
    smallpox, 421, 424, 425–6, 654

Erysipelas, 178–9
Erysipeloid, 199
Erysipelothrix, 29, 199
Erythema chronicum migrans, 350
Erythema infectiosum, 452
Erythema multiforme, 402–3, 426
Erythema nodosum, 144
Erythema nodosum leprosum, 212
Erythrasma, 194
Erythrocytes, mycoplasmas on, 384
Erythrocytic schizogony, 590
Erythrogenic toxins, 177
Erythromycin, 52
    diphtheria prophylaxis, 676
    Legionnaires' disease, 320
    ophthalmia neonatorum, 247
    pertussis, 314
    Streptococcus, 186
    syphilis, 348
Erythroviruses *see* B19 erythrovirus
Escape mutants, hepatitis B, 441–2
Eschar, malignant pustule, 226
Escherichia blattae, 273
Escherichia coli, 265–74
    adhesion, 86
    antibiotics, 644 (Tables), 645
    antigenic structure, 265–6
    attaching and effacing, 268, 272
    D value, 75
    enteritis, 267–73
    entero-aggregative, 267, 272–3
    entero-invasive, 267, 270
    enteropathogenic, 267, 268
    enterotoxigenic, 267, 268–70
        heat-labile toxins, 90
    F factor, 66
    fimbrial adhesins, 85–6
    lac operon, *63*, 66
    motility, 16
    transformation, 65
    see also Verocytotoxin-producing
        Escherichia coli
Espundia, *598*, 599
Essential mixed cryoglobulinaemia, 510
ETEC *see* Enterotoxigenic *Esch. coli*
Ethambutol, 207, 208
Ethnicity, *H. influenzae*, 308
Ethylene oxide, 74, 78
Ethylhydrocupreine, *Str. pneumoniae*
        sensitivity, 185
Eubacterium, *341*, 342
Eugonic colonies, 201
Eukarya, 10, 25, *28*
Eumycetoma, 578
Europe, rabies, 555
Evolution
    myxomatosis and rabbits, 427–8
    pathways (Woese), 9, 10
    see also Endosymbiosis; Phylogenetics
Exanthem subitum, 418
Exhaust ventilation, 668
Exogenous infections, 7
Exophiala werneckii, 577
Exopolysaccharides, bacterial, 86
Exospores, 19
Exosporium, 18, *19*

Exotoxin A, *Pseudomonas aeruginosa*,
        283, 284
Exotoxins, 90–1
    pyrogenic, *91*, 177
Expatriates, 633, 634
Experimental infections, rhinoviruses,
        465–6
Explosive outbreaks, 657
Exponential phase of growth, 38, 39
Extremophiles, 42
Extrinsic allergic alveolitis, 221
Exudates, 130, 161–2
Eye, 631
    adenoviruses, 395–6, 398
    Bacillus cereus, 229
    Candida, 586
    Chlamydia trachomatis, 362–3
    congenital rubella, 502
    herpes simplex virus, 403
    leprosy, 211–12
    Pseudomonas aeruginosa infections,
        283, 285
    specimen collection, *637*
    zoster, 409–10

F factor, *Escherichia coli*, 66
F protein
    measles virus, 96
    paramyxoviruses, 476
    RSV, 481
    Str. pyogenes, 176
Fab regions, 113, 115
Factor VIII, HIV, 535
Factor H, *Str. pyogenes*, 177
Facultative anaerobes, 41, *42*
Faecal antigen test, *Helicobacter pylori*,
        294
Faecal–oral transmission, 7
    bacillary dysentery, 262–3
    calicivirus infections, 544
    cholera, 299
    enteroviruses, 462
Faeces
    adenoviruses, 396–7
    bacteria, 338
    Campylobacter, 290
    cholera, 297
    detection using *Esch. coli*, 265
    dysentery, 261
    enteroviruses, survival, 456
    Salmonella, 255
Falciparum malaria, 590–1, 592, 633, 638
        see also Plasmodium falciparum
Fallopian tubes *see* Salpingitis
Famciclovir, *55*, 56, 406
Familial prion diseases, 563
Far Eastern subtype TBEV (Russian
        spring–summer encephalitis), 497
Farm workers
    anthrax, 228–9
    Leptospira, 356
Fasciola hepatica, 608, *609*
Fasciolopsis buski, 608–10
Fatal familial insomnia, 563
Fatty acids, identification of bacteria, 31

Favus, 574
Fc receptors, 116
Fc regions, 113, 115
Feedback control of immune response,
        140
Feline infectious peritonitis virus (FIPV),
        546, 548
Feline parvoviruses, 448, 449, 450
Feline spongiform encephalopathy, *559*
Fermentation, 41
Fernandez reaction, 213
Fetus
    B19 erythrovirus, 451, 453, 454
    cytomegalovirus, 415
    immune system, 131–2
    mycoplasmas, 386
    rubella, 502
    varicella syndrome, 409
Fever *see* Pyrexia
Fever blisters, 402
Fibres, adenoviruses, 393–4
Fibrinolysin, 178
Fibronectin, 86, 107, 176
Field's method (malaria diagnosis), 590
Fifth disease, 452
Filamentous bacteria, 10, 11, 18, 28
Filamentous fungi, 28, 568–9
Filariasis, 604–7
Fildes' peptic digest agar, 305
Filoviruses, 517–20
Filtration
    disinfection, 79
    sterilization, 73–4, 78
Fimbriae, 11, 17–18
    adhesins, 85–6
    antigens, *Esch. coli*, 85, 266, 269
    Bordetella pertussis, 315
    Klebsiella, 277
    Neisseria, 243
    Salmonella, 253
Fimbrillins, 85–6, 88
Fingerprinting, plasmids, 68
Finland, poliomyelitis, 462
Fish, toxins, 628
Fish fancier's finger, 215, 217
Fish tank granuloma, 215, 217
Fish tapeworm *see Diphyllobothrium
        latum*
Fitz-Hugh–Curtis syndrome, 247, 364,
        631
Fixation, for microscopy, 21
Fixed rabies virus, 553
F-*lac* plasmid, 66
Flagella, 11, 16–17
    as adhesins, 86
    antigens
        Escherichia coli, 265
        Salmonella, 251, 255
        Leptospira, 353
Flagellates, *589*, 595–9
Flagellin, 16
Flame sterilization, 78
Flaviviridae, 484, *485*, 506
Flaviviruses, *485*, 486–7, *489*, 495–7, *506*
Flavobacterium meningosepticum, 287
Flea-borne rickettsial fevers, 372, 374

Fleas, 617
  plague epidemiology, 331
Flies, 616, 617–19
  see also Sandflies
Flinders Island spotted fever, *370*
Floppy child syndrome, 240
Flucloxacillin, 47, *646*
Fluconazole, 54, 571, 572
Flucytosine, *55*, 571, 572, 587, 648
Flukes, 607–10
Fluorescein
  Bordetella pertussis, 313
  Pseudomonas aeruginosa, 283–4
Fluorescence
  Porphyromonas, 339
  see also Immunofluorescence
Fluorescence microscopy, 33
  fungi, 571
  Mycobacterium tuberculosis, 205
Fluorescent treponemal
    antibody-absorption test, 347, 348
5-Fluorocytosine, 54
Fluoroquinolones, 53, *646*
  Neisseria gonorrhoeae, 248
Focal epithelial hyperplasia, 433
Folic acid metabolism, antibacterial
    agents on, 53
Fomites, 6
  diphtheria, 192
  human papillomavirus, 434
Fomivirsen, *55*, 57
Food poisoning, 627–8
  Bacillus, 230
  Bacillus cereus, 229
  Botulism (*Clostridium botulinum*), 239,
      240
  calicivirus, 544, 545
  Campylobacter, 290, *291*
  Clostridium perfringens, 234–5
  fish toxins, 628
  health education, 258–9
  investigation, 637
  Listeria monocytogenes, 195, 197-8
  Salmonella, 254, 255, 257–9, 650–1
  Staphylococcus aureus, 168, 169
  Vibrio parahaemolyticus, 300
Foods
  Brucella, 323
  enteroviruses, survival, 456
  Escherichia coli, 272, 273
  hepatitis A virus, 464
Formaldehyde, 74, 78, 79, 80, 456
Formyl-methionyl peptides, 163
Forssman antigen, 112
Foscarnet, *55, 56*, 57, 417
Fosfomycin, 51
F-primes, 66
Fracastoro, Girolamo, 4
Fraction 1 protein capsular antigen,
    Y. pestis, 329
Francisella, 329, 335–6
Francisella tularensis, 335–6
  Brucella ELISA false positive, 324
  epidemiology, 336
Free slime, bacteria, 15–16
Freezing, specimens, 638

Frequent-cutting endonucleases, 34
Friedländer's pneumonia, 276
FTA-Abs test (fluorescent treponemal
    antibody-absorption test), 347, 348
Fungi, 568–88
  agents *vs*, 54, 55, 648
  classification, 28
  growth and physiology, 37
  historical aspects, 4
Fungus ball (aspergilloma), 584
Furazolidone, 54
Furious rabies, 553
Fusidic acid, *46*, 52, *646*
Fusion peptides, influenza viruses, 470
Fusion protein *see* F protein
Fusobacterium, 339

G glycoprotein, RSV, 481
G serotypes, rotaviruses, 524
Gag gene, retroviruses, 528
Gallbladder, *Salmonella* carriage, 256
Gametocytes, *Plasmodium*, 590
γ-globulins, 112
  see also Antibodies; Immunoglobulins
γ-interferon *see* Interferon-γ
Ganciclovir, *55*, 57, 648
  cercopithecine herpesvirus 1, 419–20
  cytomegalovirus, 57, 414, 417
Ganglia, latent HSV infection, 401, 402
Gardnerella vaginalis, 302
Gas gangrene, 231–4, 235, 630
Gastric carcinoma, *H. pylori*, 293
Gastric mucosa, *H. pylori*, 292
Gastritis, *H. pylori*, 292–3
Gastro-enteritis
  listerial, 197
  outbreaks, guidelines, 545
  Salmonella, 254, 256
  see also Diarrhoea
Gastro-intestinal tract, 627–8
  anthrax, 226
  antimicrobial therapy, 650–1
  caliciviruses, 542
  Campylobacter, 289–91
  Escherichia coli, 267–73
  flukes, 608–10
  hospital organisms, *663*
    guidelines for outbreaks, 545
  nematodes, 601–4
  rotaviruses, 525
  specimen collection, *636*
  spirochaetal infections, 346
  see also Enteritis
GB virus-B, 506
GB virus-C, 506
Gel electrophoresis
  bacterial typing, 34
  pulsed-field, 34, *35*
Gelatin, *Mycoplasma hominis* culture, 388
Gender
  leptospirosis, 356
  susceptibility to infection, 123
  syphilis, 348
Gene probes, 31–2, 34, 69, 71, 639
  Mycobacterium tuberculosis, 206

Gene therapy vectors, 392, 451
Gene transfer, 65–7
  virulence determinants, 84
  see also Transferable antibiotic
    resistance
Generalized transducing phages, 67
Genes, 62–3
  interferons, 146
Genetics
  bacteria, 61–72
  immunoglobulin variability, 114–15
Genital tract infections, 630–1
  adenovirus-associated virus, 450
  antimicrobial therapy, 651
  herpes simplex virus, 404
  specimen collection, *636*
  see also Cervix; Pelvic inflammatory
    disease; Urethritis
Genital warts, 432–3, 435
Genomes
  bacteria, 61
  chlamydiae, 360
  Epstein–Barr virus, 412
  hepatitis B virus, 438–9
  hepatitis C virus, 504–5
  herpesviruses, 400
  human papillomavirus, 430–1
  Mycoplasma genitalium, 382
  poxviruses, 422
  variability, rotaviruses, 526
Genomic species, 26
Genomovars, 26
Genotypes
  hepatitis B virus, 439
  hepatitis C virus, 508
    treatment response, 511
  retroviruses, 528-9
    HIV subtypes, 529, 536
Genotypic assays, antiviral agents, 59–60
Genotypic mutation, 64
Genotyping, *B. pertussis*, 315–16
Gentamicin, 51, *52*
Germ theory of disease, 4
Germ tubes, *Candida albicans*, 576
Germination of spores, 19
Gerstmann–Straussler–Scheinker
    syndrome, 563
Ghon focus, 201
Giant cells
  cell-mediated hypersensitivity, 144
  cytomegalovirus infection, 415
Giardia lamblia, 58, *594*, 595
Gingivitis
  herpes simplex virus, 403
  Treponema, 346
  Vincent's, 339, 346
Glandular fever *see* Infectious
    mononucleosis
Glomerulonephritis, 179–80
  diagnosis, 186
  membranoproliferative, 510
Glossina (tsetse flies), 618
Gloves, 80
Glucocorticoids, susceptibility to
    infection, 123
Glucose non-fermenters, 287

Glucose 6-phosphate dehydrogenase
deficiency
primaquine risk, 592
Rocky Mountain spotted fever, 372
Glutaraldehyde, 74, 80
on hepatitis B virus, 440
Glycopeptides, *46*, 51, 193, *646*
Glycoproteins of viruses, 101–2
herpesviruses, 401–2
varicella-zoster virus, 407
GM₁ ganglioside, heat-labile enterotoxin
detection, 270
Gonorrhoea, 247–9, 630
antimicrobial therapy, 651
assessment of penicillin treatment, 643
epidemiology, 248–9
see also Neisseria gonorrhoeae
Gram stain, 14, 21–2
Gram-negative bacilli, 29, 339–40
hospital environments, 663, 665
Gram-negative bacteria
antibodies *vs*, 162–3
cell walls, *13*, 14
outer membranes, 14–15
spheroplasts, 20
staining, 21–2
type III protein secretion systems, 15
Gram-negative cocci, anaerobic, 341
Gram-positive bacilli, 29, 341–2
Gram-positive bacteria, *13*, 14, 21–2
Gram-positive cocci, 340–1, 663
Granulocyte–macrophage
colony-stimulating factor, *138*, 157
Granulocytes, 122
Granulocytic ehrlichiosis, 376
Granuloma inguinale, 310
Granulomas
intracellular bacteria, 164, 165
parasitic infections, 155
tuberculosis, 202
Granulomatous cerebral angiitis, 409–10
Graunt, John (1620-74), epidemiology,
653
Griseofulvin, 54, *55*, 571, 575, 648
Group C vaccines, *Neisseria meningitidis*,
247, *675*, 676
Growth
bacteria, 18, 37–8
vs resistance to sterilization, 76
transformed cells, 105–6
Growth cycle, chlamydiae, 361–2
Growth factors (bacterial culture), 39
Growth hormone, Creutzfeldt–Jakob
disease, 563
Gruby, David, work on fungi, 4
Gruinard (Scotland), anthrax, 228
Guanarito virus, 515
Guanine plus cytosine content, DNA, 27
Guillain–Barré syndrome, 290
Guinea pig virulence, *C. diphtheriae*, 191
Guinea worm, *604*, 607
Gulf War syndrome, 229

H antigens *see* Flagella, antigens
H₅N₁ influenza, 469, 472, 473

Haemadsorption, 33
para-influenza viruses, 476
Haemagglutination, 17, 33
arboviruses, 486
echoviruses, 456
Escherichia coli, 266
Haemagglutinins, 86
influenza viruses, 468–9
paramyxoviruses, 476
rubella virus, 500
viral adsorption, 94
viral infections, 103
see also Isohaemagglutinins
Haemin (X factor), *Haemophilus
influenzae* culture, 304, 307
Haemoglobinopathies, *Streptococcus
pneumoniae* prophylaxis, 188
Haemolysins
Escherichia coli, 266
Str. agalactiae, 180–1
see also Streptolysins
Haemolysis
Streptococcus, 175
Vibrio parahaemolyticus, 300
Haemolytic anaemia
mycoplasmal pneumonia, 385
Salmonella, 144
Haemolytic uraemic syndrome, 260, 267,
271
Haemophilus, 304–10
Haemophilus aphrophilus, 305
Haemophilus ducreyi, 309
Haemophilus influenzae, 304–9
antibiotics, *644*, 650
meningitis, 305, 308, 629
see also Hib
Haemorrhage, filoviruses, 519
Haemorrhagic colitis, 267, 271
Haemorrhagic conjunctivitis, 459
Haemorrhagic cystitis, 396
Haemorrhagic fevers, *489*, 497
arenaviruses, 515
with renal syndrome, 498
Hafnia, 278
Hair
fungi, 574, 577
Hairbrush sampling, ringworm, 575
Hairpin loops, parvovirus replication,
450
Hairy leucoplakia, oral, *413*, 530
Halofantrine, 592
Halophilicity, *Vibrio*, 295, *296*, 300
Hand, foot and mouth disease, 459
Handwashing, 7, 263, 667
Hanging drop preparations, 31
Hantaan virus, 498
Hantavirus, 484, *485*, 498–9
pulmonary syndrome, 490, 498–9
Haptens, 110
mycoplasmas, 384
Hard ticks *see* Ixodid ticks
Haverhill fever, 328
Hayflick limit, 106
Hazardous substances/organisms
Bartonella, 326
botulinal toxin, 240

Burkholderia, 286
Coccidioides immitis, 580
filoviruses, 519
Francisella tularensis, 336
Histoplasma capsulatum, 581
rabies virus, 554
Rickettsia, 373
sterilization and disinfection policies,
82
vaccines, 673
Venezuelan haemorrhagic fever viruses,
516
Yersinia pestis, 330
HBcAg variants, 442
HBeAg, 439, 442–3
HBIG *see* Anti-HBs; Hyperimmune
immunoglobulins, hepatitis B
HBsAg, 441–2
Heaf test, 205, 677
Health care personnel, 668
hepatitis B, 444–5
vaccination, 446
HIV, 535
infection prevention, 537
Health education, food poisoning, 258–9
Heart
congenital rubella, 502
rheumatic fever, 180
Heat
disinfection, 74, 79
on hepatitis B virus, 440
Legionella isolation, 320
see also Heat sterilization
Heat resistance
Clostridium spores, 231
Escherichia coli, 265
Heat shock proteins, 43
chlamydiae, 360–1
Heat sterilization, 73, 76–8
spores, 18
anthrax, 226
Heat-labile enterotoxin, 90, 268
detection, 270
Heat-stable enterotoxin, 268–9
detection, 270
Heavy chains, antibodies, 112
Heck's disease, 433
HeLa cells, Verocytotoxin binding, 271
Helical symmetry, viruses, 22
Helicobacter, 292
Helicobacter pylori, 288, 291–5
adhesion, 86
treatment 294-5
urease, 92, 292, 294
Helminths, 601–14
agents *vs*, 58, *59*
specimen transport, *637*
type III hypersensitivity, 144
Helper T cells *see* CD4+ T cells; Tₕ cells
Hemiparesis, zoster, 409–10
Hemiptera (bugs), 616–17
Hendra virus, 475, 483
HEp-2 cells, adhesion of entero-
aggregative *Esch. coli*, 272
HEPA filters, 79
Hepacivirus, 506

Hepadnaviruses, 438–47
 enzymes, 24
 nucleic acids, 24
 replication, 101
Hepatitis A, 455, 463–4
 immunoglobulins, 671
 vaccines, 464
Hepatitis B, 438–47
 disinfectant resistance, 80, 444
 epidemiology, 444–5
 interferon-α on, 57
 lamivudine on, 57, 444
 vaccines, 445–6, 677
 see also HBsAg
Hepatitis C, 504–11
Hepatitis D virus (delta agent), 24, 446–7
Hepatitis e antigen, 439, 442–3
Hepatitis G, 506
Hepatocellular carcinoma
 hepatitis B virus, 441, 443
 hepatitis C virus, 509–10
Hepatomegaly, parasites, 159
Hepatovirus see Hepatitis A
Herd immunity, 317, 655, 673–4
Herodotus (484–425 BC), 653
Herpangina, 459
Herpes simplex virus, 401–7
 aciclovir on, 406, *644*
  plaque reduction assay, 59
 latent infection, 105, 401–2
 replication, 97
Herpesviruses, *23*, 399–420
 aciclovir action, 55–6
Herpetic whitlow, 403
Heterologous antibody preparations, 670
Heterologous antitoxins *see* Equine
  antitoxins
Heterophile antigens, 112
Heterotrophs, 40
Hexachlorophane, 80, 81
Hexamine, 6
Hexons, 24, 393
Hfr strains (high-frequency recombination
  strains), 66
Hib (*Haemophilus influenzae* type b)
 infections, 305–6
 vaccines, 308, 309, 675, 676
High-density oligonucleotide arrays, 32
High-efficiency particulate air filters, 79
High-frequency recombination strains,
  66
Hill, Bradford, association *vs* causation,
  660
Hippocrates (460–361 BC), 653
Hippurate, *Campylobacter*, 289
Histamine, 129, *130*
Histiocytes, 127
Histoplasmosis, 580–1
Historical aspects, 3–7
 Bacterium aerogenes, 275
 epidemiology, 7, 653–4
 leprosy, 209–10
 rabies, 5, 551
HIV *see* Human immunodeficiency
  virus
HLA (human leucocyte group A), 117–20

Hodgkin's disease
 Epstein–Barr virus, *413*
 immunodeficiency, 143
Hold times, sterilization, *76*
Homologous antibody preparations, 670
Homologous antitoxin, 237, 239
Homosexuality,
 coronaviruses, 550
 hepatitis B, 444
 HIV, 535, 536
Honey, botulism, 240
Hong Kong influenza, 469, 472, 473
Hookworms, *602*, 603
Horses, arboviruses, 494
Hospital infections, 2, 659, 662–9
 bacillary dysentery, 263
 Escherichia coli enteritis, prevention,
   273
 gastro-enteritis outbreaks, guidelines,
   545
 Klebsiella, 277
 Pseudomonas aeruginosa, 283, 285
 resistant organisms, 645
 Serratia, 279
Hospitals, sterilization and disinfection
  policies, 81–2
Host factors, infections, 654–5
Host ranges, plasmids, 68
Host ribosomes, arenaviruses, 513
Host-adapted *Salmonella*, 252
Hot air sterilizers, 78
House dust mites, 616
Household outbreaks, 656
Housekeeping genes, multilocus sequence
  typing, 35
HPV *see* Human papillomaviruses
HSV *see* Herpes simplex virus
HTLV-1 *see* Human T lymphotropic virus
  1
HTLV-2 *see* Human T lymphotropic virus
  2
Human bot fly, 619
Human coronavirus, 547–50
Human cytomegalovirus, 414
Human enteric coronavirus, 550
Human growth hormone, CJD, 563
Human herpesvirus 6, 418
 receptors, *95*
Human herpesvirus 7, 418
Human herpesvirus 8, 419
Human immunodeficiency virus, 527,
  530–4
 agents *vs*, 57–8
  susceptibility testing, 59
 antigenic variation, 152
 BCG contraindication, 209
 chancroid and, 309
 control, 536–7
 cytomegalovirus interaction, 415
 diagnosis, 532–3
 disinfectants on, 527
 epidemiology, 536
 genital herpes, 404
 isolation, 533
 Kaposi's sarcoma, 419
 mycoplasmas, 387

 pathogenesis, 531–2
 progression to AIDS, 532
 receptors, 95
 stage of infection, virus changes *vs*, 532
 surveillance reporting, 641
 temperatures, survival, 527
 transmission, 535
 treatment, 533–4
 vaccines and, 672
 vaccines for, 537
 varicella-zoster virus, 410
 see also AIDS
Human leucocyte group A, 117–20
Human normal immunoglobulin, 671
Human papillomaviruses, 429–35
 cell transformation, 107, 433
 cervix, 630
Human T lymphotropic virus 1, 107, 527,
   528, 529–30, 533, 534–5
Human T lymphotropic virus 2, 527, 528,
   535
Human tetanus immunoglobulin, 237, 239
Humoral immunity, 116–17, 131, 135–6
 antigen recognition, 110–11
 bacterial infections, 162–3
 innate immunity, 124–7
 parasitic infections, 156–7
 viral infections, 148–9
Hyaluronic acid, *Streptococcus pyogenes*,
   177
Hyaluronidase
 Clostridium perfringens, 233
 Str. pyogenes, 177–8
Hybrid Capture® assay, cervical biopsies,
   435
Hybridization
 DNA homology, 27
 genetic mapping, 69
Hybridoma technique, 32, 136
Hydatid cysts, 154, 613
Hydrochloric acid, enteroviruses, 456
Hydrogen donor types, 40
Hydrogen peroxide
 catalase on, 41
 disinfection, 81
 mycoplasmas, 383
Hydrophobia, 551
Hydrops fetalis, 451, 453
5-Hydroxytryptamine, 129
Hygiene, *Streptococcus*, 187
Hymenolepis diminuta, 613, 616
Hymenolepis nana, 611–13
Hymenoptera, 616
Hyperbaric oxygen, 234
Hyperimmune immunoglobulins
 hepatitis B, 445
  see also Anti-HBs
 respiratory syncytial virus, 482
Hyperinfection, *Strongyloides stercoralis*,
   603
Hypersensitivity, 143–5
 type I *see* Anaphylaxis
 type II (cytotoxic), 143–4
 type III *see* Immune complexes
 type IV *see* Delayed-type
  hypersensitivity

Hypervariable regions, 114
Hyphae, 28, 568
Hypnozoites, *Plasmodium*, 590
Hypochlorites *see* Chlorine-releasing
 disinfectants
Hypogammaglobulinaemias, 142
 mycoplasmas, 387, 388
 X-linked infantile, 142
 vaccination danger, 149
Hypopyon, 631
Hypothrombinaemia, cephalosporins, 48

Iatrogenic CJD, 563
Iatrogenic diseases, 161
ICAM-1, rhinovirus adsorption, 95
Icosahedral symmetry, 22–4
 adenoviruses, 392–3
 herpesviruses, 399–400
Id reactions, 574
Identification of micro-organisms, 25,
 30–3, 639, *640*
IgA, 113, *114*, *115*
 bacterial infections, 162
 deficiency, 143
 influenza virus antigenic variation,
 152
 proteases, 88–9
 Str. pneumoniae, 182
 vs viruses, 148, 149
IgD, *113*, 114, *115*
IgE, *113*, 114, *115*, 143, 156
IgG, 113, *115*
 chronic hepatitis B, 443
 neonate, 131–2
 response to antigen, 135
 rubella, 503
 vs viruses, 148
IgM, 113–14
 agglutination, 116
 B19 erythrovirus infection, 453
 hepatitis B, 443
 neonate, 131–2
 response to antigen, 135, 136
 rubella, 503
 vs viruses, 148
IgM antibody capture ELISA, 33
Imidazoles, *55*, *646*
Imipenem, 49, 224, *646*
Imiquimod, warts, 435
Immune complexes, 115
 hepatitis B, 440
 hypersensitivity, 144, 164
 parasitic infections, 159
 viral antigens, 151
Immune electron microscopy,
 caliciviruses, 542
Immune response
 chlamydiae, 365–6
 Epstein–Barr virus, 412–13
 hepatitis B, 440–1
 treatment results, 443, 444
 herpes simplex virus, 401
 regulation by T_H cells, 141
 vaccines, 671–2
 viral infections, 150–2

see also Cell-mediated immune
 responses; Immunity; Innate
 immunity
Immune response genes, 140
Immune system, 121–2
Immunity
 bacteria, 161–5
 chlamydial infection, 365–6
 cholera, 299
 herpes simplex virus, 401
 historical aspects, 5–6
 influenza, 472
 rhinoviruses, 466
 viral infections, 146–53
 see also Acquired immunity; Herd
 immunity; Innate immunity
Immunization, 670–9
 hepatitis B, 441–2, 445–6
 herd immunity, 655
 historical aspects, 5–6
 outbreaks of infection, 659
 Pseudomonas aeruginosa, 285
 varicella-zoster virus, 411
 see also Tetanus, immunization;
 Vaccines
Immunization programmes, 674–5
 age of commencement, 672
Immunoblastic lymphoma, *413*
Immunocompromise
 adenoviruses, 392, 396
 B19 erythrovirus, 453, 454
 cytomegalovirus, 416
 hepatitis C, 509
 antibodies, false negatives, 507
 herpes simplex virus, 402–3
 hospital infections, 662–3
 mycoplasmas, 387
 progressive multifocal
 leucoencephalopathy, 436
 tuberculosis, 205
 varicella-zoster virus, 410
Immunodeficiency, 141–3
 caused by viruses, 150–2
 danger of polio vaccines, 149
 enteric viruses, 542
 Str. pneumoniae, 183
Immunofluorescence, 33, 639
 indirect, arboviruses, 491
 influenza virus detection, 472
 rabies diagnosis, 554
 see also Micro-immunofluorescence
 test
Immunoglobulin supergene family, 118,
 119
Immunoglobulins, 112–16, 671
 B cell receptors, 115, 117, 132–3
 deficiencies, 142–3
 hepatitis A, 671
 hepatitis B, 445, 671
 human normal, 671
 human tetanus immunoglobulin, 237,
 239
 maternal, 503, 671
 neonate, 131–2, 503, 671
 rabies, 556
 varicella-zoster, 411

see also Hyperimmune
 immunoglobulins
Immuno-polymerase chain reaction,
 33
Immunoprophylaxis, rabies, 556–7, 557
Immunosuppression
 by parasites, 159
 therapeutic, *142*
 persistent viral infections, 152
Immunotherapy
 arenavirus infections, 516
 Epstein–Barr virus, 414
Impetigo, 178, *179*, 630
Imported infections, 633–4
Inactivated vaccines, 5, 671
 polio, 462, 676
Inactivation, measurement, 74–5
Incineration, 77–8
Inclusion blennorrhoea *see* Ophthalmia
 neonatorum, chlamydial
Inclusion bodies, 103
Inclusion conjunctivitis, 362–3
Inclusion granules, bacteria, 10
Incompatibility testing, plasmids, 68
India ink, *15*,
 Cryptococcus neoformans, 583
 Str. pneumoniae, 186
Indicator media, 39–40
 mycoplasmas, 387
Indinavir, AIDS, 534
Indirect immunofluorescence, arboviruses,
 491
Indolamine dioxygenase, *Toxoplasma
 gondii* resistance, 147
Inducers, gene transcription, 63
 interferon genes, 146
Industrial anthrax, 229
Infant mouse test, heat-stable enterotoxin,
 270
Infantile paralysis, 463
Infection control committees, hospital
 infection, 666, 669
Infection rates, tuberculosis, 208
Infections
 antibiotic-induced, 240–1, 647, 663
 defined, 3
 factors, 654–6
 syndromes, 624–34
Infectious bronchitis virus, avian, 546
Infectious hepatitis, 463–4
 see also Viral hepatitis
Infectious mononucleosis, 145, 413, 414
 ampicillin, 626
 X-linked recessive lymphoproliferative
 syndrome, 150
 see also Mononucleosis syndrome
Infective doses, *Salmonella*, 252
Infective endocarditis *see* Endocarditis
Infectivity
 enteroviruses, 462
 Q fever, 377
Inflammation, 129–30, 161–2
 chlamydial infection, 365
Influenza, 471–4
 epidemiology, 472–4
 neuraminidase inhibitors, 57

pandemics, 304, 472, 473
vaccines, 149, 474, 678
Influenza viruses, 468–74
antigenic variation, 152
endocytosis, 95
replication, 99–100, 470
Ingestion, *Salmonella*, 252
Injection sites, vaccines, 673
BCG, 677
Innate immunity, 121, 122–30, 161
deficiency, 142
parasitic infections, 155
Insects, *615*, 616–20
bacillary dysentery, 263
historical aspects, 7
Insertion mutations, *64*
Insertion sequences, gene probe typing, 34
In-situ hybridization, cervical biopsies, 435
Institutions
bacillary dysentery, 263
see also Hospital infections; Military camps
Integrins, bacterial adhesion, 87
Integrons, 70
Intensive care, *171*
Pseudomonas aeruginosa, 285
resistant organisms, 645
Interference contrast microscopy, 21
see also Phase-contrast microscopy
Interferon-α, *55*, 57, *138*
hepatitis C virus, 510
Interferon-β, *138*
Interferon-γ, 138–9
parasitic infections, 158
T. gondii resistance, 147
Interferons, 57, 125, 146–8
abortive viral infections, 105
hepatitis B treatment, 443
influenza, 471
warts, 435
Interleukin-1, *138*, 139
acute phase protein, 124
Interleukin-2, *138*
deficiency, 157
HTLV-1, cell transformation, 107
Leishmania, 159
T cell growth factor, 134
Interleukin-3, 157
Interleukin-4, *138*
on B cells, 135
Interleukin-8, *138*
Helicobacter pylori adhesion, 86
Interleukin-13, *138*
Internalin, *Listeria*, 195
Intestinal flukes, 608–10
Intestinal nematodes, 601–4
Intestine
caliciviruses, 542
rotaviruses, 525
Intimin, 268
Intracellular bacteria, 86–7, 163–4
Burkholderia pseudomallei, 286
chlamydiae, 359–60, 361–2
Legionella, 319
Listeria monocytogenes, 195

phagocytes, 88
Rickettsia, 370
Intracellular parasites, 158
Intranasal vaccine, influenza, 149
Intrapartum infection
hepatitis C virus, 509
herpes simplex virus, 404–5
Intravenous fluids
antibiotics, 647
Serratia contamination, 279
Intussusception, 396, 526
In-use concentrations, disinfectants, 79
In-use tests, disinfectants, 81
Invasion, bacteria, 86–7
Invasive aspergillosis, 584–5
Invasive meningococcal disease, 242
Inversion mutations, *64*
Involution, bacteria, 19
Iodamoeba bütschlii, *594*
Iodine
disinfectants, 81
Gram stain, 21, 22
Ionizing irradiation, sterilization, 73, 78
Ipecacuanha, 6
IPV (inactivated polio vaccine), 462, 676
Ir genes (immune response genes), 140
Iron
on bacterial protein production, 84
bacterial scavenging, 89
chelation, 87, 129
Escherichia coli, 266
Klebsiella, 277
Pseudomonas aeruginosa, 283
Serratia, 279
Iron overload, *Vibrio vulnificus* infection, 301
Irradiation, sterilization, 73, 78
Isogenic mutants, virulence determinants, 84
Isohaemagglutinins, 112
Isolates (bacteria), 33
Isolation
infectious sources, 658, 668
protective, 668
Isoniazid, 51, 207, 208, 209
Isospora belli, 593
Italy, hepatitis D virus, 447
Itch mite (*Sarcoptes scabei*), 620
Itraconazole, 54, 571, 575
Ivermectin, 58, *59*, 606–7, 620
Ixodid ticks, 350, 620–1
arboviruses, 486
flaviviruses, 497

J chain, IgA, 113, *114*
Jacuzzis, *Ps. aeruginosa*, 285
James' stippling, *591*
Jamestown Canyon virus, 497
Japanese encephalitis, 490
epidemiology, 495
vaccine, 499–500, 678
Japanese seafood
fish toxins, 628
Vibrio parahaemolyticus, 300

Japanese spotted fever, *370*
Jarisch–Herxheimer reaction, 348, 350, 351
JC virus, 429, 435–7
Jellison biovars, *Francisella tularensis*, 335
Jenner, Edward, 424
Jiggers, 617
Joblot, L., 3
Jopling reactions, leprosy, 212
Junin virus, 515, 516

K antigens
Escherichia coli, 265, *266*
Klebsiella, 276
K88 fimbrial antigen, *Escherichia coli*, 85, 266, 269
Kala azar, *598*, 599
Kanagawa phenomenon, 300
Kanamycin, *52*
Kaposi's sarcoma, 419, 531
Kaposi's sarcoma-related herpesvirus, 419
Kaposi's varicelliform eruption, 403
Kauffmann–White classification, *Salmonella*, 251
Keratin, dermatophytes, 573
Keratitis, 631
Acanthamoeba, 595
mycotic, 578
Kerions, 574
Ketodeoxyoctonate, 89, *90*
Killer cells, 136
Killing, measurement, 74–5
Kingella, 249
Kinins, *130*
Kirby–Bauer test, 59
Kissing bugs, 617
Kitchens, gastro-enteritis outbreaks, guidelines, 545
see also Catering
Klebsiella, 275–7, 644
Klebsiella pneumoniae, 275
Koala bears, chlamydia, 366
Koch phenomenon, 202
Koch, Robert, 3, 4
Haemophilus, 304
postulates, 4, 660
work on anthrax, 4, 225
Koch–Weeks bacillus, 309
Koilocytes, 434
Koplik's spots, 479
Kuru, 563
Kyasanur Forest disease, 497

La Crosse virus, 490, 497
Laboratory procedures, 635–40
Lac operon, *Esch. coli*, *63*, 66
Lachrymal canaliculitis, 342
Lactobacillus, 29, *341*
Lactoferrin, 87, 128–9
bacterial receptors, 89
Lag phase of growth, 38, 39
Lamivudine, *55*, 57, *58*, 444, 534

Lanarkshire, *Esch. coli*, 272
Lancefield grouping, 175
Langerhans cells
  arbovirus infection, 487
  contact hypersensitivity, 145
  viral infections, 150
Large T antigens, 435, 436
Larva migrans, visceral, 603
Larvae
  mosquitoes, control, 499
  Strongyloides stercoralis, 602
Laryngotracheobronchitis, 627
  see also Croup
Larynx, human papillomavirus, 433
Lassa fever, 515, 516–17
Latamoxef, 49
Late polypeptides, poxvirus, 422
Latent heat, 77
Latent infections
  syphilis, 345
  viral, 93, 105, 151, 399, 401–2, 408
Lateral flagella, bacteria, 16
Latex agglutination, 32
  Cryptococcus neoformans, 584
  rabies diagnosis, 554
Lectin pathway, complement, 125
Lectins, 133
Leeuwenhoek, Antony van, 3
Legionella, 318–21
Legionella pneumophila, 318–21
  metalloprotease, 92
  receptors for, 87
Legionnaires' disease, 318, 319–21, 627,
    658–9
Leishman-Donovan bodies, *596*
Leishmania, 596, 598–9
  agents *vs*, 58
  immunosuppression by, 159
  interleukin-2, 159
  intracellular parasitism, 158
  lymphokines, 158
  macrophages, 155
Lentiviruses, 528
Lepidoptera, 617
Lepromatous leprosy, 210–11
Lepromins, 213
Leprosins, 213
Leprosy, 164–5, 209–13
  treatment, 212-3
Leptospira, 29–30, 352–7
Leptotrichia buccalis, 339
Lethal factor, *Bacillus anthracis*, 227
Leucocytes, 121–2
Leukaemia, polyomavirus, 436
Leukotrienes, *130*
Levamisole, *59*, *604*
Levinthal agar, 305
L-forms, 20
LGV biovar, *Chl. trachomatis*, 358
Lice, 619–20
Light chains, antibodies, 112
Lincosamides, *46*, 52
Linezolid, 52
Linnaean classification, 25
Lipid A, 89, 90
Lipodystrophy syndrome, 534

Lipopolysaccharides
  chlamydiae, 361
  complement resistance, 89
  Gram-negative bacteria, 14, 15
  Salmonella, 250–1
  see also Endotoxin
Lipoproteinase, *Str. pyogenes*, 178
Lipoteichoic acid, 14
Liquid media *see* Broth media
Lister, Joseph, 7
Listeria, 29, 195–8
Listeria monocytogenes, 195–8
  intracellular parasitism, 163
  invasion, 87
  iron acquisition, 89
  meningitis, treatment, 650
Lithotrophs, 40
Live-attenuated vaccines, 5, 671
  contra-indications, 672
  influenza, 149
  measles, 480
  polio, 462–3, 676–7
Liver
  abscesses, 593, 651
  hepatitis C histology, 509
  infections, treatment, 651
  transplantation
    hepatitis B, 444, 445
    hepatitis C, 511
  see also Fitz-Hugh–Curtis syndrome
Loa loa, 604–6
Lobar pneumonia, 627
Loboa loboi, 579
Lockjaw, 237
Log phase of growth, 38, 39
Long terminal repeats, retrovirus
    replication, 100
Loose slime, bacteria, 15–16
Louping ill, 497
Louse *see* Lice
Louse-borne relapsing fever, 349–50
Löwenstein–Jensen medium, 200–1
Low-temperature steam, 79
L-phase variants, *Streptobacillus
    moniliformis*, 327
Lumbar puncture, 629
Lung fluke *see Paragonimus westermani*
Lupus vulgaris, 204
Lyme disease, 350–1
Lymph nodes, 132
  antigen-presenting cells, *134*
  viral infections, 150
Lymphadenopathy
  environmental mycobacteria,
    216–17
  HIV, 530
  see also Mesenteric lymphadenitis
Lymphoblastoid cell lines, 412
Lymphocytes, 121–2
  EBV infection, 411, 412
  epitopes, 111
  Plasmodium falciparum on, 159
  trafficking, 132
Lymphocytic choriomeningitis virus, 513,
    515
Lymphocytosis, pertussis, 314

Lymphogranuloma venereum, 364
  see also LGV biovar, *Chl. trachomatis*
Lymphoid tissues, 131–2
  enteroviruses, 460
  PrP^{sc}, variant CJD, 564
Lymphokine-activated killer cells, 136
Lymphokines, 122, 136, 137, 150
  bacterial infections, 163
  Leishmania, 158
Lymphomas *see* Body cavity lymphomas;
    specific lymphomas
Lymphoproliferative disorders, 143
L-lysine, Gram-negative bacteria, 14
Lysis
  bacteria, 13, 127
  immune cytotoxicity, 136–7
  see also Cytolysis
Lysogenic conversion, 67
Lysogeny, 34, 61, 67
Lysosomal granules, phagocytes, 88
Lysosomes, 128
Lysozyme, 87, 124, 128
  resistance of Gram-negative bacteria,
    15
Lyssavirus, 551, 552
  see also Rabies
Lytic phages, 34

M proteins, *Streptococcus pyogenes*, 88,
    176–7
  typing, 186
MAC-enzyme-linked immunosorbent
    assay (IgM antibody capture
    ELISA), 33
McFadyean's reaction, 227
Machupo virus, 515
Macrolides, *46*, 51–2, *646*
Macrophages, 122, 127
  AIDS, 531
  antigen-presenting, 134
  bacterial infections, 163
  cell-mediated immunity, 137–8
  delayed hypersensitivity, 144
  interferons on, 147
  Leishmania, 155
  parasites, 155, 158
  viral infection of, 151
Madura foot, 223
Maedi (sheep disease), 528
Maggots, 615
Magnesium chloride, 456
Maintenance hosts, *Leptospira*, 356
Major histocompatibility complex,
    117–20
  cell activation, 133–4
  class I molecules, 118, 140, 147, 163–4,
    441
  class II molecules, 118, 139, 140, 147,
    163
  T cell antigen recognition, 117
Malaria, 589–92
  Burkitt's lymphoma, 414
  colony-stimulating factors, 157
  discovery of parasites, 5
  immunopathology, 160

imported, 633
resistance
  Duffy blood groups, 155, 592
  sickle cell disease, 123, 155, 592
  see also Antimalarials; *Plasmodium*
Malassezia furfur, 569, 576–7
Malathion, 620
Male fern, 6
Malignant pustule, 226
Malnutrition, *142*, 154
MALT lymphoma, *H. pylori*, 293
Maltster's lung, 584
Mannheimia haemolytica, 335
Mannose-resistant haemagglutination,
  Escherichia coli, 266
Mannose-sensitive, mannose-resistant
  fimbriae, 85
Mansonella, *604*, 606
Mantoux test, 205, 677
Marburg virus, 517–20
Mast cells, 121, 122
  immunoglobulin binding, *115*, 116
  parasitic infections, 156
Mastadenoviruses, 394
Matching coefficient, Adansonian
  classification, 26
Maternal immunoglobulins, 503, 671
Mathematical modelling, epidemiology,
  659–60
Matrix-assisted laser desorption/ionization
  time of flight spectrometers, 35
Maurer's spots, *591*
Mazotti reaction, 606
MBC *see* Minimum bactericidal
  concentration
McFadyean's reaction, 227
Measles, 479–81
  F protein, 96
  receptors, *95*
  vaccines, 480–1
    developing countries, 675
    killed, 153
    receptors, *95*
  virus, 475, 479
Measles, mumps and rubella vaccine, 479,
  480, 504, 677
  controversy, 673
  UK scheduling, *675*
Mebendazole, 58
  activity spectrum, *604*
MecA gene, MRSA, 171
Medusa head colonies, 225
Mefloquine, 592
Melioidosis, 286
Melting temperature, DNA, 27
Membrane attack complex, 126–7
Membrane immunoglobulins, 115
  B cell receptors, 115, 117, 132–3
Membranes *see* Cytoplasmic membranes;
  Outer membranes
Membranoproliferative
  glomerulonephritis, 510
Memory cells, 132, 135, 139
MenC vaccine, *675*, 676
Meningitis

arboviruses, 488
coxsackieviruses, 459
Cryptococcus neoformans, 583
echoviruses, 458
emergency diagnosis, 638
Escherichia coli, 266, 267
Flavobacterium meningosepticum,
  287
H. influenzae, 305, 308, 629
herpes simplex virus, 404
IgA proteases, 89
listeriosis, 197, 198
mumps, 477, 478
mumps vaccine, 677
Neisseria meningitidis, 242, 244, 245,
  629
neonate, 281, 629
Salmonella, treatment, 256
Str. agalactiae, 181
Str. pneumoniae, 183, 185, 629
  penicillin resistance, 186
  see also Lymphocytic choriomeningitis
    virus; Meningococcal group
    C vaccine
Meningococcal disease, invasive, 242
Meningococcal group C vaccine
  (MenC vaccine), *675*, 676
Mercaptoethanol test, 324
Meropenem, 49
Merozoites, *Plasmodium*, 590
Mesangial cells, 127
Mesenteric lymphadenitis
  adenoviruses, 396
  Yersinia pseudotuberculosis, 333
Mesophiles, 41, *42*
Messenger RNA, 12
  adaptive responses, 43
  binding studies, 27
  synthesis by viruses, 96–7
Metabolism, bacteria, 42–3
Metalloprotease, *Legionella*, 92
Metastatic infection, *Salmonella*, 254
Methenamine, 6
Methicillin-resistant *Staphylococcus
  aureus*, 48, 171–2, 645, 663–4
Methyl violet, Gram stain, 21, 22
Metriphonate, *59*, 610
Metronidazole, 54, 58, 302, 342
MHC *see* Major histocompatibility
  complex
MIC *see* Minimum inhibitory
  concentration
Mice
  arenaviruses, 516
  Bordetella pertussis, 312–13
  coxsackieviruses, 457
  Streptobacillus moniliformis, 327, 328
  see also Suckling mice
Microaerophilic organisms, 41, *42*
  Campylobacter, 288, 290
Microarrays, DNA, 72
Microcapsules, bacteria, 11, 15
Micrococcus, 29
Microfilariae, 604, *605*, 606
Microglia, 127
Micro-immunofluorescence test, 366

Microscopic agglutination test
  leptospirosis, 355
Microscopy, 9–10, 20–2, 31, 638
  aspergillosis, 585
  Candida, 586
  fungi, 571, 575
  historical aspects, 3
  L-form bacteria, 20
  spirochaetes, 29–30
  Treponema, 347
  see also Electron microscopy;
    Fluorescence microscopy
Microsporidia, 599
Microsporum, 572, 575
Microwave ovens, 78
Midges, 618
Miliary tuberculosis, 202
Military camps
  adenoviruses, 395, 398
  coxsackieviruses, 459
  meningococcal epidemics, 246
Milk
  Brucella, 323
  Campylobacter enteritis, 290
  Staph. aureus infection, 170
  tuberculosis, 208
Milk (human), HIV, 535
Milker's nodes, 426
Millipedes, 621
Miltefosine, leishmaniasis, 599
Milzbrandbazillus, 226
Minimal media, 40
Minimum bactericidal concentration, 59
Minimum inhibitory concentration, 59,
  643
Mink
  parvoviruses, 450
  see also Transmissible mink
    encephalopathy
Mink enteritis virus, 450
Minute virus of mice, 448
Miracidia, 607–8
Miscarriage *see* Abortion
Mite-borne rickettsial fevers, 372–3, 374
Mites, 620
  house dust mites, 616
Mitis group, *Streptococcus*, 175, 184
Mitochondria, origin, 13
Mitogens, 133, 156
Mitsuda reaction, 213
MMR vaccine *see* Measles, mumps and
  rubella vaccine
Mobiluncus, 301–2, 630, 651
Moist heat, 76, 77, 79
Molecular classification, 9
Molecular weights
  antigens, 110
  viruses, 24
Mollicutes, 379
Molluscum contagiosum, 424–6
Molluscum contagiosum virus, *423*
Monkeypox, 426
Monkeys
  cercopithecine herpesvirus 1, 419, 420
  coxsackieviruses, 457
  Marburg virus, 517

Monkeys (*contd*)
  polioviruses, 456
  simian parvoviruses, 450
  simian T lymphotropic viruses, 528
Monobactams, 49
Monoclonal antibodies, 136
  defined, 6
  organism identification, 32
  para-influenza viruses, 477
  Treponema pallidum, 348
Monocytes, 127–8
Monocytic ehrlichiosis, 376
Monokines, 122, 137–8, 139, 155
Mononuclear phagocytes, 122, 415
Mononucleosis syndrome, 416
  see also Infectious mononucleosis
Montagu, Lady Mary, variolation, 5
Moraxella, 249
Moraxella catarrhalis, 242, 249
Morbillivirus, 475, 479
Morganella, 279–81
Morphogenesis, viruses, 101
Morphological index, *Mycobacterium leprae*, 212
Morphology
  bacteria, 10, 11
  classification by, 9
  study methods, 20–2
  viruses, 23
Morulae (*Ehrlichia*), 375
Mosquito cells, arboviruses, 486, 491
Mosquitoes, 618
  arboviruses, 492
  avoidance measures, 592
  control, 499
  flaviviruses, 495–7
Motility, bacteria, 16
Moulds, 28, 568–9
Mouse *see* Mice
Mouse footpad, *M. leprae*, 210
Mouse hepatitis virus, 546–7, 548
Mucocutaneous candidosis, 576
Mucocutaneous leishmaniasis, 598, 599
Mucopeptides *see* Peptidoglycans
Mucormycosis, 587
Mucosa, candidosis, 575–6
Mucosa-associated lymphoid tissue
    lymphoma, *H. pylori*, 293
Mucus, 124
Multibacillary leprosy, 212
Multidrug-resistant tuberculosis, 208
Multilocus sequence typing, 35
Multiple sclerosis, measles virus, 479
Multisite mutations, 64
Mumps, 152, 475–6, 477–9
Mupirocin, 53
Muramyl dipeptide, 163
Murein sacculi, 14
Murine typhus, 374
Murray Valley encephalitis, 490, 495–6
Muscle, *Clostridium perfringens* toxins
    on, 233
Mutans group, *Streptococcus*, 175, 184
  Str. mutans, 86
Mutations
  antigenic variation, 88

bacteria, 64–5
  antibiotic resistance, 70
  viruses, abortive infections, 104–5
Mx protein, 146–7
Mycelia, 28, 568
  bacterial, 18
Mycetoma, 223, 224, 578
Mycobacteria, 28, 200–14
  agents *vs*, 54
  cell envelopes, 15
  on immune system, 164–5
  intracellular parasitism, 163
  see also Environmental mycobacteria
Mycobacterium avium complex, 215–16
  treatment, 220
Mycobacterium bovis, 200
  culture, 201
  see also Bovine tuberculosis
Mycobacterium chelonae, 216, 217
  immunosuppressed patients, 219
  treatment, 219–20
Mycobacterium fortuitum, 216, 217
  treatment, 219–20
Mycobacterium leprae, 209–13
Mycobacterium tuberculosis, 200–9
  aminoglycosides *vs*, 52
  antibacterial agents
    activities *vs*, 46
    resistance mutations, 70
  doubling time, 38
  receptors for, 87
  see also Tuberculosis
Mycobactin, 216
Mycolic acids, mycobacteria, 15
Mycoplasmas, 28, 30, 379–89
  antibiotics, 644
  pneumonia, 385, 387, 388
Mycoses, 569–88
  subcutaneous, 569, 570
  systemic, 570, 579–88
  see also Dermatophytosis
Mycotic keratitis, 578
Myeloid pathway, 121, 122
Myeloperoxidase, 128
Myiasis, 616, 619
Myocarditis, coxsackie B, 459
Myopericarditis, coxsackie B, 459
Myositis
  coxsackieviruses, 457
  Str. pyogenes, 179
Myriapods, 615
Myxomatosis, 427–8

NAD, *H. influenzae* culture, 304–5
Naegleria, 595
Nagler reaction, 231
Nails
  candidosis, 576
  dermatophytosis, 54, 574, 575
  non-dermatophyte moulds, 577
Nairovirus, 485, 489, 498–9
Nalidixic acid, 53
Naps, mycoplasmas, 379
Nasal carriage, *Staphylococcus aureus*,
    169, 170

Nasal swabs, 636
  pernasal swabs, 313
Nasopharyngeal carcinoma, 413
Natural killer cells, 121, 129, 136, 137,
    147–8
NDV (Newcastle disease virus), 475–6
Necator americanus (hookworm), 601,
    602, 603, 604
Necrotizing fasciitis, 179, 186
Needle stick injuries
  hepatitis B vaccination, 677
  HIV, 535, 537
Needles, intravenous infection, 7
'Negative'('–') single-stranded RNA
    viruses, replication, 99–100
Negative staining, 21
Negri bodies, 553
Neisseria, 29, 88, 242–9
Neisseria gonorrhoeae, 242, 243, 247–9,
    630
  auxotyping, 243–4
  carriage, 247
  pharyngitis, 626
  see also Gonorrhoea
Neisseria lactamica, 242, 243
Neisseria meningitidis, 242, 243–7
  carriage, 244, 245
  epidemiology, 246
  group C vaccine, 247, 675, 676
  meningitis, 242, 244, 245, 629
  porin variation, 88
  vaccines, 246–7
  virulence, 83
Nelfinavir, AIDS, 534
Nematodes, 601–7
Neomycin, 52
Neonate
  BCG vaccination, 209
  conjunctivitis, 631
    see also Ophthalmia neonatorum
  coxsackieviruses, 459
  cytomegalovirus, 415–16
  diphtheria immunity, 191
  echoviruses, 458
  hepatitis B, 441, 442, 446
  herpes simplex virus, 404–5, 406–7
  HIV, 532, 535, 537
  immunoglobulins, 131–2, 503, 671
  listeriosis, 196–7, 198
  meningitis, 281, 629
  mycoplasmas, 385, 386
  Pseudomonas aeruginosa, 285
  Staph. aureus carriage, 170
  Str. agalactiae, 181, 187
  tetanus, 237–8
  vaccines, 671
  varicella, 409
  viral susceptibility, 151–2
Neorickettsia, 375
Neorickettsia sennetsu, 375, 376
Nephritis
  streptococcal, 145
  see also Glomerulonephritis
Nephropathia epidemica, 498
Nephrotoxicity, aminoglycoside, 52
Nerves, leprosy, 210

Netilmicin, *52*
Neuralgia, postherpetic, 409
Neuraminidase inhibitors, 57
Neuraminidases, 468, 469, 476
Neuromuscular junctions, rabies virus
    attachment, 553
Neurones
  herpes simplex virus, 401–2
  prion transmission, 559
  rabies, 553-4
Neurosyphilis, treatment, 348
Neurotoxins
  botulism, 92, 239, 240
  Clostridium tetani, 91, 236
  puffer fish, 628
Neutralization, 115–16
Neutrophils, 122, 128, 130, 156
Nevirapine, *56*, 58
New Guinea
  enteritis necroticans, 235
  kuru, 563
New World arenaviruses, 513, *514*
Newcastle disease virus, 475–6
Newcastle upon Tyne, adenoviruses,
    395
Newly-discovered pathogens, 2
Niclosamide, *59*, 611
Nicotinamide adenine dinucleotide,
    H. influenzae culture, 304–5
Nidovirales, 547
Nipah virus, 475, 483
Nitrofurans, *46*, 54
Nitroimidazoles, *46*, 53–4, 58
Nits, 619
NNN medium, 599
Nocardia, 28, 221, 222–4
Nomarski interference contrast
    microscopy, 21
Nomenclature, 25
Non-capsulate *H. influenzae*, 306
Non-chromogens, *Mycobacterium*,
    215–16
Non-culturable bacteria, 44
Non-fermenters, of glucose, 287
Non-fimbrial adhesins, 18, 86
Non-gonococcal urethritis
  mycoplasmas, 385–6, 388
  see also Non-specific urethritis
Non-Hodgkin's lymphoma, human
    T lymphotropic virus 1, 529
Non-lactose fermenters, 265
Non-nucleoside reverse transcriptase
    inhibitors, 58, 534
Non-O1 *Vibrio cholerae*, 297, 299
Non-specific urethritis
  chlamydial, 363
  see also Non-gonococcal urethritis
Non-sporing anaerobes, 337–42
Non-sporing Gram-positive bacilli, 29,
    341–2
Non-structural proteins *see* NS proteins
Non-toxigenic *C. diphtheriae*, 190
Normal specimens, 638
North Asian tick typhus, *370*
N⹁walk-like viruses, 539–45
I⹁wegian s⹁vies, 620

Nose
  leprosy, 211
  rhinocerebral zygomycosis, 587
  Staph. aureus carriage, 169, 170
  swabs, *636*
    pernasal swabs, 313
Nosocomial infections *see* Hospital
    infections
Notifiable diseases, 641
Novobiocin, 54
Novy, MacNeal and Nicolle's medium,
    599
NS (non-structural) proteins
  flaviviruses, 487
  hepatitis C virus, 504, 505
Nucleases, *Staph. aureus*, 169
Nucleic acids
  viral, 24
  see also DNA; RNA
Nucleocapsids, 22
Nucleoids, bacteria, 11
Nucleoproteins, paramyxoviruses, 476
Nucleoside analogues, 55–7
  AIDS, 534
  hepatitis B, 444
Nucleoside reverse transcriptase
    inhibitors, 58
Numerical classification, 26
Nutrition, infection and, 123–4
Nystatin, *55*, 648

O antigens
  Klebsiella, 276
  Salmonella, 250–1, 255
  V. cholerae serogroups, 296–7
O chain lipopolysaccharides, complement
    resistance, 89
O139 *Vibrio cholerae*, 299
O157 VTEC, 272
  on *Brucella* ELISA, 324
Obligate aerobes, 41, *42*
Obligate anaerobes, 41, *42*
OC43 human coronavirus, 547, 549
Occupational diseases
  anthrax, 228–9
  respiratory, on immunity, *142*
  see also Farm workers; Health care
    personnel
Oculo-glandular tularaemia, 336
Oedema factor, *B. anthracis*, 227
Ofloxacin, 53
Ogston, Alexander, 4
Old tuberculin, 202
Old World arenaviruses, 513, *514*
Oligoadenylate synthetase, 146
Oligonucleotides *see* Gene probes
OmpA, OmpB, *Rickettsia*, 370
OmpX, *Enterobacter cloacae*, 278
Omsk haemorrhagic fever, 497
Onchocerca volvulus, *604*, 606
Oncogenicity
  hepatitis B virus, 441
  herpes simplex virus and, 407
  papillomaviruses, 429, 431, 433–4
  polyomaviruses, 436

O'nyong-nyong virus, 494
Oocysts, *Toxoplasma gondii*, 593
Oocysts, ookinetes, *Plasmodium*, 590
Oophoritis, mumps, 478
Opacity factor, *Str. pyogenes*, 178
Open reading frames, caliciviruses, 541
Operators, gene transcription, 63
Operons, 62–3
Ophthalmia neonatorum, 247, 630
  chlamydial, 363, 367
Ophthalmic zoster, 409–10
Opisthorchis felineus, 608
Opisthorchis sinensis see Clonorchis
    sinensis
Opisthotonus, 237
Opportunist pathogens, 3, 83, 124, 664
  anaerobes, 338
  Bacillus, 230
  Clostridium, 231
  Corynebacterium jeikeium, 193
  environmental mycobacteria, 215–20
  glucose non-fermenters, 287
  Nocardia, 223
  see also AIDS; Endogenous infections;
    Immunocompromise
Opsonins, 128
Opsonization, 116
  parasitic infections, 157
Optochin, *Streptococcus pneumoniae*
    sensitivity, 185
OPV (oral polio vaccine), 462–3, 676–7
Oral candidosis, 575–6
Oral contraceptives, rifampicin on,
    207–8
Oral hairy leucoplakia, *413*, 530
Oral papillomatosis, 433
Oral polio vaccine, 462–3, 676–7
Oral rehydration therapy, 299
Orbiviruses, 521, 522
Orchitis, mumps, 478
Orf, 426
Organ culture, OC43 human coronavirus,
    549
Organotrophs, 40
Oriental sore, *598*, 599
Orientia, 369
Orientia tsutsugamushi, 370, 374
  polymerase chain reaction, 373
Original antigenic sin, 472–3, 476
Ornithodorus, 621
Ornithosis, 358, 364
ORO fever, 498
Oropouche, 498
Oroya fever, 325–6
Ortho assays, hepatitis C virus
  core protein assay, 507
  recombinant immunoblot assay, 506
Orthomyxoviruses, *23*, 24, 94, 468–74,
    484, *485*
Orthopoxviruses, morphology, *23*
Orthoreoviruses, 521, 522
Oseltamivir, *55*, 57, 474, 648
Osteoclasts, 127
Osteomyelitis, 52, 254
Otitis media, 183, 185, 306, 626
Otogenic tetanus, 237

Otomycosis, 577–8
Ototoxicity, aminoglycosides, *52*, 647
Outbreaks of infection, 656–9
Outer membrane proteins
　chlamydiae, 358, 360
　Rickettsia, 370
Outer membranes
　Gram-negative bacteria, 14–15
　spirochaetes, 343
Outgrowth, bacteria, 19
Oxa-cephems, 49
Oxamniquine, *59*, 610
Oxazolidinones, *46*, 52
Oxidizing agents, disinfection, 81
Oxygen
　hyperbaric, gas gangrene, 234
　see also Reactive oxygen intermediates
Ozaena, 277

P antigen, B19 erythrovirus, 451–2
P serotypes, rotaviruses, 524
P1 protein, mycoplasmas, 384
P24 antigen, AIDS, 531, 533
P53 protein, human papillomavirus cell
　　transformation, 107, 431
Paediatric AIDS, 531, 532, 537
Paenibacillus, 29
Paget, James, on *Trichinella spiralis*, 4
Paget's disease of bone, measles virus,
　　479
Pancreatitis, mumps, 478
Pandemics
　cholera, 298
　defined, 657
　influenza, 304, 472, 473
Papillomaviruses, 429–35
　see also Human papillomaviruses
Papovaviruses, *23*, 24, 150, 429–37
Papua New Guinea *see* New Guinea
Parachlamydiae, 359
Paracoccidioidomycosis, 582–3
Paracrine action, interleukin-2, 134
Paraffin baiting, 224
Paragonimus, sites, 154
Paragonimus westermani, 608, *609*
Para-influenza viruses, 475, 476–7
Paralysis, polio, 457–8, 460, 461
Paramyxoviruses, *23*, 24, 94, 475–83
Paranasal granuloma, 585
Parapoxviruses, *23*, *423*, 426
Parasites
　agents *vs*, 58
　defined, 3
　ectoparasites, 3, 616
　eosinophils on, 129
　evasion mechanisms, 158–9
　immune defence *vs*, 155–8
　immunopathology, 159–60
　pathogenesis, 154
　vaccination, 160
Paratopes, 111, 112–13, 114
Paratrachoma, 362–3
Paratyphoid fever, 254, 633
Parechovirus, 456
Paronychia, candidosis, 576

Parotitis
　melioidosis, 286
　mumps, 478
Partial double-stranded DNA viruses,
　　replication, 101
Parturition
　Clostridium perfringens, 233
　hepatitis C virus, 509
　herpes simplex virus, 404–5
Parvovirinae, 448
Parvoviruses, *23*, 24, 98, 448–54
　see also B19 erythrovirus
Passive immunity, 131
　diphtheria, 191
　viral infections, 149
Passive immunization, 670–1
Pasteur, Louis, 3, 5, 225, 229, 556
Pasteurella, 329, 334–5
Pathogenicity, bacteria, 83–92
Pathogenicity isles, DNA, 84
　Helicobacter pylori, 293
　Salmonella, 253
Pathogens
　definitions, 3–5
　newly-discovered, 2
Paucibacillary leprosy, 212
Paul-Bunnell test, 414
PCR *see* Polymerase chain reaction
Peak serum levels, antibiotics, 643
Pediculus humanus, 619
Peginterferon, 57
Peliosis, bacillary, 327
Pelvic inflammatory disease, 631
　antibiotics, 388
　antimicrobial therapy, 651
　chlamydial, 364
　mycoplasmas, 386
　Neisseria gonorrhoeae, 247
Pemphigus neonatorum, 170
Penciclovir, 55–6, 406
Penicillin, *646*
　anthrax, 228
　for *Burkholderia cepacia*, 287
　contact hypersensitivity, 145
　gonorrhoea, 248, 643
　historical aspects, 6
　phenoxymethylpenicillin, *646*
　procaine penicillin, 47
　resistance, meningitis, 186
　Staph. aureus, 644–5
　Str. pyogenes, 644
　syphilis, 348
　see Phenoxymethylpenicillin
Penicillin G, 47, *646*
Penicillin V *see* Phenoxymethylpenicillin
Penicillinase gene, 67
Penicillins, 47–8, *646*
　activity spectrum, *46*
　non-sporing anaerobes, 342
　Streptococcus, 186
　upper respiratory tract infections, 650
Penicillium marneffei, 588
Penis, warts, 432
Pentamidine, 588
Pentastomes, *615*, 621
Pentons, adenoviruses, 393

Peplomers, coronaviruses, 546
Peptic ulceration, *H. pylori*, 293
Peptide nucleic acids, assay of
　　antimicrobial resistance genes,
　　32
Peptidoglycans, 14
　antibacterial agents on, 47
Peptidoglycolipid I, *Mycobacterium
　　leprae*, 210
Peptostreptococcus, 340–1
Perforin, 137
Pericarditis, *Str. pneumoniae*, 183
Perihepatitis, 247, 364, 631
Perinatal infection
　cytomegalovirus, 415
　HIV, 532, 533, 535, 537
Periodontal disease, 288, 342, 346
Peritonitis, 193, 233, 651
Peritrichous flagella, 16
Permissive host cells, 93
Pernasal swabs, 313
Persistent generalized lymphadenopathy,
　　HIV, 530
Persistent infections
　chlamydial, 362
　viral, 152
　　hepatitis B, 441
　　see also Latent infections
Person-to-person spread, 656, 657
　calicivirus infections, 543
Pertussis, 312–17, 627
　adenoviruses and, 395
　epidemiology, 314–16
　triple vaccine, 671, *675*
　vaccines, 315, 316–17, 673, 676
　see also Bordetella pertussis
Pesticides, *Burkholderia cepacia*, 286–7
Pestiviruses, 484, *506*
Pet Travel Scheme, 555–6
Petroff method, *Mycobacterium
　　tuberculosis*, 206
Pfeiffer, *Haemophilus*, 304
pH
　Leptospira, 356
　phagolysosomes, 129
　rhinoviruses, 465
Phaeohyphomycosis, 579
Phage typing, 34
　Staph. aureus, 171
Phagocytes, 127–8
　bacterial infections, 162
　complement receptors, 127
　immunoglobulin binding, *115*, 116
　inflammation, 130
　intracellular bacteria, 88
　Listeria monocytogenes, 195
　see also Mononuclear phagocytes
Phagocytosis, 127–9
　bacteria, 162
　bacterial capsules *vs*, 87–8
　parasites, 156
Pharyngitis, 625–6
　Arcanobacterium haemolyticum,
　　194
　infectious mononucleosis, 413
　Str. pyogenes, 178, 625–6

Pharyngoconjunctival fever, 395, 396
Phase variation, 65
    Coxiella burnetii, 377
Phase-contrast microscopy, 21
    endospores, 18
Phenolics, 81
Phenotypic assays, antiviral agents, 59
Phenotypic variation, 64
Phenoxymethylpenicillin, 47, *646*
Phenylalanine, *Proteus*, 280
Phenylpyruvic acid test *see* PPA test
Pheromones, 84
Phlebovirus, *485*, 487, *489*, 498
Phospholipase C, 233
Phosphonoformate *see* Foscarnet
Photochromogens, 215
Phototrophs, 40
Phthirus pubis, 619–20
Phycomycosis, 587
Phylogenetics, 25
    hepatitis C virus, *508*
    human papillomaviruses, 430
    retroviruses, *528*
Physiology, bacteria, 37, 40–5
Pickles, William, 653
Picornaviruses, *23*, 455–67
Piedraia hortae, 577
Pig-bel, 235
Pigeons, *Cryptococcus*, 583
Piglet enteritis, K88 antigen, 269
Pigments
    Bordetella parapertussis, 311
    Pseudomonas aeruginosa, 282–3
    Serratia, 278–9
Pigs
    brucellosis, 325
    porcine parvovirus, 450
    Salmonella, 258
Pili, 11, 17, 66, 68, 85–6
Pilins *see* Fimbrillins
Pinocytosis, 127
Pinta, 346
Piperacillin, 47
Piperazine, *59*, *604*
Pityriasis versicolor, 569, 576–7
Pityrosporum ovale, 577
Placental transfer
    herpes simplex virus, 404
    immunoglobulins, *115*, 116
    rubella, 502
Plague, 329, 330–2, 653
Plane warts, 432
Planktonic growth, 38
Plantar warts, 431–2
Plaque reduction assay, HSV, aciclovir on, 59
Plasma membranes *see* Cytoplasmic membranes
Plasma products, hepatitis C virus inactivation, 506
Plasmids, 26, 61, 67–9
    chlamydiae, 360
    enteroinvasive *Esch. coli*, 270
    gene transfer, 66
    myc   asm s, 382
    {p   i   71

Shigella, 260
Yersinia pestis, 329
Plasmin, *130*
Plasminogen, streptokinase on, 178
Plasmodium, 158–9, 589–92
    see also Antimalarials; Malaria
Plasmodium falciparum, 589-92
    on lymphocytes, 159
    see also Falciparum malaria
Platelets, 122
    parasitic infections, 156
Platyhelminths, 601
Pleconaril, 57, 463
Pleomorphism, bacteria, 18, 19
Plesiomonas shigelloides, 301
Pleural fluid, *636*
Pneumococcus *see Streptococcus pneumoniae*
Pneumocystis carinii, 54, 531, 587–8, 588
Pneumolysin, 182
Pneumonia, 627
    adenoviruses, 395
    antimicrobial therapy, 650
    chlamydial, 364
    influenza, 471–2
    Klebsiella, 276, 277
    mycoplasmas, 385, 387, 388
    Staph. aureus, specimens, 170
    Str. pneumoniae, 182–3
    varicella, 409
    see also Legionnaires' disease; Respiratory tract infections
Pneumonic plague, 330, 331
Pneumonitis, rubella, 502
Pneumovirus, 475, 481
Podophyllin, warts, 435
Point mutations, 64–5
Point sources, 657
    calicivirus infections, 543
Pol gene, retroviruses, 528
Polar flagella, bacteria, 16
Poliomyelitis, 457–8, 460–1
    environment on, 655–6
    vaccine-associated, 462–3
    vaccines *see* Polioviruses, vaccines
Polioviruses, 456, 457–8
    antibodies *vs*, 149
    cell adsorption, 94–5
    magnesium chloride, 456
    replication, 98–9
    vaccines, 462–3, 676–7
        danger, 458
        immunity mechanisms, 149
        immunodeficiency danger, 149
        inactivated, 462, 676
        live-attenuated, 462–3, 676–7
        tropics, 463
        UK scheduling, *675*
        virulence, 462–3
Polyarthritis, epidemic, 494
Polyclonal B cell activators, 145
Polyenes, 54
Polymerase chain reaction, 35, 71–2, 639
    Bordetella pertussis, 313
    Brucella, 324
    enteroviruses, 461

gene probes, 32
Helicobacter pylori, 294
hepatitis B virus, 442
hepatitis C virus, 507, 510
HIV, 533
HSV encephalitis, 404
immuno-polymerase chain reaction, 33
Mycobacterium tuberculosis, 206
mycoplasmas, 388
organism typing, 35
real time PCR, 32
ribosomal genes, classification by, 27
Rickettsia, 373
Polymerase variants, hepatitis B virus, 442
Polymicrobial infections, 339
Polymorphonuclear leucocytes, 122
Polymyxins, 54
Polyomaviruses, 429, 435–7
Polyprotein, hepatitis C virus, 504, 505
Polysaccharides
    extracellular, 15–16
    Lancefield grouping, 175
Polysomes, bacteria, 12
Pontiac fever, 318, 319, 321
Porcine parvovirus, 450
Porins
    Gram-negative bacteria, 14
    N. meningitidis, variation, 88
Porous-load sterilizers, 77
Porphyromonas, 339, 340
Portal pyaemia, antibiotics, 651
'Positive'('+') single-stranded RNA viruses, replication, 98–9
Postherpetic neuralgia, 409
Post-injection abscesses, 217
Postnatal rubella, 500–1
Post-operative tetanus, 237
Post-primary tuberculosis, 203–4
Pott's disease, 202
Poultry
    Campylobacter enteritis, 290
    Salmonella, 257–8
Povidone iodine, 81, 234
Powassan virus, 490, 497
Poxviruses, 421–8
    enzymes, 24
    immune response, 150
    morphology, *23*, 24
    replication, 97
    uncoating, 96
PPA (phenylpyruvic acid) test, *Proteus*, 280
Praziquantel, 58, *59*, 610
Precipitin test, histoplasmosis, 581
Predictable sensitivity, 644
Pregnancy
    adenovirus-associated virus, 451
    AIDS prevention, 537
    B19 erythrovirus, 451, 453
    chlamydial infection, 364
    HIV, 532, 535, 537
    influenza, 472
    Lassa fever, 515
    listeriosis, 196
    mycoplasmas, 386
    poliomyelitis, 458
    polyomaviruses, 436

Pregnancy (*contd*)
rubella vaccination, 503, 677
Str. agalactiae, 181, 187
varicella, 409
see also Abortion; Puerperal infections
Premature rupture of membranes,
Streptococcus agalactiae, 181
Presentation, antigens, 133–4
Pressure ventilation, 668
Prevotella, 340
Primaquine, 592
Primary tuberculosis, 201–2, *203*
Primates
hepatitis B virus, 439
polioviruses, 456
Primers, PCR, 35, 71
Prion protein gene
disease susceptibility, 560, *561*, 562
Gerstmann–Straussler–Scheinker
syndrome, 563
variant CJD, 563
Prions, 9, 24, 25, 76, 558–65
Pristinamycin, 53
Procaine penicillin, 47
Proctitis, chlamydial, 364
Prodigiosin, *Serratia*, 279
Pro-drugs, erythromycin, 52
Productive viral infections, 93
Proglottids, 611
Progressive multifocal
leucoencephalopathy, 152, 436,
437
Progressive rubella subacute
panencephalitis, 502
Proguanil, 53, 592
Prokaryotes, 10, 25, *28*, 61
Promastigotes, *596*, 598
Promoters, 63, 65
Prontosil, 6
Properdin, 125
Prophages, 67
Prophylaxis
AIDS, 537
antifungal, 571–2
cercopithecine herpesvirus 1, 420
diphtheria, erythromycin, 676
gas gangrene, 234
malaria, 592
rabies, 556, 557
Str. pneumoniae, 188
see also Chemoprophylaxis
Propionibacterium, 221, *341*, 342
Prosector's wart, 201
Prostaglandins, *130*
HSV reactivation, 402
Prostatitis, antibiotics, 649–50
Protease inhibitors, 58, 534
Proteases, of IgA, 88–9
Str. pneumoniae, 182
Protective antigen, *Bacillus anthracis*,
227
Protective clothing, hospital infections,
667–8
Protective isolation, 668
Protein kinase, antiviral, 146

Protein typing, bacteria, 34
Proteinase K, *561*
Protein-conjugated group C vaccines,
Neisseria meningitidis, 247
Proteins
bacterial, 12, 61–2
secretion, 15
synthesis inhibitors, 12, 61–2
chlamydial, 360–1
viral, 24
Proteomics, 43
Proteus, 279–81, *644*
Proton pump inhibitors, 295
Protoplasts, bacteria, 10, 19–20
Protozoa, 4–5, 27, 589–600
agents *vs*, 58
specimen transport, *637*
Providencia, 279–81
Proviruses, retroviruses, 100–1
Prozone effect, *Brucella*, 324
PrP^c (prion protein), 559
PrP^{sc} (prion protein), 559, 564
Pseudomembrane, diphtheria, 190
Pseudomembranous colitis, 240–1
Pseudomonads, 282–7
Pseudomonas aeruginosa, 282–5
aminoglycosides *vs*, 52, 285
antibiotics, *46*, *644*, 650
carriage, 285
electron micrograph, *16*
epidemiology, 285
Pseudomycelia, *568*, 569
Pseudopeptides, 32
Pseudopodia, 27
Pseudotuberculosis, 332
Psittacosis, 358, 364
Psoriasis, 180
Psychiatric disorders, arthropods and,
615–16
Psychrophiles, 41, *42*
Public Health Laboratory Service, on
gastro-enteritis, 545
Puerperal infections
Clostridium perfringens, 233
see also Parturition
Puffer fish neurotoxin, 628
Pulsed-field gel electrophoresis, 34, *35*
Punch actinomycosis, 222
PUO *see* Pyrexia of unknown origin
Purified protein derivative, 205
Puumala virus, 498
Pyocyanin, 283
Pyoderma (impetigo), 178, *179*, 630
Pyogenic group, *Streptococcus*, 175
Pyogenic infections
Staphylococcus, *168*
see also Septicaemia
Pyrantel pamoate, *59*, *604*
Pyrazinamide, 207, 209
Pyrexia, 129, 148, 253, 631, 633
Pyrexia of unknown origin, 631
sites of infection, 634
Pyrimethamine, 53, 592
Pyrogenic exotoxins, *91*, 177
Pyrolysis mass spectrometry, 35

Q fever, 376–8
Quarantine, 658
historical aspects, 653
pertussis and, 316
rabies, 555
Quaternary ammonium compounds, 81
Queensland tick typhus, *369*
Quellung reaction, 186, 304
Quinine, 592
Quinolones, *46*, 53
Quinupristin, 53
Quorum sensing, 15, 84

R plasmids, 70, 71
Rabbits, myxomatosis, 427–8
Rabies, 551–7
epidemiology, 554–6
historical aspects, 5, 551
receptor binding by virus, 94
vaccines, 145, 427, 556–7, *557*
Racecadotril, 526
Radiation, sterilization, 73, 78
Ramsay–Hunt syndrome, 410
Random applied polymorphic DNA
typing (RAPD), 35
Rapid growers, *Mycobacterium*,
215, 216
Rashes, 630
B19 erythrovirus, 452
coxsackieviruses, 459
infectious mononucleosis, 413
rat-bite fever, 303
Rocky Mountain spotted fever, 372
rose spots, 253–4
roseola infantum, 418
rubella, 500
varicella, 408
see also Erythema multiforme
Raspberries, hepatitis A, 464
Rat fleas, 617
Rat-bite fever, 303, 327
Rats
Leptospira, 356, 357
plague epidemiology, 331
typhus, 374
Rats, lice and history (Zinsser), *369*
Rb protein, cell transformation, HPV,
431
Reactivation
cytomegalovirus, 415
herpes simplex virus, 402
varicella-zoster virus, 408
Reactive arthritis
Campylobacter, 289–90
ureaplasmas, 386–7
Reactive oxygen intermediates, 41
phagocytosis, 88, 128
Reagin antibodies, 347
Real time PCR, 32
RecA gene, ribosomal, 27
Reception, specimens, 638
Recombinant HIV, 536
Recombinant immunoblot assay (Ortho),
hepatitis C virus antibodies, 5 6

Recombinant vaccines, 426–7
  Lassa fever, 516–17
  rabies, 427, 557
Recombinant virus strains
  B19 erythrovirus, 453–4
  human papillomavirus, 435
Recombination, outer membrane proteins,
    chlamydiae, 358
Recrudescent typhus, 372, 374
Rectal swabs, dysentery, 261
Recurrence, HSV, 402–3
Recurrent genital herpes, 404
Recurrent respiratory papillomatosis,
    433
Reduviid bugs, 617
Refrigeration
  cold chains, 673
  Listeria monocytogenes, 195
  psychrophiles, 41
  specimens, 638
Registrars General, 653
Regulons, 44
Rehydration therapy, 299
Re-infections, rubella, 500–1
Relapses
  malaria, 590
  urinary tract infections, 649
Relapsing fevers, 345, 349–50
Renal transplantation, 432, 436–7
Reoviridae, 484, *485*, 521–6
Reoviruses, 521–6
  macrophage infection, 151
  morphology, *23*
  nucleic acids, 24
Replication of viruses, 96–101
  adenoviruses, 394
  arboviruses, 486–7
  arenaviruses, 514–15
  hepatitis B virus, 440
  hepatitis C virus, 504–5
  herpesviruses, 400–1
  human papillomavirus, 430–1
  influenza viruses, 99–100, 470
  parvoviruses, 98, 449–50
  rabies virus, 552–3
  retroviruses, 100–1, 529
Reports, laboratory results, 640
Repressors, 63
Request cards, 635, 638
Resistance
  to antifungal agents, 572
  to fluconazole, 572
  to flucytosine, 572
  of hepatitis B virus, 80, 444
  to malaria, 123, 155, 592
  to sterilization processes, 75–6
  see also Antibiotics, resistance; Heat
    resistance
Resistance-ratio method, antituberculosis
    drugs, 206
Resistotyping, 34
Respiration, bacteria, 41
Respiratory bursts, 128
Respiratory syncytial virus, 152, 475,
)481–3, 483, 627

Respiratory tract infections, 626–7
  antimicrobial therapy, 650
  hospital organisms, *663*
  human papillomavirus, 433
  mycoplasmas, 385
  para-influenza viruses, 477
  rhinoviruses, 466
  RSV, 481–2
  specimen collection, *636*
  transmission, 7
  viruses, antibodies, 149
  see also Pneumonia; Upper respiratory
    tract infections
Restricted transduction, 67
Restriction, antibiotics use, 645
Restriction endonucleases
  bacterial typing, 34
  classification of plasmids, 68
  Pseudomonas aeruginosa, 283
Reticular dysgenesis, 142
Reticulate bodies, chlamydiae, 359–60,
    361, 362
Retina
  choroidoretinitis, 631
  cytomegalovirus, 416, 417
  herpes simplex virus, 403
Retinoblastoma protein, HPV cell
    transformation, 107
Retortamonas intestinalis, 595
Retroviruses, 527–38
  agents *vs*, 55–6, 57–8
    rifampicin *vs*, 208
    see also specific drugs
  nucleic acids, 24
  replication, 100–1, 529
Rev gene, HIV, 528
Reverse transcriptase
  hepadnaviruses, 101
  retroviruses, 100, 528-9
Reverse transcriptase inhibitors, 58, 533–4
Reverse transcriptase PCR
  arboviruses, 490–1
  arenaviruses, 516
  caliciviruses, 543
Rhabdoviruses, 551–7
  arboviruses, 484, *485*
  morphology, *23*
Rheumatic fever, 145, 164, 179–80
  diagnosis, 186
Rhinocerebral zygomycosis, 587
Rhinoscleroma, 277
Rhinosporidiosis, 579
Rhinoviruses, *455*, 464–6
  receptors, 95
Rhizopus, 587
Rhodococcus equi, *192*, 194
Ribavirin, *55*, *56*, 57, 648
  arboviruses, 491
  arenavirus infections, 516
  respiratory syncytial virus, 482
Ribonuclease activity, reverse transcriptase
    complex, retroviruses, 100
Ribosomal RNA, sequencing, 27
Ribosomes, bacteria, 12
  antibacterial agents, 51–3

Ribotyping, 34
Rice water stools, 297
Rickettsia, 28, 30, 369–75, *644*
Rickettsialpox, *369*, 372, 374
Rifabutin, 54
Rifampicin, 54
  H. influenzae prophylaxis, 309
  leprosy, 212
  Neisseria meningitidis, 246
  tuberculosis, 206, 207–8, 209
Rifamycins, *46*, 54
Rifapentine, 54
Rift Valley fever, 498
Rimantadine, *55*, 57, 474, 648
Ring vaccination, 659
Ringworm, 569, 570, 572–5
  specimen collection, 570–1, 574
  see also Dermatophytosis
River blindness, 606
RNA
  diagnostic probes, 639
  hepatitis B virus, 440
  influenza virus replication, 470
  interferon inducer, 146
  ribosomal, sequencing, 27
  small subunit rRNA nucleotide
    sequences, 12
  transcriptome, 43
  viral, 24
  see also Messenger RNA
RNA copy number, AIDS, 531, 532, 533,
    534
RNA polymerases, 98, 468, 476
RNA viruses, 98, 455–67
RNA-dependent RNA polymerase, 98, 468
Rocky Mountain spotted fever, *370*, 372,
    375
Rodents
  arenaviruses, 516
  filoviruses, 520
Rolling hairpin model, parvovirus
    replication, 450
Rose Bengal plate test, 324
Rose spots, 253–4
Roseola infantum, 418
Ross River virus, 494
Rotational policies, antibiotics, 646
Rotaviruses, 521, 522–6, 526
Rothia dentocariosa, 195
Roundworms
  Toxocara canis, *601*, 603
  see also Ascaris lumbricoides
RP4 plasmid, 66
RRV-TV (rotavirus vaccine), 526
RSV *see* Respiratory syncytial virus
Rubella, 452, 484, 500–4
  vaccines, 503–4, 677
  see also Measles, mumps and rubella
    vaccine
Russian spring–summer encephalitis, 497

Sabia virus, 515
Sabin vaccine, 462–3, 676–7
Sabin–Feldman test, 593

Saddleback fever, 489
Safety *see* Hazardous substances/organisms
Saliva, rabies virus, 554, 556
Salivarius group, *Streptococcus*, 175
Salk vaccine, 462, 676
Salmonella, 250–9
  on *Brucella* ELISA, 324
  carriage, 254–5, 256–7
  haemolytic anaemia, 144
  intracellular parasitism, 163
  invasion, 87
  serotyping, 34
Salmonella Enteritidis, 250
Salmonella Paratyphi, 252
Salmonella senftenberg, *D* value, 75
Salmonella Typhi, *17*, 252
Salmonella Typhimurium, antibiotic
      resistance typing, 252
Salpingitis, 630–1
  antimicrobial therapy, 651
  chlamydial, 364
  mycoplasmas, 386
  Neisseria gonorrhoeae, 247
Salt *see* Halophilicity
Salvarsan (arsphenamine), 6
Samples *see* Specimens
Sandflies, 618
  Bartonella, 325, 326
Sandfly fever group viruses, 498
Sanitation, enteric fever prevention, 257
Sanitization, 73
Sapporo-like viruses, 539–45
Saprophytes, 3
Sarcina, 29
Sarcocystis, 593
Sarcoptes scabei, 620
Satellitism, *Haemophilus influenzae*
      culture, 305
Scabies, 620
Scalded skin syndrome, 170
Scalp, ringworm, 574
Scarlet fever, 178
Schick test, 190
Schistosoma, *608*, *609*, 610
  immunosuppression by, 159
Schistosoma haematobium, 5, *608*, *609*,
      610
Schistosomiasis
  immunopathology, 160
  treatment, hepatitis C virus, 509
Schizogony, 27, 590
Schools, bacillary dysentery, 263
Schüffner's dots, *591*
Scopulariopsis brevicaulis, 577
Scorpions, 621
Scotochromogens, 215
Scrapie, 558–9
Screening
  vs cross-infection, 668–9
  Helicobacter pylori, 293–4
  rubella, 503
Scrofula, 201, *202*
Scrofuladerma, 204
Scrub typhus, 370, 372–3, 374
  vaccines, 375
Scytalidium, 577

Seafood, *Vibrio parahaemolyticus*, 300
Sealed containers, sterilization, 77
Seasonal incidence
  cholera, 299
  coronavirus infections, 549
  para-influenza viruses, 477
  respiratory syncytial virus, 482
Sebaceous secretions, 124
Seclusion, parasites, 158
Secretory IgA, 113, *114*
Selective media, 39–40
Selective toxicity, 47
Self-antigens, 88
Self-infection, 665, 666
  see also Endogenous infections
Self-tolerance, 141
Semen, *Corynebacterium*
      glucuronolyticum, 193
Semmelweis, Ignaz, 7
Semple vaccine, rabies, 556
Sendai virus, 476
Sensitivity (of organisms)
  antimicrobial agents, 58–60, 185, 640,
      643–5
  antiviral agents, 59–60
Sepsis
  mycoplasmas, 387
  see also Pyogenic infections,
      Septicaemia
Septa, bacterial cell division, 13
Septicaemia, 632–3
  Burkholderia pseudomallei, 286
  candidaemia, 586
  Mycoplasma hominis, 387
  Neisseria meningitidis, 242, 246
  Vibrio vulnificus, 300
Septicaemic plague, 330
Sequential epitopes, 111
Sequestering, chlamydiae, 362
Serény test, 270
Seroconversion illness, HIV, 530
Serogroups, *N. meningitidis*, 243
Serology, 639
  hepatitis C virus, 506–7
  Lyme disease, 350–1
  Treponema, 347
  see also Antibodies; *specific organisms*
Serotherapy, 6
Serotypes
  Salmonella, 34, 250
  Str. pneumoniae, 182
Serotyping
  bacteria, 34
  Str. pyogenes, 186
Serpentine cords, *Mycobacterium*
      tuberculosis, 200
Serratia, 278–9
Serum, 112
  antibiotics, assay, 643
  B19 erythrovirus detection, 453
  mycoplasma culture, 382
Serum sickness, 6, 144
Sessile growth, 38
Severe combined immunodeficiency
      disease, enteric viruses, 542
Sewage, *Leptospira*, 356

Sex pili, 17–18
Sexual intercourse
  HIV, 535, 536
  human papillomavirus, 434
Sharps injuries *see* Needle stick injuries
Shedding, *Staph. aureus*, 170
Shedding of viruses, 151
  caliciviruses, 544–5
  cytomegalovirus, 415
  Epstein–Barr virus, 412
  polioviruses, 461
  rhinoviruses, 466
Sheep, chlamydial infection, 366
Shellfish
  caliciviruses, 544
  hepatitis A virus, 464
Shiga toxin, 261, 262, 271
Shigella, 260–4
  Escherichia coli vs, 265
  invasion, 87
Shipyard eye, 395–6
Shock
  anthrax, 226, 227
  dengue, 488, 490
  septic, 632
    antimicrobial therapy, 648–9
    see also Endotoxin; Toxic shock
        syndrome
Sickle cell disease, malaria resistance,
      123, 155, 592
Siderophores, 89
  Escherichia coli, 266
  Klebsiella, 277
  Pseudomonas aeruginosa, 283
  see also Iron
Signal sequences, viral envelope proteins,
      101–2
Silkworms, fungal disease, 4
Silver impregnation, 21
Simian immunodeficiency virus, 528
Simian parvoviruses, 450
Simian T lymphotropic viruses, 528
Simian virus 5, 475, 476
Simian virus 40, 429
  hybrids with adenoviruses, 396
Similarity coefficient, 26
Similarity matrices, 26
Simkania negevensis, 359
Simulium, 618, 619
Sin Nombrevirus, 498–9
Single-stranded DNA viruses, 98
Single-stranded RNA viruses
  'negative', replication, 99–100
  'positive', replication, 98–9
Sinusitis, 306, 626
Sinus-lining macrophages, 127
Sissomicin, *52*
Sjögren's syndrome, hepatitis C virus and,
      510
Skin, 630
  antimicrobial therapy 651–2
  blastomycosis, 582
  candidosis, 576
  as defence, 124
  delayed hyper   y,
  diphtheria, 19

disinfection, 667
environmental mycobacteria, 217–18
herpes simplex virus, 403
hospital organisms, *663*
hypersensitivity reactions, 144
    leprosy, 212
Listeria monocytogenes, 198
Lyme disease, 350
Neisseria gonorrhoeae, *248*
non-dermatophyte moulds, 577
preparation for surgery, 234
Pseudomonas aeruginosa, 283
specimen collection, *636*
toxins affecting, *91*
tuberculosis, 204
warts, 431–2
    see also Dermatophytosis; Rashes
Slapped cheek syndrome, 452
S-layers, 16
Sleeping sickness, 596–7
Slim disease, 531
Slime, bacteria, 15–16
Slit-skin smears, leprosy, 212
Small round structured viruses *see*
    Caliciviruses
Small subunit rRNA nucleotide
    sequences, bacteria, 12
Small t antigens, 435
Smallpox, 5, 421, 423–4, 424, 425–6, 654
Smears, leprosy, 212
Smoking
    chickenpox, 409, 411
    on immunity, *142*
Snow, John, 7, 653, 660
Snowshoe hare virus, 497
Sodium chloride, *Staph. aureus*, 169
Sodium polyanethol sulphonate, blood
    cultures, 387–8
Sodoku, 303
Soft sore, 309
Soft ticks, 620, 621
Soil
    anthrax, 228
    Clostridium tetani, 236
    Leptospira, 356
Solid phase immune electron microscopy,
    caliciviruses, 542
Somatic antigens, *Salmonella*, 250–1, 255
Sonne dysentery, epidemiology, 262
Sorbitol, VTEC, 272
Sore throat, 625–6
Sources of infection, 6–7, 84–5, 658, 668
    see also Point sources
South American haemorrhagic fever, 515
South American trypanosomiasis *see*
    Chagas' disease
South-east Asia, AIDS, 536
'Spanish fly', 616
SPE (pyrogenic exotoxins), *91*, 177
Specialized transduction, 67
Species complexes, 26
Species specificity, innate immunity, 123
Specimens, 635–7
    freezing, 638
    ringworm, 570
    transport, 637–8, 639

upper respiratory tract, *625*
    see also Sputum specimens
Spermidine, 124
Spermine, 124
Spheroplasts, 19–20
Spider colonies, 222
Spiders, 621
Spiramycin, 52
Spirilla, 11, 29
Spirillum minus, 302–3
Spirochaetes, 10, 16, 28, 29–30, 343–51
Spiroplasmas, culture, 382
Spleen
    animal anthrax, 226
    parasitic infections, 159
    prions, 559
Splenectomy, *Streptococcus pneumoniae*
    prophylaxis, 188
'Spoligotyping', *Mycobacterium*
    tuberculosis, 206
Spongiform encephalopathies,
    transmissible, 558–65
Spontaneous generation, 3
Sporadic cases, 656
Sporadic CJD, 560–3
Spores, 18–19
    Aspergillus, 584
    Bacillus anthracis, 225, 226
    Clostridium, 231
    Clostridium botulinum, 239
    dermatophytes, 573
    elementary bodies, chlamydiae, 359,
        360, *361*, 362
    Gram-negative bacilli, 29
    moulds, 568–9
    resistance to sterilization, 76
Sporogony, protozoa, 27
Sporothrix schenkii, 579
Sporotrichoid spread, swimming pool
    granuloma, 217
Sporotrichosis, 579
Sporozoa, 589–93
Sporozoites, 589–90, 590
Spotted fevers, 369–70, 372, 374
    cell invasion, 371
Spumaviruses, 528
Sputum specimens, 184–5, *636*
    Aspergillus, 585
    Haemophilus influenzae, 307
Squamous cell carcinoma, 434
SSrRNA (small subunit rRNA) nucleotide
    sequences, 12
St Louis encephalitis, 490, 492, *493*, 495
Stacked-brick formation, entero-
    aggregative *Esch. coli*, 272
Staining, bacteria, 21–2
    acid-fast, 15, 22
    fluorescent, 33
Staphylococcus, 29, 168–73
    antibacterial agents, *46*, 644–5
Staphylococcus aureus, 168–72
    antibiotic resistance, 48
    bronchopneumonia treatment, 650
    carriage, 170
    D value, 75
    fibronectin binding, 86, 176

hospital infections, 663–4
    see also Methicillin-resistant
        Staphylococcus aureus
Staphylococcus epidermidis, 75
    D value, 172
Staphylococcus haemolyticus, teicoplanin
    resistance, 173
Staphylococcus saprophyticus, urinary
    tract infections, 173
Stationary phase of growth, 38
Stavudine, 58
Steam, 77, 78, 79
Stem cells, immunodeficiencies, 142
Stenotrophomonas maltophilia, 282
Sterilization, 73–4, 666
    anthrax spores, 226
    historical aspects, 3
    hospital policies, 81, 82
    performance measurement, 77
    resistance, 75, 77–8
    spores, 18
    test bacilli, 230
    see also Heat sterilization
Sterilizers, 77
Steroids, infection and, 123
Sterol-dependent mycoplasmas, 383
Stimulons, 43–4
Stokes' method, 59
Stomatitis, HSV, 403
Strains, bacteria, defined, 33
Strawberry tongue, 178
Street rabies virus, 553
Streptobacillus moniliformis, 327–8
Streptococcus, 29, 174–88
    antibacterial agents, *46*, 644
    Arcanobacterium haemolyticum with,
        194
    group A, cross-reacting antigens, 145,
        164
    group C and G, 181–2
    group R, 182
    vaccines, 187–8
    see also Viridans streptococci
Streptococcus agalactiae, 180–1, 181,
        186, 187
Streptococcus mitis, 184
Streptococcus mutans,
    exopolysaccharides, 86
Streptococcus pneumoniae, *174*, 182–3
    antibiotic resistance, 186–7, 644
    cerebrospinal fluid, 185
    meningitis, 183, 185, 629
        penicillin resistance, 186
    optochin sensitivity, 185
    typing, 186
    vaccines, 187–8, 678
Streptococcus pyogenes, *174*, 175–80
    carriage, 178
    diagnostic kits, 185
    fibronectin binding, 86
    pharyngitis, 178, 625–6
    sensitivity (antibiotics), 644
        bacitracin, 185
    typing, 88, 186
    vaccines, 187
    see also M proteins

Streptococcus salivarius, 183, 184
Streptococcus suis, 182
Streptogramins, *46*, 52–3
Streptokinase, 178
Streptolysins
  Str. pyogenes, 177
  see also ASO test
Streptomyces, 28
Streptomycin, 51, *52*, 207, 330
Stress responses, 43–4
Strict aerobes, 41, *42*
Strict anaerobes, 41, *42*
Strongyloides stercoralis, *601*, *602*, 603, *604*
Subacute bacterial endocarditis *see* Endocarditis
Subacute sclerosing panencephalitis, 152, 479
  viral antigen capping, 151
Subcutaneous mycoses, 569, 570
Substitution mutations, *64*
Subunit vaccines, 671
Suckling mice, arbovirus isolation, 491
Suckling mouse brain vaccine, rabies, 556
Sudden infant death syndrome, RSV, 481
Sulbactam, 51
Sulphonamides, *46*, 53, 373, *646*
Sulphones, 51
Sulphur granules, 222
Superantigens, 92, 169–70, 177, 180
Superoxide anion, 128
Superoxide dismutase, 41
Suppressor T cells, 141
Suppurative arthritis, mycoplasmas, 387
Suramin, 606
Surface phagocytosis, 87
Surface-active disinfectants, 81
Surgery
  gas gangrene, 232, 233
  infection mechanisms, 665–6
  infection prevention, 667–8
  see also Wound infections
Surgical catgut, *Cl. tetani*, 236
Surveillance, 654
  AIDS, 641
  hospital infections, 669
  notifiable diseases, 641
Survival curves, 75
Susceptibility *see* Sensitivity
Swabs, *636*
  candidosis, 576
  pernasal, 313
  rectal, dysentery, 261
  Staph. aureus, 170
  throat, *636*
    epiglottitis danger, 307
Swarming, *Proteus*, 280
Sweat, 124
Swimmer's itch, 610
Swimming pool granuloma, 215, 217
Switching, phase variation, 65
Sylvatic plague, 329
Sylvatic rabies, 555
Sylvatic yellow fever, 496

Symmetry, viruses, 22–4
Syncytia
  HIV inducing, 532
  viral infections, 103
Synergy, antibiotics, 647
Syphilis, 345–6, 347–9
Systemic infections, antimicrobial therapy, 648–52
Systemic mycoses, 570, 579–88

T cell lymphoma, EBV, *413*
T cell receptors, 117, 132–3, 140
T cells, 122
  activation, 133, 134
  on antibody responses, 135
  antigen recognition, 117
  cytomegalovirus infection, 415
  defects, 143
  human herpesviruses 6 and 7, 418
  immune function, 136
    vaccines for, 153
  vs intracellular bacteria, 163–4
  parasitic infections, 157–8
  tolerization, 141
  Trypanosoma cruzi, 158
  viral infections, 149–50
  see also CD4+ T cells; CD8+ T cells; Cytotoxic T cells
TAB (typhoid, paratyphoid) vaccines, 257
Tacaribe virus, 516
Tachyzoites, *T. gondii*, 593
Taenia, 610–11, *612*
Tahyna virus, 497
Tapeworms, 610–13
Taq polymerase, 41
Tat gene, HIV, 528
Tax gene, HTLV-1, 530
Tax protein, HTLV-1, cell transformation, 107
Taxonomy *see* Classifications; Identification of micro-organisms
Tazobactam, 51
TC-83 (Venezuelan equine encephalitis vaccine), 499
TCBS agar, 297
Td vaccine, *675*, 676
Teguments, herpesviruses, 400
Teichoic acid, 14
Teicoplanin, 51, 171–2, 173
Telithromycin, 52
TEM β-lactamases, 47
Temperate phages, 34, 67
Temperature
  bacterial requirements, 41, *42*
  innate immunity, 129
  sterilization, *76*
Temperature-sensitive mutants, viruses, 104–5
Terbinafine, 54, *55*, 571, 575, 648
Terminal ileitis, *Yersinia pseudotuberculosis*, 333
Tertian malaria, benign, 589
Tertiary syphilis, 345–6
Test kits, bacteria, 31

Tetanus
  absence of herd immunity, 674
  chemoprophylaxis, 239
  epidemiology, 237–8
  immunization, 238–9
    adsorbed toxoid, 238, 675–6
    triple vaccine, 671, 675–6
    UK scheduling, *675*
  toxins, 91, 236
  see also Clostridium tetani
Tetracycline, 299, 331, 367
Tetracyclines, *46*, 51, 248, 373, *646*, 650
T-even coliphages, morphology, *23*
T$_H$ cells, 139
  erythrogenic toxin on, 177
  on immune response, 141
  subtypes, 137
  see also CD4+ T cells
Thermophiles, 41, *42*
Thiabendazole, *604*
Thiamphenicol, 51
Thiosulphate–citrate–bile salts–sucrose agar, 297
Thogotoviruses, 468
Threadworms *see Enterobius vermicularis*
Throat swabs, *636*
  danger, epiglottitis, 307
Thrush
  vaginal, 630
  see also Candida
Thymidine kinase
  deficiency, HSV resistance to aciclovir, 406
  gene, vaccinia virus, 427
Thymus
  DiGeorge syndrome, 143
  T cell selection, 140
Thymus-dependent antigens, 133
Ticarcillin, 47
Tick paralysis, 620–1
Tick-borne encephalitis viruses, epidemiology, 497
Tick-borne relapsing fever, 349–50
Ticks, 620–1
  ehrlichiosis, 376
  flaviviruses, 497
  historical aspects, 7
  Q fever, 377
  rickettsial fevers, 372, 374–5
  see also Ixodid ticks
Tine tests, 205
Tinea *see* Dermatophytosis
Tissue culture
  cytotoxicity assay, *C. diphtheriae*, 190–1
  see also Cell culture
Tissue nematodes, 604–7
Titrations *see* Dilution MIC titrations
Tobacco mosaic virus, *23*
Tobramycin, 51, *52*, 285
Togaviruses, *23*, 484, 485
  see also Alphaviruses
Tolerance, to antigens, 140, 141
Tongueworms, 6, 621
Tonsillar abscess, *Streptococcus pyogenes*

Tonsillectomy, poliomyelitis, 458
Topical treatment
    ringworm, 575
    skin, 652
Topics in international health (Wellcome Trust CD-ROM), viii
Toroviruses, 547
Toscana virus, 498
Tospovirus, 487
Tourists, 633, 634
Tox gene, *C. diphtheriae*, 191
Toxic shock syndrome, 169, 172
    Streptococcus pyogenes, 179
Toxic shock syndrome toxin 1, 92, 169–70
Toxicity, antimicrobial agents, 647
Toxins, 89–92
    Bacillus anthracis, 227
    Clostridium difficile, 240–1
    defined, 3
    food poisoning, 628
Toxocara canis, *601*, 603
Toxoids, 5, 91, 671, 675–6
    adsorbed tetanus toxoid, 238, 675–6
    anthrax vaccine, 229
    botulism, 240
Toxoplasma gondii, 592–3
    HIV, 531
    macrolides *vs*, 52
    in macrophages, 158
    resistance, interferon-γ, 147
TPHA (*Treponema pallidum* haemagglutination assay), 347
Trachoma, 362–3, 367
Trafficking, lymphocytes, 132
Transcription
    bacteria, 12, 61
    regulation, 63
Transcription errors (clerical), 638
Transcriptome, 43
Transduction, gene transfer, 66–7
Transferable antibiotic resistance, 70
Transferrin, 87, 89
Transformation
    of bacteria, 65–6
    cells by viruses, 105–7, 431, 436
Transmissible mink encephalopathy, *559*
Transmissible spongiform encephalopathies, 558–65
Transmission of infection, 6–7, 84, 656, 659
    air-borne, 664–5, 668
        see also Aerosols
    anthrax, 225, 226–7
    by contact, 665
    historical aspects, 3–4
    HIV, 535
    hospital infections, 664–6
    Rickettsia prowazekii, 374
    Staph. aureus, 170
    surgery, prevention, 667–8
    see also Arthropods; Faecal–oral transmission; Foods; Water-borne infections
Transovarial transmission, 621
Transplacental *see* Placental transfer

Transplantation
    cytomegalovirus, 416, 417, 418
    polyomaviruses, 436–7
    warts, 432
    see also Cornea, transplants; Liver, transplantation
Transport, specimens, 637–8
Transport media, 637
Transposons, 70
Trans-stadial transmission, 621
Travellers
    immunization, 678
    imported infections, 633–4
Travellers' diarrhoea, 628, 634
    ETEC, 269–70
Trehalose dimycolate, 163
Trematodes, 607–10
Trench fever, 326–7
Trench mouth, 346
Treponema, 29, 343–9
    mixed infections, 342, 346
Treponema pallidum, *343*, *344*, 345–9
    fibronectin binding, 86
    haemagglutination assay, 347
    skin penetration, 630
Trials, vaccines, 672
Triazoles, activity spectrum, *55*
Tribavirin *see* Ribavirin
TRIC agents, 358
Trichinella spiralis, 4, 155, 159, *604*, 607
Trichomonas hominis, 595
Trichomonas vaginalis, 4, 595–6
Trichophyton, 572, 575
Trichostrongylus, *601*, 603
Trichuris trichiura, *601*, *602*, 603, *604*
Triclosan, 81
Trimethoprim, 53, *646*
Triple diphtheria, tetanus and pertussis vaccine, 671, 675–6
Trivalent antimonials, *59*
Tropheryma whippelii, 221, 224
Trophozoites, *Plasmodium*, 590, *591*
Tropical fevers, arboviruses, *489*, 490
    see also named diseases
Tropical spastic paraparesis, 529
Tropical ulcer, 347
Tropics
    measles, 480
    poliomyelitis vaccination, 463
Trough serum levels, 643
True bacteria, 28, 29
Trypanosoma, 158, 159, 596–8
Trypanosoma cruzi, 58, 158
Trypomastigotes, *596*, 597
ts mutants, viruses, 104–5
Tsetse flies, 618
Tsutsugamushi disease *see* Scrub typhus
Tuberculin reaction, 137, 144, 202
Tuberculin tests, 205, 677
Tuberculoid leprosy, 210
Tuberculomas, 203
Tuberculosis, 201–9
    environment and, 655
    epidemiology, 208
    HIV, 531

mortality, 2
vs opportunist mycobacterial disease, 219
twin studies, 123
vaccines, 209
see also Mycobacterium tuberculosis
Tuftsin, 183
Tularaemia, 335–6
Tumbu fly, 619
Tumour necrosis factor, *138*, 139, 147
Tumours
    of immune cells, *142*, 143
    progressive multifocal leucoencephalopathy, 436
    transformed cells, 107
    see also Carcinoma; *specific lymphomas*
Tunga penetrans, 617
Turicella otitidis, 195
Twin studies, susceptibility to infection, 123
Type III protein secretion systems, Gram-negative bacteria, 15
Type b polysaccharide antigen, *Haemophilus influenzae*, 307
Typhlitis, 235
Typhoid fever, 253, 633, 653
'Typhoid Mary', 256
Typhus, 369, 371, 372, 374, 375
Typing, 33–5, 639
Tzanck cells, 401

UL97 gene, CMV infection, 414
Ulcero-glandular tularaemia, 336
Ultraviolet radiation, 74, 79
Uncoating, 96
    antiviral agents on, 57
Undulant fever, 322
United Kingdom
    agricultural anthrax, 228
    bacillary dysentery, 262
    immunization policies, 675
        pneumococcal vaccine, 188
        rubella, 503–4
        tetanus, *238*
    leptospirosis, 356
    Lyme disease, 351
    Public Health Laboratory Service on gastro-enteritis, 545
    rabies regulations, 555–6
    see also England and Wales
United States
    bacillary dysentery, 262
    pneumococcal vaccine, 188
'Universal precautions', 668
Upper respiratory tract infections, 625–6
    adenoviruses, 395
    antimicrobial therapy, 650
    diphtheria, 189
    human coronavirus, 548
    Str. pneumoniae, 183
    Str. pyogenes, 178
    see also specific diseases
Urban plague, 329
Urban rabies, 555

Urban yellow fever, 492, 496
Urea breath test, 294
Ureaplasma urealyticum, 384, 630
Ureaplasmas, 379
  abortion, 386
  antibiotics, 388
  biochemistry, 383
  neonatal respiratory infections, 385
  reactive arthritis, 386–7
  urinary tract infections, 386
Ureases, 92
  Helicobacter pylori, 92, 292
    test, 294
  Proteus, 280
Ureteric stenosis, 436
Urethritis, 628, 630
  chlamydial, 363, 364
  mycoplasmas, 385–6, 388
  see also Non-specific urethritis
Urinary tract infections, 628–9
  antimicrobial therapy, 649–50
  Candida, 586
  Corynebacterium urealyticum, 193
  Escherichia coli, 266–7
  hospital organisms, *663*
  Klebsiella, treatment, 277
  mycoplasmas, 386, 387–8
  Proteus, 280–1
  Staph. saprophyticus, 173
  see also Cystitis
Urine
  animals, *Leptospira*, 356
  antibiotics, assay, 643
  Escherichia coli counts, 267
  Salmonella, 255
  Schistosoma eggs, 610
  specimen collection, *636*
    transport, 637

V factor, *Haemophilus influenzae* culture,
    304, 305, 307
Vaccines, 671–9
  contra-indications, 672–3
  danger
    poliomyelitis, 458
    X-linked infantile
        hypogammaglobulinaemia,
        149
  herd immunity, 655
  historical aspects, 5
  parasites and, 160
  poxviruses in research, 421
  vaccinia virus as vector, 426–7
  viral, 152–3
  see also Measles, vaccines
Vaccinia virus, 5, 421, 424, 426–7
Vacuolating toxin, *H. pylori*, 293
Vacuoles
  enteroinvasive *Esch. coli*, 270
  intracellular bacteria, 87
Vacuum pulsing, porous-load sterilizers, 77
Vagina
  candidosis, 576
  warts, 432, 435

Vaginitis, 630
  antimicrobial therapy, 651
  Neisseria gonorrhoeae, 247
  Trichomonas vaginalis, 596
Vaginosis *see* Bacterial vaginosis
Valaciclovir, 55, 56, 406
Vampire bats, rabies, 555
Vancomycin, 51, 171–2
Variable antibiotic sensitivity, 644–5
Variant CJD, *561*, 563–4
Variants, classification of organisms, 25
Varicella, 152, 408–9, 410–11, 411, 678–9
Varicella-zoster immunoglobulin (VZIG),
    411
Varicella-zoster virus, 407–11
Variola *see* Smallpox
Variolation, 5, 424
Vascular injury, *Rickettsia* and *Orientia*,
    372
Vasculitis, type III hypersensitivity, 144
VDRL test, 347, 348
Vegetative phase, 18
Veillonella, 29, 341
Venereal Disease Research Laboratory
    test, 347, 348
Venezuelan equine encephalitis, 492, *493*,
    494, 499
Venezuelan haemorrhagic fever, 515
Ventilation, isolation rooms, 668
Ventricular shunts, 650
Vero cell cultures, 382–3
Verocytotoxin, 271–2
Verocytotoxin-producing *Escherichia
    coli*, 267, 271–2
  epidemiology, 272
  infection prevention, 273
  O157, 272
    on Brucella ELISA, 324
Verruga peruana, 326
Vesicles
  differential diagnosis, 410
  herpes simplex virus, 401
  intracellular bacteria, 87
  varicella, 408
Vesiculovirus, 551
Vesiculovirus, syndromes, *489*
Viability
  bacteria, 44–5
Viable but non-culturable bacteria (VNC),
    44
Vibrio, 11, 29, 295–301
Vibrio cholerae, 296–300
  carriage, 299
  doubling time, 38
  VNC hypothesis, 44
Vincent's gingivitis, 339, 346
Viral capsid antigen, EBV, antibodies, 413
Viral hepatitis, 440–7
  see also specific diseases
Viridans streptococci, 175, 183–4
  antibiotic resistance, 186–7
  endocarditis, 649
Virions, 22
  Dane particles, 438–9
  poxviruses, 421–2

Viroids, 9, 24, 25
Virulence, 654
  bacteria, 83
  determinants, 83–4
  Staph. aureus, 169–70
  vaccines, polio, 462–3
  vaccinia virus, 427
Virulent phages, 67
Viruses, 9, 22–4, 25, 30
  antibodies *vs*, 148–9, 151
  antigenic variation, 152
  cell transformation, 105–7, 431, 436
  conjunctivitis, 631
  disinfectants, 79–80
  escape mechanisms, 149
  as haemagglutinins, 33
  Haemophilus influenzae and, 306
  historical aspects, 5
  immunosuppressive, *142*, 150
  interactions with cells, 93–108
  in mycoplasmas, 382
  receptors for, 94–5
  specimen transport, *637*
  taxonomic authorities, 26
  see also Bacteriophages; Shedding of
      viruses
Visceral larva migrans, 603
Visceral leishmaniasis, *598*, 599
Visna (sheep disease), 528
VNC *see* viable but non-culturable
    bacteria, 44
Vomiting, 628
  Bacillus cereus, 229
  caliciviruses, 542
  staphylococcal food poisoning, 169
VTEC *see* Verocytotoxin-producing
    Escherichia coli
Vulva, warts, 432
Vulvovaginitis, *Neisseria gonorrhoeae*,
    247
VZIG *see* varicella-zoster
    immunoglobulin

Waddlia chondrophila, 359
Wagatsuma's agar, 300
Wars, infections, 656
Warts, 151, 431–3, 434
Water fleas (copepods), 621
Water-borne infections, 7
  bacillary dysentery, 263
  cholera, 298–9
  Dracunculus medinensis, 607
  enteric fever, 257
  enteroviruses, 462
  environmental mycobacteria, 220
  Legionella, 320–1
  Leptospira, 356, 357
  Schistosoma, 628, 610
  see also Snow, John
Waterhouse–Friderichsen syndrome,
    246
Web sites, viii
Weil-Felix test, 372
Weil's disease, 356

Wellcome Trust, CD-ROM, viii
West Nile virus, 495
Western equine encephalitis, 490, 492–3, 499
Wet films, microscopy, 31
Whipple's disease, 224
Whipworm *see Trichuris trichiura*
White piedra, 577
Whitewater Arroyo virus variant, 515
Whitlow, herpetic, 403
Whooping cough *see* Pertussis
Wild plague, 329
Wild rabies virus, 553
Winterbottom's sign, 596
Wiskott–Aldrich syndrome, 142–3
Woese, Carl, 9, 10
Wood's lamp, 574
Wool-sorter's disease, 226
World Health Organization
  arboviruses defined, 484
  immunization programmes, 675
  influenza virus nomenclature, 469
  poliomyelitis eradication, 463

rabies vaccination, 556
  smallpox eradication, 424, 654
Wormseed, 6
Wound cleaning, rabies prophylaxis, 556
Wound infections, 630, 651
  botulism, 240
  gas gangrene, 232–4
  hospital organisms, *663*
  tetanus, 238
  Vibrio vulnificus, 301
Wuchereria bancrofti, 604, *605*

X factor, *Haemophilus influenzae* culture, 304, 307
X-adhesins, *Escherichia coli*, 85
Xenodiagnosis, *Tr. cruzi*, 597–8
Xenopsylla cheopsis, 617
X-linked infantile hypogammaglobulinaemia, 142
  vaccination danger, 149
X-linked recessive lymphoproliferative syndrome, 150

Yaws, 346
  syphilis serology, 348
Yeast-like fungi, 28
Yeasts, 28, *568*, 569, 571
Yellow fever, 488, *489*, 492, 496, 499
Yersinia, 329–34
Yersinia enterocolitica, 333–4
  on *Brucella* ELISA, 324
Yersinia pestis, 21, 329–32
Yersinia pseudotuberculosis, 332–3
  receptors for, 87

Zanamivir, *55*, 57, 474, 648
Zidovudine, *56*, 58, 533–4, 537, 648
Ziehl–Neelsen method, 22, 205
Zinsser, H., *Rats, lice and history*, 369
Zoonoses
  anthrax as, 228–9
  brucellosis, 322
  defined, 7, 656
Zoster, 408, 409–10, 411
Zygomycosis, 587